PATHOLOGY	FIGURES
Developmental dysplasia of the hip	4-96, 4-106, 4-107
Diastrophic dysplasia	10-5
Diffuse idiopathic skeletal hyperostosis	6-24, 11-69 through 11-74
Disc herniation	9-3; 11-84; figures on p. 487, p. 488, and p. 489, *top;* 11-89 through 11-95
Disc hypoplasia	6-32, 11-64, 11-88
Dyschondrosteosis	8-24
Elbow dislocation	Figure on p. 548, *bottom*
Enchondroma	7-21, 7-22, 7-58, 8-43, 15-27, 15-31 through 15-34, 15-37
Enthesis fracture	Figure on p. 546, *bottom*
Eosinophilic granuloma	5-2, 5-7, 6-39, 6-74, 7-45, 7-65, 17-7 through 17-13
Epiphyseal dysplasia	7-16, 10-12, 10-13, 10-28
Ewing's sarcoma	7-46, 15-92 through 15-95
Facet dislocation/ subluxation	Figures on p. 531, *middle;* p. 532, *top*
Facet tropism	4-103
Femur fracture	Figure on p. 561, *top*
Fibrosarcoma	7-47, 15-9, 15-99, 15-101
Fibrous cortical defect	4-120, 4-121, 15-39
Fibrous dysplasia	5-6, 5-13, 5-23, 5-49, 6-9, 6-40, 6-41, 7-27 through 7-29, 7-63, 8-31, 15-44 through 15-48
Fibrous histiocytoma	15-10, 15-96, 15-100, 15-102
Fibula fracture	Figures on p. 519, *bottom right;* p. 561, *bottom*
Fluorosis	8-32
Gaucher's disease	17-2 through 17-5
Giant cell tumor	6-10, 6-42, 7-30, 7-31, 15-50 through 15-55
Gibbous configuration	14-6
Glenoid labral tears	Figure on p. 543, *bottom*
Gout	8-7, 8-53, 11-48 through 11-50
Greenstick fracture	Figure on p. 521, *bottom;* p. 522, *top*
Hemangioma	5-20, 6-11, 6-43, 15-56 through 15-60
Hemivertebra	4-88, 6-18, 6-71, 17-44
Hemochromatosis	8-8
Hemophilia	13-17 through 13-19
Hereditary multiple exostosis	15-68
Homocystinuria	6-1, 8-26
Humeral head fracture	Figures on p. 539, *middle* and *bottom*

PATHOLOGY	FIGURES
Humerus dislocation	Figures on p. 542
Hydatid cyst	6-44
Hydroxyapatite crystal deposition disease (HADD)	8-49
Hyperparathyroidism	5-9, 7-1, 16-5 through 16-13
Hypervitaminosis A	16-24, 16-25
Hypervitaminosis D	16-26 through 16-28
Hypothyroidism	16-18
Infantile cortical hyperostosis	17-15
Infection	6-33 through 6-35, 6-45, 6-46, 7-32, 7-49, 7-66 through 7-68, 8-9 through 8-12, 9-2, 14-1 through 14-14, 14-16 through 14-25
Inflammatory bowel disease	11-9
Intervertebral canal stenosis	11-99 through 11-101
Intervertebral disc calcification	6-29, 6-30
Intraosseous ganglion	7-43
Jaccoud's arthritis	11-10
Jefferson's fracture	Figure on p. 528, *bottom*
Juvenile rheumatoid arthritis	6-7, 8-19, 11-11, 11-12
Klippel-Feil syndrome	6-5, 6-6, 6-28, 10-7, 10-8
Knife clasp deformity	4-94
Kyphoscoliosis	17-20
Lead intoxication	17-6
LeFort I fracture	Figure on p. 525
Legg-Calvé-Perthes disease	7-10, 7-13, 13-12
Leukemia	13-20
Ligamentum flavum calcification	9-10
Limbus bone	6-79
Lipoma	7-33, 15-61 through 15-66
Liposarcoma	15-103 through 15-105
Lunate dislocation	
Lymphoma	
Maffucci's syndrome	
Marfan's syndrome	
Mastocytosis	17-16
Mauclaire's disease	7-11

Continued

Bone, Joints, and Soft Tissues—cont'd

PATHOLOGY	FIGURES	PATHOLOGY	FIGURES
Medial collateral ligament tear	9-22	Os odontoideum	10-14 through 10-18
Medullary bone infarction	13-3, 13-4	Os peroneum	4-128
		Os tibiale externa	4-130
Melorheostosis	7-61		
Meniscal tear/ injury	9-23, 9-24, figures on p. 566	Os trigonum	4-129
		Ossification of the posterior longitudinal ligament	11-75
Metaphyseal corner fracture	12-1		
Metastatic bone disease (mixed density)	15-114, 15-115, 15-127, 15-130, 15-138, 15-142		
		Osteitis condensans ilii	4-109, 6-68
Metastatic bone disease (osteoblastic)	6-58, 6-59, 8-35 through 8-37, 8-46, 15-112, 15-113, 15-117 through 15-119, 15-125, 15-126, 15-128, 15-129, 15-134	Osteoblastoma	6-48, 15-77, 15-78
		Osteochondritis dissecans	Figures 12-7 through 12-12
Metastatic bone disease (osteolytic)	5-21, 5-22, 5-24 through 5-27, 6-47, 7-51 through 7-54, 15-110, 15-111, 15-116, 15-120 through 15-124, 15-131 through 15-133, 15-135, 15-136, 15-140	Osteochondroma	6-53, 15-67, 15-69 through 15-72
		Osteogenesis imperfecta	10-19
		Osteoid osteoma	7-64, 15-73 through 15-76
Metatarsal dislocation	Figures on p. 572, *bottom*	Osteoma	5-14, 15-21 through 15-23
		Osteomalacia	16-29, 16-30
Modic (vertebral marrow) changes	Figures on p. 468, p. 469	Osteopetrosis	6-62, 6-63, 6-82, 6-83, 8-38, 9-1, 10-20
		Osteopoikilosis	15-18
Mucopolysaccharidosis	10-11	Osteoporosis	8-27 through 8-30, 16-20 through 16-22
		Osteosarcoma	7-57, 7-69, 15-151 through 15-153, 15-155 through 15-157
Multiple myeloma	7-36, 7-55, 7-56, 8-48, 15-149		
		Osteosclerosis	8-34, 8-40, 8-41, 8-47
Myelofibrosis	6-56	Paget's disease	5-28, 6-12, 6-49, 6-60, 7-62, 8-39, 17-25 through 17-38
Myositis ossificans	12-5, 12-6		
		Paracondylar process	4-56
Nasal fracture	Figures on p. 526, *bottom;* p. 527, *top*		
Negative ulnar variance	4-115	Pars interarticularis fracture	Figure on p. 529, *top;* 12-18
		Patella fracture	9-27; figure on p. 562, *top*
Neuroblastoma	6-52	Pectus carinatum	4-89
Neurofibroma	9-4, 17-21 through 17-23		
Neurofibromatosis	9-7, 17-17 through 17-19, 17-24	Pectus excavatum	4-87
Neurotrophic arthropathy	11-77 through 11-83	Pellegrini-Stieda disease	8-50
Nonossifying fibroma	7-23 through 7-26, 15-40 through 15-43	Pelvic fracture	Figures on p. 559
		Periosteal chondroma	15-28, 15-35, 15-36
Nuclear impression	6-2, 6-80	Phalanx dislocation	Figure on p. 558, *bottom*
Occipitalization	4-48		
Ochronosis	6-31	Phalanx fracture	Figures on p. 519, *bottom left;* p. 520, *top;* p. 558, *top;* p. 571, *bottom*
Odontoid fracture	Figures on p. 529, *middle* and *bottom;* p. 530, *top*	Pigmented villonodular synovitis	17-39 through 17-43
Odontoma	5-30		
Ollier's disease (multiple enchondromatosis)	15-29	Plasmacytoma	7-37, 15-143 through 15-148
		Platyspondylia	4-69
		Polydactyly	4-131
		Ponticulus posticus	4-58
Oppenheimer's ossicle	4-97	Posterior cruciate ligament tear	9-21, figure on p. 565
Orbital fracture	Figure on p. 527, *bottom*		
Os acetabuli	4-110		

Bone, Joints, and Soft Tissues—cont'd

PATHOLOGY	FIGURES
Proatlas ossicle	4-54
Protrusio acetabulum	4-108, 8-1 through 8-4
Pseudo-hypopara-thyroidism	16-14 through 16-16
Pseudopseudo-hypothyroidism	16-17
Psoriatic arthritis	6-27, 8-14, 8-15, 11-13, 11-14, 11-16
Pyknodysostosis	5-12, 7-4, 10-21
Radial fracture	Figures on p. 522; p. 547; p. 553, *top;* p. 555, *top*
Radiation necrosis	6-84, 6-85
Red marrow reconversion	9-25
Reiter's disease	6-26, 8-16, 11-20 through 11-22
Renal osteodystrophy	16-35
Reticulohistio-cytosis	8-13
Rheumatoid arthritis	6-8, 6-22, 8-17, 8-18, 11-15, 11-23 through 11-25, 11-27 through 11-34, 11-40
Rib fracture	Figures on p. 535, *top*
Rib synostosis	4-62, 4-78
Rickets	7-17, 7-77, 16-31 through 16-34, 16-36
Rotator cuff tendonopathy	Figures on p. 544; p. 545, *top*
Sacroiliitis	6-66, 6-67, 6-69, 6-70, 11-1, 11-60
Salter-Harris fracture	12-2; figures on p. 520, *bottom*
Sarcoidosis	8-20
Scaphoid fracture	Figures on p. 551; p. 552, *top left* and *bottom*
Scaphoid subluxation	Figure on p. 555, *bottom left*
Scapula fracture	Figures on p. 540
Scheuermann's disease	6-86, 10-22 through 10-27
Schmorl's nodes	6-87, figures on p. 464
Scleroderma	8-55, 8-56, 11-41, 11-42
Scoliosis	6-72, 17-48
Scurvy	7-18, 7-78, 16-37 through 16-39
Sesamoid bone fracture	Figure on p. 557, *bottom*
Shoulder impingement syndrome	Figure on p. 545, *bottom*
Sickle cell anemia	6-3, 6-78, 6-88, 13-21 through 13-23
Simple bone cyst	7-39; 7-40; figures on p. 523, *right;* 15-80 through 15-84
Sinusitis	5-18
Situs inversus	4-101
Six lumbar vertebrae	4-105
Skull fracture	Figures on p. 521, *top;* p. 526, *top*
Slipped capital femoral epiphysis	12-13, 12-14
Spina bifida occulta	4-59, 4-73
Spondyloepiphy-seal dysplasia	6-73
Spondylolisthesis	12-15 through 12-17, 12-19 through 12-24, 12-26
Sprung pelvis	Figure on p. 560, *bottom*
Sternal fracture	Figure on p. 535, *bottom*
Straight back syndrome	4-85, 4-86
Stress fracture	Figures on p. 517; p. 518; p. 524, *bottom*
Sturge-Weber syndrome	5-15
Stylohyoid ligament ossification	4-61
Subchondral cysts	7-41, 7-42
Subchondral sclerosis	13-16
Subperiosteal hemorrhage	7-71
Supracondylar process	4-113
Suprapatellar effusion	Figure on p. 562, *bottom right*
Swan-neck deformity	11-25, 11-26
Synovial inflammation	11-38, 11-39
Synovial osteochondro-matosis	7-8, 7-9, 8-44, 17-52 through 17-54
Synovial sarcoma	15-158, 15-159
Syphilis	7-72, 14-1, 14-2
Syringomyelia	9-11
Systemic lupus erythematosus	8-21
Talus fracture	Figures on p. 571, *bottom*
Tarlov cyst	4-99
Teardrop fracture	Figure on p. 531, *top*
Tethered cord syndrome	9-9
Thalassemia	5-8, 8-25, 8-42, 13-24
Thickened heel pad	4-126
Thyroid cartilage calcification	4-60
Tibia fracture	Figures on p. 562, *bottom left;* p. 568
Torus fracture	Figures on p. 522, *bottom;* p. 553, *bottom*
Transitional segments	4-74, 4-80, 4-93, 4-105
Triquetrum fracture	Figure on p. 554, *top*

Continued

Pathology Quick Reference—cont'd

Bone, Joints, and Soft Tissues—cont'd

PATHOLOGY	FIGURES	PATHOLOGY	FIGURES
Tumoral calcinosis	8-58, 8-59	Venous clefts	4-79
Ulna fracture	Figures on p. 549, *bottom;* p. 575	Vertebral compression fracture	6-20; 6-21; 6-75 through 6-77; figures on p. 523, *bottom left,* p. 536, and p. 537, *top*
Uncinate process degeneration	11-56, 11-57	Wrist fibrocartilage tears	Figure on p. 556, *bottom*
Vacuum phenomena	Figures on p. 462, p. 463		

Chest

PATHOLOGY	FIGURES	PATHOLOGY	FIGURES
Adult respiratory distress syndrome	24-1	Pneumothorax	24-6 through 24-9
		Pulmonary abscess	19-48
Asbestosis	24-3, 24-4	Pulmonary aneurysm	19-22, 21-2, 21-4, 21-5
Aspergillosis	22-5		
Atelectasis	19-1 through 19-3, 20-1 through 20-3, 24-5	Pulmonary arteriovenous malformation	19-51, 21-8
Azygous fissure	18-2		
Bronchiectasis	20-4		
Bronchogenic carcinoma	17-14, 19-11, 19-17, 19-26, 19-45, 19-52, 19-53, 19-59, 23-1 through 23-7, 23-10, 23-12 through 23-15, 23-17, 23-18	Pulmonary cavity	19-23 through 19-25
		Pulmonary consolidation	19-12
Coarctation of aorta	21-6, 21-7	Pulmonary cyst	19-7, 19-29, 20-6
Congestive heart failure	21-9, 21-11	Pulmonary edema	19-9, 19-49, 19-50
Cysticercosis	8-54	Pulmonary infarct	19-13
Cystic fibrosis	19-14		
Emphysema	19-5, 20-7, 20-8	Pulmonary nodules	23-8, 23-9
Extrapleural sign	19-4	Sarcoidosis	19-16, 19-19 through 19-21, 24-10, 24-11
Ganglioneuroma	19-44		
Granuloma	19-57, 19-60, 22-11	Septic emboli	19-27
Hamartoma	23-15	Silicosis	19-36
Hemothorax	19-37	Substernal thyroid	19-40, 23-22
Histoplasmosis	19-56		
Lipoma	19-38	Teratoma	19-41, 23-21
Lipomediastinum	19-43	Thymoma	23-23
Lymphoma	19-18, 19-39, 23-16	Tracheal carcinoma	20-2
Mesothelioma	23-20		
Pericardial calcification	19-33, 19-34	Tuberculosis	22-10, 22-12
Pleural effusion	19-46, 19-47, 21-1, 21-12, 22-1	Wegener's granulomatosis	19-28, 19-62
Pneumonia	22-1 through 22-4, 22-6 through 22-9		
Pneumoperitoneum	19-6		

Abdomen

Brain and Spinal Cord

CLINICAL
IMAGING

With Skeletal, Chest, and Abdomen
Pattern Differentials

CLINICAL IMAGING

With Skeletal, Chest, and Abdomen
Pattern Differentials

DENNIS M. MARCHIORI, DC, MS, DACBR

Assistant Professor,
Palmer Center for Chiropractic Research;
Coordinator of Clinical Research,
Palmer Chiropractic Clinics,
Palmer College of Chiropractic,
Davenport, Iowa

With illustrations by Mike Rekemeyer

with 15 contributors
with 2453 illustrations and photos

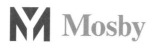 Mosby

St. Louis Baltimore Boston Carlsbad Chicago Minneapolis New York Philadelphia Portland
London Milan Sydney Tokyo Toronto

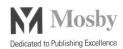 Mosby

Dedicated to Publishing Excellence

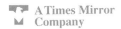 A Times Mirror
Company

Publisher: John Schrefer
Executive Editor: Martha Sasser
Senior Developmental Editor: Amy Christopher
Project Manager: Linda McKinley
Senior Production Editor: Catherine Comer
Designer: Renée Duenow
Manufacturing Manager: Betty Mueller
Cover Design: Elizabeth Rohne Rudder

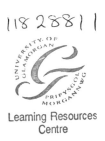
Composition by Top Graphics
Printing/binding by Walsworth Publishing Co.

Mosby, Inc.
11830 Westline Industrial Drive
St. Louis, MO 63146

Library of Congress Cataloging-in-Publication Data
Marchiori, Dennis M.
    Clinical imaging : with skeletal, chest, and abdomen pattern
differentials / Dennis M. Marchiori; with 15 contributors; with
illustrations by Mike Rekemeyer.
        p.   cm.
    Includes bibliographical references and index.
    ISBN 0-8151-8616-9
    1. Diagnostic imaging.   2. Diagnosis, Differential.   I. Title.
    [DNLM: 1. Diagnostic Imaging.   2. Diagnosis, Differential.   WN
180 M317c 1998]
RC78.7.D53M367   1998
616.07′4—dc21
DNLM/DLC
for Library of Congress   98-23694
                                                                            CIP

98 99 00 01 02/9 8 7 6 5 4 3 2 1

Contributors

TAWNIA ADAMS, DC, DACBR
Private Practitioner,
Northern Exposure Radiology Consultants,
Anchorage, Alaska

RICHARD ARKLESS, MD
President,
Advanced Diagnostic Imaging Services, PC,
Seabeck, Washington;
Instructor in Radiology,
Western States Chiropractic College,
Portland, Oregon

VINCENT DE BONO, RT, DC
Attending Clinician,
National College of Chiropractic,
Lombard, Illinois

DEBORAH M. FORRESTER, MD
Director,
Residency Training Program,
Los Angeles County and University of
    Southern California Medical Center,
Los Angeles, California

BEVERLY L. HARGER, DC, DACBR
Director of Clinical Radiology,
Western States Chiropractic College,
Portland, Oregon

LISA E. HOFFMAN, DC, DACBR
Assistant Professor, Clinical Radiology,
Western States Chiropractic College,
Portland, Oregon

D. ROBERT KUHN, AS, DC, DACBR
Assistant Professor, Department of Radiology,
Logan College of Chiropractic,
St. Louis, Missouri

DENNIS M. MARCHIORI, DC, MS, DACBR
Assistant Professor,
Palmer Center for Chiropractic Research;
Coordinator of Clinical Research,
Palmer Chiropractic Clinics,
Palmer College of Chiropractic,
Davenport, Iowa

IAN D. McLEAN, DC, DACBR
Associate Professor,
Palmer Chiropractic Clinics;
Director, Clinical Radiology,
Palmer College of Chiropractic,
Davenport, Iowa

TIMOTHY J. MICK, DC, DACBR
Associate Professor and Chair,
Department of Radiology;
Director, Radiological Consultation Service,
Northwestern College of Chiropractic,
Bloomington, Minnesota

ROBERT PERCUOCO, DC
Professor, Department of Radiology;
Dean of Academic Affairs,
Palmer College of Chiropractic,
Davenport, Iowa

CYNTHIA PETERSON, RN, DC, DACBR, MMEd
Head, Department of Radiology,
Anglo-European College of Chiropractic,
Bournemouth, England

RUTH G. RAMSEY, MD
Professor of Radiology;
Chief, Section of Neuroradiology,
University of Chicago,
Chicago, Illinois

DAVID J. SARTORIS, MD
Professor of Radiology;
Director, Quantitative Bone Densitometry,
University of California School of Medicine,
San Diego, California

GARY D. SCHULTZ, DC, DACBR
Professor and Chairman,
Clinical Sciences Division,
Los Angeles College of Chiropractic,
Whittier, California

RAJIV SHAH, MD
Metro Health Medical Center,
Assistant Professor of Clinical Radiology,
Case Western Reserve University,
Cleveland, Ohio

Reviewers

MURRAY SOLOMON, MD
Medical Director,
Los Gatos MRI and Redwood City MRI,
Los Gatos, Redwood City, California

JAMES C. REED, MD, FACR
Professor of Radiology;
Chair, Department of Radiology,
University of Kentucky, College of Medicine,
Chandler Medical Center,
Lexington, Kentucky

To Cheryl Lynn (Gray) Marchiori,
a loving wife, devoted mother, and trusted friend.

Foreword

Although many excellent books deal with the several phases of radiology, this book takes a unique approach that is particularly valuable to students and nonradiologists.

Dr. Marchiori's *Clinical Imaging* is based on a gamut, or pattern, approach to radiology. The interpreter begins by using radiological signs to develop a differential list of possible diagnoses and then progresses to traditional discussions of the several diseases or conditions that are within that differential list. Until now, there has not been a book available that incorporates both pattern differentials and detailed traditional discussions of diseases in such a comprehensive format. This is the approach that I have tried to teach to students, particularly radiology residents, over the years. This book follows the approach to radiological interpretation that is usually used in clinical practice and is therefore valuable for students and helpful for practitioners who do not have the depth of radiological knowledge possessed by those whose primary practice is in radiological interpretation.

By enlisting the skills of contributors to cover areas in which they have particular expertise, Dr. Marchiori has produced a book that I feel will be welcomed by teachers, students, and many clinicians. The chapter outlines and quick-reference features make it easy to use. The approach to pattern recognition is simplified over that found in other books that deal with this subject. The disease chapters have sufficient depth to meet the needs of those in general clinical practice.

I congratulate Dr. Marchiori and his contributors on producing a book that will find its way into the libraries of many clinicians, chiropractic colleges, and students in training.

JOSEPH W. HOWE, DC, DACBR, FACCR, FICC
Professor of Radiology;
Former Chairman, Radiology Department,
Los Angeles College of Chiropractic,
Whittier, California;
Former Chairman, Radiology Department,
National College of Chiropractic,
Lombard, Illinois

Advances in medical imaging have revolutionized diagnostic capabilities over the past 2 decades. The explosion in imaging technology has vastly improved diagnostic accuracy and thus benefitted patient management. However, the negative aspect of this burgeoning technology has been the increasing cost of health care delivery. Even though medical imaging accounts for approximately only 4% of the total health care budget in the United States, rising costs and over-utilization of medical imaging concerns federal agencies, third-party payors, and politicians alike. Current medical practice and reimbursement schemes no longer permit all available tests to be performed on every patient. As radiologists, we have the responsibility to ensure that the different imaging methods are not indiscriminately used but selectively chosen according to their cost effectiveness and benefit for the patient's management.

Subspecialization leads to progress in medical imaging and provides expertise in the performance and interpretation of examinations in particular areas of radiology. However, when individuals need examinations in multiple areas, subspecialization requires many more radiologists than are needed. Under present financial constraints, subspecialization has become a luxury that is only affordable in a few major academic centers, even if it is recognized that radiology would be best served by individuals with expertise in a single area. With subspecialists participating in after-hours call, coverage within their department and consultation in areas outside their expertise become problematic. A subspecialty can be compared to a "feather in a cap" that is of little use without the cap.

A variety of excellent texts in all subspecialties dealing either with a specific imaging modality or a selective organ system is currently available. Texts in general radiology are fewer in number and tend to be either disease or pattern oriented. An imaging pattern is for a radiologist what a symptom is for a clinician. *From the Symptom to the Diagnosis* is a German text written by my former teacher, Walter Hadorn, Chairman of Internal Medicine at the University of Bern, Switzerland, that impressed me as a medical student by its practicality and usefulness. The book survived its author and is now in its eighth edition.

Correlation of an imaging pattern with clinical and laboratory findings was introduced by Fraser and Paré in 1970 with the original edition of their outstanding text entitled *Diagnosis of Diseases of the Chest.* These authors added a chapter to their text that comprised 17 tables of differential diagnosis with all the basic roentgenographic patterns of chest disease. Descriptions of specific imaging findings to be expected for a specific diagnosis as well as differential points aided the radiologist in arriving at a likely diagnosis and reasonable differential diagnosis. Using this concept, Martti Kormano and I introduced the first text covering the entire field of conventional radiology. This imaging pattern approach in tabular form has since been adopted by many authors, and we feel complimented by the old cliché, "Imitation is the sincerest form of flattery."

In his text, Dennis Marchiori has garnered contributions from an outstanding group of radiologists who represent the broad areas of subspecialization. The book is a successful attempt to combine the elements of a standard disease-oriented text with the pattern-oriented approach. Until Dennis Marchiori undertook this task, no publication fulfilled this need. The text provides a basic approach to both performance and interpretation of various imaging studies and can be recommended as an introductory text for the first year resident as well as reference book for a general radiologists or a subspecialists outside their area of expertise. Dennis Marchiori is to be congratulated on recognizing this need and carrying out the task of putting together such an outstanding text that combines the pattern with the more traditional disease-oriented approach.

FRANCIS A. BURGENER, MD
Professor of Radiology,
University of Rochester Medical Center,
Rochester, New York

A s we enter the third century of clinical imaging, practitioners worldwide rely on noninvasive examinations of internal structures to diagnose disease and guide treatment. Popular tomographic methods, computer processing, and alternative forms of energy have not replaced the basic method used to depict Frau Roentgen's hand in 1895.

Recognition of anatomical silhouettes and tissues' characteristic patterns of x-ray absorption changed clinical practice forever. Simple x-ray photography remains by far the most important diagnostic technique for examination of the skeleton, chest, and abdomen.

Clinical Imaging: With Skeletal, Chest, and Abdomen Pattern Differentials builds its clinical teachings on the foundation of introductory chapters, efficiently covering the fundamentals of modern imaging technology. The strengths, weaknesses, pitfalls, and artifacts of clinical imaging are illustrated well.

This text usefully organizes the basic image patterns that must be recognized to accurately distinguish between diseased and normal anatomy. Basic principles of image interpretation are reduced into themes that can be applied over and over during academic training and in clinical practice.

The book is organized into four body regions that have distinctive clinical problems and imaging characteristics. Common, important, and diagnostic image findings are beautifully illustrated and summarized throughout this well-organized text.

This will be a most memorable introduction to practical clinical imaging for students and clinicians alike. Enjoy!

DAVID D. STARK, MD, FACR
Professor and Chairman,
Department of Radiology,
University of Nebraska Medical Center,
Omaha, Nebraska

Preface

The goal of this book is to assist students and practitioners of the health sciences with developing a better understanding of diagnostic imaging. The content of this book emphasizes plain film radiology and integrates it with magnetic resonance imaging and computed tomography. It includes comprehensive coverage of skeletal imaging in addition to imaging of the chest, abdomen, brain, and spinal cord. Although many excellent radiology books are available, the approach of this book is unique. The majority of currently available books employ a traditional approach. That is, diseases are presented individually within chapters that are devoted to broad categories (e.g., congenital, arthritide, tumor, trauma). However, a traditional design does not parallel strategies of diagnostic image interpretation.

In clinical practice, interpreting radiographs or other diagnostic images begins with scanning the studies to detect abnormalities. An identified abnormality is classified into broad patterns that can be used to develop a list of differential diagnoses. Unfortunately, most traditional books do little to bridge the transition from image to differential diagnosis. This is a particularly serious deficit for nonradiologist interpreters, who are less familiar with the possible causes of particular imaging presentations. In contrast, this book is structured to help students and clinicians recognize abnormal patterns and develop a list of viable diagnostic possibilities. This is accomplished by allowing the reader to begin with an image presentation and progress to determining the responsible disease rather than requiring the reader begin with a disease and progress to the image presentation. The few books currently on the market that utilize this "pattern approach" leave out crucial details about particular diseases. To avoid this limitation, we have *combined* the utility of a pattern approach with the detailed descriptions of disease entities found in more traditional designs. This provides an easy-to-use, comprehensive radiology resource for clinicians and students.

This book is divided into five parts: "Introduction to Imaging"; "Bone, Joints, and Soft Tissues"; "Chest"; "Abdomen"; and "Brain and Spinal Cord." Thumbnail tabs along the borders of the pages demarcate each part and allow for quick referencing. "Bone, Joints, and Soft Tissues"; "Chest"; and "Abdomen" are further subdivided into pattern chapters and disease chapters. Disease chapters follow a traditional design, presenting selected entities of a disease category (e.g., tumors, infections, trauma). Most disease entities are listed alphabetically and in a structured format that includes *Background, Imaging Findings, Clinical Comments,* and *Key Concepts,* facilitating the reader's use of these chapters. The pattern chapters, found toward the beginning of the parts, comprise multiple tables of disease entries grouped by similarity of imaging appearance.

The pattern, or gamut, approach of these chapters functions in two ways. First, it facilitates the development of correlations between diseases of similar imaging appearance. For instance, if the book is to be used as a textbook, readers can begin in the disease chapters. After becoming familiar with the individual disease topics, readers can then consult the pattern chapters as a capstone to their learning and integrate similar appearances of individual diseases. Second, the pattern chapters assist clinicians in developing a workable list of possible diseases that may be responsible for particular imaging presentations. The list of differentials can be narrowed by reading the short comments that accompany each table entry. In addition, a page number accompanying most entries in the pattern chapters refers the reader to a section in the disease chapters in which more detailed descriptive information can be found. Clinicians will find the *Clinical Comments* in the disease chapters to be particularly useful for patient management decisions.

Each chapter begins with an outline of chapter content and includes elements such as tables, boxes, case studies, suggested readings, and numerous high-quality illustrations and photographs—more than 2400 are included in the book. A comprehensive glossary at the end of the book can be used as a guide to radiological terms. A pathology quick-reference list containing corresponding figure numbers can be found on the front inside cover. In addition, the back inside cover contains a list of radiology mnemonics. These elements should prove to be excellent learning tools for students and clinicians.

We have resisted the tendency to become repetitious in our writing. Rather, we have produced a concise, user-friendly resource for those in training, as well as those in clinical practice.

DENNIS M. MARCHIORI

Acknowledgments

The completion of this project is due to the unselfish efforts of many individuals. My wife, Cheryl, is first and foremost on the list of those I would like to acknowledge. Although she is not listed as a contributor, her involvement was certain and necessary. She assumed responsibility for nearly everything in our lives, allowing me to concentrate on this book. This task became especially arduous following the birth of our daughter, Isabella, near the beginning of this 3-year effort. Without the contributors, this book would not be worth reading, but without Cheryl, there would not be a book.

I am especially fortunate to have been raised by very nurturing and loving parents, Phillip Valentino Marchiori and M. Judy Wymer. My late father was truly an inspiring man. He worked very hard to give his children opportunities that were not available to him. No one would be more proud of this book than my dad. We all miss him very much. All children need someone in their lives who is irrationally devoted to them. I am lucky enough to be my mother's son and receive this kind of love.

There were few surprises during this project. Going into it, I thought it might be a lot of work. No surprise, it was. However, working with the contributors has been surprising. All of the contributors have been extremely enthusiastic and steadfast in their commitment. It was always a bit puzzling to me why many of them were so anxious to spend hundreds of hours working on their contributions for so little conventional reward. I have concluded that they understand the importance of scholarship and are dedicated to their professions and the topic of radiology. Each contributor has added an integral part to this book. Their contributions vary in size but not importance. I would also like to acknowledge their families and colleagues, whose efforts and sacrifices are certainly nested within each contribution. The contributors' efforts have done more than produce a book, they have formed friendships and other collaborations that will extend into the future.

Ian McLean has written the sections dealing with magnetic resonance imaging, but his influence is far greater. Ian introduced several of us who have worked on this project to the topic of radiology. Sometimes it is difficult to know where information gained from his teachings end and our own thoughts begin.

Martha Sasser, Amy Christopher, Cathy Comer, and all of the staff at Mosby–Year Book, Inc. deserve special recognition. From my first phone conversation with Martha to review of the last page proofs with Amy and Cathy, I found the entire experience to surpass any preconceived ideal I held going into the project.

Mike Daiuto is my research workstudy, and along with my wife, was the closest thing to a staff we had on the book. He was particularly helpful in obtaining the citations for each chapter. His cheerful, easy manner was always appreciated. Mike Rekemeyer produced the line art illustrations. He turned the assignments around quickly and his rendition was always better than what I had envisioned. Jim Bandes photographed and developed a third of the halftone illustrations; his dedication to detail is appreciated.

Most of the imaging studies in this book came from three sources. The first is Palmer Chiropractic Clinics. The second and third are personal libraries compiled by Joseph Howe and the combined efforts of Steven Brownstein and William Litterer. These individuals deserve tremendous recognition for compiling these superb collections that have assisted me and so many other students and authors over the past years.

Don Betz, Iftikar Bhatti, Robert (Bucky) Percuoco, Bill Meeker, and Clay McDonald provided the environment in which this project was conceived and completed. I admire each of these individuals for their strong commitment to educational excellence, faculty development, and our institution. As with most projects I am involved in, I found advice and inspiration from my friend and colleague Chuck Henderson to be of particular value. I would like to thank Don Gran, Robin Canterbury, Ron Firth, and Robert Tatum for their helpful comments on several chapters.

Palmer College has a proud tradition of excellence in chiropractic. The Palmers and other early fathers of the chiropractic profession underwent tremendous personal sacrifice to bring chiropractic to the world. It is in this proud tradition that we present this book. We hope this book helps students better serve their studies, teachers better serve their students, and practitioners better serve their patients.

DENNIS M. MARCHIORI

Contents

PART THREE   Chest

PART FOUR   Abdomen

PART FIVE   Brain and Spinal Cord

CLINICAL IMAGING

With Skeletal, Chest, and Abdomen
Pattern Differentials

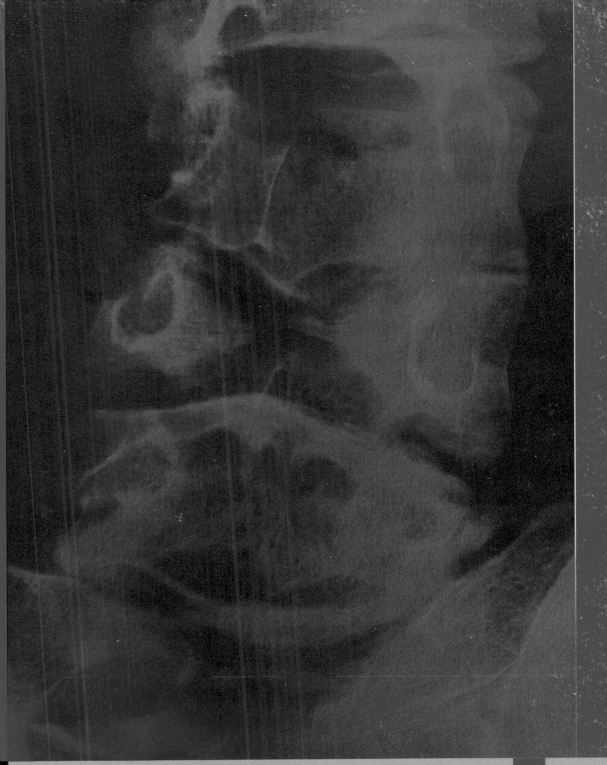

PART **ONE**

Introduction
to Imaging

chapter 1

Plain Radiographic Imaging

ROBERT PERCUOCO

Concepts of Radiation

X-RAY DISCOVERY

X-rays were discovered by Wilhelm Konrad Roentgen on November 8, 1895, in Wurtzburg, Germany. As he activated a simple cathode ray tube, called *Crookes' tube,* he happened to observe visible light emanating from a nearby plate coated with a phosphorescent substance, barium platinocyanide. Light emission increased as he brought the plate closer to the tube. He found that the newly discovered ray passed through objects of various composition. Roentgen named the strange phenomenon *x-light,* with *x* representing the unknown. The name *x-ray* was later adopted, although some called it a "roentgen ray" in honor of Roentgen.

PROPERTIES OF X-RAYS

Within months of Roentgen's discovery, he had uncovered nearly every property of x-rays known today. X-rays have the following properties:

- They are a type of electromagnetic radiation with neither mass nor charge that travel in straight lines at the speed of light.
- They travel in packets, or bundles, called *photons* or *quanta.*
- They produce chemical and biological effects in matter because of their ionizing capability.
- They cause certain materials to fluoresce.
- They sensitize radiographic and photographic film.
- They cannot be detected by human senses.
- They produce secondary and scatter radiation.
- They obey the inverse square law.
- They are absorbed by heavy, dense materials, such as lead and cement.
- They have a wave/particle dual nature.
- Because of their extremely short wavelengths, they penetrate materials that normally absorb or reflect light.
- They cannot be focused by a lens.
  - X-ray is a form of electromagnetic radiation that is produced when high-speed electrons in an electric circuit interact with a hard metal surface. The interaction takes place at the subatomic level and involves the electrical attributes of an atom.

ATOMIC STRUCTURE

In 1913 German physicist Niels Bohr compared the atom with a miniature solar system. Current theories have evolved beyond the Bohr atom; however, Bohr's theory works well for illustrating and understanding atomic forces. Basically, Bohr described the atom as having a dense core, or *nucleus,* made up of neutrons and positively charged protons. Negatively charged electrons, spinning on their axes, orbit the nucleus at fixed distances called *quantum shells* or *energy levels.* Quantum shells are assigned the letters *K, L, M, N,* and so on, with *K* being the innermost shell (Fig. 1-1). Electrons occupying shells farther away from the nucleus have greater *potential energy* than those found closer to the nucleus.

In a neutral atom the number of protons in the nucleus, or *atomic number (Z),* is equal to the number of orbiting electrons. The maximum number of electrons occupying a given shell is determined by the formula $2n^2$, where *n* is the quantum shell number. The quantum shell number is obtained by counting the shells outward from the nucleus. The *K* shell ($n = 1$) can hold $2(1)^2$, or 2 electrons, the *L* shell ($n = 2$) can hold $2(2)^2$, or 8 electrons, and so on. The outermost shell, or *valence shell,* never exceeds 8 electrons at one time in a stable atom.

Positively charged nuclear protons exert an electrostatic attractive force that binds electrons to their orbit. Electron spin velocity counters the attractive force and keeps electrons at discrete distances from the nucleus. Electrons occupying shells closer to the nucleus are bound tighter. The amount of energy needed to remove an electron completely from its orbit is called *electron binding energy.* Electron binding energy is measured in *electron volts (eV),* the same units used to describe x-ray energy. A free electron is assumed to have zero binding energy; therefore, a bound electron is in a negative energy state, because it takes positive energy to unbind or raise the binding energy to zero. Electrons occupying shells closer to the nucleus have greater binding energy than those found farther away from the nucleus. The binding energy for any given electron increases as atomic number increases (Fig. 1-2).

RADIATION

Energy is defined as the ability to do work. When energy is transmitted through space and/or matter, it is called *radiation.* Radiation takes on many forms, such as heat, light, and sound. Its energy is often described in the ability or inability to ionize matter. *Ionizing radiation* possesses sufficient energy to remove an orbital electron from a stable atom or molecule. X-rays, gamma rays, and alpha and beta particles are examples of ionizing radiation. *Nonionizing radi-*

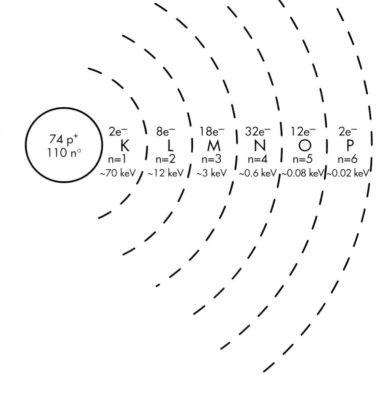

FIG. 1-1 The closer an electron is to the nucleus, the stronger its attraction to the nucleus.

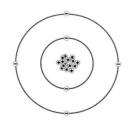

FIG. 1-2 Atomic shell levels and approximate electron binding energies for carbon and tungsten. Inner shell electrons are more tightly bound than are the outer shell electrons.

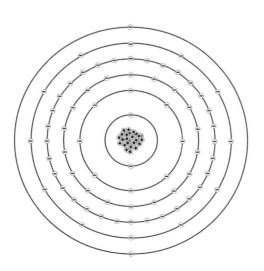

CARBON $\left(^{12}_{6}C\right)$		
Shell	Number of electrons	Approximate binding energy (keV)
K	2	0.284
L	4	0.006

TUNGSTEN $\left(^{184}_{74}W\right)$		
Shell	Number of electrons	Approximate binding energy (keV)
K	2	69.525
L	8	12.100
M	18	2.820
N	32	0.595
O	12	0.077
P	2	-

ation falls short of causing an ionization; however, it may excite stable atoms by raising an orbital electron to a higher energy state. This type of radiation includes visible light, infrared rays, microwaves, and radio waves. Ionizing radiation is categorized as either *particle* or *electromagnetic* radiation.

Particle radiation. Particle radiation is made up of any subatomic particles, such as subatomic protons, neutrons, and high-speed electrons, capable of causing ionization. Alpha and beta particles are two of the more common types of particle radiation. They come from the nuclei of radioactive atoms through radioactive decay. They have a mass component, may have a charge, and travel at varying speeds (slower than the speed of light).

Electromagnetic radiation. Electromagnetic radiation (EM) is an electric and magnetic disturbance traveling through space at the speed of light (2.998×10^8 m/s). It contains no mass nor charge but travels in packets of radiant energy called *photons,* or *quanta.* Examples of EM radiation include radio waves, TV waves, and microwaves, as well as infrared, ultraviolet, gamma, and x-rays. Some sources of EM radiation include the cosmos (such as the sun and the stars), radioactive elements, and man-made devices. Electromagnetic radiation exhibits a dual *wave/particle nature.*

Electromagnetic radiation travels in a waveform at a constant speed. The wave characteristics of EM radiation are found in the relationship of *velocity* to *wavelength* (the straight line distance of a single cycle) and *frequency* (cycles per second, or hertz, Hz), expressed in the formula

$$c = \lambda\nu$$

where c = velocity, λ = wavelength, and ν = frequency.

Because the velocity is constant, any increase in frequency results in a subsequent decrease in wavelength. Therefore, wavelength and frequency are *inversely proportional.* All forms of EM radiation are grouped according to their wavelengths into an electromagnetic spectrum, seen in Fig. 1-3.

The particlelike nature of EM radiation manifests in the interaction of ionizing photons with matter. The amount of energy *(E)* found in a photon is equal to its frequency *(ν)* times Planck's constant *(h):*

$$E = \nu h$$

Photon energy is *directly proportional* to photon frequency. Photon energy is measured in eV or keV (kilo electron volts). The energy range for diagnostic x-rays is 40 keV to 150 keV. Ultraviolet rays, x-rays, and gamma rays possess sufficient energy (greater than 10 keV) to cause ionizations.

The energy of EM radiation determines its usefulness for diagnostic imaging. Gamma rays and x-rays, because of their extremely short wavelengths, are capable of penetrating large body parts. Gamma rays are used in radionuclide imaging. X-rays are used for plain film and computerized tomographic (CT) imaging. Visible light is applied to observe and interpret images. Magnetic resonance imaging (MRI) uses *radiofrequency* EM radiation as a transmission medium (see Fig. 1-3).

RADIATION UNITS OF MEASUREMENT

Four units used to measure radiation are the *roentgen (R),* the *rad,* the *rem,* and the *curie.* The roentgen is a measurement of *radiation exposure,* or intensity, which will create 2.08×10^9 ion pairs in a cubic centimeter (cm^3) of air. The SI system (Systéme Internationale d'Unités) is a modernized metric system based on meters-kilograms-seconds or centimeters-grams-seconds. The SI units are used more broadly in science and most countries of the world than

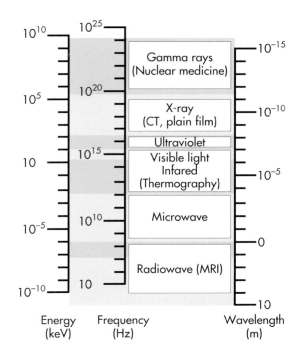

FIG. 1-3 The energy, frequency, and wavelength of the electromagnetic spectrum and their associated imaging modalities.

are the British, or Customary, units of feet-pounds-seconds. The SI unit for radiation exposure is coulombs/kilogram (C/kg); 1 roentgen is equal to 2.58×10^{-4} C/kg. Radiation exposure emitted from x-ray machines is measured in roentgens or C/kg.

The *rad* is the unit that measures *absorbed dose.* It is a measure of energy (expressed in ergs) deposited into a mass of tissue (expressed in grams or kilograms) and is often related to the biological effects of radiation. One rad is equal to 100 ergs in 1 gram of irradiated tissue. The SI unit for absorbed dose is the *gray (Gy).* One gray is equal to 100 rads. One rad is equal to 1/1000 of a gray, or 1 centigray (cGy).

The unit that defines *absorbed dose equivalent* for man is the *rem (rad equivalent man).* The rem is used exclusively for radiation protection reporting of occupational exposure. It is a measure of the biological effectiveness of different types of radiation. Compared with x-rays and gamma rays, radiation such as alpha and beta particles and fast neutrons produces different magnitudes of biological effects, even at the same absorbed dose.

The National Council on Radiation Protection and Measurements (NCRP) is the governing body responsible for reporting guidelines for radiation protection and measurements. The most recent report, *NCRP No. 116: Limitations of Exposure to Ionizing Radiation,* which succeeds NCRP report No. 91, replaces the term *dose equivalent (H)* with the term *equivalent dose ($H_{T,R}$).* The change goes beyond word semantics. Dose equivalent *(H)* is a measurement of absorbed dose at some certain location in tissue. Equivalent dose *($H_{T,R}$)* is a measurement of an *average absorbed dose* in tissues and organs. Equivalent dose is the product of the average absorbed dose *($D_{T,R}$)* of radiation *(R)* in a tissue *(T)* and a radiation weighting factor *(W_R):*

$$H_{T,R} = W_R D_{T,R}$$

The weighting factor replaces the previously used *quality factor (QF)* and accounts for the biological effectiveness of specific types of radiation. The weighting factor for x-rays and gamma rays is 1; 1 rad of x-rays is equal to 1 rem. Alpha particles have a W_R of 20; 1 rad of alpha particles is equal to 20 rems. The SI unit for the rem is the *sievert (Sv)*. A sievert is the product of the absorbed dose in grays and the radiation weighting factor. One Sv is equal to 100 rems, and 1 rem is equal to 10 mSv.

The curie (Ci) is a quantitative measure of *radioactive material.* It is defined as the amount of radioactive material in which 3.7×10^{10} atoms disintegrate every second. The radiation emitted from a curie of radioactive material is measured in roentgens, rads, and rems. The SI unit is the *becquerel (Bq),* defined as 1 disintegration per second. Millicurie (mCi) and microcurie (μCi) amounts are common in nuclear medicine procedures. The reporting units used in the radiological sciences are listed in Table 1-1.

TABLE 1-1
Units of Measure in the Radiological Sciences

Quantity	Customary unit	SI unit
Exposure	Roentgen (R)	Coulomb/kilogram (C/kg)
Absorbed dose	Rad (rad)	Gray (Gy)
Dose equivalent	Rem (rem)	Sievert (Sv)
Activity	Curie (Ci)	Becquerel (Bq)

X-Ray Tube

Producing x-rays requires a source of electrons, a means to rapidly accelerate them, and a means to rapidly decelerate them. These factors are built into the x-ray apparatus. The three principle components of an x-ray machine are the *x-ray tube,* the *generator,* and the *control console.*

TUBE HOUSING

The *tube housing* is a grounded, lead-lined metal shelter that protects and supports the glass x-ray tube insert (Fig. 1-4). X-rays are emitted multidirectionally from the tube, but only those rays passing through an opening, or *window,* in the housing expose the patient. All other rays are trapped in the housing wall, thereby decreasing unnecessary exposure to patients and/or x-ray personnel. Radiation emitted from the tube housing is called *primary radiation.*

Several high-voltage electrical cables connect through the back of the housing to the tube. The housing is factory packed with industrial grade oil to provide thermal and electrical insulation. Many modern x-ray tubes have protection circuitry hooked into an expansion bellows inside the housing. As the oil expands with heating, the bellows trips a switch, which prohibits further exposure until the tube cools sufficiently. Industrial x-ray tubes may have a large heat exchanger that circulates and cools the oil.

GLASS ENVELOPE

X-rays are produced when high-speed electrons are rapidly decelerated in an x-ray tube. The x-ray tube is a device composed of two

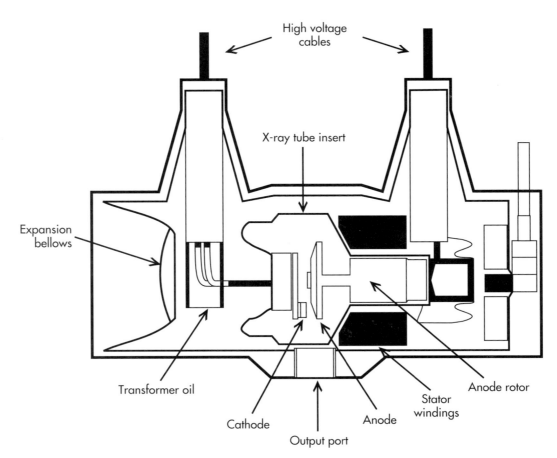

FIG. 1-4　A rotating anode x-ray tube with housing assembly.

electrodes, *cathode* and *anode,* sealed in an evacuated borosilicate glass envelope. Electrons in an electric circuit, generated at the cathode, are accelerated toward and strike an anode target, resulting mostly in heat energy and some x-ray energy. Approximately 1% of the kinetic energy of high-speed electrons produces x-rays.

Cathode. The cathode is the negative electrode and contains a filament embedded in a shallow depression called the *focusing cup.* Most diagnostic x-ray tubes are dual focus because they have two filaments: a large filament for large exposures and a small filament for small exposures.

The cathode *filament* supplies a controlled number of electrons to the anode. The filament is a thoriated tungsten wire drawn into a small, thin coil. Tungsten is used because its high atomic number (74) makes it electron rich. Current running through the filament heats it to white incandescence, which results in electrons being "boiled off" the tungsten by a process called *thermionic emission.* A cloud of electrons, or *space charge,* forms around the filament (Fig. 1-5). The space charge size is controlled by the amount of current running through the filament. Filament current is regulated by

the *mA (milliamperage) selector* on the control console. The space charge generates *tube current,* current between the cathode and anode. The tube current is directly proportional to radiation exposure or quantity of x-rays produced.

Electrons travel in only one direction in the tube, from cathode to anode. As the space charge builds, electrons repulse each other. This causes them to diverge, covering an unacceptable area on the anode. A *focusing cup* surrounding the filament carries a negative potential that tends to condense or "focus" the electron stream onto the anode target.

Anode. The anode is the positive electrode in the x-ray tube.

The anode (1) produces x-rays, (2) conducts electricity, and (3) conducts heat away from the anode surface.

There are two types of anodes: *stationary* and *rotating.* Most diagnostic applications require the rotating type. The stationary anode is most applicable when a smaller electrical load is required for imaging (e.g., mammographic and dental x-rays).

A stationary anode consists of a copper shaft with a tungsten-rhenium target imbedded into a beveled surface (Fig. 1-6). Tungsten

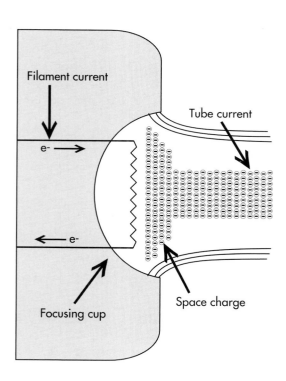

FIG. 1-5 Electrons that "boil off" the heated filament create a space charge surrounding the filament producing the tube current.

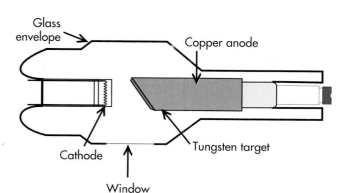

FIG. 1-6 Stationary anode x-ray tube.

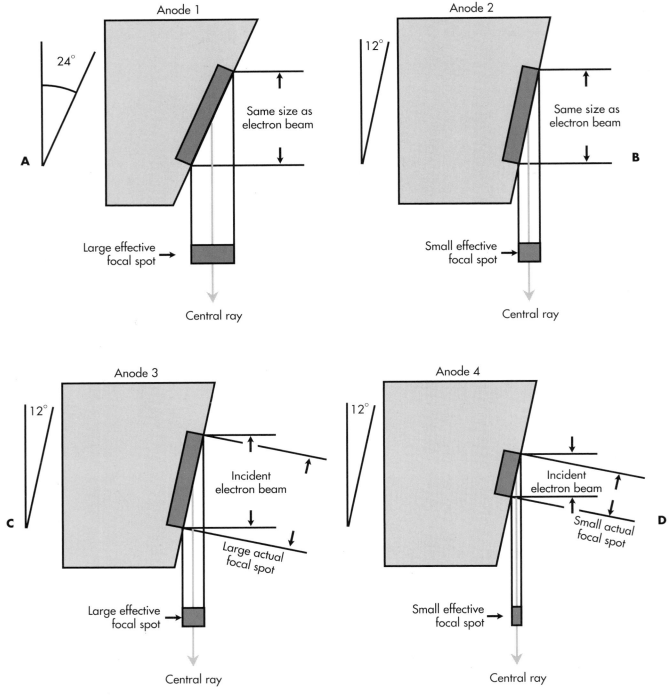

FIG. I-7   The line-focus principle results in a smaller effective focal spot than the actual focal spot. **A** and **B,** The larger the angle of the anode is, the larger the effective focal spot is. **C** and **D,** The larger the actual focal spot is, the larger the effective focal spot.

is used because of its high melting point (3410° C) and its high atomic number (74). The atomic number affects the ability of tungsten to produce x-rays in the diagnostic range. The beveled or angled surface affects the electron-loading capacity of the anode by providing more surface area for heat conduction. The angle on stationary anodes ranges from 30 degrees to 45 degrees. The most common angle used on rotating anodes is 12 degrees with a useful range of 7 to 17 degrees.

A rotating anode allows for significantly greater electron loading by providing a much larger surface area, or *focal track,* for heat conduction. The rotating anode consists of three component parts: (1) the disc or target, (2) the stem, and (3) the rotor.

The disc is made of molybdenum and is covered with a tungsten-rhenium target material. An *electromagnetic induction motor* is used to rotate the anode disc an average of 3400 revolutions per minute (RPM) during the exposure, with high-speed anodes rotating at 10,000 RPM. Tube electron loading is directly proportional to anode rotation.

The stem connects the disc to the rotor and is made of copper for electrical conduction. The rotor is a shaftlike part composed of bars of copper and soft iron. The rotor is held in place in the tube by bearings that facilitate high-speed rotation. Outside of the evacuated glass tube and adjacent to the rotor is a series of electromagnets called a *stator.* Current running through the stator creates a magnetic field that crosses the rotor. The stator windings are sequentially energized, creating a rotating magnetic field that turns the rotor (see Fig. 1-4).

Anode rotation is initiated by pressing the rotor or "prep" switch on the control console prior to activating the exposure. The filament circuit is also wired into the rotor switch so that filament current is boosted to preset levels at the time the rotor switch is pressed. Rotor speed and space charge are generated first in anticipation of the exposure. Pressing the exposure switch causes electrons to move from cathode to anode.

With many x-ray machines, the exposure switch alone activates all functions of the tube—rotation of the anode, creation of the space charge, and movement of electrons from cathode to anode. However, two-handed operation of the rotor and exposure switches allows the operator to control exactly when exposure occurs. Single-handed operation of the exposure switch alone is best when using very fast exposure time (milliseconds).

LINE-FOCUS PRINCIPLE

Electrons strike the surface of the anode at a target site called the *actual focal spot* (Fig. 1-7). The actual focal spot size varies, based on filament size and anode angle. As the actual focal spot size increases, the electron-loading capacity of the anode increases. The entire target area emits x-rays; however, only x-rays traveling in the direction of the patient are useful. The *line-focus principle* results in a reduction of the effective area of the actual focal spot to that portion of the beam projected toward the patient. This results in an increase in recorded detail on film. The effective target area, or *effective focal spot,* is a projection from the center of the actual focal spot, along the central ray, and perpendicular to the plane of the x-ray port. The size of the effective focal spot is controlled by the size of the filament and the angle of the anode (see Fig. 1-7). Effective focal spot sizes commonly used in diagnostic radiology range from 0.6 mm to 1 mm for small focus and 1.5 to 2 mm for large focus.

Focal spot selection is linked to specific mA stations on the control console. For example, the small focal spot is coupled with the 50, 100, and 150 mA stations on some machines. This limits the load on the anode and is best used with small body parts, such as the cervical spine and extremities. The large focal spot is coupled with the 200 mA station and higher to allow for greater electron loading of the anode. It is best used with large body parts, such as the lumbar spine. The small focus produces images with better detail than the large focus.

OFF-FOCUS RADIATION

Some electrons may stray from the focal spot and interact with other internal component parts of the tube, such as the anode stem. An alternate site is created for x-ray production, and the rays produced may cause shadowing of the image. *Off-focus radiation* is controlled mainly by beam-limiting devices called *collimators.*

HEEL EFFECT

X-ray intensity emanating from the tube is not uniform across the span of the beam. Exposure intensity is greater on the cathode side of the beam than on the anode side. This is called the *anode heel effect.* Electrons penetrate the target at various depths, causing x-rays to be emitted with equal intensity in all directions. Those x-rays traveling into the substance of the anode are immediately absorbed. The angle at which x-rays emerge from the target surface toward the patient varies and causes some x-rays to be absorbed in the heel of the anode. The heel attenuates a portion of the x-ray beam and leaves less exposure (intensity) on the anode side of the beam (Fig. 1-8).

The heel effect can be used to advantage when imaging body parts of different thicknesses by placing the cathode portion of the beam over the thicker part of the patient. The heel effect is less noticeable with smaller film sizes (8-inch × 10-inch) and longer tube distances (72-inch), because more of the central, uniform portion of the beam is used.

FILTRATION

Very-low-energy x-rays, or *soft rays,* add no diagnostic information to the image, because they are completely absorbed by the pa-

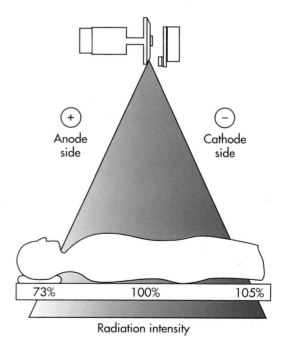

FIG. 1-8 Because of the anode heel effect, the x-ray beam is more intense on the cathode side.

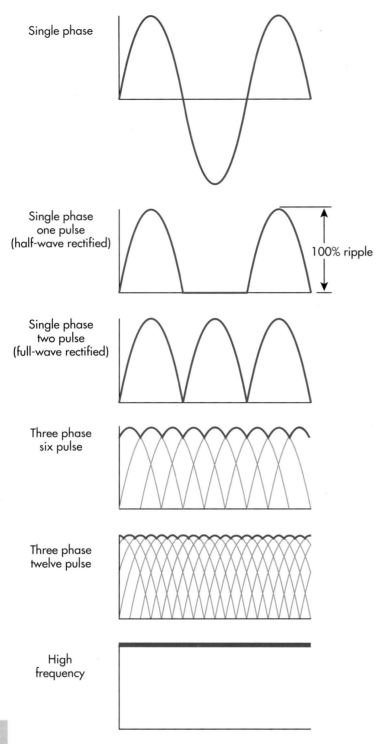

Single phase

Single phase
one pulse
(half-wave rectified)

100% ripple

Single phase
two pulse
(full-wave rectified)

Three phase
six pulse

Three phase
twelve pulse

High
frequency

FIG. 1-9   Voltage waveforms for various types of x-ray generators. Single-phase generators experience 100% ripple, whereas high-frequency generators deliver a near-constant potential with less than 1% to 2% ripple.

tient. To reduce patient dose from soft radiation, federal law requires a minimum of 2.5 mm, equivalent of aluminum (equiv/Al) filtration for a beam greater than 70 kVp. Aluminum absorbs many of the low-energy photons while transmitting a large proportion of high-energy photons. The glass port window and oil within the tube housing provide *inherent filtration* of approximately 0.5 mm equiv/Al The silver-coated mirror in the collimator is placed so that the x-ray beam must pass through it. It may supply another 1 mm equiv/Al of inherent filtration.

Another 2 mm of aluminum are *added* to most diagnostic x-ray machines to meet federal guidelines for total filtration. Inherent filtration plus added filtration equals *total filtration*. Compensating filters, used to offset variations in patient density, are not calculated into the total filtration needed to decrease the soft x-ray dose.

Generator (The Power to Generate X-rays)

The electrical potential needed to accelerate electrons to high speed in the tube is provided by *single phase, 3-phase,* and *constant potential (high-frequency) generators.* The scope of this chapter does not permit a detailed discussion on how these generators work; however, it is important to understand that the output waveform affects average x-ray energy, exposure time, and patient dose from soft radiation.

Alternating current (AC) is dispensed to the x-ray machine from an external source, but it is changed to direct current (DC) before it reaches the tube. AC manifests in electrons oscillating back and forth in a circuit and is graphically represented in Fig. 1-9 by a sine wave. Each cycle of single-phase AC comprises a positive and negative pulsation. Running AC through the tube would create two problems: (1) it would destroy the cathode when electrons reverse polarity during the negative pulsation, and (2) a secondary site for x-ray production would be generated and negate any advantage of increased image detail produced by the line-focus principle.

AC is changed to DC through a process called *rectification.* For our purposes, how rectification occurs is less important than why it occurs. Suppressing the negative pulsation of alternating current protects the tube and results in a type of pulsating DC called *half-wave rectification* (see Fig. 1-9). X-ray energy is produced at the peak of these pulsations (Fig. 1-10). Reversing the negative pulsation to a positive direction provides *full-wave rectification,* resulting in twice the number of pulsations per unit of time. This reduces the exposure time by half when compared with half-wave rectified circuits.

X-rays are produced when electrons strike the target at or near their peak potential, or *kVp.* In the case of full-wave rectified circuits, bursts of diagnostic x-rays are produced when the electrical potential reaches its peak with periods of no x-rays produced between the peaks. The voltage drop from peak kilovoltage (kVp) is called *ripple* and represents the efficiency at which x-rays are produced. The greater the ripple, the less efficient the x-ray production. A kVp of zero accompanies 100% ripple. A voltage potential that drops below peak kilovoltage produces x-ray photons with a spectrum of energies.

SINGLE-PHASE GENERATORS

Single-phase, full-wave rectified generators utilize a 220-volt, 100-amp, single-phase AC line source to produce two pulsations per cycle (120 pulsations per second), with 100% voltage ripple. With a constantly changing voltage potential, a spectrum of x-ray energies is produced with an average energy somewhere below peak kilo-

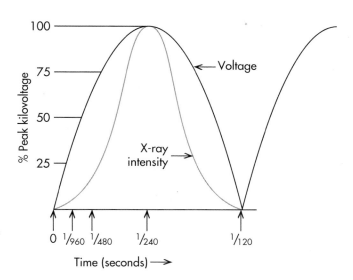

FIG. 1-10 Following a slight lag, x-ray intensity increases rapidly as the voltage across the x-ray tube increases from zero to its peak value.

voltage. This pulsating beam results in an inefficient use of electricity, longer exposure time, and greater patient dose from lower-energy *soft x-rays* compared with more efficient generators that deliver a nonpulsating, constant electrical potential.

THREE-PHASE GENERATORS

A three-phase generator utilizes a three-phase AC line source for the purpose of creating more pulsations per unit time. This effectively reduces voltage ripple and increases efficiency of x-ray production. Three-phase power is best understood by imagining three single-phase line sources electrically intertwined to create greater incoming power. A *six-pulse generator* delivers six pulsations per cycle, which reduces voltage ripple to 13% of peak kilovoltage (see Fig. 1-9). Changing the wiring configuration produces 12 pulses per cycle *(12-pulse generator),* reducing voltage ripple to 3% of peak kilovoltage. Using three-phase power results in greater photon output per unit of electrical input (mR/mAs) with higher average energy compared with single-phase units. Three-phase generators are expensive, relying on costly power line installations.

CONSTANT POTENTIAL GENERATORS

Medium- and high-frequency generators operate on either single-phase or three-phase power and through rectification and smoothing circuits virtually eliminate voltage ripple. Medium-frequency generators produce an electrical frequency in the 6 to 30 kHz range, and high-frequency generators produce an electrical frequency of approximately 100 kHz. Medium- and high-frequency generators allow more accurate control of tube voltages. Tube voltage regulates penetration of the x-ray beam. High-frequency generators produce the greatest mR/milliampere-seconds output, the lowest soft radiation dosage to patients, the highest average (effective) x-ray energy and the shortest exposure time.

TIMER CONTROL

Every x-ray exposure requires a certain predetermined tube current (mA) for a specific period of time. Both the timer and timer circuit are located on the control console and are electrically connected to the exposure switch.

Timers are described as *mechanical, synchronous,* or *electronic.* A simple *mechanical timer* is spring-loaded and unwinds at a set rate. Mechanical timers are used with single-phase, low-output x-ray generators such as those seen in dental offices. They are not very accurate and are limited to exposure times faster than ¼ second.

Synchronous timers operate from a synchronous motor running at 60 Hz. The time increments are in multiples of ¹⁄₆₀ second, such as ¹⁄₃₀, ¹⁄₂₀, and ¹⁄₁₀. The shortest exposure time is ¹⁄₁₂₀ second. Synchronous timers are not as accurate as electronic timers and cannot be used with serial exposures because they require a short recycling time.

An *electronic timer* is the most common timer in use today. It is accurate to less than 1 millisecond (msec) and to greater than 1 second. Electronic timers operate on sophisticated electronic circuitry by energizing a silicon-controlled rectifier (SCR), which activates the exposure. The combination of constant potential generators and very fast imaging systems (rare earth) requires the need for an accurate timer in milliseconds.

The product of mA and time, milliampere-seconds (mAs), determines the number of x-ray photons emitted and hence, the relative darkness of the film. Patient part size and density govern how much milliampere-seconds is needed to produce a diagnostic image. Calculating exposure by using units of milliampere-seconds is common in a clinical setting. A *mAs timer* accurately provides the highest safe tube current with the shortest exposure time for a given milliampere-seconds. Independent control of mA and time may not be possible with some milliampere-seconds timers.

AUTOMATIC EXPOSURE CONTROL (AEC)

Automatic exposure control (AEC), often referred to as *phototiming,* terminates the exposure when a predetermined amount of film density (darkness) is reached by x-rays passing through the patient to the image receptor. The radiographer selects the appropriate beam penetration (peak kilovoltage) and desired tube current (mA) for the part under examination. The phototiming device senses the exposure and, in response, creates an electronic signal that breaks the timer circuit.

Automatic exposure devices include the earlier photomultiplier tube and the more common ionization chamber. The photomultiplier tube converts a light signal from a fluorescent screen exposed to x-rays to an electronic signal that feeds back to terminate the exposure. The radiation-sensitive ionization chamber creates an electronic signal proportional to the number of ions produced by radiation exposure and feeds back to terminate the exposure.

The phototiming circuit usually has one, two, or three photocells of different shapes and positions in relation to the image receptor. From the control console, the operator may choose to use one or more photocells to determine exposure. When using more than one photocell, the exposure is averaged between them. A manual backup timer is set to approximately 1½ times the anticipated exposure to prevent tube overload and excessive patient dose. Setting the backup time too short may result in a risk of underexposure.

AEC decreases the need for repeat radiographs by compensating for patient density and reducing human error in exposure calculation. However, positioning the body part under examination precisely over the photocell(s) is paramount to producing adequate exposure. Malposition results in over- or underexposure. The calibration of the phototimer must be matched with the sensitivity of the image receptor (film/screen).

TUBE FAILURE

X-ray tubes can fail in a number of different ways. Most tube failure occurs as the result of thermal wear on the internal component parts. The wear usually develops over a period of time; however, an

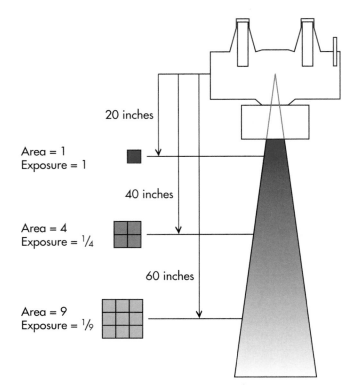

20 inches

Area = 1
Exposure = 1

40 inches

Area = 4
Exposure = ¼

60 inches

Area = 9
Exposure = ⅑

FIG. 1-11   Inverse square law. The intensity of the x-ray beam decreases with increasing distance from its source. The magnitude of intensity is inversely proportional to the square of the distance.

3. *Exposure time* is another factor controlling the number of x-rays (*quantity*) produced. Time is measured from milliseconds to seconds and is given the abbreviation *s*. Longer exposure time allows more electrons to be generated from the filament. Exposure time is also linear in that as time is doubled, exposure is doubled.

   In clinical settings, exposure intensity (quantity) is commonly described by the product of milliamperes and time, or milliampere-seconds. Ascribing milliampere-seconds to a particular body part size is helpful in determining the total exposure needed to produce an acceptable image. Once the measurement of milliampere-seconds is determined, any combination of milliamperage and time to produce that same measurement of milliampere-seconds yields a similar exposure. Kilovoltage is responsible for supplying the penetration required to produce adequate subject contrast on the image receptor.

4. *Distance,* the fourth exposure parameter, is often expressed as *FFD* (focal-spot-to-film distance), *SID* (source-to-image receptor distance), and *TFD* (target-to-film distance). Distance affects the number of x-rays reaching the image receptor (film). As the x-ray tube is moved farther away from the film, the beam diverges and offers less x-ray photons per unit area. The number of x-ray photons striking the film is inversely proportional to the square of the distance. This is called the *inverse square law* and is expressed as

$$I = 1/d^2$$

where I = x-ray intensity and d = tube distance. If the distance is doubled, approximately ¼ of the number of x-rays reaches the film (Fig. 1-11).

An increase in distance mandates an increase in exposure proportional to the square of the distance. Exposure increase is expressed by the formula

$$\text{New mAs} = \text{Old mAs} \times (FFD_2/FFD_1)^2$$

where FFD_1 is the original distance, FFD_2 is the new distance, *old mAs* is the exposure at the original distance, and *new mAs* is the exposure at the new distance.

Control Console

Basic single-phase operating consoles (Fig. 1-12) provide selectors for *power (on/off), line-voltage compensation, peak kilovoltage, milliamperage, time, focal spot, bucky, AEC, rotor,* and *exposure.*

Control consoles have evolved with the use of computer technology. Manufacturers have reduced console size by replacing copper wiring, steel construction, and knob controls with micro circuitry. Menu-driven push-button controls, preprogrammed anatomical techniques, and AEC have dramatically reduced human error in the calculation and selection of exposure parameters.

Modern single-phase 300 mA/125 kVp x-ray machines may offer any or all of the following:
- Automatic line-voltage compensation (surge protection)
- Kilovoltage selection by units of 1 kV, from 40 to 125 kVp
- Milliamperage selection normally ranging from 25 mA to 300 mA and as high as 600 mA in 50 to 100 mA increments
- Automatic focal spot selection based on milliampere designation
- Electronic SCR timers with milliampere-seconds readout
- AEC with photocell selector and plus and minus density control
- Bucky selection
- Single-switch or double-switch operation of rotor control and exposure control
- Tube protection circuitry to safeguard against overload

instantaneous load significantly above the tube rating can immediately cause a tube to fail. Common types of tube failure include worn rotor bearings, a cracked or pitted anode, gassing of the tube, and open cathode filament.

To better prepare the tube to receive a high heat load, it is best to perform a *tube warm-up* procedure. Performing a couple of low-load exposures puts some heat into the anode and reduces the stress of an instantaneous large load on a cold anode. An example of a warm-up technique is an initial exposure of 50 kVp, 100 mA, at 1/10 second, followed by a second exposure where the mA is raised to 200.

PRIMARY FACTORS CONTROLLING X-RAY EXPOSURE

Four primary exposure factors control the quantity and quality of x-rays produced: peak kilovoltage, mA, time (seconds), and distance.
1. *Kilovoltage* (expressed in peak kilovolts, or kVp) directly controls the speed of electrons traveling from cathode to anode. As electrons strike the target, their kinetic energy is transformed into x-ray and heat energy. X-ray *quality,* or *penetration power,* is directly proportional to peak kilovoltage. Kilovoltage is the only controlling factor affecting x-ray beam energy (quality).
2. *Milliamperage* (measured in milliamperes, or *mA*) is a measure of tube current generated from the filament by thermionic emission. The number of electrons available to produce x-rays is directly proportional to milliamperage. Changes in milliamperage affect the *quantity* of x-rays produced. Milliamperage is linear in that as it is doubled, exposure is doubled.

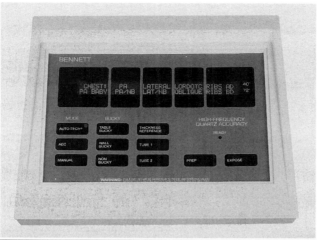

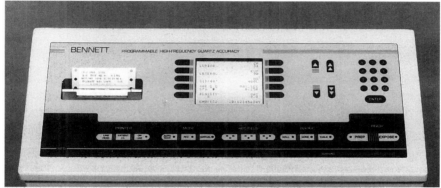

FIG. 1-12 X-ray consoles. (From Guebert G: *Radiologic science for the chiropractor,* St Louis, 1995, Mosby.)

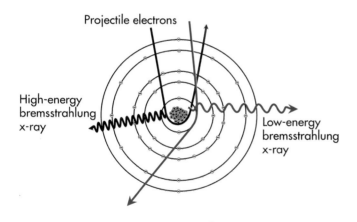

FIG. 1-13 Bremsstrahlung x-rays are emitted when the speed and direction of a projectile electron is altered secondary to interaction with the target's nucleus.

X-Ray Production

X-rays are generated by two different yet simultaneous processes as high-speed electrons lose energy at the target. One reaction involves high-speed electrons interacting with the nucleus of tungsten target atoms to generate what is called *bremsstrahlung radiation.* The other involves collisions of high-speed electrons with inner shell electrons of target atoms to produce what is called *characteristic radiation.*

BREMSSTRAHLUNG X-RAYS

Bremsstrahlung is the German word for *braking,* or slowing down. When a high-speed projectile electron from the cathode passes the nucleus of a tungsten atom in the target, the nucleus exerts a strong attractive force that causes the electron to decelerate and change direction (Fig. 1-13). This deceleration results in a loss of kinetic energy, which is converted into electromagnetic radiation (x-rays). The quality (or energy) of radiation released is contingent upon the amount of deceleration and the amount of kinetic energy possessed by the incoming electron (measured in peak kilovolts, or kVp). Deceleration is affected by the proximity in which electrons randomly approach the nucleus and the size of the nucleus. Electrons directly striking the nucleus and giving up 100% of their kinetic energy generate the highest-energy x-rays.

Bremsstrahlung x-rays have a spectrum of energies, with an average energy somewhere below, but proportional to, the peak kilovolts used. Primary control of x-ray quality, or overall penetrating power, is a result of the effect of peak kilovolts on bremsstrahlung

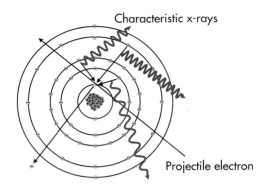

FIG. 1-14   Characteristic x-rays are emitted when outer shell electrons fill the K-shell vacancy created by the projectile electron.

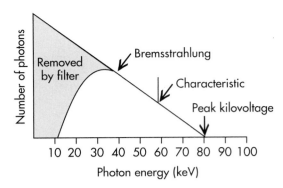

FIG. 1-15   Photon energy spectrum typical for a machine operating at 80 kVp.

interactions. The quantity of bremsstrahlung x-rays is related more to milliampere-seconds (tube current) than to peak kilovolts. Higher values of milliampere-seconds release more electrons to the target. Most of the x-rays produced in a diagnostic beam are of bremsstrahlung origin.

CHARACTERISTIC X-RAYS

When a high-speed electron from the cathode interacts with an inner shell electron in the tungsten target and the kinetic energy of the projectile electron exceeds the binding energy of the electron it interacts with, the orbital electron is ejected, leaving a vacancy in the inner shell (Fig. 1-14). Immediately, an outer shell electron fills the vacancy, resulting in a release of a discrete amount of electromagnetic radiation (x-ray). The amount of energy released is equal to the difference in the binding energies of the orbital shells involved. For tungsten, atomic number 74, the following applies:

$$E_{Kshell} - E_{Lshell} = 69.5 \text{ keV} - 12.1 \text{ keV} = 57.4 \text{ keV x-ray}$$

A cascade effect causes all inner shell vacancies to be filled and lower energy photons to be released. The total amount of energy released equals the input energy required to remove the inner shell electron.

Binding energies are unique to each element. The x-ray released is "characteristic" of the atom it is generated from, hence the name *characteristic x-ray*. A *K*-characteristic x-ray of tungsten is 57.4 keV. A *K*-characteristic x-ray of molybdenum is 17.4 keV. It takes at least 70 keV (kVp) of input energy to release a *K*-shell electron in tungsten. Kilovoltage has no effect on the quality (energy) of characteristic radiation. The energy of characteristic x-rays increases, however, as atomic number increases. Characteristic x-rays make up approximately 10% of the radiation emitted in the 80 to 100 kVp range. Fig. 1-15 illustrates a filtered beam of bremsstrahlung and characteristic x-rays at 80 kVp.

Diagnostic X-Ray Interactions with Matter

One of three things can happen to a diagnostic x-ray as it encounters matter. It can (1) be totally absorbed, (2) be partially absorbed and scattered, or (3) pass through unaffected. The quality of the image produced is greatly affected by all three events.

PHOTOELECTRIC EFFECT

The *photoelectric effect* is a total absorption reaction, where moderate- to lower-energy x-rays interact with inner shell electrons of an absorbing medium to cause ionizations (Fig. 1-16). The x-ray gives up all of its energy to overcome the binding energy of an inner shell electron and the x-ray ceases to exist. The empty shell is filled with an electron from an upper orbit resulting in the release of characteristic radiation. The characteristic ray is called *secondary radiation* and is emitted randomly like scatter radiation. Most of these rays are reabsorbed in the body.

A photoelectric interaction is dependent upon the atomic number of the absorbing medium and the energy of the x-ray. The tighter an electron is bound, the more likely it is to be involved in a photoelectric interaction. Also, the closer the x-ray energy is to the binding energy of an inner shell electron, the greater the chance is for a photoelectric effect. Absorption probability is inversely proportional to the cube of the x-ray energy (E) ($\frac{1}{E^3}$) and it is directly proportional to the cube of the atomic number (Z), or Z^3.

The photoelectric effect is responsible for subject contrast seen on a radiograph. The x-ray beam is *attenuated,* or weakened, through absorption as it encounters tissues of different densities and atomic numbers. The resulting *differential absorption* produces subject contrast. With higher energy x-rays (high peak kilovoltage), subject contrast is decreased as a result of an overall decrease in absorption.

COMPTON SCATTERING

Compton scattering is a partial absorption reaction that involves moderate-energy x-rays. As photon energy increases with a higher number of peak kilovolts, the x-ray gives up some of its energy as it strikes an outer shell electron in an absorbing medium (Fig. 1-17). The electron is ejected and the x-ray deflects from its original path. The photon energy loss results in a longer wavelength x-ray that is scattered. The angle of deflection is proportional to the energy loss. Radiation that scatters 180 degrees back in the direction of the tube is called *backscatter.* Scatter radiation delivers misinformation to the image receptor, which fogs the film and decreases image visibility. Scatter increases the overall darkness of the film, but not in a way that provides useful information.

The probability that an x-ray will undergo a Compton effect depends upon the density of the absorbing medium and the energy of the x-ray. Water density tissues (e.g., muscle, blood, and solid organs) create the greatest amount of scatter radiation in the body. Tissues of greater density, such as bone, tend to completely absorb x-rays. Low-density tissues that contain air (e.g., lung and large bowel) allow a greater amount of complete penetration. Higher-energy x-rays tend toward complete penetration, medium-energy x-rays tend toward scattering, and lower-energy x-rays tend toward complete absorption.

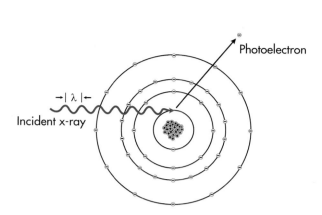

Photoelectric effect describes total absorption of the incident x-ray and ejection of an electron, known as a *photoelectron* once it is ejected. The empty shell is filled with an electron from an upper orbit, resulting in the release of characteristic radiation.

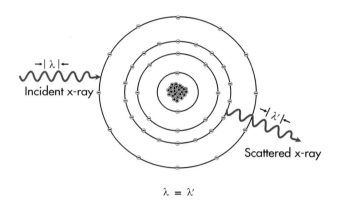

Compton's effect describes the interaction between medium-energy x-rays and outer shell electrons. The interaction results in ionization of the target atom (with ejection of a Compton electron), deflection of the incident x-ray, and higher energy in the scattered x-ray.

CLASSICAL (RAYLEIGH) SCATTERING

Classical scattering involves very-low-energy x-rays (10 keV) and matter. An incoming, or incident x-ray, photon interacts with an atom, causing its electrons to vibrate at the same frequency as the photon (Fig. 1-18). The excited atom releases the excess energy in the form of a new photon. The new photon is randomly emitted as scatter and has a wavelength and energy equal to the incident photon. Rayleigh scattering accounts for less than 5% of scatter in the diagnostic range and does not significantly impact image quality.

FACTORS CONTRIBUTING TO SCATTER RADIATION PRODUCTION

Beam energy, field size, patient size, and tissue type are the major contributors to scatter radiation production. As *beam energy* is increased, for example, from 70 to 90 kVp, fewer x-rays are completely absorbed. This leaves more photons to scatter. The percentage of Compton interactions increases as peak kilovolts increases. As *field size* is increased, scatter increases by expanding the area of tissue that interacts with primary radiation. As *patient size* increases, augmented by an increase in *soft tissue* water density, more scatter is produced.

METHODS OF SCATTER CONTROL

As previously mentioned, scatter radiation fogs a radiograph, thereby decreasing overall film contrast. Controlling scatter helps to increase contrast. Scatter may be regulated in the production phase or, once it is produced, by constraining it from reaching the film. Limiting peak kilovolts, minimizing beam size, and utilizing patient recumbency, air-gap technique, and grids are all viable methods for controlling scatter.

Although the kilovoltage range for diagnostic x-rays is between 40 and 150 kVp, scatter is best controlled by limiting peak kilovolts to 70 to 90 for the axial skeleton. The presentation of an obese patient may tempt the radiographer to drive the peak kilovolts higher; however, for scatter control, it is better to limit the peak kilovolts and increase the milliampere-seconds.

Classical scattering describes an interaction between lower energy x-rays and atoms. The wavelengths of the incident and scattered x-rays are the same.

Limiting the exposure area helps to minimize patient dose and scatter radiation. Field size is regulated by beam restrictors.

The simplest type of beam restrictor is an *aperture diaphragm*. An aperture diaphragm is a flat sheet of lead with a prescribed opening size to cover a certain film size; it is attached to the tube housing at the port. The aperture diaphragm is used in situations where film size and tube distance are constant, such as head or chest radiography.

Cones and *cylinders* are extension tubes attached to the tube housing to control beam size. Flared cones (Fig. 1-19) are designed to resemble a divergent x-ray beam, but they are often flared wider than the beam. The effectiveness is reduced to that of an aperture diaphragm. A cylinder provides true beam restriction as the field size is controlled by the constricted outer opening, which is farther away from the focal spot. Some cylinders are adjustable, which enhances versatility and effectiveness.

A *collimator* is a variable-aperture beam-limiting device. It contains two sets of lead shutters, fixed upper shutters and adjustable lower shutters (Fig. 1-20). The upper shutters serve

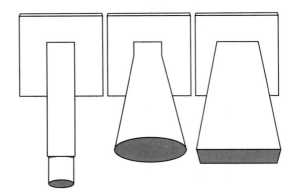

FIG. 1-19   Cones and cylinders.

Adjustable   Circular   Rectangular
cylinder   flare   flare

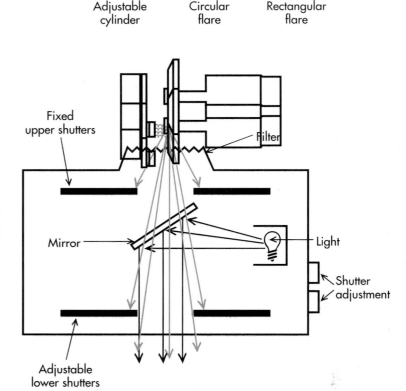

FIG. 1-20   A collimator restricts the primary beam with fixed upper and adjustable lower shutters. An interposed mirror is used to reflect light through the opening created by the moveable shutters to yield a representation of the beam size during patient positioning.

as an aperture diaphragm, controlling off-focus radiation. The lower shutters adjust in the vertical and horizontal directions to control the exposure area. A light field is projected through the lower shutter opening to help the radiographer approximate the exposure field. The light comes from a high-intensity lamp that reflects off a mirror strategically placed within the collimator. Collimators must be periodically checked to ensure that the light field and exposure field coincide.

PBL (positive beam limitation) collimators are manufactured to automatically adjust field size to film size. Distance and film size sensors regulate a motorized mechanism in the collimator to automatically adjust the lower shutters to the film size. An automatic collimator "locks out" an exposure if the beam size exceeds the film size.

Patient recumbency. When a patient is placed in a recumbent (lying down) position, soft tissue is more evenly distributed and the overall thickness of the patient is decreased. The decreased thick-ness results in production of less scatter. Accurate measurement of exposure factors requires that the patient be in the recumbent position.

Air-gap technique. If the OFD (object-to-film distance) is increased to create an air space between the patient and the film, some scatter traveling obliquely will miss the film. Fig. 1-21 shows the effect of a patient/film air-gap in reducing the scatter that reaches the film.

Compression devices. Different types of compression devices help decrease the thickness of tissue the x-ray beam must pass through. With a wider and flatter distribution of tissue, primary beam-tissue interaction decreases, resulting in less scatter.

Grids. A *grid* is a selective lead filter used to increase film contrast. It is designed to absorb a large percentage of scatter radiation, tracking obliquely as it exits the patient. The grid is located behind the patient but in front of the film, and it absorbs scatter before it reaches the film.

Today's modern grid apparatus is derived from the combined in-

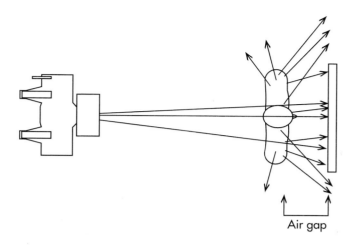

FIG. 1-21   Because scatter radiation travels in many directions, a 6-inch to 10-inch air gap between the patient and the film reduces the amount of scatter that contacts the film.

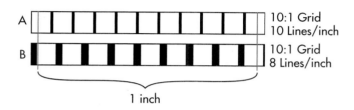

FIG. 1-22   Grid frequency is calculated by the number of grid lines per inch or centimeter. Grids A and B have the same grid ratio, but because B has thicker grid lines, it has a lower grid frequency.

ventions of medical radiologists Gustav Bucky and Hollis Potter in the early 1900s. Bucky designed a grid with lead lines spaced 2 cm apart, arranged in a cross-hatched pattern. Although the grid increased contrast, unsightly grid lines appeared on the film. Potter improved on the concept by reconfiguring the lines in a vertical direction only and laterally moving the grid during the exposure. Moving the grid caused the lead lines to blur and disappear from the film. Potter's invention is known as the *Potter-Bucky diaphragm,* or *bucky.*

Grid design.   Contemporary grids have thin lead strips configured in a linear or cross-hatched pattern with a *radiolucent interspacing* material between the strips (Fig. 1-22). Ideally, the interspacing is designed to allow maximum penetration of the beam. Interspacing materials include cardboard, plastic, carbon fiber, and aluminum. Carbon fiber and aluminum are commercially available. Aluminum has a higher atomic number than carbon fiber. At higher peak kilovoltage, aluminum improves contrast by absorbing more lower-energy x-rays. At lower peak kilovoltage, however, aluminum absorbs more primary radiation than fiber, which leads to higher patient dose. Carbon fiber grids are preferred in situations where low peak kilovoltage techniques are employed and their use can contribute to lower patient dose.

Beyond the linear and cross-hatched patterns, grids are designed with parallel or focused lead strips. In a *parallel grid,* the lead strips and interspacing run parallel to one another (Fig. 1-23). A significant amount of cutoff of the primary beam at the periphery of the grid results when using a short tube distance (40 inches); therefore, parallel grids are best used with a long distance (72 inches) where more of the central, or perpendicular, part of the beam is used.

Focused grids are used more commonly than parallel grids. In a *focused grid,* the lead strips and interspacing are angled toward the center of the grid to accommodate a divergent x-ray beam (Fig. 1-24). The intent is to reduce peripheral cutoff. The focus is deter-

mined by the angle of the divergent beam, which is governed by the distance between the grid and the focal spot. If the lead lines were extended in space beyond the grid, they would converge at a focal point called the *grid radius.* When the x-ray tube is set at the grid radius distance, the grid is in optimum focus. The tube can be moved a short distance from the grid radius without significant peripheral cutoff. *Focal range* describes the distance plus or minus the grid radius where the cutoff is not significant. Making exposures outside of the focal range results in noticeable cutoff. A focused grid must be accurately aligned to ensure that the center of the beam (central ray) is positioned in the middle of the grid. A misaligned grid results in peripheral cutoff to one side of the film and gives the appearance of underexposure.

Grid ratio.   Scatter cleanup is directly related to *grid ratio (GR).* Grid ratio is described as the height of the lead strips *(h)* divided by the distance *(d)* between each lead strip, or

$$GR = h/d$$

The ratio is taken on the edge of the grid where the height of the lead strip is actually a measurement of the thickness of the grid plate (Fig. 1-25). Grid ratio can be increased by increasing the height of the lead or by decreasing the space between the lines (see Fig. 1-25). Scatter radiation approaching at an angle that is not accommodated by the interspacing is trapped by the grid. Common grid ratios for diagnostic radiology include 6:1, 8:1, 10:1, and 12:1. Unfortunately, grids also absorb a significant amount of primary rays. Increasing exposure is necessary to get enough primary rays to the film. Patient dose is three to five times higher when using a grid versus not using a grid.

Grid frequency.   *Grid frequency* is a measure of the number of lead lines per inch (lines/inch) or per centimeter (lines/cm). Grids are manufactured with a frequency range between 60 and 200 lines/inch. For diagnostic imaging, frequencies between 85 and 103

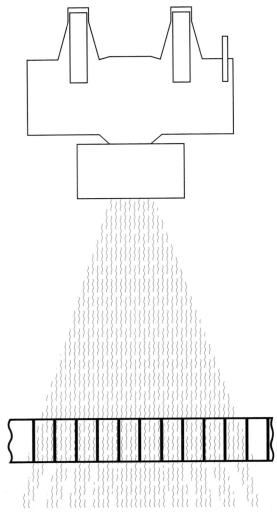

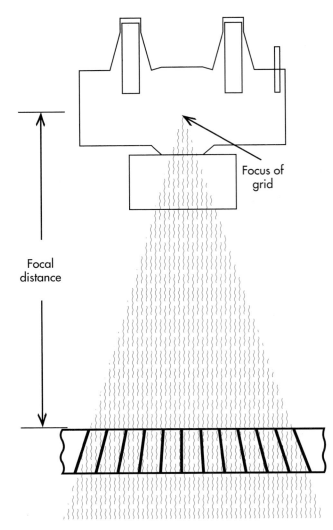

FIG. 1-23   A parallel (or linear) grid is constructed with parallel grid lines, which may result in peripheral cutoff at a short SID caused by a divergent x-ray beam.

FIG. 1-24   A focused grid accommodates the divergence of the x-ray beam. However, cutoff occurs as the SID deviates from the focal range.

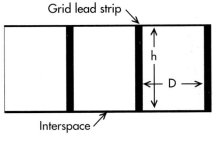

FIG. 1-25   Grid ratio is defined as the height of the lead strip (h) divided by the distance (D) between the lead strips (interspace).

$$\text{Grid ratio} = \frac{h}{D}$$

lines/inch are most common. Fine line grids (103 lines/inch) are best used in a stationary mode where the grid plate does not move during the exposure. The lines are thin and so close together that they become virtually invisible. At higher frequencies (more than 103 lines/inch), the lead strips become too thin to be effective when using high peak kilovoltage techniques. Grids with 200 lines/inch can be used in mammography, because the peak kilovoltage range is 20 to 30 kVp. Lower-frequency grids (85 lines/inch) show lead lines on a film and should be used in a Potter-Bucky diaphragm. The diaphragm moves a linear grid in a reciprocating (back-and-forth) motion during exposure and blurs the lead lines. A cross-hatch grid requires an oscillating motion to blur all lines.

Application. Typically a grid is indicated if the body thickness measures greater than 10 cm or if greater than 60 kVp is needed. Using grids may increase the contrast 1.5 to 3.5 times.

X-Ray Film

Of all image receptors used in diagnostic imaging, plain radiographic film is still the most common. Film is photosensitive, which causes it to respond to wavelengths of light in the electromagnetic spectrum, particularly visible light and x-rays.

CONSTRUCTION

Radiographic film comprises two primary layers: a support layer (base) and a radiosensitive layer (emulsion) (Fig. 1-26). The *base* layer is made of polyester and is tinted with blue dye to reduce eyestrain for the interpreter. The base layer is unreactive to processing chemistry. The *emulsion* layer consists of a gelatinous matrix embedded with silver halide crystals, predominantly silver bromide. Silver halide is the photoactive ingredient in the emulsion. The gelatin provides a means for even distribution of silver halide crystals. It is water soluble, which allows easy penetration of processing chemistry to reach and act on the silver. The emulsion layer is attached to the base with a thin *adhesive* and is covered with a protective *supercoating.* Typically, radiographic film is coated with emulsion on both sides to increase film sensitivity and reduce patient dose.

FILM CHARACTERISTICS

Speed. *Film speed,* or sensitivity, is a measure of the response time of film to a minimal x-ray exposure. Film is blackened proportionally to exposure. A faster film requires less exposure time to sensitize. Film speed is governed by the thickness of the emulsion layer, the size of the silver grains, whether the emulsion is coated on one or both sides, and processing.

Contrast. *Contrast* is the difference between adjacent exposure densities (darkness) on a film; it is described in gray scale from black to white. *Radiographic contrast* includes both subject contrast and detector contrast. *Subject contrast* is determined by attenuation of the beam by the patient, or subject, and is controlled by peak kilovoltage. *Detector contrast* refers to inherent film response characteristics in recording high and low contrast. Depending on clinical need, detector contrast varies. Chest radiography often requires a film type with less contrast compared with bone imaging.

Latitude. *Latitude* is the range of exposures over which the film responds with densities in the diagnostic range. *Latitude and contrast are inversely related.* Film with wide exposure latitude is low contrast. High-contrast film has narrow exposure latitude.

Spectral response. The *spectral response* of a film describes its sensitivity to different wavelengths (colors) of light.

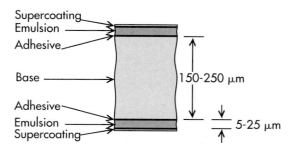

FIG. 1-26 Cross-section of x-ray film. The majority of the film is base. The emulsion contains the image.

Screen film is manufactured to respond primarily to blue and green light. Calcium tungstate intensifying screens emit blue light; blue sensitive film is matched with these screens. Rare earth intensifying screens emit light in both the blue and green range. Orthochromatic film is sensitive to green light.

FILM TYPES

Direct-exposure film. Film that is exposed to only x-ray is called *direct-exposure,* or *nonscreen,* film. Direct-exposure film is used for *high-detail imaging.* In general, film is much more sensitive to visible light than to x-ray photons. It takes considerable exposure to sensitize direct exposure film, limiting its use in general radiography. The emulsions are significantly thicker and contain more fine-grain silver than screen film. Limited medical applications include dental radiography (bite-wing), imaging of occult (hidden) fractures of the small bones of the face and extremities, and localization of foreign objects. Its greatest application today is in industrial radiography, where dose is not a concern.

Screen film. *Screen film* is the most common film used in medical imaging. It is matched with intensifying screens that convert the energy of x-rays into visible light. Approximately 95% of exposure to screen film is by visible light. A double-emulsion film is routinely sandwiched between two intensifying screens. Screen film emulsions are considerably thinner than nonscreen film; however, when used in combination with intensifying screens, they are substantially faster. Resolution (detail) is diminished with screen film as compared with nonscreen film. Screen film is commercially available in a wide variety of speeds, contrasts, spectral responses, and detail.

Single-emulsion film. Certain radiographic exams, such as mammography and extremity imaging, utilize a single-emulsion, fine-grain film in conjunction with a single intensifying screen. The single emulsion/single screen combination offers better detail than a dual system and at a lower dose than a nonscreen film. Care should be taken to ensure that the emulsion side of a single-emulsion film is placed against the screen. Failure to do so results in some loss of speed.

Duplicating film. Radiographs are often duplicated for teaching files or for medicolegal reasons. The process involves a film duplicator that uses ultraviolet light. Regular x-ray film is a negative. *Duplicating film* is a single-emulsion positive film. Because duplicating film is exposed mostly in areas that are clearer on the original film and least exposed where the original film is darker, duplicating film reacts to exposure in an opposite manner to that of regular x-ray film. The silver crystals respond to light in an opposite fashion. To lighten a dark original, more exposure time is needed. To darken a light original, less exposure time is needed.

Storage and handling. X-ray film is sensitive to light, x-rays, heat, moisture, pressure, fumes, and aging, all of which are capable of fogging the film or producing artifacts. Film should be stored in a cool, dry place (50° to 70° F, 30% to 50% relative humidity), safe from light and x-ray exposure. Film boxes should sit on end to decrease pressure sensitization. Stock should be rotated for use before the expiration date.

Intensifying Screens

An intensifying screen converts the energy of x-ray into visible light for the purpose of decreasing patient dose.

CONSTRUCTION

An intensifying screen consists of a protective coating, a phosphor layer, an undercoating layer, and a base layer (Fig. 1-27). The outer *protective coating* helps minimize abrasions of the sensitive phosphor layer. The *phosphor layer* is the photoactive layer of the screen. A *phosphor* is a phosphorescent substance that emits light when energized by x-rays. Tiny phosphor crystals are evenly distributed in a polymer matrix. When energized, light is emitted isotropically (in all directions). The *undercoating layer* can be reflective or absorptive. Light traveling away from the film is reflected back to the film by a *reflective layer*. Screen speed is increased when a reflective layer is used. An absorptive undercoat decreases light flare from the screen, resulting in increased detail. The base, made of plastic or paper, is a support layer that is coated with an anticurl backing.

PHOSPHORS

Modern intensifying screens most frequently use blue-emitting calcium tungstate and blue- and green-emitting rare earth phosphors. Rare earth phosphors are named according to the family of elements from which they are formed. Lanthanum oxysulfide, lanthanum oxybromide, and gadolinium oxysulfide come from the lanthanide series of elements in the periodic table, otherwise known as the *rare earth elements.*

A suitable phosphor should have a high absorption capability, called *quantum detection efficiency (QDE)*. Atomic number determines the QDE. Phosphors should also have a high *conversion efficiency,* or ability to convert the energy of x-rays into visible light. At the instant an exposure is terminated, light emission should stop. Persistence of luminance is called *screen lag,* or *afterglow,* and should be minimal.

SCREEN SPEED

The amount of light emitted per unit of exposure defines *screen speed.* A faster screen emits more light per photon of x-ray. Arbi-

trary numbers are assigned to screens based on their performance against other screens. The term *relative speed (RS)* is used. Relative speed is determined by the type of phosphor used, the thickness of the phosphor layer, phosphor crystal size, the presence of a reflective layer, and peak kilovoltage. Rare earth phosphors have a higher QDE and conversion efficiency than calcium tungstate, which makes rare earth phosphors faster. The increase in speed does not significantly diminish image detail. A 400-speed gadolinium oxysulfide screen produces an image with approximately the same resolution as a 250-speed calcium tungstate screen.

Screen speed varies across the useful peak kilovoltage range. With kilovoltage measurements below what is needed to ionize K-shell electrons in the phosphor, a noticeable decrease in light emission occurs because of a decrease in characteristic photon production. This is called the *K-shell absorption edge phenomenon.* The K-shell absorption edge varies for each phosphor. To compensate for the drop-off in light emissions, milliampere-seconds is increased. An increase in peak kilovoltage causes an increase in screen speed.

Speed is often referred to in respect to both film and screen, or film/screen speed. Matching film sensitivity to screen emission is the goal in maximizing speed, contrast, and resolution. Not all matches are perfect. Mixing and matching films with screens creates *working speed.* Working speed is one of the true indicators of how much exposure is needed; it is directly proportional to milliampere-seconds. Patient dose and image detail are *inversely related* to speed. Typical working speeds for calcium tungstate film/screens are 40 to 250; for rare earth, 40 to 1200. The slower speeds (40 to 80) are used in extremity radiography. Extremities are less radiosensitive than other organs of the body, so the increased dose is considered acceptable for the increase in detail. The most common working speed for rare earth imaging of the axial skeleton is 400.

Cassettes

Unexposed film must be housed in a light-tight holder to be handled in daylight conditions. The most common film holder is a *cassette.* Cassettes are designed specifically for screen film (Fig. 1-28). Two rigid surfaces are hinged together to support intensifying screens that are attached to the cassette with a compressive foam or felt. It is important to have tight film-to-screen contact to reduce blurring of the image. Many modern cassettes are made with biconcave surfaces to squeeze air out when closed. This helps maintain tight film-to-screen contact. The front cover is made of a radiolucent substance to minimize x-ray absorption by the cassette. *Bakelite* (i.e., lightweight) *plastic* and *carbon fiber* are the two substances most often used. Carbon fiber absorbs less radiation than the Bakelite,

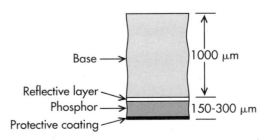

FIG. 1-27   Cross-section of an intensifying screen.

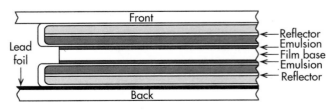

FIG. 1-28   Cross-section of a cassette, two intensifying screens, and radiographic film. A thin sheet of lead foil is often mounted behind the second intensifying screen to absorb backscatter.

minimizing patient dose. The back cover is often made of a light-weight metal, such as magnesium, with a thin foil of lead just inside the cover to absorb backscatter radiation.

Direct-exposure film is not used with intensifying screens and therefore does not need an expensive film holder such as a cassette. Nonscreen film is placed in a cardboard holder or is individually wrapped in light-tight paper.

The Latent Image

When light and x-ray expose a film, a physical change takes place. The change is invisible to the naked eye. A *latent (hidden) image* is formed.

GURNEY-MOTT THEORY OF LATENT IMAGE FORMATION

The most accepted theory on latent image formation was proposed by Gurney and Mott in 1938. Silver halide crystals are manufactured in a lattice of silver, bromine, and iodine atoms. Ionic bonds couple positively charged silver (Ag^{++}) to negatively charged bromine and iodine (Br^- or I^-). The crystalline structure allows for some migration of free silver ions and free electrons within the crystal. An impurity, called a *sensitivity speck,* is built into the surface of many crystals and becomes an electrode for attracting free silver ions in the latent image process (Fig. 1-29).

When light or x-ray interacts with the film, the input energy causes bromine and/or iodine to release an electron. The electron is free to wander and eventually may be trapped by the sensitivity speck. The more electrons that migrate to the sensitivity speck, the more electrically negative it becomes. The negatively charged speck attracts free silver ions, reducing them to atomic silver. A small mass of atomic silver begins to form at the sensitivity speck, invisible to the naked eye. Chemical development further reduces the silver in the latent image, causing the invisible image to become manifest.

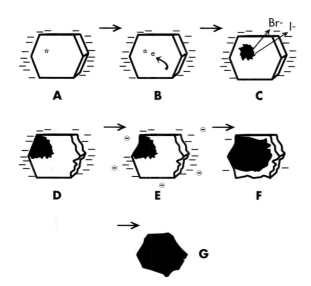

FIG. 1-29 Steps in producing and converting the latent image into a manifest image. **A,** Normal silver halide crystal. **B,** Following irradiation of silver halide crystals, electrons migrate to the sensitivity speck. **C,** Atomic silver is formed at the sensitivity speck. **D,** The process is repeated many times, decreasing the amount of negative surface electrification and increasing the amount of silver atoms. **E** and **F,** The presence of a developing agent assists further reduction to atomic silver. **G,** The process ends with the crystal completely converted to black atomic silver.

Processing the Latent Image

DARKROOM ENVIRONMENT

The darkroom should be located as close to the exposure room as possible. The environment should be conducive to safe operations for both film and radiographer. The darkroom must be light tight and safe from x-ray exposure. Common areas of light leaks include single-door thresholds and jambs and around drop ceilings. Using a double door or a light-tight revolving door may help remedy light leaks around the darkroom entrance. Contrary to popular belief, a darkroom need not be painted black. Rooms that are painted black may require more intense safelighting to provide ample visibility. Safelight fog is directly related to safelight intensity. A light pastel color (preferably yellow) reflects low levels of light and helps minimize *postexposure fog.*

The darkroom should be properly ventilated to reduce the build-up of chemical fumes. Eye protection (goggles), rubber gloves, and aprons are basic protection apparel for darkroom workers. Chemical contact with skin must be minimized. A water source is needed for film processing and darkroom maintenance.

Lighting. Two types of lighting are typically installed in a darkroom, *safelight* and *white light.* The white light is for general lighting when films are not being handled. White light is used when mixing chemicals, cleaning the automatic film processor, and for normal room maintenance. It is wise to strategically place the white light switch higher on the wall than a standard switch so that a conscious effort is made to turn on the white light.

The safelight switch should be installed at a standard height. Safelighting is "relatively safe" for the film. Film sensitivity corresponds to a certain wavelength (color) of light. Safelight emissions are found at the other end of the visible light spectrum. A blue- or green-sensitive film is least sensitive to red light. Kodak's *GBX-2* red filter is commonly used with both green- and blue-sensitive film. Exposed film is many times more sensitive to light of any wavelength than unexposed film. Postexposure fog is directly proportional to safelight intensity. The type of filter, the intensity of the bulb, the number of safelights, the distance between the safelight and the film handling area, and handling time all affect the relative safeness of the light. Bulb wattage should not exceed 15 W; 7.5 W is preferred. The minimum distance between light and work area (and film processor) is 4 feet. By the inverse square law, light intensity is inversely proportional to the square of the distance.

CHEMICAL PROCESSES

The latent image is made manifest by running the film through a series of chemical processes. The procedure may be done by hand or in an automatic film processor. The two main solutions are *developer* and *fixer.* Each solution is composed of several chemicals responsible for different functions in the chemical-film interaction. The sequential steps in auto processing are as follows: *developing, fixing, washing,* and *drying.*

Developing. The critical phase in film processing is developing. Developer action is controlled by immersion *time,* solution *temperature,* and chemical concentration *(activity).* The developer contains *reducing agents,* an *activator,* a *restrainer,* a *hardener,* and a *preservative,* all mixed in water.

A *reducing agent* readily gives up electrons to silver ions attached to the sensitivity speck in the latent image. The reducing agents amplify the latent image more than a million times by completely reducing (neutralizing) the silver to black atomic silver. Fig. 1-29 shows the interaction of the reducing agents with silver halides. Rapid process (RP) chemistry used in automatic film processing contains two reducing agents, *hydroquinone* and *phenidone.* Hydroquinone is slow-acting and is responsible for the *heavy black densities.* Phenidone is fast-acting, building *shades of gray* in the areas of lighter exposure on the film. Metol is used in manual processing chemistry in lieu of phenidone.

If a film is left in solution too long, or if the developer temperature is too high, unexposed silver ions are reduced, producing a *chemical fog* density, which leads to a darker film with decreased contrast. Oxidation (weakening) of the reducing agents through use or exposure to air, heat, light, and contaminants results in underdevelopment. A film developed in weak developer appears light with low contrast. Increasing the milliampere-seconds to compensate for the lack of density should be avoided because it results in a higher patient dose. To offset oxidation of reducing agents, a replenishment solution is periodically added to the developer. With an automatic film processor, replenishment is metered into the chemical tanks per inch of film travel. Changing chemicals monthly helps control underdeveloping because of weak developer.

In addition to reducing agents, other agents affect the end result of development. A sodium carbonate *activator,* or accelerator, increases the permeability of the emulsion by causing the gelatin layer to swell. This allows the reducing agents to reach the silver halides within the emulsion. A potassium bromide (KBr) *restrainer* serves as an *antifogging agent.* It restrains the reducing agents from reducing unexposed silver. A glutaraldehyde *hardener* keeps the emulsion from *overswelling,* preventing scratches and abrasions in automatic processing. Glutaraldehyde helps maintain a uniform film thickness for easy travel through the roller transport system of an automatic processor. A sodium sulfite *preservative* minimizes *developer oxidation* caused by exposure to air.

Fixing. The fixer stops the developing process, removes undeveloped silver halides, and shrinks and hardens the emulsion. It contains an *acidifier,* a *clearing agent,* a *hardener,* a *preservative,* and water as a solvent. Acetic acid acts as a stop bath in neutralizing the alkaline developer. Ammonium thiosulfate is the agent that clears the film of unexposed silver. The film takes on a milky white appearance if the unexposed silver is not completely removed. Aluminum chloride and potassium alum are hardeners that shrink and harden the emulsion. The preservative, sodium sulfite, ionizes the silver from the clearing agent so that it may remove more silver from the film. The buildup of silver ions in the fixer makes it environmentally unsafe. The silver must *first* be removed from the solution *before* the fixer can be discarded.

Washing. Water is used to wash developer and fixer from the film. Water should be of drinking quality. Relative hardness should be moderate, 40 to 150 ppm of calcium carbonate. Insufficient washing may result in brown, yellow, or green staining of the emulsion after several years. In an automatic processor, the environment may be conducive to algae growth in the wash water. Algae appear as black flecks on a radiograph. Adding 3 to 6 ounces of bleach to the wash tank at shutdown should eradicate the algae. If the problem persists, this procedure should be repeated two to three times per week. The tank should be thoroughly washed and the bleach eliminated before processing films. Draining the wash tank when the processor is shut down helps prevent algae growth.

Drying. Hot air forced over both sides of the film dries the film as it exits the processor. Air temperature varies from 110° to 160° F, with 120° F being the average temperature. Films may emerge wet if the heater or blower is not functioning. Chemical-induced wetness may result from depleted hardener in the developer. Developer temperature may also affect film wetness. If the devel-

oper temperature exceeds 95° F, the emulsion may swell beyond the hardener's ability to control it.

TIME-TEMPERATURE METHOD
Film processing is based on *time* and *temperature. Optimum developer temperature is 68° F for manual processing.* Processing at this temperature provides latitude for human error. The higher the temperature, the greater the activity of the developer, and a compensatory decrease in developing time is needed. Strict adherence to manufacturers' time-temperature charts is necessary. Manual processing times range from 15 to 35 minutes before drying.

Automatic processing dictates no such single developer temperature at which all films are processed. Optimum temperature is determined by the manufacturer and is contingent upon processing time, film, and chemistry. The temperature range is between 92° F and 96° F for a 90-second processor and lower for 2- and 3-minute processors. Automatic processing has distinct advantages over manual processing in reduced time and increased consistency of results. A film dropped into an auto processor emerges dry in 90 to 180 seconds and is ready for analysis or storage.

MANUAL PROCESSING APPARATUS AND PROCEDURE
Before the advent of automatic film processors in 1942, the time-consuming method of manually dipping films in chemical solutions predominated. Fig. 1-30 shows a typical setup for manual processing. Equipment needs include the following:
1. Master tank filled with free-flowing water
2. In-line mixing valve to mix hot and cold water in the master tank; the circulating water is used to control chemical temperatures and to wash films
3. Two insert tanks with lids, one for developer and one for fixer
4. Thermometer to read chemical temperatures
5. Darkroom clock to set processing times
6. Separate stir paddles for developer and fixer
7. Time-temperature chart
8. Drying bin or area
9. Film hangers

Before a film is processed, chemicals must be stirred, developer temperature checked, clock set for the appropriate time, and the film placed on a hanger. Processing times are set according to film type and chemistry. Once a film is placed in the developer, depending on the type of chemistry, agitation may be required. The film should not be taken out of solution before the development time has expired. The lid should be kept on the developer tank when the film is not being agitated. As the film is removed from the developer, chemicals running off the film should *not* be "dripped back" into the tank. This oxidized developer weakens the main volume of chemistry. At the end of development, the film is immersed in a rinse bath of water for approximately 15 seconds. The clock is reset for fixing time and the film, placed in the fixer, is agitated. Once the fixing time has expired, the film is removed and the excess fixer allowed to drip back into the fixer tank. This ensures that ionic silver dripping off the film is retained in the fixer tank. The film is then placed in the wash water to remove fixer from the emulsion. Once the film is in the final wash, the white light may be turned on for wet viewing. Finally, the film will be air-dried from 15 minutes to more than an hour, depending on the temperature and humidity of the drying area.

Replenishment should be added at the end of each day of film processing. Chemical manufacturers set mixing concentrations for

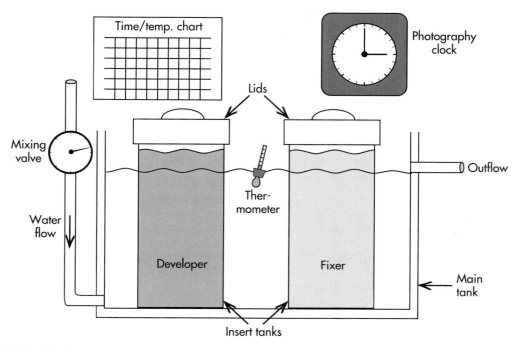

FIG. 1-30 Typical setup for manual processing. The developer and fixer tanks are seated into a larger tank filled with flowing water. The flowing water serves to maintain the temperature of the smaller tanks and also doubles as a wash.

replenishment and determine replenishment rates based on film size.

AUTOMATIC FILM PROCESSOR

The automatic processor is a collection of electrical and mechanical systems that control temperature, time, and chemical activity in a way that results in rapid processing of film (Fig. 1-31).

1. The auto processor has a *roller transport system* composed of rollers and deflector plates that transport film through the different tanks. A drive motor attached to a worm gear with a drive chain controls the feed rate.

2. Heaters controlled by thermostats make up the *temperature control system.* Developer, fixer, water, and dryer temperatures all come under control of the temperature control system. Depending on the size of the developer tank, it takes between 15 and 30 minutes for developer temperatures to stabilize once the machine is turned on.

3. The *replenishment system* replenishes chemicals that are depleted through use, oxidation, or evaporation. Film sensors activate a pump to inject fresh chemicals from reservoirs outside the processor to regenerate volume and chemical activity.

4. The *circulation/filtration system* (composed of pumps, filters, and tubing) filters and circulates the chemicals to maintain uniform activity and to stabilize temperatures.

5. Films are dried through a *dryer system,* which includes a blower, heater, and thermostat in addition to exhaust ducts.

6. The *electrical system* provides power to the other systems. Most processors are designed to partially shut down if a certain amount of time elapses between films being processed. When in

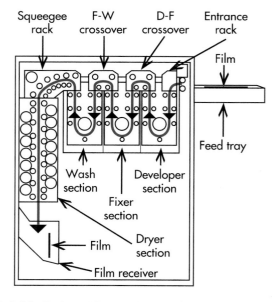

FIG. 1-31 Design and film path *(blue arrow)* of an automatic processor.

"standby" mode, the drive motor and drying system (blower fan and heater) shut down to conserve energy. The developer heater coil remains active at all times when the machine is on. This ensures that developer temperature is ready any time a film is processed. Placing a film in the processor activates all systems and takes the machine off standby.

Silver Recovery

Silver is a heavy metal that renders the fixer a hazardous waste, which causes damage to biological systems. For this reason, silver must be recovered from spent fixer before it is discarded. Approximately 10% of the silver from a fresh film is recoverable, which may also generate a monetary return.

Residual silver is recovered from fixing solutions through *metallic exchange, electrolysis* or *electroplating,* and *chemical precipitation.* Metallic replacement and electroplating can be performed in house. Currently only commercial silver dealers use chemical precipitation. The fixer collecting system in the processor is directly attached to the silver recovery unit. The unit has an outflow tube connected to the drain.

A *metallic exchange unit* is a plastic bucket filled with steel wool or a steel screen. It has an inflow that accepts silver-laden fixer and outflow that passes silverless fixer to the drain. It is usually used in low-volume situations. No electricity is used. The iron in the steel gives up electrons to the silver, which causes silver to attach to the steel. Efficiency decreases with age based on total gallons of fixer treated or total silver exchanged. The useful life of a metallic exchange unit is approximately 6 months to 1 year.

An *electrolytic unit* utilizes an electric current passing between an anode and a cathode. The cathode offers electrons to ionic silver, converting it to atomic silver. The silver attaches to the cathode. Electrolytic units are designed for higher-volume situations. A properly sized electrolytic cell can recover 97% of the silver from the fixer.

Chemical precipitation requires the use of chemicals such as zinc chloride and sodium sulfite to precipitate metallic silver. The chemical reaction produces toxic chlorine gas and volatile hydrogen gas. The hazardous nature of the process requires a controlled environment not usually found in a radiology facility.

Silver may also be recovered from processed film through an industrial chemical process.

Image Quality

The goal of radiography is to maximize the amount of clearly defined anatomy on a film while maintaining a minimum dose to the patient. To realize this, the film must have adequate density (darkness/brightness), contrast (gray scale) and detail (resolution), with a minimum of distortion (aberrant size and shape). Film quality characteristics can be divided into *photographic properties* (image visibility), which include density, contrast, noise and fog factors, and *geometric properties* (structural sharpness), which include recorded detail and size and shape distortion.

PHOTOGRAPHIC PROPERTIES

Film density. *Film density* is described as the overall blackness seen on a finished radiograph. It results from the development of exposed silver halide crystals in the film emulsion. The greater the concentration of developed silver halide on a film, the less light is transmitted through the film, giving the appearance of a very dark area or image. From a photographic perspective, film may appear too dark, or *overexposed,* which demonstrates too much density; too light, or *underexposed,* which demonstrates too little density; or adequate exposure, which represents proper density (Fig. 1-32).

Film density is *inversely related* to patient density. The greater the patient density is, the lesser, or lighter, the film density is. The body comprises tissues of different densities (expressed in g/cm^3), which allow disparate amounts of x-ray radiation to penetrate. Radiographic contrast results from shades of these different film densities. Five observable radiographic densities result from x-ray interaction with patient density. They range from *radiolucent* (black) to *radiopaque* (white)—*air, fat, water, bone,* and *metal* (Fig. 1-33).

Film density is controlled by *milliampere-seconds,* because controlling milliampere-seconds regulates exposure. In a similar manner in which the brightness control knob on a black-and-white television controls overall darkness and lightness, milliampere-seconds controls the relative darkness of a radiograph. Individual film den-

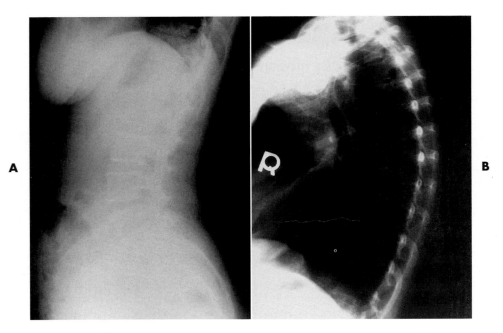

FIG. 1-32   **A,** Underexposed lateral lumbar film. **B,** Overexposed lateral thoracic film.

sities represented by tissues such as bone, muscle, and fat are affected more by peak kilovoltage than milliampere-seconds, because peak kilovoltage controls x-ray beam penetration. X-ray absorption is determined by beam penetration. Controlling factors and affecting factors for density can be seen in Box 1-1.

Under normal conditions, affecting factors are standardized so that milliampere-seconds can be used to predictably control density. Milliampere-seconds is adjusted according to patient size and density. If affecting factors such as processing and/or peak kilovoltage become variable, then milliampere-seconds, and therefore film density, become less predictable.

The minimum change in milliampere-seconds necessary to cause a visible change in film density is 30%. Clinically repeating a radiograph for a 30% change in milliampere-seconds is rarely justified. Most commonly, films repeated for density require a doubling or halving of the milliampere-seconds. Within the useful range for film density, density is *doubled* when milliampere-seconds is *doubled* and reduced to *half* when milliampere-seconds is *halved*. Kilovoltage also has a direct effect on film density. According to the *15% rule for peak kilovoltage*, a 15% increase in peak kilovoltage doubles film density. Conversely, a 15% decrease in peak kilovoltage reduces the density by half. Changes in peak kilovoltage affect density by altering the absorption-to-penetration ratio. Hence, low-density tissues appear significantly darker than high-density tissues when peak kilovoltage is increased.

Film contrast. As discussed previously, *radiographic contrast* includes both subject and detector contrast. *Subject contrast* is determined by attenuation of the beam by the patient or subject and is controlled by peak kilovoltage. *Detector contrast* refers to inherent film response characteristics in recording high and low contrast. Subject contrast is variable.

Contrast is the difference between adjacent film densities and is described in gray scale from black to white (Fig. 1-34). A *high-contrast* radiograph demonstrates a *short gray scale*, or black and white, and is achieved with low peak kilovoltage. At lower peak

kilovoltage, high-density tissues absorb more x-ray radiation, which produces a very white appearance. Low-density tissues absorb little x-ray radiation and appear very dark. A *low-contrast* radiograph portrays a *long gray scale,* or many shades of gray, and is achieved with high peak kilovoltage. High peak kilovoltage increases penetration to tissues of all densities, thereby decreasing the difference in blackening between tissues of various thicknesses and densities. Fig. 1-35 compares films of different contrast.

The primary controlling factor of contrast is *peak kilovoltage.* The kilovoltage selector works similarly to a contrast knob on a black-and-white television. An increase in peak kilovoltage with a subsequent decrease in milliampere-seconds decreases contrast. A

BOX 1-1
Film Density

Controlling factors
Milliampere-seconds

Primary factors
Peak kilovoltage
Film processing
Film/intensifying screens
Source-image distance (SID)
Patient size, shape, and pathology

Secondary factors
Filtration
Grid
Beam limitation
Fog
Contrast media
Anode heel effect

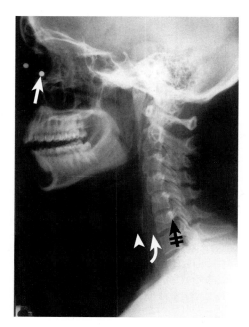

FIG. 1-33 Lateral cervical projection demonstrating four of the five radiographic densities: metal *(arrow)*, bone *(crossed arrow)*, water or muscle *(curved arrow)*, and air *(arrowhead)*.

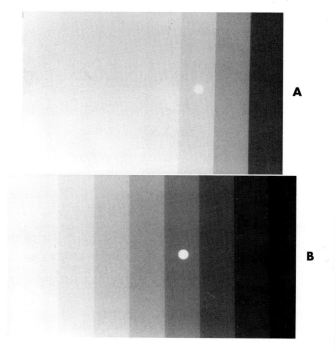

FIG. 1-34 Contrast describes the range of shades of gray in an image. **A** demonstrates higher contrast and a shorter scale of contrast than **B** because it progresses from white to dark with fewer shades of gray.

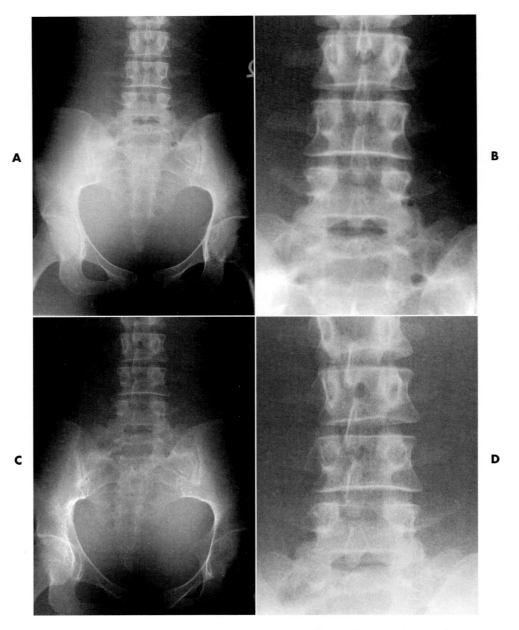

FIG. 1-35   **A** and **B,** These films demonstrate higher contrast (few shades of gray, shorter scale) than films **C** and **D.**

decrease in peak kilovoltage with a compensatory increase in milliampere-seconds increases contrast. Milliamperage-seconds alone plays no significant role in contrast because it has no effect on the absorption-to-penetration ratio. (Controlling factors and affecting factors for contrast can be found in Box 1-2.) Aberrant film processing and various fog factors can significantly compromise film contrast.

Noise and fog factors. The term *noise* is often used to describe static found in audio systems. Visual systems such as television manifest noise as "snow." Radiographic "noise" is undesirable background information that causes fluctuations in film density, but it does not contribute to the quality of the image. Noise affects the *visibility of detail,* or the visible perception of the structural details

transferred to the film. Types of radiographic noise include *film graininess, structural mottle,* and *quantum mottle.*

Film graininess results from the size and distribution of silver halide crystals in the emulsion. *Structural mottle* is the intensifying screen version of film graininess and results from the size and distribution of phosphor crystals in the screen. *Quantum mottle* results from the random interaction of x-ray photons with the image receptor and is somewhat under the control of the technologist. With a very fast imaging system, where a small amount of x-ray is needed to expose the film, the photons interact randomly, causing an incomplete distribution of exposure and leaving a mottled appearance. With slower imaging systems, or if a large number of photons are used as with a high milliampere-seconds/low peak kilo-

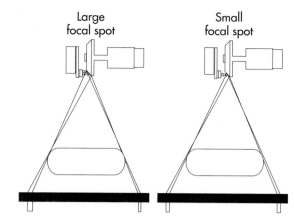

FIG. 1-36 A larger focal spot results in less detail than a smaller focal spot. The area of unsharpness, or penumbra, is more on the cathode side of the x-ray beam.

BOX 1-2
Film Contrast

Controlling factors
Peak kilovoltage

Primary factors
Fog
Grid
Film processing
Beam limitations
Patient size, shape, and pathology
Pulsations in waveform
Contrast media
Filtration

Secondary factors
Film/intensifying screens
Compression devices
Object-to-film distance (OFD)

BOX 1-3
Film Detail

Factors affecting visibility of detail
Density
Contrast
Noise
Fog

Factors affecting recorded detail
Motion
SID
OFD
Focal spot size
Intensifying screen
Object shape and density

Factors affecting distortion
OFD
SID
Patient thickness
Central ray centering
Object plane
Film plane

---

metric sharpness can be found in Box 1-3. X-rays do not emanate from a point source but rather from an area called a *focal spot.* Not all x-rays emitted from the focal spot hit a locus on an object at the same projectional angle (Fig. 1-36). The distinct core of the object is defined as the *umbra,* or area of geometric sharpness. The image may demonstrate an area of geometric unsharpness, or *penumbra,* adjacent to the umbral shadow. A large focal spot inherently produces a larger penumbra than a small focal spot.

Penumbra can be minimized by using a small focal spot, a long focal spot-to-film distance (FFD), and short object-film distance (OFD). The penumbral effect contributing to geometric unsharpness may be calculated using the following formula:

$$\text{Geometric unsharpness (penumbra)} = (\text{Focal spot size}) \times (\text{OFD})/(\text{FFD})$$

Other factors affecting image sharpness include motion unsharpness, intensifying screen unsharpness, and absorption unsharpness. *Motion unsharpness* most commonly results from patient movement during the exposure and compromises recorded detail. A less common source of motion is vibration of the imaging equipment. Patients exhibit voluntary (gross movement) and involuntary motion (cardiac and respiratory motion). Radiographers have learned to control the effects of patient motion by using reliable immobilization techniques, short exposure time, and specific breathing instructions.

Intensifying screen unsharpness, also called *inherent unsharpness,* increases with larger phosphor crystals, thicker phosphor layers, use of a reflective layer, and poor contact between film and screen.

Variation in the absorption of the beam by the structural edges of an object may lead to *absorption unsharpness.* The shape and density of an object, in addition to the angle of incidence of the x-ray beam, may cause the edges to appear well defined or fuzzy. Absorption unsharpness gives the appearance of increased penumbra.

Distortion. *Distortion* is an exaggeration of the size and/or shape of an object because of unequal magnification of different parts of the object. *Shape distortion* occurs when any combination of film, object, and central ray do not lie in the same plane (Fig. 1-37). Angulation of the film, object, or central ray (Fig. 1-38) causes

---

voltage technique, quantum mottle is decreased and the blackening of the film appears smoother. All film/screen imaging systems inherently produce quantum mottle, with higher levels found in the faster systems.

Image visibility is intimate to contrast. Low contrast caused from such phenomena as increased scatter, safelight fog, and chemical fog decreases visibility of detail.

GEOMETRIC PROPERTIES

Recorded detail. An image that appears "in-focus" with sharply defined structural borders and clarity of minute internal structures has good *recorded detail.* Various factors affecting geo-

an unequal elongation of the object, changing its shape. Off-centering of the object to the central ray also causes shape distortion (Figs. 1-39 and 1-40). Simple *magnification,* where the object size is increased, results in *size distortion.* Maintaining a short object-film distance and a long focal-film distance minimizes magnification. Recorded detail is increased as size and shape distortion are reduced (Fig. 1-41).

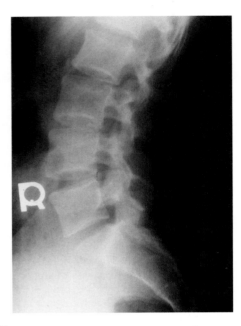

FIG. 1-37   Distortion of the lumbar spine with noted "hourglassing" effect. In this case, the convexity of the lumbar curve was not adjacent to the bucky. If the side of the patient with the convexity of a curve were placed against the bucky, the divergence of the x-ray beam would be better accommodated by the spinal curvature.

TROUBLESHOOTING IMAGE QUALITY

Common image problems seen in radiography include inadequate density, poor contrast, and loss of detail. A myriad of causes exists; however, some occur with greater frequency than others. Algorithms have been created to help troubleshoot the more common causes of poor image quality.

Technique

The art of radiography is seen through the ability of the radiographer to select proper exposure factors for a given examination. Although many influences exist, results are most predictable when many of the variables are standardized while varying a single factor. The two more common exposure theories in use today are *fixed peak kilovoltage/variable milliampere-seconds* and *variable peak kilovoltage/fixed milliampere-seconds* techniques.

FIXED PEAK KILOVOLTAGE/VARIABLE MILLIAMPERE-SECONDS TECHNIQUE

Kilovoltage affects many factors, such as contrast, density, patient dose, detail, penetration power, and scatter radiation. These outcomes are more predictable when applying a fixed peak kilovoltage technique. In a fixed peak kilovoltage system, optimum kilovoltage is held constant for a given range of patient densities, and milliampere-seconds is varied to attain the proper film density. Optimum peak kilovoltage is the *maximum kilovoltage* that will consistently produce an image with contrast within acceptable limits. Optimum peak kilovoltage provides greater penetration than what is minimally needed to penetrate the part. This ensures adequate penetration of a larger population of subjects without varying peak kilovoltage. With a fixed peak kilovoltage, milliampere-seconds changes with the patient measurement. The smallest increment of milliampere-seconds change on the technique chart is 30%, because significant visible changes cannot be detected below 30%. On av-

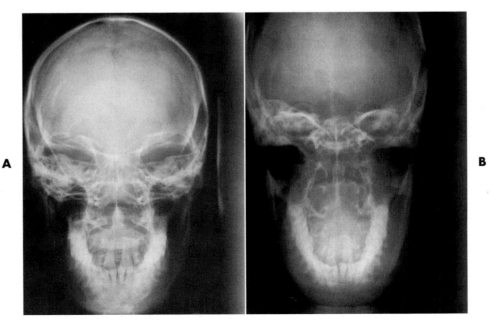

FIG. 1-38   Distortion caused by tube tilt: **A,** which was taken with 15-degree tube tilt, is sharper and less distorted than **B,** which was taken with 35-degree tube tilt.

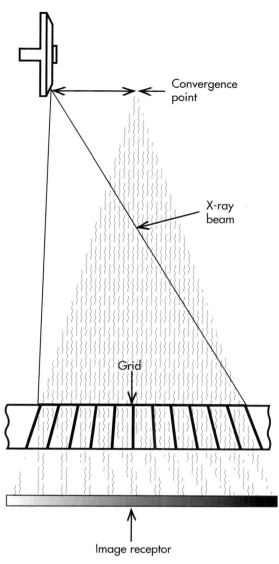

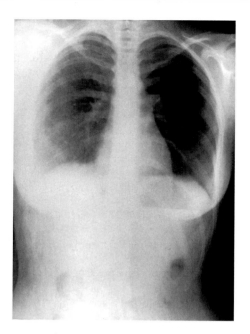

FIG. 1-40 Unequal density across the thorax secondary to misalignment of the bucky and tube (grid cutoff).

FIG. 1-39 An off-center grid error results in uneven grid cutoff. Cutoff manifests as a lighter density on one side of the film.

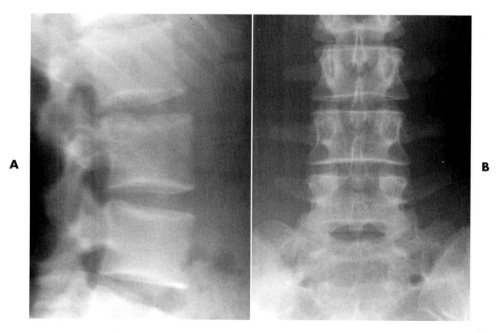

FIG. 1-41 **A,** Decreased detail caused by motion. **B,** No motion artifact, resulting in higher detail.

erage, milliampere-seconds doubles for every 5-cm increase in patient measurement.

Advantages of a fixed kilovoltage technique include reduced patient dose, a wider exposure latitude, and longer gray scale. Those who prefer high-contrast films may negatively perceive the lower contrast. A disadvantage of optimum kilovoltage is an increase in scatter radiation. Some subjectivity is involved in selecting optimum peak kilovoltage because of contrast preference of the radiologist. Table 1-2 lists suggested optimum peak kilovoltage for different body parts using single-phase and high-frequency technology.

VARIABLE PEAK KILOVOLTAGE/FIXED MILLIAMPERE-SECONDS TECHNIQUE

With variable peak kilovoltage technique, milliampere-seconds is fixed and peak kilovoltage varies, based on patient thickness. The size of the patient part determines the change in penetration of the beam. A range of kilovoltages from high to low can potentially be used for any given body part. *Milliamperage values are based primarily on film/screen speed, grid ratio, and body part size.* The quantity of radiation (mAs) remains constant from the smallest to the largest part.

Historically, with variable peak kilovoltage technique it is common practice to change peak kilovoltage by 2 for every 1 cm of patient tissue thickness. The formula

$$\text{Peak kilovoltage} = 2 \text{ kVp} \times \text{Part size} + \text{A base number}$$

is applied. The base number varies, based on the minimum peak kilovoltage needed to penetrate the body part. For small extremities, the base number is 30; for cervical and thoracic spine and large extremities, 40; and for lumbar spine and pelvis, 50.

Variable peak kilovoltage techniques, by design, use lower peak kilovoltage than variable peak kilovoltage systems. Advantages include high-contrast films and incremental changes in peak kilovoltage to compensate for variations in patient thickness. The disadvantages are high patient dose, low exposure latitude, and variable contrast for the same body part as thickness changes.

TABLE 1-2
Suggested Optimum* Peak Kilovoltage (kVp) for Body Parts

Anatomy	Optimum kVp	
	Single phase	High frequency
Small extremity**	55-65	55-65
Large extremity**	65-70	65-70
Lateral cervical spine	75	70
AP cervical spine	70	70
AP open mouth	75	70
Lateral thoracic spine	80	80
AP thoracic spine	75	70
Lateral lumbar spine	90	80
AP lumbar spine	80	75
AP pelvis	80	75
Abdomen	80	80
Ribs	70	70
Skull	80	75
Chest	110	110

*Pragmatic technique charts may list a small range of kVp settings accounting for extremes of body size.

TECHNIQUE APPLICATION

Multiple mechanisms exist to apply technique. AEC provides automated density control once peak kilovoltage is selected. Accuracy of exposure correlates to accuracy of positioning the anatomy over the photosensors. *Technique charts,* constructed based on fixed or variable peak kilovoltage, are customized to individual x-ray machines and imaging systems. Exposure accuracy is based on precise caliper measurements of the patient part. Charts are not easily transferable from one facility to another without some tinkering. The SuperTech technique calculator is a pocket-sized slide rule device with the versatility to provide accurate exposure information for many clinical situations. It can easily be applied to any x-ray setup. The newest innovation in technique application is the *anatomical preprogrammed technique.* The control console is outfitted with a software package that provides push-button selection of predetermined techniques based on anatomy and part thickness. All technique systems possess inherent error that must be monitored and eliminated. Fine tuning is essential to minimizing repeat radiographs and therefore patient dose.

Radiation Protection

Ionizing radiation exposures should be kept *As Low As Reasonably Achievable (ALARA).* ALARA is the overriding principle in radiation protection of patients and personnel.

PROTECTION OF THE PATIENT

The radiographer is responsible for understanding and applying safe radiological procedures that minimize dose to the patient. Unfortunately, many factors that contribute to producing a diagnostic image also increase patient dose. Such factors must be properly applied to minimize the dose while producing acceptable quality images. Recommendations to reduce patient dose are as follows:

1. *Technique.* Techniques that utilize high peak kilovoltage and low milliampere-seconds decrease patient dose. Proper attention ensures that the contrast is acceptable for the peak kilovoltage used.
2. *Grids.* Exposure must be increased when using a grid because both primary and scatter radiation are absorbed by the grid. Using the lowest acceptable grid ratio to improve contrast helps minimize dose.
3. *Beam restriction.* The exposure field size should be limited to the area of interest whenever possible and should never exceed the film size.
4. *Shielding.* To protect against genetic effects on the progeny of irradiated individuals, especially during childbearing years, use of *gonad shields* is recommended whenever their use does not compromise diagnostic information. Collimation, properly applied, may minimize gonadal dose. Other radiosensitive organs such as eyes, thyroid, and female breasts should be shielded when appropriate.
4. *Filtration.* Inherent filtration plus added filtration help reduce soft radiation exposure to the patient. Compensating filters, such as wedge filters, help even out exposure to the film and at the same time reduce patient dose over the areas filtered.
5. *PA radiography.* Many radiosensitive organs (such as eyes, thyroid, breasts, and gonads) are located anteriorly in the patient. Projecting the beam through the patient posterior-to-anterior helps reduce organ exposure as the beam is attenuated in the patient.
6. *Image receptors.* The film/intensifying screen combination plays a pivotal role in reducing patient dose. Faster systems linearly reduce dose. A 400-speed system requires approximately one

half the exposure of a 200-speed system. However, factors such as quantum mottle and film graininess must be considered when trying to balance patient dose with acceptable recorded detail.

7. *Repeat radiographs.* Common reasons for repeating radiographs include poor positioning of the patient, film, or tube; improper technique selection; inadequate film processing; artifacts; and patient motion. Patient dose increases any time a film is repeated. Many repeats could be avoided by effectively communicating with the patient initially and by being cognizant of the common errors that result in repeat films.

PROTECTION OF PERSONNEL

Laws entitle occupational radiation workers to a radiation-safe environment. A state inspector scrutinizes each facility for radiation safety annually or biannually. Basic principles of radiation protection for personnel include *time, distance,* and *shielding. Time* spent in the vicinity of x-ray exposure should be kept to a minimum. In accordance with the inverse square law, radiation exposure decreases significantly as *distance* is increased. Whenever possible, workers should maintain a safe distance from sources of ionizing radiation. Unfortunately, radiographers work very close to the x-ray machine, especially the fluoroscope, and fluoroscopic exposures run intermittently for minutes to an hour or more. In this case *shielding* is best applied. Shielding includes anything from a lead apron and gloves to a protective barrier placed between the source of radiation and the exposed individual.

For personal radiation protection, radiographers should follow these guidelines:

- Apply the rules of time, distance, and shielding.
- Maintain the smallest collimation field appropriate for the examination.
- Always wear a radiation monitoring device (i.e., film badge, thermoluminescent dosimeter (TLD), pocket dosimeter) to detect exposure.
- Avoid holding a patient during a radiographic examination. If using a restraining device is not possible and a patient must be held, no person should *routinely* hold patients.
- Ensure that anyone holding a patient is properly protected with a full lead apron and lead gloves.

Dose limits. The federal government of the United States sets dose limits for radiation workers and the general public. The federal agency that enforces radiation safety laws and dose limits is the Nuclear Regulatory Commission (NRC). Dose limits are reported in the National Council on Radiation Protection and Measurements' (NCRP) publications. NCRP Report No. 116, *Limitation of Exposure to Ionizing Radiation* (1993), provides the most up-to-date information on dose limits.[2] A summary of Report No. 116 can be found in Table 1-3. These dose limits do *not* pertain to patients receiving medical exposures for diagnostic or therapeutic purposes. The *annual* effective dose limit for occupational exposures is *5 rem (50 mSv) per year.* The *cumulative* effective dose limit for occupational exposures is

$$1 \text{ rem} \times \text{Age of worker.}$$

Dose limits are established primarily to minimize the risks of *stochastic* and *nonstochastic* radiation effects. A *stochastic effect* is an effect in which the probability of occurrence, rather than severity, increases as the dose increases. No threshold dose exists below which risk is eliminated. Examples of stochastic effects are cancer and genetic effects.

A *nonstochastic* effect is one that manifests with certainty following a certain dose and the severity increases as the dose increases. A threshold dose exists below which nonstochastic effects do not manifest. Examples include sterility changes, radiation burns, and cataract formation in the lens of the eye.

X-RAY AND PREGNANCY

Because of the radiosensitive nature of the embryo-fetus, especially in the first 14 weeks after conception, radiation exposure to the pregnant or potentially pregnant patient or worker should be reduced.

According to NCRP Report No. 54, *Medical Radiation Exposure of Pregnant and Potentially Pregnant Women,* the decision to x-ray a pregnant patient is relegated to the judgment of the physician.[1] Where the protection of the patient's health requires a radiological examination at a specific time, and adequate radiological equipment and technique are used, in most cases, the potential benefits of the procedure outweigh the risks of the exposure. One in 1000 of all radiological examinations (excluding fluoroscopy), performed properly, exposes the embryo-fetus to 1 rad or more of radiation. The NCRP Report No. 54 states that human embryo-fetus exposures below 5 rad are considered to be an acceptable risk when compared with the medical benefit of the radiological examination to the patient.[1] Diagnostic procedures rarely result in a dose to the uterus as high as 5 rad. *The equivalent dose limit* (excluding medical exposure) *for the embryo should not exceed 0.05 rem (0.5 mSv) per month.*

TABLE 1-3
Estimated Exposures*

Exposure	SI	Customary
Occupational exposures		
Effective dose limit		
Annual	50 mSv	5 rem
Cumulative	10 mSv × age	1 rem × age
Annual equivalent dose limits for tissues and organs		
Lens of eye	150 mSv	15 rem
Skin, hands, and feet	500 mSv	50 rem
Public exposures (annual)		
Effective dose limit		
Continuous or frequent exposure	1 mSv	0.1 rem
Infrequent exposure	5 mSv	0.5 rem
Equivalent dose limits for tissues and organs		
Lens of eye	15 mSv	1.5 rem
Skin, hands, and feet	50 mSv	5 rem
Education and training exposures (annual)		
Effective dose limit	1 mSv	0.1 rem
Equivalent dose limits for tissues and organs		
Lens of eye	15 mSv	1.5 rem
Skin, hands, and feet	50 mSv	5 rem
Embryo-fetus exposures (monthly)		
Effective dose limit	0.5 mSv	0.05 rem

*From National Council on Radiation Protection and Measurements: Report No. 116, *Limitations of exposure to ionizing radiation* (supercedes NCRP report No. 91), Bethesda, Md, 1993, NCRP.

PART ONE Introduction to Imaging

Pregnant patients. Performing radiography of pregnant patients requires precisely collimated x-ray beams and properly positioned protective shields.

In the past, elective (nonemergency) radiological procedures to the abdominal area of patients of child-bearing potential were recommended to be scheduled at a designated time to minimize exposure to an embryo in the early days of pregnancy. The *10-day rule* was applied to the 10-day period following the onset of menses, when the probability of pregnancy is low. The 10-day rule is now obsolete for medical procedures.

The pregnancy status of females of child-bearing potential should always be predetermined so that appropriate radiation protection measures may be taken. When pregnancy is not known, it is common practice to solicit the date of the patient's last menses. If pregnancy is suspected, the exam may be rescheduled.

Pregnant workers. As stated previously, radiation exposure to the fetus of a pregnant worker must be limited. Pregnant workers should minimize or avoid rotations in fluoroscopy, portable work, and special procedures. Radiation protection practices such as time, distance, and shielding, should be reviewed and strictly enforced. Fetal dose may be monitored by having the worker wear a second personnel-monitoring device below a lead apron covering the abdomen. The annual effective dose limit for the worker is reduced to the equivalent dose limit for the fetus, 0.05 rem per month, while the worker is pregnant.

Problem Solving

The following charts are designed to assist radiographers in problem solving commonly encountered errors of image quality. Each radiograph warrants critical evaluation for density, contrast, and detail. If the radiograph is of diagnostic quality, close observation will demonstrate areas that can be improved upon for future studies. If the radiograph is not of diagnostic quality, the following charts will assist the radiographer in determining which factors can be altered to improve the image prior to repeat radiography.

Pictorial Summary

Figs. 1-42 through 1-67 (see pp. 35-41) illustrate selected artifacts that are often encountered in clinical practice.

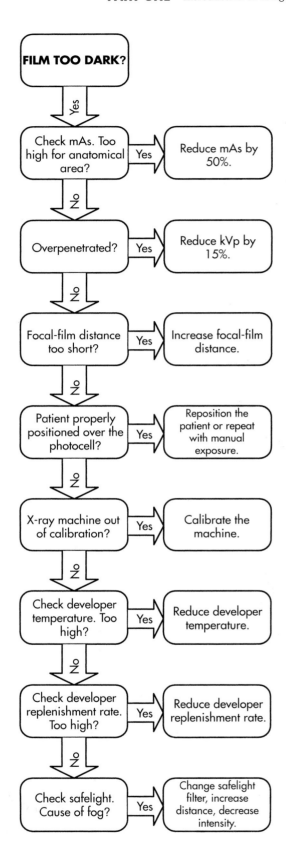

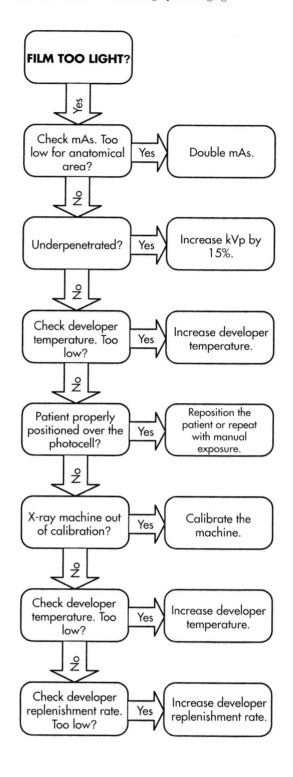

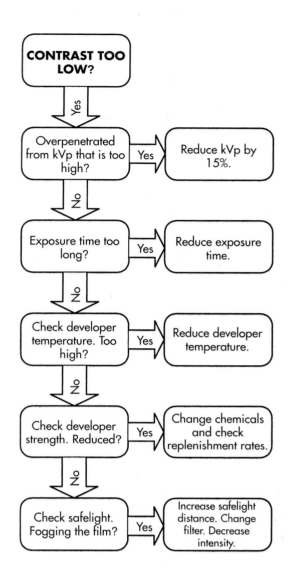

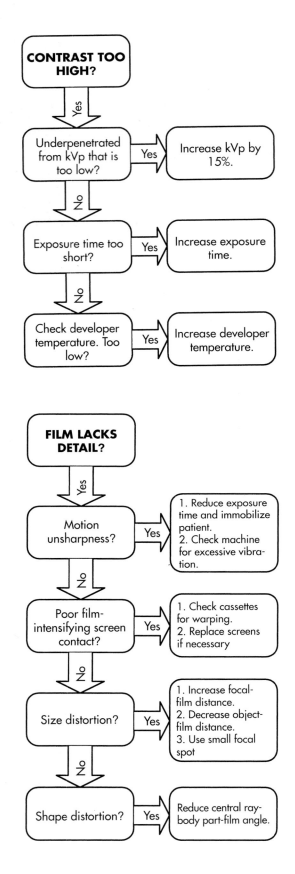

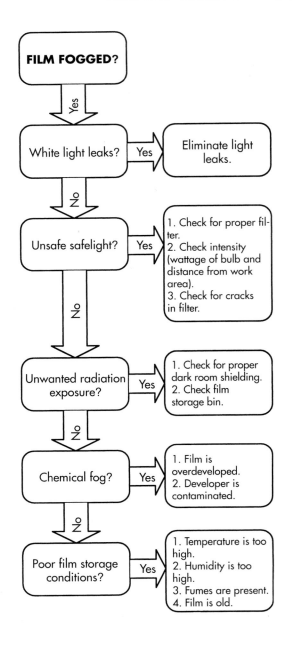

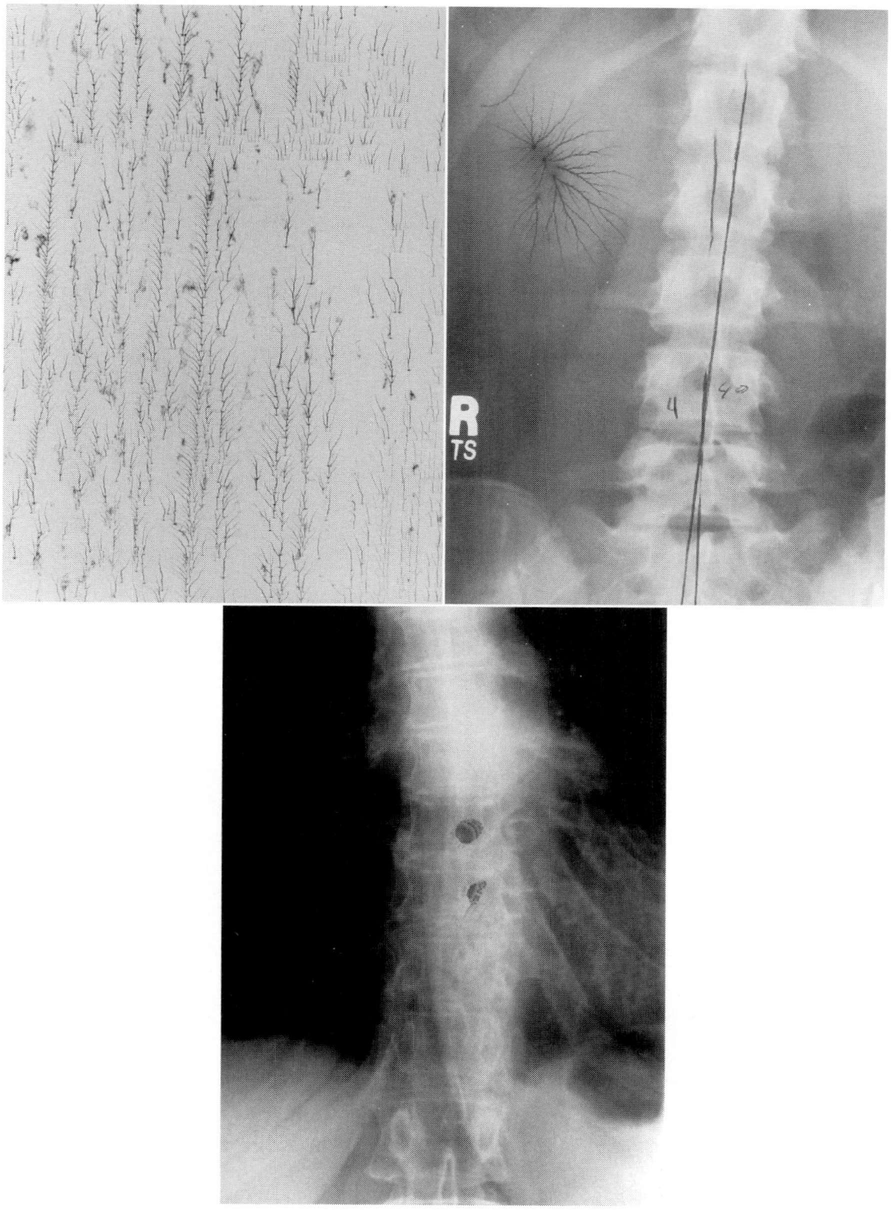

FIG. 1-42   Various static electricity markings.

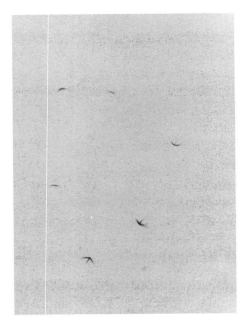

FIG. 1-43 Crescent artifacts that result from kinked film.

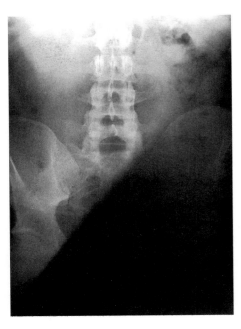

FIG. 1-44 Overexposed lower corner of the film secondary to light leak.

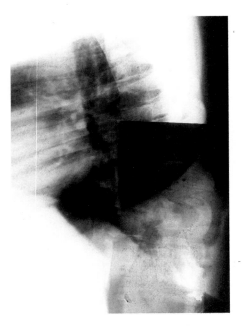

FIG. 1-45 Two films adhered together during processing.

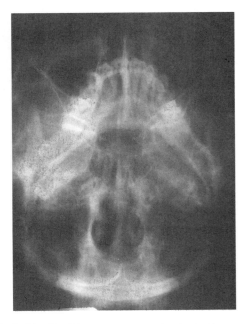

FIG. 1-46 Blurred appearance secondary to double exposure.

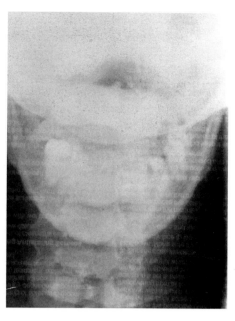

FIG. 1-47 Protective contact paper adhered to the screen of a new cassette that was not removed before cassette use.

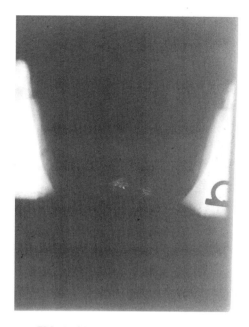

FIG. 1-48 Duplication film in cassette.

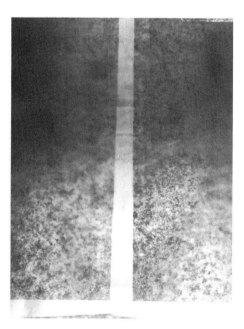

FIG. 1-49 Exposed film was left in a paper film envelope in a lighted room while the radiographer went to lunch. Following development, the light leaked through the paper envelope, creating this mottled appearance.

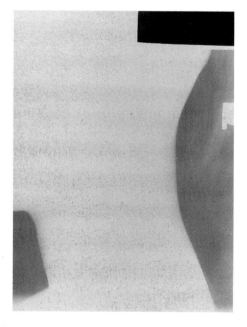

FIG. 1-50 Grossly underexposed film caused by single-emulsion extremity film that was mistakenly placed in the cassette.

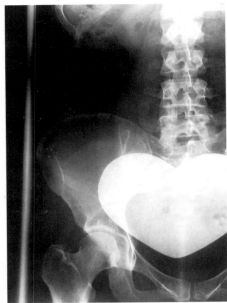

FIG. 1-51   Cassette not fully pushed into the bucky.

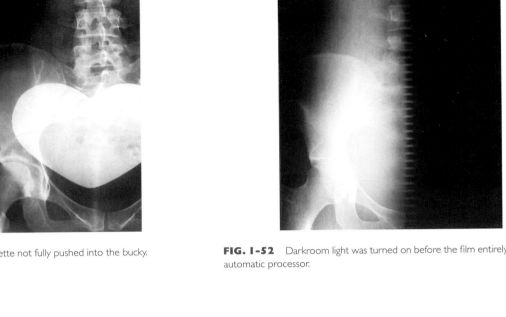

FIG. 1-52   Darkroom light was turned on before the film entirely entered the automatic processor.

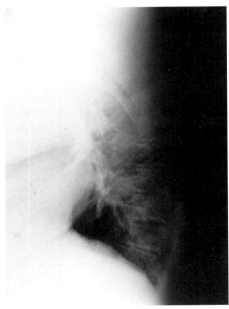

FIG. 1-53   Film fog because of a light leak.

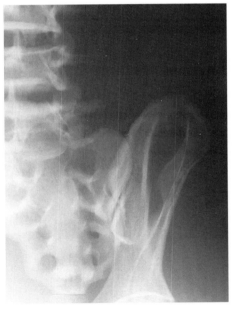

FIG. 1-54   Linear artifacts from processor's crossover rack.

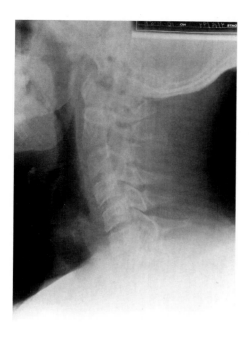

FIG. 1-55   Chemical streaks.

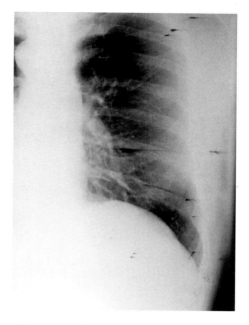

FIG. 1-56   Dark streaks from debris on rollers.

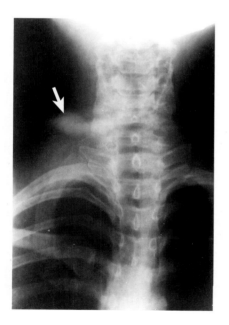

FIG. 1-57   Hair braid artifact *(arrow)*.

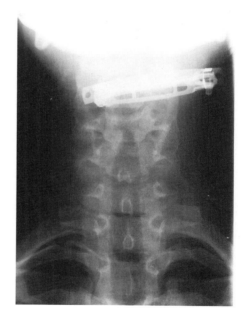

FIG. 1-58   Barrette artifact.

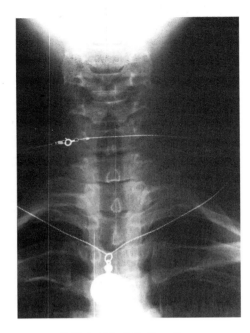

FIG. I-59   Patient's necklace.

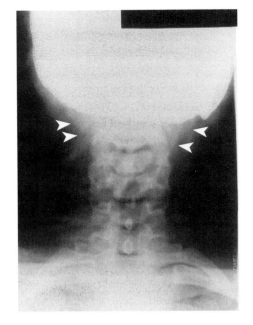

FIG. I-60   Hair cornrow artifact. *(arrowheads).*

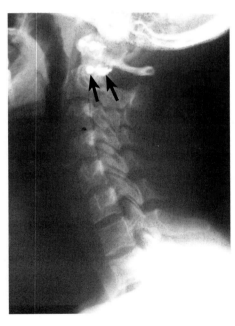

FIG. I-61   Earring artifact. *(arrows).*

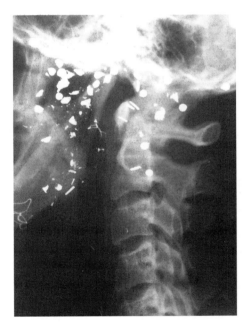

FIG. I-62   Gunshot to the face.

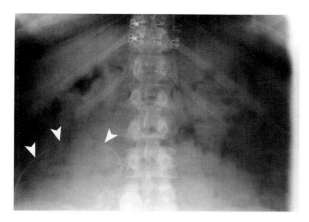

FIG. 1-63 Bra clasp and infant's skull artifacts. *(arrowheads).*

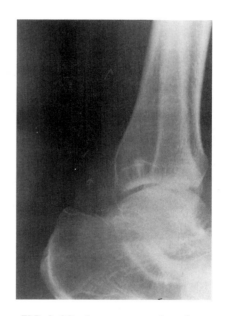

FIG. 1-64 Bra clasp and underwire artifacts.

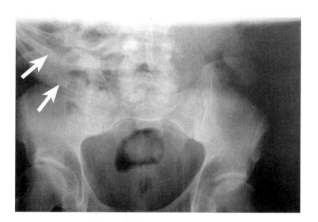

FIG. 1-65 Hand artifact. *(arrows).*

FIG. 1-66 Acupuncture needle artifacts.

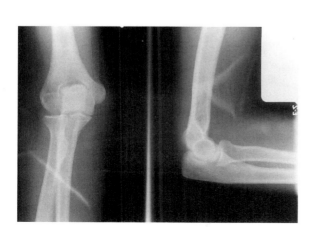

FIG. 1-67 Clothing artifact.

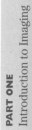

References

1. National Council on Radiation Protection and Measurements: Report No. 54, *Medical radiation exposure of pregnant and potentially pregnant women,* Bethesda, Md, 1977, NCRP.
2. National Council on Radiation Protection and Measurements: Report No. 116, *Limitations of exposure to ionizing radiation* (supersedes NCRP Report No. 91), Bethesda, Md, 1993, NCRP.

Suggested Readings

Burns EF: *Radiographic imaging. A guide for producing quality radiographs,* Philadelphia, 1992, WB Saunders.

Bushberg JT et al: *The essential physics of medical imaging,* Baltimore, 1994, Williams & Wilkins.

Bushong SC: *Radiologic science for technologists: physics, biology, and protection,* ed 5, St Louis, 1993, Mosby.

Carlton RR, Adler AM: *Principles of radiographic imaging: an art and science,* ed 2, Albany, 1996, Delmar Publishers.

Cullinan AM: *Producing quality radiographs,* Philadelphia, 1987, JB Lippincott.

Curry TS, Dowdey JE, Murry RC: *Christensen's introduction to the physics of diagnostic radiology,* ed 4, Philadelphia, 1990, Lea & Febiger.

Eastman Kodak Company: *The fundamentals of radiography,* ed 12, Rochester, 1980, Health Sciences Markets Division.

Grigg ERN: *The trail of the invisible light: from x-Stahlen to radio(bio)logy,* Springfield, Ill, 1965, Charles C. Thomas.

Lauer OG, Mayes JB, Thurston RR: *Evaluating radiographic quality. The variables and their effects,* Mankato, Minn, 1990, Burnell.

Selman J: *The fundamentals of x-ray and radium physics,* ed 7, Springfield, Ill, 1985, Charles C. Thomas.

Sprawls P: *Principles of radiography for technologists,* Rockville, Md, 1987, Aspen.

Statkiewitcz-Sherer MA, Visconti PJ, Ritenour ER: *Radiation protection in medical radiography,* St Louis, 1993, Mosby.

Tortorici M: *Concepts in medical radiographic imaging,* Philadelphia, 1992, WB Saunders.

chapter 2

Specialized Imaging

IAN D MCLEAN

Magnetic Resonance Imaging
Computed Tomography

Myelography
Discography

Radionuclide Imaging

Magnetic Resonance Imaging

HISTORY

Contemporary magnetic resonance imaging (MRI or MR) developed from the nuclear magnetic resonance (NMR) technology that chemists use to evaluate the chemical composition of laboratory samples. Laboratory use of NMR began in 1946, when Felix Bloch proposed that nuclei could behave as small magnets in the presence of a strong magnetic field.[1] Nearly 3 decades later, Raymond Damadien first utilized this technology as an imaging tool when he produced a crude image of a rat tumor in 1974.[1] He produced a successful image of a full body in July of 1976.

MRI offers advantages over other diagnostic imaging modalities. In particular, MRI provides superior tissue contrast when compared with computed tomography (CT) and conventional radiography. The image contrast achieved in CT scanning is based on x-ray attenuation properties. Instead, MRI spatially analyzes the magnetic spin properties of tissue nuclei, principally hydrogen. Analysis of this information results in greater sensitivity to subtle differences among tissue types than is possible with imaging systems based on x-ray attenuation.

Notably, MRI does not use ionizing radiation in the process of obtaining an image, and therefore, its use is not associated with the potential harmful effects of ionizing radiation. MRI uses high magnetic fields and radiofrequencies to analyze the magnetic spin properties of hydrogen nuclei. Although minimal bioeffects have been associated with high magnetic fields and radiofrequencies, the parameters of their application in MRI are without significant health hazard.

EQUIPMENT

On casual observation, the MRI scanner appears similar to a CT unit. Each is composed of a gantry, a couch for the patient, and a computer. The gantry of an MRI unit is longer than that of a CT scanner. The MRI gantry contains a large primary magnet to create a net magnetization of the hydrogen nuclei within the patient. Three principle types of magnets are used to generate the high magnetic fields needed for MRI imaging.

1. *Superconducting* magnets consist of primary magnetic coils supercooled by cryogens such as liquid helium or liquid nitrogen. These types of magnets are most commonly used in current MRI systems (Fig. 2-1).
2. *Permanent* magnets are not able to obtain the high magnetic fields of superconductive systems, but they are very popular because of their "open" and "nonclaustrophobic" design.
3. *Resistive electromagnets* are large, classical electromagnets. Although these systems are perhaps of lower initial cost than superconducting magnets, and of lower weight than permanent magnets, the power consumption is very high.

Gradient magnetic coils are located within the gantry and allow "slicing" of the patient's anatomy along sagittal, coronal, or transverse planes (Fig. 2-2). During the examination these coils switch on and off very rapidly, which produces the characteristic, sometimes quite loud, tapping noise associated with an MRI scan. Radiofrequency (RF) coils are placed on or near the area of the patient's anatomy being investigated. They are used to excite and receive information pertaining to the location of the hydrogen nuclei (Fig. 2-3).

IMAGE PRODUCTION

MRI image production is based on the system's ability to spatially localize hydrogen atoms within body tissues. Within the body, the nuclei of hydrogen atoms are charged particles that generate small magnetic fields, similar to tiny bar magnets. Normally, the hydrogen atoms are randomly oriented, their magnetic vectors cancel out, and no net magnetism of the tissue is produced (Fig. 2-4). Hydrogen is particularly useful because it is plentiful, representing 80% of all atoms found in the body.[1]

The MRI unit creates a strong magnetic field. Magnetic field strengths are measured in units of gauss (G) and tesla (T). One tesla is equal to 10,000 gauss. In comparison, the earth's magnetic field is approximately 0.5 gauss. Consequently, a 1.5 T MRI magnet is about 30,000 times the strength of the earth's magnetic field. The strength of electromagnets used to pick up cars in junkyards (1.5 to 2 T) is approximately the same field strength of an MRI magnet.

When the patient is placed in the MRI scanner, each of the small magnetic fields of the patient's hydrogen atoms tends to orient itself with, or less often against, the stronger external magnetic field of the MRI unit. The hydrogen atoms are not statically polarized by the strong external magnetic force of the MRI unit; rather, they wobble like a child's top.

Hydrogen wobbling is a phenomenon known as *precession.* In MRI, the rate of precession is intimately dependent on the element (in this case hydrogen) and the strength of the external magnetic field created by the MRI. A strictly linear relationship exists between the frequency of precession and the strength of an external magnetic field, known as the *gyromagnetic ratio,* and is measured in megahertz/tesla (MHz/T). When hydrogen is placed in a magnet of 1 T, it assumes a characteristic precession frequency of 42.6 MHz. The relationship between the gyromagnetic ratio and mag-

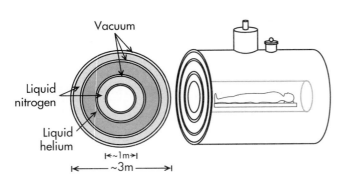

FIG. 2-1 Cross-section of a superconducting magnet.

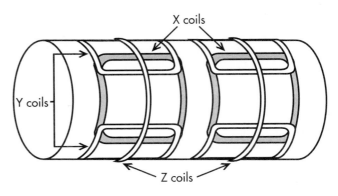

FIG. 2-2 The location of the three sets of gradient coils relative to the primary magnet. Gradient coils produce inhomogeneities of the magnet field that permit selection of slice thickness and pixel location within a slice.

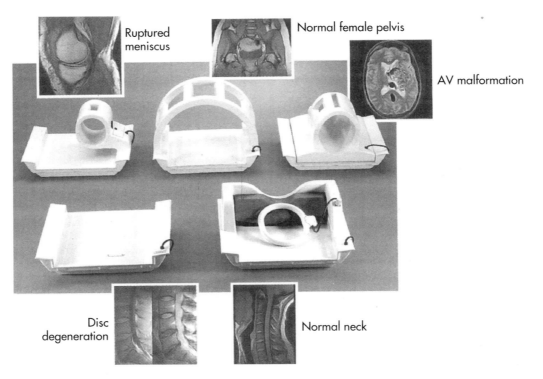

FIG. 2-3 RF coils are used to excite and receive information about the location of the hydrogen nuclei. (Courtesy Picker International, Inc, Cleveland Ohio.)

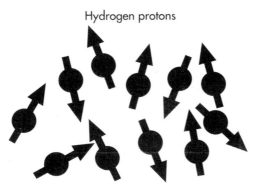

FIG. 2-4 Hydrogen protons within a patient are randomly oriented and behave like tiny bar magnets.

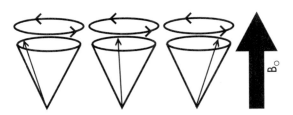

FIG. 2-5 When a patient is placed in the strong magnet field (B$_o$) of the MRI unit, some of the patient's hydrogen atoms align themselves with the strong magnetic field as they precess or spin about a central axis. The individual spins of the hydrogen atoms are synchronized but are out of phase, until a radiofrequency (RF) pulse occurs.

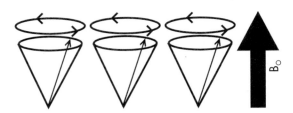

FIG. 2-6 Following the application of a radiofrequency (RF) pulse identical to the Larmor frequency, the hydrogen atoms precess in phase.

netic field strength is described by the Larmor equation and forms the basis for MRI imaging (Fig. 2-5). The following is the Larmor equation:

$$\text{Frequency of precession} = \text{Gyromagnetic ratio} \times \text{Strength of the external magnetic field}$$

To obtain images, a radiofrequency (RF) identical to the Larmor frequency of precession is pulsed into the patient. If, for instance, the hydrogen nuclei have spins of 40 MHz, these nuclei can be "excited" only by a 40 MHz radiofrequency pulse. This is the concept of resonance, similar to the vibration of a guitar string when a tuning fork of the same frequency is placed next to the instrument (Fig. 2-6). When the RF pulse is turned off, the excited nuclei undergo "relaxation," where the accumulated energy is released in the form of RF and is detected by the surface coil acting as an antenna system for the MRI equipment. The MRI signal received from the tissues is used to reconstruct an image.

IMAGING TECHNIQUES

As presented in the previous chapter, the production of a radiographic image is dependent upon two principal controls that cover technique selection. These controls are kVp (peak kilovoltage) and mAs (milliampere-second). By carefully selecting peak kilovoltage and milliampere-seconds selections, radiographers can optimize the appearance of an image.

In MRI, image appearance is manipulated by controlling the timing of radiofrequency pulses sent into the patient and the echo of the signal from the patient. The most commonly utilized MRI imaging technique is referred to as a *spin echo sequence*. During this process RF pulses are transmitted into the patient. Following nuclear excitation, the RF pulses are discontinued and the hydrogen nuclei relax. As they relax, radiofrequency is emitted from the tissue. This emitted MRI signal is received by the surface coil and used to reconstruct an image of the tissues being studied. The appearance of the image reflects the intensity of the emitted signal. A high signal intensity appears bright on the image, and a low signal intensity appears dark.

Signal intensity is dependent upon the population of hydrogen atoms and two magnetic relaxation times (T1 and T2) of the tissue. By manipulating the repetition of RF pulses (repetition time, TR) and the collection of the emitted signal (echo time, TE), an operator can dramatically influence which of these three factors are emphasized in the image. In other words, the resultant image can be based on the population of hydrogen (proton density), or emphasized to either the T1 (T1-weighted) or T2 (T2-weighted) properties of the tissue. The appearance, or signal intensities, of various tissues

TABLE 2-1
Signal Intensities of Various Tissues

Signal	T1-weighting	T2-weighting
Bright	Fat Yellow bone marrow Subacute hemorrhage White matter of brain	CSF-water Cysts Edema Normal nucleus pulposus Tumor
Medium	Fluid IVD Muscle Red bone marrow Spinal cord Tumor	Dehydrated nucleus pulposus Fat Gray matter of brain Muscle Spleen
Dark	Air Calcification Cerebrospinal fluid Cortical bone Fast-moving blood Fibrous tissue Ligaments, tendons	Air Calcification Cortical bone Fast-moving blood Fibrous tissue Ligaments, tendons

are listed in Table 2-1. Further elaboration on how these sequences are obtained is beyond the scope of this discussion, and the reader seeking additional information is referred to the Suggested Readings listed at the end of this chapter.

PATIENT PREPARATION

As far as is known, no harmful effects result from an MRI examination. In most circumstances, the steps are routine, and no preparation of the patient is required. Claustrophobia is the most common reason for not completing a study. It is estimated to complicate up to 5% of MRI studies. Although reassurance works for most patients, a mild tranquilizer can be very effective in alleviating high anxiety.

The length of the MRI examination can vary from 30 to 90 minutes, with an average examination taking 45 minutes. The length of the examination depends on the imaging sequences, which are gathered over 2- to 10-minute periods. Because of these prolonged examination times, it is critical that patients lie absolutely still for the duration of each imaging sequence. Referring physicians may find it beneficial to visit the MRI facility so that they can adequately

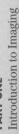

PART ONE Introduction to Imaging

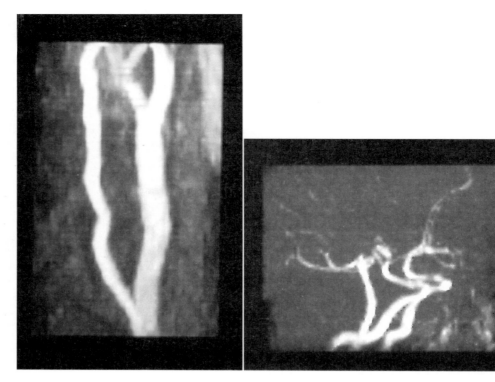

FIG. 2-7   Magnetic resonance angiography (MRA) of the carotid and intracranial circulation.

explain the procedure to their patients. A well-informed patient is less likely to be overly anxious about the examination.

CONTRAINDICATIONS

Prior to the MRI examination a thorough history must be obtained from the patient, with particular attention given to surgical intervention and industrial exposure to metals. Patients with pacemakers or other implanted electronic devices (including certain ear implants) generally cannot be examined. Many intracranial aneurysm clips are ferromagnetic and as a result experience a torque or twisting in a magnetic field. Therefore, MRI examinations are contraindicated in patients with vascular clips within the brain. Some types of heart valves are also affected; however, this torque is usually less than the stresses that normally occur as a result of blood flow. Therefore, the presence of heart valves is not necessarily an absolute contraindication for an MRI examination. Orthopedic devices, although not usually a contraindication to the MRI examination, can lead to considerable image degradation by causing significant alteration to the magnetic field homogeneity. In all circumstances, the presence of surgical devices should be made known to the MRI facility staff and radiologist.

MRI CONTRAST AGENTS

MRI can obtain most anatomical information simply by relying on the inherent contrast of the body's tissues; however, under certain clinical circumstances an artificial contrast medium may be required. MRI contrast media are based on gadolinium (Gd). Gadolinium is a T1-shortening agent that causes tissues containing this element to appear bright on T1-weighted images. Gadolinium is especially useful in the detection of various CNS pathologies such as tumors and multiple sclerosis. Most commonly, chiropractic patients may require gadolinium to help differentiate recurrent disc

herniation from scar formation in those patients with failed low back surgery. Gadolinium is not an iodinated contrast media such as is used in CT examinations and angiography; subsequently adverse reactions are quite rare.

MRI ANGIOGRAPHY

MRI angiography (MRA) is a developing alternative to conventional angiography for the evaluation of vascular disease. This examination has the specific advantage of being totally noninvasive, because no contrast media is used. However, the spatial resolution of MRA is lower than routine angiographic examinations. Presently this examination should be used only to study larger vessels (Fig. 2-7).

Computed Tomography

HISTORY

Until the advent of computed tomography (computerized tomography, CT), many areas of the body could not be evaluated by usual radiographic methods. For instance, examination of the brain for suspected lesions required extraordinary and often very invasive procedures such as pneumoencephalography, a procedure that involved a spinal puncture along with the injection of contrast material and air. Not only would this leave the patient with a serious headache, often requiring hospitalization, but it could also result in a transtentorial or foraminal herniation of the brain. Similar examinations in the form of myelography were required as routine examination for spinal disc herniation.

Although early attempts to construct computerized tomographic equipment occurred during the late 1950s, the first practical working model of a CT system was developed by Geoffrey Hounsfield in 1970. Hounsfield, a computer engineer working at the Central Research Laboratory for Electric and Music Industry (EMI) in Eng-

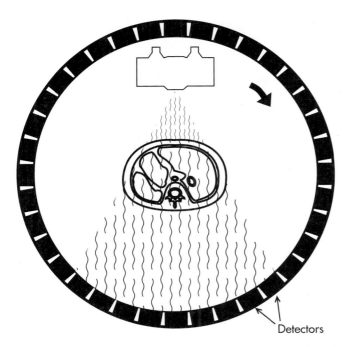

FIG. 2-8 CT does not use x-ray film as the image receptor system but relies on an array of detectors.

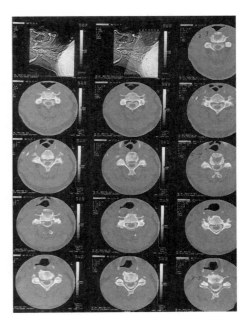

FIG. 2-9 A typical layout of CT cervical spine images with the scout, or localizer, images in the upper left corner.

land, (the British company most famous for recording the Beatles), later went on to win the Nobel Prize for Medicine and Physiology in 1979.

IMAGE PRODUCTION

The CT scanner utilizes a radiographic tube contained within a gantry that emits x-rays as it rotates about the patient. An array of detectors on the opposite side of the tube intercepts those x-rays transmitted through the patient. Importantly, CT does not use x-ray film as the image receptor system but relies on an array of detectors and computer algorithms (a mathematical set of instructions) to create digitized axial tomographic images of the body (Fig. 2-8).

Critical to the image quality of CT scans are collimators. As in conventional radiography, collimation reduces patient dose by restricting the volume of tissue being irradiated and importantly decreases the unwanted effects of scatter radiation. CT utilizes at least two collimator systems. The prepatient collimator is located adjacent to the tube housing; the predetector collimator restricts the x-ray field that will be intercepted by the detector array. Collectively, the collimators define the thickness of the image slice.

In conventional radiography, anatomy is displayed in an analog form, that is, directly by the radiographic film, which acts as the radiation detector. In CT, however, the x-ray beam that traverses the patient's body is subsequently attenuated and is ascribed a coefficient of attenuation. The coefficient of attenuation, also referred to as a *CT number* or a *Hounsfield unit,* represents the density of a volume of tissue (voxel). The CT number for water is designated 0, air is −1000 and dense bone is +1000, approximately. Consequently, all the various tissues within the examined area are assigned Hounsfield units and corresponding gray scales. Each voxel with its Hounsfield unit is displayed in a two-dimensional manner as a pixel on a CRT (cathode ray tube), an image monitor.

The radiologist or the radiologic technologist has the ability to alter the appearance of the images on the CRT by manipulating the contrast (window width) and density of selected tissues (window level). For the best visual appearance of bone lesions, for example, a wide window width and a high window level are appropriate. Finally, the images are printed on radiographic film.

In musculoskeletal imaging, especially of the spine, image formats usually include both a soft tissue and a bone image for each axial slice. Examinations of the lumbar spine, for example, usually include 12 axial images along with a scout image on a 14-inch by 17-inch sheet of radiographic film (Figs. 2-9 and 2-10).

IMAGING TECHNIQUES

A commonly used CT examination technique of the lumbar spine utilizes contiguous axial slices parallel to the angle of each disc interspaces, with each slice being approximately 3 to 5 mm thick. The slices are angled to conform to each disc interspace. At the L5-S1 level, often the slice angle cannot be parallel to the disc plane line because the gantry of the CT scanner cannot be tilted sufficiently.

The actual axial examination of the spine is preceded by digitized frontal or lateral scout views with appropriate numerical annotations, allowing for accurate localization of the subsequent axial slices (see Fig. 2-9).

Another commonly used technique utilizes consecutive axial slices obtained perpendicular to the tabletop. These axial slices can then be reformatted by the computer as sagittal or coronal images. Although reformatted images do have the advantage of displaying anatomy in another plane line, rarely do these images contribute much more information in routine examinations (Fig. 2-11). On occasion where there are lesions such as complex fractures, sagittal or coronal reformatted images may prove useful. Three-dimensional reformatted images are also possible (Fig. 2-12).

Advantages of CT over conventional radiography include its much greater ability to discriminate low-contrast objects, the cross-sectional display of anatomy and possible reconstruction of the image in additional planes (sagittal and coronal). The spatial resolution

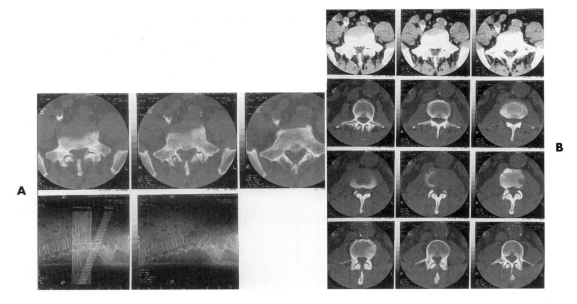

FIG. 2-10   A, The scout, or localizer, image allows for accurate localization of the axial slices. **B,** Typical skeletal CT examinations comprise two arrays of images; those that emphasize soft tissues (soft tissue window) *(top row)* and those that emphasize the bone anatomy (bone window) *(bottom three rows).*

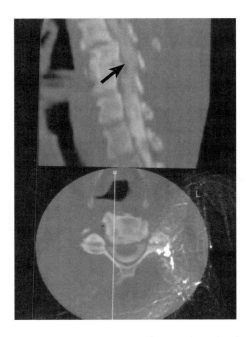

FIG. 2-11   Reformatted planar images of the cervical spine demonstrating hypertrophic spinal changes effacing the column of contrast *(arrow).*

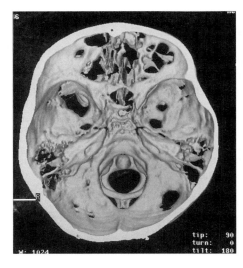

FIG. 2-12   Three-dimensional reconstructed CT image of the base of the cranium.

of CT, however, is less than that of conventional radiography. Further, the radiation dose is considerably higher, often 3 to 5 rads to the skin within the collimated area.

CT MYELOGRAPHY

CT myelography (CTM) describes a CT study made after the injection of contrast media into the subarachnoid space. With the advent of high-resolution CT and MRI, CT myelography is not considered

to be a routine examination procedure of the spine. On occasion, where MRI nor CT does not provide the necessary information to resolve a clinical problem, CTM may be helpful (Fig. 2-13).

CT ARTHROGRAPHY

CT examination of a joint usually requires the administration of a contrast media. CT arthrography is a distinctly less common procedure in recent times, in part because of the popularity of MRI. MRI

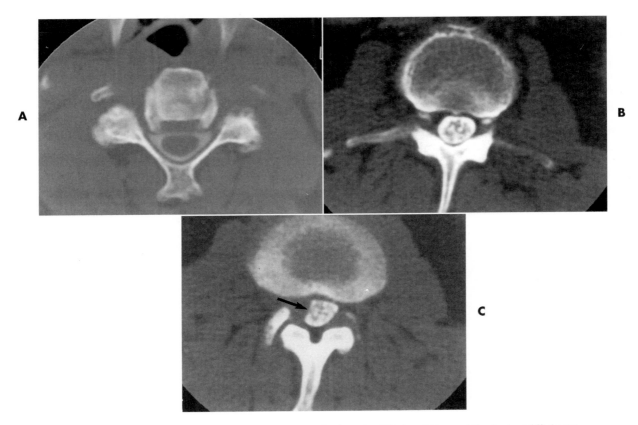

FIG. 2-13 CT myelography of the cervical spine **(A)** and lumbar spine **(B)**. An axial image at the disc level **(C)** demonstrates effacement of the contrast filled dural sac secondary to disc herniation (*arrow*).

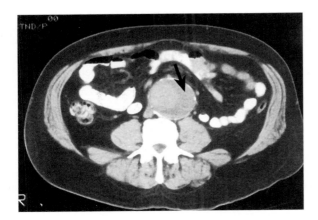

FIG. 2-14 Aneurysm of the abdominal aorta. Note the differences in density between the contrasted lumen of the vessel and the adjacent thrombus (arrow).

has the advantage of being noninvasive; furthermore, the inherent high soft tissue contrast makes this examination ideal for the evaluation of most major joints. Some joints, however, are perhaps arguably still best evaluated with CT arthrography; the most outstanding examples of this are the labrum of the shoulder and the hip.

CLINICAL APPLICATIONS

Trauma. The principal indication for CT today is in the evaluation of trauma, mainly of the spine but also for the evaluation of complex fractures of the hip and shoulder.

Tumors. MRI is the imaging modality of choice in evaluation of soft tissue tumors. However, CT continues to be valuable in the evaluation of tumors that invade bone. It is likely under most clinical circumstances, particularly if both CT and MRI are available, that both of these imaging systems will be used to plan the management of bone tumors.

Bone mineral analysis. Because CT has the ability to measure the attenuation coefficient of tissue, this imaging tool is particularly valuable in acquiring an accurate, quantitative analysis of bone mineral particularly in cases of osteoporosis.

Abdomen CT. Examination of the abdomen continues to be a prevalent use of CT often in conjunction with diagnostic ultrasonography. In chiropractic practice, CT of the abdomen is commonly ordered for the evaluation of aortic aneurysms consequent to discovering dilatation of an arteriosclerotic vessel on conventional x-rays of the lumbar spine (Fig. 2-14).

Myelography

HISTORY

Jacobius of Sweden described myelography in 1921, utilizing air as a contrast medium. Over the subsequent half-century, other substances have been utilized as contrast media, including poppyseed oil and Pantopaque. Both had the major disadvantage of potentially creating arachnoiditis. Water-soluble contrast agents were available in the 1940s but were quite toxic. With the advent of nonionic water-soluble contrast agents (i.e., metrizamide) in the late 1970s, myelography has evolved into a relatively safe and reliable examination of the thecal sac and its contents. Serious side effects of myelography still occur, reflecting its invasive nature. Potentially serious but relatively rare complications include infections and arterial bleeding, the latter most likely seen with cervical puncture. Headache remains the most common side effect of myelography and is perhaps related to the leakage of cerebral spinal fluid.

IMAGE PRODUCTION

Myelography describes the injection of radiopaque substance into the subarachnoid space for radiographic visualization of the spinal cord or its extensions. Abnormality is inferred from alterations in the column of injected contrast.

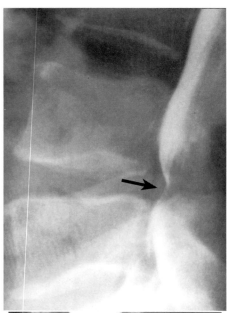

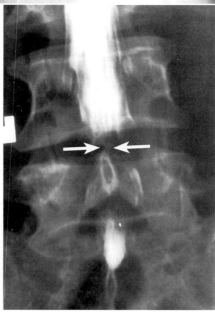

FIG. 2-15 Myelography of the lumbar spine showing an extradural defect consistent with disc herniation at the L4 level (arrows).

CLINICAL APPLICATION

MRI is now considered to be the examination of choice in spinal infection, primary and secondary malignant disease, and general lumbar disc disease. However, myelography combined with CT has been argued as the method of choice in the evaluation of lateral cervical disc herniations and cervical foraminal narrowing. Because MRI is less invasive and rapidly evolving, the use of myelography can be expected only to decrease in the immediate future. Myelography will likely continue to be performed on those patients that for one reason or another cannot undergo an MRI examination, or on patients for whom the resulting MRI images are of poor diagnostic accuracy or quality.

Disc herniations. Disc herniations displace myelographic contrast media at the level of the disc interspace and also displaces the dural sleeve about the corresponding nerve root. Diagnoses of disc bulge and disc herniation are possible. Accuracy of 97% has been recorded in distinguishing disc bulge from disc herniation. Ability to image disc herniations at the L5 level is decreased because of increased anterior epidural fat, which displays the myelographic contrast media within the subarachnoid space away from the offending disc lesion. The appearance of a disc herniation on a myelogram is marked by the following (Fig. 2-15):

- sharp angular indentation on the lateral aspect of the thecal sac
- narrowing of the disc space (a sign of disc degeneration)
- enlargement of a nerve root secondary to edema
- displacement of a nerve root secondary to nonfilling of a root sleeve

Arachnoiditis. Arachnoiditis is inflammation of the pia mater and arachnoid of the brain or spinal cord. It is a potential complication of myelography. Its presence is suggested by a blunted appearance of the nerve root sleeves.

Intradural-intramedullary lesions. An intradural-intramedullary lesion is a lesion within the spinal cord, including astrocytomas, ependymomas, and syringomyelia. Syringohydromyelia, representing cavitation within the spinal cord, is difficult if not impossible to differentiate from spinal cord intramedullary tumor and is consequently best evaluated with MRI. Characteristically, intradural-intramedullary lesions expand the spinal cord somewhat symmetrically with consequent effacement of the myelographic column.

Intradural-extramedullary lesions. Intradural-extramedullary pathologies are located within the subarachnoid space, external to the spinal cord. Common examples include meningiomas and neurofibromas. The characteristic findings of myelography are compression of the spinal cord with widening of the subarachnoid space at the site of the mass, with consequent widening of the overall thecal sac. The borders of the lesions may be sharply defined.

Extradural lesions. These lesions are lateral to the thecal sac, the most common examples of which are disc herniations and degenerative spondylosis with osteophyte formation. The most common tumor type to create extradural myelographic effacement is spinal metastasis. The characteristic finding on myelography is displacement of the myelographic column away from the adjacent bone or disc interspace; displacement is typically asymmetrical.

Discography

Discography is the injection of a contrast medium within an intervertebral disc. This is now a rarely performed procedure requiring multiple lumbar punctures. Its most common application is in conjunction with chemonucleolysis.

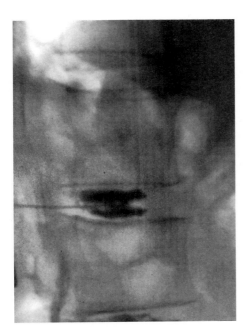

FIG. 2-16 Discography revealing normal disc structure with subtraction fluoroscopy.

The examination is able to define extravasation of contrast material extending to the periphery of the disc space. Further, the procedure has the advantage of possibly reproducing the patient's clinical symptoms. This may increase the diagnostic accuracy of whether the disc lesions are clinically important, or it may designate the symptomatic disc when multiple levels of herniation are present (Fig. 2-16).

Radionuclide Imaging

IMAGE PRODUCTION

Radionuclide imaging is a relatively noninvasive technology that utilizes radiopharmaceuticals to evaluate pathophysiological abnormalities of various organ systems. Imaging is dependent on certain substances concentrating selectively in different parts of the body. A radionuclide can be chemically tagged to these substances and consequently allow for evaluation of specific organ systems by imaging the radionuclide. The skeleton, lungs, liver, thyroid, and heart are common organ systems to be scanned with radionuclide imaging.

Skeletal radionuclide imaging is performed with 99m technetium methylene diphosphonate (^{99m}Tc-MDP), a phosphate analog that is incorporated into the hydroxyapatite crystal of bone by the osteoblasts. Increased uptake of the radiopharmaceutical is seen in conditions that produce both an increased metabolic activity and blood supply, including tumors, infections, fractures, metabolic diseases, and joint diseases. Radionuclide bone imaging is sensitive, but it is not as specific as some other imaging systems available for many presentations. Its major advantage over other imaging systems is that the whole skeleton can be imaged at one time.

The radiopharmaceutical is injected into a vein, where it is subsequently disseminated throughout the body. Images are most commonly obtained 2 to 3 hours after injection, which allows clearance of the isotope from the blood and incorporation of it into bone.

Bone scans are most often interpreted in three phases. The first phase, or *flow phase,* supplies a *radionuclide angiogram,* occurring

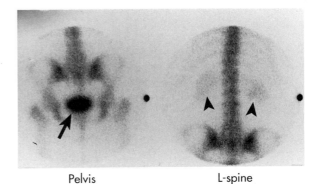

Pelvis   L-spine

FIG. 2-17 Radionuclide scintigraphy demonstrating nonpathological accumulation of the radioisotope within the bladder *(arrow)* and kidneys *(arrowheads).*

within the first minute following the injection. The second phase is noted as the *blood pool scan,* occurring 1 to 3 minutes following injection. The third phase is the *static bone scan,* occurring 2 to 4 hours following injection. With increased blood flow, the first and second phases demonstrate prominent collection. Collection of radionuclide in the third phase corresponds to osteogenic activity and blood flow.

Technetium is the most widely used radiopharmaceutical for bone scanning because it is widely available, easily prepared, and has a relatively short half-life (6 hours). Consequently, the radiation dose is very acceptable, with a whole-body dose of approximately 10 mrads/mCi.

Nonpathological increased uptake is noted in the most metabolically active regions of the body (i.e., epiphyses, costochondral junctions, the sacroiliac joints, and the sternoclavicular joints). Increased uptake is also found in the kidneys secondary to the excretion of the radioisotope; therefore, the radiologist has an opportunity to secondarily evaluate kidney anatomy and function (Fig. 2-17).

Gamma rays are emitted from the patient's body by the isotope. The gamma rays are detected by a gamma camera, which contains a sodium iodide crystal coupled to a photomultiplier system. The photomultiplier produces light to produce a radiographic image.

Single proton emission tomography (SPECT) imaging is an extension of simple planar radionuclide imaging. SPECT images may be obtained in three dimensions and provide better delineation of complex or small anatomy than is possible with conventional scanning.

CLINICAL APPLICATION

Radionuclide examinations hold negligible risk for the patient. The only health conditions for which radionuclide examinations are contraindicated are pregnancy and breastfeeding. The most common use of a bone scan is in the detection of metastatic bone disease. A common scenario that might warrant a radionuclide bone scan would be a patient with low back pain with a prior history of primary malignancy, especially of the breast or prostate. Unfortunately radionuclide bone imaging cannot always differentiate benign from malignant lesions. Ultimate differentiation depends on correlating the radiographic and clinical features and possibly biopsy.

In the spine, mild increased uptake might be created by posterior facet arthrosis and is usually easily differentiated from more serious pathology such as metastatic bone disease by the typical distribution of the "hot-spot" in the region of the facet joints. Occult frac-

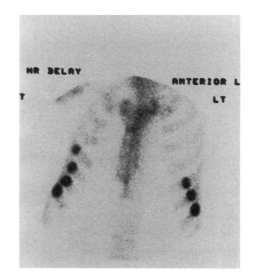

FIG. 2-18   Radionuclide scintigraphy revealing the typical linear distribution of "hot-spots" diagnostic of multiple rib fractures.

TABLE 2-2
Appropriate Imaging Modalities Based on Pathology

Clinical presentation	MRI	CT	X-ray
Spine and spinal cord			
Disc herniation	Procedure of choice	Reasonably sensitive	Insensitive
Recurrent disc vs postoperative scar	Procedure of choice	Insensitive	Insensitive
Degenerative disc disease (DDD)	Very sensitive	Sensitive	Moderately sensitive
Radiculopathy	Procedure of choice	Reasonably sensitive	Adjunctive
Myelopathy	Procedure of choice	Insensitive	Adjunctive
Multiple sclerosis	Procedure of choice	Insensitive	Insensitive
Arnold Chiari malformation	Procedure of choice	Reasonably sensitive	Insensitive
Syringomyelia	Procedure of choice	Reasonably sensitive	Insensitive
Spinal metastasis, multiple myeloma	Very sensitive	Reasonably sensitive	Insensitive in early disease
Infections	Very sensitive	Reasonably sensitive	Insensitive in early disease
Cord tumors and "drop" metastases	Procedure of choice	Insensitive	Insensitive
Extremities (knee, shoulder, wrist, and ankle)			
Avascular necrosis	Procedure of choice	Insensitive	Insensitive in early disease
Cruciate ligament tears	Procedure of choice	Insensitive	Insensitive
Meniscal tears	Procedure of choice	Insensitive	Insensitive
Osteochondritis dessicans	Procedure of choice	Adjunctive	Insensitive in early disease
Posttrauma	Very sensitive	Sensitive	Procedure of choice
Chrondomalacia patella	Procedure of choice	Intensive	Insensitive in early disease
Rotator cuff tear	Procedure of choice	Insensitive	Insensitive
Glenoid labrum tear	Sensitive	Sensitive	Insensitive
Tendonitis	Very sensitive	Insensitive	Insensitive
Joint effusions	Procedure of choice	Adjunctive	Insensitive
Cartilage degeneration (DJD)	Very sensitive	Adjunctive	Moderately sensitive
Infection, osteomyelitis	Very sensitive	Adjunctive	Insensitive in early disease
Tumor, multiple myeloma, metastasis	Very sensitive	Adjunctive	Insensitive in early disease
Brain			
Malignancy primary/metastasis	Procedure of choice	Adjunctive	Insensitive
Infections	Procedure of choice	Adjunctive	Insensitive
Chronic headaches	Procedure of choice	Adjunctive	Insensitive
Infarction	Procedure of choice	Adjunctive	Insensitive
Aneurysms	Very sensitive angiography	Procedure of choice	Insensitive
Hematoma, hemorrhage	Very sensitive angiography	Procedure of choice	Insensitive
Congenital anomalies	Procedure of choice	Sensitive	Insensitive
Pituitary lesions, tumor, empty sella	Procedure of choice	Adjunctive	Insensitive

tures are also well discriminated by radionuclide scintigraphy; it is commonly used in the examination of the rib cage (Fig. 2-18).

Radionuclide lung scans are most commonly used to assess pulmonary embolism, liver scans to assess the presence of metastasis, and heart scans to assess myocardial function and perfusion.

Table 2-2 presents common applications of the previously discussed imaging modalities for selected clinical pathologies.

References

1. Bushong SC: *Magnetic resonance imaging,* ed 2, St Louis, 1996, Mosby.

Suggested Readings

Armstrong P et al: Magnetic resonance imaging: basic principles of image production, *Br Med J* 303:35, 1991.

Bushong SC: *Magnetic resonance imaging,* ed 2, St Louis, 1996, Mosby.

Bushong SC: *Radiologic science for technologists* ed 5, St Louis, 1993, Mosby.

Friedland GW, Thurber BD: The birth of CT, *AJR Am J Roentgenol* 167:6, 1365, 1996.

Kleinfield S: *A machine called indomitable,* 1985, Times Books.

chapter 3

Film Interpretation, Report Writing, and Roentgenometrics

Film Interpretation
DENNIS M MARCHIORI

Report Writing
CYNTHIA PETERSON

Roentgenometrics
DENNIS M MARCHIORI

▉ Film Interpretation

Obtaining the Image

Diagnostic imaging plays an integral role in the diagnosis and management of patients. For most clinical assessments, the historically dominant modality of plain film radiography continues to be the first step. In addition, the past 2 decades have given rise to the creation and evolution of more sophisticated specialized imaging systems, such as magnetic resonance imaging, that have made previously difficult and rare diagnoses relatively easy and routine. However, because plain film radiography is widely available, relatively inexpensive, and rapidly obtained, it will likely remain as the dominant imaging method in the near future.

The most effective application of diagnostic imaging for many conditions in clinical practice is widely debated. The multifaceted and unique clinical presentations of most patients make the formation of common criteria for ordering diagnostic imaging problematic at best. Yet it is a task that needs to be accomplished to limit costs, radiation exposure, and procedural complications associated with some imaging methods.

An example of a controversial issue involves the use of plain film radiography for patients experiencing low back pain. Multiple questions cloud the issue: Should radiographs be taken of patients who have acute but not chronic back pain? What are the appropriate film-ordering criteria that maximize clinical information yet minimize cost and the patient's exposure to radiation? In what way should the film-ordering criteria developed for medical physicians differ from those for practitioners who adjust or manipulate the lumbar spine using manual therapies? Parallel and similarly controversial issues surround the application of specialized imaging. (e.g., whether magnetic resonance imaging [MRI] should be ordered for a patient in whom disc herniation is suspected but neurological findings are limited).

When clinicians are deciding which diagnostic imaging modality to use, they can follow a generally accepted rule for the use of all diagnostic procedures: if the patient's diagnosis or management is likely to significantly change from information routinely provided by the diagnostic procedure in question, then the study should be performed; if the required information is not routinely provided by the procedure or knowing the information that will be obtained will not change the patient's management, then the procedure should not be performed.

Reading the Image

Although film interpretation is truly an art, several common steps can be described. The first step is for the interpreter to become familiar with the clinical rationale for the studies: Is a fracture suspected? Does the 65-year-old patient with unrelenting low back pain have a history of night pain, unexplained weight loss, or past malignancy? It has been suggested that interpreters should not immediately look at the rationale for examination because knowing this information may bias the observation. This is correct. It will create bias—and lead the interpreter to the correct diagnosis. This is a "systematic error" that most interpreters would welcome.

Next the images should be viewed completely with a specific search pattern of observation. A search pattern is used to ensure the entire image has been observed. The best search pattern is a unique one developed by the interpreter over time that compensates for the individual's inherent weaknesses in observation. For instance, if an interpreter has difficulty remembering to look at the sella turcica on a lateral radiograph of the cervical spine, the search pattern should be altered to emphasize that region; this will compensate for the interpreter's inherent tendency to underinterpret that portion of the film.

If an abnormality is found while performing the search pattern, the search pattern may be modified so it will reveal clues that correlate with the abnormality, but the original search pattern should still be completed to ensure identification of other abnormalities unrelated to the first finding are identified. Although unique elements are incorporated into each interpreter's search pattern, all search patterns should be complete, concise, and consistently employed and should emphasize regions of the image in which pathologies are commonly found or missed.

At times, imaging findings are pathognomonic for a specific condition, but more often the imaging findings are best summarized in a "pattern" of abnormality. The pattern of abnormality leads to a list of differential diagnoses that are known to cause the observed appearance. The list of differential possibilities is narrowed by testing each possibility against the images and available historical data. A definitive diagnosis cannot routinely be obtained from only plain film radiography. Specialized imaging procedures, laboratory studies, biopsies, and additional clinical data often must be obtained to reach a definitive diagnosis (Fig. 3-1).

The format of this book embraces this "pattern-based" approach to film interpretation. Certain chapters address common radiographical patterns of abnormality in bone, chest, and abdomen imaging. In addition, diseases commonly present on MRI scans are tabulated by body region. The differential list of diagnoses listed for the common patterns of abnormalities can be used to suggest further differential possibilities. The patient's clinical data, including results of additional imaging and laboratory studies, can then be consulted to narrow the differential list to a few possibilities or a single diagnosis.

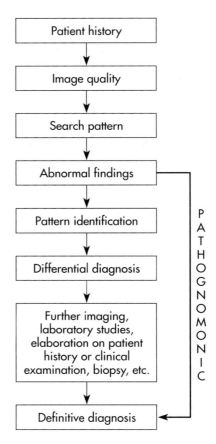

FIG. 3-1   Flowchart for film interpretation.

Report Writing

The radiological report is an integral component of the patient's medicolegal record. As such, care must be given to ensure that the information contained in this report is as accurate as possible while still being concise. Many practitioners consider the task of writing the radiological report to be unnecessarily time consuming and onerous. As a result, they either write a brief summary of their impressions or make no written record whatsoever.[22,36] Failing to report on the patient's radiographs in writing is analogous to performing a physical examination without making any written entries into the patient's file.[38] The medicolegal implications are obvious.

The radiographs should confirm or rule out a clinical suspicion. Thus an important component of the report should be the attempt to link the radiographical signs with the history and physical examination findings.[30] Radiological reports also offer opportunity to monitor radiographical quality—to act as a sort of ongoing audit.[38] They can help the practitioner maintain and improve standards of radiographical quality while keeping radiation dosages to a minimum. Other important benefits of radiological reports include the fact that they provide (1) a standard of comparison with previous or later examinations, (2) a permanent record if radiographs are lost or not immediately available, and (3) a way to expedite the treatment regime by providing a resume of important indications and contraindications for therapy.[46]

As with all components of the medical record, the radiological report is a reflection of the abilities and professionalism of the practitioner. It also serves to facilitate interprofessional and intraprofessional communication. Unfortunately, the format and terminology of radiological reports are not standardized, with the literature clearly pointing out their wide variation in length and style.[10,11,24,27]

Pitfalls in Radiological Interpretation

Before embarking directly on the task of writing the radiological report, several areas of caution in radiograph interpretation must first be addressed. Twenty to forty percent of the statements made in radiology reports by medical radiologists or radiology residents have been found to be erroneous, with many of these errors having life-threatening consequences.[16,34,39] Not surprisingly, the error rate is higher among less experienced radiology residents.[7,8,34] Non–radiologist practitioners should keep these concepts in mind when choosing to interpret their own radiographs. In contrast, chiropractic and medical radiologists were shown to demonstrate significantly superior radiological interpretative abilities as compared with non–radiologist practitioners in the evaluation of skeletal radiographs.[41] Although the debate about who should carry out radiological reporting continues,[42] the fact remains that many chiropractors choose to report on the majority of cases within their own practices.

Because all non–radiologist practitioners may be held legally responsible for failing to properly interpret radiographs,[15] increasing numbers are choosing to use the facilities of either chiropractic or medical radiologists for radiographical diagnosis and reporting. Although the use of these specialists should increase diagnostic accuracy and decrease the potential for litigation, no human being is infallible, and all practitioners should double-check all radiographs and reports themselves.

Radiographs of each patient must be evaluated in the proper environment.[46] The radiographs should *never* be read for the first time in front of a patient or a member of a patient's family. If a serious pathology is found, the clinician may inadvertently say something that is inappropriate and cannot easily be retracted. Similarly, significant pathology may be missed and then discovered later when sufficient time is allocated for the interpretation. Radiographs cannot be read quickly. A quiet, dark room that is free of distractions is necessary.[46] The patient's file containing the history and physical examination information should be readily available for correlation with the radiographical findings. Make sure that the identification labels and film dates are correct. Comparison of current radiographs with old films is extremely valuable when these are available.

Errors in radiological diagnosis can be caused by several factors. These errors are commonly classified as either errors of observation or errors of interpretation. Another way of classifying these radiological errors is *false positive* or *false negative*. A false negative error occurs when a significant abnormal finding is not detected or is detected but interpreted as normal. False positive errors are those in which a significant abnormality is "found" (hallucinated) in a radiographical region that is actually normal.[34] Faulty and incomplete search patterns are responsible for many of the errors in radiological diagnosis.[30] Errors of interpretation often reflect practitioners' lack of knowledge of the significance of abnormal radiographical signs or the inability to link the signs with the clinical information.[30]

Practitioners who are aware of potential pitfalls in radiological interpretation, as well as their own abilities in radiological interpretation, and are determined to provide the best diagnostic service to the patient are better able to determine which cases they would like to interpret themselves and which may benefit from a second opinion.

Generating the Radiological Report

GENERAL

Many practitioners dictate the radiological report, which is then typed by a transcriptionist.[5] Although this method is quick and efficient for the clinician, it requires careful proofreading once the report is completed, as well as the services of a typist. *Computer macros*—parts of reports and common phrases that are preprogrammed into the computer—can decrease transcription time, but a typist is still needed.[5] The need for a transcriptionist can be eliminated by using automated radiology reporting systems with software that presents radiological findings and anatomical terms in graphic form and allows the desired terms to be selected using a trackball or touch-sensitive screen.[5] However, these systems do require more of the clinician's time than simply dictating the report. Another drawback of the automated reporting system is that the clinician must frequently look away from the radiographs to the computer screen, which could potentially increase the error rate in interpretation.

Standard, or "canned," radiology reports have been available within the medical profession for many years.[3] They are very economical and can be created easily on the computer for normal studies. However, standard reports for abnormal studies are not currently practical. Speech recognition by computers may have a major role in the future of radiology reports.[3] This would eliminate transcription and allow immediate proofreading and signing of the form. Preliminary studies have demonstrated that the accuracy of the speech recognition system for chest radiological reports is between 96% and 99%.[3] At the opposite extreme a few practitioners may still prefer to hand write their radiological reports. Regardless of the way in which the radiological report is generated, it should always contain the following components[7,24,27,42,46]:

  I. Heading (preliminary information)
 II. Clinical Information (brief)
III. Findings
IV. Conclusions
 V. Recommendations (optional)
VI. Signature

Heading. The radiological report should be written on the clinician's stationery and should include the name and address of the individual or clinic. Additional information contained in the heading includes the following[13,32,42,46]:

• Date of the actual report
• Patient information
  1. Name
  2. Date of birth (or age)
  3. Gender
  4. Date the radiographs were taken
  5. X-ray number (if available)
  6. Physician (if other than the person writing the report)
• Radiographical information
  1. Part imaged
  2. Views obtained

NOTE: It may be advantageous to write separate reports for each region that has been radiographed to improve the clarity and reduce potential reading and reporting errors. For example, if radiographs are taken of both the cervical and lumbar regions, two separate reports may be written rather than one that combines all the information. Including the technical parameters into the heading of the report is optional.

Variation in the heading for reports on computed tomography scans. Special imaging procedures should come complete with the radiologist's report to the practitioner ordering the study. It should be rare for a non–radiologist practitioner to be required to report on these images without a second opinion. However, the following information may prove useful in the interpretation of computed tomography (CT) scan reports or for cases in which the clinician does not have access to the original report.

1. Part imaged: Note the exact area imaged by referring to the longitudinal scan view (e.g., L3 to S1 contiguous slices).
2. Views obtained: Record the imaging plane (e.g., axial) and whether there was gantry angulation to the slices. It may also be useful to note the thickness of the slices; include reformatted coronal and sagittal images if applicable. Also state which windows are included. Both bone and soft tissue windows should be provided. The use of intrathecal contrast agent must also be mentioned (e.g., "with myelogram").

Summary of information included in the heading of a CT report

A. Levels imaged
B. Contiguous or interrupted slices
C. Slice thickness*
D. Plane of imaging
E. Angulation of the gantry
F. Reformatting*
G. Windows provided
H. Use of contrast agent*

Variations in the heading for reports on MRI scans. As with CT scanning the clinician should not be expected to provide original reports on MRI scans. The following information is unique to the heading of these reports and may help the practitioner understand some of the differences between CT and MRI.

1. Area imaged: MRI has the advantage over CT scanning of being able to image an entire region (e.g., the entire cervical or lumbar spine at the very least).
2. Imaging planes: Most scans provide at least the sagittal plane, with axial images of areas of interest. Coronal scans can also be included. These imaging planes are not reformatted (reconstructed) images as they are in CT scans, so these terms should not be used. As a result, the detail of MRI images of the sagittal and coronal planes is superior to CT reformatted images.
3. Imaging sequences: T1- and T2-weighted spin echo pulse sequences are the most commonly used. However, each imaging center has its own parameters, which may include gradient echo pulse sequences. Do *not* use the terms "bone" or "soft tissue" windows in the description of MRI images.

Clinical information. Although some authors do not include the clinical information within the radiology report, it has been proven that practitioners who can easily link clinical information with radiographical findings are significantly more accurate in their radiological diagnoses.[27,30,42] Providing a brief summary of the relevant features in the history, physical examination, and laboratory analysis may help the clinician focus more attention on certain areas of the radiograph (while still considering others) or interpret the radiological signs more precisely.[46]

----

*Optional considerations.

The following information should be included in the radiological report after *Heading*[31]:

1. Location, duration, onset, and type of symptoms
2. History of traumatic injury and exact dates received
3. Positive orthopedic or neurological tests
4. Abnormal laboratory studies
5. Any other abnormal physical examination findings that may be related to the area imaged

SKELETAL RADIOLOGY REPORTS

Findings. *Findings* is the body of the report and contains the relevant abnormal (and occasionally normal) radiographical signs. It is written in narrative form using professional terminology, complete sentences, and proper grammar. This is the portion of the report in which the clinician should describe abnormalities, not state diagnoses.[42,46] However, occasional exceptions to this rule exist, especially in cases involving fractures and dislocations. A tumor or other destructive lesion should be described in *Findings* and diagnosed under *Conclusions*. The erosions or osteophytes associated with an arthritic condition should be described in *Findings* and the specific diagnosis included in *Conclusions*. *Findings* is the most controversial section of the report in the literature. The choice of terminology has often been determined by personal preference,[27] with subjectivity being the order of the day. In the *Handbook of Radiologic Dictation,* it is recommended that this section of the report be kept short (but complete) and simple with minimal use of pompous terms.[28]

It may be appropriate to occasionally comment on normal radiographical appearances if some peculiarity of positioning or superimposition could lead to misinterpretation of the normal appearance as pathological. It is also important to indicate the level of certainty about the presence or absence of abnormal radiographical signs[42]; however, clinicians should not purposely and unnecessarily make noncommittal statements about the findings. If the findings are "equivocal," it should not be the result of insufficient knowledge or experience on the part of the interpreter.

Several authors recommend dividing *Findings* into paragraphs.[28,42,46] These paragraphs may reflect the organization of the various findings into related categories. One commonly used method of organizing reports for skeletal radiology is the ABC'S approach[42,46]:

A = Alignment
B = Bone
C = Cartilage
S = Soft Tissues

The ABC'S format is often taught to students as a search pattern approach for thoroughly evaluating a set of skeletal radiographs. Yochum and Rowe[46] recommend using a "step-by-step sequential evaluation" of the radiographs; the ABC'S approach is such a step-by-step format. However, recent research has revealed that the students who are most successful at radiological diagnosis do not follow a rigid search pattern exclusively but rather are flexible in their evaluation and look for related radiographical signs.[30] However, this does not mean that these students are performing an incomplete evaluation. They use the various aspects of the ABC'S but modify their search pattern to fit the specific clinical information and abnormal radiographical signs detected. Therefore although a rigid ABC'S format may at times be inadequate as a search pattern approach for evaluating the radiographs, it can work very well in most situations as a guide for actually writing an organized report.

Clinicians should feel free to be flexible regarding the order in which the various radiological findings are organized in the report.

It may be more appropriate to record the findings of a patient with a large abdominal aortic aneurysm who also has signs of diffuse idiopathic skeletal hyperostosis (DISH) in the order SBCA. This organizes the radiological findings by priority or severity. In addition, segregating the findings strictly into the ABC'S categories may be not only burdensome but also confusing. Arthritic conditions usually present with both cartilaginous and bony abnormalities at the very least. Organizing together the various findings that relate to a particular condition may make more sense than separating them. For example, consider the following two excerpts from reports on the same set of lumbopelvic radiographs:

Version 1. Erosions and sclerosis of both sacroiliac joints are noted with a marginal syndesmophyte at the adjacent left lateral body margins between L1-L2. Moderate narrowing of the L5-S1 disc space is present with an approximate 10% anterolisthesis of L5 and hypertrophy of the L5-S1 facet articulations.

Version 2. An approximate 10% anterolisthesis of L5 is noted. (Alignment)

There is hypertrophy of the L5-S1 facet articulations. (Bone)

Erosions and sclerosis of both sacroiliac joints are noted. Moderate narrowing of the L5-S1 disc space is present. (Cartilage)

There is a marginal syndesmophyte at the adjacent left lateral body margins between L1-L2. (Soft tissues)

Both versions are technically correct and acceptable. Version 2 will most likely be easier for a student beginning the process of radiological report writing to record. Its rote format can be followed, ensuring no important radiological signs are missed. However, advanced students and practicing clinicians should recognize that version 1 logically organizes the related abnormal findings together. It is also clear from the way in which the report is written that the practitioner is aware these findings are related, which shows that the practitioner is thinking like an expert diagnostician.[30] Paragraphs can still be used with version 1; the current example has them organized according to pathological processes rather than ABC'S.

For the sake of simplicity in this book the detailed description of the way various findings should be written into the body of the report will use the ABC'S approach. Modifications can be made at the clinician's discretion.

Alignment. Roentgenometric lines, angles, and various measurements should be included in the report when appropriate. Include a normal or an abnormal measurement if it helps substantiate or refute a clinical suspicion based on the history and examination.[13,31] As a general rule of thumb, also include a measurement if it falls significantly outside the accepted normal range. This section should include information such as alterations of spinal curves, listheses, apparent leg length discrepancies, joint misalignments due to arthritic conditions, and the alignment of fracture fragments.[42,46] Marked static vertebral malpositions may also be mentioned in this section. However, the recognition of these malpositions does not necessarily confirm a clinically significant finding.[46] They must be correlated to the patient's symptoms and other examination results.

It is critical to know that visual estimation of spinal curves should be avoided. Actual measurements help prevent this part of the report from being discredited at a later date. The interexaminer and intraexaminer reliability of chiropractors and students visually estimating cervical and lumbar lordosis has proven to be poor.[4,43] Furthermore, the validity (i.e., accuracy) of visually estimating these curves is equally inadequate.[4,43] Boxes 3-1 through 3-3 include guidelines for incorporating various spinal measurements into the radiological report.[13,31,46]

If no abnormalities are detected, a negative statement attesting to this fact should be included under the heading *Alignment* (e.g.,

---

BOX 3-1

Guidelines for Cervical Spine Roentgenometrics

Lordosis
- Assess patient positioning by evaluating Chamberlain's line. A horizontal Chamberlain's line indicates a neutral lateral position. Poor patient positioning gives false impressions of hyperlordosis or hypolordosis.
- Evaluate the architecture of the articular pillars on the lateral view. Hyperplasia causes a local loss of lordosis due to a structural alteration.[19,21]
- There are at least nine different roentgenometric methods of evaluating cervical lordosis. They do not all appear to have concurrent validity.[4,21]
- The angle of cervical lordosis is commonly measured using the atlas plane line and the inferior end plate of C7; normal is 35 degrees to 45 degrees.[46] This method seems to be overly influenced by the tilt of the atlas; the depth method is probably a better alternative.

Chamberlain's line
- Assess this line to evaluate patient positioning.

McGregor's line
- This is an important line to evaluate for basilar invagination/impression.
- Only mention results if they are positive.

Atlantodental interval
- Give particular attention to all patients with inflammatory arthropathy, who have suffered a traumatic injury, or who have Down syndrome.
- Normal <3 mm in adults and <5 mm in children.[46]

Sella turcica size
- Mention the size only if the sella turcica is enlarged (i.e., more than 12 × 16 mm).
- Enlargement may be associated with increased intracranial pressure.

George's line
- Evaluation is used to assess for the presence of anterolisthesis, retrolisthesis, or instability.

Posterior spinal (spinolaminar) line
- Evaluation is used to assess for anterolisthesis, retrolisthesis, or instability.

Prevertebral soft tissues
- Retropharyngeal <5 mm. Retrotracheal <20 mm.
- Tissues may become enlarged because of trauma, infection, or tumor.

Flexion/extension studies
- Template flexion/extension studies are used to assess for the following:
  Anterolisthesis/retrolisthesis >3 mm from flexion to extension
  Hypomobility/hypermobility
  Evidence of instability
  Aberrant motion at levels other than C0/C1

BOX 3-2
Guidelines for Thoracic Spine Roentgenometrics

Scoliosis evaluation
- Five components of each abnormal curvature must be mentioned:
  Configuration of curve (S or C)
  Direction of curve (right or left)
  Area of involvement (e.g., lumbar, thoracolumbar)
  Apex (apices)
  Cobb's or Risser Ferguson's angle if greater than 10 degrees.

Kyphosis evaluation
- The method of measurement is similar to Cobb's method for scoliosis evaluation.
- The superior end plate of T1 is usually difficult to see.
- The upper limit of normal is 56 degrees in women and 66 degrees in men.[46]

"Alignment of the visualized osseous structures is within normal limits.") Another way of saying the same thing is "There are no abnormalities in alignment detected." Including a negative statement about a particular component in the radiological report indicates that the clinician actually evaluated this aspect of the films.

Bone. Descriptions of any congenital or acquired osseous abnormalities are included under the heading *Bone* in the report. In general, no conclusions should be made in this section of the report. The exception to this rule occurs in the event of a patient with a fracture. It is much more clear to state that "There is an oblique fracture through the distal one third of the shaft of the left radius" than "There is an oblique lucent line that disrupts the cortices of the distal one third of the left radius."

Concise descriptions using appropriate radiological terminology are written to describe any abnormalities in the size, shape, density, or number of bones or cortical disruption or osseous destruction.[42,46] Advanced students and practitioners should report on more serious bone abnormalities first, before including less significant abnormalities.[13,31]

BOX 3-3
Guidelines for Lumbar Spine Roentgenometrics

Lordosis evaluation
- Several different roentgenographic methods using different anatomical landmarks have been used.[45]
- The full significance of hyperlordosis/hypolordosis has not been determined.
- A common procedure is to use the superior end plate of L1 and superior end plate of S1; average is 50 to 60 degrees. Because L1 is commonly wedge shaped, this is probably not appropriate. The inferior end plate of L1 may be preferred.[44]

Sacral base (Ferguson's) angle
- This is the most researched angle of the lumbopelvic region.
- The normal range is 27 to 56 degrees (standard deviation = 2). The mean is 41 degrees in the upright position.
- Persons with spondylolytic spondylolistheses have a statistically significantly higher sacral base angle.[32,37]
- Increased angles may be associated with increased compressive forces at the facets or transverse shearing forces at the disc.[46]
- Decreased angles may be associated with increased axial loading of the disc or increased axial shearing forces at the facets.

Lumbosacral disc angle
- The normal range is 10 to 20 degrees.
- Larger angles may be associated with facet syndrome.
- Smaller angles may be associated with acute disc injuries and transitional segments.

Gravitational line from L3
- The line normally intersects the anterior one third of the sacral base. It may also fall anterior to the sacral base a distance equal to one third of the sacral base sagittal diameter and still be normal.

- The posterior line may be associated with increased axial forces to the facet joints.
- The anterior line may be associated with increased transverse forces to the facet joints and anterior compressive forces to the disc.

Anterolisthesis
- Evaluate the extent of anterior slippage using either the Meyerding classification system or preferably the percentile measurement.
- State whether pars defects can be observed.

Retrolisthesis/lateral listhesis
- Evaluate the severity of slippage using percentile measurement.

Sagittal canal diameter
- A value of <15 mm may indicate spinal stenosis (according to Eisenstein's method).
- The measurement should be given serious consideration if associated findings such as hypertrophy of the facets or posterior vertebral body osteophytes are detected.

Flexion and extension studies
- Displacement of >3 mm from full flexion to full extension may indicate instability.
- Up to 5 mm translation may be normal at L3-L4 and L4-L5.[40]
- Up to 4 mm translation may be normal at L5-S1.[40]
- There is a large range of variation in normal.
- Greater than 25 to 26 degrees of angular motion at L5-S1 is abnormal.[40]
- If one motion segment translates significantly more than the adjacent segments, it is probably abnormal.

If no abnormalities are noted under the heading *Bone* in the report, a negative statement regarding this should be included to confirm that the practitioner thoroughly evaluated this area should any future medicolegal questions arise. Because the radiographs should confirm or rule out a clinical suspicion, negative statements can be targeted specifically to the clinical concerns. For example, the statement "No evidence of osseous destruction or focal sclerotic or lytic lesions are detected" could be included in the report for a patient being evaluated for possible metastatic bone disease. "No evidence of recent fracture or dislocation is evident" can be stated in the report on a patient with a history of recent trauma. A generic negative statement may read "There are no abnormalities visualized in the osseous structures."

Cartilage.   Articular cartilage is not normally visible on a radiograph. Instead the clinician evaluates the joint spaces. Abnormalities in joint space width, symmetry, subchondral bone, fusion, and joint congruity are described in this section.[42,46] It is important for the practitioner to evaluate the apophyseal, uncovertebral, costotransverse and costovertebral joints as well as the disc spaces on spinal radiographs.[46] It is too easy for the clinician to evaluate the obvious disc spaces while ignoring or missing significant abnormalities in the synovial spinal joints.

As previously stated for the other components of the radiological report, if all joint spaces visualized are normal, a statement to that effect needs to be included (e.g., "The visualized joint/disc spaces are within normal limits.")

Soft tissues.   *Soft Tissues* is a very important section in the skeletal radiological report because it is a commonly overlooked area by clinicians who are concerned primarily with skeletal structures.[46] Clinicians must be aware of this potentially dangerous omission and discipline themselves to always evaluate these structures. Success in correctly identifying abnormalities within the soft tissues depends on a thorough knowledge of structures expected to be seen in the region and their normal radiographical appearance. Organ enlargement or displacement, displacement of normal structures (e.g., the trachea), abnormal accumulations of gas, abnormal soft tissue calcifications, prevertebral or paraspinal soft tissue swelling, foreign bodies (including surgical clips and sutures), masses, and displacement or blurring of fat or fascial planes are the soft tissue abnormalities that should be described in this section. Diagnostic conclusions should not be included.

If no abnormalities are observed within the visualized soft tissues, a negative statement is included as proof that these structures were thoroughly evaluated. This negative statement can be targeted specifically to a clinical suspicion or can be generic. Examples could include "No abnormalities are detected within the visualized soft tissues," "The visualized soft tissues are within normal limits," or "The splenic shadow does not project below the twelfth rib with no displacement of the gastric air bubble. The remainder of the soft tissues are unremarkable."

Conclusions.   Although some authors recommend the use of the term *Impressions* for this section of the report, it has been strongly argued that the word is inappropriate in the radiological report because it ". . . suggests knowledge is vague, subjective, and unreliable."[27] The suggested words to use are *Conclusions, Diagnosis, Judgment, Interpretation,* or *Reading.*[27]

The section of the report called *Conclusions* is a point-by-point summation of *Findings* (and includes all of the ABC'S components). Complete sentences are not necessary in this section, and it is expected that diagnostic terminology will be used. This section is the appropriate portion of the report in which to *label* the condition or conditions (e.g., lytic metastatic disease, rheumatoid arthritis,

new compression fracture). The diagnoses should be listed in the order of severity, starting with the most serious condition. For example, "metastatic disease" would be listed before "osteoarthritis". If the entire radiographical series reveals no abnormalities, *Conclusions* may simply read "Radiographically negative (cervical, thoracic, lumbar, etc.) series."

Recommendations.   The section *Recommendations* is optional and should only be included if specific follow-up procedures are indicated.[42,46] Additional plain radiographs (i.e., "spot" or supplementary views), special imaging procedures, laboratory evaluations, and referrals to other health care providers are examples of appropriate recommendations. If recommendations are included, they must be very specific and appropriate for the conditions diagnosed or suspected from the original radiographs. It is not acceptable to simply state "Further laboratory tests are indicated" without explaining exactly which laboratory procedures are needed.

Recommendations regarding improvement of quality of the original radiographs can also be included in this section. Comments referring to improved patient positioning or altered technical factors for repeat radiographs can be mentioned.

Signature.   All reports must be signed by the author and include credentials. Box 3-4 summarizes the sections in the skeletal radiology report.

CHEST X-RAY REPORTS

Controversy exists within the medical profession regarding the quantity of detail desired in chest x-ray reports.[24] Due to the work load of medical radiologists, a common chest x-ray report simply

---

BOX 3-4
Template for Writing Skeletal Radiology Reports

Heading
Practitioner and clinic information
Patient information
X-ray details

Clinical information
Relevant history
Pertinent examination findings
Abnormal laboratory studies

Findings (body of report)
ABC'S format in appropriate order
Starts with most serious pathology first

Alignment	*or*	Bone	*or*	Soft tissues
Bone		Cartilage		Alignment
Cartilage		Alignment		Bone
Soft Tissues		Soft tissues		Cartilage

Conclusions
Diagnosis or differential diagnosis

Recommendations*
Follow-up plain radiographs
Special imaging procedures
Specific laboratory tests
Technical comments

Signature

*Optional.

states that the examination is normal (if that is true), with no other remarks. However, for patients with specific chest complaints, referring physicians are not satisfied with these one-line reports; they prefer detailed reports targeting the specific symptoms.[24] Unfortunately, physicians cannot agree on how much detail should be included or the format of the reports. For those in chiropractic practice, it is better to err on the side of caution and include comments on all aspects of the chest radiograph.

The ABC'S format is not applied to chest radiological reports in the same way that it is applied to skeletal reports. The purpose of taking chest radiographs is to evaluate the various soft tissue structures rather than the osseous components. Therefore much more detail regarding these soft tissues needs to be included in the body of the report. The *Heading* and *Clinical Information* for a chest x-ray report follow the same format as the one included previously for skeletal radiographs. Box 3-5 contains a suggested template for writing chest x-ray reports.

Findings. The body of the chest x-ray report can use the ABC'S format, but the section *Soft Tissues* is significantly expanded and usually starts the report. The soft tissues expected to be evaluated on these radiographs include the following:

- Heart and mediastinum
- Lung parenchyma
- Pleura and costophrenic angles
- Infradiaphragmatic soft tissues
- Soft tissues of the chest wall

Once comments have been included for each of the soft tissue areas, the skeletal structures should be examined. Because chest radiographs are primarily taken to assess the heart, mediastinum, lungs, and pleura, clinicians may forget to evaluate the osseous structures, missing significant abnormal pathological processes. Thus there is no substitute for a thorough search pattern. Being forced to write an x-ray report may help the clinician to thoroughly evaluate all aspects of each film.

If no abnormalities are detected in each of the components of the soft tissue analysis, negative statements attesting to these facts should be included within the body of the report. An example of a normal chest report follows:

> The PA projection demonstrates a full inspiration with no signs of pathology in the heart or mediastinum. The lung parenchyma are symmetrical in density with normal pulmonary markings and no masses evident. There is no pleural thickening and the costophrenic angles are sharp. No abnormalities are detected in the visualized infradiaphragmatic structures or soft tissues of the chest wall. The thoracic cage is symmetrical with no evidence of pathology in the ribs or other visualized osseous structures.

This example may seem rather lengthy for a normal chest radiological report. However, by using computer macros, the generation of such a report takes only a few seconds. In addition, the report indicates that the person evaluating the radiographs was thorough in assessing all aspects of the films.

PLAIN FILM ABDOMINAL RADIOLOGY REPORTS

The chiropractor should rarely be called on to write radiological reports on plain films of the abdomen. These radiographs should initially be taken in the recumbent position with technical factors chosen to enhance visualization of the abdominal soft tissues rather than the osseous structures. The plain abdominal radiograph is often used as a "scout" (preliminary search) film preceding various contrast studies. However, plain radiographs of the abdomen may be used alone to identify abnormalities in gas patterns, evaluation of

the size and location of certain organs, the presence or absence of foreign bodies, and the identification of abnormal calcifications.

While writing the radiological report for abdominal films, it is important to remember which anatomical structures can and cannot normally be visualized:

Normally seen	Not normally seen
Liver shadow	Pancreas
Spleen	Uterus
Kidneys	Prostate
Large bowel gas pattern	Small bowel gas (in ambulatory adult)
Gastric air pattern	Aorta (and other vessels)
Bladder (if full)	
Psoas muscle shadows	
Flank stripe (properitoneal fat stripe)	
Phleboliths (if present—age related)	
Calcified costal cartilages (if present—age related)	

The radiological report should reflect the purpose of the abdominal study that was performed. If a plain abdominal radiograph is taken because a patient has the signs and symptoms of a kidney stone, the first statement within the body of the report should reflect this concern and comment on the presence or absence of a calcific density in the region of the kidney or ureter. If the clinician

---

BOX 3-5
Template for Writing Chest Radiology Reports

Heading
Practitioner and clinic information
Patient information
X-ray details

Clinical information
Relevant history
Pertinent examination findings
Abnormal laboratory studies

Findings (body of report)
Emphasis on *soft tissues*
Starts with most serious pathology first
   Soft tissues
   Heart and mediastinum
   Lung parenchyma
   Pleura and costophrenic angles
   Soft tissues of chest wall
   Bone
   Cartilage
   *Alignment**

Conclusions
Diagnosis or differential diagnosis

Recommendations*
Follow-up plain radiographs
Special imaging procedures
Specific laboratory tests
Technical comments

Signature

*Optional.

palpates a pulsating abdominal mass, the radiological report must address this finding by noting whether a dilated, calcified abdominal aorta or iliac artery is present.

As in the chest radiological report, the ABC'S format does not strictly apply to abdominal reports. The section *Soft Tissues* is emphasized and expanded, including appropriate negative statements added for the various organs and anatomical structures normally visualized. Although this process may seem unusually lengthy and cumbersome, computer macros allow these reports to be completed in minimal time while enhancing thorough scrutiny of the radiographs and professional competence. Box 3-6 offers a template for the creation of plain film abdominal radiology reports. Although abdominal radiology reports emphasize the soft tissue component of the anatomy, it is imperative that the clinician evaluate the entire radiograph, including the osseous and cartilaginous structures. Alignment should also be considered, even though these radiographs are usually taken in the recumbent position.

REPORTS ON CT OR MRI OF THE SPINE

No consensus exists about the proper length or content of special imaging reports. As mentioned previously, general practice chiropractors should not be expected to report on special imaging procedures. However, they frequently must interpret a radiologist's report and explain abnormalities seen on special imaging procedures to the patient.

Both CT and MRI reports on the spine should contain information regarding the presence or absence of disc herniation. If a herniation is detected, the exact location, size, and type of herniation should be mentioned using standard, universally accepted terminology. Displacement or obliteration of the spinal cord, thecal sac, or nerve roots must also be stated. If no encroachment onto these structures is visible, this information should be included. Stenosis of the central spinal canal, lateral recess, or intervertebral foramina should be mentioned, as well as an identification of the anatomical structures responsible for the stenosis and the severity of the stenosis.

Reports for both CT and MRI scans should address the clinical concern (as should all other radiology reports). If a tumor or infectious disease is suspected because of the history or examination findings, the special imaging procedure should confirm or rule out the clinical suspicion, with appropriate statements appearing in the body of the report.

Abnormalities of signal intensity, their specific anatomical location and imaging sequence, and the significance of these alterations must also be mentioned in MRI reports. For example, decreased signal intensity of intervertebral discs is seen with dehydration of the disc associated with degenerative disc disease. This same finding is not seen on CT scans.

Summary

The quality and thoroughness of the radiological report is a reflection of the professionalism and competence of the clinician. As an important component of the medicolegal record, information contained in these reports is vital to the current and ongoing care of the patient, facilitates interprofessional and intraprofessional communication, and may help protect the patient and clinician in litigious circumstances. Each report should be tailored to the individual patient and clinical suspicions. However, because of the development of computer macros, individualized reports are no longer extraordinarily time-consuming tasks.

Sample Radiology Reports

The following case studies provide examples of radiographic, CT, and MRI written reports.

BOX 3-6

Template for Writing Plain Film Abdominal Radiology Reports

Heading
Practitioner and clinic information
Patient information
X-ray details

Clinical information
Relevant history
Pertinent examination findings
Abnormal laboratory studies

Findings (body of report)
Focus on *soft tissues* component
Start with most serious abnormality first
  Soft tissues
  • Abnormal size, location, or orientation of the following:
  Liver
  Spleen
  Kidneys
  Gastric air bubble
  Large bowel gas pattern
  Bladder
  • Blurring of the following:
  Flank stripe
  Psoas shadows
  • Abnormal calcific densities
  • Foreign bodies
  • Abnormal accumulation of gas
    Bone
    Cartilage
    *Alignment**

Conclusions
  • Diagnosis or differential diagnosis

Recommendations*
  • Follow-up plain radiographs
  • Special imaging procedures
  • Specific laboratory tests
  • Technical comments

Signature

*Optional.

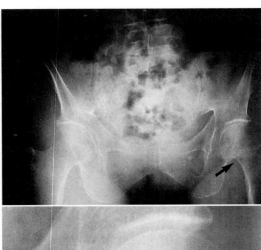

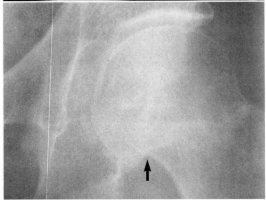

FIG. 3-2   Recent impaction fracture of the left femoral neck *(arrows)*.

CASE STUDY 1

Report date:	December 2, 1992
Clinician:	Dr. Marc Adams
Patient:	Mrs. I. Stepson
Age/sex:	61/F
X-ray number:	A4291
Imaging date:	12/02/97
Part:	Pelvis
Views:	Recumbent anteroposterior (AP)

CLINICAL INFORMATION

Fell two weeks ago and has had left hip pain since the fall. Was diagnosed with degenerative joint disease (DJD) by a general practitioner (GP) and an orthopedist. Has had no previous radiographs. Has been on corticosteroids for the past 2 years because of asthma.

FINDINGS

A sclerotic line is noted traversing the neck of the left femur with disruption of the cortex medially at the junction of the femoral head and neck (Fig. 3-2). The remainder of the cortices are intact. The bone density reveals a marked generalized osteopenia.

No abnormalities are detected in the hip joints, sacroiliac articulations, or symphysis pubis.

There is a slight right lateral listhesis of L3.

Several amorphous calcific densities are noted in the vicinity of the midsacrum (most likely superimposed over the sacrum). The remainder of the visualized soft tissues are unremarkable.

CONCLUSIONS

1. Recent impaction fracture of the left femoral neck.
2. Marked osteoporosis, most likely due to a combination of age, gender, and long-term use of corticosteroids.
3. Mild degenerative right lateral listhesis of L3.
4. Sclerotic densities in the region of the sacrum—most likely calcified lymph nodes from an old healed infectious process.

RECOMMENDATIONS

1. The patient should receive an immediate orthopedic referral for consideration of surgical pinning.
2. Long-term monitoring is needed to detect possible development of avascular necrosis of the femoral head.

Cynthia Peterson, RN, DC, DACBR, MMEd

CASE STUDY 2

Report date:	July 27, 1997
Clinician:	Dr. Denise Marcos Adams
Patient:	Mr. D. Smith
Age/sex:	62/M
X-ray number:	B9393
Imaging date:	7/26/97
Part:	Cervical spine
Views:	Upright AP and lateral

CLINICAL INFORMATION

Long history of progressive neck pain and stiffness.

FINDINGS

Thick, flowing hyperostosis is noted along the adjacent anterior body margins of C3-C7. Thin, nonmarginal syndesmophytes are visualized at the adjacent anterior body margins of C2-C3. There is a thick longitudinal osseous band extending from the posterior odontoid process to the posterior inferior body margin of C3 (Fig. 3-3), with apparent fusion to the posterior aspect of C3 and separation from the body of C2 and the dens. This osseous band occupies approximately 32% of the sagittal diameter of the spinal canal at the C3 level. Mild/moderate hypertrophy and sclerosis of the facet articulations is present bilaterally at the C3-C7 levels.

The visualized disc spaces are well preserved. The uncovertebral joints are difficult to evaluate because of underpenetration of the AP radiograph.

Calcific densities are present at the tips of the spinous processes of C6, C7, and T1.

No abnormalities of alignment are detected.

CONCLUSIONS

1. DISH with ossification of the posterior longitudinal ligament (OPLL). Significant encroachment into the spinal canal. Calcific densities at the tips of the spinous processes: common with DISH; represent calcification/ossification of the supraspinous ligament.
2. Mild/moderate facet arthrosis of C3-C7.

RECOMMENDATIONS

1. If any neurological deficits are detected, CT or MRI of the cervical spine is indicated to evaluate the severity of canal stenosis caused by the OPLL.
2. Test for the possibility of diabetes mellitus, which has been associated with DISH.

Cynthia Peterson, RN, DC, DACBR, MMEd

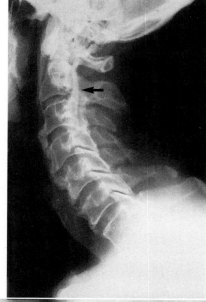

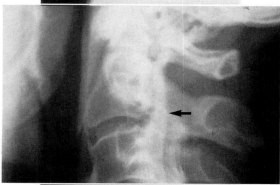

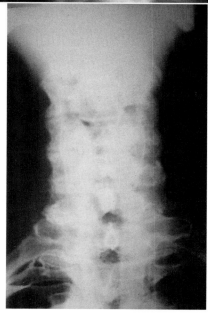

FIG. 3-3   DISH with ossification of the posterior longitudinal ligament *(arrows).*

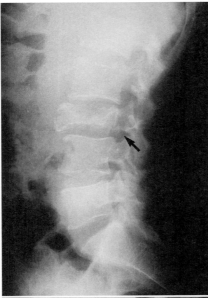
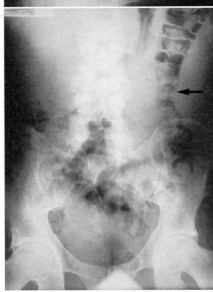

FIG. 3-4   Malignant pathological fracture of L3. Arrows point to the osseous fragment at the posterior inferior corner of L3 and the medial displacement of the colon.

CASE STUDY 3

Report date:	April 12, 1996
Clinician:	Dr. Prospero Antonuccio
Patient:	Mr. M. Melvin
Age/sex:	43/M
Imaging date:	4/12/96
X-ray number:	B8050
Part:	Lumbar spine
Views:	Recumbent AP and lateral

CLINICAL INFORMATION

8 months of increasing low back pain. "Electric" type of pain radiating into both posterior legs. Numbness in groin, testicles, and penis. Difficulty urinating. Atrophy of quadriceps, hamstrings, and calf muscles. Has been treated by a physical therapist with no improvement.

FINDINGS

There is lytic destruction of the vertebral body of L3 with pathological collapse and elongation (Fig. 3-4). A separate osseous fragment is noted at the posterior inferior body of L3. No other lytic lesions are detected.

Marked medial displacement of the descending colon is evident because of the presence of a large soft tissue mass within the lateral aspect of the left side of the abdomen. A marked quantity of gas and fecal material is noted within the large bowel. A small, round osseous dense region is present adjacent to the superolateral margin of the right acetabulum.

The visualized disc spaces, hips, and sacroiliac joints are within normal limits.

No significant abnormalities of alignment are noted.

CONCLUSIONS

1. Malignant tumor of L3 with abdominal mass, which may represent a primary abdominal malignancy with metastatic spread to L3. However, may also be lymphoma, considering the patient's age and the radiographical findings. Malignant destruction of L3 responsible for the patient's clinical presentation of cauda equina syndrome.
2. Os acetabulum right hip.

RECOMMENDATIONS

1. The patient should receive immediate referrals for an abdominal CT, a spinal MRI, and a biopsy.

Cynthia Peterson, RN, DC, DACBR, MMEd

CASE STUDY 4

Report date:	January 30, 1998
Clinician:	Dr. Doug Smith
Patient:	Mr. R. Hinley
Age/sex:	40/M
Imaging date:	1/12/98
Part:	Lumbar spine
Views:	Upright AP and lateral

CLINICAL INFORMATION

Long history of low back pain with recent severe, colicky left flank pain.

FINDINGS

There is a small, oval calcific density in the left upper quadrant, lateral to the L2 to L3 disc space (Fig. 3-5). This is also suggested on the lateral view superimposed over the L2 to L3 disc space. No other abnormalities are noted within the visualized soft tissues.

The lower two thirds of both sacroiliac joints are sclerotic with joint space narrowing and ill-defined subchondral bone. The remainder of the osseous and cartilaginous structures are within normal limits.

No significant abnormalities of alignment are detected.

CONCLUSIONS

1. Kidney stone on the left (nephrolithiasis).
2. Bilateral sacroiliitis. Differential diagnosis: includes ankylosing spondylitis, enteropathic spondylitis, Reiter's syndrome, and psoriatic arthritis. Clinical correlation indicated.

RECOMMENDATIONS

1. The patient should receive an immediate referral to a urologist for management of the kidney stone.
2. Spot angled lumbosacral radiograph should be obtained to better visualize the sacroiliac joints.
3. Erythrocyte sedimentation rate (ESR) and HLA-B27 lab tests may be useful.

Cynthia Peterson, RN, DC, DACBR, MMEd

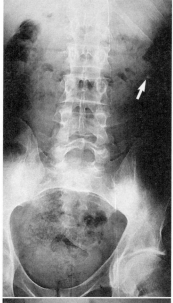
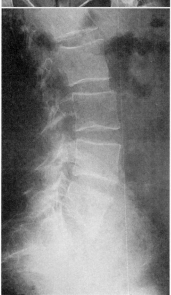

FIG. 3-5   Bilateral sacroiliitis with kidney calculus *(arrow).*

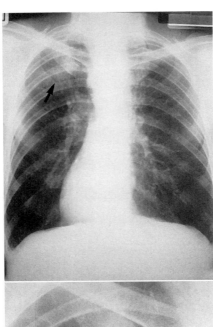

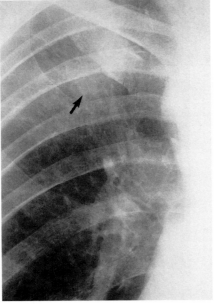

FIG. 3-6   Chronic obstructive airway disease with enlarged left hilus and mass in the left upper lung field *(arrow)*.

CASE STUDY 5

Report date:	March 10, 1998
Clinician:	Dr. Nancy Dafner
Patient:	Mr. Anthony Charminster
Age/sex:	62/M
Imaging date:	3/9/98
Part:	Chest
Views:	Upright PA

CLINICAL INFORMATION

Increasing dyspnea and long history of cigarette smoking.

FINDINGS

An ill-defined area of partial consolidation measuring approximately 2 cm × 3 cm barely appears in the left upper lung field between the posterior aspects of the fifth and sixth ribs, partially superimposed over the fifth rib (Fig. 3-6). The left hilar region appears enlarged.

The hemidiaphragms are low and flat bilaterally, at the level of the twelfth ribs. The lung fields appear hyperlucent.

The heart and mediastinal structures other than the left hilus appear to be within normal limits.

The costophrenic angles are sharp, and there is no pleural thickening.

No abnormalities are detected in the infradiaphragmatic or chest wall soft tissues.

The visualized osseous and articular structures are unremarkable. The thoracic cage is symmetrical.

CONCLUSIONS

1. Left upper lobe infiltrate combined with prominent left hilus: must be considered malignant until proven otherwise. Most likely diagnosis (because of patient's long smoking history): bronchogenic carcinoma with possible metastatic spread. Primary neoplasm: may be hilar with peripheral spread to the lung parenchyma or parenchymal infiltrate may represent primary lesion with spread to mediastinum.
2. Chronic obstructive pulmonary disease.

RECOMMENDATIONS

1. The patient should receive an immediate referral for CT of the chest, a cytology examination of sputum, a possible bronchoscopy, and a biopsy.

Cynthia Peterson, RN, DC, DACBR, MMEd

CASE STUDY 6

Report date:	April 9, 1997
Clinician:	Dr. Abraham Weir
Patient:	Mrs. J. Van der Veer
Age/sex:	44/F
Imaging date:	3/14/97
Part:	Lumbar spine
Procedure:	CT scan of L3-S1 intervertebral discs; angled gantry; soft tissue window only

CLINICAL INFORMATION

Signs and symptoms of right-sided radiculopathy into the lateral aspect of the foot.

FINDINGS

There is a very large right posterolateral disc protrusion at the L5-S1 level that is best seen on slices 16 and 17 (Fig. 3-7). This encroaches posteriorly on approximately 64% of the sagittal canal diameter with displacement of the thecal sac without visualization of the right S1 nerve root.

Accurate assessment of the lateral recesses and osseous structures cannot be achieved without the corresponding "bone" windows.

No other abnormalities are detected.

CONCLUSIONS

1. Large right posterolateral disc herniation L5-S1 affecting the right S1 nerve root and thecal sac, which correlates with the patient's clinical complaints.

Cynthia Peterson, RN, DC, DACBR, MMEd

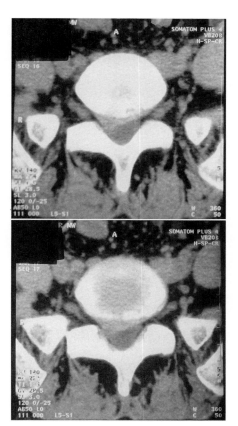

FIG. 3-7   Right posterolateral disc herniation at L5-S1.

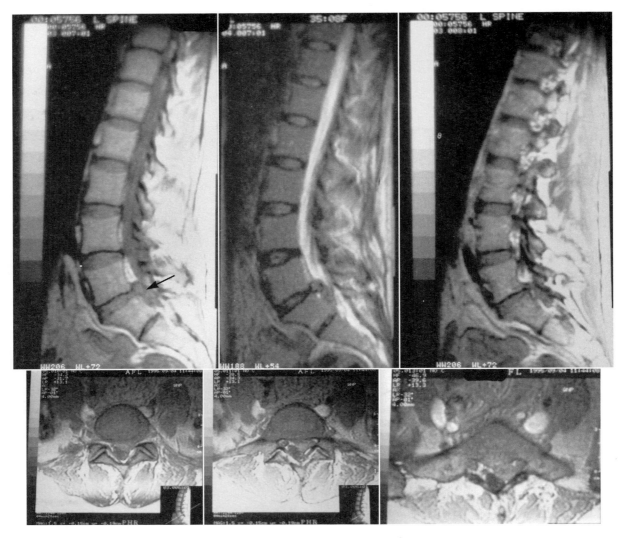

FIG. 3-8   Huge posterocentral disc herniation with sequestration *(arrow)*.

CASE STUDY 7

Report date: April 12, 1997
Clinician: Dr. Michelle Hansell
Patient: Miss J. Adams
Age/sex: 35/F
Imaging date: 4/9/97
Part: Lumbar spine
Procedure: T1- and T2-weighted sagittal scans. T1-weighted axial scans.

CLINICAL INFORMATION

Acute onset of severe low back and leg pain with neurological deficits after lifting heavy glider wing.

FINDINGS

A large left posterocentral intervertebral disc extrusion is noted at the L5-S1 level with inferior migration of the large discal fragment posterior to the body of S1 (Fig. 3-8). The discal fragment extends posteriorly approximately 75% of the sagittal canal diameter. Marked posterior and right displacement of the thecal sac is present at this level. The left S1 nerve root is still faintly visualized.

Slight decreased signal intensity of the L4-L5 and L5-S1 discs is noted.

S1 appears to be somewhat transitional, with a remnant S1-S2 disc.

No other abnormalities are detected.

CONCLUSIONS

1. Huge left posterocentral disc herniation with inferior migration of the sequestered fragment. Encroachment on approximately 75% of the sagittal canal diameter.
2. Decreased signal intensity at the L4-L5 and L5-S1 levels that is consistent with early degenerative disc disease.

RECOMMENDATIONS

1. Neurosurgical consultation should be strongly considered.

Cynthia Peterson, RN, DC, DACBR, MMEd

Roentgenometrics

Roentgenometrics play an important role in film interpretation by allowing quantification of observed structural and biomechanical alterations. Roentgenometrics should be used but not overemphasized in film interpretation. Many sources of error and anatomical variation exist, and results should be interpreted in light of all clinical data. The reliability, validity, and clinical usefulness of each measure should be considered. However, when carefully utilized, roentgenometrics provide a useful tool for image interpretation.

The measures listed in Tables 3-1 through 3-4* are stratified by anatomical location.

---

*References 1, 2, 6, 9, 12, 14, 17, 18, 20, 23, 25, 26, 32, 33, 35, 43, 46.

TABLE 3-1
Skull Measures

Description	Significance	
Basilar angle On the lateral skull or cervical projection, two lines are drawn. The first connects the frontal-nasal junction (nasion) to the center of the sella turcica. The second connects the anterior margin of the foramen magnum (basion) with the center of the sella turcica. The angle of intersection *(x°)* should not exceed 152 degrees, with a minimum value of 137 degrees.	Abnormally high angle measurements indicate an elevation of the skull base in relation to the anterior portion of the skull. This occurs with basilar invagination/impression secondary to congenital bone deformity or acquired bone softening disease (e.g., Paget's disease, fibrous dyplasia).	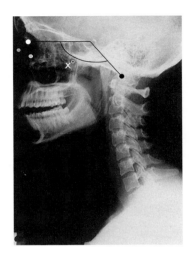
Chamberlain's line On the lateral skull or cervical projection a line is drawn from the posterior aspect of the hard palate to the posterior aspect of the foramen magnum (opisthion). The tip of the odontoid should not extend more than 7 mm above the line *(x).*	Elevation of the odontoid tip suggests basilar invagination/impression or upward deformity of the skull base. This may occur secondary to congenital or acquired bone softening disorders (e.g., Paget's disease, fibrous dysplasia).	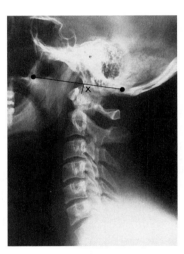
Digastric line On the frontal skull or cervical projection a line is drawn connecting the right and left digastric grooves (just medial to the mastoid processes). The tip of the odontoid should not project above this line.	Elevation of the odontoid tip suggests basilar impression or upward deformity of the skull base. This may occur secondary to congenital or acquired bone softening disorders (e.g., Paget's disease, fibrous dysplasia).	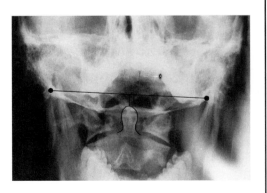

TABLE 3-1
Skull Measures—cont'd

Description	Significance
McGregor's line On the lateral skull or cervical projection a line is drawn from the posterior aspect of the hard palate to the inferior surface of the occiput. The tip of the odontoid should be below the line *(x)* and is always abnormal if it extends more than 8 mm above the line in men and 10 mm in women.	Elevation of the odontoid tip suggests basilar impression or upward deformity of the skull base. This may occur secondary to congenital or acquired bone softening disorders (e.g., Paget's disease, fibrous dysplasia). McGregor's method is considered the best method to assess for basilar impression.	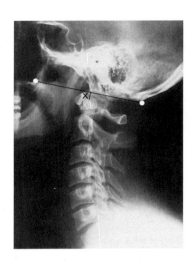
McRae's line On the lateral skull or cervical projection a line is drawn between the anterior (basion) and posterior (opisthion) margin of the foramen magnum. The posterior portion of the occiput should be below this line. In addition, a vertical line extended from the tip of the odontoid process should intersect in the anterior fourth of the foramen magnum line.	If the posterior occiput is convex upward or extends above the foramen magnum line, an upward deformity of the skull surrounding the foramen magnum is present. This occurs with basilar impression secondary to congenital or acquired bone softening disorders (e.g., Paget's disease, fibrous dysplasia). If the tip of the odontoid is found posterior to the anterior fourth of the foramen magnum line, fracture or dislocation is suspected.	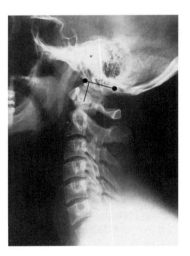
Occipitoatlantal alignment On the lateral skull or cervical projection, two lines are constructed: a foramen magnum line *(FML)* is drawn along the inferior margin of the occiput, and an atlas plane line *(APL)* is drawn through the center of the anterior tubercle and the narrowest portion of the posterior arch of atlas. The FML and APL should be parallel.	Divergence of the FML and APL anteriorly suggests anterior-superior malposition of the occiput. Divergence of the lines posteriorly suggests posterior-superior malposition of the occiput.	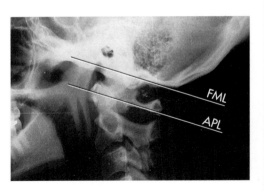

Continued

TABLE 3-1
Skull Measures—cont'd

Description	Significance
On the frontal open-mouth cervical projection, two lines are constructed: a transverse condylar line *(TCL)* is drawn connecting the grooves on the medial aspect of the mastoid processes bilaterally, and a transverse atlas line *(TAL)* is drawn connecting the lower junctions of the transverse processes and the lateral masses. The TCL and TAL should be parallel.	Divergence of the TCL and TAL to the right suggests right occiput laterality. Divergence of the TCL and TAL to the left suggests left occiput laterality. 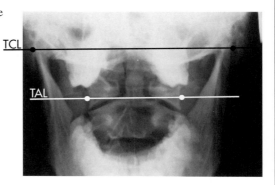
On the frontal open-mouth cervical projection, atlas rotational malposition is suggested by asymmetry in the width of the lateral masses. Occiput rotation is assumed to occur opposite atlas rotation.	The lateral mass with the wider measure is the side with anterior rotation of the atlas and posterior rotation of the occiput. Often the medial margin of the anteriorly rotated lateral mass appears more radiopaque.
Sella turcica size In the lateral skull projection (40 inches focal film distance [FFD]), the greatest horizontal dimension of the sella turcica should not exceed 16 mm, and the depth should not exceed 12 mm.	An enlarged sella turcica may represent a normal variant or suggest the presence of a space-occupying lesion or condition (e.g., pituitary tumor, carotid aneurysm, and empty sella syndrome). 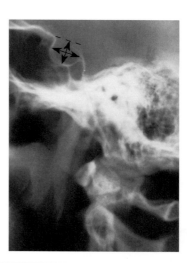

TABLE 3-2
Spine Measures

Description	Significance	

Atlantoaxial "overhang" sign

On the anteroposterior open-mouth projection the lateral margin of the lateral masses of atlas should not appear more lateral than the superior articular processes of the axis.

Lateral displacement suggests fracture (atlas or odontoid process) or dislocation. A mild degree of "overhanging" of the atlas may be a normal variant in children.

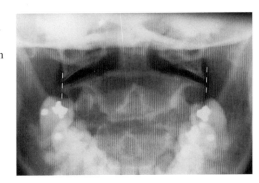

Atlantodental interval (ADI)

On the lateral cervical projection the distance *(x)* between the posterior surface of the anterior tubercle of atlas and the anterior surface of the odontoid process of axis should not exceed 3 mm in adults and 5 mm in children. The flexion lateral projection places the most stress on the atlantoaxial joint and would be most likely to reveal an abnormality. The ADI may appear V-shaped. In such cases the smallest portion of the joint space should be measured to limit false positives.

An enlarged atlantodental interval may result from congenital absence or weakness of the transverse atlantal ligament (e.g., Down syndrome, Morquio's syndrome, Larsen's syndrome), trauma, infection, or an inflammatory arthritide (e.g., rheumatoid arthritis, ankylosing spondylitis).

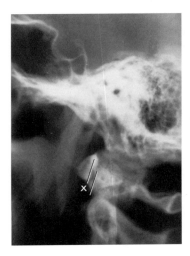

Atlas alignment

On the lateral cervical projection, two lines are constructed. An atlas plane line *(APL)* is drawn through the anterior tubercle and the narrowest portion of the posterior arch. Next an odontoid line *(OL)* is drawn to bisect the odontoid process. It is thought a line drawn perpendicular to the odontoid line (odontontoid perpendicular line *[OPL]*) should be parallel to the APL.

Anterior divergence of the lines suggests an anterior-superior malposition of the atlas in relation to the axis. Anterior convergence of the lines suggests an anterior-inferior malposition of the atlas.

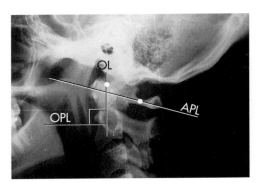

On the frontal open-mouth cervical projection, two line are constructed: a transverse atlas line *(TAL)* is drawn connecting the lower junction of the transverse processes and the lateral masses, and an axis plane line *(AxPL)* is drawn between the lamina-pedicle junctions bilaterally. The TAL and AxPL should be parallel.

Right atlas lateral malposition is suggested if the TAL and AxPL diverge to the right. Left atlas lateral malposition is suggested if the TAL and AxPL diverge to the left.

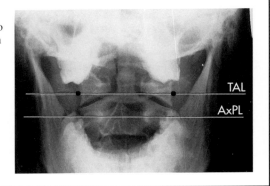

TABLE 3-2
Spine Measures—cont'd

Description	Significance

Atlas alignment—cont'd

On the frontal open-mouth cervical projection, atlas rotational malposition is suggested by asymmetry in the width of the lateral masses.

The lateral mass with the wider measure is the side with anterior rotation. Often the medial margin of the anteriorly rotated lateral mass appears more radiopaque.

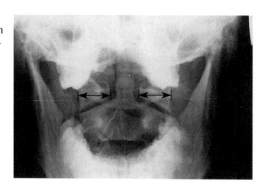

Cervical gravity line

In the lateral cervical projection, a vertical line drawn from the tip of the odontoid should intersect the seventh cervical vertebral body.

An anterior weight-bearing posture is noted if the line is found anterior to C7 (as shown in figure), and a posterior weightbearing posture is noted if the line is behind C7.

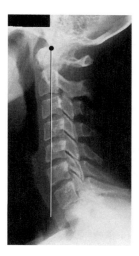

Cervical Jackson's stress lines

On the lateral cervical flexion and extension projections, lines are drawn along the posterior aspect of C2 and C7. The posterior body lines should intersect the C5-C6 intervertebral disc space on the flexion film and C4-C5 intervertebral disc space on the extension film.

The intersection of the lines is postulated to occur at the levels of greatest stress. Degeneration, muscle spasm, aberrant intersegmental mechanics, and other conditions may alter the levels of intersection.

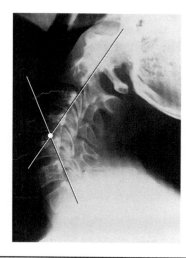
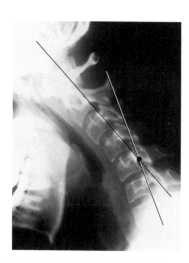

TABLE 3-2
Spine Measures—cont'd

Description	Significance

Cervical lordosis
Visual assessment
On the lateral cervical projection a subjective appraisal of the cervical curve is made. Well maintained anterior convexity is lordosis, exaggerated anterior convexity is hyperlordosis, slight anterior convexity hypolordosis, lack of curvature is alordosis, and posterior convexity is kyphosis.

Altered cervical lordosis may be caused by factors such as trauma, degeneration, muscle spasm, and aberrant intersegmental mechanics.

Depth method
On the lateral cervical projection a line is drawn from the tip of the odontoid process to the posterior surface of C7. A horizontal measure is taken from the vertical line to the posterior surface of the C4 body *(X)*. The average depth is 12 mm.

Negative values indicate kyphosis, and largest values indicate hyperlordosis. The depth method provides a more accurate assessment of cervical lordosis than the angle method. Lower measurements may result from factors such as trauma, degeneration, muscle spasm, and aberrant intersegmental mechanics.

Angle of curve
On the lateral cervical projection a line is drawn connecting the anterior and posterior tubercles of the atlas, and a second line is drawn along the inferior endplate of C7. Perpendicular lines are drawn from the atlas and C7 lines, and their angle of intersection is recorded as the cervical lordosis *(X°)*. The average value is 40 degrees, although a variety of average values has been reported in the literature.

Negative values indicate kyphosis, and large values indicate hyperlordosis. This method of measuring cervical lordosis is more common but less accurate than the depth method. Because the measurements depend only on C1 and C7, a kyphotic curve with compensatory extension of C1 will have the measurement of a lordotic curve. Reduced cervical curvature may be caused by factors such as trauma, degeneration, muscle spasm, and aberrant intersegmental mechanics.

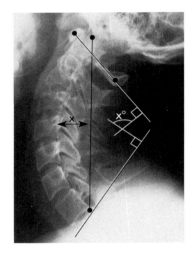

Cervical prevertebral soft tissues
On the lateral cervical projection the distance between the anterior aspect of C2 and the pharyngeal air shadow should not exceed 5 mm, and the distance between C6 and the tracheal air shadow should not exceed 20 mm.

Posttraumatic hematoma, tumor, abscess, or other space-occupying lesion of the prevertebral space may distend these measures beyond their normal values.

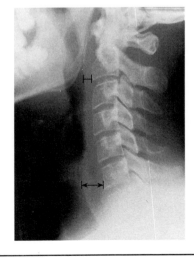

TABLE 3-2
Spine Measures—cont'd

Description	Significance
Cervical spinal canal On the lateral cervical projection the horizontal width of the spinal canal between the posterior surface of the vertebral body (or odontoid) and the spinolaminar line should be at least 16 mm at C1, 14 mm at C2, 13 mm at C3, and 12 mm at C4-C7. (These measurements are for adults.)	Sagittal canal widths less than these values indicate spinal canal stenosis. Spinal stenosis is more accurately assessed on the axial images provided by MRI or CT.	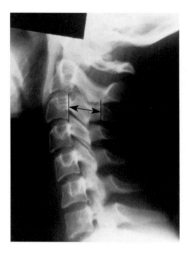
Cervical spinolaminar line On the lateral cervical projection a curvilinear line is drawn along the spinous process and lamina junctions. The curve should have a smooth contour without segmental disruption.	Disruption is caused by segmental anterolisthesis or retrolisthesis. Disruptions at multiple consecutive levels may be caused by normal flexion and extension patterns. Care should be taken not to interpret this as abnormal.	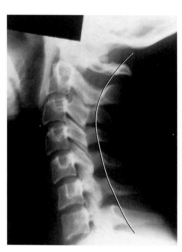
Cervical, thoracic, and lumbar endplate lines On the lateral cervical projection, lines are drawn along the inferior endplate of the C2-T1 vertebrae and extended posteriorly to the cervical spine. The cervical endplate lines should all intersect at a common point located posterior to the spine.	Lack of convergence suggests alterations in the normal lordotic cervical spine curve or intersegmental malpositions. Lines that cross closely to the spine suggest extension malposition of the superior segment. Lines that diverge sharply suggest flexion malposition of the superior segment.	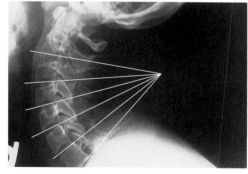

TABLE 3-2
Spine Measures—cont'd

Description	Significance	

Cervical, thoracic, and lumbar endplate lines—cont'd

On the frontal cervical, thoracic, and lumbar projections, lines are drawn to approximate the inferior vertebral endplates. The lines at adjacent levels should be parallel.

Divergence of the endplate lines drawn on the frontal projection suggests lateral flexion malposition opposite the side of divergence.

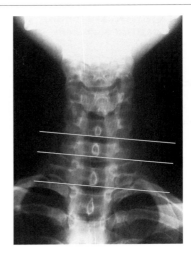

Cervical, thoracic, and lumbar vertebral rotation

Body width method

On the frontal cervical, thoracic, and lumbar projections, the distance from the lateral margins of the vertebral bodies to the origin of the spinous process (*a* and *b*) should be equal bilaterally.

If the distances from the base of the spinous process to the lateral margins of the vertebra are not equal, vertebral rotation is suggested, with spinous process deviation to the side of the smaller distance. A better analysis of vertebral rotation would probably incorporate the rotation of the vertebra above and below the segment in question. For instance, if a vertebra demonstrates 5 mm rotation to the right, and the segment below demonstrates 7 mm rotation to the right, the first segment demonstrates 2 mm of relative rotation to the left. Analysis of relative rotation attempts to limit spurious measurements of vertebral rotation caused by errors in patient positioning.

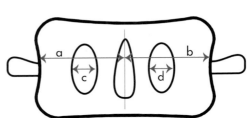

Pedicle method

On the frontal cervical, thoracic, and lumbar projections the appearance of the pedicle shadows may suggest vertebral rotation. It is expected the pedicle shadows demonstrate bilateral symmetry (*c* and *d*).

If the width of a pedicle shadow appears narrower than the contralateral pedicle shadow, it suggests (1) segmental rotation with the spinous process deviated to the side of the narrower pedicle shadow and (2) posterior vertebral body rotation to the side of the wider pedicle shadow.

Continued

TABLE 3-2
Spine Measures—cont'd

Description	Significance

Cervical, thoracic, and lumbar vertebral sagittal alignment

George's line

On the lateral cervical, thoracic, and lumbar projections, a curvilinear line is drawn along the posterior surfaces of the vertebral bodies. The curve should maintain a smooth contour throughout the spinal region without segmental disruption.

Disruption is caused by segmental anterolisthesis or retrolisthesis. Disruptions at multiple consecutive levels may be caused by normal flexion and extension patterns. Care should be taken not to interpret this as abnormal. However, the adjacent posterior body lines should not demonstrate more than 3 mm of net translation in a comparison of the flexion and extension radiographs.

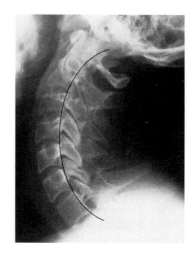

Barge's "e" space

On the lateral lumbar projection, lines are drawn along the superior and inferior vertebral endplates of each segment. Lines perpendicular to each endplate line are then drawn and extended across the intervertebral disc space. The distance between the perpendicular lines at the inferior endplate of each lumbar segment is measured as the "e" space. The space should not exceed 3 mm.

A larger Barge's "e" space suggests retrolisthesis of the segment above. Negative values indicate anterolisthesis. A more complete assessment would include the "e" space measurements at adjacent levels to determine relative retrolisthesis or anterolisthesis, thereby reducing spurious measurements that are caused by patient posture.

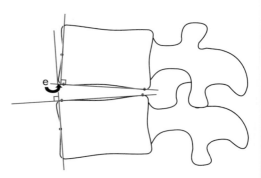

Visual method

Segmental retrolisthesis may be indicated by the presence of the following:

- Intervertebral disc degeneration (osteophytes, eburnation, reduced disc space, Schmorl's nodes, endplate irregularity)
- The lowest segment of a "stack" of three or more vertebrae that do not contribute to a sagittal curvature may be posterior
- The lowest involved segment of three or more consecutive segments that appear to be flexed or extended during neutral patient posture may be posterior
- Segmental rotation in a coronal plane that produces an hourglass appearance
- Narrowed sagittal diameter of the intervertebral foramen
- Visual disparity of segmental alignment when comparing the margins of adjacent vertebrae

Retrolisthesis of L5 is often seen as a normal variant, accompanying short pedicles.

TABLE 3-2
Spine Measures—cont'd

Description	Significance

Cervical toggle analysis

Atlas tilt

On the lateral cervical projection, three lines are constructed: an occipital condyle line *(OCL)* is drawn along the base of the occipital condyles, an atlas plane line *(APL)* is drawn through the center of the anterior tubercle and the narrowest portion of the posterior arch of the atlas, and a listing line *(LL)* is drawn parallel to the occipital condyle line and through the narrowest portion of the posterior arch of the atlas. The atlas plane line should be 4 degrees above the listing line.

If the APL is more than 4 degrees above the listing line, a superior malposition of the atlas is suspected; if the measure is less than 4 degrees, an inferior malposition of atlas is suspected. (NOTE: The malposition of the atlas is described with four letters. The first letter is always "A," the second indicates superior [S] or inferior [I] malposition, the third letter designates to right [R] or left [L] laterality, and the fourth letter designates whether the lateral malposition is anteriorly [A] or posteriorly [P] rotated.)

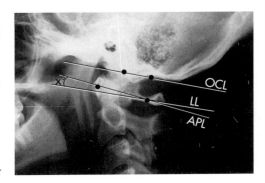

Atlas laterality

On a frontal cervical projection taken horizontal to the atlas (nasium projection), four lines are constructed: a horizontal ocular orbit line *(OOL)* is drawn through similar matched points of the orbits, a superior basic line *(SBL)* is drawn parallel to the OOL through the tip of the most superior occipital condyle, an inferior basic line *(IBL)* is drawn through the inferior tips of the lateral masses, and a vertical median line *(VML)* is drawn perpendicular to the OOL and through the center of the foramen magnum. The distances between the inferior lateral tip of each lateral mass and the VML should be equal.

The atlas is lateral toward the side of the greater measurement when the distances between the lateral inferior tip of each lateral mass and the VML are not equal. In addition, the SBL and IBL lines are thought to converge to the side of atlas laterality 70% of the time.

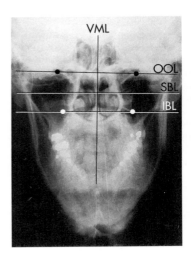

Atlas rotation

On a cervical film whose projection is directed vertical to the atlas (base posterior), two lines are constructed: a transverse atlas line *(TAL)* is drawn through the transverse foramen bilaterally, and a perpendicular skull line *(PSL)* is drawn through points representing the centers of the nasal septum and the basal process of the occiput. The angle of intersection of the two lines should be approximately 90 degrees.

The atlas is rotated posteriorly on the side of the larger angle created by the intersection of the PSL and TAL. In addition, 70% of the time the atlas is posteriorly rotated to the side of the diverging superior basic line (SBL) and inferior basic line (IBL) on the frontal open mouth projection.

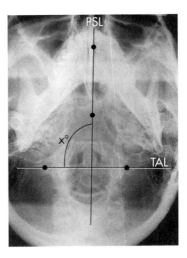

TABLE 3-2
Spine Measures—cont'd

Description	Significance

Axis malposition

On the frontal open-mouth projection, four lines are constructed: an ocular orbit line (OOL) is drawn through a set of similar points of the orbit (see Atlas Laterality), a superior basic line *(SBL)* is drawn bilaterally through the jugular processes, the inferior basic line *(IBL)* is drawn through the lateral inferior tip of both lateral masses, a vertical median line *(VML)* is drawn perpendicular to the OOL through the center of the foramen magnum. The VML should approximate the center of the odontoid process base.

If the VML does not bisect the odontoid, the axis is laterally malpositioned to the side opposite the VML. In addition, the center of the odontoid process base is compared with the center of the spinous process to assess for possible spinous deviation. The direction and magnitude of spinous process lateral malposition may be different from the lateral malposition of the axis body (i.e., the body of the axis may be exhibit right laterality with left spinous deviation).

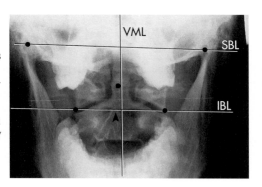

Cobb's method for scoliosis

On the frontal cervical, thoracic, or lumbar projection, lines are drawn along the superior endplate of the upper and inferior endplate of the lower vertebrae involved in the curvature. The end vertebrae chosen for measurement are the ones that tilt the most severely toward the scoliosis concavity. Perpendicular lines are constructed from the endplate lines, and the superior angle at their intersection is measured.

This is the preferred method of quantifying the degree of scoliosis.

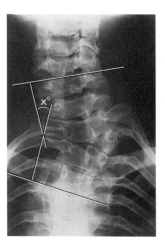

Coupled spinal motion sign

Spinal motion is not pure and occurs in directions other than the primary direction of movement. For example, on frontal cervical, thoracic, or lumbar lateral bending projections, the lateral tilting of each vertebra is accompanied by concurrent vertebral rotation. In the cervical and upper thoracic region the spinous processes rotate to the convexity of the curve. In the lumbar and lower thoracic region the spinous processes rotate to the concavity of the curve. The amount of coupled motion may be small and therefore radiographically imperceptible.

Alteration of the normal coupled motion occurs with aberrant intersegmental mechanics, muscle spasm, and vertebral fusion.

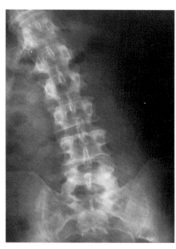

TABLE 3-2
Spine Measures—cont'd

Description	Significance

Interpedicular distance

On the frontal cervical, thoracic, or lumbar projections, the width *(x)* between opposing paired pedicles is typically 30 mm in the cervical spine, 20 mm in the thoracic spine, and 25 mm (L1-L3) to 30 mm (L4-L5) in the lumbar spine.

Narrowed interpedicular distance results from congenital maldevelopment (e.g., achondroplasia) and is an indicator of spinal stenosis. Enlargement of the interpedicular distance occurs secondary to expanding canal lesions (e.g., tumor).

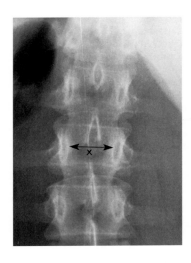

Thoracic cage dimension

On the lateral chest radiograph the distance *(x)* between the posterior surface of the sternum and the anterior margin of T8 should be at least 9 cm in females and 11 cm in males.

Narrowed anteroposterior dimension of the thoracic cage may result in cardiac compression.

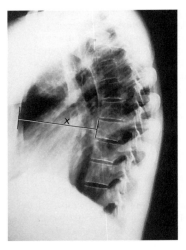

Thoracic spine kyphosis

On the lateral thoracic projection, lines are drawn along the superior endplate of T1 and the inferior endplate of T12. Vertical perpendicular lines are extended from these endplate lines, and the angle of intersection *(x°)* is measured, with values averaging near 30 degrees. The upper limit of normal is 56 degrees in women and 66 degrees in men.

Measures of thoracic kyphosis are largely age dependent. Younger patients demonstrate less kyphosis, and older individuals greater kyphosis.

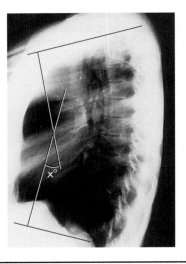

Continued

TABLE 3-2
Spine Measures—cont'd

Description	Significance

Lumbar intervertebral disc angles

On the lateral projection, lines are drawn along the superior and inferior vertebral endplates. The lines corresponding to each disc level intersect posterior to the lumbar spine. The disc angles *(x°)* increase with descending lumbar levels: L1—8 degrees, L2—10 degrees, L3—12 degrees, L4—14 degrees, L5—14 degrees.

Alterations of the lumbar disc angles occur with postural changes, aberrant intersegmental mechanics, muscular imbalances, and intervertebral disc pathology (e.g., herniations).

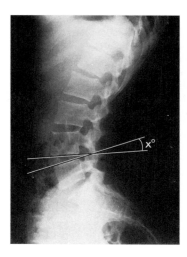

Lumbar intervertebral disc height
Visual assessment

On the lateral projection a subjective appraisal is made of the disc height compared with the adjacent levels and past experience.

Narrowing of the intervertebral disc space usually indicates degeneration. If narrowing occurs at the L5 level without concurrent findings of degeneration, underdevelopment is most probable. More aggressive pathology (e.g., infection) or surgery may narrow the disc space.

Ratio method

On the lateral projection the anterior *(a)* and posterior *(b)* heights of the intervertebral disc space are averaged and divided by the horizontal width *(c)* of the middle portion of the disc. Therefore the disc height is expressed as a ratio of the disc width and height, which offers a method to control for differing patient sizes. In the lumbar spine, normal disc ratios increase with descending lumbar levels: L1—0.17, L2—0.18, L3—0.20, L4—0.25, L5—0.28.

Narrowing of the intervertebral disc space usually indicates degeneration. If narrowing occurs at the L5 level without concurrent findings of degeneration, underdevelopment is most probable. More aggressive pathology (e.g., infection) or surgery may narrow the disc space.

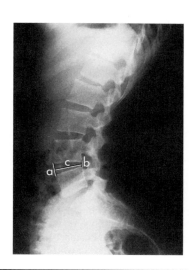

TABLE 3-2
Spine Measures—cont'd

Description	Significance	

Lumbar facet (Hadley's "S") curve

On the lateral or oblique lumbar projection, it should be possible to construct a smooth curve along the inferior margin of a transverse process that extends along the lateral margin of the inferior articular process, across the facet joint, and along the lateral margin of the superior articular process of the segment below.

Alterations in the smooth progression of the curve suggest facet arthrosis or malposition.

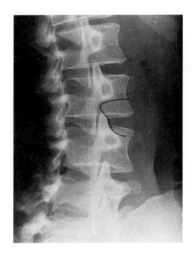

Lumbar gravity line

On the lateral lumbar projection a vertical line is drawn from the center of the L3 vertebral body inferiorly. Normally the vertical line will pass through the anterior third of the sacral base.

If the line falls more than 1-2 cm anterior to the sacrum, it suggests anterior weight-bearing with increased shear stress on the lower lumbar discs and facet joints (see figure). Posterior weight-bearing may lead to more weight distribution on the facet joints.

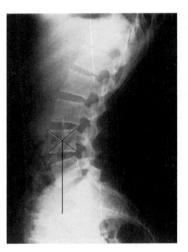

Continued

TABLE 3-2
Spine Measures—cont'd

Description	Significance	
Lumbar instability (Van Akkerveeken's) lines On the neutral or extension lateral lumbar projection, lines are drawn along the superior and inferior vertebral endplates adjacent to the same disc space. The distance between the posterior margin of each vertebra and the intersection of the two lines is measured (*a* and *b*). The presence of an abnormality is suggested if the measurements differ by more than 3 mm.	Ligamentous injury to the disc or other spinal ligaments may result in increased translation and abnormal measurements. The extension radiograph is more likely to demonstrate an abnormality.	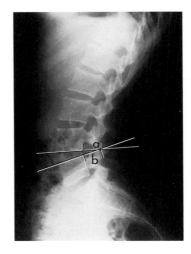
Lumbar spine lordosis On the lateral lumbar projection, lines are drawn along the superior endplate of L1 and the base of sacrum. Vertical perpendicular lines are drawn from the endplate and sacral lines, and the angle of intersection (*x*°) averages 50 to 60 degrees.	Wide variations in lordosis measurements have been noted. Alterations have been related to low back pain, disc herniations, altered posture, and other findings.	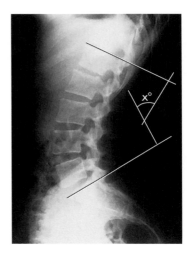
Lumbar spinal canal *Eisenstein's method* On the lateral lumbar projection a line is drawn connecting the tips of the superior and inferior articular processes of the same segment. The canal width (*x*) is expressed as the distance from the posterior body margin to the middle portion of the facet line. The canal dimension should not fall below 15 mm (although some use 14 mm or 12 mm as the cutoff).	Smaller measurements may indicate spinal stenosis. However, spinal stenosis is more accurately assessed on axial MRI and CT images, which provide additional information regarding canal shape.	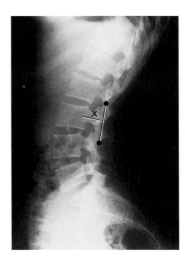

TABLE 3-2
Spine Measures—cont'd

Description	Significance

Ratio method

On the frontal lumbar projection the interpedicular distance is multiplied by sagittal width obtained using Eisenstein's method as described previously on the lateral lumbar projection. Next, on the frontal lumbar projection the coronal width of the vertebrae is multiplied by the sagittal width of the vertebrae obtained from the lateral lumbar projection. The product of the two canal measures is divided by the product of the two vertebral measures, expressing the canal size as a ratio of the vertebral body. In the lumbar spine, the canal ration should not fall below 1:3.

Smaller measurements may indicate spinal stenosis. However, spinal stenosis is much more accurately assessed on axial MRI and CT images, which provide additional information regarding canal shape.

Meyerding's grading for spondylolisthesis

On the lateral lumbar projection the sacral base is divided into four quadrants. A line drawn along the posterior surface of the L5 vertebra should not intersect the sacral base.

If spondylolisthesis is present, the posterior body line will intersect the sacral base. The sacral base quadrant that is intersected is used to qualify the amount of anterior displacement into Grades I-IV. (The figure shows a Grade I spondylolisthesis.) The method can be used at other spinal levels by dividing the segment below the spondylolisthesis into quadrants.

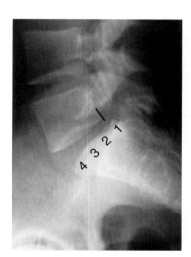

Risser-Ferguson method for scoliosis

On the frontal, cervical, thoracic, or lumbar projection, lines are drawn from the center of the upper vertebra to the center of the vertebra at the apex of the lateral curvature (apical vertebra) and from the center of the lower vertebra to the center of the apical vertebra. The inferior angle (x°) at the intersection of these lines is measured. The apical vertebra is the one that is the most laterally deviated. The end vertebrae are most severely tilted to the concavity of the curve.

This method is not used as often as Cobb's method to quantify scoliosis.

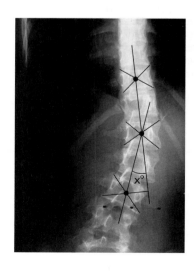

Continued

TABLE 3-2
Spine Measures—cont'd

Description	Significance

Sacral angle

Barge's angle (a)

On the lateral weight-bearing lumbar projection a line is drawn along the sacral base. The inferior angle of intersection between the sacral base line and a vertical line drawn parallel to the vertical edge of the film average 53 degrees, with a standard deviation of 4 degrees.

Smaller Barge's angles and larger Ferguson's angles are associated with increased compressive forces at the facets or transverse shearing forces at the disc. Larger Barge's angles and smaller Ferguson's angles are associated with increased axial loading of the disc of increased axial shearing forces at the facets.

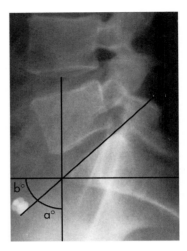

Ferguson's angle (b)

On the lateral lumbar projection a line is drawn along the sacral base. The inferior angle of intersection between the sacral base line and a horizontal line drawn parallel to the horizontal edge of the film average 41 degrees, with a standard deviation of 2 degrees and average values of between 27 and 56 degrees.

Ulmann's line

On the lateral lumbar projection a line is drawn along the sacral base. A second line is drawn perpendicular to the sacral base line just anterior to the sacrum. Normally the L5 vertebra is found posterior to the perpendicular line.

If the L5 vertebra crosses the perpendicular line, spondylolisthesis may be present. Ulmann's line is less sensitive to spondylolisthesis than George's posterior body line.

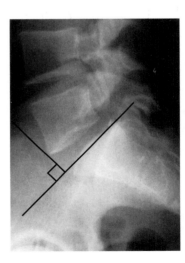

TABLE 3-3
Upper Extremity Measures

Description	Significance	
Shoulder		
Acromioclavicular joint space		
On the anteroposterior shoulder or acromioclavicular projection, the space *(x)* between the distal clavicle and proximal acromion process averages 3 mm.	An enlarged space suggests fracture, traumatic ligament tears, or bone resorption (e.g., due to hyperparathyroidism). A narrowed space is associated with degeneration.	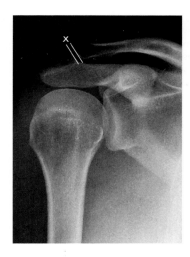
Acromiohumeral joint space		
On the anteroposterior shoulder projection, the distance *(x)* from the inferior surface of the acromion to the humeral head averages 10 mm.	A narrowed space is indicative of superior shoulder displacement, which is often secondary to shoulder impingement syndrome with rotator cuff tendonopathy. An enlarged space is associated with dislocation, joint effusion, and paralysis.	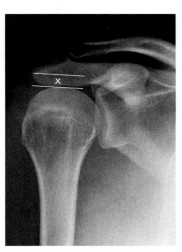
Glenohumeral joint space		
On the anteroposterior shoulder projection, the distance *(x)* from the glenoid to the humeral head averages 5 mm.	An enlarged glenohumeral space is suggestive of joint effusion, acromegaly, and posterior humeral dislocation. A narrowed space is often secondary to degeneration and rheumatoid arthritis.	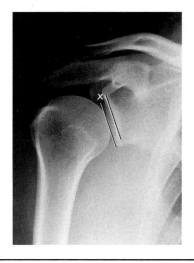

Continued

TABLE 3-3
Upper Extremity Measures—cont'd

Description	Significance	
Elbow		
Anterior humeral line		
On the lateral elbow projection a line drawn along the anterior surface of the humerus should intersect the middle third of the lateral condylar ossific center.	If the line passes anterior or posterior to the middle third of the lateral condyle, a fracture may be present.	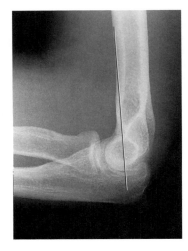
Radiocarpal line		
On the lateral elbow projection a line is drawn through the center of the radius to approximate its long axis. The line should pass through the elbow joint to intersect the center of the capitellum.	Assessment assists in determining the presence of fracture or dislocation.	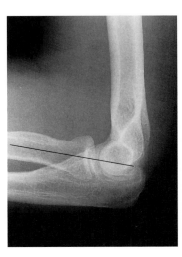
Hand		
Capitolunate sign		
On the lateral wrist projection, lines are drawn to approximate the long axes of the lunate and capitate. Their angle of intersection (x°) should be less than 20 degrees.	Carpal instability is suggested if the angle exceeds 20 degrees.	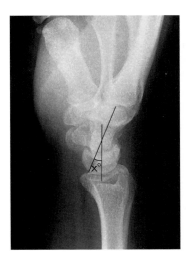

TABLE 3-3	
Upper Extremity Measures—cont'd	
Description	**Significance**

Hand—cont'd

Metacarpal sign

On the posteroanterior hand projection, an oblique line drawn along the distal articular surfaces of the fourth and fifth metacarpals should also intersect the distal articular surface of the third metacarpal.

If the oblique line intersects the third metacarpal at a more proximal point than the distal articular surface, the fourth metacarpal may be abnormally short. This finding is often seen in gonadal dysgenesis (Turner's syndrome) or metacarpal fracture.

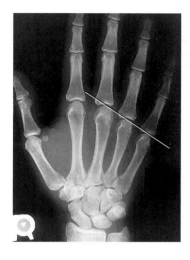

Radiolunate angle (lunate tilt)

On the lateral wrist projection, lines drawn to approximate the long axes of the radius and lunate should be parallel.

If the lunate is flexed more than 15 degrees, volar intercalated segment instability (VISI) is suggested. If the angle is greater than 10 degrees in extension, dorsal intercalated segment instability (DISI) is suggested. Occasionally VISI and usually DISI occur with scapholunate dissociation; VISI is also related to triquetrolunate dissociation.

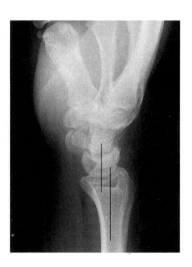

Radioulnar variance

On the anteroposterior wrist projection, the distal ulnar articular surface should align with the inner portion of the distal radial articular surface.

A short ulna (i.e., negative ulnar variance) is associated with avascular necrosis of the lunate (Kienböck's disease) and greater carpal stress distribution to the radius. A long ulna (i.e., positive ulnar variance) is associated with greater carpal stress distribution to the ulna. Differences of less than 5 mm are probably not significant.

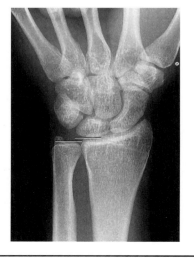

Continued

TABLE 3-3
Upper Extremity Measures—cont'd

Description	Significance
Hand—cont'd	
Scapholunate angle (scaphoid tilt)	
On the lateral wrist projection, lines are drawn to approximate the long axes of the scaphoid and lunate. Their angle of intersection *(x°)* averages 47 degrees with variance between 62 and 32 degrees.	If the angle is greater than 80 and the lunate is also extended (dorsiflexed), dorsal intercalated segmental instability (DISI) is suggested.

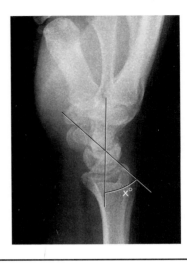

TABLE 3-4
Lower Extremity Measures

Description	Significance

Hip

Acetabular (Wiberg's) center-edge angle

On the anteroposterior pelvic or hip projection, a vertical line is drawn from the center of the femoral head superiorly through the acetabulum. A second line is drawn from the lateral aspect of the acetabulum to the center of the femoral head. The angle (x°) formed by the two lines is normally between 20 and 35 degrees.

The angle serves as a width measure of the amount of coverage the acetabular roof provides. A shallow angle (i.e., less than 20 degrees) may be caused by acetabular dyplasia and is associated with hip dislocation and hip degeneration.

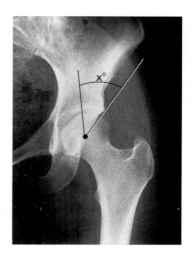

Acetabular index

On the anteroposterior pelvic projection, a horizontal line (a) is drawn through the right and left triradiate cartilage (Y-Y or Hilgenreiner's line). Another line is drawn along each of the acetabuli (b) to intersect the horizontal triradiate cartilage line. The angles of intersection (x°) should not exceed standards based on age: at birth—less than 36 degrees in females, less than 30 degrees in males; 6 months—less than 28 degrees in females, less than 25 degrees in males; 1 year—less than 25 degrees in females, 24 degrees in males; 7 years—less than 19 degrees in females, less than 18 degrees in males.

An enlarged angle is associated with acetabular dysplasia and possible lateral congenital dislocation of the hip. A shallow angle is seen in patients with Down syndrome.

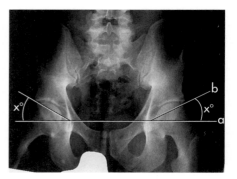

Acetabular protrusion (Kohler's) line

On the anteroposterior pelvic projection, a nearly vertical line is drawn from the outer border of the obturator foramen superiorly to the lateral cortical margin of the pelvic inlet. The floor of the acetabulum should not extend medially to this line.

If the floor of the acetabulum extends medially to Kohler's line, protrusio acetabuli is present. Protrusio acetabuli is secondary to rheumatoid or degenerative arthritis, Paget's disease, osteogenesis imperfecta, and idiopathic or other bone softening disorders.

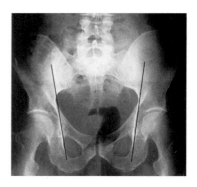

Continued

TABLE 3-4
Lower Extremity Measures—cont'd

Description	Significance	

Hip—cont'd
Femoral neck angle
On the anteroposterior pelvic or hip projection, a near vertical line is drawn approximating the femoral shaft *(a)*. A second line is drawn through the center of the femoral neck *(b)*. The angle of intersection *(x°)* is normally 124 degrees and should not be less 110 degrees or more than 130 degrees.

An angle of less than 110 degrees is termed *coxa vara*. A measure greater than 130 degrees is termed *coxa valga*.

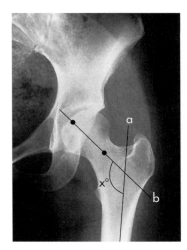

Hip joint space
On the anteroposterior pelvic or hip projection, the hip joint between the cortex of the femoral head and the acetabulum should not exceed 6 mm superiorly *(s)*, 7 mm axially *(a)*, or 13 mm medially *(m)*.

A wider hip joint distance is associated with hip joint effusion. The superior joint space is usually narrowed by degeneration. The axial space is more commonly affected by an inflammatory arthritide (e.g., rheumatoid arthritis). The medial joint space is narrowed by degeneration and an inflammatory arthritide.

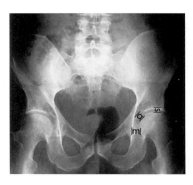

Iliofemoral line
On the anteroposterior pelvic or hip projection, it should be possible to draw a smooth curve along the outer surface of the lower ilium that extends inferiorly along the femoral neck. The line should be bilaterally symmetrical.

Disruption of the smooth line is associated with hip dislocation, femoral neck fracture, and slipped capital femoral epiphysis.

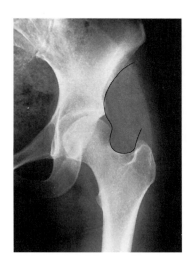

TABLE 3-4
Lower Extremity Measures—cont'd

Description	Significance	
Hip—cont'd		
Kline's (femoral epiphysis) line On the anteroposterior pelvic, antero-posterior hip, or frogleg hip projection, a line drawn along the outer border of the femoral neck should intersect the femoral capital epiphysis.	Slipped capital femoral epiphysis is suspected if the femoral capital epiphysis is found medial to the femoral neck line or if the line transects less of the epiphysis than is found on the contralateral side.	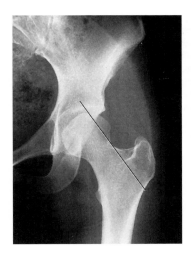
Shenton's hip line On the anteroposterior pelvic or hip projection, it should be possible to draw a smooth curve along the medial and superior surface of the obturator foramen to the medial aspect of the femoral neck.	Disruption of the smooth line is associated with hip dislocation, femoral neck fracture, and slipped capital femoral epiphysis.	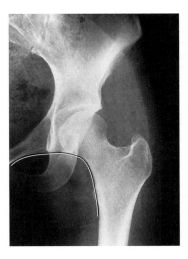
Skinner's (femoral angle) line On the anteroposterior pelvic or hip projection, a near vertical line is drawn approximating the femoral shaft. A second line is drawn perpendicular to the first line at the level of proximal tip of the greater trochanter. The fovea capitus should be found at the level of or above the perpendicular line.	If the fovea capitus is found below the perpendicular line, fracture or bone softening conditions causing coxa vara are suspected.	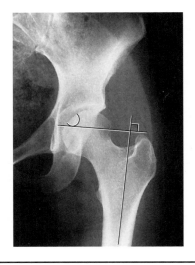

Continued

TABLE 3-4
Lower Extremity Measures—cont'd

Description	Significance	

Hip—cont'd

Teardrop distance

On the anteroposterior pelvic projection, the distance between the most medial portion of the femoral head and the most lateral portion of the teardrop at the inner acetabulum should not exceed 11 mm or differ from the contralateral side by more than 2 mm (which is Waldenstrom's sign).

A wider teardrop distance is associated with hip joint effusion.

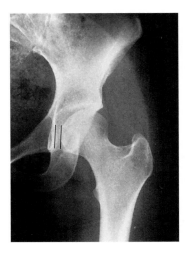

Pelvis

Iliac angle

On the anteroposterior pelvic projection, a horizontal line is drawn through the right and left triradiate cartilage. Two additional lines are drawn. One along the lateral margin of each ilium. The sum of the right and left angles (x°) of intersection (the iliac index) should not be less than 60 degrees in a newborn.

A sum (iliac index) of less than 60 degrees is indicative of Down syndrome. A sum of between 60 and 68 degrees is suggestive of Down syndrome.

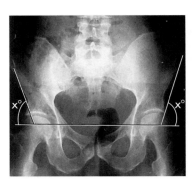

Pelvic misalignment

Innominate rotation. On the weight-bearing frontal pelvic projection, a femoral head line *(FHL)* is drawn along the superior margins of the femoral heads bilaterally. A perpendicular line from the FHL is constructed to intersect the second sacral tubercle and should pass through the center of the pubic symphysis when extended inferiorly.

If the perpendicular line intersects the pubic bone instead of the symphysis, the innominate is externally rotated on the side the line crosses through. The innominate on the opposite side is internally rotated. Rotation can be double-checked by measuring the width of the ilium *(a)* and the obturator foramen *(b)*. External rotation of the innominate, using the posterior superior iliac spine (PSIS) as a reference point, is accompanied by a narrower ilium width and a wider obturator foramen on the ipsilateral side. Internal rotation is associated with a wider ilium and narrower obturator width ipsilaterally.

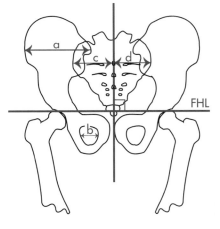

TABLE 3-4
Lower Extremity Measures—cont'd

Description	Significance

Pelvis—cont'd

Pelvic misalignment—cont'd

Innominate flexion-extension. On the weight-bearing frontal pelvic projection, the distance from the top of the iliac crest to the inferior margin of the ischial tuberosity should be bilaterally similar.

Sacrum rotation. On the weight-bearing frontal pelvic projection, the distances from the lateral margins of the sacrum to the second sacral tubercle (*c* and *d*) are measured parallel to the FHL and should be similar.

Leg length inequality. On the frontal weight-bearing pelvic projection, a line is drawn parallel to the lower margin of the film to the superior margin of the highest femoral head. The line should approximate both femoral heads if the legs are of equal length.

The vertical measurement of the innominate is larger on the flexed side (the posterior superior iliac spine [PSIS] has moved posterior and inferior) and smaller on the extended side (the PSIS has moved anterior and superior).

The sacrum is rotated posteriorly on the wider side and anteriorly on the narrower side.

If the line constructed parallel to the bottom of the film does not approximate the femoral heads bilaterally, the line is drawn to the higher femoral head, and the distance from the line to the lower femoral head estimates the measured leg length deficiency. The clinical interpretation of a measured deficiency is dependent on accompanying pelvic misalignment. It is believed that a flexed (PI) or externally rotated (EX) innominate will decrease the leg length discrepancy when the innominate misalignment is corrected on the ipsilateral side of the short leg. In other words, correction of flexed or externally rotated innominate raises the ipsilateral femoral head. Conversely, an extended (AS) or internally (IN) rotated innominate will increase the leg length discrepancy when corrected on the ipsilateral side of the short leg. The opposite will be noted if the short leg is on the contralateral side of the innominate misalignment. It has been estimated that the magnitude of leg length change is anticipated to be 40% of the measured misalignment of the innominate. Consideration of the pelvic misalignment will allow an estimation of the actual leg length deficiency.

Continued

TABLE 3-4
Lower Extremity Measures—cont'd

Description	Significance

Pelvis—cont'd
Presacral space
On the lateral sacral projection the space *(x)* between the anterior sacral cortex and the posterior margin of the rectal gas should not exceed 2 cm in the adult and 5 mm in children.

An enlarged presacral space is associated with expansile lesion of the sacrum, soft tissue masses associated with abnormality of the sacrum, sacral trauma, or abnormalities of the bowel.

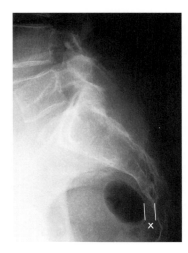

Symphysis pubis
On the anteroposterior pelvic projection the pubic symphysis *(x)* should not exceed 6 mm in females and 7 mm in males.

A widened space occurs with cleidocranial dysostosis, trauma, hyperparathyroidism, bladder exstrophy, and secondary to an inflammatory arthritide.

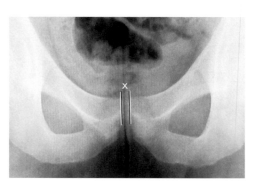

Knee
Lateral patellofemoral angle
On a tangential or Merchant's knee projection, a line is drawn along the femoral condyles. A second line is drawn along the lateral margin of the patella. The angle of intersection *(x°)* of these two lines usually opens laterally.

If the lines are parallel or their angle opens medially, recurrent patellar subluxation is likely.

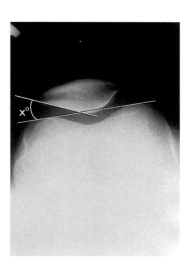

TABLE 3-4
Lower Extremity Measures—cont'd

Description	Significance	
Knee—cont'd		

Patellar displacement (Insall ratio)

On the lateral knee projection a ratio of the greatest height of the patella *(a)* to the distance from the inferior pole of the patella to the tibial tubercle *(b)* should be 1:1; a 20% variation is often seen.

A high patella (1:1.2, patella alta) may be the result of trauma or chondromalacia patella. A low patella (1:0.8, patella baja) is seen in patients with achondroplasia, polio, or juvenile rheumatoid arthritis.

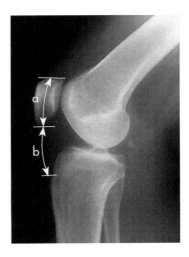

Patellar sulcus

On a tangential or Merchant's knee projection, a sulcus angle *(x°)* is formed by drawing a line from the highest portion of the medial femoral condyle to the lowest portion of the intercondylar notch; the line is also drawn for the lateral femoral condyle. The intersection of these lines forms the sulcus angle. The angle ranges from 126 to 150 degrees, with the average being 138 degrees.

Larger sulcus angles are associated with subluxation or dislocation of the patella.

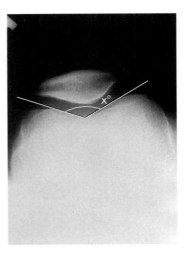

Foot
Boehler's angle

On the lateral foot or calcaneous projection, an angle *(x°)* formed along the superior margin of the calcaneous is normally between 30 and 35 degrees; a measurement of less than 28 degrees is abnormal.

The angle is decreased or increased by calcaneal dysplasia or fracture.

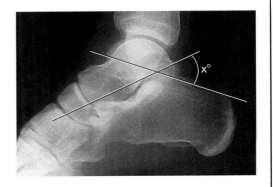

Continued

TABLE 3-4
Lower Extremity Measures—cont'd

Description	Significance

Knee—cont'd

First metatarsal angle

On the anteroposterior foot projection, lines drawn to approximate the long axes of the first metatarsal and proximal first phalanx should form an angle *(x°)* of less than 15 degrees.

An increased angle indicates a hallux valgus deformity.

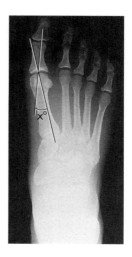

Heel pad measurement

On the non–weight-bearing lateral foot or calcaneous projection, the soft tissue of the heel inferior to the calcaneous should not exceed 23 mm in females and 25 mm in males.

Increased heel pad thickness is associated with acromegaly, obesity, and edema.

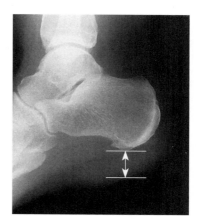

Meary's angle

On the lateral foot projection, lines drawn to approximate the longitudinal axis of the first metatarsal and talus should be parallel.

If the lines are not parallel and form an angle that is greater than 0 degrees, forefoot cavus deformity is indicated.

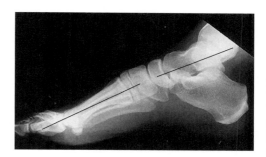

References

1. Armbruster JG et al: The adult hip: an anatomic study. I. The bony landmarks, *Radiology* 128(6):1, 1978.
2. Barge FH: *Chiropractic technique: tortipelvis, the slipped disc syndromes: its causes and correction,* ed 4, Davenport, Iowa, 1986, Bawden Bros.
3. Bauman RA: Reporting and communications, *Radiol Clin North Am* 34(3):597, 1996.
4. Beck C: *Accuracy and reliability of chiropractors and AECC students at visually estimating the cervical lordosis from radiographs,* student project, Bournemouth, England, 1997, Anglo-European College of Chiropractic.
5. Bluemke DA, Eng J: An automated radiology reporting system that uses hypercard, *AJR* 160:185, 1993.
6. Brant WE, Helms CA: *Fundamentals of diagnostic radiology,* Baltimore, 1994, Williams and Wilkins.
7. Christensen E et al: The effect of search time on perception, *Diag Radiol* 138:361, 1981.
8. Doubilet P, Herman P: Interpretation of radiographs: effect of clinical history, *Am J Roentgenol* 137:1055, 1981.
9. Eyring EJ, Bjornson DR, Peterson CA.: Early diagnostic and prognostic signs in Legg-Calve-Perthes disease, *AJR* 93:392, 1965.
10. Friedman C et al: A general natural-language text processor for clinical radiology, *JAM Med Inform Assoc* 1(2):161, 1994.
11. Friedman C, Cimino JJ, Johnson SB: A schema for representing medical language applied to clinical radiology, *J Am Med Inform Assoc* 1(3):233, 1994.
12. Hak DJ, Gautsch TL: A review of radiographic line and angles used in orthopedics, *Am J Orthoped* 24:590, 1995.
13. Harger BL, Taylor JAM, Peterson CK: *Radiology report writing guidelines,* Class notes, 1997, Western States Chiropractic College.
14. Hellems HK, Keats TE.: Measurement of the normal lumbosacral angle, *AJR* 113(4):642, 1971.
15. Hirtle RL: Chiropractic malpractice, *ACAJ Chiro* 24:35, 1987.
16. Holman BL et al: Medical impact of unedited preliminary radiology reports, *Radiology* 191:519, 1994.
17. Hubbard MJ: The measurement and progression of protrusio acetabuli, *AJR* 106(3):506, 1969.
18. Insall J, Salvati E.: Patella position in the normal knee joint, *Radiology* 101(1):101, 1971.
19. Isdahl M: *Inter- and intra-examiner reliability in determining hyperplasic articular pillars on lateral cervical radiographs,* chiropractic student project, Bournemouth, England, 1997, Anglo-European College of Chiropractic.
20. Keats TE: *Atlas of roentgenographic measurement,* ed 6, St Louis, 1990, Mosby.
21. Kirk R: *Effect of hyperplastic articular pillars on cervical lordosis,* chiropractic student project, Bournemouth, England, 1997, Anglo-European College of Chiropractic.
22. Mackintosh CE: Radiology: is reporting important? *Br J Hosp Med* 24:259, 1980.
23. Marchiori DM et al: A comparison of radiographic findings of degeneration to corresponding MRI signal intensities in the lumbar spine, *J Manipulative Physiol Ther* 17(4):238, 1994.
24. McLoughlin RF et al: Radiology reports: how much descriptive detail is enough? *AJR* 165:803, 1995.
25. Meyerding HW: Spondylolisthesis, *Surg Gynecol Obstet* 54:371, 1932.
26. Nelson SW: Some important diagnostic and technical fundamentals in the radiology of trauma with particular emphasis on skeletal trauma, *Radiol Clin North Am* 4(2):241, 1966.
27. Orrison WW et al: The language of certainty: proper terminology for the ending of the radiologic report, *AJR* 145:1093, 1985.
28. Paris A Jr: *Handbook of radiologic dictation,* Cincinnati, 1995, MRI-EFI Publications.
29. Peterson CK, Haas M, Harger BL: A radiographic study of sacral base, sacrovertebral and lumbosacral disc angles in persons with and without defects in the pars interarticularis, *J Manip Physiol Ther* 13(9):491, 1990.
30. Peterson CK: *Factors associated with success or failure in diagnostic radiology,* master's thesis, Scotland, 1996, University of Dundee Centre for Medical Education.
31. Peterson CK: *Outline for radiological report,* class notes, Bournemouth, England, 1997, Anglo-European College of Chiropractic.
32. Petersson CJ, Redlund-Johnell I: Joint space in normal glenohumeral radiographs, *Acta Orthop Scand* 54(2):274, 1983.
33. Plaugher GP: *Textbook of clinical chiropractic: a specific biomechanical approach,* Baltimore, 1993, Williams & Wilkins.
34. Rhea J, Potsaid M, Deluca S: Errors of interpretation as elicited by a quality audit of an emergency radiology facility, *Radiology* 132:277, 1979.
35. Rigler LG, O'Laughlin BJ, Tucker RC: Significance of unilateral enlargement of hilus shadow in early diagnosis of carcinoma of the lung with observations on method of mensuration, *Radiology* 59:683, 1952.
36. Rose JF, Gallivan S: Plain film reporting in the UK, *Clin Radiol* 44:192, 1991.
37. Rosok G, Peterson CK: Comparison of the sacral base angle in females with and without spondylolysis, *J Manip Physio Ther* 16(7):447, 1993.
38. Saxton HM: Should radiologists report on every film? *Clin Radiol* 45:1, 1992.
39. Swensson R, Hessel S, Herman R: Omissions in radiology: faulty search or stringent reporting criteria? *Radiology* 123:563, 1977.
40. Tallroth K, Alaranta H, Soukka A: Lumbar mobility in asymptomatic individuals, *J Spinal Disord* 5(4):481, 1992.
41. Taylor JAM et al: Interpretation of abnormal lumbosacral spine radiographs: a test comparing students, clinicians, radiology residents and radiologists in medicine and chiropractic, *Spine* 20(10):1147, 1995.
42. Taylor JAM: Writing radiology reports in chiropractic, *JCCA* 34(1):30, 1990.
43. Tuck AM, Peterson CK: Accuracy and reliability of chiropractors and AECC students at visually estimating the lumbar lordosis from radiographs, *J Chiro Tech,* 1997 (in press).
44. Vix VA, Ryu CY: The adult symphysis pubis: normal and abnormal, *AJR* 112(3):517, 1971.
45. Worrill NA, Peterson CK: Effect of anterior wedging of L1 on the measurement of lumbar lordosis: comparison of two roentgenological methods, *J Manip Physiol Ther* 20:459, 1997.
46. Yochum TR, Rowe LJ: *Essentials of skeletal radiology,* ed 2, 1996, Baltimore, Williams and Wilkins.

chapter 4

Radiographic Positioning

Radiographic Positioning
VINCENT DE BONO

Anatomy
DENNIS M MARCHIORI

Anatomical Variants
TIMOTHY J MICK

Radiographic Positioning

The first section of this chapter is a quick-reference guide to radiographic positioning and technique. Technical tips and supplemental views are provided to aid in obtaining optimal film quality using the most appropriate views. The basic study is highlighted in blue; this is the minimal study that must be performed to accomplish a complete evaluation of the area in question. For further information the reader is referred to a textbook dedicated to radiographic positioning. A list of suggested readings is included at the end of this chapter.

Radiographic Technique

The radiographic techniques listed in (Tables 4-1 through 4-27) were derived within the following parameters:
- 300/125 kVp Single-phase generator
- 400-Speed rare earth screens with matched film
- Extremity detail screens with matched films
- 10:1 Stationary grids
- Automatic processor

The suggested technique is within a fixed kilovoltage range per body part. In smaller patients the lower spectrum of the kilovoltage range is used; in larger patients the upper range of kilovoltage is used. In this system the milliampere-seconds setting is variable, and corrections in exposure factors require changing the amount of milliampere-seconds only. The exposure factors in a film that is underexposed can be corrected by raising the milliampere-seconds by at least 30% to have a detectable change or by 100% to have a significant change.

The reverse is true for films that are overexposed. The use of a fixed kilovoltage system requires that only one exposure factor, the milliampere-seconds, needs to be changed to correct for errors. The techniques contained in the following tables provide a starting point and should produce adequate exposures if used with any radiographic system similar to the one described above. Corrections for individual variations in machines are made by adjusting the milliampere-seconds setting only, because the table was formulated using the fixed kilovoltage technique.

The tables are also applicable to practitioners using high-frequency generators by applying the following correction factor to all the techniques:
- Lower kilovoltage range by 5
- Decrease the milliampere-seconds by 50%

Using this correction factor ensures that the tables will provide an accurate starting point in radiographic techniques and that corrections for individual variations among machines can be accomplished by adjusting the milliampere-seconds.

Patient Preparation

The patient should be informed of the study about to take place and what is to be expected during the examination. Patients should be properly gowned and all artifacts should be removed before the radiographic examination begins. Female patients of childbearing years should be assessed for possible pregnancy. If the patient may be pregnant, the exam should be delayed, if possible, until it can be determined the patient is not pregnant by either a negative human chorionic gonadotropin (HCG) test or the start of menses. If possible, all radiographic examinations of the lumbar lower abdomen and pelvis should be scheduled during the first 10 days following the onset of the patient's menstruation because the possibility of pregnancy is at its minimum during this time. Both male and female patients require appropriate gonadal shielding.

Using the Tables

The following 27 tables describe commonly performed radiographic projections sorted by body region (Tables 4-1 through 4-27). Entries of each table are categorized by anatomical region.

- The basic study is outlined in blue. This list contains the minimum series of views that must be accomplished to obtain a complete study of the area. Additional views are included in most sections and can be added to the basic study. These views are usually added to better demonstrate an area in question or to assess motion or stability.
- The view section of each table explains the position setup, central ray placement, tube angulation, optimal film size, and focal-film distance for each view.

- The position section of each table contains a picture demonstrating the position and central ray placement.
- The structure section lists the anatomy best illustrated by the view.
- The kilovoltage and milliampere-seconds section lists the type of film-screen combination used and whether the study is performed with the use of a grid or tabletop. If *grid* is listed, this suggests a fast-film screen combination such as rare earth. The word *detail* in this column suggests a slow speed-film screen combination, such as those found in extremity cassettes. A suggested kilovoltage and milliampere-seconds range is also provided for systems described in the previous section.
- The supplemental view section describes other views that may be done to better demonstrate the desired anatomy. Technical tips are also included to aid in obtaining optimal studies.

Text continued on p. 169.

TABLE 4-1
Skull

BASIC STUDY: PA Caldwell
AP Towne
Lateral skull

View	Position	Structures	kV range	mAs range	Supplemental studies and technical tips
PA Caldwell Patient facing film holder. Rest patient's nose and forehead against film holder so that orbitomeatal line is perpendicular to the film. Center the cassette to the nasion. Central ray is then centered to the cassette with a 15-degree caudal tilt. Optimal film size = 10 × 12 FFD = 40"	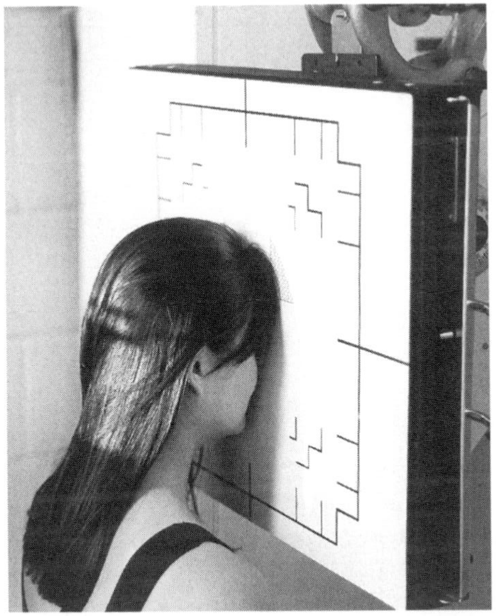	Frontal bone, frontal and ethmoid sinuses, greater and lesser wing of the sphenoid, superior orbital fissure, foramen rotundum, and orbital margins	Grid 70 to 80	20 to 40	Caudal tube angle may be increased to 30 degrees to better define the inferior orbital rim area. Petrous pyramids should be projected in the lower ⅓ of the orbit with 15-degree tilt. Petrous pyramids will be projected below the inferior orbital rim on the 30-degree tilt. Study may be done on table with patient prone. Shield gonads. Suspend respiration on exposure.
AP Towne Patient with back of head against film holder. Tuck the chin so that the orbitomeatal line is perpendicular to the film. Central ray enters the superciliary arch (2" above the glabella) with a 30-degree caudal tilt. Optimal film size = 10 × 12 FFD = 40"	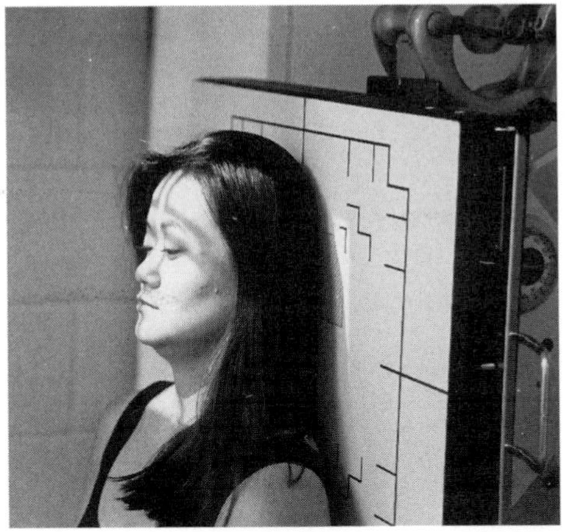	Occipital bone, petrous pyramids, foramen magnum with dorsum sellae and posterior clinoids projected through it	Grid 70 to 80	30 to 60	If patient is unable to tuck chin sufficiently, line up infraorbitomeatal line to film and increase caudal angle to 37 degrees. Procedure may be done on table with patient supine. Shield gonads. Suspend respiration on exposure.

Continued

PA, Posteroanterior; *AP*, anteroposterior; *kV*, kilovolt; *mAs*, milliampere-seconds; *FFD*, focal film distance.

TABLE 4-1
Skull—cont'd

BASIC STUDY: PA Caldwell
AP Towne
Lateral skull

View	Position	Structures	kV range	mAs range	Supplemental studies and technical tips
Lateral skull Place head in lateral position with side of interest closest to the film holder. Oblique the patient's body to obtain position comfortably. Central ray enters 1" superior and anterior to external auditory meatus (EAM). Optimal film size = 10 × 12 FFD = 40"	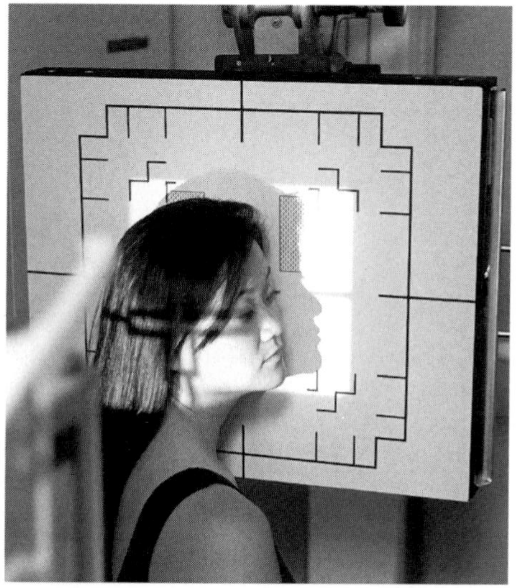	Lateral cranium closest to the film, sella turcica, anterior and posterior clinoids, ethmoid sinus	Grid 70 to 80	20 to 40	Making sure that the interpupillary line is perpendicular to the film can prevent head tilt. Palpating the external occipital protuberance and the nasion to make sure that the two points are equidistant from the film can prevent head rotation. Study may be done on table with patient in lateral recumbent position. Shield gonads. Suspend respiration on exposure.

TABLE 4-2
Facial Bones

BASIC STUDY: PA Waters
PA Caldwell
Lateral facial bones

View	Position	Structures	kV range	mAs range	Supplemental studies and technical tips
PA Waters	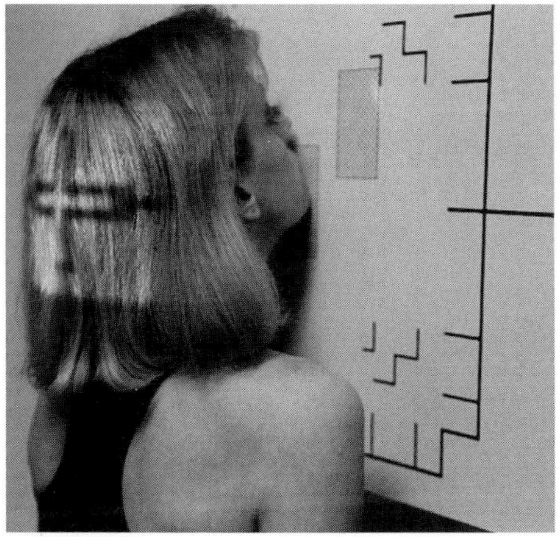	Floor of the orbits, maxillary sinuses	Grid 70 to 80	20 to 40	Projections are excellent for evaluation of possible "blow-out" orbit fractures. Should be done upright to evaluate air fluid level in maxillary sinuses. Petrous ridges should be projected in the lower half of the maxillary sinus below the inferior orbital rim. Shield gonads. Suspend respiration on exposure.
Patient facing film holder. Extend neck and rest patient's chin and nose against film holder so that orbitomeatal line forms a 55-degree angle to the film. Center the cassette to the acanthion. Central ray is then centered to the cassette. Optimal film size = 8 × 10 FFD = 40"					
PA Caldwell		Orbital rim, maxillae, nasal septum, and zygomatic bones	Grid 70 to 80	20 to 40	Caudal tube angle may be increased to 30 degrees to better define the inferior orbital rim area. Petrous pyramids should be projected in the lower $\frac{1}{3}$ of the orbit with 15-degree tilt. Petrous pyramids will be projected below the inferior orbital rim on the 30-degree tilt. Study may be done on table with patient prone. Shield gonads. Suspend respiration on exposure.
Patient facing film holder. Rest patient's nose and forehead against film holder so that orbitomeatal line is perpendicular to the film. Center the cassette to the nasion. Central ray is then centered to the cassette with a 15-degree caudal tilt. Optimal film size = 8 × 10 FFD = 40"	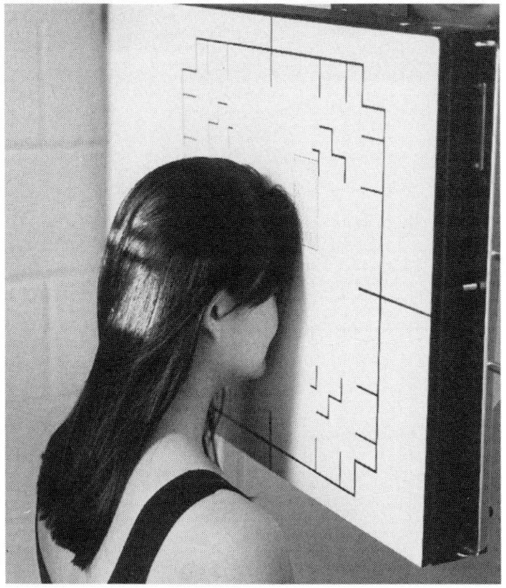				

Continued

PA, Posteroanterior; *kV,* kilovolt; *mAs,* milliampere-seconds; *FFD,* focal film distance.

TABLE 4-2   **BASIC STUDY: PA Waters**
Facial Bones—cont'd   **PA Caldwell**
                                                              Lateral facial bones

View	Position	Structures	kV range	mAs range	Supplemental studies and technical tips
Lateral facial bones Place patient's head in lateral position with side of interest closest to the film holder. Oblique the patient's body to obtain position comfortably. Central ray enters ½" posterior to the outer canthus. Optimal film size = 8 × 10 FFD = 40"	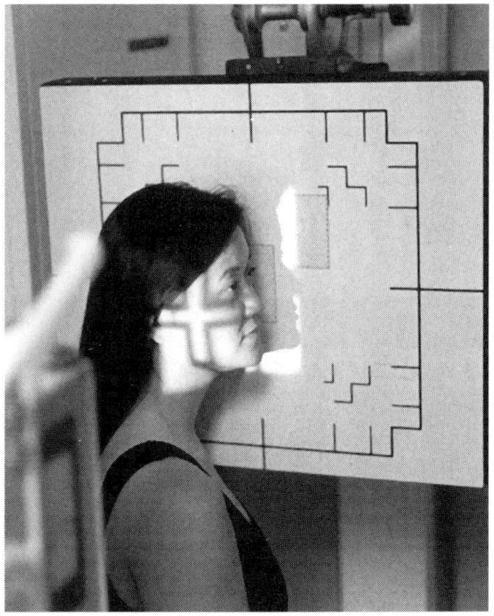	Ethmoid, frontal, sphenoid, and maxillary sinuses in the lateral projection	Grid 70 to 80	10 to 20	Study should be accomplished upright to evaluate for air fluid levels. Shield gonads. Suspend respiration on exposure.

TABLE 4-3 Cervical Spine		BASIC STUDY:	**AP open mouth** **AP lower cervical** **Lateral cervical**		
View	**Position**	**Structures**	**kV range**	**mAs range**	**Supplemental studies and technical tips**
AP open mouth Central ray to midpoint of open mouth, line up upper occlusal plate to occiput. Optimal film size = 8 × 10 FFD = 40″	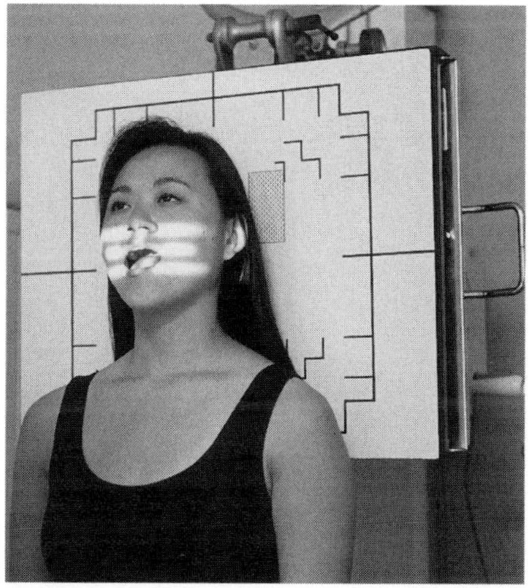	Lateral masses, anterior and posterior arches of C1, odontoid process, pedicles, lamina, and spinous process of C2	Grid 70 to 80	10 to 15	If odontoid is poorly visualized, oblique odontoid or Fuch's view may better demonstrate anatomy. Teeth obscure odontoid if head is not tilted back enough; occiput obscures odontoid if head is tilted back too much.
AP lower cervical Central ray to mid thyroid cartilage, 15-degree cephalic tilt, slightly elevate chin. Optimal film size = 8 × 10 FFD = 40″	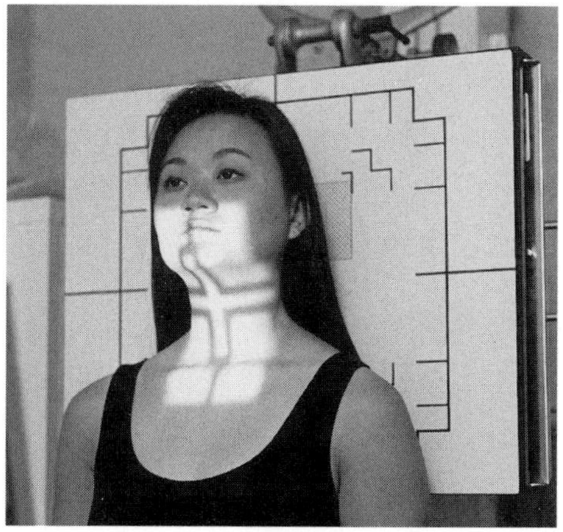	Pedicles, lamina, transverse processes, vertebral bodies, and uncinate processes of C3 to C7 Lung apices are also visualized	Grid 65 to 75	6 to 12	If mandible obscures C3 and C4, elevate chin more or increase cephalic angulation on tube. If a lesion is suspected in visualized lung apices, PA and lateral chest should be performed.

Continued

AP, Anteroposterior; *kV,* kilovolt; *mAs,* milliampere-seconds; *FFD,* focal film distance.

TABLE 4-3
Cervical Spine—cont'd

BASIC STUDY: AP open mouth
AP lower cervical
Lateral cervical

View	Position	Structures	kV range	mAs range	Supplemental studies and technical tips
Lateral cervical (neutral position) Central ray directed horizontally to C4-C5 disc level, relax and drop shoulders as much as possible. Optimal film size = 8 × 10 FFD = 72"	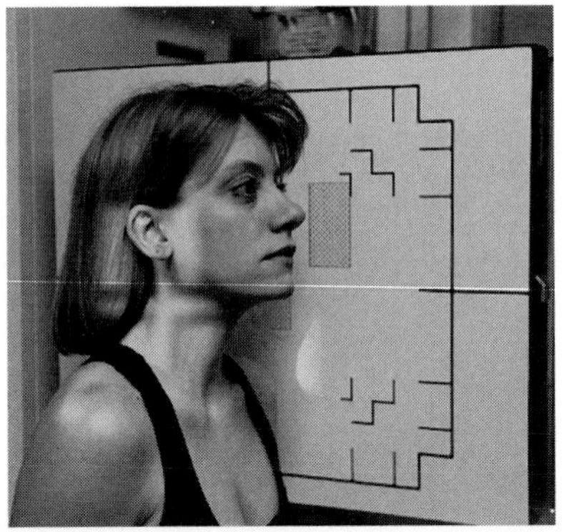	Vertebral bodies, intervertebral disc spaces, articular pillars, spinous processes, and anterior and posterior arch of atlas	Grid 70 to 80	15 to 30	This is the single most important view in evaluation of cervical spine trauma. Lateral film should be checked before continuing with the rest of the cervical series in trauma cases. If C7 is poorly visualized, swimmers' view may be utilized.

Continued

Flexion or extension views should not be accomplished until lateral cervical film is evaluated for a gross instability.

If patient is very flexible, 10 × 12 film may be turned sideways in flexion view.

15 to 30

Grid
70 to 80

Additional views used to evaluate excessive or diminished inter-segmental mobility of the cervical spine

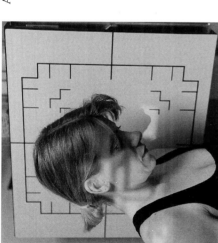

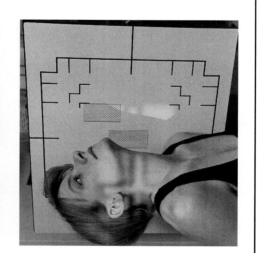

Lateral cervical (flexion and extension)
Same as neutral lateral but with neck in flexion or extension.
Optimal film size = 10 × 12
FFD = 72"

TABLE 4-3
Cervical Spine—cont'd

BASIC STUDY: AP open mouth
AP lower cervical
Lateral cervical

View	Position	Structures	kV range	mAs range	Supplemental studies and technical tips
Oblique cervical (posterior oblique) 15-degree cephalic tilt to the C4-C5 disc interspace. Anterior oblique 15-degree caudal tilt to C4-C5 disc interspace. Optimal film size = 8 × 10 FFD = 72″	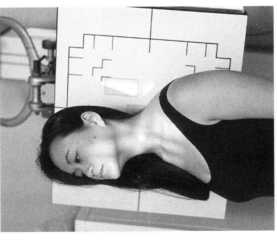 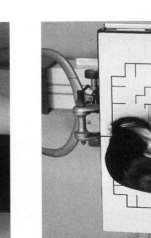	Additional views used to evaluate the borders of the intervertebral foramen—pedicles, facet joints, uncinates, and posterior vertebral bodies	Grid 70 to 80	15 to 30	This is the optimal view for evaluation of bony foraminal effacement resulting from cervical spine spondylosis. Also best plain film view for evaluation of pedicles for possible fracture and relationship of superior and inferior facet joints for possible dislocation in trauma cases. Suspend respiration during exposure.

Continued

**Oblique odontoid
(Kasabach method)**

Turn head 45 degrees to either side, direct central ray 15 degrees caudal to enter midway between the outer canthus and auditory meatus.
Optimal film size = 8 × 10
FFD = 40"

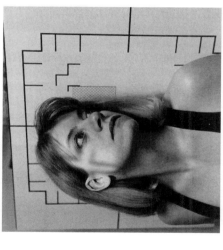

Supplemental view used to better evaluate the odontoid process. Demonstrates an oblique view of the odontoid process.

Grid
75 to 85

15 to 25

Study should be done when odontoid cannot be demonstrated after repeated attempts of AP open mouth view. In cases of trauma or in patients with decreased range of motion, the entire body may be turned 45 degrees.

Fuchs

Central ray to enter 1" below the chin with angulation of 0 to 15 degrees, depending upon ability to extend neck.
Optimal film size = 8 × 10
FFD = 40"

AP projection of the odontoid process lying within the shadow of the foramen magnum

Grid
70 to 80

10 to 15

This is a supplemental view used when the upper half of the dens is not visualized on the AP open mouth view.
Because of neck extension required for this view, it should not be attempted if fracture of upper cervical spine is suspected. Linear tomography may be used to better visualize odontoid in cases of suspected fracture.

TABLE 4-3
Cervical Spine—cont'd

BASIC STUDY: AP open mouth
AP lower cervical
Lateral cervical

View	Position	Structures	kV range	mAs range	Supplemental studies and technical tips
Pillar The AP view is positioned as you would an AP lower cervical except that there is a 25-degree caudal angulation on the tube. Central ray enters mid thyroid cartilage. For oblique views the head is rotated 45 degrees. Central ray enters about 3" below the EAM. Optimal film size = 8 × 10 FFD = 40"	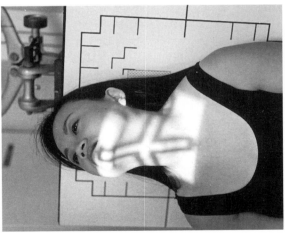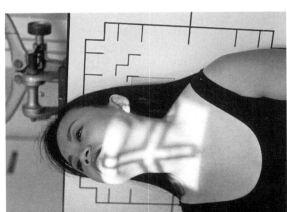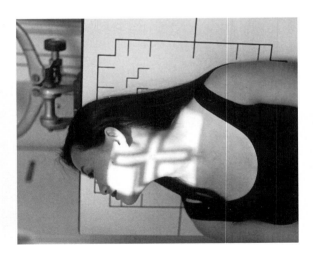	The shape and height of each pillar can be assessed. AP oblique views are taken. May be the only view in which articular pillar fractures are visualized	Grid 70 to 80	10 to 15	With the advent of computerized tomography (CT), this view is rarely performed. If a pillar fracture is suspected clinically, CT is the exam of choice to demonstrate these types of fracture. To better demonstrate lower facet joints (below C6) on oblique views, rotate the head 60 to 70 degrees. Suspend respiration during exposure.

Nasium*

Patient is seated AP with head in neutral position. Film holder is angled to touch back of head and shoulders. Central ray is angled caudally to enter glabella and exit base of occiput. Caudal angle is determined by measurement obtained from the lateral cervical film.

Optimal film size = 8 × 10
FFD = 40"

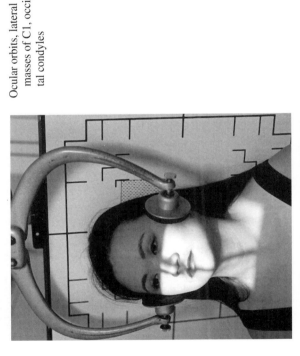

Ocular orbits, lateral masses of C1, occipital condyles

Grid
70 to 80

15 to 30

Filter is used over ocular orbits.
Suspend respiration during exposure. Head clamps may be used to hold head in neutral position.
Film is used in determining atlas laterality.

Base posterior*

Patient is seated AP with head in neutral position, vertex of skull is centered to film holder, which is angled 45 degrees. Central ray is tilted cephalically so that it enters 1" below chin and passes ½" anterior to the EAM.

Optimal film size = 8 × 10
FFD = 40"

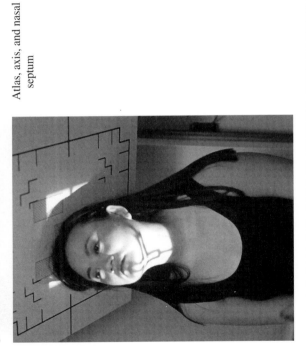

Atlas, axis, and nasal septum

Grid
75 to 85

20 to 30

Filter is used over ocular orbits.
Suspend respiration during exposure.
Film is used in determining atlas rotation.
Vertex may be used as an alternate view.

Continued

*Special view used for Palmer upper cervical technique analysis.

TABLE 4-3
Cervical Spine—cont'd

BASIC STUDY: AP open mouth
AP lower cervical
Lateral cervical

View	Position		Structures	kV range	mAs range	Supplemental studies and technical tips
Palmer open mouth* Patient is seated AP with head in neutral position; film holder is angled to touch back of head and shoulders. Central ray is angled to be even with upper occlusal plate and enters midpoint of open mouth. Optimal film size = 8 × 10 FFD = 40"	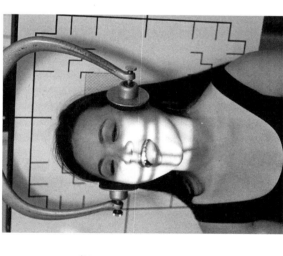		Lateral masses, anterior and posterior arches of C1, odontoid process, pedicles, lamina and spinous process of C2, ocular orbits	Grid 70 to 80	10 to 15	Collimation is to film size. Filter is used over ocular orbits. Suspend respiration during exposure. Film is used in determining axis listings.
Palmer lateral* Patient in true lateral position with head in neutral position. Central ray to enter C1 transverse process. Optimal film size = 10 × 12 FFD = 72"	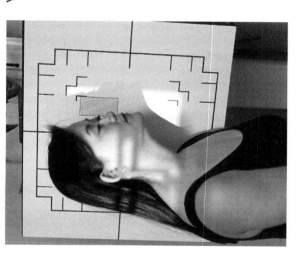		Vertebral bodies, intervertebral disc spaces, articular pillars, spinous processes, and anterior and posterior arch of atlas	Grid 70 to 80	15 to 30	Film in this series is used to evaluate atlas superiority or inferiority. Measurements are also taken off this film to determine caudal tube tilt on the nasium view.

Vertex*

Patient is seated PA with film holder tilted 45 degrees. Patient rests chin on film holder so that central ray exits 1" below chin. Central ray enters vertex of skull with a caudal tilt so that it passes ½" anterior to the EAM.

Optimal film size = 8 × 10

FFD = 40"

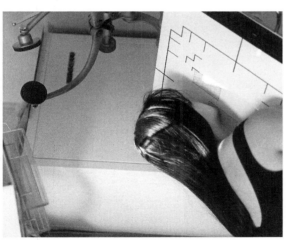

Atlas, axis, and nasal septum

Grid
75 to 85

20 to 30

Filter is used over ocular orbits.
Suspend respiration during exposure.
Film is used in determining atlas rotation.
This view is used as an alternate to the base posterior view.

*Special view used for Palmer upper cervical technique analysis.

TABLE 4-4
Thoracic Spine and Chest

BASIC STUDY: AP thoracic spine
Lateral thoracic spine
PA chest*

View	Position	Structures	kV range	mAs range	Supplemental studies and technical tips
AP thoracic spine Central ray to T6-T7 level; enters approximately 3″ to 4″ below sternal angle. Film should be 2″ above upper border of shoulders. Optimal film size = 7 × 17 FFD = 40″	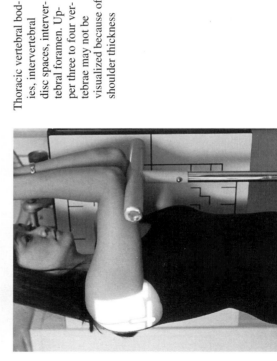	Thoracic vertebral bodies, intervertebral disc spaces, pedicles, spinous and transverse process, posterior ribs and costovertebral joints. Paraspinal lines (pleural interface) also seen	Grid 70 to 80	20 to 40	X-ray tube should be positioned so that anode is up (toward patient's head) and the cathode is down for more uniform density on the film by taking advantage of the "heel effect." Wedge filtration down to the mid sternum may also be used to achieve a more uniform density. Hold on full inspiration for exposure.
Lateral thoracic spine Central ray to T6-T7 level along midaxillary plane. Patient's arms elevated to right angles and supported. Optimal film size = 14 × 17 FFD = 40″		Thoracic vertebral bodies, intervertebral disc spaces, intervertebral foramen. Upper three to four vertebrae may not be visualized because of shoulder thickness	Grid 75 to 85	40 to 60	Filtration up to the inferior aspect of shoulder may be used for a more uniform density. Breathing technique (shallow, even breaths during exposure with an increase in exposure time) will obscure rib, allowing better visualization of thoracic spine.

Swimmer's

Central ray to T1-T2 level with patient along midaxillary plane. Patient's arm nearest to the film is elevated over the head. Arm and shoulder nearest x-ray tube is pressed downward, and shoulder is rolled posteriorly.
Optimal film size = 8 × 10
FFD = 40"

Grid 80 to 90

80 to 120

Lower cervical and upper thoracic vertebral bodies and intervertebral disc spaces projected between the shoulders

A caudal angulation of 5 degrees may help to separate the shoulders on this view. May be done as supplemental view to either a cervical spine series or thoracic spine series. In cases of trauma all seven cervical vertebrae must be visualized.
Suspend respiration during exposure.

PA chest

Central ray to enter approximately the T6-T7 level. Film should be 2" to 3" above patient's shoulder. Hands on hips and roll shoulders forward. Elevate patient's chin.
Optimal film size = 14 × 17
FFD = 72"

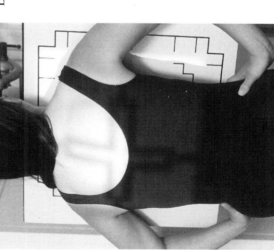

Grid 110 to 120

1 to 4

Lungs, including both apices, air-filled trachea, heart and great vessels, and diaphragm to include the costophrenic angles, bony thorax. The vertebral column behind the heart should be faintly visible

High kVp technique is used to lower contrast and increase scales of gray on the radiograph.
Study must be performed on full inspiration with 10 posterior ribs on the right visible. Poor inspiratory efforts will alter cardiothoracic ratio. In suspected apical lesions or right middle lobe infiltrates, lordotic view may be performed to better define these areas.
If pneumothorax is suspected, a film on full expiration may be done because this will accentuate the visceral-parietal pleural interspace.

Continued

PA, Posteroanterior; *AP,* anteroposterior; *kV,* kilovolt; *mAs,* milliampere-seconds; *FFD,* focal film distance.
*In patients over 50 years of age with thoracic complaints, a PA chest should be included in series.

PART ONE
Introduction to Imaging

TABLE 4-4
Thoracic Spine and Chest—cont'd

BASIC STUDY: AP thoracic spine
Lateral thoracic spine
PA chest*

View	Position	Structures	kV range	mAs range	Supplemental studies and technical tips
Lateral chest Central ray to enter approximately the T6-T7 level in the midsagittal plane. Film is 2″ above patient's shoulders. Optimal film size = 14 × 17 FFD = 72″	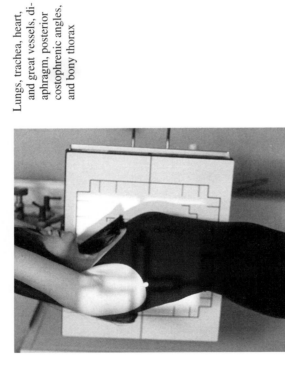	Lungs, trachea, heart, and great vessels, diaphragm, posterior costophrenic angles, and bony thorax	Grid 110 to 120	4 to 16	Left lateral is standard position to reduce magnification of the heart shadow. Arms are raised and crossed above head; chin is elevated. Study must be performed on full inspiration.
Apical lordotic Patient in AP position standing about 1 foot from film holder. Have patient lean back with shoulders against the film holder. Hand on patient's hips and roll shoulders forward. Central ray enters midsternum. Optimal film size = 14 × 17 FFD = 72″	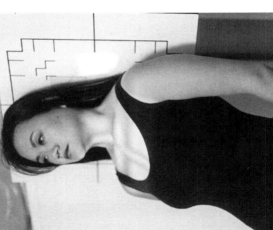	Demonstrates the apices of the lung free of superimposition of the clavicles. This view will also better demonstrate interlobar effusions if present	Grid 110 to 120	1 to 4	If apical lesion is suspected on PA radiograph, apical lordotic view may help to localize and better define the lesion, especially if the suspected lesion is posterior to the clavicle. View may also be useful in demonstrating infiltrates within the right middle lobe. Study is performed on full inspiration.

Lateral decubitus

Patient lying on affected side, right side down for right lateral decubitus, left side down for left lateral decubitus. Raise both arms above head. Patient is positioned on table or cart so that shoulders are 2″ to 3″ from top of film. Central ray is directed horizontally to the center of the film.

Optimal film size = 14 × 17

FFD = 72″

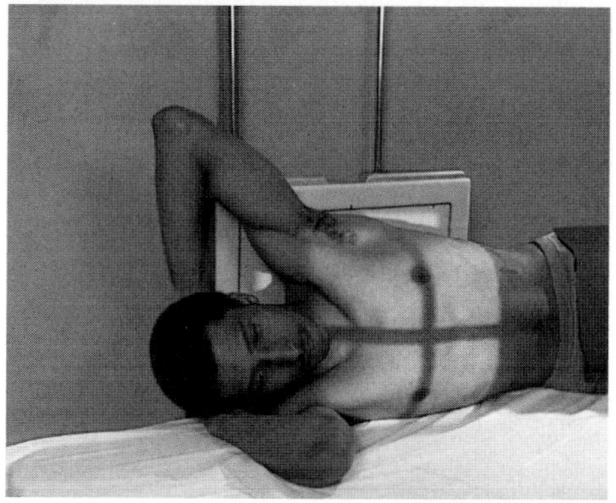

Grid
110 to 120

2 to 5

Supplemental view done when pleural effusion is suspected. Because the side down is now the dependent portion of the chest, small pleural effusions may be demonstrated. Will also be helpful in determining if apparent pleural effusion is truly an effusion or scar tissue formation

Exposure is taken on full inspiration. Flex knees slightly, and be sure that pelvis and shoulders are parallel to the film and that no body rotation is present.

Pleural effusions under 300 cc usually cannot be seen on PA chest radiographs. Pleural effusions as small as 50 cc can be seen on lateral decubitus films. In cases where pleural effusions are suspected, lateral decubitus should be included.

*In patients over 50 years with thoracic complaints, a PA chest should be included in series.

TABLE 4-5
Ribs and Bony Thorax

BASIC STUDY: AP of affected sides
              Oblique of affected side
              PA chest

View	Position		Structures	kV range	mAs range	Supplemental studies and technical tips
AP bilateral upper Central ray to enter midsternum, exits T7 level, top of film 2″ above patient's shoulders. Internally rotate arms to remove scapula from lung fields, place hands on hips or in back of head if possible. Optimal film size = 14 × 17 FFD = 40″	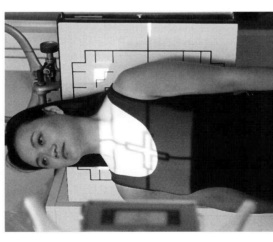		Ribs above the diaphragm, especially the posterior aspect of the ribs	Grid 65 to 75	20 to 40	Exposure is taken on full inspiration. Most common area of rib fracture is within the axillary margin of the rib, which is not clearly seen on this projection. Oblique views are required to adequately visualize the axillary margin of the rib. In cases of suspected rib fracture, PA chest should also be performed to help in exclusion of pneumothorax.
AP bilateral lower Place cassette crosswise so that the bottom of the cassette is 1″ below the iliac crest. Central ray enters 1½″ below xiphoid and exits T12 level. Optimal film size = 14 × 17 FFD = 40″	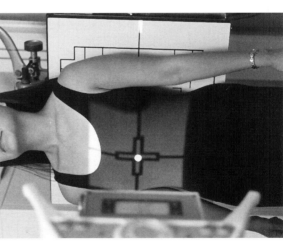		Ribs below the diaphragm	Grid 70 to 80	30 to 60	Exposure is taken on full expiration because it is below the diaphragm. Cassette must be placed crosswise because the rib cage is widest at the eighth and ninth ribs. Fracture of lower ribs may be indicative of damage to internal organs, such as the liver, spleen, or kidneys. CT of the abdomen is warranted if this is suspected.

AP unilateral

Midclavicular line is centered to film, top of film 2" above patient's shoulder.
Optimal film size = 14 × 17
FFD = 40"

Ribs above the diaphragm on the affected side. Film should include from costovertebral joints to the axillary border of the ribs

Grid
65 to 75

20 to 40

Exposure is taken on full inspiration. View may be used when the patient presents with rib complaints on one side only.
Oblique view must also be included with this view to best visualize axillary margin of the ribs.

Oblique ribs

Patient is placed in AP position; affected side is rotated 45 degrees towards the film. Right-sided rib injuries require RPO; left-sided rib injuries require LPO. Central ray enters just lateral to midsternum.
Optimal film size = 14 × 17
FFD = 40"

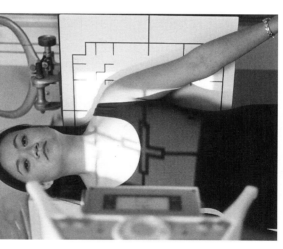

Axillary margin of ribs on the affected side

Grid
70 to 80

20 to 40

Exposure is taken on full inspiration. If films cannot be accomplished with the patient in the posterior oblique position, anterior oblique may be done, but the affected side is away from the film. In right-sided rib injuries, an LAO would be required; in left-sided rib injuries, an RAO would be required.

Continued

PA, Posteroanterior; *AP,* anteroposterior; *kV,* kilovolt; *mAs,* milliampere-seconds; *FFD,* focal film distance.

TABLE 4-5
Ribs and Bony Thorax—cont'd

BASIC STUDY: AP of affected sides
Oblique of affected side
PA chest

View	Position	Structures	kV range	mAs range	Supplemental studies and technical tips
Costal joints Patient is in AP position; central ray is angled 30 degrees to enter the lower aspect of sternum and exit at T6 level. Optimal film size = 11 × 14 FFD = 40"	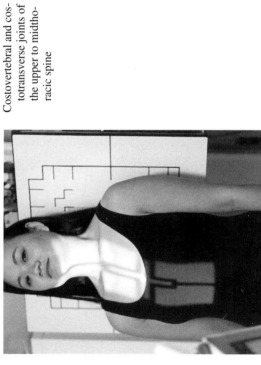	Costovertebral and costotransverse joints of the upper to midthoracic spine	Grid 70 to 80	20 to 40	Exposure is taken on full inspiration. This view is useful in demonstrating changes to this joint from entities such as rheumatoid arthritis and degenerative joint disease.
RAO sternum Patient is placed in 20-degree RAO position. Long axis of sternum is centered to film. Central ray enters just left of the spine at approximately the T6 level. Optimal film size = 10 × 12 FFD = 40"	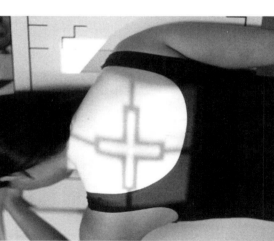	Slightly oblique PA projection of the sternum	Grid 75 to 85	30 to 40	Exposure is taken using breathing method. Patient takes even, shallow breaths, and a long exposure time is used. RAO position is used, because this will superimpose the sternum over the heart, providing a homogeneous background, and allowing better visualization.

Lateral sternum

Patient placed in lateral position, arms clasped behind back. Central ray enters midsternum. Film placed 1" above suprasternal notch. Optimal film size = 8 × 10 FFD = 40"

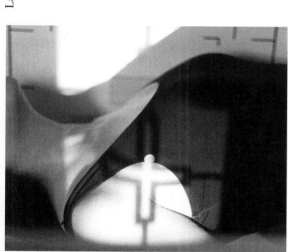

Lateral projection of the entire length of the sternum

Grid
75 to 85

40 to 60

Exposure is taken on full inspiration. If patient is in lateral recumbent position, raise arms above head.
In female patients the breasts should be moved to the side and secured with a wrap so that their shadows do not obscure the lower aspect of the sternum.

TABLE 4-6
Lumbar Spine

BASIC STUDY: AP lumbopelvic
Lateral lumbar

View	Position	Structures	kV range	mAs range	Supplemental studies and technical tips
AP lumbar spine Align midsagittal plane to center of film holder. Central ray enters in the midline 1″ below the iliac crest and exits L3 disc interspace. Optimal film size = 14 × 17 FFD = 40″	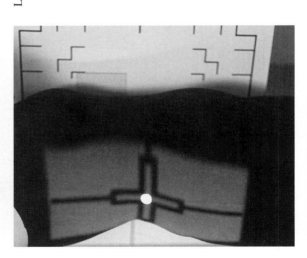	Lumbar vertebral bodies and intervertebral disc interspaces, lumbar spinous and transverse processes, lamina, pars interarticularis, SI joints, sacral ala, pelvis	Grid 75 to 85	30 to 80	Exposure is taken on full expiration. Gonad shielding should be used on these views. Heart (female) or bell (male) type shielding should be used for minimum obstruction of anatomy. In larger patients, methods such as abdominal compression or perforance of exam recumbent help to improve film quality.
Lateral lumbar spine Align midaxillary plane to center of film holder; central ray enters 1″ above iliac crest and passes through L3 disc interspace. Optimal film size = 14 × 17 FFD = 40″		Lumbar vertebral bodies and intervertebral disc interspaces, lumbar spinous processes, intervertebral foramina, sacrum, and coccyx	Grid 80 to 90	90 to 180	Exposure is taken on full inspiration. If L5-S1 area is not well visualized, an L5-S1 spot shot is warranted. This view may be accomplished in lateral recumbent position in larger patients to improve film quality.

L5-S1 lateral

Midaxillary plane centered to film; central ray enters 2″ below iliac crest.
Optimal film size = 8 × 10
FFD = 40″

L5-S1 disc interspace

Grid
80 to 90

120 to 200

Exposure is taken on full expiration.
5-degree caudal angle may be used to better demonstrate the lumbosacral joint space.
In larger patients, lateral recumbent view improves film quality.

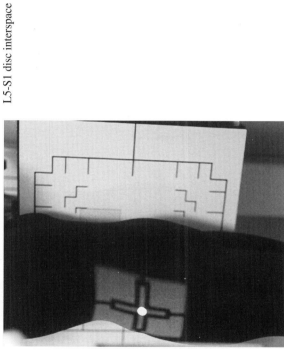

L5-S1 AP

Align midsagittal plane to film holder, 30-degree cephalic angle on the central ray to enter at the level of the anterior superior iliac spine (ASIS) and exit L5 disc space.
Optimal film size = 8 × 10
FFD = 40″

Projection opens up the L5-S1 disc interspace. SI joints are also visualized

Grid
75 to 85

30 to 80

Exposure is taken on full expiration.
In females, increase the cephalic angulation to 35 degrees.
This view better demonstrates L5 transitional vertebra. Also, it better demonstrates SI joints than the standard AP lumbopelvic view.

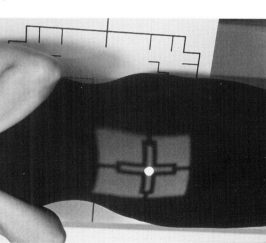

Continued

AP, Anteroposterior; *kV,* kilovolt; *mAs,* milliampere-seconds; *FFD,* focal film distance.

TABLE 4-6
Lumbar Spine—cont'd

BASIC STUDY: AP lumbopelvic
Lateral lumbar

View	Position	Structures	kV range	mAs range	Supplemental studies and technical tips
Oblique lumbar spine Patient is AP with body rotated 45 degrees toward film holder for posterior oblique. Central ray enters 2″ superior and 2″ medial from the iliac crest (area of inferior rib margin) and exits at the L3 level. Optimal film size = 10 × 12 FFD = 40″	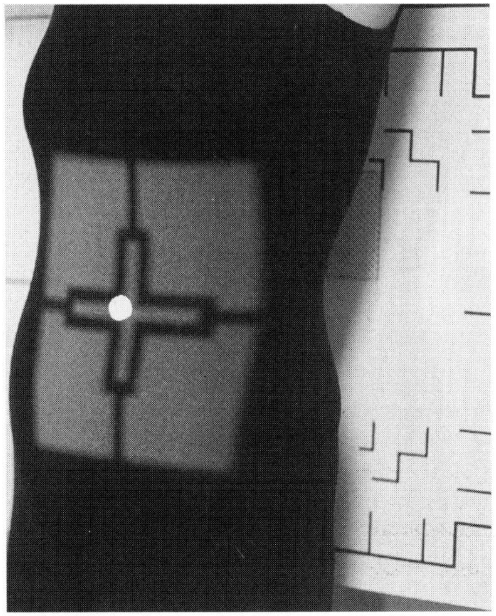	Lumbar vertebral bodies and intervertebral disc interspaces, lumbar spinous and transverse processes, lamina, pars interarticularis, apophyseal joints. Properly positioned oblique will demonstrate the "Scotty dog" appearance formed by the pedicle, transverse process, superior and inferior articular facets, and pars interarticularis.	Grid 75 to 85	30 to 80	Exposure is taken on full expiration. Cases of suspected spondyloloysis warrant this view because it yields optimal visualization of the pars interarticularis. Apophyseal joints of the lower lumbar spine, (L5-S1), may be demonstrated by 30-degree posterior oblique.

TABLE 4-7
Sacrum and Coccyx

BASIC STUDY: **AP sacrum**
Lateral sacrum
AP coccyx
Lateral coccyx

View	Position	Structures	kV range	mAs range	Supplemental studies and technical tips
AP sacrum Align midsagittal plane to center of film holder; central ray directed 15 degrees cephalic to enter midway between the symphysis pubis and a line connecting the ASISs. Optimal film size = 10 × 12 FFD = 40″	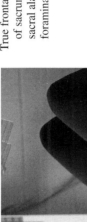	True frontal projection of sacrum, SI joints sacral ala, and sacral foramina	Grid 75 to 85	30 to 80	Exposure is taken on full expiration. Fecal material in rectosigmoid colon may obscure detail; it may be helpful to x-ray patients soon after they evacuate.
Lateral sacrum Patient in lateral position; central ray enters at level of ASIS and 2″ anterior to posterior surface of sacrum. Optimal film size = 10 × 12 FFD = 40″	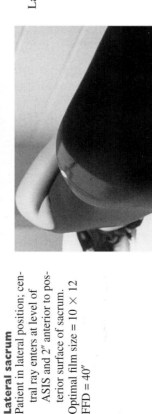	Lateral projection of sacrum and coccyx	Grid 75 to 85	90 to 180	Exposure is taken on full expiration. Bowel gas in the rectal vault may be helpful in this view because displacement of the rectal shadow is useful in evaluating trauma to the sacrum. Lead strip placed on film holder behind patient helps to absorb scatter radiation, improving quality of film.

Continued

AP, Anteroposterior; *kV,* kilovolt; *mAs,* milliampere-seconds; *FFD,* focal film distance.

TABLE 4-7
Sacrum and Coccyx—cont'd

BASIC STUDY: AP sacrum
Lateral sacrum
AP coccyx
Lateral coccyx

View	Position	Structures	kV range	mAs range	Supplemental studies and technical tips
Sacroiliac (SI) joints Patient is positioned PA, and unaffected side is rotated 25 degrees away from film holder to perform an anterior oblique. In an RAO position the right SI joint is visualized; in LAO the left is visualized. Central ray enters the SI joint of the side that is against the film holder at the level of the ASIS. Optimal film size = 8 × 10 FFD = 40"	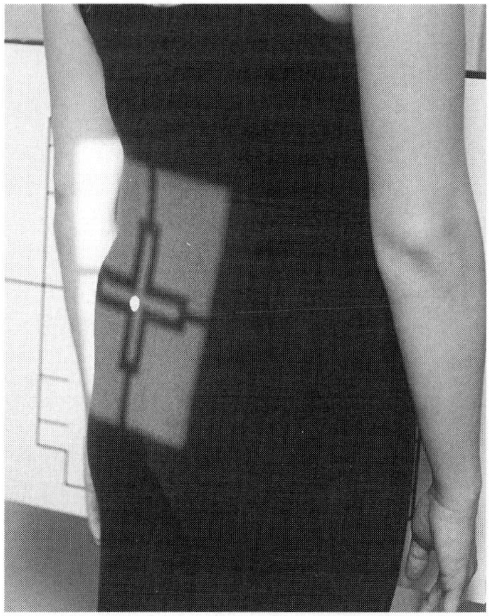	Profile image of the SI joint nearest the film. Both sides should be done for comparison	Grid 75 to 85	30 to 80	Exposure is taken on full expiration. Posterior oblique may be done in patients unable to perform anterior oblique. The posterior oblique will demonstrate the SI joint that is farthest from the film.
AP coccyx Align midsaggital plane to center of film; central ray enters with a 10-degree caudal tilt 2" superior to the symphysis pubis. Optimal film size = 8 × 10 FFD = 40"	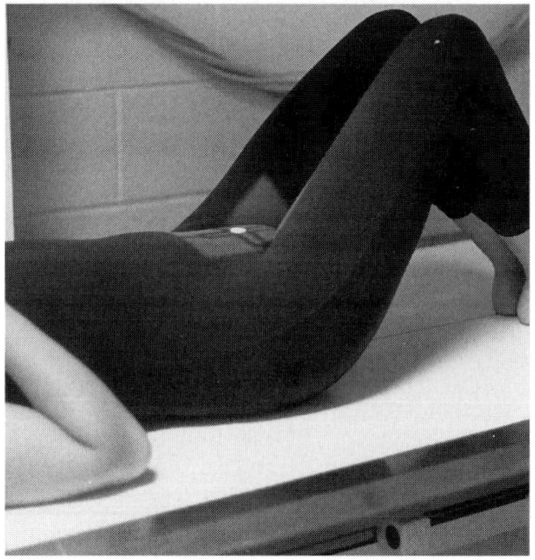	True AP projection of the coccyx free of superimposition of the symphysis pubis	Grid 70 to 80	30 to 50	Exposure is taken on suspended respiration. Fecal material in rectosigmoid colon may obscure the coccyx.

Lateral coccyx

Patient in lateral recumbent position with knees flexed.

Central ray to enter ½" superior to coccyx.

Optimal film size = 8 × 10

FFD = 40"

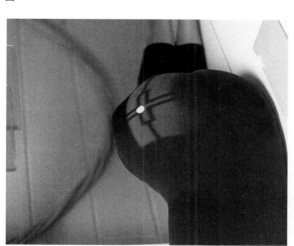

Lateral projection of the coccyx

Grid
70 to 80

30 to 50

Exposure taken on suspended respiration.

Lead strip placed behind patient helps to absorb scatter radiation, improving film quality.

TABLE 4-8
Full Spine

BASIC STUDY: AP full spine
Lateral sectionals

View	Position	Structures	kV range	mAs range	Supplemental studies and technical tips
AP full spine Patient with back against film holder with arms at sides and slightly abducted to bring the hands out of the collimation field. Center film so that the bottom of the cassette is 1″ below the gluteal fold. Central ray is then centered to the film. Open mouth and align head to obtain C1-C2 level. Optimal film size = 14 × 36 FFD = 72″	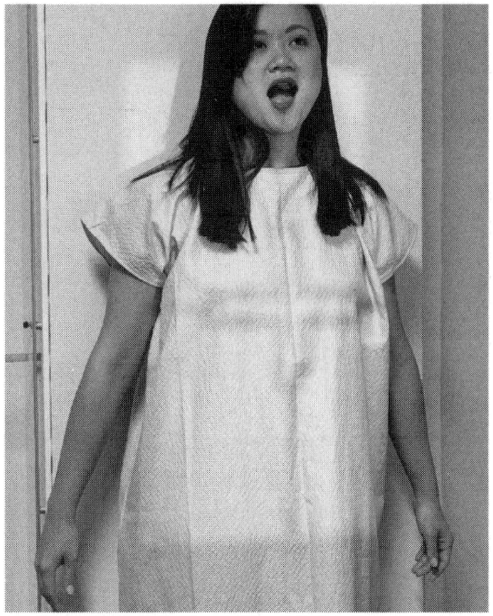	AP projection of the entire vertebral column, including the pelvis	Grid 80 to 90	50 to 100	Exposure is taken on full expiration. Use filtration down to the midsternum to accommodate for differences in thickness of anatomy. This view should not be attempted on large patients because technical factors prevent a quality radiograph. Large patients should be done as a sectional series. This view is useful in scoliosis evaluation. May be done PA to reduce breast and gonadal dose.
Lateral full spine Because of technical limitations and resultant poor film quality, this view is not recommended. Lateral sectional series should accompany AP full spine for a complete study.		Refer to lateral views in sectional series	—	—	—

AP, Anteroposterior; *kV,* kilovolt; *mAs,* milliampere-seconds; *FFD,* focal film distance.

TABLE 4-9
Shoulder Nontraumatic Series*

BASIC STUDY: AP external rotation
AP internal rotation
AP glenoid fossa

View	Position	Structures	kV range	mAs range	Supplemental studies and technical tips
AP internal rotation Patient with back against film holder, rotated slightly towards affected shoulder. Central ray enters coracoid process. Internally rotate arm until distal humeral epicondyles are perpendicular to the film. Optimal film size = 10 × 12 FFD = 40″	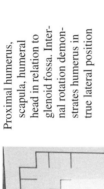	Proximal humerus, scapula, humeral head in relation to glenoid fossa. Internal rotation demonstrates humerus in true lateral position	Grid 70 to 80	8 to 16	Suspend respiration on exposure. This view clearly demonstrates area of subdeltoid bursa. If the shoulder is too painful to internally rotate, turn affected shoulder away from film to obtain a similar view.
AP external rotation Patient with back against film holder, rotated slightly toward affected shoulder. Central ray enters coracoid process. Externally rotate arm until epicondyles of distal humerus are parallel to the film. Optimal film size = 10 × 12 FFD = 40″	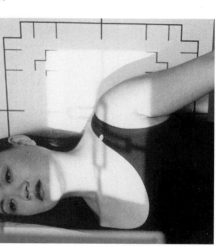	Proximal humerus, scapula, humeral head in relation to glenoid fossa. External rotation demonstrates proximal humerus in the true AP position	Grid 70 to 80	8 to 16	Suspend respiration on exposure. This view demonstrates calcified deposits in tendon insertions and the greater tuberosity of proximal humerus in profile, which is the site of insertion of the supraspinatus tendon.

Continued

AP, Anteroposterior; *kV,* kilovolt; *mAs,* milliampere-seconds; *FFD,* focal film distance.
*If fracture or dislocation is suspected, do not attempt to rotate the shoulder. Suspected fracture warrants traumatic shoulder series.

TABLE 4-9
Shoulder Nontraumatic Series*—cont'd

BASIC STUDY: AP external rotation
AP internal rotation
AP glenoid fossa

View	Position	Structures	kV range	mAs range	Supplemental studies and technical tips
AP glenoid fossa Patient with back against film holder. Rotate patient 35 to 40 degrees toward affected side so that scapula is parallel to the film. Arm is in neutral position and abducted slightly. Place top of film 2″ above shoulder. Central ray enters glenohumeral joint space. Optimal film size = 10 × 12 FFD = 40″	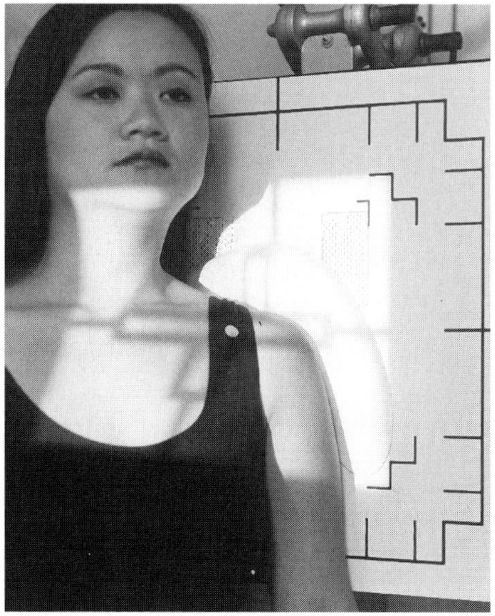	Glenoid fossa in profile projection. Joint space between the humeral head and glenoid fossa	Grid 70 to 80	8 to 16	Suspend respiration on exposure. Degree of patient rotation will depend upon how round-shouldered the patient is. Angle will increase the more round-shouldered the patient is. This view may be used with internal and external rotation in place of standard AP internal and external rotation views.

AP, Anteroposterior; *kV,* kilovolt; *mAs,* milliampere-seconds; *FFD,* focal film distance.
*If fracture or dislocation is suspected, do not attempt to rotate the shoulder. Suspected fracture warrants traumatic shoulder series.

TABLE 4-10
Shoulder Traumatic Series

BASIC STUDY: AP neutral position
Transthoracic lateral

View	Position	Structures	kV range	mAs range	Supplemental studies and technical tips
AP neutral position Patient with back against film holder, rotated slightly toward affected shoulder. Place top of film 2" above shoulder. Central ray enters coracoid process. Arm at side in neutral; position with no rotation. Optimal film size = 10 × 12 FFD = 40"	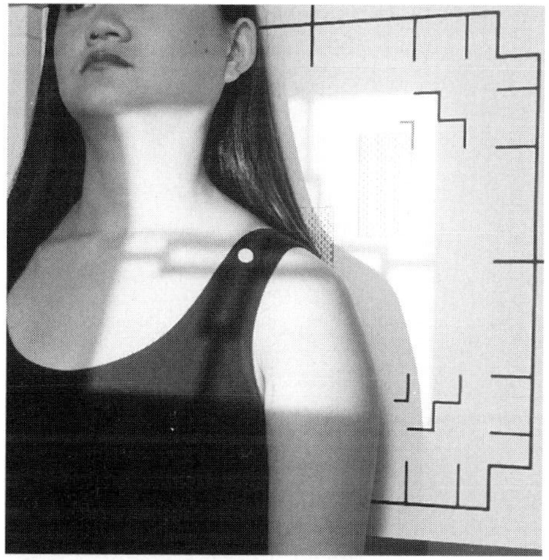	Proximal humerus, scapula, humeral head in relation to glenoid fossa	Grid 70 to 80	8 to 16	Suspend respiration on exposure. This view is used in patients suspected of having a fracture or dislocation within the shoulder girdle. Do not attempt to rotate the arm in cases of suspected fracture.
Transthoracic lateral Affected side placed against film holder, patient raises opposite arm above head. Film is positioned 3" above top of shoulder; center affected humerus to film. Central ray enters the opposite axilla with a 10- to 15-degree cephalic tilt to exit the surgical neck of the humerus of the affected side. Optimal film size = 10 × 12 FFD = 40"	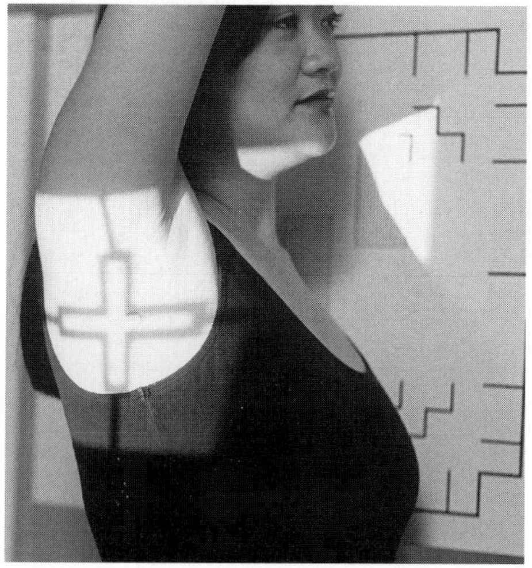	Upper half of the humerus in relation to glenoid fossa projected through the thorax	Grid 75 to 85	40 to 60	Suspend respiration on exposure or use breathing technique and long exposure time with patient taking even, shallow breaths. It is important to have patient in true lateral position because otherwise overlapping thoracic spine will obscure humerus. This is an excellent view for demonstrating anterior or posterior displacement of surgical neck fractures of the humerus. An alternate view is a lateral scapula with arm hanging by patient's side.

AP, Anteroposterior; *kV,* kilovolt; *mAs,* milliampere-seconds; *FFD,* focal film distance.

TABLE 4-11
Acromioclavicular Joints

BASIC STUDY: AP unweighted
AP weighted

View	Position		Structures	kV range	mAs range	Supplemental studies and technical tips
AP unweighted Patient with back against film holder. Adjust film height so that AC joint is in the middle of the film. Direct central ray to AC joint with a 5-degree cephalic tilt. Optimal film size = 8 × 10 FFD = 40″	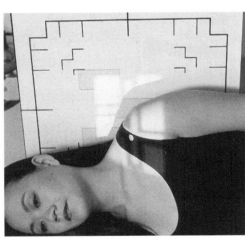		Relationship of distal clavicle to the acromion. Integrity of acromioclavicular joint	Grid 60 to 70	6 to 12	Suspend respiration on exposure. Cephalic angle may be increased to 15 degrees to elongate the AC joint in relation to the acromion.
AP weighted Patient with back against film holder. Adjust film height so that AC joint is in the middle of the film. Direct central ray to AC joint with a 5-degree cephalic tilt. Have patient hold a 10-pound sandbag to stress AC joint. Optimal film size = 8 × 10 FFD = 40″	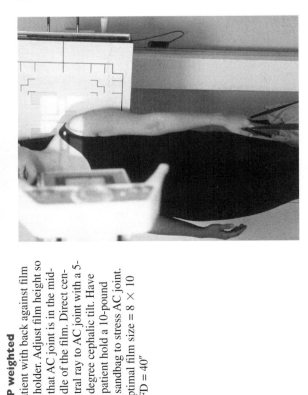		Relationship of distal clavicle to acromion. Integrity of acromioclavicular joint under stress	Grid 60 to 70	6 to 12	Suspend respiration on exposure. Cephalic angle may be increased to 15 degrees to elongate the AC joint in relation to the acromion. The inferior aspect of the acromion is compared with the distal clavicle in evaluating AC joint separation because the superior aspect of the clavicle is normally raised with respect to the acromion.

AP, Anteroposterior; *kV,* kilovolt; *mAs,* milliampere-seconds; *FFD,* focal film distance.

TABLE 4-12
Clavicle

BASIC STUDY: PA clavicle
AP axial clavicle

View	Position		Structures	kV range	mAs range	Supplemental studies and technical tips
PA clavicle Front of patient against film holder. Turn head away from affected side and center clavicle to film. Central ray enters midclavicle. Optimal film size = 10 × 12 FFD = 40″			Frontal projection of the clavicle and acromioclavicular joint	Grid 60 to 70	8 to 16	Suspend respiration on exposure. Detail is increased when film is taken PA because of decreased object-film distance.
AP axial clavicle Patient with back against film holder. Turn head away from affected side and center clavicle to film. Central ray enters midclavicle. Optimal film size = 10 × 12 FFD = 40″			Axial projection of the clavicle free of superimposition of underlying structures	Grid 60 to 70	8 to 16	Suspend respiration on exposure. To further exaggerate the axial view, place patient in lordotic position, 1 foot away from film holder, leaning backwards so that affected side is touching the film holder.

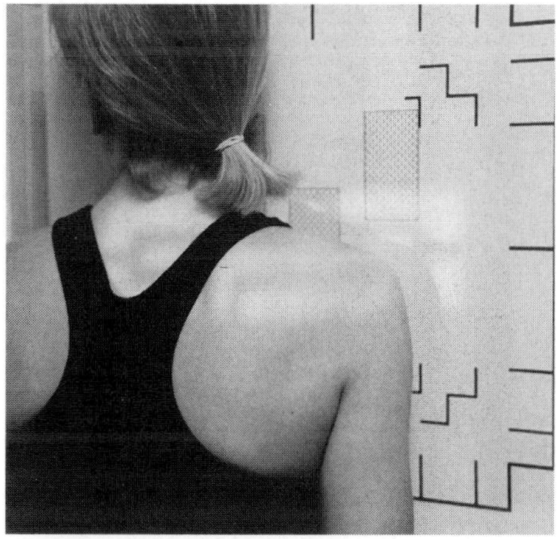

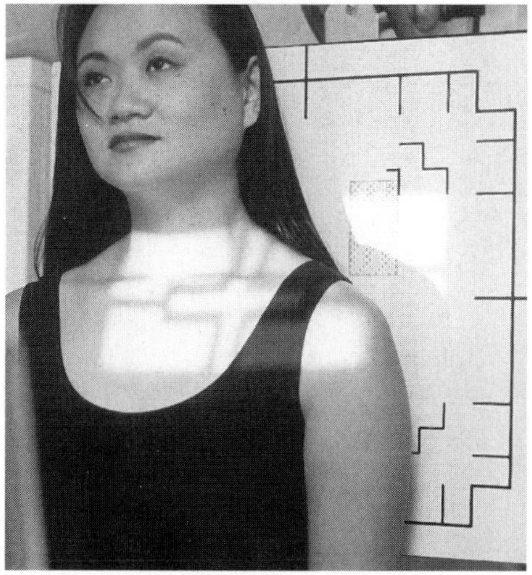

PA, Posteroanterior; *AP*, anteroposterior; *kV*, kilovolt; *mAs*, milliampere-seconds; *FFD*, focal film distance.

TABLE 4-13
Scapula

BASIC STUDY: AP scapula
Lateral scapula

View	Position	Structures	kV range	mAs range	Supplemental studies and technical tips
AP scapula Patient with back against film holder. Center affected scapula to the midline of film, abduct arm to 90 degrees to draw the scapula laterally, and flex elbow to support hand in a comfortable position. Central ray is directed to enter 2″ below coracoid and exit midscapula. Optimal film size = 10 × 12 FFD = 40″	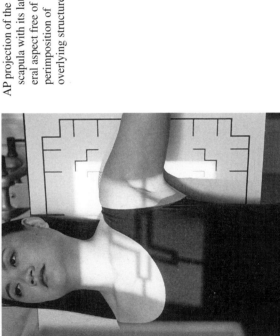	AP projection of the scapula with its lateral aspect free of superimposition of overlying structures	Grid 70 to 80	15 to 25	Suspend respiration on exposure. Do not rotate toward affected side in this view because this will superimpose lateral border of scapula over bony thorax. Shoulder series is usually done in conjunction with scapula series.
Lateral scapula Front of patient against film holder, in anterior oblique position with affected side against film. Have patient grasp opposite shoulder with affected arm so that scapula is in a true lateral position to the central ray. Place top of film 2″ above shoulder. Central ray enters midvertebral border of scapula. Optimal film size = 10 × 12 FFD = 40″	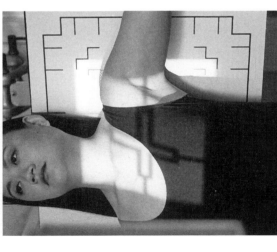	Lateral view of the scapula free of superimposition of the ribcage	Grid 70 to 80	20 to 40	Suspend respiration on exposure. Average patient will be in a 60-degree anterior oblique. This is the best view for demonstrating fractures within the body of the scapula. For better demonstration of the acromion and coracoid process, extend patient's arm upward and rest arm on head. For better demonstration of humeral head in relation to the glenoid fossa, hang patient's arm along body so that the wing of the scapula superimposes it. This view can be used as an alternate to the transthoracic view in a traumatic shoulder series.

AP, Anteroposterior; *kV,* kilovolt; *mAs,* milliampere-seconds; *FFD,* focal film distance.

TABLE 4-14
Humerus

BASIC STUDY: AP humerus
Lateral humerus
Transthoracic lateral*

View	Position	Structures	kV range	mAs range	Supplemental studies and technical tips
AP humerus Patient with back against film holder. Rotate patient toward affected side so that humerus is in contact with film holder. Supinate hand and slightly abduct arm. Center film to midshaft of humerus to include both shoulder and elbow joints if possible. Direct central ray to midshaft of humerus. Optimal film size = 7 × 17 FFD = 40"	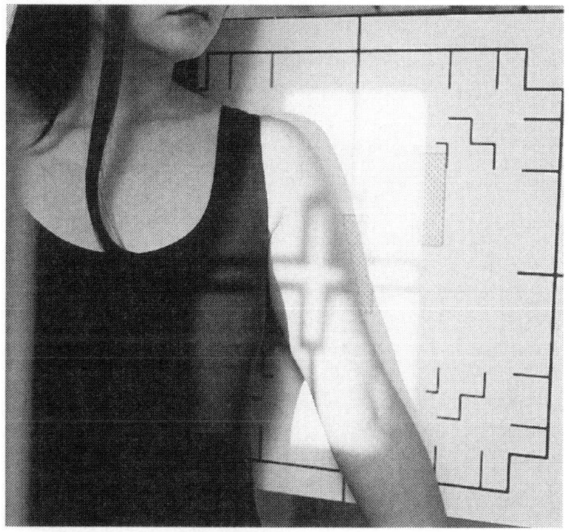	Frontal projection of the humerus	Grid 60 to 70	5 to 10	Suspend respiration on exposure. If patient is in severe pain or if fracture is suspected, do not attempt to supinate the hand. Instead take AP humerus in neutral position without rotating the patient's arm.
Lateral humerus Patient with back against film holder. Rotate patient toward affected side so that humerus is in contact with film holder. Flex elbow to 90 degrees with hand supinated to internally rotate humerus. Optimal film size = 7 × 17 FFD = 40"	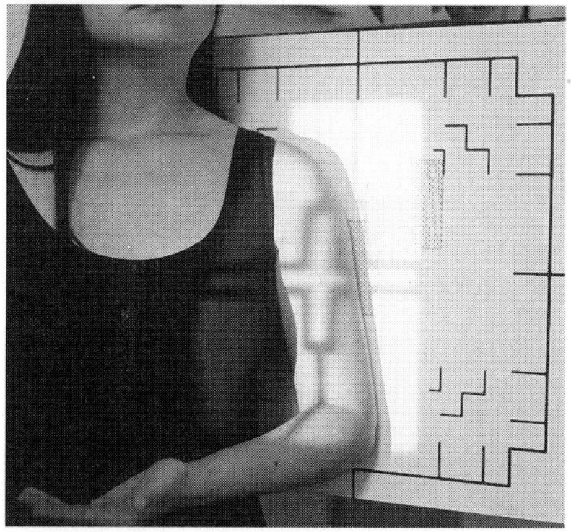	Lateral projection of the humerus	Grid 60 to 70	5 to 10	Suspend respiration on exposure. If patient is in severe pain or if fracture is suspected, do not attempt to internally rotate humerus for lateral position.*

AP, Anteroposterior; *kV,* kilovolt; *mAs,* milliampere-seconds; *FFD,* focal film distance.
*Cases of suspected fracture of the proximal humerus warrant substitution of a transthoracic lateral.

Continued

TABLE 4-14
Humerus—cont'd

BASIC STUDY: AP humerus
Lateral humerus
Transthoracic lateral*

View	Position	Structures	kV range	mAs range	Supplemental studies and technical tips
Transthoracic lateral Affected side placed against film holder; opposite arm raised above head. Film is positioned 3″ above top of shoulder; center affected humerus to film. Central ray enters the opposite axilla with a 10- to 15-degree cephalic tilt to exit the surgical neck of the humerus of the affected side. Optimal film size = 10 × 12 FFD = 40″	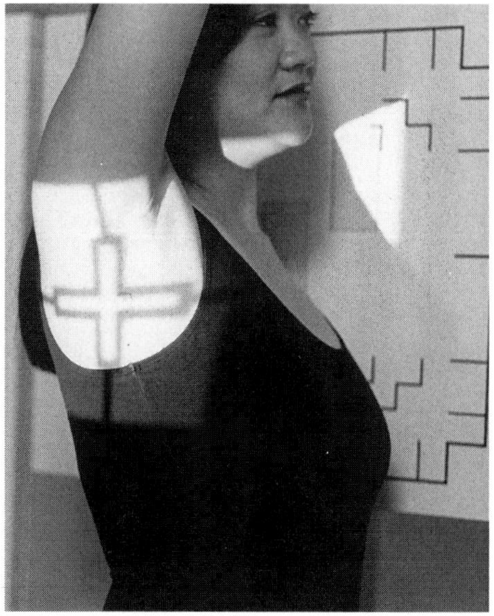	Upper half of the humerus in relation to glenoid fossa projected through the thorax	Grid 75 to 85	40 to 60	Suspend respiration on exposure or use breathing technique, long exposure time with patient taking even, shallow breaths. It is important to have patient in true lateral position because overlapping thoracic spine will otherwise obscure humerus. This is an excellent view for demonstrating anterior or posterior displacement of surgical neck fractures of the humerus. An alternate view is a lateral scapula with patient's arm hanging by his or her side.

*Cases of suspected fracture of the proximal humerus warrant substitution of a transthoracic lateral.

TABLE 4-15
Elbow

BASIC STUDY: AP elbow
Lateral elbow

View	Position		Structures	kV range	mAs range	Supplemental studies and technical tips
AP elbow	Patient seated with elbow fully extended with hand supinated. Lower shoulder to same plane as tabletop. Central ray passes through the elbow joint. Optimal film size = ½ 10 × 12 FFD = 40″		AP projection of elbow joint, proximal radius and ulna, distal humerus	Nongrid detail 55 to 65	15 to 30	Divide 10 × 12 film in half to fit both AP and lateral on one film. Place sandbag over wrist to prevent motion. If patient can only partially extend elbow, take two AP views in the partial flexed position: one with the forearm resting on the film and one with the humerus resting on the film. Drape lead shield over patient's lap.
Lateral elbow	Patient seated with elbow flexed 90 degrees. Drop shoulder to rest humerus on tabletop. Hand must be in lateral position, thumb up. Central ray passes through the elbow joint. Optimal film size = ½ 10 × 12 FFD = 40″		Lateral projection of elbow joint, proximal radius and ulna, distal humerus. Clearly demonstrates olecranon process	Nongrid detail 55 to 65	15 to 30	Divide 10 × 12 film in half to fit both AP and lateral on one film. This is an important view for evaluating elevation of distal humeral fat pads. Elevation of distal humeral fat pads is indicative of intraarticular effusion, such as hemarthrosis from fracture, especially radial head fractures. External oblique view of the elbow may demonstrate radial head fracture that is not readily apparent on AP or lateral views. Drape lead shield over patient's lap.

Continued

AP, Anteroposterior; *kV*, kilovolt; *mAs*, milliampere-seconds; *FFD*, focal film distance.

TABLE 4-15
Elbow—cont'd

BASIC STUDY: AP elbow
Lateral elbow

View	Position	Structures	kV range	mAs range	Supplemental studies and technical tips
External oblique Patient seated with elbow fully extended and hand supinated. Lower shoulder to same plane as tabletop. Laterally rotate arm so that elbow joint is 45 degrees to film. Central ray to elbow joint. Optimal film size = ½ 10 × 12 FFD = 40″	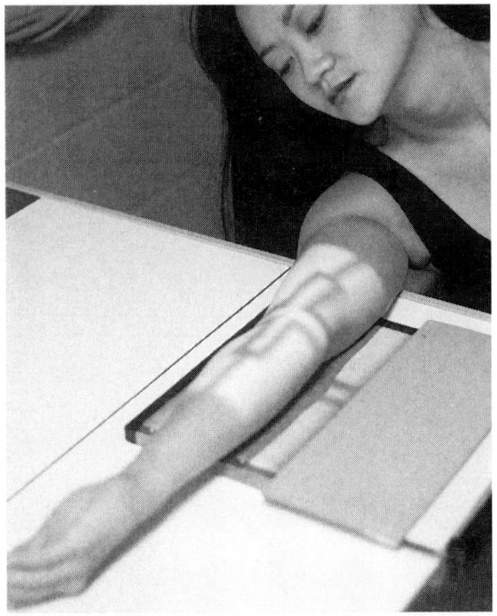	Oblique projection of the elbow joint, proximal radius and ulna, distal humerus. Clearly demonstrates radial head, free of superimposition	Nongrid detail 55 to 65	15 to 30	Divide 10 × 12 film in half to fit both external and internal oblique on one film. This is the view used in cases where radial head fracture is suspected, elevation of distal humeral fat pads is noted on lateral view, and fracture line is not readily apparent. If patient cannot externally rotate elbow, angle tube 15 to 20 degrees from medial to lateral for similar view. Drape lead shield over patient's lap.
Internal oblique Patient seated with elbow fully extended. Lower shoulder to same plane as tabletop. Pronate hand into natural palm down position. Central ray to elbow joint. Optimal film size = ½ 10 × 12 FFD = 40″	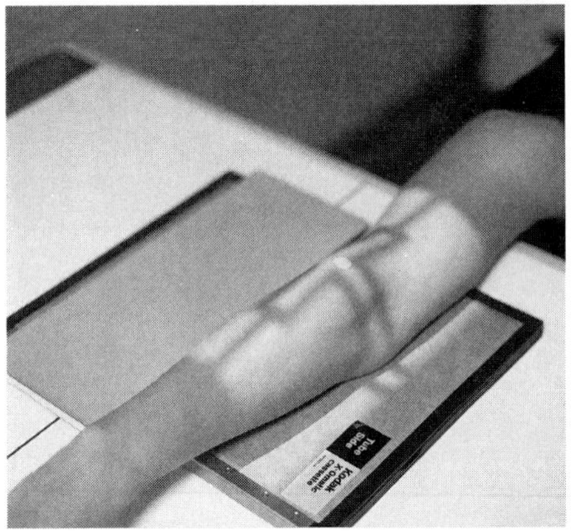	Oblique projection of the elbow joint, proximal radius and ulna, distal humerus. Clearly demonstrates coronoid process, free of superimposition of the radial head	Nongrid detail 55 to 65	15 to 30	Divide 10 × 12 film in half to fit both external and internal oblique on one film. This is a useful view in evaluating coronoid process. Drape lead shield over patient's lap.

Axial projection

Patient placed in Jones position, complete flexion of the elbow, with elbow joint centered to film. Central ray enters the elbow joint.
Optimal film size = 8 × 10
FFD = 40″

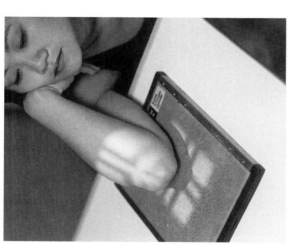

Superimposed distal humerus and proximal radius and ulna. Very clear image of the olecranon process

Nongrid
detail
55 to 65

15 to 30

If the distal humerus is the area of concern, direct the central ray perpendicular to film with no angle. If distal forearm is the area of concern, angle central ray to be perpendicular with radius and ulna.
Drape lead shield over patient's lap.

TABLE 4-16
Forearm

BASIC STUDY: AP forearm
Lateral forearm

View	Position		Structures	kV range	mAs range	Supplemental studies and technical tips
AP forearm	Patient seated with elbow fully extended with hand supinated. Lower shoulder to same plane as tabletop. Central ray to midshaft of forearm. Include joint nearest injury site. Optimal film size = ½ 10 × 12 FFD = 40"	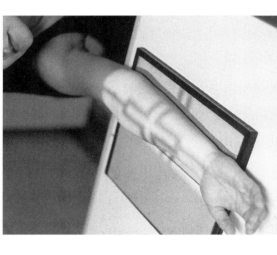	AP projection of the radius and ulna, elbow joint and proximal row of carpals	Nongrid detail 55 to 65	15 to 30	Divide 10 × 12 film in half to fit both AP and lateral on one film. Place sandbag over patient's hand to prevent motion. For AP projection of forearm, hand must be supinated because pronation will result in an oblique view of forearm with the radius crossed over the ulna. Drape lead shield over patient's lap.
Lateral forearm	Patient seated with elbow flexed 90 degrees. Drop shoulder to rest humerus on tabletop. Hand must be in lateral position, thumb up. Central ray to midshaft of forearm. Include joint nearest injury site. Optimal film site = ½ 10 × 12 FFD = 40"	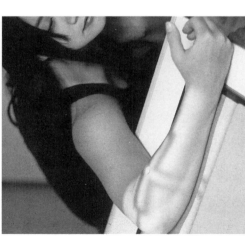	Lateral projection of the superimposed radius and ulna, elbow joint and proximal row of carpals	Nongrid detail 55 to 65	15 to 30	Divide 10 × 12 film in half to fit both AP and lateral on one film. Drape lead shield over patient's lap.

AP, Anteroposterior; *kV,* kilovolt; *mAs,* milliampere-seconds; *FFD,* focal film distance.

TABLE 4-17
Wrist

BASIC STUDY: PA wrist
Oblique wrist
Lateral wrist

View	Position	Structures	kV range	mAs range	Supplemental studies and technical tips
PA wrist	Patient seated with hand and forearm parallel to long axis of film. Partially flex fingers and arch hand so that wrist makes close contact with the film. Central ray enters midcarpals. Optimal film size = ⅓ 10 × 12 FFD = 40"	PA projection of the carpals, distal radius and ulna, proximal metacarpals	Nongrid detail 55 to 60	12 to 24	Divide 10 × 12 cassette into thirds to fit PA, oblique, and lateral views on one film. When midcarpal area is difficult to locate because of swelling, ask patient to flex wrist slightly and center to the point of flexion. Drape lead shield over patient's lap.
Oblique wrist	Patient seated with hand and forearm parallel to long axis of film. Partially flex fingers and arch hand for stability. From lateral position, rotate wrist medially to form a 45-degree angle with film. Central ray enters midcarpals. Optimal film size = ⅓ 10 × 12 FFD = 40"	Better demonstrates carpals on lateral aspect of the wrist. Navicular projected free of superimposition of itself	Nongrid detail 55 to 60	12 to 24	Divide 10 × 12 cassette into thirds to fit PA, oblique, and lateral views on one film. Drape lead shield over patient's lap.

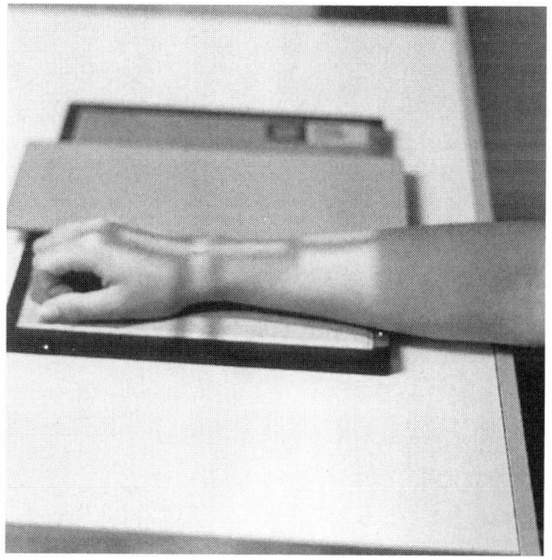

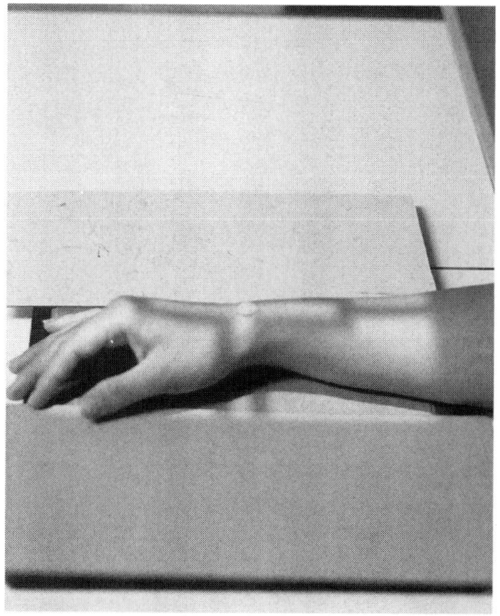

PA, Posteroanterior; *kV,* kilovolt; *mAs,* milliampere-seconds; *FFD,* focal film distance.

Continued

TABLE 4-17
Wrist—cont'd

BASIC STUDY: PA wrist
Oblique wrist
Lateral wrist

View	Position	Structures	kV range	mAs range	Supplemental studies and technical tips
Lateral wrist Patient seated with elbow flexed 90 degrees and rotate wrist to lateral position. Central ray enters the wrist joint. Optimal film size = ½ 10 × 12 FFD = 40″		Lateral projection of the carpals, distal radius and ulna, proximal metacarpals	Nongrid detail 55 to 60	12 to 24	Divide 10 × 12 into thirds to fit PA, oblique, and lateral views on one film. Drape lead shield over patient's lap. Make sure wrist is in true lateral position because patients tend to place wrist in slight flexion when in the lateral position.
PA ulnar flexion Patient seated with hand and forearm parallel to long axis of film. Hand in PA position, without moving forearm radial; deviate (ulna flex) as far as possible without lifting forearm. Central ray enters navicular area. Optimal film size = 8 × 10 FFD = 40″	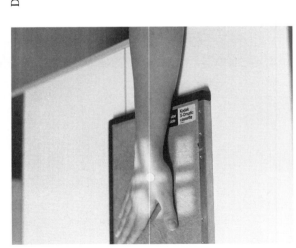	Demonstrates the navicular without the foreshortening that is present on the direct PA position	Nongrid detail 55 to 60	12 to 24	Clearer delineation of the navicular may be obtained with a 15- to 20-degree central ray tilt towards the elbow. Drape lead shield over patient's lap.

Carpal canal

Patient seated with hand and forearm parallel to long axis of film. Hand in PA position, hyperextend the wrist and center film to level of radial styloid. Rotate hand slightly toward radial side. Central ray enters with a 25- to 30-degree angulation 1″ above the base of the fourth metacarpal.

Optimal film size = 8 × 10

FFD = 40″

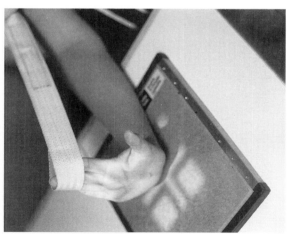

Projection of carpal canal, palmar aspect of greater multangular, lesser multangular, tuberosity of navicular, capitate, hook of hamates, and entire pisiform

Nongrid
detail
55 to 60

12 to 24

This is a useful view in demonstrating fractures of the pisiform and hook of the hamate.

Have patient use strap around fingers and grasp with opposite hand to aid in hyperextension of wrist.

Drape lead shield over patient's lap.

TABLE 4-18
Hand and Fingers

BASIC STUDY: PA hand
Oblique hand
Lateral fingers

View	Position		Structures	kV range	mAs range	Supplemental studies and technical tips
PA hand Patient seated with hand and forearm parallel to long axis of film. Pronate hand with palmar surface in contact with film. Central ray enters third metacarpophalangeal joint. Optimal film size = ½ 10 × 12 FFD = 40"	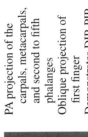		PA projection of the carpals, metacarpals, and second to fifth phalanges Oblique projection of first finger Demonstrates DIP, PIP, and MP joints	Nongrid detail 55 to 60	12 to 24	Divide 10 × 12 in half to fit PA and oblique views on one film. Drape lead shield over patient's lap. Ensure that all fingers are included on the radiograph.
Oblique hand Patient seated with hand and forearm parallel to long axis of film. From lateral position, rotate wrist medially to form a 45-degree angle with film with fingers slightly flexed so that fingertips rest on film. Central ray enters third metacarpophalangeal joint. Optimal film size = ½ 10 × 12 FFD = 40"	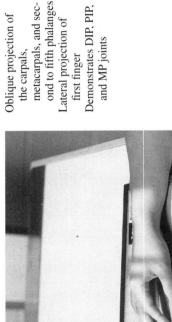 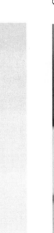		Oblique projection of the carpals, metacarpals, and second to fifth phalanges Lateral projection of first finger Demonstrates DIP, PIP, and MP joints	Nongrid detail 55 to 60	12 to 24	If fingers are primary area of interest, use a 45-degree wedge sponge to extend fingers on this view. Drape lead shield over patient's lap.

Continued

Lateral finger

Individual lateral projection of second to fifth fingers. Extend affected finger and fold rest of fingers. Place second to third with radial side down and fourth to fifth with ulna side down in lateral position. Central ray enters PIP.

Optimal film size = 8 × 10 or corner of film on hand series

FFD = 40"

Lateral projection of phalanges of affected finger

Nongrid
detail
50 to 55

6 to 12

Exposure is taken in conjunction with hand series.

Use tape or tongue depressor to aid patient in holding affected finger in extension.

Small avulsion fractures of phalanges can lead to permanent deformity and are best seen on lateral films.

Drape lead shield over patient's lap.

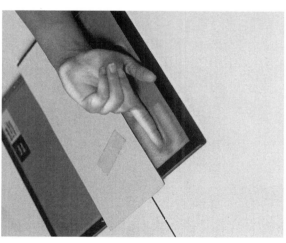

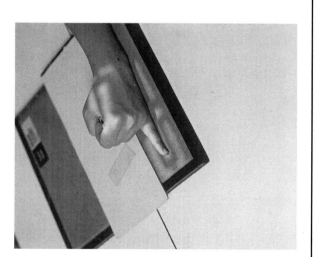

PA, Posteroanterior; *kV,* kilovolt; *mAs,* milliampere-seconds; *FFD,* focal film distance.

TABLE 4-18
Hand and Fingers—cont'd

BASIC STUDY: PA hand
Oblique hand
Lateral fingers

View	Position	Structures	kV range	mAs range	Supplemental studies and technical tips
AP thumb Individual AP projection of thumb. Internally rotate hand until posterior surface of thumb is in contact with the film. Hold fingers back with opposite hand. Central ray enters first metacarpophalangeal (MP) joint. Optimal film size = 8 × 10 or corner of film on hand series FFD = 40″	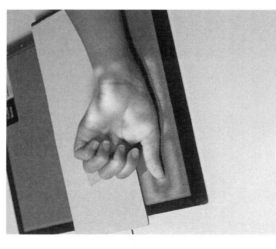	AP projection of phalanges of first finger and MP and PIP joints	Nongrid detail 50 to 55	6 to 12	Exposure is taken in conjunction with hand series. This view is taken because first finger is in an oblique and lateral position on the standard hand series. Drape lead shield over patient's lap.
Lateral hand Patient seated with hand in lateral position. Completely extend fingers and place ulnar aspect of hand against film. Central ray is directed to metacarpophalangeal joints. Optimal film size = 8 × 10 FFD = 40″	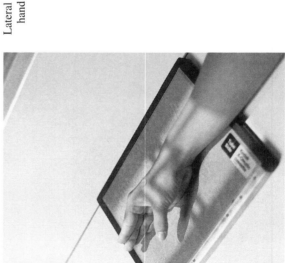	Lateral projection of the hand in extension	Nongrid detail 55 to 60	12 to 24	This view is used mainly for localization of foreign bodies within the hand. Drape lead shield over patient's lap.

Norgaard method

Seat patient at end of radiographic table with both hands in half-supinated position on film. Fingers should be extended and thumbs slightly abducted to prevent superimposition of the fingers. Central ray enters midway between both hands at the level of the MP joints.

Optimal film size = 10 × 12

FFD = 40″

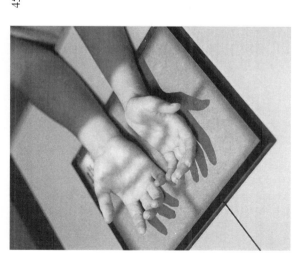

AP, Anteroposterior.

45-degree oblique position of the hands

Nongrid detail 55 to 60

12 to 24

This view is useful in detecting the early radiological changes associated with rheumatoid arthritis because it clearly demonstrates the medial aspect of the metatarsal heads, one of the first areas affected. Also, this view clearly demonstrates the pisiform, another sight of early erosions in rheumatoid arthritis.

Shield gonads.

TABLE 4-19
Pelvis and Hip

BASIC STUDY: AP pelvis
AP hip
Frog leg lateral

View	Position	Structures	kV range	mAs range	Supplemental studies and technical tips
AP pelvis Patient with back against film holder or supine on radiographic table. Place center of film 2″ above greater trochanter. Central ray enters midway between the symphysis pubis and iliac crest. Rotate both legs internally 15 to 20 degrees to reduce the femoral anteversion. Optimal film size = 14 × 17 FFD = 40″	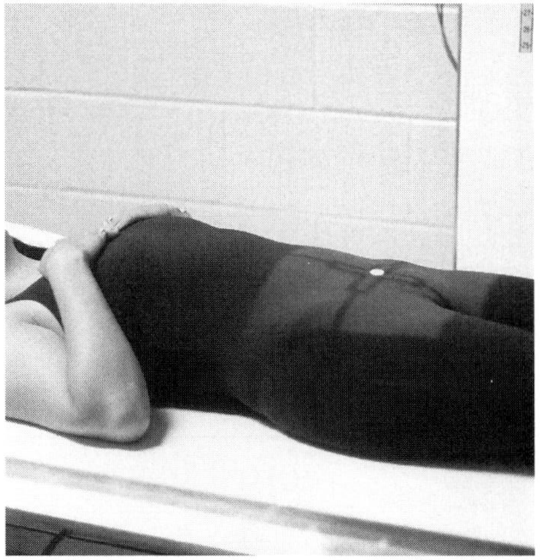	AP projection of the pelvis and head, neck, trochanter, and proximal third of the femora	Grid 75 to 85	30 to 80	Gonadal shielding should be used if possible. Suspend respiration on exposure. Internally rotating legs allows better visualization of the femoral neck by reducing anteversion. Do not attempt to internally rotate the legs if femoral neck fracture is suspected.
AP hip Patient with back against film holder or supine on radiographic table. Center femoral head to film 2½″ below midpoint of line between the ASIS and symphysis pubis. Central ray enters femoral head. Rotate leg internally 15 to 20 degrees to reduce the femoral anteversion. Optimal film size = 10 × 12 FFD = 40″	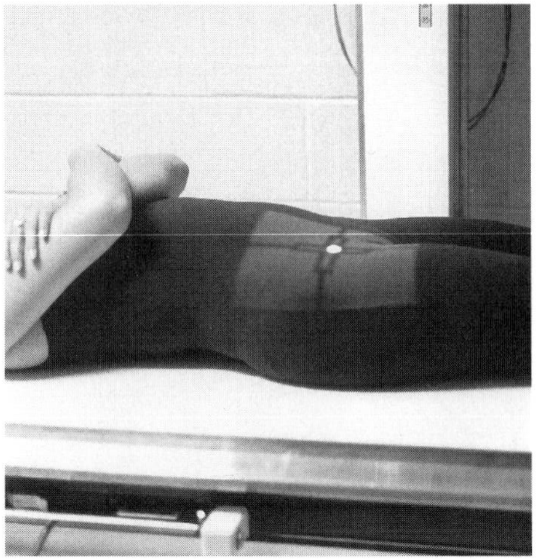	Femoral head, neck and greater trochanter, acetabulum	Grid 75 to 80	20 to 50	Suspend respiration on exposure. Internally rotating legs allows better visualization of the femoral neck by reducing anteversion. Do not attempt to internally rotate the legs if femoral neck fracture is suspected. Gonadal shielding should be used if possible. Unilateral AP hip is usually done as a follow-up study. The AP pelvis is included in the initial examination of a patient with suspected hip pathology.

Frog leg lateral

Patient with back against film holder or supine on radiographic table. Center femoral head to film 2½″ below midpoint of line between the ASIS and symphysis pubis. Central ray enters femoral head. Have patient flex knee and draw up thigh. Rotate pelvis towards affected side slightly so that affected femoral shaft is parallel to the table.
Optimal film size = 10 × 12
FFD = 40″

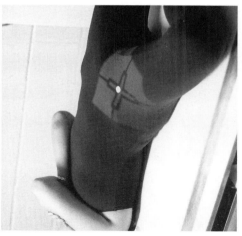

Lateral view of femoral head, neck and greater trochanter, acetabulum

Grid
75 to 80

20 to 50

Suspend respiration on exposure.
In upright position, have patient flex knee and draw the leg up while stabilizing self with a chair.
This position should never be attempted when hip fracture is suspected.
Gonadal shielding should be used if possible.
A 20-degree cephalic tilt may be added to the central ray to better demonstrate the femoral neck.

AP, Anteroposterior; *kV,* kilovolt; *mAs,* milliampere-seconds; *FFD,* focal film distance.

TABLE 4-20
Femur

BASIC STUDY: AP femur, Lateral femur

View	Position		Structures	kV range	mAs range	Supplemental studies and technical tips
AP femur	Patient supine on radiographic table. Center affected thigh to midline of film. Rotate leg internally 15 to 20 degrees to reduce the femoral anteversion. Leg must be in AP position with femoral epicondyles parallel to the table. Direct central ray to midshaft of femur. Take into account that the proximal and midfemur are in the lateral portion of the thigh. Optimal film size = 7 × 17 FFD = 40"	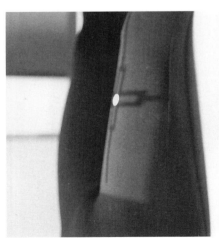	AP projection of the femur including knee and/or hip joint	Grid 75 to 85	20 to 40	Suspend respiration on exposure. Internally rotating legs allows better visualization of the femoral neck by reducing anteversion. Do not attempt to internally rotate the legs if femoral neck fracture is suspected. If femur is too long to fit on one film, include the knee joint and take a separate film of the hip. Shield gonads.
Lateral femur	Patient in lateral recumbent position on radiographic table with affected side down. Center the affected thigh to the midline of the film. Flex the knee approximately 35 degrees; femoral epicondyles should be perpendicular to the film. Direct central ray to the midshaft of the femur to include the knee. Optimal film size = 7 × 17 FFD = 40"	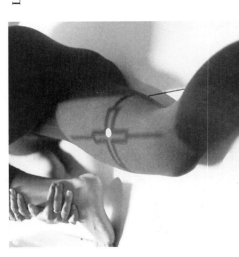	Lateral view of the femur to include the knee joint	Grid 75 to 85	20 to 40	Suspend respiration on exposure. Separate frog leg lateral of the hip may be included to obtain complete lateral of the femur. Shield gonads.

AP, Anteroposterior; *kV*, kilovolt; *mAs*, milliampere-seconds; *FFD*, focal film distance.

TABLE 4-21
Knee

BASIC STUDY: AP knee
Lateral knee
Open joint

View	Position		Structures	kV range	mAs range	Supplemental studies and technical tips
AP knee	Patient supine on radiographic table. Internally rotate the leg slightly (5 degrees). Central ray enters ½" below the apex of the patella with a 5-degree cephalic tilt. Optimal film size = 8 × 10 FFD = 40"	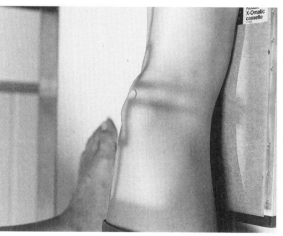	AP projection of the knee	Nongrid detail 60 to 65	20 to 40	If knee measures greater than 14 cm, should be done in bucky with high-speed film. The most common positioning error for the knee is to center too high; make sure central ray is entering the knee joint. Shield gonads.
Lateral knee	Patient in lateral recumbent position on radiographic table with affected side down. Center the affected thigh to the midline of the film. Flex the knee approximately 20 to 30 degrees; femoral epicondyles should be perpendicular to the film. Direct central ray to the knee joint, approximately 1" distal to the medial epicondyle with a 5-degree cephalic tilt. Optimal film size = 8 × 10 FFD = 40"	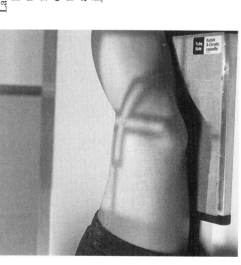	Lateral projection of the knee joint to include the distal end of the femur, the proximal end of the tibia and fibula, the patella, and patellofemoral joint	Nongrid detail 60 to 65	20 to 40	Knee should only be flexed 20 to 30 degrees because further flexion will tighten muscles and tendons, causing the patella to be drawn into the intercondylar sulcus. This may obscure diagnostic information such as fat pad displacement resulting from effusion. Shield gonads.

AP, Anteroposterior; *kV,* kilovolt; *mAs,* milliampere-seconds; *FFD,* focal film distance.

Continued

TABLE 4-2 I
Knee—cont'd

BASIC STUDY: AP knee
Lateral knee
Open joint

View	Position	Structures	kV range	mAs range	Supplemental studies and technical tips
Open joint (Homblad method) Patient kneeling on radiographic table. Place cassette against anterior surface of knee and flex the knee 70 degrees from full extension. The shaft of the femur should form a 20-degree angle with the central ray. Central ray enters the popliteal fossa. Optimal film size = 8 × 10 FFD = 40"	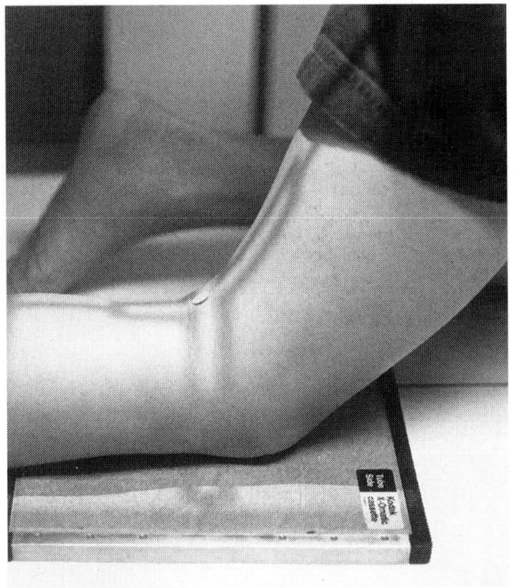	Intercondylar fossa, medial and lateral intercondylar tubercles of the intercondylar eminence in profile	Nongrid detail 65 to 70	20 to 40	A variation on the Homblad method includes resting the affected knee on a stool while patients support themselves against the radiographic table of film holder. The open joint view is helpful in evaluation for radiopaque loose bodies within the knee joint. Also useful in evaluation of femoral condyles in entities such as osteochondritis dissecans. Shield gonads. Alternate view is the Camp-Coventry method.
Open joint (Camp-Coventry method) Place patient in prone position on radiographic table. Flex the knee to a 40-degree angle and rest the foot on support. Direct the central ray perpendicular to the long axis of the leg, 40-degree caudal tilt, entering the popliteal fossa. Optimal film size = 8 × 10 FFD = 40"	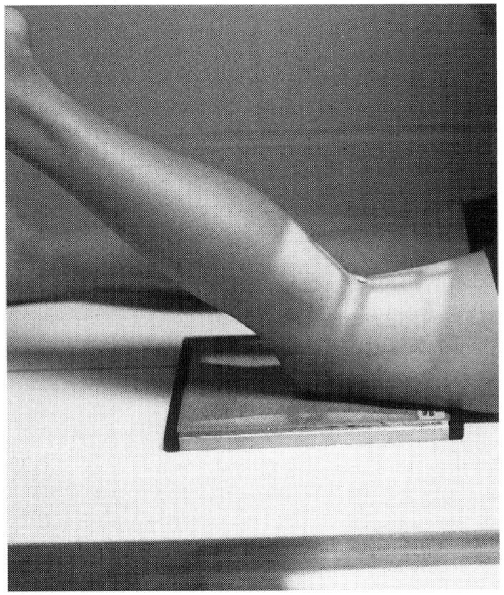	Intercondylar fossa, medial and lateral intercondylar tubercles of the intercondylar eminence in profile	Nongrid detail 65 to 70	20 to 40	The open joint view is helpful in evaluation for radiopaque loose bodies within the knee joint. Also useful in evaluation of femoral condyles in entities such as osteochondritis dissecans. Shield gonads.

Continued

Bilateral AP weight bearing

Patient with back against film holder. Center knees to film. Have patient stand with toes straight ahead and knees fully extended with weight equally distributed. Central ray to center of film midway between the knees at the level of the apices of the patellae.

Optimal film size = 14 × 17
FFD = 40"

Evaluates joint spaces of both knees. Also useful in evaluation of varus and valgus deformities of the knee joint

Grid
60 to 70

10 to 20

This view is useful in evaluation of the arthritic knee. Weight-bearing studies often reveal joint space narrowing that is not apparent on non–weight-bearing studies.
Shield gonads.

Axial patella (Settegast method)

Place patient in prone position on radiographic table. Flex the knee to a 90-degree angle and rest the foot on support. Direct the central ray perpendicular to the patellofemoral joint with a 10- to 20-degree cephalic tube tilt dependent upon the amount of knee flexion accomplished by patient.

Optimal film size = 8 × 10
FFD = 40"

Axial view of the patella and patellofemoral joint, including the intercondylar sulcus in profile. Will demonstrate vertical patella fractures

Detail
65 to 70

20 to 40

Acute flexion of the knee should not be attempted in this view until fractures of the patella have been ruled out by other projections.
If patient is unable to flex knee to 90 degrees, flex knee to 55 degrees and increase angle on central ray to 45 degrees.
Quadriceps femoris is contracted in this view, pulling the patella into the intercondylar sulcus, making evaluation of patellar subluxation difficult. Suspected patellar subluxation warrants use of Merchant's view.
Shield gonads.

TABLE 4-21
Knee—cont'd

BASIC STUDY: AP knee
Lateral knee
Open joint

View	Position	Structures	kV range	mAs range	Supplemental studies and technical tips
Merchant Patient supine with knees flexed 45 degrees over edge of table and resting on Merchant board support. Place knees together and secure legs below the knee. Place cassette in Merchant holder and direct central ray midway between the patellae with a 30-degree tube tilt. Optimal film size = 14 × 17 FFD = 40″	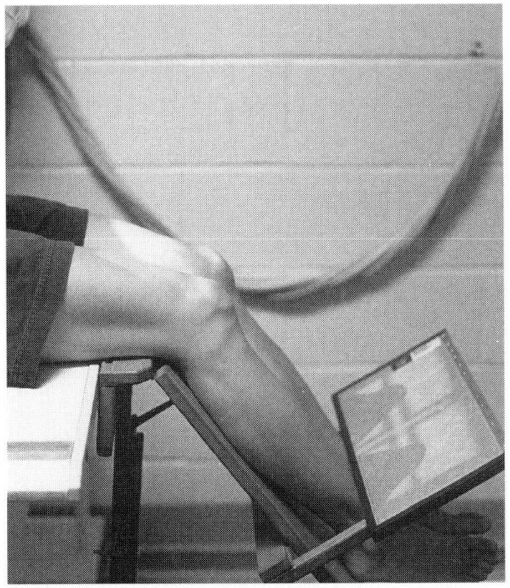	Bilateral axial projection of the patellae. Patellofemoral joint space without distortion of quadriceps femoris contraction	Nondetail 60 to 65	5 to 10	The quadriceps femoris muscle must be relaxed to aid in accurate diagnosis of patellar subluxation. Merchant board/film holder must be used to properly accomplish this radiograph. Shield gonads.
PA patella Patient prone on radiographic table. Center patella to film. Central ray enters popliteal fossa, passing through patella. Optimal film size = 8 × 10 FFD = 40″	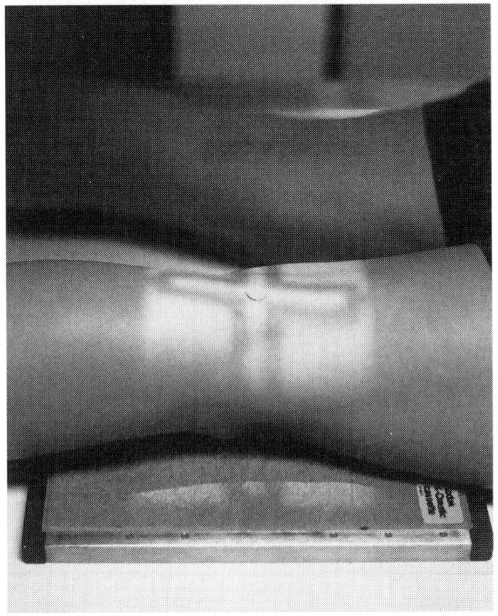	PA projection of the knee with better demonstration of the patella than in AP knee view	Nongrid detail 64 to 68	20 to 40	If potential fracture of the patella is present, do not place direct pressure on patella against radiographic table; provide support under thigh to minimize pressure or take film in AP knee position. Shield gonads.

Lateral patella
Patient in lateral recumbent position on radiographic table with affected side down. Center the affected thigh to the midline of the film. Flex the knee approximately 20 to 30 degrees; femoral epicondyles should be perpendicular to the film. Direct central ray to the patellofemoral joint.
Optimal film size = 8 × 10
FFD = 40"

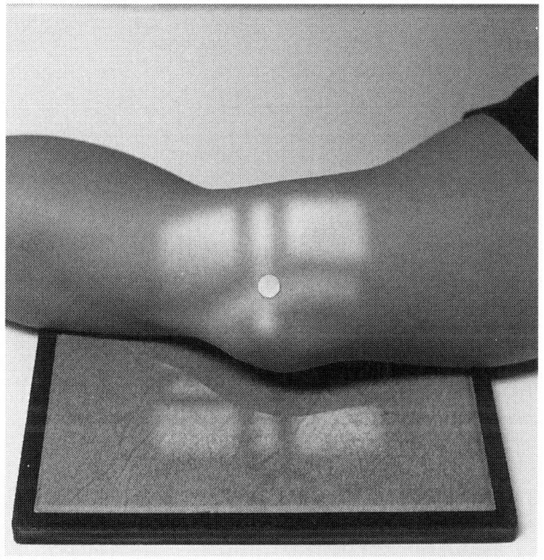

Lateral projection of patella and patellofemoral joint space

Nongrid detail 56 to 62

20 to 40

If potential fracture of the patella is present, flex knee only 5 to 10 degrees because further flexion may distract fracture fragments. Shield gonads.

PA, Posteroanterior.

TABLE 4-22
Tibia and Fibula

BASIC STUDY: AP leg
Lateral leg

View	Position		Structures	kV range	mAs range	Supplemental studies and technical tips
AP leg	Patient supine on table with leg fully extended. Internally rotate leg 5 degrees and dorsiflex foot. Center leg to film to include both knee and ankle joints. If unable to include both joints, center film to joint closest to area of interest. Direct central ray to midshaft of tibia. Optimal film size = 7 × 17 FFD = 40″	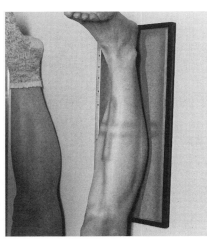	AP projection of the tibia and fibula	Nondetail tabletop 60 to 65	3 to 5	If fracture of the distal leg is discovered, it is important to include the proximal tibiofibular joint because it is common to have an accompanied fracture at this site. Anode should be over distal leg to take advantage of heel effect. A sandbag may be placed against ball of foot to aid in stabilization. Shield gonads.
Lateral tibia	Patient in lateral recumbent position on radiographic table with affected side down. Center the affected leg to the midline of the film in true lateral position with ankle in dorsiflexion. If unable to include both joints, center film to joint closest to area of interest. Central ray enters the midshaft of the tibia. Optimal film size = 7 × 17 FFD = 40″	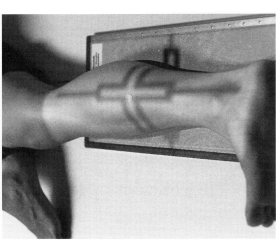	Lateral projection of the tibia and fibula	Nondetail tabletop 60 to 65	3 to 5	If fracture of the distal leg is discovered, it is important to include the proximal tibiofibular joint because it is common to have an accompanied fracture at this site. Anode should be over distal leg to take advantage of heel effect. Shield gonads.

AP, Anteroposterior; *kV,* kilovolt; *mAs,* milliampere-seconds; *FFD,* focal film distance.

TABLE 4-23
Ankle

BASIC STUDY: AP ankle
Oblique ankle
Lateral ankle

View	Position		Structures	kV range	mAs range	Supplemental studies and technical tips
AP ankle	Patient supine on table with leg fully extended. Internally rotate leg 5 degrees. Dorsiflex foot so that plantar surface is perpendicular to the film. Center ankle joint to unmasked side of the cassette. Central ray enters the ankle joint. Optimal film size = ½ 10 × 12 FFD = 40″	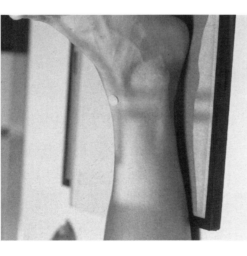	AP projection of the ankle joint, including distal tibia and fibula and proximal talus	Detail 65 to 70	15 to 30	Lateral portion of ankle mortise will not appear open on a true AP because the malleoli are not the same distance from the film in this position. If the lateral portion of the mortise joint appears open on a true AP, it is suggestive of spread of the ankle mortise resulting from rupture ligaments. Oblique view is done on other half of the film. Shield gonads.
Oblique ankle (Mortise view)	Patient supine on table with leg fully extended. Internally rotate leg 15 to 20 degrees until intermalleolar line is parallel to the film. Dorsiflex foot so that plantar surface is perpendicular to the film. Center ankle joint to unmasked side of the cassette. Central ray enters the ankle joint. Optimal film size = ½ 10 × 12 FFD = 40″	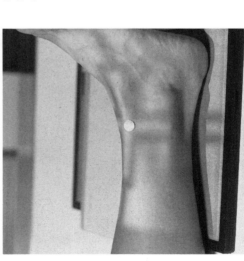	Ankle mortise without superimposition of the lateral malleolus on the talus	Detail 65 to 70	15 to 30	In cases of suspected ligament ruptures or instability, stress view may be accomplished. AP view is done on other half of the film. Shield gonads.

Continued

AP, Anteroposterior; *kV,* kilovolt; *mAs,* milliampere-seconds; *FFD,* focal film distance.

TABLE 4-23
Ankle—cont'd

BASIC STUDY: AP ankle
Oblique ankle
Lateral ankle

View	Position	Structures	kV range	mAs range	Supplemental studies and technical tips
Lateral ankle Patient in lateral recumbent position on radiographic table with affected side down. Center the affected ankle to the midline of the film in true lateral position in dorsiflexion. Central ray enters medial side of ankle joint. Optimal film size = 8 × 10 FFD = 40"	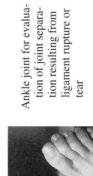	Lateral projection of the ankle joint to include the distal tibia and proximal fibula, proximal talus, calcaneus, and base of fifth metatarsal	Detail 65 to 70	15 to 30	Base of fifth metatarsal should be included on lateral ankle view because this is a common area of fracture in ankle inversion injuries. Shield gonads.
AP ankle inversion stress Patient supine on table with leg fully extended. Dorsiflex foot so that plantar surface is perpendicular to the film. Center ankle joint to cassette. Stabilize lower leg and with opposite hand, apply inversion stress to ankle. Central ray enters the ankle joint. Optimal film size = ½ 10 × 12 FFD = 40"	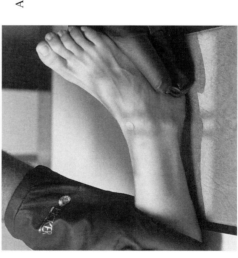	Ankle joint for evaluation of joint separation resulting from ligament rupture or tear	Detail 65 to 70	15 to 30	Stress should be applied only by physician because further damage to ankle ligaments may occur if too great a stress is applied. Physician should wear lead gloves and apron during exposure. Shield gonads.

TABLE 4-24
Foot

View	Position	Structures	kV range	mAs range	Supplemental studies and technical tips
AP foot	Patient supine on table with knee flexed and plantar surface of affected foot flat on cassette. Center foot to half of cassette. Central ray enters base of third metatarsal with a 10-degree cephalic tilt. Optimal film size = ½ 10 × 12 FFD = 40"	AP projection of the tarsals anterior to the talus, metatarsals, and phalanges	Detail 60 to 65	15 to 30	In patients with pes planus (flat feet), the cephalic angle may be reduced; in cases of pes cavus (high arch), the angle may be increased. Medial oblique foot is done on the other half of the film. Shield gonads.
Medial oblique foot	Patient supine on table with knee flexed and plantar surface of affected foot flat on cassette. Internally rotate the foot until the plantar surface forms a 30-degree angle to the cassette. Center foot to half of cassette. Central ray enters perpendicular to the base of the third metatarsal. Optimal film size = ½ 10 × 12 FFD = 40"	Joint spaces of the cuboid articulations, joint space between the navicular and talus, oblique projection of the metatarsals and phalanges, including the tuberosity of the base of the fifth. The sinus tarsus is well demonstrated on this view	Detail 60 to 65	15 to 30	Increasing the obliquity to 45 degrees may better demonstrate separation at the bases of the second to fifth metatarsals and in individual tarsals. AP foot is done on other half of the film. Shield gonads.

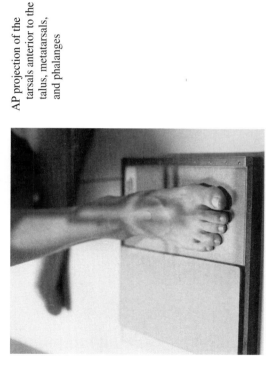

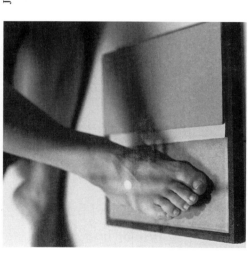

Continued

AP, Anteroposterior; *kV,* kilovolt; *mAs,* milliampere-seconds; *FFD,* focal film distance.

TABLE 4-24
Foot—cont'd

BASIC STUDY: AP foot
Oblique foot
Lateral foot

View	Position	Structures	kV range	mAs range	Supplemental studies and technical tips
Lateral foot	Patient in lateral recumbent position on radiographic table with affected side down. Center the affected foot to the midline of the film in true lateral position in dorsiflexion. Central ray enters first cuneiform. Optimal film size = 8 × 10 FFD = 40"	Lateral projection of the foot, ankle joint, and distal tibia and fibula	Detail 60 to 65	15 to 30	Cassette may be angled so that heel is in one corner and the toes in the opposite corner to allow entire foot to be included in study. In patients with larger feet, a 10 × 12 cassette should be used. Shield gonads.

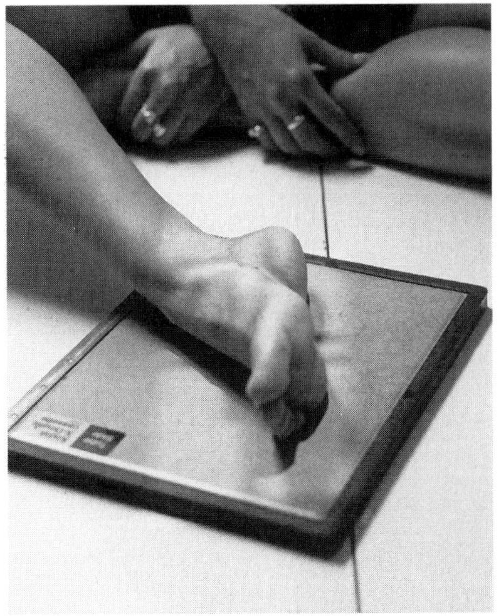

TABLE 4-25
Calcaneus

BASIC STUDY: Axial calcaneus
Lateral calcaneus

View	Position	Structures	kV range	mAs range	Supplemental studies and technical tips
Axial calcaneus Patient supine on table with leg fully extended. Dorsiflex foot so that plantar surface is perpendicular to the film. Patient may use loop around foot to assist in bringing foot into dorsiflexion. Center foot to half side of cassette. Central ray enters at the level of talocalcaneal joint with a 40-degree cephalic angle. Optimal film size = ½ 8 × 10 FFD = 40″	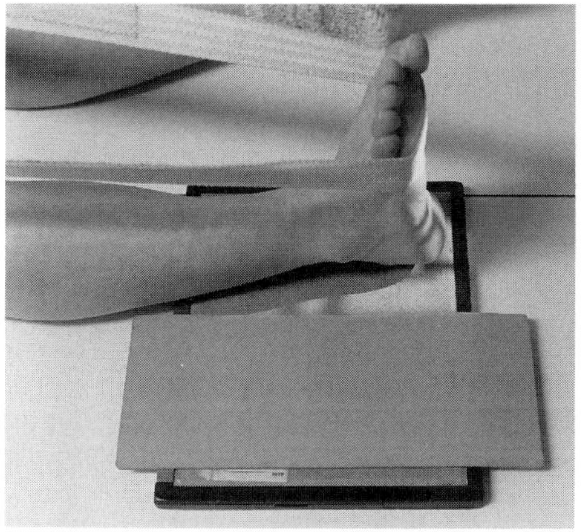	An axial projection of the calcaneus from the tuberosity to the talocalcaneal joint. The sustentaculum tali will appear to profile	Detail 65 to 70	15 to 30	Avoid rotation of the ankle; the base of the first or fifth metatarsals should not be visible on either side. Lateral calcaneus is done on other half of the film. Shield gonads.
Lateral calcaneus Patient in lateral recumbent position on radiographic table with affected side down. Center the affected heel to half of the cassette in true lateral position with ankle in dorsiflexion. Central ray enters 1″ below medial malleolus. Optimal film size = 8 × 10 FFD = 40″	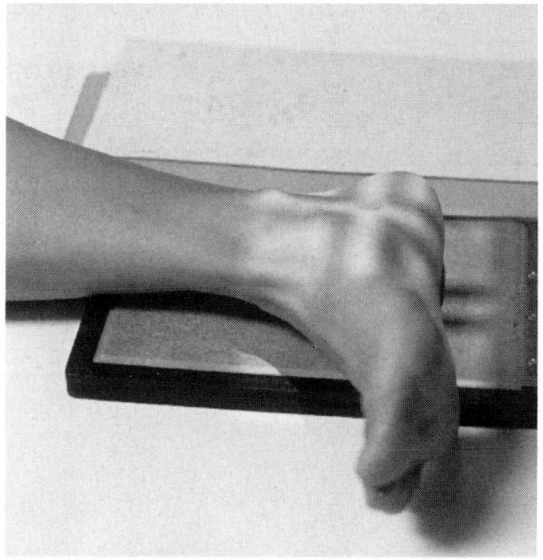	Lateral projection of the calcaneus to include the calcaneocuboid and talonavicular joint spaces	Detail 65 to 70	15 to 30	Axial calcaneus is done on other side of the film. Shield gonads.

kV, Kilovolt; *mAs*, milliampere-seconds; *FFD*, focal film distance.

TABLE 4-26
Abdomen—Acute Abdomen Series*

BASIC STUDY: AP abdomen supine
AP abdomen upright
PA chest

View	Position	Structures	kV range	mAs range	Supplemental studies and technical tips
AP abdomen supine Place patient in supine position, with knees flexed to relieve strain. Patient's hands are placed over the chest so that arms are out of collimator field. Center the cassette to the level of the iliac crest. Direct the central ray to the level of the crest. Optimal film size = 14 × 17 FFD = 40"		AP projection of the abdomen demonstrating size and shape of liver, spleen, and kidneys. Also demonstrates intraabdominal calcifications, bowel gas patterns, and evidence of tumor masses	Grid 70 to 80	40 to 60	Suspend respiration at the end of full expiration. Film should exhibit a long scale of gray (low contrast) to demonstrate outlines of internal organs. Shield gonads.
AP abdomen upright Place patient in upright position with back against film holder. Center the film 2" to 3" above iliac crest to include the diaphragm. Direct the central ray 2" to 3" above the crest. Optimal film size = 14 × 17 FFD = 40"		AP projection of the abdomen demonstrating size and shape of liver, spleen, and kidneys. Also demonstrates intraabdominal calcifications, bowel gas patterns, and evidence of tumor masses Upright will also demonstrate intraperitoneal free air under the diaphragm, as well as air fluid levels within the bowel	Grid 70 to 80	60 to 80	Suspend respiration at the end of full expiration. Diaphragm must be included in upright abdomen for evaluation of free air. If intraperitoneal free air is suspected clinically, lay patient in left lateral position for 10 to 20 minutes before performing upright radiograph. This position allows free air to rise into the area under the right hemidiaphragm, where it will not be superimposed by the gastric air bubble. If entire pelvic area cannot be included because of height of the patient, a second radiograph to include the bladder should be obtained. This view may be done on a 10 × 12 film. Shield gonads.

PA chest

Central ray to enter approximately the T6-T7 level. Film should be 2″ to 3″ above patient's shoulder. Hands on hips and roll shoulders forward. Elevate patient's chin.

Optimal film size = 14 × 17

FFD = 72″

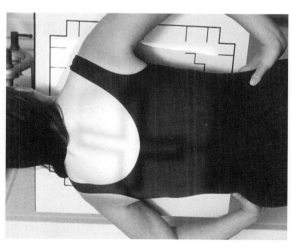

Lungs, including both apices, air-filled trachea, heart and great vessels, and diaphragm to include the costophrenic angles, bony thorax. The vertebral column behind the heart should be faintly visible

Grid
110 to 120

1 to 4

High kV technique is used to lower contrast in increasing scales of gray.

Study must be performed on full inspiration with 10 posterior ribs on the right visible. Poor inspiratory efforts will alter cardiothoracic ratio.

In suspected apical lesions or right middle lobe infiltrates, lordotic view may be performed to better define these areas.

Be sure to include diaphragm for evaluation of possible free air.

PA, Posteroanterior; *AP,* anteroposterior; *kV,* kilovolt; *mAs,* milliampere-seconds; *FFD,* focal film distance.

*Series used in cases of suspected bowel obstruction or perforation.

TABLE 4-27
Abdomen—Localization Series*

BASIC STUDY: AP supine abdomen / Oblique abdomen

View	Position	Structures	kV range	mAs range	Supplemental studies and technical tips
AP supine abdomen Place patient in supine position, with knees flexed to relieve strain. Patient's hands are placed over the chest so that arms are out of collimator field. Center the cassette to the level of the iliac crest. Direct the central ray to the level of the crest. Optimal film size = 14 × 17 FFD = 40″	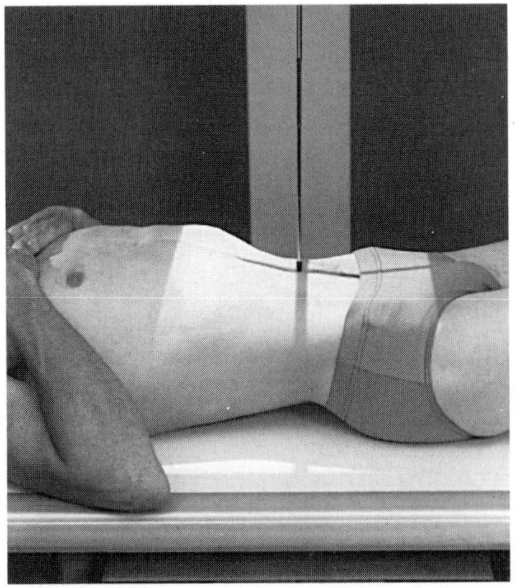	AP projection of the abdomen demonstrating size and shape of liver, spleen, and kidneys. Also demonstrates intraabdominal calcifications, bowel gas patterns, and evidence of tumor masses	Grid 70 to 80	40 to 60	Suspend respiration at the end of full expiration. Film should exhibit a long scale of gray (low contrast) to demonstrate outlines of internal organs. Shield gonads.
Oblique abdomen Place patient in supine position on radiographic table. Oblique patient toward affected side, elevating unaffected side 30 degrees from the tabletop. Patient's hands are placed over the chest so that arms are out of collimator field. Center the cassette to the level of the iliac crest. Direct the central ray to the level of the crest. Optimal film size = 14 × 17 FFD = 40″	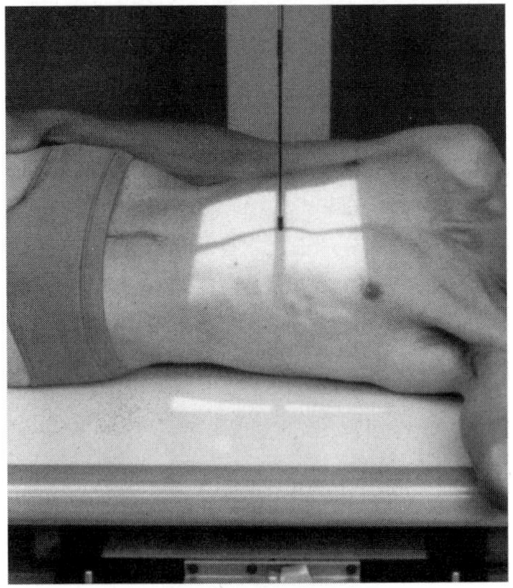	Oblique projection of the abdomen demonstrating aperpendicular renal shadow of the side down perpendicular, while the renal shadow on the elevated side will be projected in profile	Grid 70 to 80	40 to 60	Suspend respiration at the end of full expiration. Film should exhibit a long scale of gray (low contrast) to demonstrate outlines of internal organs. Helpful in localizing intraabdominal radiopacities. By placing the affected side down, anteriorly located radioopacities such as gallstones will be projected further away from the spine in the RPO position as compared with the AP abdomen. Posterior radioopacities such as kidney stones will be projected closer to the spine in the posterior oblique projection as compared with the AP abdomen. Shield gonads.

AP, Anteroposterior; kV, kilovolt; mAs, milliampere-seconds; FFD, focal film distance.
*Series used for localization of abdominal calcifications such as nephrolithiasis or cholelithiasis.

Anatomy

The second section of this chapter provides an overview of the anatomical structures emphasized on imaging studies.

Embryology

The fertilized ovum migrates down the uterine tube and implants itself on the uterine mucosa. Implantation is followed by a period of rapid mitosis, passing through morula, blastocyst, and two-layer (endoderm and ectoderm) embryonic disc stages. A portion of the ectoderm extends ventrally, proliferates, and gives rise to the mesoderm, which separates the endoderm and ectoderm.

The neural plate of the ectoderm involutes to form the neural tube (future spinal cord). A rod of cells, known as the *notochord,* is situated between the developing gut and neural tube. The notochord guides the development of the spine.

The dorsal portion of the mesoderm located on either side of the notochord begins to condense and segment into 42 to 44 pairs of somites (4 occipital, 8 cervical, 12 thoracic, 5 lumbar, 5 sacral, and 8 to 10 coccygeal). Within each somite exist cells that form the sclerotomal tissues (bone and dense connective tissues). These cells are guided by the notochord to form the vertebrae and ribs with further lateral migration to form the limb buds and extremities. The sclerotomal cells forming the vertebral bodies develop intervertebral fissures, filled with mesenchymal, that become the intervertebral disc. The notochordal elements within the disc become the nucleus pulposus. The somite also gives rise to myotomal (muscles) and dermatomal (dermis) structures.

Bone

BONE DEVELOPMENT

Bone functions to protect and support the body. Bone is a connective tissue and is composed of fibers, cells, and noncellular matrix material (ground substance). Bone is truly a remarkable substance that offers high tensile and compressive strength, while maintaining some degree of elasticity. Bone is a relatively lightweight and resilient tissue. Contrary to popular belief, bone is not dead; it is highly dynamic and metabolically active. Bone provides a storehouse of calcium, phosphorus, and other minerals. It is constantly remodeling; atrophy occurs in areas of understress, and hypertrophy in areas of overstress.

BONE COMPOSITION

Like any connective tissue, bone is composed of cells and matrix. The matrix is composed of fibers, inorganic salts, and ground substance. The fibers are mostly collagen; elastic fibers are minimal. Collagen fibers are present to a greater degree than in other tissues, giving bone strength and resiliency. Organic salts give bone hardness and rigidity. Organic salts are present in crystal as hydroxyapatite crystals, a form of calcium phosphate. The ground substance consists of glycosaminoglycans (GAGs), namely chondroitin sulfate, keratan sulfate, and hyaluronic acid.

BONE FORMATION

The cellular constituents and chemical reactions are the same for all bones formed in the body. Bone always forms by replacing some other preexisting material. The histogenesis of bone is dichotomized into bones that form in preexisting cartilage and bones that form from preexisting embryonic mesenchyme. The two types

of bone production are not mutually exclusive. Often, both processes may occur within the same bone. For instance, the femoral bone is lengthened by enchondral bone formation at its metaphyses, but increased width of the bone occurs from intermembranous bone in the periosteum.

Enchondral ossification

Enchondral bone formation represents bones formed in a hyaline cartilage template. This is the most common method by which bones form. Examples include the femur, tibia, vertebrae, and metacarpals. The process begins in centers of ossification located in the embryonic skeleton and continues into the late teen years. Lengthening of the bone occurs in the epiphyseal growth plate. Cells on the metaphyseal side are ossifying (zone of provisional calcification), and cells on the epiphyseal side are multiplying (zone of proliferation).

Intermembranous ossification

Intermembranous bone formation occurs when embryonic mesenchyme condenses into highly vascular connective tissue, which produces a thin layer of matrix and collagen. Peripheral connective tissue cells differentiate into osteoblasts, which produce additional matrix and collagen. Calcification of the matrix occurs, trapping the osteoblasts within the newly formed bone, thereby converting them to osteocytes. Examples include the mandible and bones of the cranium.

BONE STRUCTURE

Macroscopic structure. Inspection of a longitudinal section of a long bone reveals two different types of bone structure: compact (substantia compacta) and spongy (substantia spongiosa), or cancellous, bone. Compact bone is found at the outer border of a bone; cancellous bone is the latticelike network within a bone. Both compact and cancellous bone are lamellar. Woven bone represents immature bone, which will be replaced with lamellar bone over time.

A typical long bone is divided into a diaphysis (shaft), metaphysis, and epiphysis. The diaphysis is the central portion or shaft of the long bone, with a hollow inner medullary cavity (marrow cavity) encased by a thick, compact bony cortex. The ends of a long bone are capped by epiphyses, representing secondary centers of ossification.

In the immature skeleton, epiphyses are separated from the shaft of the long bone by a thin, cartilaginous epiphyseal plate. Cartilaginous epiphyseal plates are attached to the bony diaphysis by a transitional region, known as the *metaphysis.* The epiphysis and portions of the metaphysis contain a lattice of small bone spicules known as *trabeculae.*

In the adult, once the cartilaginous plates ossify, the medullary cavity of the diaphysis is continuous with the intertrabecular spaces of the metaphysis and epiphysis. At each end of the bone, a thin layer of articular cartilage covers the thin cortex of the epiphyses.

The periosteum represents a specialized connective tissue that covers the bone. It is composed of two layers: an inner layer with the ability to form bone through intramembranous ossification and an outer fibrous layer that anchors into the compact bone by Sharpey's fibers. Periosteum does not cover the ends of the bone where articular cartilage exists, nor does it extend under joint capsules. The femoral neck and talus are examples of bone structures that lack periosteum. Clinically, fractures in these areas heal more precariously because of the absence of the osteogenic capabilities of the inner layer of the periosteum. Periosteum is also absent on

TABLE 4-28
Classification of Joints by Function and Structure

Classification	Description	Examples
Function		
Synarthrosis	Fixed joints, no motion	Skull sutures
Amphiarthrosis	Deformable joints, slight motion	Intervertebral disc
Diarthrosis	Free joints, wide range of motion	Knee
Structure		
Fibrous	Apposing elements are connected by fibrous tissue; no joint cavity	Skull sutures; teeth
Cartilaginous	Apposing elements are connected by hyaline cartilage (synchondrosis) or fibrocarcartilage (symphysis); no joint space	Costochondral, intervertebral disc
Synovial	Apposing elements are separated by a joint space, surrounded by a fibrous joint capsule, may contain articular disc or meniscus, and are lined by a synovial membrane	Knee, ankle, elbow

bones formed within tendons (i.e., sesamoids, patella) and at ligament and tendon insertions.

The medullary cavity and interspaces of the cancellous bone are lined with endosteum. Endosteum lacks the tough fibrous nature of the periosteum, but similar to the periosteum, it possesses osteogenic properties.

In the flat bones of the skull the cortex forms two thick layers of bone (inner and outer table), which sandwich an interposed layer of spongy bone (diploë). The periosteum is known as *pericranium,* and the inner surface of the bone is lined by dura mater.

Microscopic structure

Compact bone. The basic anatomic unit of compact bone is the *osteon.* An osteon consists of 4 to 20 lamellae surrounding a central osteonal canal. Osteocytes are located within lacunae found between adjacent lamellae. Adjacent osteocytes communicate through tiny canals extending radially from the lacunae, known as *canaliculi.* Blood vessels are found in the osteonal canals with radial branches extending through lateral canals to reach the periphery of the osteon. Between each osteon are partially resorbed or restructured osteons known as *interstitial systems.*

Cancellous bone. Cancellous bone does not form an orderly osteon, as compact bone. Cancellous bone is found in sheets or layers. Osteocytes are found in lacunae orderly aligned in rows. Osteocytes are nourished by nutrient diffusion through canaliculi. An osteonal system is not needed because of the proximity of the rich blood supply in the bone marrow.

Cells. Osteoblasts form bone; they produce the matrix and collagen fibers. Once the bone is formed, osteoblasts become trapped and are known as *osteocytes. Osteoclasts* are large multinucleated cells responsible for the breakdown of bone by secreting osteolytic enzymes.

Joints

Joints, or articulations, represent connections between adjacent skeletal structures. The connections are maintained by connective tissues. The movement of the joint is largely dependent upon its structure and the nature of surrounding connective tissues. Joints are classified by either their degree of motion or the type of intervening connective tissue (Table 4-28).

Anatomical Figures

Figs. 4-1 through 4-45 present normal anatomy by body region.

■ Anatomical Variants

Figs. 4-46 through 4-131 present anatomical variants by body region.

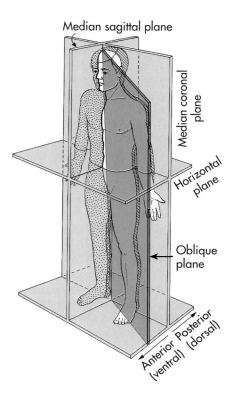

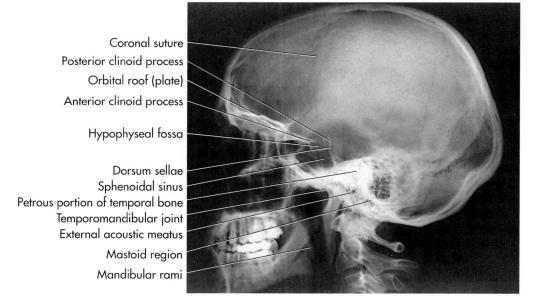

FIG. 4-1 Planes of the body. (From Ballinger PW: *Merrill's atlas of radiographic positioning and radiologic procedures*, ed 8, St Louis, 1995, Mosby.)

FIG. 4-2 Lateral skull. (From Ballinger PW: *Merrill's atlas of radiographic positioning and radiologic procedures*, ed 8, St Louis, 1995, Mosby.)

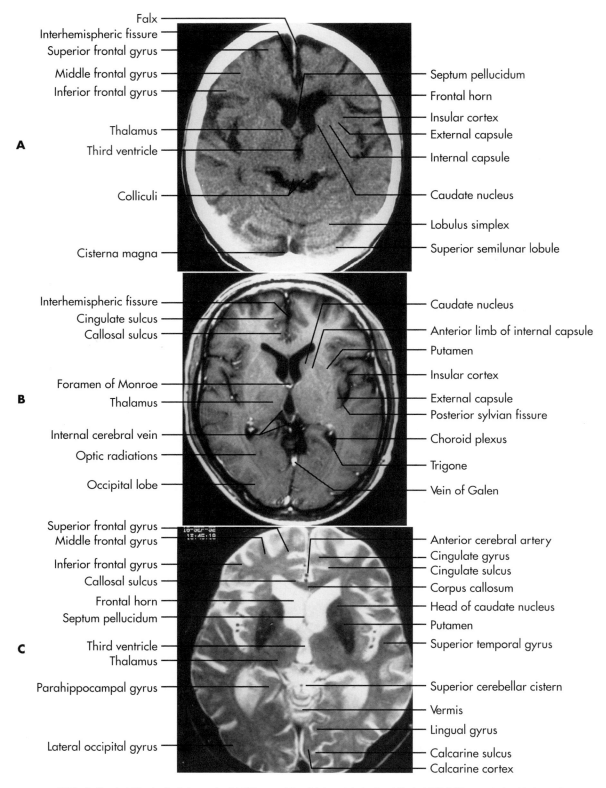

FIG. 4-3   Axial brain. **A,** Enhanced axial CT scan at the third ventricular level. **B,** Axial T1 MRI scan at the third ventricular level. **C,** Axial T2 MRI scan at the third ventricular level. (From Haaga JR: *Computed tomography and magnetic resonance imaging of the whole body,* ed 3, vol I, St Louis, 1994, Mosby.)

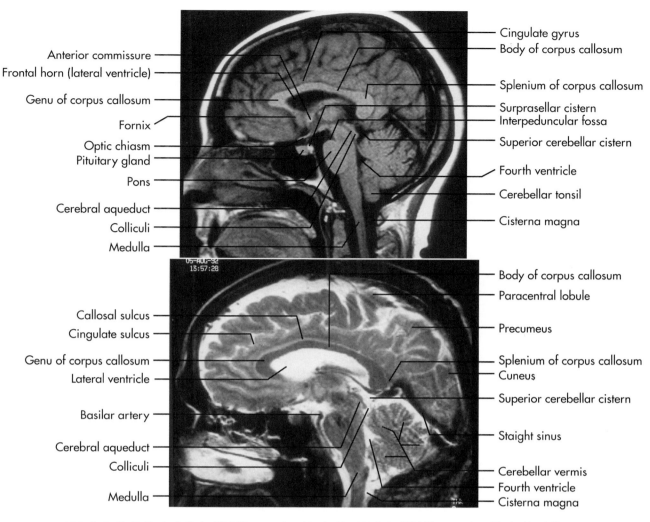

Anterior commissure

Frontal horn (lateral ventricle)

Genu of corpus callosum

Fornix

Optic chiasm

Pituitary gland

Pons

Cerebral aqueduct

Colliculi

Medulla

Cingulate gyrus

Body of corpus callosum

Splenium of corpus callosum

Surprasellar cistern

Interpeduncular fossa

Superior cerebellar cistern

Fourth ventricle

Cerebellar tonsil

Cisterna magna

Callosal sulcus

Cingulate sulcus

Genu of corpus callosum

Lateral ventricle

Basilar artery

Cerebral aqueduct

Colliculi

Medulla

Body of corpus callosum

Paracentral lobule

Precumeus

Splenium of corpus callosum

Cuneus

Superior cerebellar cistern

Staight sinus

Cerebellar vermis

Fourth ventricle

Cisterna magna

FIG. 4-4   Sagittal brain. **A,** Sagittal T1 MRI scan at the midsagittal level. **B,** Sagittal T2 MRI scan at the midsagittal level. (From Haaga JR: *Computed tomography and magnetic resonance imaging of the whole body,* ed 3, vol I, St Louis, 1994, Mosby.)

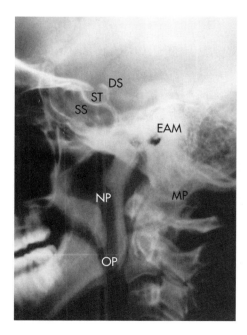

FIG. 4-5   Lateral skull and cervical vertebrae: *ST,* sella turcica; *DS,* dorsum sella; *EAM,* external auditory meatus; *SS,* sphenoid sinus; *NP,* nasopharynx; *OP,* oropharynx; *MP,* mastoid processes.

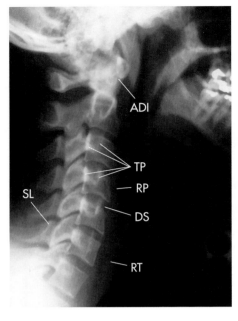

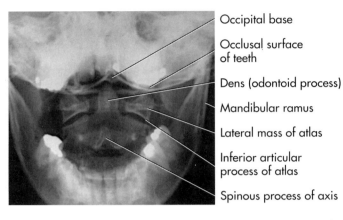

FIG. 4-6 Lateral cervical vertebrae: *ADI*, atlantodental interval; *TP*, transverse process; *RP*, retropharyngeal space; *RT*, retrotracheal space; *DS*, intervertebral disc space; *SL*, spinolaminar line.

FIG. 4-7 Open-mouth atlas and axis. (From Ballinger PW: *Merrill's atlas of radiographic positioning and radiologic procedures,* ed 8, St Louis, 1995, Mosby.)

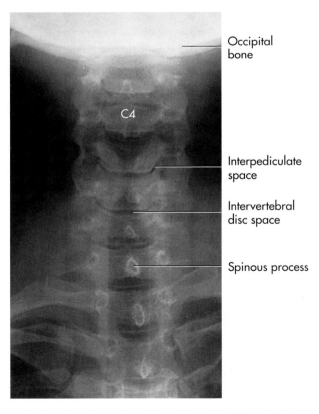

FIG. 4-8 AP axial cervical vertebrae. (From Ballinger PW: *Merrill's atlas of radiographic positioning and radiologic procedures,* ed 8, St Louis, 1995, Mosby.)

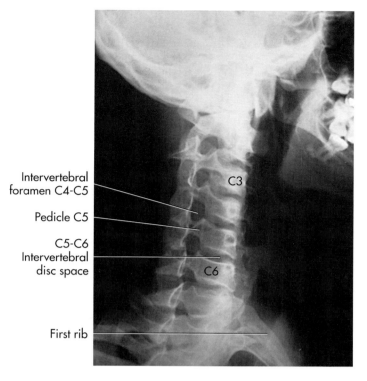

FIG. 4-9 AP axial oblique intervertebral foramina. (From Ballinger PW: *Merrill's atlas of radiographic positioning and radiologic procedures*, ed 8, St Louis, 1995, Mosby.)

Intervertebral foramen C4-C5

Pedicle C5

C5-C6 Intervertebral disc space

First rib

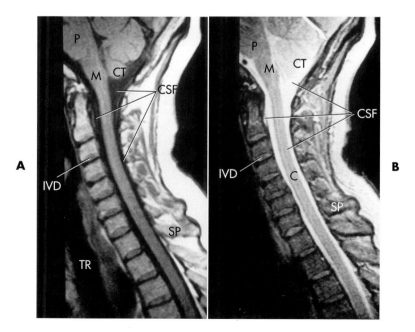

FIG. 4-10 Sagittal T1-weighted, **A,** and T2-weighted, **B,** MR images of the cervical spine: *P,* pons; *M,* medulla oblongata; *CT,* cerebellar tonsils; *CSF,* cerebral spinal fluid; *C,* cervical spinal cord; *IVD,* intervertebral disc; *TR,* trachea; *SP,* spinous process.

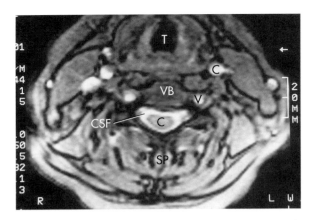

FIG. 4-11   Axial T2-weighted cervical MR image: *T*, trachea; *C*, carotid artery; *V*, vertebral artery; *VB*, vertebral body; *C*, cervical spinal cord; *CSF*, cerebral spinal fluid; *SP*, spinous process.

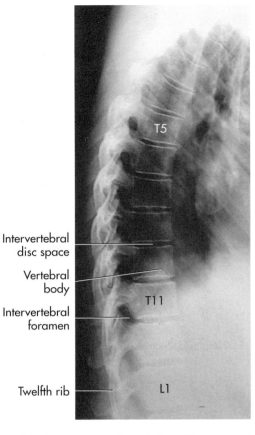

FIG. 4-12   Lateral thoracic spine. (From Ballinger PW: *Merrill's atlas of radiographic positioning and radiologic procedures,* ed 8, St Louis, 1995, Mosby.)

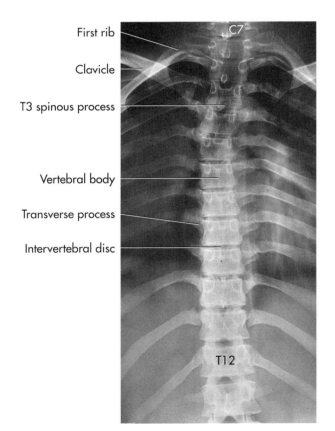

FIG. 4-13   AP thoracic spine. (From Ballinger PW: *Merrill's atlas of radiographic positioning and radiologic procedures,* ed 8, St Louis, 1995, Mosby.)

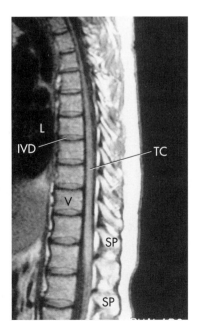

FIG. 4-14   Sagittal T1-weighted thoracic MR image: *L*, heart and lung; *IVD*, intervertebral disc; *V*, vertebral body; *TC*, thoracic spinal cord; *SP*, spinous process.

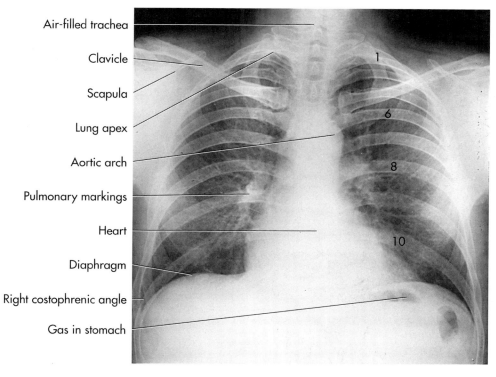

Air-filled trachea
Clavicle
Scapula
Lung apex
Aortic arch
Pulmonary markings
Heart
Diaphragm
Right costophrenic angle
Gas in stomach

1
6
8
10

FIG. 4-15 PA chest. (From Ballinger PW: *Merrill's atlas of radiographic positioning and radiologic procedures,* ed 8, St Louis, 1995, Mosby.)

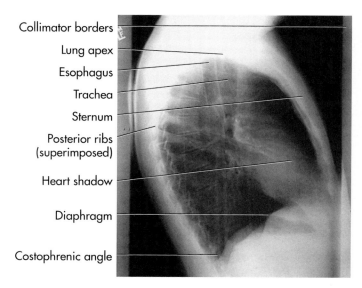

Collimator borders
Lung apex
Esophagus
Trachea
Sternum
Posterior ribs (superimposed)
Heart shadow
Diaphragm
Costophrenic angle

FIG. 4-16 Lateral chest. (From Ballinger PW: *Merrill's atlas of radiographic positioning and radiologic procedures,* ed 8, St Louis, 1995, Mosby.)

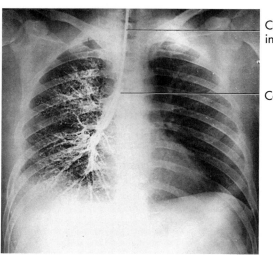

Catheter in trachea
Carina

FIG. 4-17 PA for right lung. (From Ballinger PW: *Merrill's atlas of radiographic positioning and radiologic procedures,* ed 8, St Louis, 1995, Mosby.)

PART ONE Introduction to Imaging

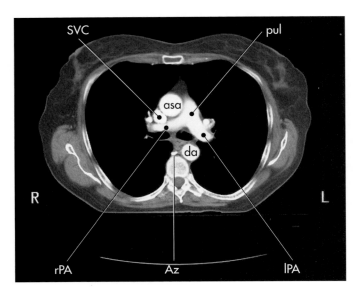

FIG. 4-18 Axial CT scan of chest with pulmonary trunk: *asa*, ascending aorta; *Az*, azygous vein; *da*, descending aorta; *lPA*, left pulmonary artery; *pul*, pulmonary trunk; *rPA*, right pulmonary artery; *SVC*, superior vena cava). (From Kelley LL: *Sectional anatomy for imaging professionals,* St Louis, 1997, Mosby.)

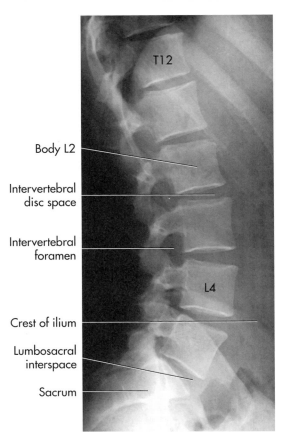

FIG. 4-19 Lateral lumbar spine. (From Ballinger PW: *Merrill's atlas of radiographic positioning and radiologic procedures,* ed 8, St Louis, 1995, Mosby.)

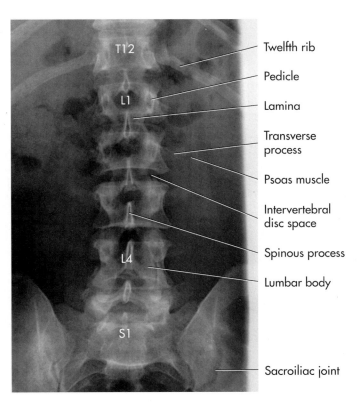

FIG. 4-20 AP lumbar spine. (From Ballinger PW: *Merrill's atlas of radiographic positioning and radiologic procedures,* ed 8, St Louis, 1995, Mosby.)

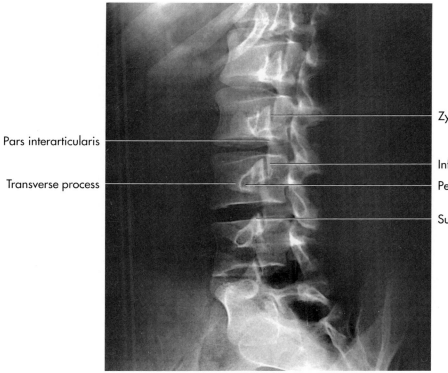

Pars interarticularis

Transverse process

Zygapophyseal joint

Inferior articular process

Pedicle

Superior articular process

FIG. 4-21 Oblique lumbar spine. (From Ballinger PW: *Merrill's atlas of radiographic positioning and radiologic procedures,* ed 8, St Louis, 1995, Mosby.)

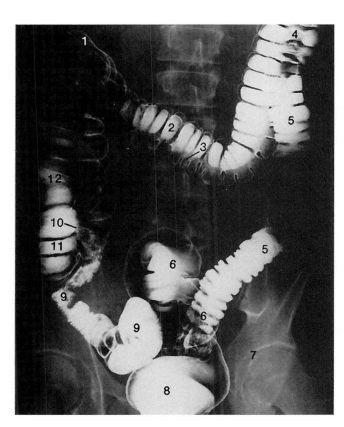

FIG. 4-22 Large intestine. *1,* Right colic (hepatic) flexure; *2,* transverse colon; *3,* sacculations; *4,* left colic (splenic) flexure; *5,* descending colon; *6,* sigmoid colon; *7,* hip joint; *8,* rectum; *9,* terminal ileum; *10,* ileocecal junction; *11,* cecum; *12,* ascending colon. (From McMinn RMH: *Color atlas of human anatomy,* ed 3, St Louis, 1993, Mosby.)

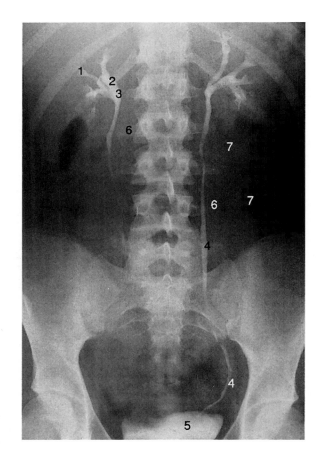

FIG. 4-23 Upper urinary tract. *1,* Minor calyx; *2,* major calyx; *3,* renal pelvis; *4,* ureter; *5,* bladder; *6,* transverse processes of lumbar vertebrae; *7,* psoas muscle. (From McMinn RMH: *Color atlas of human anatomy,* ed 3, St Louis, 1993, Mosby.)

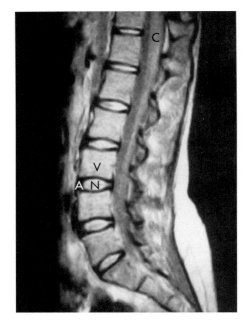

FIG. 4-24 Sagittal T1-weighted lumbar MR image: *C,* spinal cord; *V,* vertebral body; *A,* annulus fibrosus; *N,* nucleus pulposus.

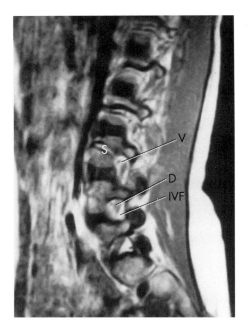

FIG. 4-25 Parasagittal T1-weighted lumbar MR image: *S,* segmental vessel; *V,* radicular vessel; *D,* dorsal root ganglion; *IVF,* intervertebral foramen with high signal intensity epidural fat.

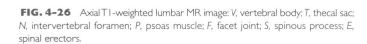

FIG. 4-26 Axial T1-weighted lumbar MR image: *V,* vertebral body; *T,* thecal sac; *N,* intervertebral foramen; *P,* psoas muscle; *F,* facet joint; *S,* spinous process; *E,* spinal erectors.

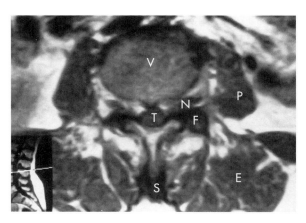

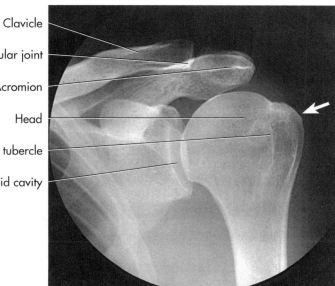

Clavicle

Acromioclavicular joint

Acromion

Head

Lesser tubercle

Glenoid cavity

FIG. 4-27 AP shoulder. (From Ballinger PW: *Merrill's atlas of radiographic positioning and radiologic procedures,* ed 8, St Louis, 1995, Mosby.)

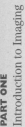

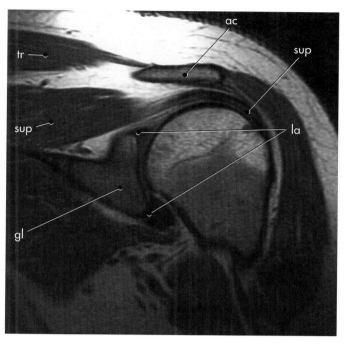

FIG. 4-28   Coronal oblique MR scan of shoulder with glenoid labrum: *ac,* acromion process; *gl,* glenoid; *la,* labrum; *sup,* supraspinatus; *tr,* trapezius. (From Kelley LL: *Sectional anatomy for imaging professionals,* St Louis, 1997, Mosby.)

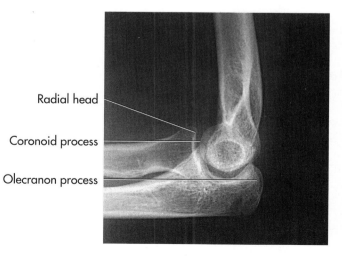

Radial head

Coronoid process

Olecranon process

FIG. 4-29   Lateral elbow. (From Ballinger PW: *Merrill's atlas of radiographic positioning and radiologic procedures,* ed 8, St Louis, 1995, Mosby.)

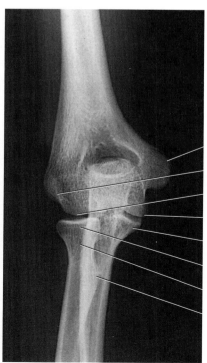

Medial epicondyle

Lateral epicondyle

Capitulum (capitellum)

Trochlea

Proximal ulna

Radial head

Radial neck

Radial tuberosity

FIG. 4-30   AP elbow. (From Ballinger PW: *Merrill's atlas of radiographic positioning and radiologic procedures,* ed 8, St Louis, 1995, Mosby.)

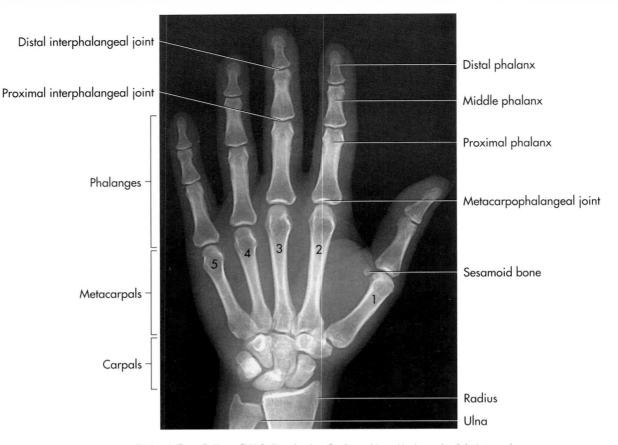

Distal interphalangeal joint

Proximal interphalangeal joint

Phalanges

Metacarpals

Carpals

Distal phalanx

Middle phalanx

Proximal phalanx

Metacarpophalangeal joint

Sesamoid bone

Radius

Ulna

FIG. 4-31 PA hand. (From Ballinger PW: *Ballinger's atlas of radiographic positioning and radiologic procedures,* ed 8, St Louis, 1995, Mosby.)

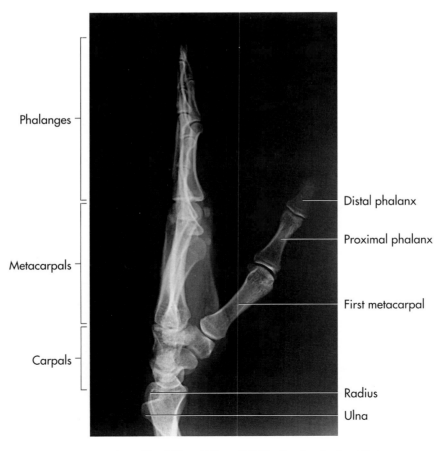

Phalanges

Metacarpals

Carpals

Distal phalanx

Proximal phalanx

First metacarpal

Radius

Ulna

FIG. 4-32 Lateral hand. (From Ballinger PW: *Merrill's atlas of radiographic positioning and radiologic procedures,* ed 8, St Louis, 1995, Mosby.)

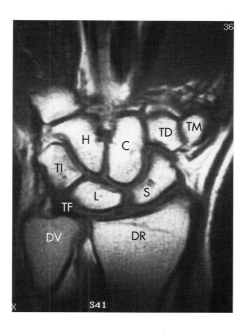

FIG. 4-33   Coronal wrist MRI: *DR*, distal radius; *DU*, distal ulna; *S*, scaphoid (navicular); *L*, lunate; *Tl*, triquetral; *TM*, trapezium; *TD*, trapezoid; *C*, capitate; *H*, hamate; *TF*, triangular fibrocartilage.

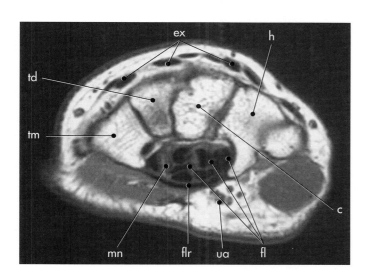

FIG. 4-34   Axial MR scan with neurovasculature of wrist: *c*, capitate; *ex*, extensor tendons; *fl*, flexor tendons; *flr*, flexor retinaculum; *h*, hamate; *mn*, median nerve; *td*, trapezoid; *tm*, trapezium; *ua*, ulnar artery. (From Kelley LL: *Sectional anatomy for imaging professionals*, St Louis, 1997, Mosby.)

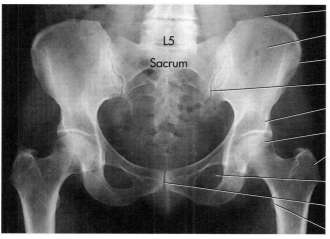

Crest of ilium

Wing of ilium

Anterosuperior iliac spine

Sacroiliac articulation

Anteroinferior iliac spine

Femoral head

Greater trochanter

Obturator foramen

Symphysis pubis

Lesser trochanter

FIG. 4-35   AP pelvis. (From Ballinger PW: *Merrill's atlas of radiographic positioning and radiologic procedures*, ed 8, St Louis, 1995, Mosby.)

PART ONE
Introduction to Imaging

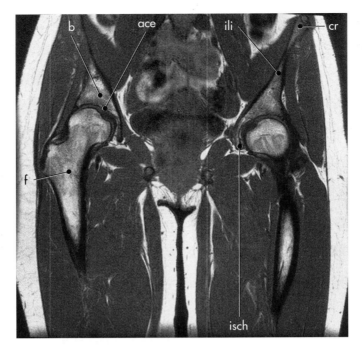

FIG. 4-36   Coronal MR scan of acetabulum: *ace,* acetabulum; *b,* body of ilium; *cr,* crest; *f,* femur; *ili,* iliac fossae; *isch,* ischium. (From Kelley LL: *Sectional anatomy for imaging professionals,* St Louis, 1997, Mosby.)

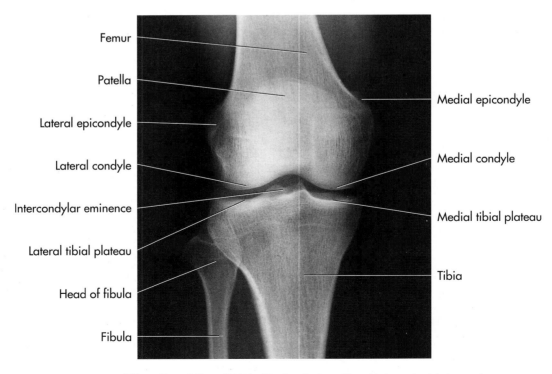

FIG. 4-37   AP knee. (From Ballinger PW: *Merrill's atlas of radiographic positioning and radiologic procedures,* ed 8, St Louis, 1995, Mosby.)

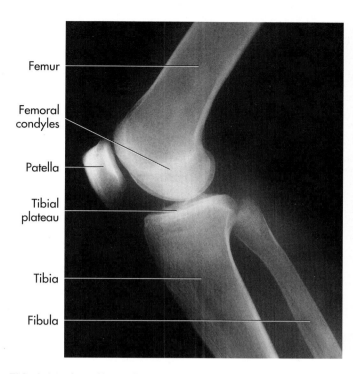

FIG. 4-38 Lateral knee. (From Ballinger PW: *Merrill's atlas of radiographic positioning and radiologic procedures*, ed 8, St Louis, 1995, Mosby.)

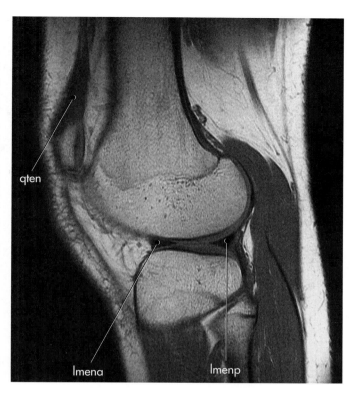

FIG. 4-39 Sagittal MR scan of knee with meniscus and ligaments of knee: *lmenp*, lateral meniscus posterior horn; *lmena*, lateral meniscus anterior horn; *qten*, quadriceps tendon. (From Kelley LL: *Sectional anatomy for imaging professionals*, St Louis, 1997, Mosby.)

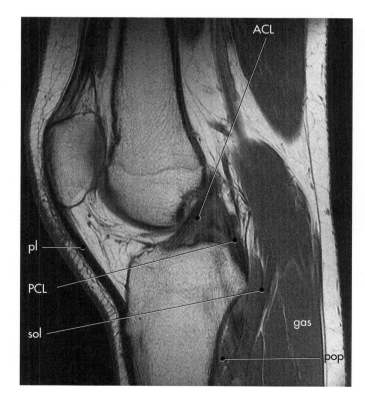

FIG. 4-40 Sagittal MR scan of knee with anterior cruciate ligament: *ACL*, anterior cruciate ligament; *pl*, patellar ligament; *PCL*, posterior cruciate ligament; *sol*, soleus muscle; *gas*, gastrocnemius muscle; *pop*, popliteus muscle. (From Kelley LL: *Sectional anatomy for imaging professionals*, St Louis, 1997, Mosby.)

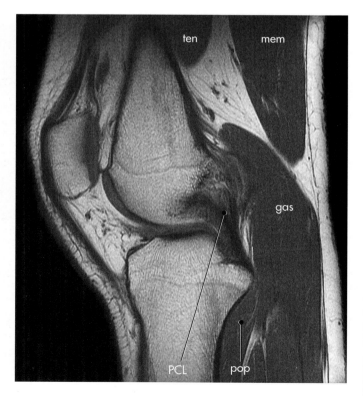

FIG. 4-41 Sagittal MR scan of the knee: *ten*, semitendinosus; *mem*, semimembranosus; *gas*, gastrocnemius; *PCL*, posterior cruciate ligament; *pop*, popliteus. (From Kelley LL: *Sectional anatomy for imaging professionals*, St Louis, 1997, Mosby.)

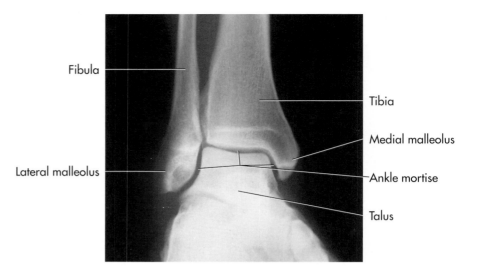

FIG. 4-42   AP oblique ankle, 15- to 20-degree medial rotation, for demonstration of the ankle mortise. (From Ballinger PW: *Merrill's atlas of radiographic positioning and radiologic procedures,* ed 8, St Louis, 1995, Mosby.)

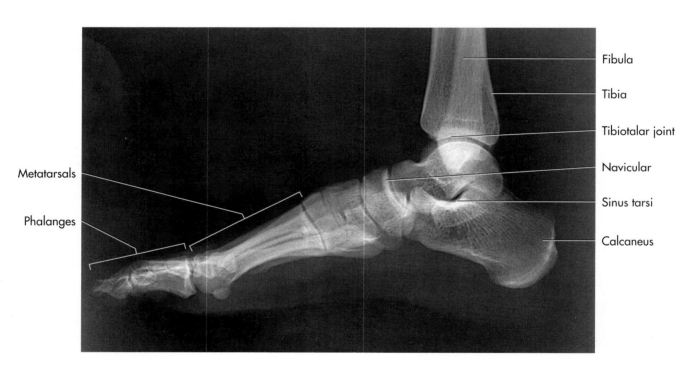

FIG. 4-43   Lateral foot. (From Ballinger PW: *Merrill's atlas of radiographic positioning and radiologic procedures,* ed 8, St Louis, 1995, Mosby.)

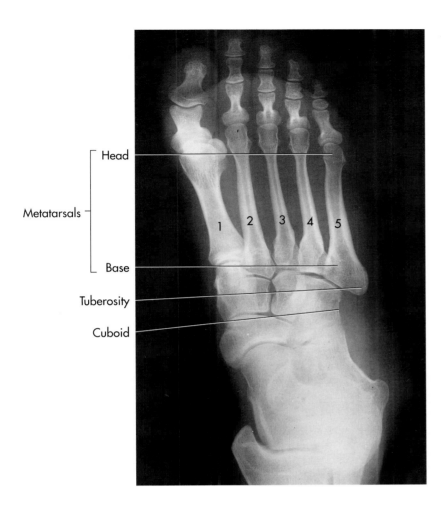

Metatarsals — Head

Base

Tuberosity

Cuboid

FIG. 4-44 PA oblique foot. (From Ballinger PW: *Merrill's atlas of radiographic positioning and radiologic procedures,* ed 8, St Louis, 1995, Mosby.)

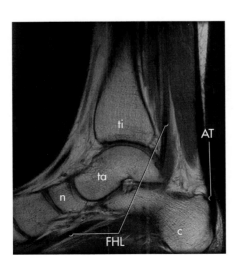

FIG. 4-45 Sagittal ankle MR scan of lower leg with posterior group of tendons: *ti,* tibia; *ta,* talus; *n,* navicular; *FHL,* flexor hallucis longus; *AT,* Achilles tendon; *c,* calcaneous. (From Kelley LL: *Sectional anatomy for imaging professionals,* St Louis, 1997, Mosby.)

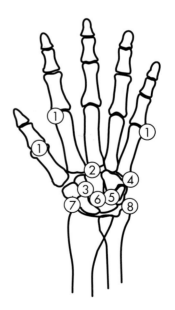

FIG. 4-46 Accessory ossicles of the hand: *1,* sesamoid bones; *2,* os styloideum; *3,* os centrale; *4,* os vesalianum manus; *5,* epipyramis; *6,* epilunatum; *7,* os radiale externum; *8,* os triangulare.

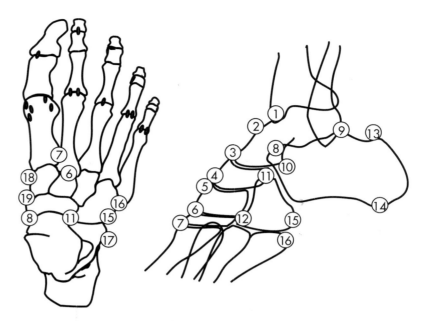

FIG. 4-47   Accessory ossicles of the foot: *1*, os talotibiale; *2*, os supratalare; *3*, os supranavic- ulare; *4*, os infranaviculare; *5*, os intercuneiforme; *6*, os cuneometatarsale; *7*, os intermetatarsale; *8*, os tibiale externum; *9*, os trigonum; *10*, calcaneus secundarius; *11*, secondary cuboid; *12*, os unci; *13*, os accessorium supracalcaneum; *14*, os subcalcis; *15*, peroneal bone (os peroneum); *16*, os vesalianum; *17*, os trochleare calcanei; *18*, sesamum tibiale anterius; *19*, os cuneonaviculare mediale.

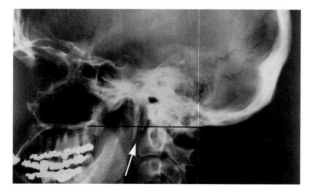

FIG. 4-48   Complete bony assimilation of C1 to occiput (occipitalization) and congenital basilar impression. This is diagnosed by observing the tip of the dens sig- nificantly above MacGregor's line (in this case more than 15 mm). This may be as- sociated with Chiari type 1 malformation, and MRI is often indicated. Note also the accessory ossicle inferior to the C1 anterior tubercle (*arrow*), not to be confused with the pro-atlas ossicle. Other normal variables here include calcification of the di- aphragma sella, of no clinical relevance and a prominent but normal diploic pattern.

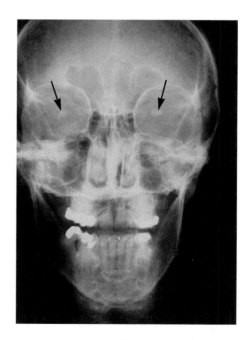

FIG. 4-49   Cataracts (*arrows*).

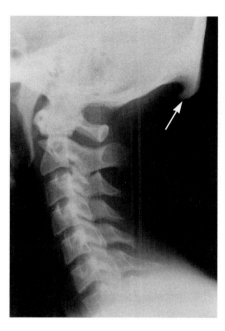

FIG. 4-50 Enlarged appearance of the external occipital protuberance (inion) *(arrow)*.

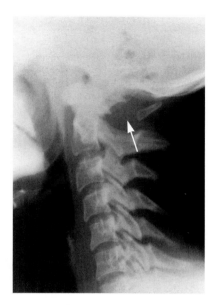

FIG. 4-51 Partial agenesis of the posterior arch of atlas *(arrow)*.

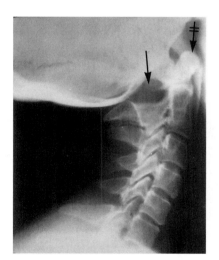

FIG. 4-52 Agenesis of the posterior arch of atlas *(arrow)* with compensatory sclerosis and hypertrophy of the anterior tubercle *(crossed arrow)*. Associated congenital nonsegmentation of C2-3. Note remarkable close approximation of occiput to C2 on this extension lateral view, without focal symptoms. Flexion/extension cervical projections would help in the assessment for associated instability.

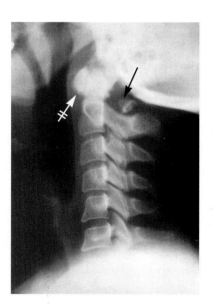

FIG. 4-53 Partial agenesis of the C1 posterior arch *(arrow)*. Increased stress transferred to the anterior tubercle results in sclerosis and hypertrophy *(crossed arrow)* similar to that seen more commonly with spina bifida occulta. The lucent defects are generally occupied by nonossified fibrocartilage. Note that the space available for the cord is narrowed to less than 15 mm, well below the lower limits of normal. MRI is indicated to assess for cord compromise.

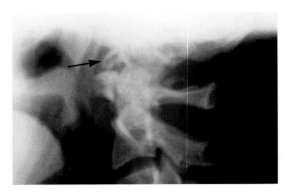

FIG. 4-54 Pro-atlas ossicle and posterior ponticle at C1 (arrow). The pro-atlas ossicle represents partial persistence of a lower occipital somite, a form of the so-called "third condyle."

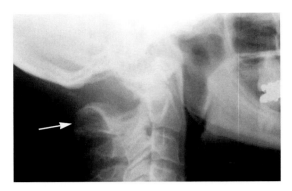

FIG. 4-55 Agenesis of the C1 posterior arch. In actuality the posterior tubercle of C1 has been assimilated to the C2 spinous process, creating the so-called "megaspinous" appearance (arrow).

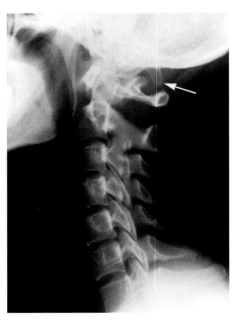

FIG. 4-56 Paracondylar process (arrow).

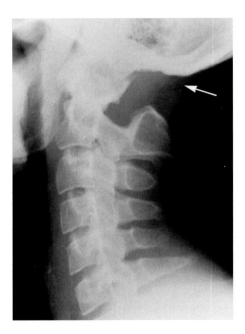

FIG. 4-57 Aplasia of the posterior arch of atlas (arrow).

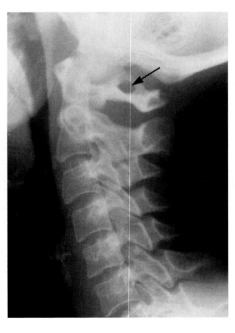

FIG. 4-58 Ponticulus posticus (posterior ponticle) (arrow).

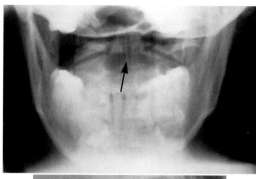

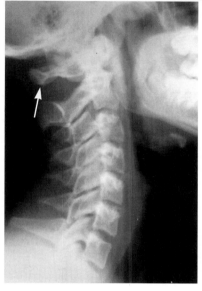

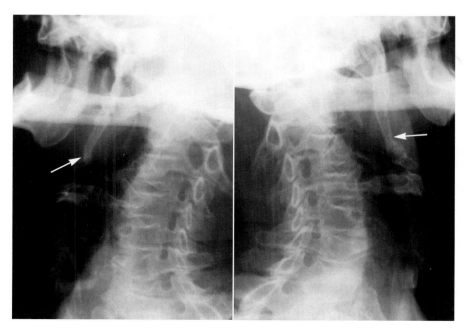

FIG. 4-60   Calcification of the thyroid cartilage *(arrowheads)* and carotid vessels *(arrows)*.

FIG. 4-59   Cleft dens and double spina bifida occulta of the atlas. Note bulbous, indistinct appearance of the anterior tubercle, characteristic of an anterior cleft of C1 *(arrows)*. The dens develops from two ossification centers, with persistence of a midline synchondrosis representing a rather rare anomaly.

FIG. 4-61   Ossification of the stylohyoid ligament *(arrows)*.

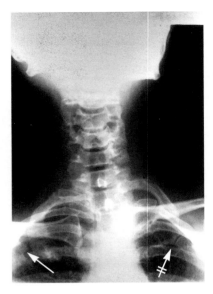

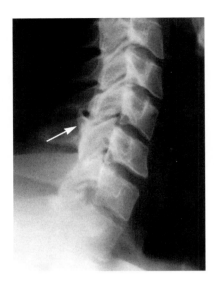

FIG. 4-62 Srb's anomaly. Accessory articulation between the left first rib and a prominent tubercle arising from the anterosuperior margin of the second rib *(crossed arrow)*. The mild left structural scoliosis is typical. Note severe uncovertebral arthrosis focally on the left at C5-C6. This 43-year-old cook had sudden onset of left upper extremity radiculopathy after reaching for and lowering a bag of potatoes from a shelf. It may be difficult to isolate the source of the radiculopathy because both the uncovertebral arthrosis and the Srb's anomaly could produce neurovascular compression syndromes of the upper extremity. Note also the prominent scalene tubercle at the superior margin of the right second rib, a prominent insertion for the anterior scalene muscle of no clinical significance *(arrow)*.

FIG. 4-63 Prominent tubercle at the origin of the semispinalis capitus, near the junction of the C6 articular pillar and lamina *(arrow)*. This may be mistaken for a large facet osteophyte or osteochondroma, but it is actually of no clinical significance.

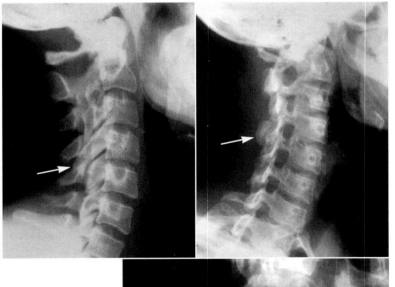

FIG. 4-64 Lateral **(A)**, oblique **(B)**, and pillar **(C)** radiographic projections demonstrating an unusual anomaly of the left C4 articular pillar, apparently representing partial duplication *(arrows)*. The differential diagnosis might include posttraumatic ossification, although there was no history of trauma in this 25-year-old female with no focal symptoms.

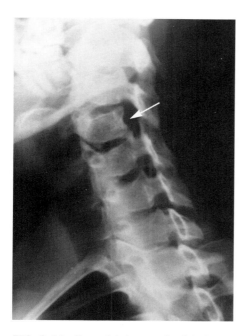

FIG. 4-65 Congenital absence of pedicle *(arrow)*.

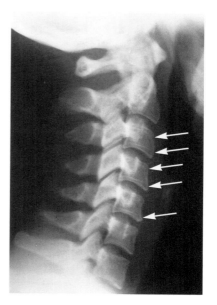

FIG. 4-66 Growth resumption lines in a normal healthy young adult *(arrows)*. These resemble the bone-within-a-bone appearance of osteopetrosis. Growth resumption lines, or "growth arrest" lines, which they were initially called, are more often seen in the metaphyses of long bones, generally bilaterally and symmetrically. These may be multiple, especially when there is cessation and resumption of growth because of exacerbation and remission of serious childhood illness. When found singly, they are typically an incidental finding of no clinical relevance.

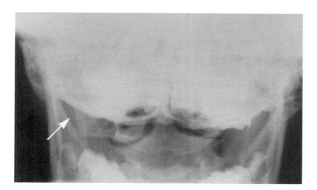

FIG. 4-67 Multiple craniovertebral junction and upper cervical anomalies. Note the right epitransverse process at C1 *(arrow)* and double spina bifida occulta of C1 in this 10-year-old female x-rayed for generalized neck pain following a motor vehicle accident.

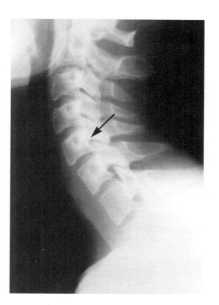

FIG. 4-68 Prominent posterior vertebral body scalloping *(arrow)*. More often seen in the lumbar spine, this may represent a developmental variant, but clinical correlation and advanced imaging may be necessary to rule out pressure erosion from such phenomena as cord or nerve root mass lesion, dural ectasia, or hydrocephalus.

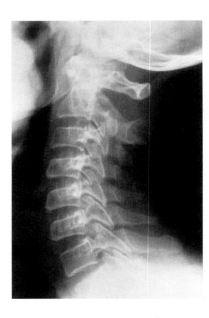

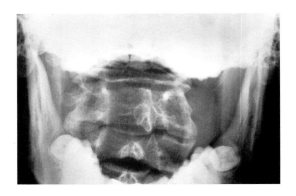

FIG. 4-70   Prominent but normal trabecular pattern in normal young adult female, which could resemble a permeative bone destruction or marrow infiltrative process.

FIG. 4-69   Marked developmental platyspondylia in a generally healthy 51-year-old male with neck pain and headaches. This should be a clinically insignificant, incidental finding.

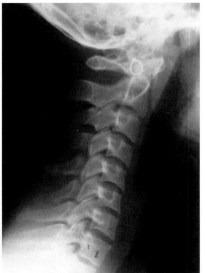

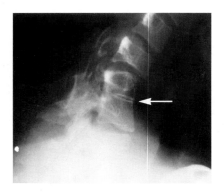

FIG. 4-71   Congenital nonsegmentation (block vertebra) C6-7 *(arrow)*. Note the rudimentary, nonfunctional disc space and fusion across the facet joints and laminae, along with a common spinolaminar junction line, but separate spinous processes. Lack of motion at this level may contribute significantly to development of instability at C5-6 on flexion. Hypermobility and early advanced degenerative changes are more common both immediately above and below a congenital nonsegmentation. Some have considered a single block vertebra to be a normal variant of no clinical relevance. However, this case refutes this idea and indicates the importance of consideration of altered biomechanics that may not be readily apparent on static plain films.

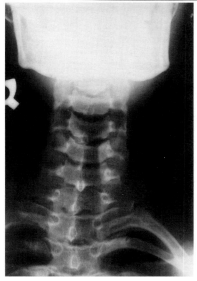

FIG. 4-72   Eight true cervical vertebrae. This is a rare segmentation anomaly, with the cervical spine demonstrating the least variability in segmentation of the three spinal regions.

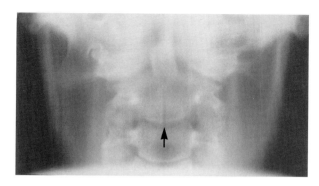

FIG. 4-73 Cleft dens and double spina bifida occulta of the atlas. Note bulbous, indistinct appearance of the anterior tubercle, characteristic of an anterior cleft of C1. The dens develops from two ossification centers, with persistence of a midline synchondrosis representing a rather rare anomaly.

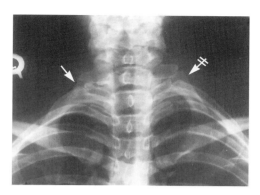

FIG. 4-74 Evidence of the transitional nature of C7. The right half of C7 resembles a C7 segment with a small cervical rib (arrow), whereas the left half resembles T1 with a well-formed thoracic-type rib (crossed arrow).

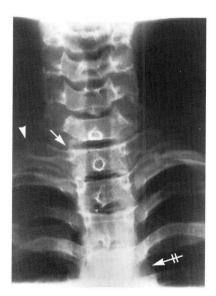

FIG. 4-75 Developmental asymmetry of the C7 uncinate processes, with hypoplasia on the right (arrow). The clinical relevance is questionable. Note also the normal persistent transverse process apophyses in the upper thoracic spine (arrowhead) in this 15-year-old male. The manubrium is superimposed on the upper thoracic spine (crossed arrow), frequently mistaken for an upper mediastinal mass.

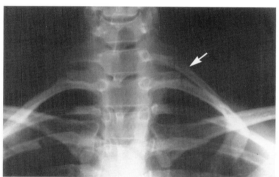
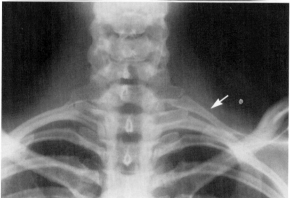

FIG. 4-76 Left cervical rib in two cases (arrows).

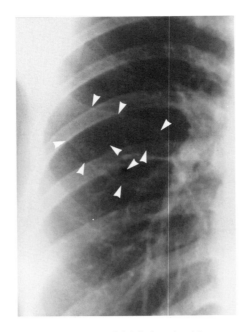

FIG. 4-77   Bifid rib *(arrowheads).*

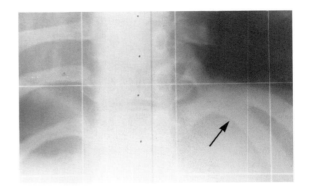

FIG. 4-78   Rib synostosis *(arrow).*

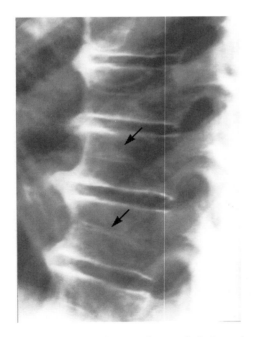

FIG. 4-79   Venous (Hahn's) clefts most often seen in the lower thoracic spine *(arrows).*

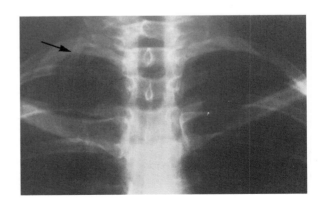

FIG. 4-80   Transitional first thoracic segment. Typically, T1 may be identified by the cephalically oblique orientation of its transverse processes, as opposed to the caudally oblique orientation of the transverse processes at C7. Taking note of this distinction is important in this case because the transitional T1 is somewhat ambiguous, bearing a cervical-type rib on the right *(arrow)* and a typical first thoracic rib on the left.

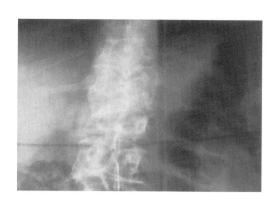

FIG. 4-81 Butterfly vertebrae at T12 and L2, with typical associated endplate anomaly at T11 and L1. The L2 butterfly vertebra is incomplete. Note only four true non–rib-bearing lumbar-type vertebrae.

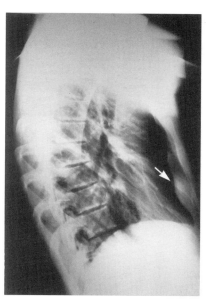

FIG. 4-82 Prominent internal thoracis muscle, which may be mistaken for a retrosternal soft tissue mass *(arrow)*. This will appear to be even more prominent with slight obliquity of the patient on the lateral view.

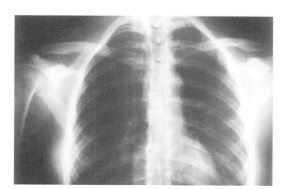

FIG. 4-83 Stress-related hypertrophy of the right clavicle and apparent hyperlucency of the right lung field resulting from agenesis of the right pectoral muscle (Poland's syndrome).

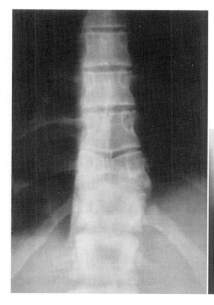

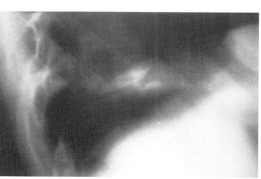

FIG. 4-84 Butterfly vertebra at T11 with typical anteriorly wedged vertebral body on the lateral view. Patient had been told this represented a compression fracture. This mistake may have been avoided, had there been an appreciation of the accompanying angular deformity of the adjacent vertebral endplates and slightly widened interpeduncular distance at T11, characteristic of a butterfly vertebra. This anomaly results from deficient central ossification related to incomplete notochordal regression.

PART ONE Introduction to Imaging

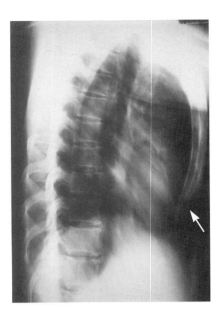

FIG. 4-85   Straight back syndrome. Marked thoracic hypokyphosis and pectus excavatum (invagination of the distal sternum) *(arrow)* narrows the anteroposterior dimension of the thorax. This may be associated with distortion and magnification of heart sounds to the anterior chest wall, which may mimic murmurs resulting from organic heart disease. The heart is typically displaced to the left and not actually compressed. Patients may be greatly relieved to know that their "heart problem" is functional rather than an intrinsic cardiac disease.

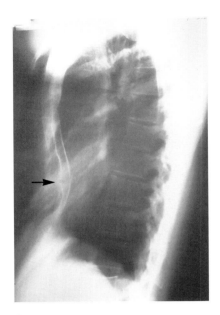

FIG. 4-86   Straight back syndrome. Typical plain film findings in a 29-year-old male with chronic back pain and report of infrequent heart palpations, discovered only upon directed questioning following the radiographs. The minimal anteroposterior thoracic dimension at the distal sternum was just over 5 cm. Pectus excavatum is also noted *(arrow)*.

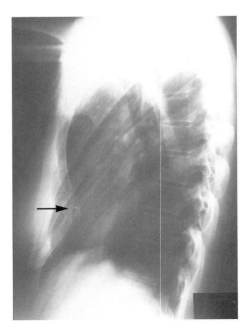

FIG. 4-87   Pectus excavatum *(arrow)*.

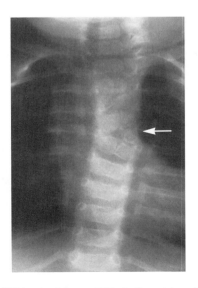

FIG. 4-88   Left T5 hemivertebra and T4 butterfly vertebra with mild left structural scoliosis *(arrow)*. Note 11 right ribs and 12 left ribs.

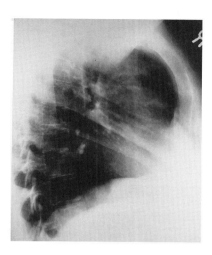

FIG. 4-89 Pectus carinatum (also known as "pigeon chest" or "keel chest").

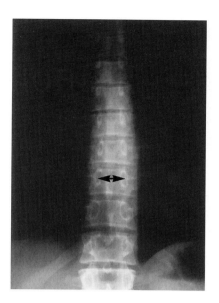

FIG. 4-90 Unusually small interpedicular distance *(arrows)*. At T8 and T9 this measured 16 mm. No obvious related signs or symptoms existed, and this presumably was of no clinical relevance. The term *strabismic*, or *hyperteloric*, vertebra may be used because "one-eyed," "winking," and "blind" are often used to to describe absence of one or both pedicle shadows.

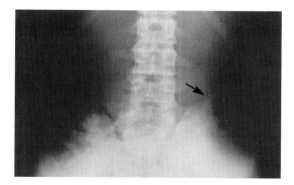

FIG. 4-91 Normal unfused iliac crest apophysis that has completed its "excursion" of ossification from the lateral iliac crest near the anterior superior iliac spine *(arrow)*. Full excursion without evidence of fusion indicates a Risser grade of 4+. The iliac crest is divided into four quadrants from lateral to medial, and the apophyseal excursion is graded based upon its relationship to these quadrants. As soon as any portion fuses to the parent ilium, a grade 5+ is given. This may be largely academic because a wide range of normal exists in terms of onset, progression, and fusion of the apophyseal ossification. In recent years, it has been determined that the Risser index is not the most accurate method for determining skeletal maturity. A more accurate method is to compare the posteroanterior view of the left wrist to the standard atlas of skeletal development like Greulich and Pyle's.[2] Note the pelvic unleveling on this upright film. A possible right lower extremity deficiency may be better assessed using a film performed at a 72-inch tube-to-film distance (TFD) and the central ray placed at the height of the femoral heads. This is only slightly less accurate than an orthoroentgenogram as a quick and inexpensive screen for a lower extremity deficiency (anisomelia).

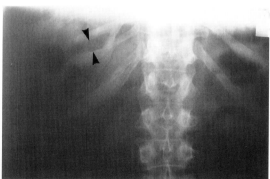

FIG. 4-92 Unusual lower rib anomaly with supernumerary rib and synostosis on the right at T11 and fenestrated rib (rib foramen) *(arrowheads)* at T12. No history of trauma existed, and the findings were noted incidentally on an AP lumbopelvic film obtained for low back complaints.

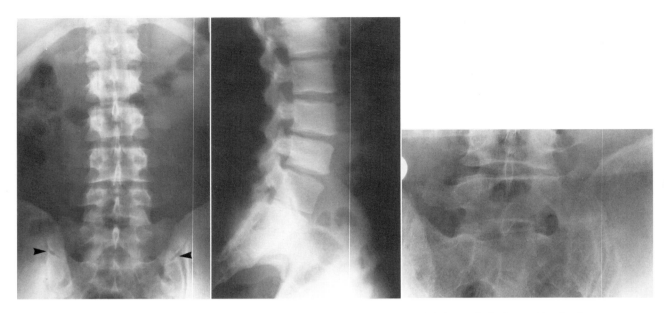

FIG. 4-93   Transitional L1 and lumbosacral segments with bilateral accessory articulations at the lumbosacral junction *(arrowheads)*. Note rudimentary lumbar ribs at L1 that are frequently described, incorrectly, as persistent transverse process apophyses or even mistaken for transverse process fractures. Describing the lumbosacral transitional segment as either a lumbar vertebra or a sacral segment is often arbitrary and subjective, especially where features are ambiguous, with approximately equal lumbar and sacral characteristics. Some might describe this as L6, and others as S1. Adding further confusion, authors have introduced the terms *lumbarization, sacralization, pseudolumbarization,* and *pseudosacralization.* It is clearer to simply designate the segments as L6 or S1 and thoroughly describe the morphology. The only transitional segment to be clearly associated with back pain (and an especially high incidence of disc lesions at the adjacent cephalic level) is one with a unilateral accessory articulation with the sacral ala. This type has been implicated in the so-called *Bertolotti syndrome,* in which there are sciatica and antalgic scoliosis in conjunction with the asymmetric transitional segment. Note the rudimentary transitional disc, which has been designated L6-S1. This is frequently mistaken for degenerative disc disease on the lateral view. Note also moderate degenerative disc space narrowing at L4-5 and L5-6 as well as hypoplasia and tropism (facet joint plane asymmetry) at the lumbosacral junction.

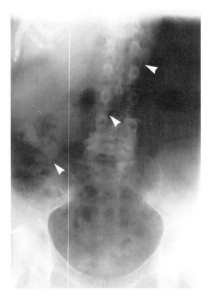

FIG. 4-94   Right breast shadow superimposed on the abdomen and mimicking hepatomegaly or an abdominal mass *(arrowheads)*.

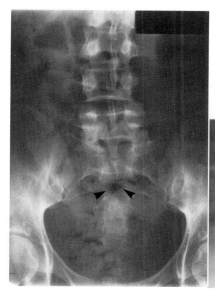

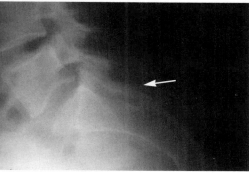

FIG. 4-95 Knife clasp (also known as *clasp knife*) deformity *(arrowheads)*. This consists of apparent elongation of the L5 spinous process resulting from assimilation of the upper sacral posterior tubercles, combined with spina bifida occulta of the upper sacrum. Note the variant here with a pseudoarthrosis in the midportion of the L5 spinous *(arrow)*.

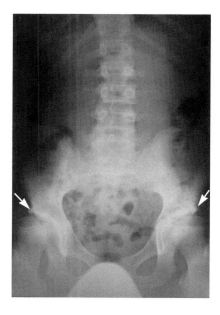

FIG. 4-96 Developmental dysplasia of the hips in a 16-year-old male, over-looked in infancy and early childhood *(arrows)*. This patient may have benefited from diagnostic ultrasound examination at birth.

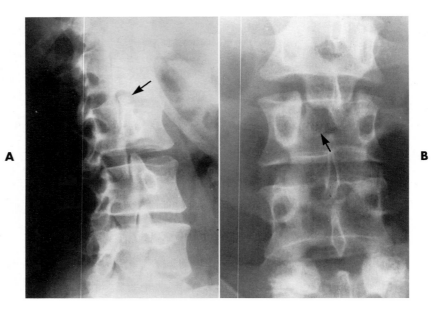

FIG. 4-97   Oppenheimer's ossicle. **A,** Persistent apophysis at the tip of the superior articular process of L2, typical in appearance but atypical in location *(arrow)*. Most of these are found at the tip of the inferior, rather than superior, articular process of a lumbar vertebra, **B** *(arrow)*. These resemble ununited fractures and may be multiple. Any relationship to symptoms, especially low back pain, is questionable.

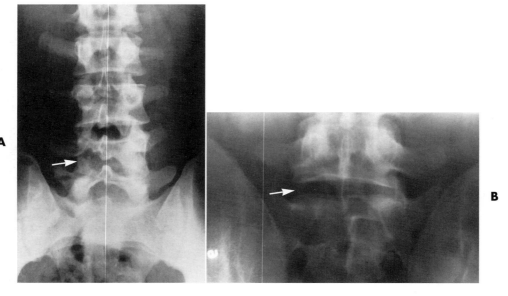

FIG. 4-98   A, Agenesis of right L4 inferior articular process *(arrow)*. **B,** Agenesis of the right L5 articular process *(arrow)*.

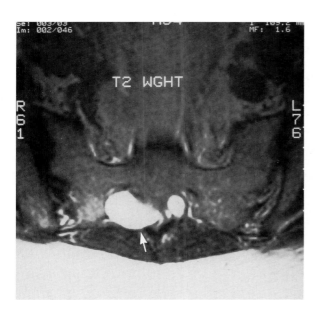

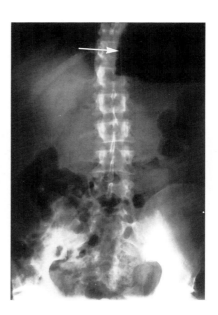

FIG. 4-99   Tarlov (perineural) cyst, cystic dilation of the right S2 nerve root sheath with associated long-standing pressure erosion of the adjacent sacrum *(arrow)*. Smaller Tarlov cysts are a common incidental finding on an MRI, but even larger Tarlov cysts may be completely asymptomatic. Others may produce signs and symptoms mimicking a disc lesion with compressive neuropathy. MRI is typically ordered in these cases with the request to "rule out herniated nucleus pulposus."

FIG. 4-100   Large gastric air bubble *(arrow)* and abundant large bowel gas in young adult male with no abdominal complaints.

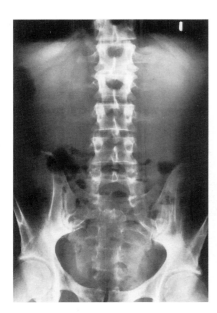

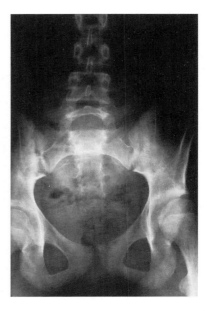

FIG. 4-101   Complete situs inversus. Asymptomatic adult male, with situs inversus discovered incidentally. Although a side marker is not visible, the identification blocker is on the left, the same side as the liver and opposite of the gastric air bubble. A consultation with the clinician was necessary to confirm that the blocker was, in fact, on the patient's left and that the film had been taken in the conventional anteroposterior projection.

FIG. 4-102   Marked physiological irregularity and apparent widening and sclerosis of the sacroiliac joints in a 14-year-old female. This may easily be mistaken for bilateral sacroiliitis of ankylosing spondylitis. The sacroiliac joints cannot be accurately assessed on plain film before age 16 and often even later in males. CT and MRI may be quite helpful in making an early diagnosis of ankylosing spondylitis, which frequently begins in the late teens and early twenties. Note also the normal ischial tuberosity apophyses.

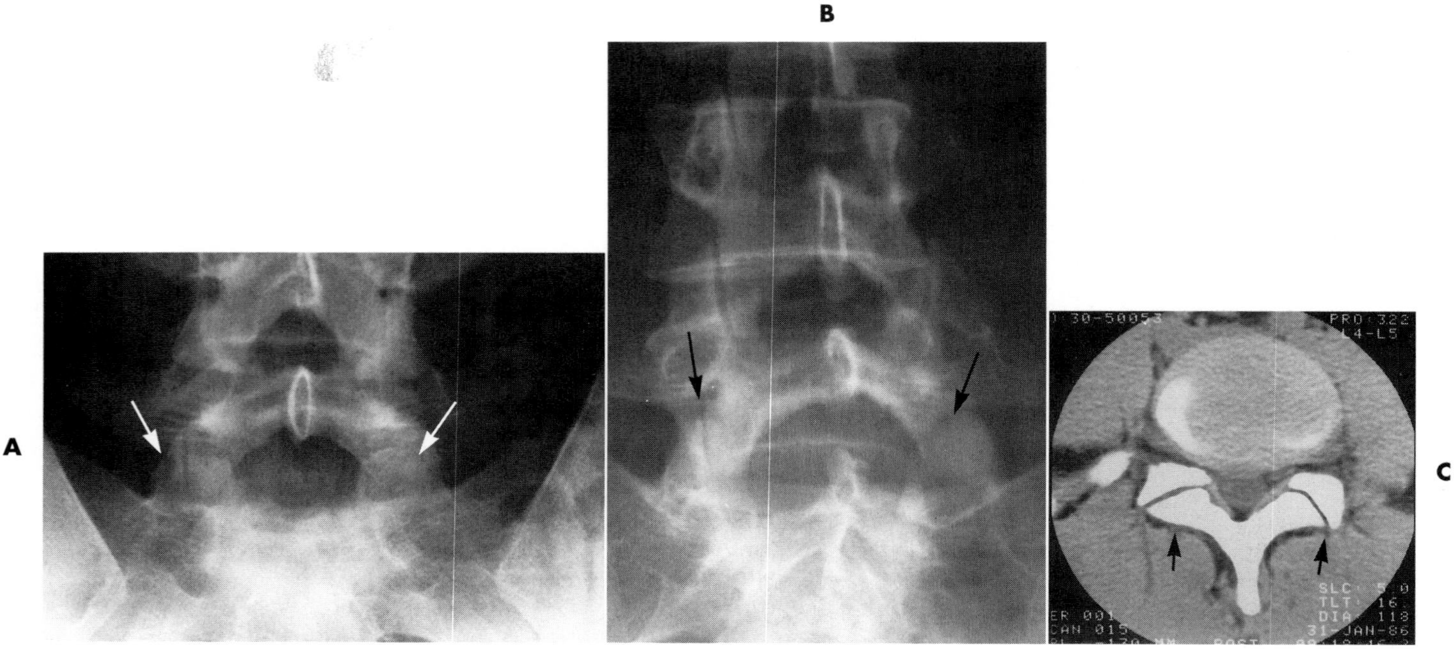

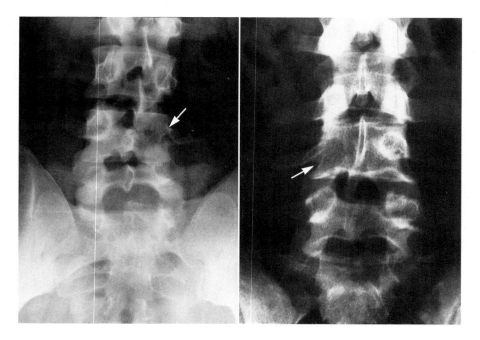

FIG. 4-103   Developmental facet joint plane asymmetry (tropism) noted on plain film (**A** and **B**) and CT (**C**) *(arrows)*. This is a common finding, much more accurately assessed on advanced imaging than on plain films, which are quite poor for assessing tropism. The clinical relevance of this finding has been debated, but there is still no evidence to clearly indicate that tropism in the lumbar spine represents an independent cause of low back pain. Tropism certainly must affect the biomechanics of the involved motion segment, but to what extent remains to be determined. Interestingly, evidence exists that facet joint tropism is developmental rather than congenital, with the actual planes of the facet joints being determined in the first years of life. Joint tropism is possibly influenced by stresses of early childhood, especially those related to crawling and, eventually, ambulation.

FIG. 4-104   Congenital absence of pedicle *(arrows)* with contralateral hypertrophy.

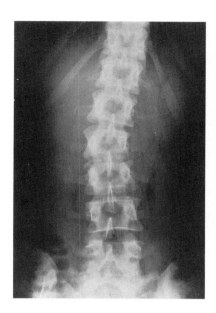

FIG. 4-105 Six lumbar vertebrae.

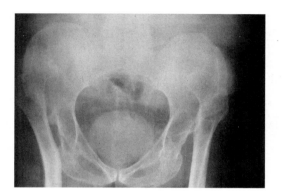

FIG. 4-106 Developmental dyplasia of the hip. A 62-year-old male with the most severe form (type 3) of development dysplasia of the hips. Note coxa valga and bowing of the femoral diaphyses resulting from altered weight-bearing and biomechanics. Remarkably little pain frequently results, but typical manifestations include restricted range of motion of the hips and a waddling, "Trendelenburg" gait.

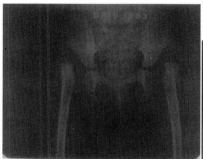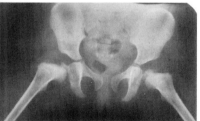

FIG. 4-107 Developmental dyplasia of the hip. Infant female postoperatively at 14 months. Note increased acetabular angles with shallow acetabula. Dislocation of the femoral heads superolaterally on the initial film has been successfully reduced. This study is from the 1950s. Today, diagnostic ultrasound is the most optimal study for identifying DDH in infants with positive dislocation/reduction orthopedic tests.

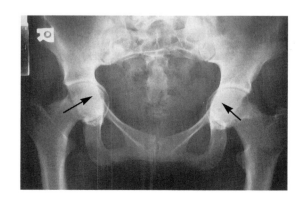

FIG. 4-108 Idiopathic protrusio acetabulum *(arrows)* in an 18-year-old female with premature osteoarthritis of the hips. Chronic hip pain was accompanied by markedly diminished range of motion. Idiopathic protrusio acetabulum is diagnosed after excluding bone-softening conditions, rheumatoid arthritis, or other underlying causes.

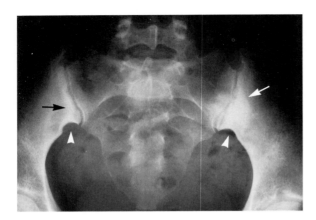

FIG. 4-109 Osteitis condensans ilii presenting as bilateral triangular radio-densities of the medial aspect of the ilia *(arrow)*. Also noted are bilateral grooves known as *preauricular* or *paraglenoid sulci (arrowheads)*. These grooves are believed to represent bone resorption secondary to stress on the anterior sacroiliac ligament, most often seen among parous women.

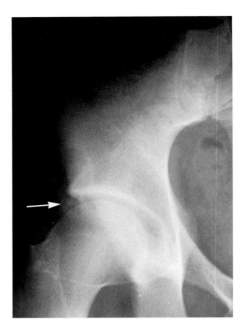

FIG. 4-110 Os acetabuli *(arrow)*.

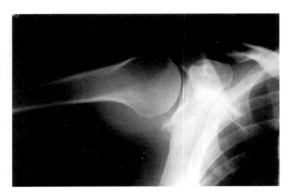

FIG. 4-111 Glenohumeral dysplasia. The glenoid appears to arise directly from the scapular body, without a neck, and is shallow and flat rather than concave. This predisposes to repeated glenohumeral dislocations and instability, as in this 46-year-old former boxer. Note the healed bony Bankart lesion just off of the inferior glenoid margin, evidence of a severe labral injury from previous anterior humeral dislocation.

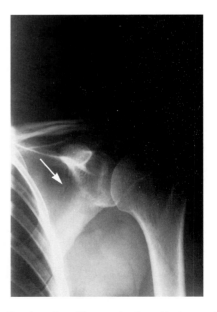

FIG. 4-112 Prominent, branching vascular channel in the scapula, which could be mistaken for a stellate (star-shaped) fracture line *(arrow)*. As with other flat or irregular bones, scapular fractures tend to be comminuted and stellate or complex in appearance.

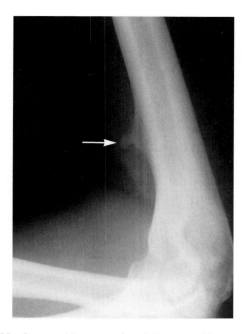

FIG. 4-113 Supracondylar process *(arrow)*. A supracondylar process is differentiated from an osteochondroma by its characteristic location and growth pattern toward the elbow joint. It may cause symptoms if fractured or if it becomes large enough to compress adjacent nerves or vessels.

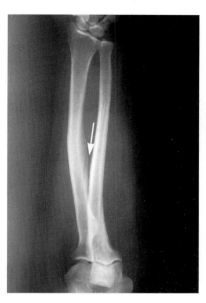

FIG. 4-114 Normal prominent channel for the nutrient artery in the radial diaphysis with normal, thickened appearance of the adjacent cortex *(arrow)*. This was misdiagnosed as a stress fracture, and multiple serial radiographs were performed unnecessarily. This might have been avoided by recalling the mnemonic "to the elbow I go and from the knee I flee." Nutrient channels are obliquely oriented such that it appears as if they are running from outside of the bone in toward the medullary bone of the metaphysis in the region of the elbow. This orientation is opposite to that in the lower extremities. As the nutrient channel appears to approach the knee, it "flees" from inside the bone to outside of the cortex, as if attempting to avoid the knee. This orientation does vary somewhat, but it is consistent enough to be frequently helpful in distinguishing nutrient channels from fractures.

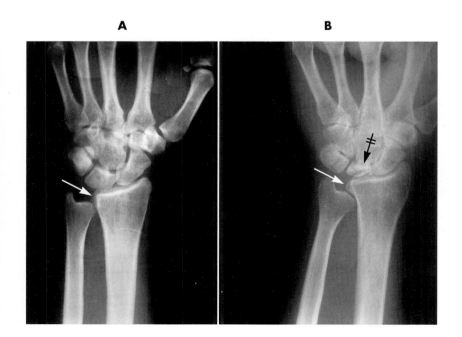

A   **B**

FIG. 4-115 Two cases of negative ulnar variance *(arrows)*. **A,** In the first case the ulnar is approximately 5 mm shorter than the radius. Although this finding is not necessarily clinically significant, a strong correlation exists between negative ulnar variance and avascular necrosis of the lunate as seen in the second case, **B** *(crossed arrow)*. As many as 75% of cases of lunate AVN have underlying negative ulnar variance. Orthopedic surgical shorting of the radius may be offered as a solution to this problem, attempting to either prevent AVN or lessen the progression and severity of symptoms in already established AVN. There may also be an association with tears of the triangular fibrocartilage complex (TFCC) in a so-called ulnar impingement syndrome.

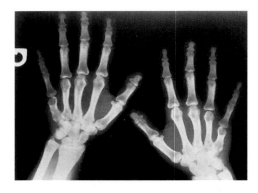

FIG. 4-116   Brachydactyly. Note developmentally short fifth metacarpals and first and third phalanges bilaterally and symmetrically, with resultant brachydactyly of the fifth ray bilaterally. The patient was normal clinically, except for short stature. The differential diagnosis includes an isolated congenital anomaly, pseudohypoparathyroidism and pseudopseudohypoparathyroidism. Note also spade-shaped distal phalangeal tufts, classically associated with acromegaly but also seen occasionally as an isolated normal variant.

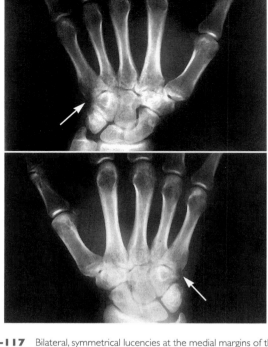

FIG. 4-117   Bilateral, symmetrical lucencies at the medial margins of the bases of the fifth metacarpals, mimicking erosions as in rheumatoid arthritis *(arrows)*. These are normal variants of no clinical relevance. This is not a common site for earliest erosions of rheumatoid arthritis, which locally favors the pisiform-triquetral joint and the ulnar styloid process.

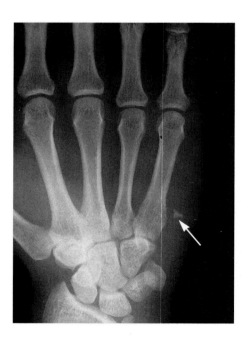

FIG. 4-118   Shard of glass located medial to the fifth metacarpal *(arrow)*.

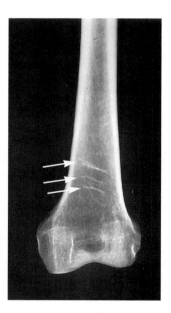

FIG. 4-119   Bone bars. These specimen radiographs of the femur demonstrate focally more prominent trabeculae described as *bone bars (arrows)*. These are of no clinical relevance but are often mistaken for growth resumption lines. They should be distinguished by their oblique orientation and the fact that they do not completely traverse the bone, as do growth resumption lines. Also unlike growth resumption lines, they may be seen outside of the metaphysis in the diaphyseal region. Bone bars are more prominent and more numerous in the presence of osteoporosis. They are not generally bilateral and symmetrical, another feature typical of growth resumption lines because of significant childhood illness.

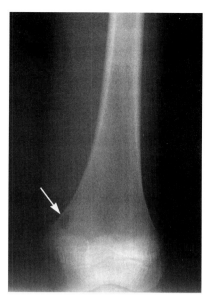

FIG. 4-120   Small fibrous cortical defect (FCD) in the distal femoral metaphysis of a 10-year-female *(arrow)*. It is estimated that as many as 50% of all individuals have at least one FCD during normal growth and development, most commonly around the knee. By definition, these will regress, usually prior to adulthood.

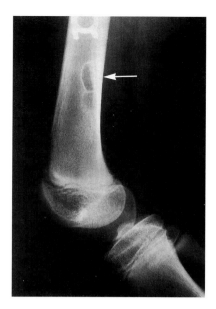

FIG. 4-121   An 11-year-old female with a small benign developmental fibrous lesion (fibroxanthoma) *(arrow)*. Similar larger lesions extending into the medullary bone and persisting into adulthood are termed *nonossifying fibromas,* whereas these smaller lesions confined to the cortex and regressing (converting gradually to normal bone, usually prior to skeletal maturity) are termed *fibrous cortical defects.* Commonly discussed along with benign tumorlike conditions, these are really not tumors but focal regions of developmental failure to convert fibrous osteoid matrix to bone. The lesions are painless, unless fracture occurs, and are usually found incidentally. These are especially common around the knee, particularly in the distal femoral metaphysis or metadiaphysis. Unless the lesion affects more than one third of the total cross-sectional area of the bone, it is unlikely to fracture and should be considered one of the "leave me alone" lesions of bone. Note the geographic nature of the lucency, which may demonstrate a "smoky," "washed out," or "ground glass" appearance similar to fibrous dysplasia. A well-defined thin cortical margin or "rind" of sclerosis and lack of cortical disruption, periosteal reaction, and soft tissue mass and geographic radiolucency all favor a benign rather than malignant process.

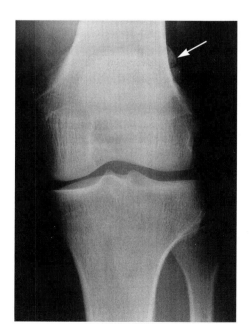

FIG. 4-122   Bipartite patella with a characteristic superolateral location of the secondary fragment *(arrow)*.

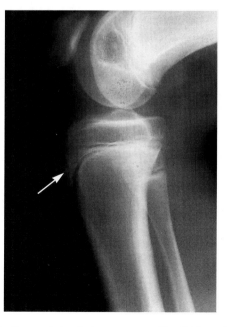

FIG. 4-123   Fragmented variant appearance of the tibial apophysis *(arrow)*. This appearance is not necessarily indicative of Osgood-Schlatter disease.

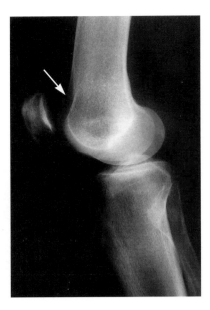

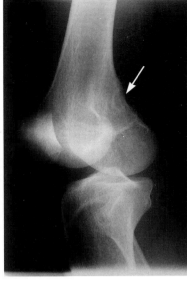

FIG. 4-124   Prominent developmental notch in the anterior aspect of the medial femoral condyle *(arrow)*. This could be mistaken for an osteochondral defect. Note also the fabella superimposed on the femoral condyle on the lateral view. This sesamoid bone in the lateral gastrocnemius tendon, could be mistaken for an intraarticular loose body, further confusing the condylar notch with osteochondritis dissecans. The fabella could also be mistaken for a bone island, superimposed on the lateral femoral condyle on an A-P view of the knee.

FIG. 4-125   Distal femoral cortical irregularity *(arrow)*. This stress-related developmental irregularity occurs at the posteromedial aspect of the distal femoral metaphysis at the site of the adductor magnus tendon insertion. This defect may demonstrate irregular margins, resembling an aggressive, spiculated periosteal reaction. In the past, this has resulted in unnecessary aggressive treatment, including amputation, resulting from misdiagnosis of osteosarcoma. Biopsy may further complicate things because of a reactive or "desmoplastic" appearance histologically that may be mistaken for neoplasm. Furthermore, focal tenderness may exist, especially in very active adolescents. The location of the irregularity is of supreme importance in rendering the correct diagnosis.

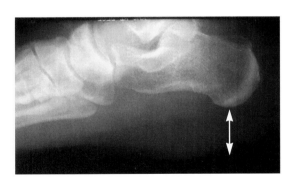

FIG. 4-126   Thickened heel pad *(arrows)* in obese 37-year-old female (measures just under 30 mm). Classically, a thickened heel pad has been associated with acromegaly or Cushing's syndrome. Heel pad thickness also tends to be greater in African-Americans than white individuals and in non–shoe-wearing populations, versus shoe wearers. The thickness increases with increased weight but tends to decrease slightly with age, although this is not statistically significant.[1]

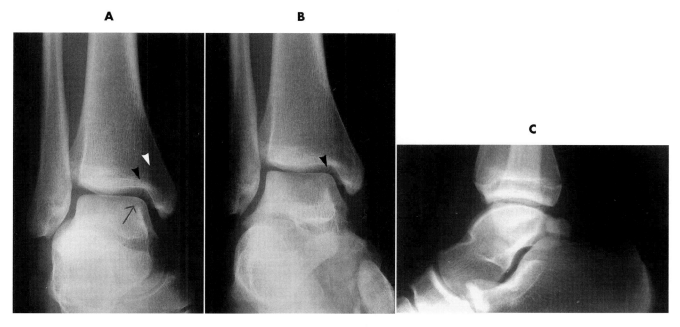

A **B** **C**

FIG. 4-127 Normal cleft distal tibial epiphysis in a 17-year-old female with recent inversion sprain *(arrowheads)*. An arrow drawn on the first film **(A),** from 1-15-93 indicates that the initial interpreter was convinced a subtle fracture of the medial malleolus. Both the soft tissue swelling and pain were mild, however. The patient was nevertheless casted, and follow-up films were obtained at 6 days, 18 days (not shown) and, finally, 40 days posttrauma. Obviously, the "fracture" has not changed, and the patient was casted unnecessarily **(B).** Consultation of a good atlas of normal radiographic variants could have avoided this mistake. The same patient had an os trigonum **(C),** an ununited apophysis of the posterior process of the talus. This may also be mistaken for a fracture and, in fact, occasionally may result from acute or stress fracture. This is most often related to forced plantar flexion, as in athletes involved in kicking sports, especially soccer.

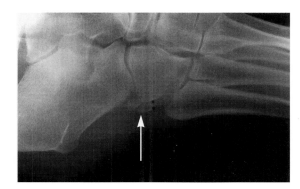

FIG. 4-128 Peroneal bones (os peroneum) *(arrow)*.

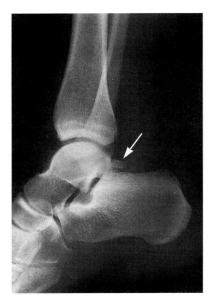

FIG. 4-129   Os trigonum *(arrow).*

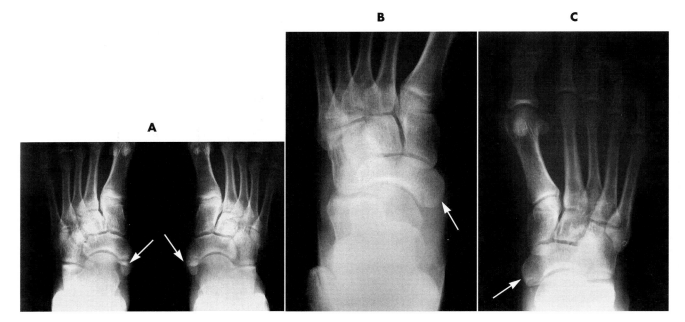

FIG. 4-130   **A,** Bilateral os tibiale externa *(arrows),* also known as "accessory navicular." There are now believed to be three types of this "variant," including a small oval ossicle not thought to be clinically relevant. The type shown in **B** may actually represent ununited stress fracture *(arrow).* The third type, **C,** *(arrow)* consists of hyperplasia of the medial navicular tubercle without a separate ossicle. The last type is believed by some to be a precursor of the type pictured in **B,** and both of these types have been associated with focal pain, especially with markedly pronated feet. There seems to be an actual causal relationship between the pronation and the anomaly, with pronation of the foot increasing stresses and leading to fatigue fracture of the tubercle. A painful, pronated foot with palpable and tender prominence over the medial navicular is frequently seen, and the os tibiale externa is now considered to be among a group of "not-so-normal" variants. Note also pronation of the first metatarsals (**A** and **B**), with the tubercles at the bases of these metatarsals rotated laterally away from the central point of the medial cuneiforms. This is believed to predispose to hallux valgus. Finally, note the bipartite medial sesamoid of the left first metatarsal, which may be mistaken for a fracture.

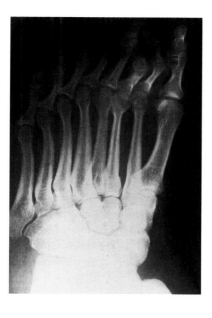

FIG. 4-131 Polydactyly.

Suggested Readings

RADIOGRAPHIC POSITIONING

Ballinger PW: *Merrill's atlas of radiographic positioning,* ed 8, St Louis, 1995, Mosby.

Bontrager KL: *Textbook of radiographic positioning and related anatomy,* ed 3, St Louis, 1993, Mosby.

Percuoco RE: *Radiographic positioning for the chiropractor,* ed 2, Grand Rapids, Mich, 1993, Colorhouse Graphics.

ANATOMY

Fleckenstein P: *Anatomy in diagnostic imaging,* Philadelphia, 1993, WB Saunders.

Kelley LL: *Sectional anatomy for the imaging professional,* St Louis, 1997, Mosby.

Weir J: *An imaging atlas of human anatomy,* St Louis, 1992, Mosby.

ANATOMICAL VARIANTS

Keats TE: *Atlas of normal roentgen variants that may simulate disease,* ed 6, St Louis, 1996, Mosby.

References

1. Bohrer SP, Ude AC: Heel pad thickness in Nigerians, *Skeletal Radiology* 5:108, 1978.
2. Greulich WW, Pyle SI: *Radiographic atlas of skeletal development of the hand and wrist,* ed 2, Stanford, Calif, Stanford University Press.

PART TWO

Bone, Joints, and Soft Tissues

Skull Patterns

DENNIS M MARCHIORI

PART TWO Bone, Joints, and Soft Tissues

217

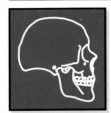

SKI | Basilar Invagination

Basilar invagination (or basilar impression) is an upward migration deformity of the base of the skull. *Platybasia* is an anthropological term describing flattening of the skull base; it should not be used synonymously with *basilar invagination.* The major causes of basilar invagination are summarized by the mnemonic *COOP,* representing the following: congenital osteogenesis imperfecta, osteomalacia, and Paget's disease.

McGregor's line is a widely used roentgenometric method to detect the presence of basilar invagination. It involves drawing a line segment from the posterior aspect of the hard palate to the inferior margin of the skull on the lateral radiograph. Basilar invagination is probable if the tip of the odontoid process is more than 8 mm above the line segment in men or 10 mm in women.

The diagnosis of basilar invagination is made with conventional radiography and is supplemented by computed tomography (CT) and magnetic resonance imaging (MRI). MRI is particularly helpful to assess possible concurrent neurological involvement.

DISEASE	COMMENTS
Achondroplasia [p. 385]	Rhizomelic dysplasia resulting from a congenital defect of enchondral bone formation; characteristics include rounded lumbar "bullet-nosed" vertebrae, lumbar spine kyphosis, posterior vertebral body scalloping, increased intervertebral disc height, flattened vertebral bodies, narrowed spinal canal, and alterations of the skull base; the pelvis may appear hypoplastic; milder expressions of the disease may occur
Arnold-Chiari malformation [p. 999]	Malformation of the skull base with caudal displacement of the cerebellomedullary region; several levels of inferior displacement are recognized
Bone softening disorders **(FIG. 5-1)**	Alterations of the skull base secondary to bone-softening diseases: osteogenesis imperfecta, rickets, osteomalacia, and Paget's disease
Cleidocranial dysplasia [p. 390]	Defect of intramembranous bone formation manifesting as osseous defects of the calvarium, clavicles, and pelvis; associated with persistence of metopic suture
Congenital anomalies	Alterations of the skull base associated with atlantooccipital fusion (occipitalization or assimilation), Klippel-Feil syndrome, and stenosis of the foramen magnum
Trauma	Posttraumatic deformity from a skull fracture

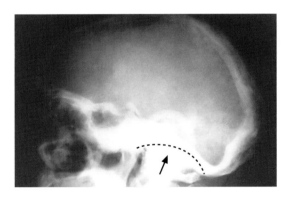

FIG. 5-1   Basilar invagination secondary to bone softening from Paget's disease of the skull *(arrow).* (Courtesy Joseph W. Howe, Sylmar, Calif.)

SK2 | Change in Size and Shape of Epiphyses

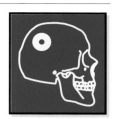

A button sequestration is a small, solitary osteolytic bone lesion that contains a central focus of calcification. Often this change represents a normal variant, particularly if it is surrounded by an osteosclerotic margin ("donut lesion"). However, aggressive pathologies need to be considered.

DISEASE	COMMENTS
Eosinophilic granuloma (FIG. 5-2) [p. 747]	Common cause of osteolytic skull defects; the inner and outer skull tables are affected—however, the defects in the skull tables do not completely superimpose, leaving an appearance of a beveled margin
Infection	Osteolytic defects secondary to *Staphylococcus,* syphilis, or tuberculosis infections; often result from contiguous spread of scalp infection
Necrosis	Osteonecrosis resulting from irradiation, electric shock therapy, or electric burns; often a latent period of several years elapses before osteolytic lesion becomes apparent
Neoplasm	Epidermoid, dermoid cyst, metastasis (especially from breast carcinoma), myeloma, meningioma, and hemangioma
Normal variant	Radiolucent defects with central calcification and surrounding sclerosis possibly representing normal variants; these defects are differentiated from true button sequestrations by the absence of reported pain and disability; these variants are usually discovered incidentally and are not clinically significant
Postsurgical	Burr hole or shunt placement

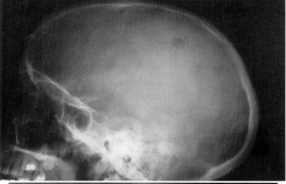

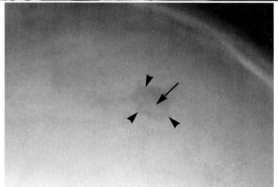

FIG. 5-2 Eosinophilic granuloma, producing an osteolytic defect of the skull *(arrowheads)* with a central radiodense sequestrum (button sequestration)*(arrow).* (Courtesy Stan Higgins, Davenport, Iowa.)

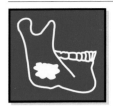

SK3 | Cystic Lesions of the Mandible

C ystic lesions of the mandible are often caused by pathologies that produce cystic lesions elsewhere in the skeleton and a variety of causes that are seen only in the mandible. Most pathologies comprising the latter group are related to pathological conditions of the teeth.

DISEASE	COMMENTS
Ameloblastoma (adamantinoma) (FIG. 5-3) [p. 673]	Multilocular radiolucent lesion with coarse inner trabeculation; it may grow very large, distorting the symmetry of the face; the condition is usually noted in patients older than 30 years of age
Aneurysmal bone cyst/osteoblastomas/hemangiomas (FIG. 5-4) [p. 634]	Benign nonodontogenic tumors, including aneurysmal bone cysts, osteoblastomas, and hemangiomas, all producing osteolytic, expansile lesion of the mandible; each is much more common in other skeletal locations
Cherubism	Bilateral, symmetrical enlargement of the mandible, histologically similar to fibrous dysplasia, although the former has a familial incidence and is limited to the jaw
Dentigerous (follicular) cyst (FIG. 5-5)	Well-circumscribed mandibular cyst that characteristically contains the crown of an unerupted tooth; this cyst is usually found in children
Fibrous dysplasia (FIG. 5-6) [p. 651]	Unilateral, expansile, usually osteolytic, well-circumscribed lesions appearing locally or in association with other skeletal lesions; the osteosclerotic form of the disease is more typical of the maxilla; craniofacial form (leontiasis ossea) of the disease is limited to the calvarium and face

Continued

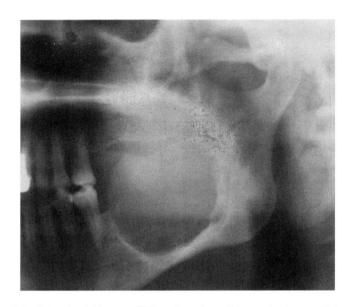

FIG. 5-3   Ameloblastoma. Oblique view of mandible reveals a large cystic lesion in body and ramus of mandible with attenuation and loss of bone superiorly. The lesion has broken through upper part of mandible. (From Som PM, Bergeron RT: *Head and neck imaging*, ed 2, St Louis, 1991, Mosby.)

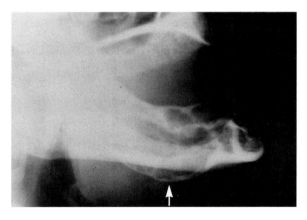

FIG. 5-4   Aneurysmal bone cyst, presenting as a cystic expansile lesion of the mandible *(arrow)*. (Courtesy William E. Litterer, Elizabeth, NJ.)

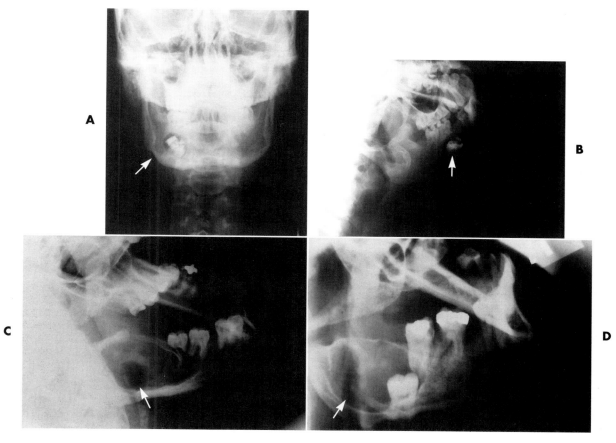

FIG. 5-5 Three patients (**A/B, C,** and **D**) all with a dentigerous cyst of the right ramus of the mandible. Each appears as a central lucency, and two exhibit a centrally located density representing the unerupted tooth *(arrows)*. (Courtesy Steven P. Brownstein, Springfield, NJ.)

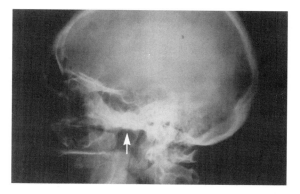

FIG. 5-6 Fibrous dysplasia of the maxilla causing an increased radiodensity of the region *(arrow)*. (Courtesy Joseph W. Howe, Sylmar, Calif.)

DISEASE	COMMENTS
Giant cell reparative granuloma	Expansile osteolytic lesion of the mandible and maxilla with thin overlying cortex; this lesion is believed to represent a nontumorous reparative process
Histiocytosis X (Eosinophilic granuloma) (FIG. 5-7) [p. 747]	Common in the mandible; the destruction may be so advanced that the teeth appear to "float" without surrounding osseous support; Ewing's tumor, metastatic neuroblastoma, and non-Hodgkin's lymphoma may produce similar appearances of "floating teeth"
Hyperparathyroidism [p. 718]	Single or multiple osteolytic lesions representing brown tumors; the lamina dura thins, as is also noted in fibrous dysplasia, Paget's disease, and osteomalacia
Metastasis [p. 687]	Osteolytic lesions similar to those of other skeletal sites; metastasis may appear secondary to hematogenous seeding or direct extension from approximate nasal, oral, cutaneous, or salivary gland primary lesions
Multiple myeloma [p. 700]	Multiple osteolytic lesions that appear well defined and of uniform size; concomitant skull changes are nearly always present

DISEASE	COMMENTS
Infection [p. 616]	Irregular osteolytic lesion, often with accompanying sequestration; infections of the mandible and maxilla may develop from hematogenous seeding or secondary to dental or sinus infection; trauma and local carcinoma have also been implicated
Paget's disease [p. 761]	Diffuse osteolytic, osteosclerotic, or mixed pattern of bone disease with bilateral enlargement; concomitant skull changes nearly always occur
Periapical granuloma	Well-circumscribed cyst in a periapical location, which may develop into periodontal cyst
Periodontal cyst	Common cyst of the jaw that develops from chronic infection; it appears as a well-defined radiolucent cyst in the periapical location and is contained within osteosclerotic margins
Solitary bone cyst (hemorrhagic bone cyst)	Poorly defined irregular cyst of the mandible; this condition is seen in children, usually accompanied with a history of trauma

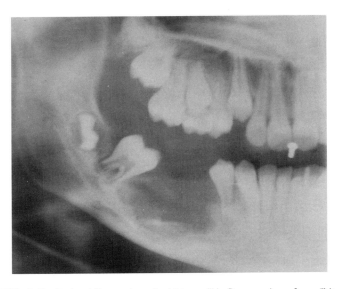

FIG. 5-7 Eosinophilic granuloma in right mandible. Panorex view of mandible reveals a lucent, irregular area that is fairly well defined in the body of the mandible between the second molar tooth and first premolar tooth. Some loss of lamina dura has occurred in the lower second molar tooth. (From Som PM, Bergeron RT: *Head and neck imaging,* ed 2, St Louis, 1991, Mosby.)

SK4 | Diffuse Demineralization

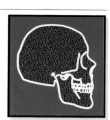

Diffuse demineralization of the skull is typically related to senile osteoporosis. Hyperparathyroidism mimics the radiographic appearance of osteoporosis, both appearing with pure patterns of diffuse demineralization. Most of the other conditions listed in the following table produce patterns of diffuse demineralization that occur in combination with larger osteolytic lesions. For example, hemolytic anemias, leukemia, and metastatic neuroblastoma may produce a classic "hair-on-end" appearance in addition to diffuse demineralization.

DISEASE	COMMENTS
Anemias **(FIG. 5-8)**	Possible diffuse osteoporosis related to marrow hyperplasia caused by sickle-cell anemia and thalassemia; other findings include a "hair-on-end" appearance involving the outer table of the calvarium
Hyperparathyroidism **(FIG. 5-9)** [p. 718]	Granular, or "salt-and-pepper," appearance of the skull as result of diffuse demineralization; rarely larger focal osteolytic lesions develop
Infection [p. 616]	Diffuse presentation of infection is uncommon; in general, infections of the skull are less common in the United States than in underdeveloped countries
Metastatic bone disease [p. 687]	Typically noted with multiple, ill-defined osteolytic lesions; this disease infrequently results in a diffuse demineralization pattern; breast, lung, and prostate origins are common in the adult; in the child, neuroblastoma and leukemia are more likely
Multiple myeloma [p. 700]	Characterized by diffuse demineralization with focal "punched-out" lesions
Osteoporosis [p. 727]	Appears with diffuse demineralization and is typically related to aging; less commonly, osteoporosis develops from steroid supplementation or endocrinopathy
Paget's disease [p. 761]	Diffuse demineralization that may accompany the more classic presentation of large osteolytic areas of bone destruction (osteoporosis circumscripta); demineralization occurs most often in the outer table of the skull during the lytic phase of the disease

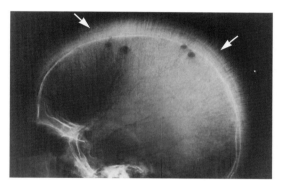

FIG. 5-8 Thalassemia (Cooley's anemia), causing diffuse demineralization and "hair-on-end" appearance (*arrows*) of the anterior calvarium related to marrow hyperplasia. (Courtesy Joseph W. Howe, Sylmar, Calif.)

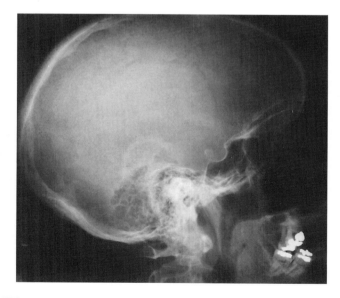

FIG. 5-9 Hyperparathyroidism. Granular deossification appearance of the calvarium, resulting in a salt-and-pepper appearance to skull. (From Deltoff MN: *The portable skeletal x-ray,* St Louis, 1997, Mosby.)

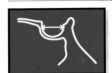

SK5 | Enlargement or Destruction of the Sella Turcica

Although variation exists, the sella turcica should not exceed an anteroposterior dimension of 16 mm or a vertical depth of 12 mm on the lateral skull radiograph. Normally the floor of the sella is well defined by a single cortical line. The appearance of two cortical lines represents a "double-floor" sign, suggesting osseous erosion of the floor by an expansile mass. Hurler's disease is associated with elongation of the posterior aspect of the sella, creating a J-shaped configuration.

DISEASE	COMMENTS
Chordoma [p. 676]	Blumenbach's clivus, representing the sloping surface of bone between the dorsum sellae and the foramen magnum (composed of the body of the sphenoid and pars basilaris of the occiput); the clivus is a target location for chordomas, which may secondarily involve the sella turcica from its posterior aspect; their appearance is marked by bone destruction and likely tumor matrix calcification; chordoma occurs most often is 30- to 60-year-olds
Craniopharyngioma	Seen in children and young adults, tumor that may produce bone destruction of the sella; most lesions calcify; gliomas of the optic chiasm may cause similar changes

DISEASE	COMMENTS
Empty sella syndrome **(FIG. 5-10)**	Appears as an enlarged sella without bone destruction or considerable deformity; the syndrome is believed to result from a congenital or acquired defect of the diaphragm sellae, which allows an intrasellar extension of the suprasellar arachnoid space; pulsations of the cerebrospinal fluid are thought to cause the sellar enlargement; the pituitary function is typically normal

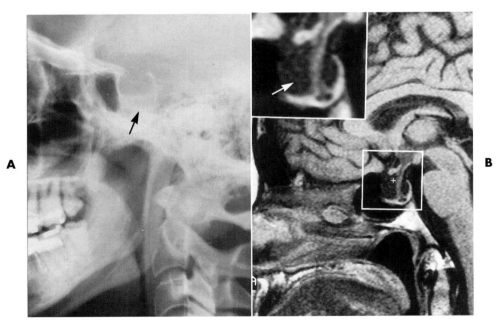

FIG. 5-10   A, The lateral cervical projection reveals an enlarged sella (beyond 12 × 16 mm on the original film) with a double density of the floor of the sella *(arrow).* **B,** The sagittal T1-weighted MRI image denotes hypointense fluid signal intensity in the sella turcica consistent with cerebrospinal fluid *(arrow).*

Increased intracranial pressure	Associated with other conditions such as hydrocephalus, intracranial tumors, and edema; chronic increased intracranial pressure may manifest as erosion and deformity of the sella, resulting from downward pressure of an enlarged third ventricle
Internal carotid artery aneurysm	Enlarged sella resulting from expanded cavernous segment of the carotid artery; linear vascular calcification is often present
Meningioma [p. 996]	Arising from arachnoid and dura mater in the area of the diaphragma sellae, not within the pituitary fossa; meningioma appears with bone destruction and sclerosis; calcification is uncommon
Pituitary tumors (FIG. 5-11)	Enlarged sella, uneven erosion of the floor, producing a "double-floor" appearance; pituitary tumors may be classified by size (microadenoma is less than 1 cm and macroadenoma is greater than 1 cm in diameter) or by their appearance after staining; eosinophilic adenoma (causing acromegaly), chromophobe adenomas (causing hypopituitarism), and basophilic adenoma (causing Cushing's disease) occur

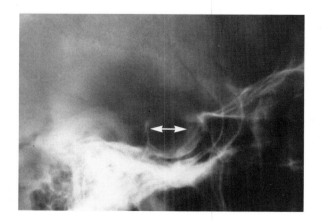

FIG. 5-11 Enlarged sella turcica *(arrow)* secondary to pituitary adenoma.

PART TWO
Bone, Joints, and Soft Tissues

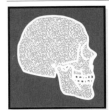

SK6 | Increased Radiodensity of the Calvarium

Increased radiodensity of the skull results from pathological thickening of the inner, outer, or both tables of the calvarium. Generally, it is difficult to determine which table is involved from plain film radiographs. At times, the diploic space may be entirely obliterated by sclerosis. Increased density may be localized or generalized throughout much of the skull. Osteomas, meningiomas, and cephalohematomas usually result in localized changes. Renal osteodystrophy, fluorosis, myelosclerosis, acromegaly, hemolytic anemias, and selected congenital diseases typically produce a generalized increase in the radiodensity of the skull. Paget's disease, fibrous dysplasia, metastasis, and hyperostosis frontalis interna may occur as localized or generalized patterns.

DISEASE	COMMENTS
Acromegaly [p. 715]	Thickening and generalized increased radiodensity of the skull; concurrent enlargement of the jaw, sella turcica, and frontal sinuses is also noted
Calcified cephalohematoma	Describes a localized calcific skull radiodensity or thickening that develops from a subperiosteal hematoma; the area of involvement is usually in a parietal location and is confined by suture borders; this condition is often associated with forceps delivery
Congenital diseases (FIG. 5-12)	Osteopetrosis, pyknodysostosis, and Pyle's disease associated with generalized increase in skull radiodensity and other skeletal changes

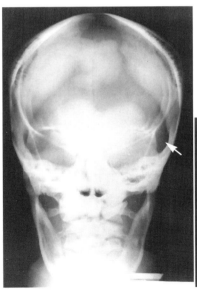
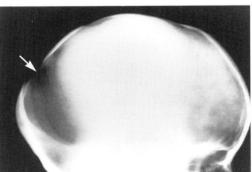

FIG. 5-12   Pyknodysostosis, demonstrating a radiodense skull and widened sutures *(arrows)*. (Courtesy Joseph W. Howe, Sylmar, Calif.)

Fibrous dysplasia (FIG. 5-13) [p. 651]	Localized or generalized increased radiodensity, typically involving the skull base or facial bones; the skull is commonly involved if multiple skeletal sites are found
Fluorosis	Generalized increase in skull radiodensity; changes are more prominent in the spine
Hematologic anemias	Hyperplastic marrow changes associated with thalassemia, hereditary spherocytosis, and sickle cell anemia leading to spicules of new bone growth; these spicules are orientated perpendicular to the calvarium ("hair-on-end" appearance), producing a generalized increase in the radiodensity of the skull
Hyperostosis frontalis interna	Localized idiopathic process more common in women over the age of 40 years; it does not cross the midline and involves the inner table of the skull; hyperostosis interna generalisata describes more widespread changes of the skull
Meningioma [p. 996]	Hyperostosis of the inner table occurring over the areas of the tumor; an exaggerated appearance of the meningeal grooves and foramen spinosum is a common result
Metastatic disease [p. 687]	Localized or, more commonly, generalized skull involvement; this disease develops from breast or prostate carcinoma following therapy; an osteolytic presentation is more common than an osteodense presentation
Myelosclerosis	Generalized increase in skull radiodensity; concurrent splenomegaly is usual
Osteoma (FIG. 5-14) [p. 637]	Most common primary calvarial neoplasm; osteoma develops only in intramembranously formed bone; this disease appears as a localized region of dense cortical hyperostosis and may arise from the inner or outer skull table; it is more common in the sinuses, particularly the frontal sinus
Paget's disease [p. 761]	Thickened trabeculae leading to a localized or, more typically, generalized increased radiodensity; eventually the delineation of an inner and outer table is lost; the osteoblastic ("cotton-wool") appearance signifies an advanced stage of the disease
Renal osteodystrophy	Generalized increase in skull radiodensity that parallels changes elsewhere in the skeleton; appearance may be similar to Paget's disease

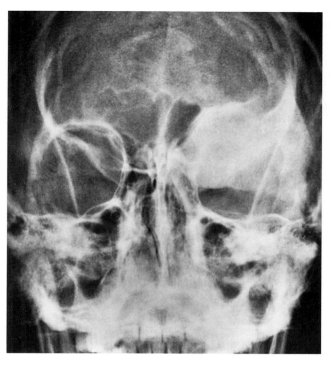

FIG. 5-13 Fibrous dysplasia of the skull on a Caldwell view shown as a very dense expansile lesion of the left frontal and zygomatic bones that has encroached on the left orbit. (From Som PM, Bergeron RT: *Head and neck imaging,* ed 2, St Louis, 1991, Mosby.)

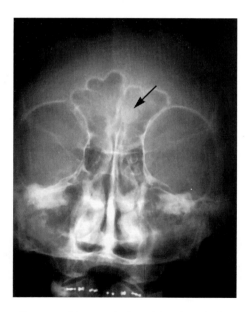

FIG. 5-14 Osteoma arising near the frontal sinus *(arrow).* (Courtesy Steven P. Brownstein, Springfield, NJ.)

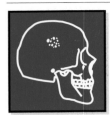

SK7 | Intracranial Calcification

Intracranial calcifications are a common finding on plain film radiographs and even more common on computed tomography scans of the skull. Although most represent physiologic calcifications of limited clinical significance, aggressive pathology (i.e., tumor, infection, vascular disturbance) is an important consideration in the differential diagnosis. Intracranial calcifications are typically localized; when they present with a scattered pattern, they are commonly associated with infections or tuberous sclerosis.

DISEASE	COMMENTS
Physiological calcifications	Those that involve the pineal and habenula commonly found in the midline in a frontal skull projection; physiological calcifications of the basal ganglia and choroid plexus are often bilateral and symmetrical in a frontal projection; physiological calcification of the dura mater typically occurs along the superior sagittal sinus, falx, and tentorium; short, nearly horizontal linear calcifications located immediately posterior to the posterior clinoids in a lateral projection are often seen in the elderly and represent calcifications of the petroclinoid ligaments; physiological calcifications are usually of no clinical significance; however, a shift in their normal location may indicate a space-occupying lesion (mass, hemorrhage, etc.); additionally, if they occur in young children, they may suggest underlying pathology; the typical age of presentation is noteworthy: pineal, older than 10 years; choroid plexus, older than 3 years; habenular, older than 10 years; petroclinoid, older than 5 years; and falx or tentorium, older than 3 years
Tumors	Oligodendroglioma, craniopharyngioma, ependymoma, choroid plexus papilloma, meningioma, teratoma, pinealoma, pituitary adenoma, etc; craniopharyngiomas are more common in children; meningiomas are more common in middle-aged adults and are rare in children
Infections	Cysticercosis, cytomegalovirus, paragonimiasis, torulosis, toxoplasmosis, tuberculomas, vi-

Infections— cont'd	ral encephalitis, etc.; infections usually occur with multiple scattered foci of calcification
Vascular	Including aneurysm, arteriosclerosis, and arteriovenous malformations (AVM), which are common vascular causes of intracranial calcification; arteriosclerotic calcifications of the internal carotid arteries are typically seen in the parasellar region where the arteries pass through the cavernous sinuses; by contrast, an aneurysm is more often in a suprasellar location and therefore is suspected when a sellar pattern of calcification extends superiorly beyond the confines of the sella
Basal ganglia	Pathologic basal ganglia calcification appears as bilateral, central scattered radiodensities occurring secondary to endocrine disorders (hypoparathyroidism, pseudohypoparathyroidism, pseudopseudohypoparathyroidism), infections (cytomegalovirus, toxoplasmosis, and cysticercosis), and toxic exposure (lead and carbon monoxide poisoning)
Phakomatosis (FIG. 5-15)	Various patterns of calcifications are produced by neurofibromatosis (meningiomas and gliomas), Sturge-Weber syndrome (parallel serpentine plaques), tuberous sclerosis (scattered nodules), and von Hippel-Lindau disease (retina and intracranial angiomas)
Trauma	Localized areas of calcification following post-traumatic hemorrhage
Artifacts	Hair braids, toupees, barrettes, and other artifacts simulating intracranial calcifications

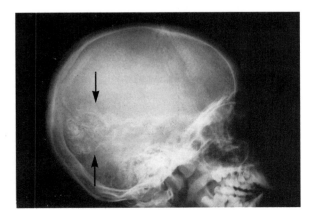

FIG. 5-15 Parallel serpentine calcifications consistent with Sturge-Weber syndrome (*arrows*).

SK8 | Mass in the Paranasal Sinuses

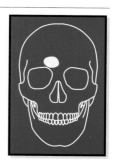

The paranasal sinuses comprise the paired frontal, ethmoid, sphenoid, and maxillary sinuses. Alteration in the normally radiolucent appearance of the sinus suggests the presence of pathology. Because of the sinuses' anatomical proximity to the brain and eye, aggressive pathology within the sinuses may have serious complications. Multiple radiographic projections and possibly computed tomography are needed to evaluate all of the paranasal sinuses.

DISEASE	COMMENTS
Benign tumors (FIG. 5-16)	Masses of varying radiodensity, ranging from the very radiodense osteomas to the more radiolucent lipomas; others include chondroma, dermoid, and hemangioma, and lesions extending from the maxilla and mandible
Fibrous dysplasia/Paget's disease	Paranasal sinus opacification related to Paget's disease or fibrous dysplasia involving the adjacent bone; leontiasis ossea is the bilateral enlargement and distortion of the facial bones secondary to fibrous dysplasia
Fracture	Paranasal sinus opacification resulting from recent trauma and hemorrhage, or less often old fracture and residual bone deformity
Infection	Typically follows dental or sinus infection; the appearance of thick mucosa with bone demineralization and destruction is suggestive; osteomyelitis involving the calvarium above the frontal sinus has been referred to as "Pott's puffy tumor"
Malignant tumors	Characterized by a soft tissue mass and bone destruction; squamous cell carcinomas are the most common, others include lymphoma, extramedullary plasmacytoma, adenoid cystic carcinomas (cylindromas), and mixed salivary tumors; the maxillary sinus is most commonly involved
Mucocele	Radiodense accumulation of mucous secretions secondary to obstruction of the involved sinus ostium; obstruction is usually the result of swollen mucosa, thick secretions, or both; mucoceles may completely opacify the sinus; most mucoceles are found in the frontal sinuses, followed by ethmoid sinuses; an infected mucocele is known as a *pyocele*

Continued

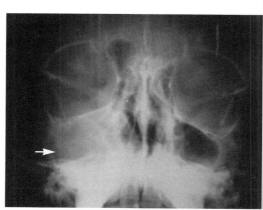

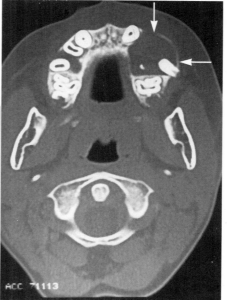

FIG. 5-16 A, The right maxillary sinus opacification on plain film *(arrow)*, resulting from **B,** fluid accumulations related to a dentigerous cyst of the maxilla, seen on CT *(arrows)*.

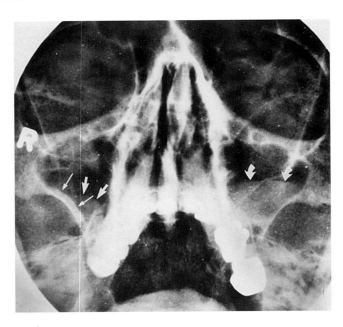

FIG. 5-17   Waters view shows a large "flat" retention cyst *(curved arrows)* in the left antrum. This can simulate an air-fluid level if careful attention is not paid to its slightly convex upper surface. The mucosa has thickened slightly in the right antrum *(thin arrows)*, and another small retention cyst is present in the lower right maxillary sinus *(arrows)*. (From Som PM, Bergeron RT: *Head and neck imaging,* ed 2, St Louis, 1991, Mosby.)

DISEASE	COMMENTS
Mucus retention cyst/serous cyst **(FIG. 5-17)**	Smooth, rounded, radiodense mass representing a plugged and consequentially expanded sinus mucous gland; the floor of the maxillary sinus is most commonly involved; the serous cyst is radiographically identical to the mucus retention cyst, representing fluid accumulation between submucosal layers; both cysts are related to chronic sinusitis
Polypoid rhinosinusitis	Complication of allergies, tobacco, and chronic nasal or paranasal sinusitis manifesting as multiple polypoid enlargements and degeneration of the mucosa
Sinusitis **(FIG. 5-18)**	Opacification, mucosal thickening, and regional bone demineralization; an air-fluid level is characteristic; sinusitis occurs secondary to acute sinus infection; the maxillary sinuses are most commonly involved with acute or chronic sinusitis; sphenoid sinuses are least involved
Wegener's granulomatosis	Autoimmune necrotizing granulomatosis usually affecting pulmonary, renal, and sinus tissues; sinus mucosal thickening with regional bone destruction is common; involvement of the mastoid sinus is characteristic

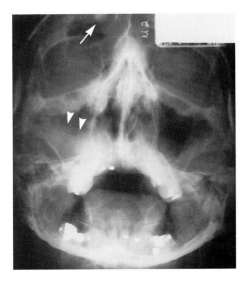

FIG. 5-18   Sinus opacification associated with sinusitis *(arrowheads)*. Incidentally noted is an osteoma near the frontal sinus *(arrow)*. (Courtesy Ian D. McLean, Davenport, Iowa.)

SK9 | Multiple Wormian Bones

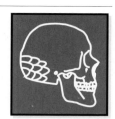

Wormian bones are intrasutural islands of bone occurring in the lambdoid, posterior sagittal, and temporosquamosal sutures. Their appearance is often a variant of normal, particularly when found when the child is younger than the age of 6 months. Wormian bones have been associated with a number of pathological conditions. Many of the conditions are described by the mnemonic *PORK CHOPS,* representing the following: *pyknodysostosis, osteogenesis imperfecta, rickets in healing phase, kinky hair syndrome, cleidocranial dysplasia, hypothyroidism* (and *hypophosphatasia*), *otopalatodigital syndrome, primary acro-osteolysis* (and *pachydermoperiostosis*), *Down syndrome.*

DISEASE	COMMENTS
Cleidocranial dysplasia (FIG. 5-19) [p. 390]	Defect of intramembranous bone formation largely involving the calvarium, clavicles, and pelvis; this disease is associated with persistence of the metopic suture
Hypoparathyroidism/hypophosphatasia [p. 722]	Metabolic disturbances resulting from low levels of parathormone or alkaline phosphatase, respectively; both are associated with delayed closure of sutures
Osteogenesis imperfecta [p. 409]	Defect of connective tissue formation; characteristics include blue sclera, brittle bones, multiple fractures, and delayed closure of sutures
Pyknodysostosis [p. 413]	Rare syndrome of bone dysplasia marked by short stature, mandibular hypoplasia, and a failure of sutures to close
Rickets [p. 735]	Defect of calcification resulting from deficiency of vitamin D (dietary or poor metabolism) associated with altered skull shape and delayed closure of sutures

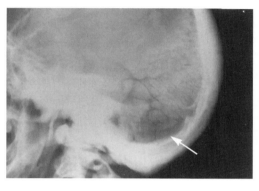

FIG. 5-19 Cleidocranial dysostosis with multiple wormian bones *(arrow).* (Courtesy Joseph W. Howe, Sylmar, Calif.)

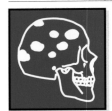

SK10 | Osteolytic Defects of the Skull

The calvarium (or skull cap) is composed of a central, marrow-filled diploic space sandwiched between inner and outer cortical tables of bone. Osteolytic lesions of the skull may involve primarily either the inner or outer skull tables or may arise from the diploic space progressively involving both the inner and outer layers equally.

Osteolytic defects of the skull may be solitary or multiple. A solitary lesion with surrounding osteosclerotic border is known as a "donut lesion"; one with a central nidus of calcification is known as a "button sequestration" and is detailed in pattern SK2 earlier in this chapter. Osteolytic defects of the skull are described by the mnemonic *HELP ME*, contained in the following list: hemangioma, epidermoid/dermoid, leptomeningeal cyst (and lambdoidal suture defect), Paget's (osteoporosis circumscripta), postsurgical, metastasis, and eosinophilic granuloma/encephalocele.

DISEASE	COMMENTS
Solitary *Donut lesion*	Defect with surrounding sclerosis of variable thickness; they are of no clinical significance
Encephalocele	Rare, representing a herniation of brain substance though a congenital defect in the skull
Epidermoid, dermoid	Benign tumors presenting with well-defined lucent defects, often with osteosclerotic borders; they form from tissues that become trapped in the diploic space secondary to a defect in the formation of the neural tube; dermoids are usually located in the midline and form from ectodermal and mesodermal tissue; epidermoids form from ectodermal tissue

Solitary—cont'd	
Hemangioma *(hemangioma cases)* **(FIG. 5-20)**	Benign solitary osteolytic lesion that demonstrates characteristic honeycomb or spoke-wheel trabecular patterns; histologically these are the same as those lesions occurring in the vertebrae
Histiocytosis X [p. 747]	Abnormal proliferation of histiocytes that encompasses several clinical entities, all of unknown origin; few bone changes are noted with Letterer-Siwe disease; Hand-Schüller-Christian disease may demonstrate bone lesions of the calvarium, skull base, and mandible; eosinophilic granuloma represents the most common and proliferative form of the disease; it is marked by osteolytic skeletal defects, most prominent in the skull; bone lesion resulting from histiocytosis X involves the inner and outer tables of the skull; the lesions do not completely superimpose, forming a characteristic beveled-edge appearance; although lesions are usually solitary, multiple lesions often occur
Infection [p. 616]	Acute infection resulting in irregular, poorly defined osteolytic margins that have a tendency to coalesce; often develop secondary to contiguous spread from paranasal or middle ear infections
Lambdoid suture	Wide appearance of the lambdoidal suture often seen in neurofibromatosis
Leptomeningeal cyst	Describes an entrapment of the arachnoid dura between the margins of an existing skull fracture; the continuous pulsations of the cerebral spinal fluid cause erosions of the skull, giving a "growing" nature to the fracture

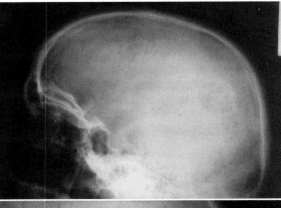
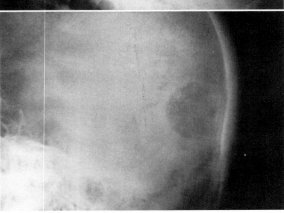

FIG. 5-20 Hemangioma of the calvarium.

Solitary—cont'd

Malignancy **(FIG. 5-21)**	Malignancies of the scalp, bone, orbit, dura, and brain
Metastases **(FIG. 5-22)** [p. 687]	Usually occur in patients older than 40 years of age; typically patients have a history of primary malignancy; breast carcinoma is a particularly common sources of skull metastasis; lesions are usually multiple
Necrosis	Radiation, electric shock therapy, or electric burns
Parietal foramina	Bilateral, symmetrical lucent defects in the posterior region of the parietal bones of no clinical significance
Postsurgical	Burr holes or shunt placement

Multiple

Cushing's syndrome [p. 717]	Demineralization and fine granular osteolytic defects similar in appearance to hyperparathyroidism
Fibrous dysplasia **(FIG. 5-23)** [p. 651]	Single or multiple defects, usually appearing with a mixed osteosclerotic and osteolytic pattern in the calvarium
Histiocytosis X **(FIG. 5-24)** [p. 747]	Abnormal proliferation of histiocytes that encompasses several clinical entities, all of unknown origin; few bone changes are noted with Letterer-Siwe; Hand-Schüller-Christian disease may demonstrate bone lesions of the calvarium, skull base, and mandible; eosinophilic granuloma represents the most common and proliferative form of the disease; it is marked by osteolytic skeletal defects, most prominent in the skull; bone lesion resulting from histiocytosis X involves the inner and outer tables of the skull; the lesions do not completely superimpose, relating a characteristic beveled-edge appearance; although lesions are usually solitary, multiple lesions often occur

Continued

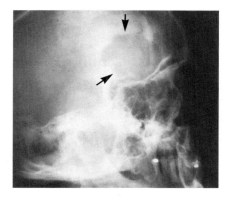

FIG. 5-21 Osteolytic defect of the skull *(arrows)* secondary to squamous cell carcinoma of the orbit. (Courtesy Steven P. Brownstein, Springfield, NJ.)

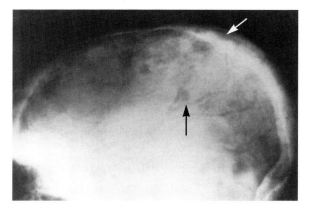

FIG. 5-23 Mixed pattern of bone sclerosis with focal osteolytic regions *(arrows)* secondary to fibrous dysplasia of the calvarium. (Courtesy Joseph W. Howe, Sylmar, Calif.)

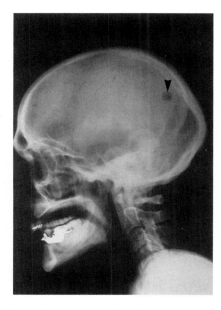

FIG. 5-22 Metastatic disease presenting with one prominent osteolytic defect *(arrowhead)*. (Courtesy Ian D. McLean, Davenport, Iowa.)

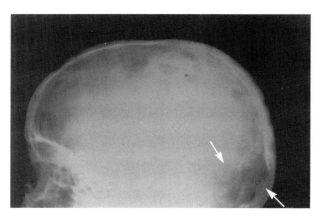

FIG. 5-24 Multiple osteolytic regions of bone destruction. In the occipital region the area of bone destruction of the inner and outer table is not identical. The lack of overlap produced a beveled-edge appearance, characteristic of histiocytosis X *(arrows)*. (Courtesy Joseph W. Howe, Sylmar, Calif.)

DISEASE	COMMENTS
Multiple—cont'd *Hyperparathyroidism* [p. 718]	Classic appearance of demineralization and fine granular or "salt-and-pepper" appearance to the skull; less commonly larger osteolytic skull defects appear
Metastasis **(FIGS. 5-25 AND 5-26)** [p. 687]	Multiple osteolytic defects of varying sizes; most patients have metastasis elsewhere in the skeleton, resulting from an increased blood supply; the calvarium is more commonly involved than the skull base; patients are usually older than 40 years of age; breast and lung primaries are most common in adults; neuroblastoma and leukemia are most common in children
Multiple myeloma **(FIG. 5-27)** [p. 700]	Characteristic presentation of demineralization with multiple, well-defined osteolytic defects of approximate uniform size (ranging between 0.5 to 4 cm); the lesions appear as "punch-out" defects without osteosclerotic borders
Neurofibromatosis [p. 755]	Single or multiple defects in the occipital and temporal bone, more commonly involving the greater wing of the sphenoid
Pacchionian bodies (arachnoid granulations or villi)	Fingerlike extensions of the arachnoid mater into the dural venous sinus; these extensions exert pressure on the thinned dura mater, forming pit or erosion defects of the supraadjacent inner table of the skull; these defects are located within several centimeters of the sagittal sinus and are of no clinical significance
Paget's disease **(FIG. 5-28)** [p. 761]	Single or multiple osteolytic areas occurring with the osteolytic phase of Paget's disease, known as *osteoporosis circumscripta;* usually begins in the frontal or occipital regions and progresses as a wave of osteoporosis; the osteolytic areas are well demarcated, often bilateral, involving the outer table more than the inner table of the skull; more common among patients older than 40 years of age
Radiation	Mixed osteosclerotic and osteolytic pattern of bone disease with widely scattered irregular defects usually presenting a year after irradiation

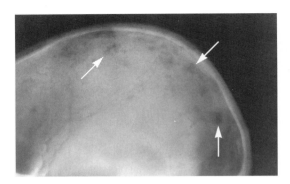

FIG. 5-26   Metastatic bone disease of the skull with multiple well-defined osteolytic defects *(arrows)*. This appearance is also strongly suggestive of multiple myeloma. (Courtesy Joseph W. Howe, Sylmar, Calif.)

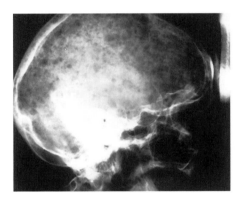

FIG. 5-27   Multiple "punch-out" osteolytic lesions of consistent size, characteristic of multiple myeloma of the skull.

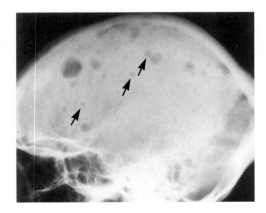

FIG. 5-25   Metastatic bone disease appearing as multiple osteolytic defects *(arrows)*. Metastatic lesions are often larger than depicted in this case. (Courtesy Ian D. McLean, Davenport, Iowa.)

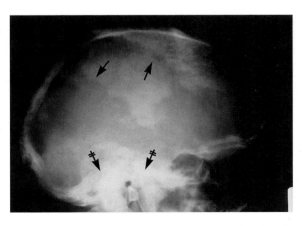

FIG. 5-28   Paget's disease of the skull. Large circumscribed regions of osteolysis (osteoporosis circumscripta) *(arrows)*, with basilar impression *(crossed arrows)*.

SKII Radiodense Mandible Lesions

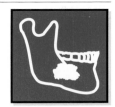

Osteosclerotic lesions of the mandible may appear solitary, multiple, or generalized throughout the bone. The appearance often changes over time. Many diseases appear originally as radiolucent osteolytic bone lesions and become osteosclerotic over time.

DISEASE	COMMENTS
Cementinoma/ cementoma	Tumor of mesodermal origin, most often involving the anterior portion of the mandible; this disease is more common among females from 30 to 40 years of age; lesions may appear solitary or multiple; in its initial stages the lesion appears as a radiolucent cyst and becomes radiodense in the late stages, having an appearance of a mass within a cyst
Fibrous dysplasia [p. 651]	Usually osteolytic; however, fibrous dysplasia may present as solitary or multiple radiodense lesions with an occasionally expansile appearance; less commonly a mixed osteolytic-osteosclerotic pattern occurs
Infantile cortical hyperostosis (Caffey's disease) **(FIG. 5-29)** [p. 754]	Bilateral, symmetrical thickening of the mandible resulting from intramembranous new bone formation; although other skeletal sites are involved (e.g., clavicle), the mandible is the most common location; clinical findings include hard, tender soft tissue enlargement over involved region; this disease occurs before 5 months of age
Odontoma **(FIG. 5-30)**	Radiodense mass with two appearances; a complex odontoma represents a single mass of maldeveloped solid dental tissues (i.e., enamel, dentin, pulp) that appear radiographically as an amorphous radiodense mass; the second type—compound odontomas—are similar, but they may contain discernable, poorly developed, misshapen teeth
Osteosarcoma/ chondrosarcoma	Similar appearance to that of lesions elsewhere in the skeleton; mandibular lesions are less common and typically follow lesions at other skeletal sites
Paget's disease [p. 761]	Appears as a radiodense, bilateral, symmetrical, enlarged appearance of bone during its blastic phase; the mandible is more commonly involved than the maxilla
Sclerosing infection	Infection of the jaw typically secondary to trauma or a dental or sinus infection; the appearance may originally be osteolytic, later forming a sequestrum and becoming osteosclerotic
Torus palatinus/torus mandibularis	(Torus palatinus) exostoses arising from the median suture of the hard palate; (torus mandibularis) bone projections from the internal, anterior portion of the mandible are similar to that of torus palatinus; both are typically bilateral and symmetrical

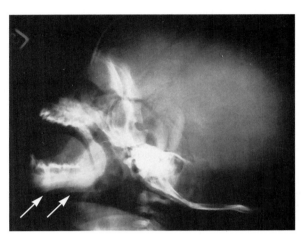

FIG. 5-29 Infantile cortical hyperostosis. Note thick and radiodense jaw (*arrows*). (Courtesy William E. Litterer, Elizabeth, NJ.)

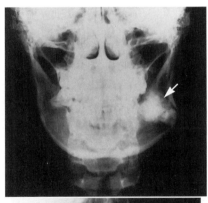

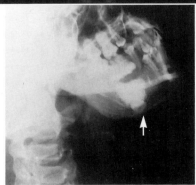

FIG. 5-30 Odontoma appearing as a radiopaque mass of the left ramus of the mandible (*arrows*). (Courtesy Steven P. Brownstein, Springfield, NJ.)

Suggested Readings

Burgener FA, Kormano M: *Differential diagnosis in conventional radiology,* ed 2, New York, 1991, Thieme Medical Publishers.

Chapman S, Nakielny R: *Aids to radiological differential diagnosis,* ed 3, Philadelphia, 1995, WB Saunders.

Dahnert W: *Radiology review manual,* Baltimore, 1991, Williams and Wilkins.

Dolan KD: Cervicobasilar relationships, *Radiog Clin N Am* 15(2):155, 1977.

Eisenberg R: *An atlas of differential diagnosis,* ed 2, Gaithersburg, 1992, Aspen Publishers.

Jacobson HG: Dense bone—too much bone: radiographical considerations and differential diagnosis, *Skel Radiol* 13:1, 1985.

Keller JD: *Basics of head and neck film interpretation,* Boston, 1990, Little, Brown and Company.

Ravin CE, Cooper C, Leder RA: *Review of radiology,* Philadelphia, 1994, WB Saunders.

Reeder MM, Bradley WG: *Reeder and Felson's gamuts in radiology,* ed 3, New York, 1993, Springer-Verlag.

Taybi H, Lachman RS: *Radiology of syndromes, metabolic disorders, and skeletal dysplasias,* ed 4, St Louis, 1996, Mosby.

Teodori JB, Painter MJ: Basilar impression in children, *Pediatrics* 74(6):1097.

Unger JM: *Head and neck imaging,* New York, 1987, Churchill Livingstone.

Weissleder R, Wittenberg J: *Primer of diagnostic imaging,* St Louis, 1994, Mosby.

chapter 6

Spine Patterns

DENNIS M MARCHIORI

PART TWO
Bone, Joints, and Soft Tissues

237

SP I | Altered Vertebral Shape

Altered vertebral shape is typically the result of congenital conditions. Although a vertebra's appearance may be altered in a myriad of ways, the following table includes some of the more commonly encountered alterations. Vertebral collapse and vertebral expansion are larger topics and therefore are discussed separately in this chapter.

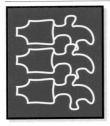

SP I a | Beaked or Hooked Vertebrae

DISEASE	COMMENTS
Achondroplasia [p. 385]	Congenital defect of endochondral bone formation, producing characteristic rounded lumbar "bullet-nosed" vertebrae, lumbar kyphosis, posterior scalloping of the vertebrae, increased intervertebral disc height, flattened vertebral bodies, and narrowed spinal canal; the pelvis may appear hypoplastic; milder forms of the disease may occur
Cretinism [p. 725]	Congenital hypothyroidism with delayed appearance of ossification centers, skeletal underdevelopment, wormian bones, and poorly developed sinuses; sail-like or tonguelike vertebrae and kyphosis at the thoracolumbar junction are common; changes may regress in adulthood
Diastrophic dysplasia [p. 393]	Autosomal, recessive, rhizomelic dwarfism secondary to a cartilage disorder; it is characterized by multiple skeletal disorders, including progressive kyphoscoliosis, anteriorly deformed vertebrae, hypoplastic first metacarpal, clubfoot, and deformed, flattened epiphyses
Mucopolysaccharidoses [p. 401]	A group of lysosomal storage diseases marked by a common disorder in mucopolysaccharide metabolism, evidenced by various mucopolysaccharides excreted in the urine; these substances collect in connective tissue, resulting in bone, cartilage, and connective tissue defects; characteristics are platyspondyly with dwarfism, kyphosis, and alterations in the appearance of the vertebrae; mucopolysaccharidosis I (Hurler syndrome) is associated with oval, posteriorly scalloped, anterior inferiorly beaked vertebrae; mucopolysaccharidosis IV (Morquio syndrome) is associated with flattened, anterior centrally beaked vertebrae
Neurofibromatosis (von Recklinghausen's disease) [p. 755]	Congenital disturbance of mesodermal and neuroectodermal tissue development, appearing clinically with cutaneous markings, bone deformity, and neurofibromas; spinal changes include posterior vertebral scalloping, enlarged intervertebral foramina, kyphoscoliosis, and anteriorly beaked or wedged vertebrae
Normal variant	Slightly beaked vertebrae, most often occurring in the thoracic spine; the vertebral defect usually appears more wedged than beaked; the vertebral body may appear anteriorly beaked before ossification of the ring epiphyses; these steplike defects contain the cartilage growth centers of the vertebral endplate; as ossification proceeds, a focus of bone fills the radiolucent defect (between 6 and 12 years of age), fusing to the vertebral body between 20 and 25 years of age

SP1b | Biconcave Vertebrae

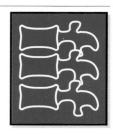

DISEASE	COMMENTS
Gaucher's disease [p. 744]	Genetic deficiency of glucocerebrosidase, with clinical findings of hepatosplenomegaly, osteopenia, osteonecrosis, focal osteolytic bone changes; biconcave vertebrae is a less common feature of the disease
Homocystinuria (FIG. 6-1) [p. 396]	Genetic disorder causing defect in collagen metabolism; it's presentation is similar to Marfan's disease; vertebrae appear osteopenic and biconcave or flattened
Notochordal persistence (FIG. 6-2)	Nonfocal, congenital, smooth, inward deformity of all or part of the superior, inferior, or both vertebral endplates; this type of deformity is less focal and involves more of the endplate than Schmorl's nodes

Continued

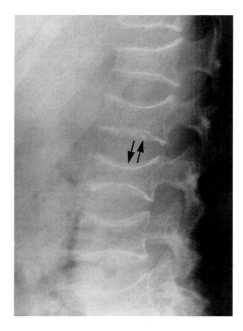

FIG. 6-1 Homocystinuria presenting with osteoporosis and biconcave vertebrae *(arrows)*. (Courtesy Steven P. Brownstein, Springfield, NJ.)

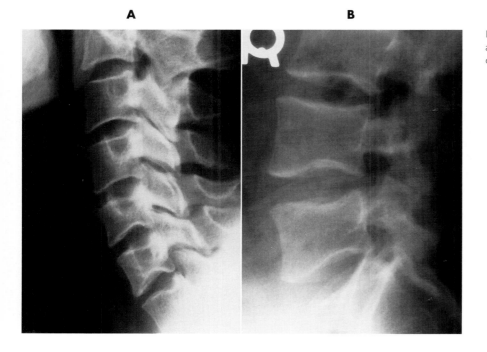

A   **B**

FIG. 6-2 Biconcave appearance of the cervical **(A)** and lumbar **(B)** vertebrae in different patients' notochordal persistency (or nuclear impression).

DISEASE	COMMENTS
Osteopenia	Deformity from decreased bone mass secondary to rickets, osteomalacia, steroid therapy, hyperparathyroidism, malnutrition, senile osteoporosis, immobilization, or postmenopausal bone alterations
Renal osteodystrophy [p. 718]	Secondary to renal glomerular disease; vertebral changes present with osteosclerosis ("rugger-jersey") and, less commonly, a biconcave appearance

DISEASE	COMMENTS
Schmorl's nodes	Prolapse of the nucleus pulposus into the vertebrae, producing abrupt, inward deformities of a focal area of the endplate; both endplates and multiple vertebrae may be involved
Sickle cell anemia (FIG. 6-3) [p. 604]	Genetic abnormality in which red blood cells assume a sickled configuration in low oxygen tension; the sickled cells may occlude small vessels with resulting ischemia; skeletal changes include osteopenia, coarse trabeculae, biconcave (more precisely, steplike or H-shaped) vertebrae, and dactylitis

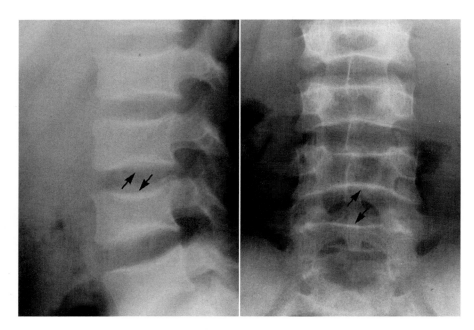

FIG. 6-3   Sickle cell anemia causing biconcave deformity of the lumbar vertebrae secondary to underperfusion of the center of the vertebrae in two patients (arrows).

SPIc | Blocked Vertebrae

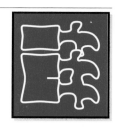

DISEASE	COMMENTS
Ankylosing spondylitis [p. 428]	Acquired interbody fusion—seronegative spondyloarthropathy characterized by involvement in the sacroiliac joints and spine; the vertebrae appear square with ossification of the annulus fibrosus; disc height maintained; the disease has a strong male predominance and always involves the sacroiliac joints
Infections	Acquired interbody fusion secondary to pyogenic (i.e., staphylococcus) or tuberculosis infections; disc height is usually decreased or absent
Isolated anomalies (FIG. 6-4)	Congenital failure of segmentation; presentation varies from slight hypoplasia of intervertebral disc space to complete fusion of adjacent vertebral bodies and neural arches; interbody fusion and neural arch fusion are most common in the lumbar spine but frequently occur in the thoracic and cervical regions as well; the sagittal diameter of the vertebrae is decreased with an inward concavity of the anterior body margins at the site of segmentation failure; fusion of posterior elements and underdevelopment of the intervertebral disc space is common and used to differentiate congenital from acquired etiology

Continued

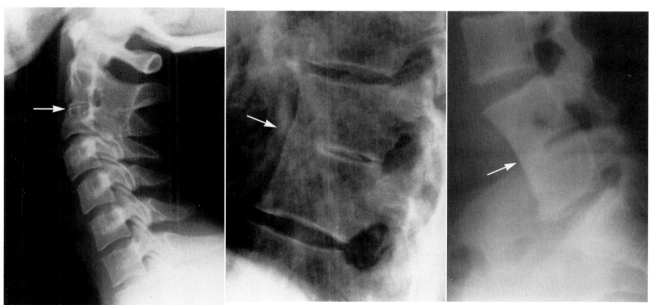

FIG. 6-4   Cervical **(A)**, thoracic **(B)**, and lumbar **(C)** congenital blocked vertebrae. All three patients exhibit hypoplasia of the intervertebral disc (*arrows*).

PART TWO Bone, Joints, and Soft Tissues

DISEASE	COMMENTS
Klippel-Feil syndrome (FIGS. 6-5 AND 6-6) [p. 397]	Congenital failure of segmentation occurring at multiple levels; associated radiographic findings may include Sprengel's deformity (elevation and medial rotation of the scapula), syndactyly, platybasia, and renal anomalies; patients usually demonstrate a clinical triad of a short neck, restricted cervical motion, and low posterior hairline
Rheumatoid arthritis (FIGS. 6-7 AND 6-8) [p. 442]	Chronic inflammatory arthritide that may demonstrate acquired interbody fusion, more commonly occurring with juvenile rheumatoid than adult presentations; the spinous processes do not fuse, but the remaining vertebral arches may fuse, particularly in the juvenile form
Surgical fusion	Acquired interbody fusion resulting from surgery; multiple levels may be involved; posterior joints are typically spared, intervertebral disc spaces are not visible; vertebral bodies may have a thick, square appearance, resulting from surgically placed paraspinal layers of bone as part of the fusion surgery
Trauma	Acquired interbody fusion from bone remodeling following severe trauma

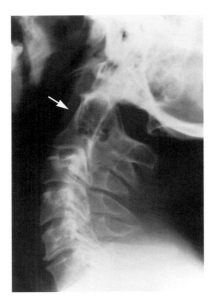

FIG. 6-5 Klippel-Feil syndrome characterized by the multiple blocked segments in the cervical spine. The occipital-atlantal space is nonexistent because of occipitalization of atlas, and the C2 and C3 levels are fused across the vertebral bodies and neural arches (*arrow*). (Courtesy Joseph W. Howe, Sylmar, Calif.)

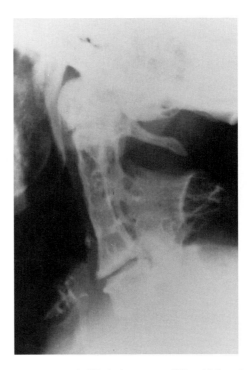

FIG. 6-6 Multiple congenital blocked segments of Klippel-Feil syndrome. Fusion is noted across the disc spaces and the vertebral arches. (Courtesy Joseph W. Howe, Sylmar, Calif.)

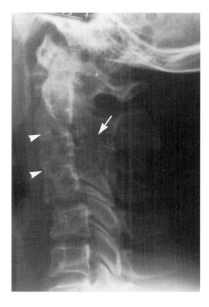

FIG. 6-7 Juvenile rheumatoid arthritis demonstrating fusion across the posterior joints of C2-4 *(arrow)* and underdevelopment of the vertebral bodies and disc spaces *(arrowheads).* (Courtesy Joseph W. Howe, Sylmar, Calif.)

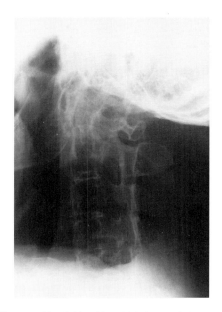

FIG. 6-8 Rheumatoid arthritis with multiple levels of disc and posterior joint fusion, appearing as blocked segments. (Courtesy Joseph W. Howe, Sylmar, Calif.)

PART TWO Bone, Joints, and Soft Tissues

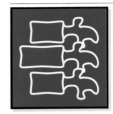

SP1d | Wide Enlarged Vertebrae

DISEASE	COMMENTS
Acromegaly [p. 715]	Pituitary eosinophilic adenoma that produces excess somatotropin, leading to increased levels of growth hormone; the disorder is marked by progressive enlargement of the hands, feet, head, jaw, and abdominal organs; vertebrae are enlarged with posterior body scalloping; patients may have diabetes mellitus
Expansile bone lesions **(FIGS. 6-9, 6-10, AND 6-11)**	Examples of expansile lesions known to develop in the vertebrae: giant cell tumor, hemangioma, aneurysmal bone cyst, osteoblastoma, Paget's disease, hydatid cyst, eosinophilic granuloma, fibrous dysplasia, chordoma, metastasis, osteosarcoma, chondrosarcoma, and angiosarcoma
Paget's disease **(FIG. 6-12)** [p. 761]	A generalized skeletal disease in which bone formation and resorption are both increased, leading to abnormally thick and soft bones with disorganized "mosaic" trabeculae; skull, pelvis, and vertebrae are common sites of involvement; vertebrae appear enlarged with thick cortices ("picture framed" vertebrae)

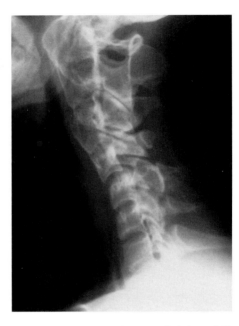

FIG. 6-9   Fibrous dysplasia causing expansile lesions of C2 and C3.

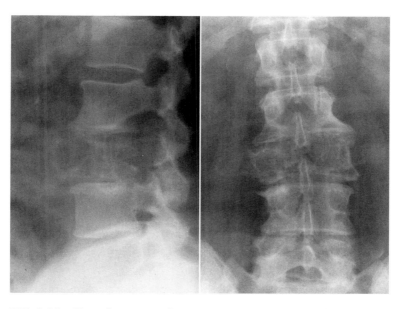

FIG. 6-10 Giant cell tumor appearing as a cystic expansile lesion of L3. (Courtesy Joseph W. Howe, Sylmar, Calif.)

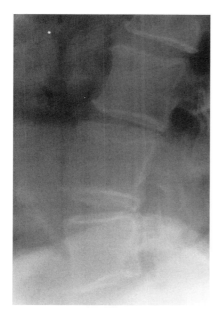

FIG. 6-11 Hemangioma of L4 presenting as an expansile body lesion. (Courtesy Joseph W. Howe, Sylmar, Calif.)

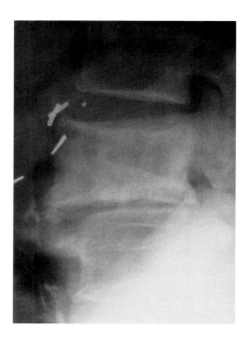

FIG. 6-12 Marked enlargement of the L3 vertebra secondary to Paget's disease.

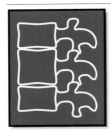

SP1e | Tall Enlarged Vertebrae

DISEASE	COMMENTS
Blocked vertebrae	If associated with congenital or acquired etiologies, may appear as single "tall" vertebrae, which is particularly true with neural arch involvement
Gibbus formation	Often has a tall vertebra at its lower end secondary to altered compressive forces on the vertebra; this formation is seen in the tuberculosis of children
Marfan's syndrome (Arachnodactyly) [p. 399]	Congenital disturbance of collagen formation primarily expressed as defects of the skeleton and heart valves; skeletal changes include tall vertebrae, posterior vertebral scalloping, wide spinal canal, scoliosis, and a long, slender appearance of the metatarsals, metacarpals, phalanges, and long narrow bones (dolichostenomelia)

SP1f | Anterior Scalloped Vertebrae

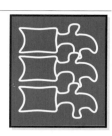

DISEASE	COMMENTS
Aortic aneurysms **(FIGS. 6-13 AND 6-14)** [p. 979]	Because of proximity, may cause erosions along the anterior left side of the vertebrae, sometimes termed *Oppenheimer erosions;* although not always present, the majority of cases will also demonstrate calcification of the dilated vessel walls; the intervertebral disc is not involved
Lymphadenopathy	Enlarged lymph nodes resulting from lymphoma, inflammatory lymphadenopathy, or metastatic lymphadenopathy that may cause pressure erosions on the anterior surfaces of the vertebrae, primarily the lumbar vertebrae
Normal variant	Mild in size; multiple levels are common; variants are most often seen in the lower thoracic and upper lumbar spine
Tuberculosis [p. 611]	Common to find infectious erosions of the vertebral margins with paraspinal masses and involvement of the intervertebral disc

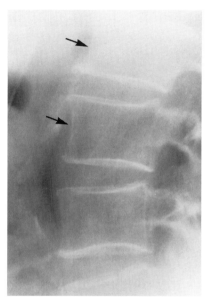

FIG. 6-13 Lateral lumbar radiograph with an increased anterior concavity of the upper lumbar vertebrae *(arrows),* which was thought to represent pressure erosions from an aneurysm later diagnosed in this patient. (Courtesy Joseph W. Howe, Sylmar, Calif.)

A

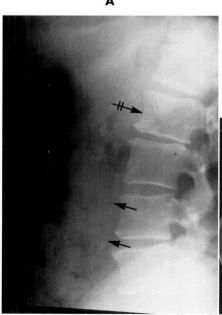

B

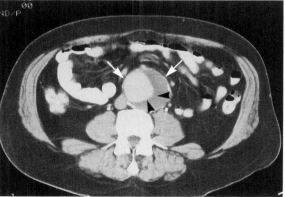

FIG. 6-14 Lateral lumbar radiographs with vascular calcification in the posterior wall of the abdominal aorta **(A)** and poor visualization of the anterior wall **(B)**. There is an exaggerated anterior concavity of the L2 vertebral body, suspicious for erosion secondary to the aneurysm *(crossed arrow).* The CT demonstrates an aneurysm of the abdominal aorta *(arrows)* with a less dense perimeter of the vessel lumen corresponding to clotting blood **(B)** *(arrowheads).*

PART TWO Bone, Joints, and Soft Tissues

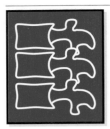

SPIg | Posterior Scalloped Vertebrae

DISEASE	COMMENTS
Achondroplasia [p. 385]	Congenital defect of endochondral bone formation resulting in the following spinal changes: posterior scalloping of the vertebrae, increased intervertebral disc height, flattened vertebral bodies, narrow spinal canal, lumbar kyphosis, "bullet-shaped" lumbar vertebrae; the pelvis may appear hypoplastic; milder forms of the disease may occur
Acromegaly [p. 715]	Excess levels of growth hormone resulting from a pituitary eosinophilic adenoma overproducing somatotropin; the disorder is marked by progressive enlargement of the hands, feet, head, jaw, and abdominal organs; vertebrae are enlarged with posterior scalloping; patients may have diabetes mellitus
Congenital syndromes (FIGS. 6-15 AND 6-16)	Arachnodactyly (see previous Enlarged Vertebra discussion), mucopolysaccharidosis syndromes (i.e., Hurler, Hunter's, Morquio, and others), Marfan syndrome, Ehlers-Danlos syndrome, and others
Increased intraspinal pressure	Increased intraspinal pressure from an ependymoma or communicating hydrocephalus may cause adjacent bone erosions
Neurofibromatosis (von Recklinghausen's disease) [p. 755]	Congenital disturbance of mesodermal and neuroectodermal tissues, appearing clinically with cutaneous markings, bone deformity, and neurofibromas; selected skeletal changes include kyphoscoliosis, enlarged intervertebral foramina, posterior vertebral body scalloping from dural ectasia or neurofibroma, bowing deformity of the lower extremities
Tumors	Bone erosion from adjacent spinal canal tumors (e.g., meningioma, ependymoma, lipoma, neurofibroma)

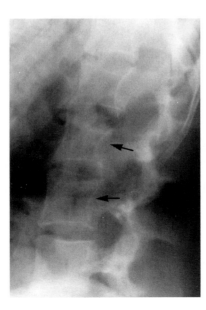

FIG. 6-15 Posterior body scalloping secondary to dural ectasia of unknown etiology (arrows). (Courtesy Joseph W. Howe, Sylmar, Calif.)

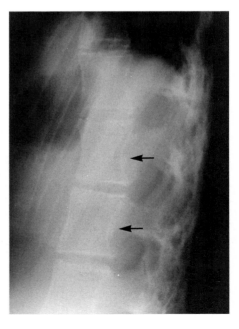

FIG. 6-16 Marfan's syndrome with prominent scalloping of the posterior vertebral bodies (arrows).

SP1h | Square Vertebrae

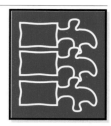

DISEASE	COMMENTS
Inflammatory arthropathies (FIG. 6-17)	Commonly associated with most characteristically square vertebrae, which is one of the earliest findings of this disease; square vertebrae may also be a feature of psoriatic arthritis, Reiter's syndrome, and rheumatoid arthritis (usually juvenile); the seronegative inflammatory arthropathies usually involve the sacroiliac joints
Paget's disease [p. 761]	A generalized skeletal disease in which bone formation and resorption are both increased, leading to abnormally thick, soft bones with disorganized "mosaic" trabeculae; skull, pelvis, and vertebrae are common sites of involvement; vertebrae usually appear enlarged and square with thick cortices ("picture-framed" vertebrae)

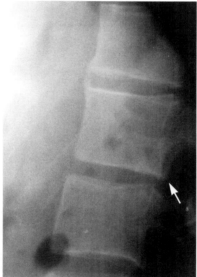

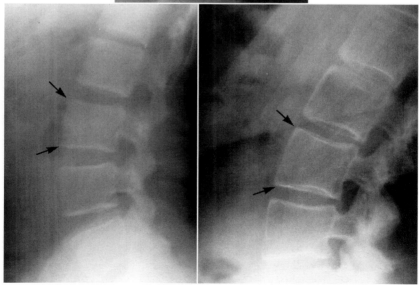

FIG. 6-17 Three cases of ankylosing spondylitis presenting with square lumbar vertebrae resulting from corner proliferations *(arrows).* (*Top* and *bottom left,* Courtesy Joseph W. Howe, Sylmar, Calif.)

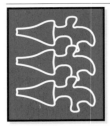

SPIi | Wedged Vertebrae

DISEASE	COMMENTS
Congenital syndromes	Possible causes of wedged congenital vertebrae and other characteristic alterations; syndromes include achondroplasia, hypothyroidism, and mucopolysaccharidoses; usually multiple levels are involved
Hemivertebrae (FIG. 6-18)	Focal vertebral hypoplasia, resulting in a lateral, anterior, or posterior wedged hemivertebra at one or multiple levels; lateral hemivertebrae produce scoliosis; posterior hemivertebrae are commonly posteriorly displaced up to 3 mm and produce a kyphosis
Infections (FIG. 6-19)	Tuberculosis and pyogenic infections (e.g., staphylococcus); clues to an infection include involvement of intervertebral disc space, paraspinal masses and calcifications, cortical demineralization, and angular kyphosis
Normal variant	Slightly wedged vertebrae that usually develop in the thoracic spine
Scheuermann's disease [p. 413]	Posttraumatic defect of vertebral endplate maturation presenting during adolescence with three or more levels of wedged vertebrae, narrowed anterior disc space, multiple Schmorl's nodes, and vertebral endplate irregularity; the disease usually develops in the middle and lower thoracic spine
Trauma (FIGS. 6-20 AND 6-21)	Compression fracture leading to wedged configuration; endplate defects, cortical offset of anterior body margin ("step defect"), horizontal zone of bone impaction within vertebrae, and history of trauma are clues to traumatic etiology

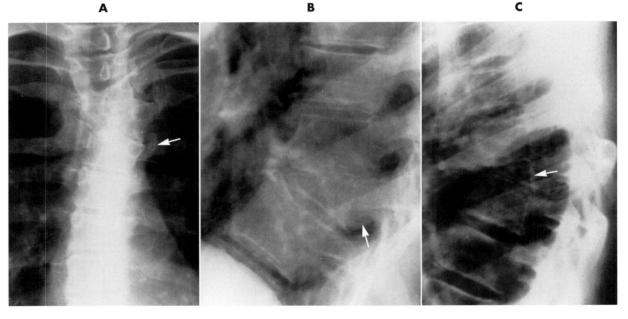

A   **B**   **C**

FIG. 6-18 Lateral **(A)** and dorsal **(B)** and **(C)** thoracic hemivertebrae *(arrows)*. (*Top* and *bottom right,* Courtesy Joseph W. Howe, Sylmar, Calif.)

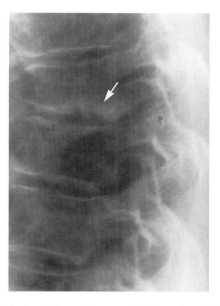

FIG. 6-19 Infection leading to the trapezoidal shape of a middle thoracic vertebra with destructive endplate changes and narrowing of the intervertebral disc space *(arrow)*. (Courtesy Joseph W. Howe, Sylmar, Calif.)

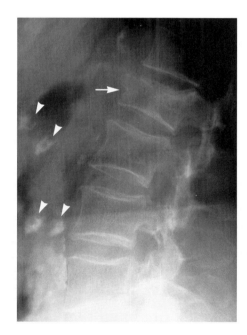

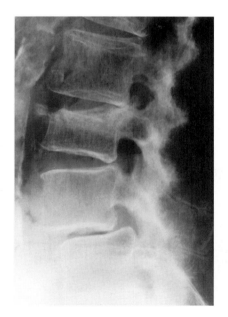

FIG. 6-20 Compression fracture in the upper lumbar spine *(arrow)* and multiple levels of costal cartilage calcification *(arrowheads)*. (Courtesy Steven P. Brownstein, Springfield, NJ.)

FIG. 6-21 Compression fracture and resulting wedged vertebral configuration. In addition, a grade I degenerative spondylolisthesis of L4 on L5 is present with degenerative vacuum phenomena at L4. Calcification of the abdominal aorta anterior to the spine can also be seen.

PART TWO
Bone, Joints, and Soft Tissues

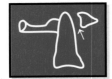

SP2 | Atlantoaxial Subluxation

The normal measurement of the atlantodental interval (ADI) is less than or equal to 5 mm in children and 3 mm in adults. A measurement beyond these limits suggests instability of the atlantoaxial articulation. Instability results from compromise of the transverse atlantal ligament or C2 odontoid process. Because the joint is most stressed during flexion, forward flexion radiographs provide a more specific measure of ADI enlargement than neutral lateral radiographs. If the anterior tubercle or odontoid process does not represent fixed, clearly defined points of mensuration, atlantoaxial instability can be assessed by choosing another point on the atlas and axis.

DISEASE	COMMENTS
Congenital conditions	Conditions that include occipitalization of atlas, Down syndrome (20% of cases), Morquio syndrome, and spondyloepiphyseal dysplasia; these are associated with atlantoaxial subluxation secondary to absence or attenuation of the transverse atlantal ligament, which may also occur as an isolated anomaly
Inflammatory spondyloarthropathy (FIG. 6-22)	Condition that includes rheumatoid (adult and juvenile types) arthritis, ankylosing spondylitis, psoriatic arthritis, Reiter's syndrome, and systemic lupus erythematosus; these are associated with synovitis, ligament attenuation, and odontoid erosions, which may lead to instability of the atlantoaxial articulation
Marfan's syndrome [p. 399]	Genetic disorder of connective development that leads to ocular, cardiovascular, and musculoskeletal abnormalities; joint instability follows ligamentous laxity
Odontoid anomalies	Aplasia, hypoplasia, or malunion of the odontoid process to axis—conditions that may lead to instability
Regional infections	Include retropharyngeal abscesses, otitis media, mastoiditis, cervical adenitis, parotitis, and alveolar abscesses
Trauma	Instability resulting from fracture or torn ligaments

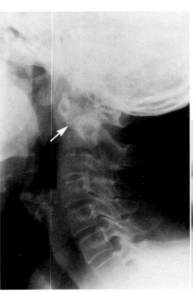
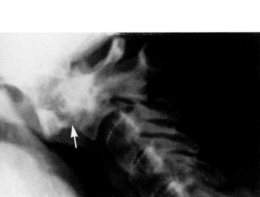
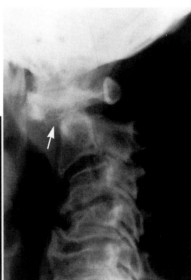

FIG. 6-22   Three patients with rheumatoid arthritis and an increased atlantodental space *(arrows)*. (Courtesy Joseph W. Howe, Sylmar, Calif.)

SP3 | Bony Outgrowths of the Spine

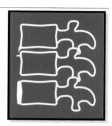

ost bony outgrowths of the spine represent osteophytes, related to degenerative arthropathy of the intervertebral disc spaces or posterior joints. An appearance of multilevel, flowing, thick, mostly anterior paravertebral outgrowths is characteristic of diffuse idiopathic skeletal hyperostosis (DISH). Large, coarse, incompletely bridging paravertebral outgrowths are associated with Reiter's syndrome and psoriatic arthropathy. In contrast, delicate, thin, completely bridging outgrowths *(marginal syndesmophytes)* are characteristic of ankylosing spondylitis.

DISEASE	COMMENTS		
Acromegaly [p. 715]	Excess levels of growth hormone resulting from a pituitary eosinophilic adenoma over-producing somatotropin; the disorder is marked by progressive enlargement of the hands, feet, head, jaw, and abdominal organs; vertebrae are enlarged with posterior scalloping and new bone growth along the anterior body margins	**Ankylosing spondylitis (FIG. 6-23)** [p. 428]	Seronegative spondyloarthropathy characterized by arthritis targeted to the sacroiliac joints and spine; bilateral, symmetrical, thin intervertebral connections, known as *syndesmophytes,* are prominent features, representing ossification of the outermost lamellae of the annulus fibrosis; posterior joint fusion is common; collectively, multiple levels produce a "bamboo spine" appearance; in addition, the anterior body margins appear straight or square

Continued

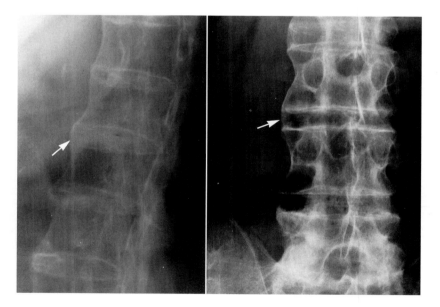

FIG. 6-23   Thin, bridging syndesmophytes characteristic of ankylosing spondylitis in four patients *(arrows)*. *(Left,* Courtesy Joseph W. Howe, Sylmar, Calif.)   *Continued*

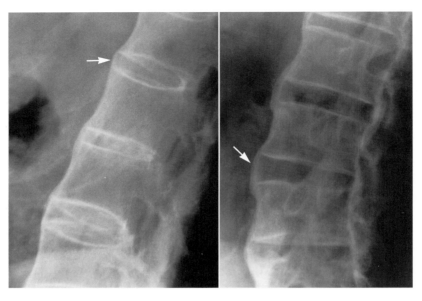

FIG. 6-23—cont'd   Thin, bridging syndesmophytes characteristic of ankylosing spondylitis in four patients (arrows). (Left, Courtesy Joseph W. Howe, Sylmar, Calif.)

DISEASE	COMMENTS
Diffuse idiopathic skeletal hyperostosis (DISH) **(FIG. 6-24)** [p. 477]	Idiopathic disease marked by thick, flowing anterior longitudinal ligament ossifications along the anterior and lateral body margins; DISH is most common in the thoracolumbar region
Fluorosis	Chronic fluoride intoxication associated with osteophytosis and vertebral hyperostosis with calcification of the paraspinal ligaments; vertebrae have increased radiodensity; fluorosis is most marked in the innominates and lumbar spine
Hypoparathyroidism [p. 722]	Inadequate parathormone from undersecretion or surgical removal of gland; skeletal changes include increased or decreased radiodensity, thickened calvarium, premature fusion of ossification centers, and ossification of the paraspinal ligaments
Neuropathic spine [p. 483]	Primarily caused by diabetes mellitus, syringomyelia, and tabes dorsalis; the radiographic appearance is marked by loss of intervertebral disc height, increased bone radiodensity, misalignment, fragmentation, and prominent osteophytosis
Ochronosis	Inherited disorder of excessive homogentisic acid production and subsequent accumulation within connective tissues; the spine is affected by multiple levels of intervertebral disc calcification and massive osteophytosis and ankylosis, especially in the elderly
Spondylosis deformans (degenerative disc disease) **(FIG. 6-25)** [p. 458]	Degenerative disease involving principally the outer portions of the intervertebral disc, is appearing as curved ("claw") or horizontal ("traction") vertebral osteophyte, with or without other findings of degenerative disc disease (i.e., endplate osteosclerosis and irregularity, narrowed disc space, misalignment, and others); osteophytes form in response to increased tension at the Sharpey's fibers anchoring the outer annulus into the cortical bone of the adjacent endplate; degenerative osteophytes are moderately thick (thicker than AS, thinner than DISH) and typically incompletely bridge the intervertebral disc space
Reiter's and psoriatic arthropathy **(FIGS. 6-26 AND 6-27)**	Inflammatory arthropathies associated with paravertebral ossifications incompletely bridging the intervertebral disc spaces; typically found at the thoracolumbar spine; the paravertebral ossifications are typically thick, but uncommonly may appear thin; the latter appearance is identical to those of ankylosing spondylitis
Trauma	May cause bony outgrowths from degenerative joint changes or dystrophic tissue calcifications

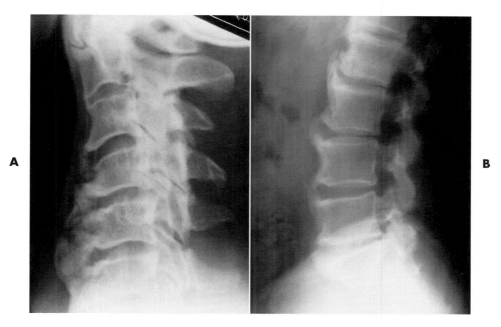

FIG. 6-24 DISH affecting the cervical **(A)** and lumbar **(B)** spines of different patients.

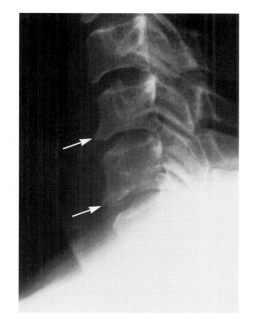

FIG. 6-25 Degenerative osteophytes projecting from the anterior vertebral body margins *(arrows)*.

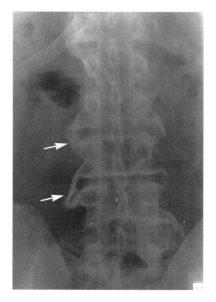

FIG. 6-26 Reiter's disease with prominent syndesmophytes at multiple lumbar levels *(arrows)*. (Courtesy Joseph W. Howe, Sylmar, Calif.)

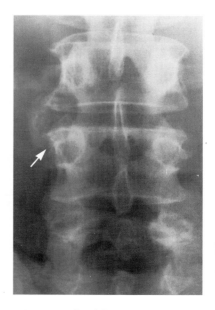

FIG. 6-27 Psoriatic spondyloarthropathy with characteristic thick syndesmophytes incompletely bridging the disc space *(arrow)*. (Courtesy Joseph W. Howe, Sylmar, Calif.)

PART TWO Bone, Joints, and Soft Tissues

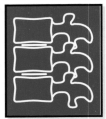

SP4 | Calcification of the Intervertebral Discs

Calcification of the intervertebral disc is noted by increased radiopacity within the normally radiolucent disc space. The appearance represents dystrophic calcification of the nucleus pulposus or surrounding annulus. The appearance is usually stable, with the notable exception of idiopathic juvenile disc calcification, which disappears by adulthood.

DISEASE	COMMENTS
Ankylosing spondylitis [p. 428]	Seronegative spondyloarthropathy characterized by involvement in the sacroiliac joints and spine; single or multiple levels of disc calcification may be seen, usually concurrent with facet ankylosis and syndesmophytes at the same level
Blocked segmentation (FIG. 6-28)	Dystrophic disc calcification occurring with congenital block segmentation, Klippel-Feil syndrome, myositis ossificans progressiva, and surgical fusion; it is probably related to a loss or reduction of intersegmental motion with consequential nutritional deprivation of tissue
CPPD crystal deposition disease (chondrocalcinosis) [p. 453]	Calcium pyrophosphate dihydrate deposition (CPPD) disease, presenting with crystal-induced synovitis (pseudogout) and cartilage calcification (chondrocalcinosis); spine involvement appears with calcification of the annulus fibrosis, reduction of the disc space, and sclerotic vertebral body margins; CPPD more commonly involves the extremities
Degenerative spondylosis	Common findings of degenerative arthropathy of the intervertebral disc: vertebral marginal osteophytosis, vertebral endplate sclerosis, Schmorl's nodes, disc vacuum phenomena, and narrowing of the disc space; another finding, particularly in the elderly, includes calcification of the posterior portion of the nucleus pulposus
Hemochromatosis [p. 600]	A disorder of iron metabolism leading to hemosiderin deposits in the visceral and connective tissues; calcification of the nucleus pulposus and annulus fibrosus may occur
Hyperparathyroidism [p. 718]	Overproduction of parathormone from primary or secondary disorders of the parathyroid glands; the disease is marked by osteopenia, osteosclerosis, bone resorption, and soft tissue and vascular calcification; both the nucleus pulposus and annulus fibrosis may become calcified; specifically, the central regions of the vertebral bodies appear osteopenic with characteristic homogeneous radiodense bands traversing horizontally at each end of the vertebra ("rugger-jersey" spine)
Idiopathic (FIGS. 6-29 AND 6-30)	Includes childhood and adult forms; the childhood variety is transient (usually of the cervical spine), restricted to the nucleus pulposus (often at only one level), and commonly associated with clinical symptoms; the adult variety is asymptomatic, persistent, and probably related to degeneration

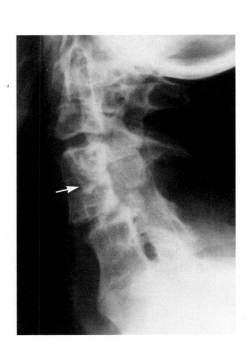

FIG. 6-28　Multiple congenital blocked segments indicative of Klippel-Feil syndrome. There appears to be a focus of intervertebral disc calcification at the C3 and C4 disc space (arrow).

Continued

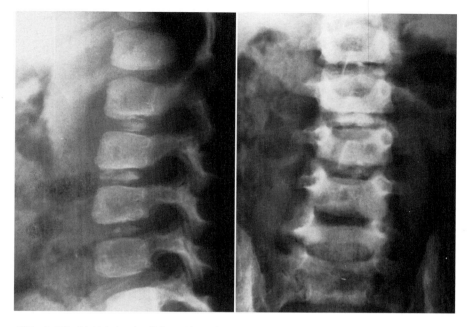

FIG. 6-29 Multiple levels of idiopathic lumbar intervertebral disc calcification. (Courtesy Steven P. Brownstein, Springfield, NJ.)

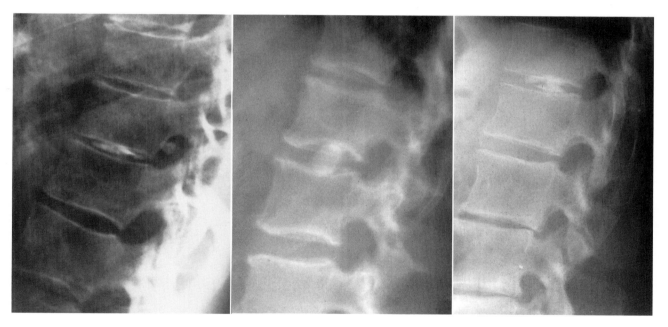

FIG. 6-30 Idiopathic disc calcification in three patients who do not demonstrate degenerative changes at the level of calcification. (Courtesy Joseph W. Howe, Sylmar, Calif.)

DISEASE	COMMENTS
Ochronosis (FIG. 6-31)	Inherited disorder of excessive homogentisic acid production and subsequent accumulation within connective tissues; degeneration of the cartilage results; multiple levels of disc calcification are essentially pathognomonic; the disease typically develops in the elderly and may be accompanied by advanced degenerative disease of the spine
Posttraumatic	Potential of developing one or more levels of disc calcification if spine has been previously injured; patients with poliomyelitis may have disc calcification, which is believed to result from trauma caused by lack of muscular support
Sequestered disc prolapse	May have dystrophic calcification in displaced portions of the intervertebral disc; more common in posterior fragments

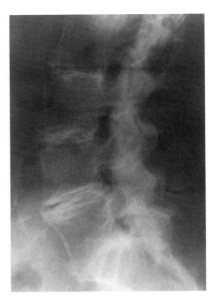

FIG. 6-31   Ochronosis marked by multiple levels of intervertebral disc calcification. In addition, advanced posterior joint arthrosis is indicated by the radiodense and irregular appearance. (Courtesy Joseph W. Howe, Sylmar, Calif.)

SP5 | Narrow Intervertebral Disc Height

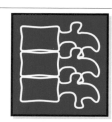

In the adult patient, narrowing of the intervertebral disc spaces is typically related to degenerative disc disease. Degenerative narrowing typically exhibits other degenerative findings (i.e., osteophytes, eburnation) and in its advanced stages involves multiple levels and the posterior joints. Grossly advanced degenerative spinal changes may be due to neuropathy. Infections represent more serious causes of a narrowed disc space, presenting with bone destruction, paraspinal mass, and less prominent degenerative findings. In particular, intradiscal vacuum phenomena are not seen with infection. The following table lists causes of narrowed intervertebral disc spaces at one or more levels.

DISEASE	COMMENTS
CPPD crystal deposition disease (chondrocalcinosis) [p. 453]	Calcium pyrophosphate dihydrate deposition (CPPD) disease, presenting with crystal induced synovitis (pseudogout) and cartilage calcification (chondrocalcinosis); spine involvement appears with calcification of the annulus fibrosis, reduction of the disc space, and sclerotic vertebral body margins; extremities are much more commonly involved than the spine
Hypoplastic disc (developmental) **(FIG. 6-32)**	Congenital underdevelopment of the intervertebral disc seen as an isolated anomaly at the L5 level or in conjunction with congenital block segmentation or Scheuermann's disease

Continued

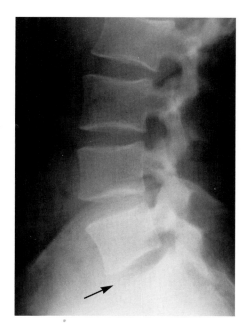

FIG. 6-32   The L5 disc space is slightly decreased *(arrow);* however, because no other signs of degeneration are present (e.g., osteophytes, vacuum phenomena), the narrowing of the L5 disc is more likely representative of disc hypoplasia. Disc hypoplasia is a common cause of a narrow disc space at the L5 level and is particularly suggested by an L5 disc space, which appears narrow in a younger patient who is not likely to exhibit degeneration.

PART TWO Bone, Joints, and Soft Tissues

DISEASE

**Infections
(FIGS. 6-33,
6-34, AND 6-35)**

COMMENTS

Spinal infections secondary to various causative agents (e.g., pyogenic, tuberculosis, brucellosis, typhoid infections) producing bone destruction, indistinct cortical margins, intervertebral disc space narrowing, and paraspinal mass; usually involve only one level, not multiple levels as occurs with a degenerative etiology

**Inflammatory
arthritides**

Seropositive (i.e., rheumatoid) or seronegative (i.e., ankylosing spondylitis) inflammatory arthritide involving the spine, which manifests with osteoporosis, osteosclerosis of the vertebral body margins, and concurrent involvement of the posterior joints; reduction of the disc spaces is uncommon, with the exception of rheumatoid arthritis in the cervical spine; ankylosing spondylitis has propensity to involve the sacroiliac joints, and rheumatoid arthritis to involve the metacarpal phalangeal joints

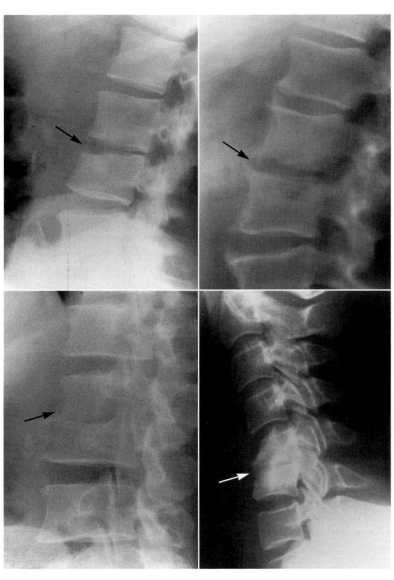

FIG. 6-33   Intervertebral disc infections in different patients indicated by narrowed disc spaces with accompanying endplate destruction *(arrows)*. (Courtesy Joseph W. Howe, Sylmar, Calif.)

Intervertebral osteochondrosis (degenerative disc disease) (FIG. 6-36) [p. 459]

Degenerative disease involving principally the inner portions of the intervertebral disc (nucleus pulposus and cartilaginous endplate), typically presenting with other degenerative findings: osteophytes, misalignment, vacuum phenomena, endplate osteosclerosis and irregularity

Neuropathic spine [p. 483]

Primary causes: diabetes mellitus, syringomyelia, and tabes dorsalis; the radiographic appearance is marked by loss of intervertebral disc height, increased bone radiodensity, misalignment, fragmentation, and prominent osteophytosis; the changes are more advanced than those of age-related degeneration

Ochronosis

Inherited disorder of excessive homogentisic acid production and subsequent accumulation within connective tissues; the spine is affected by multiple levels of intervertebral disc calcification and massive osteophytosis and ankylosis, especially in the elderly

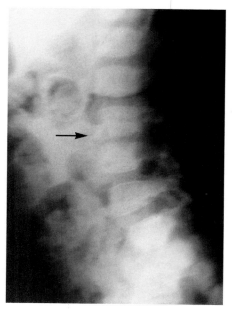

FIG. 6-35 L3 intervertebral disc infection *(arrow)*.

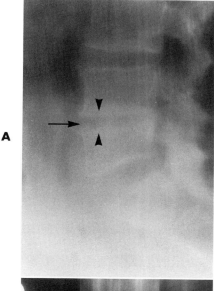

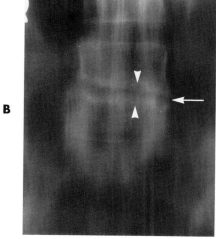

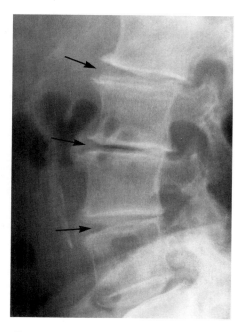

FIG. 6-34 Lumbar intervertebral disc infection seen on a lateral radiograph **(A)** and an anteroposterior linear tomogram **(B)**. Both studies demonstrate a narrowed L4 intervertebral disc space *(arrows)* with endplate irregularity following bone destruction *(arrowheads)*.

FIG. 6-36 Degenerative narrowing of the intervertebral disc space *(arrows)*.

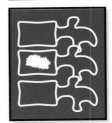

SP6 | Osteolytic Lesions of the Spine

This pattern encompasses solitary and multiple osteolytic lesions of the spine and sacrum. A lesion may involve the vertebral body, neural arch, or appendages of the segments. The list of differentials is long but can be functionally abbreviated by noting the area of the vertebrae that is primarily involved.

Lesions that more commonly involve the vertebral body include chordoma, aneurysmal bone cyst, leukemia, lymphoma, hemangioma, hydatid cyst, osteoblastoma, multiple myeloma, metastasis, and eosinophilic granuloma. A helpful mnemonic for these lesions is *CALL HOME*. Although this mnemonic is most often applied to vertebral body lesions in general, each of the entries in the mnemonic may present as osteolytic lesions.

Lesions primarily seen in the neural arch and transverse processes include giant cell tumor, osteoblastoma, aneurysmal bone cyst, plasmacytoma, and eosinophilic granuloma. A helpful mnemonic for these lesions is *GO APE*. Many of these lesions also appear expansile. The conditions that most often involve the sacrum include giant cell tumor, aneurysmal bone cyst, plasmacytoma, chordoma, chondrosarcoma, and hemophilic pseudotumor. If multiple vertebrae are involved, the list can be abbreviated to metastasis, myeloma, lymphoma, Paget's, angiosarcoma, and eosinophilic granuloma. Regardless of their location in the vertebrae, lesions most noted for their expansile tendencies include aneurysmal bone cysts, hemangioma, and osteoblastoma. Any expanding spinal lesions may encroach on the neural canal. Specialized imaging may be needed to assess the canal and assist in definitive diagnosis.

DISEASE	COMMENTS
Aneurysmal bone cysts **(FIG. 6-37)** [p. 634]	Solitary, benign osteolytic lesions that expand within a long bone or a vertebra (10% to 30%), are associated with local pain and tenderness, and usually develop before age 20 years
Angiosarcoma	A rare, malignant, expansile neoplasm occurring most often in the breast and skin, with only 10% occurring in the spine (mostly lumbar)
Chordomas **(FIG. 6-38)** [p. 676]	Rare, low-grade malignancies arising from notochord remnants; only 13% arise in the spine (above sacrum), usually at C2; appearance may include body collapse and anterior vertebral mass; tumor may cross the intervertebral disc space
Eosinophilic granuloma **(FIG. 6-39)** [p. 747]	Proliferation of eosinophils seen most commonly in children and young adults, with spine involvement in less than 10% of cases; it may appear with advanced body collapse "vertebra plana" and multiple levels
Fibrous dysplasia **(FIGS. 6-40 AND 6-41)** [p. 651]	Nonneoplastic disturbance of bone maintenance; spine involvement is uncommon; it may have nonhomogeneous "ground glass" appearance

Continued

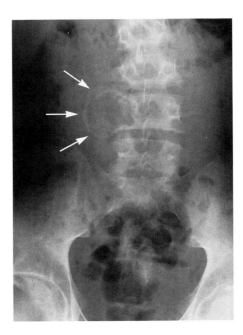

FIG. 6-37   Aneurysmal bone cyst involving the right transverse process of L4 *(arrows)*.

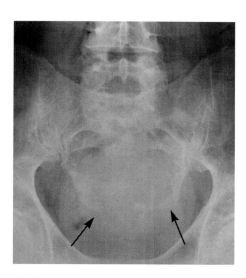

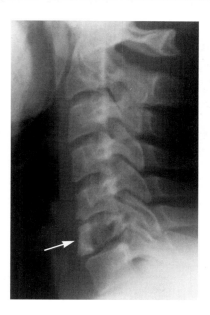

FIG. 6-38 Midline osteolytic sacrococcygeal chordoma *(arrows)*. (Courtesy Steven P. Brownstein, Springfield, NJ.)

FIG. 6-39 Osteolytic defect of the C6 vertebral body secondary to eosinophilic granuloma *(arrow)*. (Courtesy Joseph W. Howe, Sylmar, Calif.)

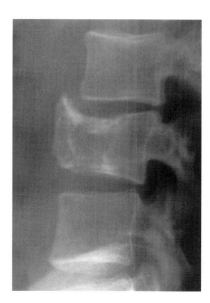

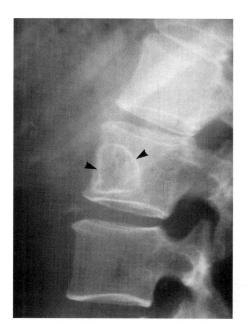

FIG. 6-40 Cystic expansile lesion resulting from fibrous dysplasia of the L3 vertebral body. (Courtesy Joseph W. Howe, Sylmar, Calif.)

FIG. 6-41 Fibrous dysplasia appearing as a well-marginated *(arrowheads)* osteolytic lesion of the vertebral body. The matrix of the lesion is not radiolucent, but it appears "smoky," or similar to ground glass. (Courtesy Steven P. Brownstein, Springfield, NJ.)

DISEASE	COMMENTS
Giant cell tumors (FIG. 6-42) [p. 654]	Occasionally malignant, well-defined, osteolytic lesions of bone; spine involvement (above sacrum) is rare
Hemangioma (FIG. 6-43) [p. 658]	Common congenital proliferation of vascular endothelium that leads to a benign osteolytic appearance, commonly with characteristic vertical struts ("jailbar" vertebrae); most occur in the vertebral bodies
Hydatid (*Echinococcus*) cysts (FIG. 6-44) [p. 979]	Cysts that may be formed in bone (but are usually formed in the liver) by the larval stage of *Echinococcus;* they appear as slow-growing, destructive lesions surrounded by sclerotic borders and are mostly limited to endemic areas

DISEASE	COMMENTS
Infections (FIGS. 6-45 AND 6-46)	Spinal infections secondary to various causative agents (e.g., pyogenic, tuberculosis, brucellosis, typhoid infections), producing bone destruction, indistinct cortical margins, intervertebral disc space narrowing, and paraspinal mass
Lymphoma [p. 685]	Primary and secondary (from systemic non-Hodgkin's lymphoma and Hodgkin's disease) lymphoma of bone that appears as permeative radiolucent lesions of the lower extremities, pelvis, and spine; less commonly the lesions appear with dense vertebral sclerosis

Continued

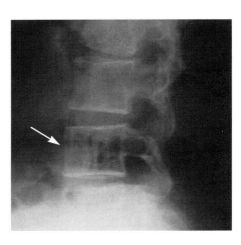

FIG. 6-43   Hemangioma of L4 with characteristic vertical striations *(arrow).* (Courtesy Ian D. McLean, Davenport, Iowa.)

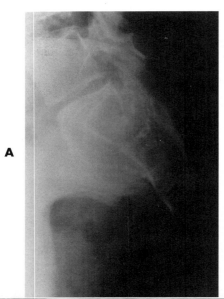

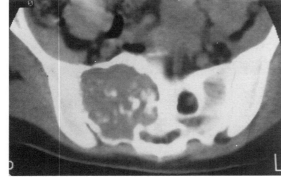

FIG. 6-42   Giant cell tumor appearing on plain film **(A)** and computed tomogram **(B)** as a cystic lesion of the sacrum. (Courtesy Joseph W. Howe, Sylmar, Calif.)

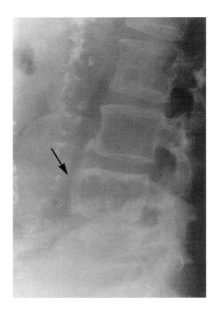

FIG. 6-44   Hydatid cyst causing an expansile osteolytic lesion of the L4 vertebral body *(arrow).* (Courtesy Joseph W. Howe, Sylmar, Calif.)

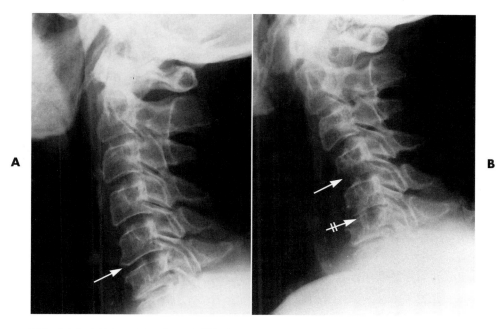

FIG. 6-45 Initial cervical radiograph **(A)** of a patient with neck pain reveals only moderated disc degeneration at C5 *(arrow)* and reduced cervical curvature. One month following, the kyphotic cervical spine **(B)** exhibits osteolytic bone destruction of the C4 vertebral body *(arrow)* and more advanced disc space narrowing at C5 *(crossed arrow)* consistent with multiple levels of infection. (Courtesy Steven P. Brownstein, Springfield, NJ.)

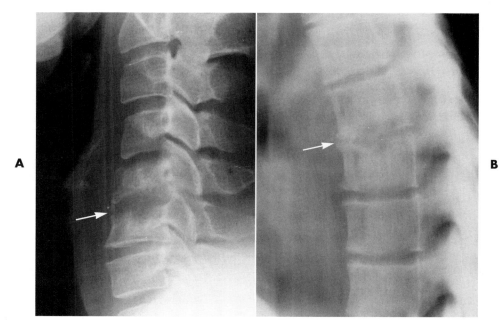

FIG. 6-46 Two patients who both exhibit narrowed intervertebral disc spaces and osteolytic endplate changes *(arrows)* consistent with infection in the cervical **(A)** and thoracic **(B)** spine. (Courtesy Steven P. Brownstein, Springfield, NJ.)

DISEASE	COMMENTS
Metastases (FIG. 6-47) [p. 687]	Bone metastases: common to the spine and rarely involves the skeleton distal to the elbows or knees (acral metastasis) and typically appears as a polyostotic, moth-eaten pattern of osteolytic bone destruction with poorly defined zones of transition; periosteal reaction and soft tissue masses are typically small or absent; this usually develops in patients over the age of 40 years; neuroblastoma, retinoblastoma, rhabdomyosarcoma, and Ewing's tumors are common causes of metastasis among infants and children
Multiple myelomas/plasma-cytomas [p. 700]	Malignant proliferations of plasma cells developing in predominately the red marrow of various bones; the skull, vertebral bodies, ribs, and proximal humeri and femora are most commonly involved

DISEASE	COMMENTS
Osteoblastomas (FIG. 6-48) [p. 667]	Benign bone lesions that have a propensity to involve the neural arches of the spine; they may be very expansile or appear as a radiodense lesion with a central nidus
Paget's disease (FIG. 6-49) [p. 761]	Chronic skeletal disease of aberrant bone remodeling, marked by bone enlargement, softening, and rarely sarcomatous changes; the lumbar spine is one of the most common areas of involvement; the enlarged and thickened vertebral cortices appear as radiodense bands around the perimeter of the vertebra ("picture frame"); less commonly it appears predominantly as a solitary osteolytic or sclerotic lesion of the vertebral body

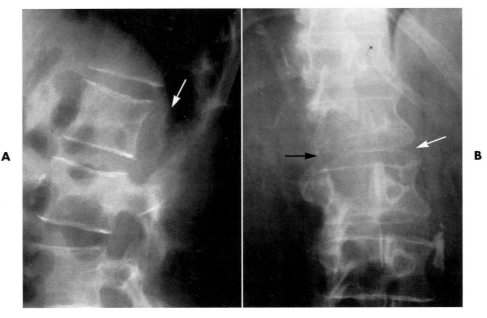

FIG. 6-47   Lateral **(A)** and anteroposterior **(B)** lumbar projections revealing osteolytic destruction of the vertebral arch of L1 *(arrows)*.

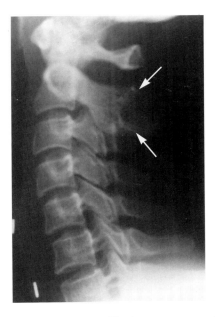

FIG. 6-48 Expansile lesion of the C2 spinous process consistent with osteoblastoma *(arrows).* An aneurysmal bone cyst may have an identical appearance. (Courtesy Joseph W. Howe, Sylmar, Calif.)

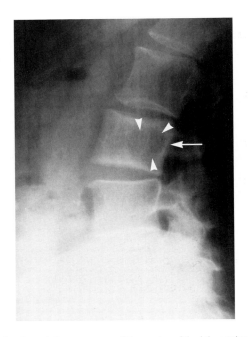

FIG. 6-49 Osteolytic appearance of the center of the L4 vertebral body *(arrowheads)* secondary to Paget's disease. The L4 vertebral body appears enlarged *(arrow)* and the cortices are thick ("picture frame" vertebra).

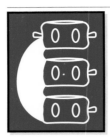

SP7 | Paraspinal Mass

The following table lists common causes of paraspinal masses. Tuberculosis is a common cause of paraspinal mass in countries where tuberculosis is prevalent. The most important differential to exclude probably is a tumor mass. Tumors in the pediatric age group include neuroenteric cysts, histiocytosis X, leukemia, neuroblastomas and tumors of the kidney. In the adults, neurofibromas, metastasis, and myeloma should be excluded.

DISEASE	COMMENTS
Aortic aneurysms (FIGS. 6-50 AND 6-51) [p. 979]	Circumscribed dilations of the aorta secondary to atherosclerosis, trauma, syphilis, etc.; the dilated segments may produce elongated paraspinal masses in the thoracic or lumbar regions; often in the lumbar region an abdominal aortic aneurysm demonstrates thin, curvilinear calcification of the vessel's walls; with increasing age, uncoiling of the aortic arch occurs, and the resulting tortuosity of the descending aorta may mimic an aneurysm
Achalasia	Esophageal motility disorder marked by failure of the lower esophageal sphincter to relax, resulting in dilatation of the upper third of the esophagus; the distended esophagus produces a paraspinal mass in the middle to upper thoracic spine in the frontal projection; an air-fluid level may be appreciated
Hiatal hernia [p. 972]	Herniation of part or all of the stomach through the esophageal hiatus of the diaphragm, possibly appearing as a largely left-sided paraspinal mass near the level of the diaphragm with an air-fluid level

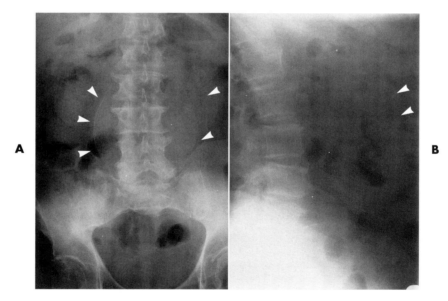

FIG. 6-50   Anteroposterior **(A)** and lateral **(B)** lumbar projections demonstrating a paraspinal **(A)** and prespinal mass **(B)** resulting from a large abdominal aortic aneurysm with calcification of the outer wall **(A)** *(arrowheads)*. (*Left,* Courtesy Joseph W. Howe, Sylmar, Calif.)

| Infections | Infectious spondylitis (tuberculosis, sarcoid, fungal, brucella, salmonella, and others) with associated paraspinal abscess; osteolytic vertebral changes and narrowed disc spaces accompany findings | **Neurogenic tumors (FIG. 6-52)** | Include neurofibroma, neurilemoma, ganglioneuroma, and neuroblastoma; because of the proximity of the intervertebral foramina and chain ganglia, they may produce a paraspinal mass |
| Lymphadenopathy | Because of their paraspinal location, enlargement of the lymph nodes from tumor (e.g., metastasis, lymphoma), infection (e.g., granuloma), or other etiologies may produce paraspinal masses | **Extramedullary hematopoiesis** | Vertebral bone marrow extrusion seen with the congenital anemias (e.g., thalassemia), producing smooth-appearing paravertebral masses in the posterior mediastinum and often associated with splenomegaly |

Continued

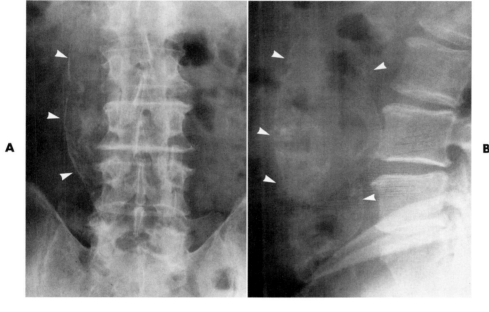

FIG. 6-51 Anteroposterior **(A)** and lateral **(B)** lumbar radiographs demonstrating an abdominal aortic aneurysm demarcated by the calcified curvilinear lines representing the anterior and posterior walls of the vessels *(arrowheads)*. (Courtesy Robert C. Tatum, Davenport, Iowa.)

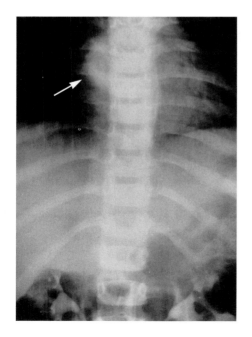

FIG. 6-52 Neuroblastoma presenting as a paraspinal mass *(arrow)*. It is not certain whether this is a primary intrathoracic lesion or metastatic lesion from the abdomen. (Courtesy Steven P. Brownstein, Springfield, NJ.)

DISEASE	COMMENTS
Trauma	May produce a focal paraspinal mass (e.g., a hematoma forming from spinal fractures or direct soft tissue injury); a history of trauma and possible evidence of fracture are clues
Expansile spine lesions (FIG. 6-53)	Expansile lesions of the vertebrae (e.g., osteoblastoma, osteochondroma, aneurysmal bone cyst, etc.)

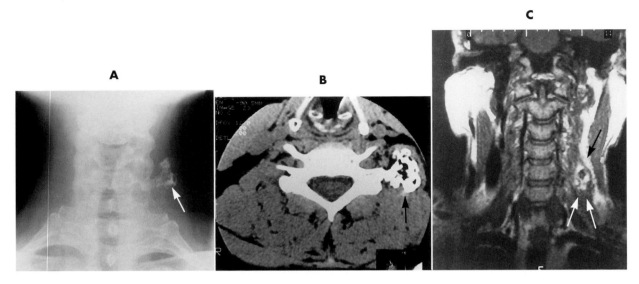

FIG. 6-53 Plain film **(A)**, CT **(B)**, and MRI **(C)** of an osteochondroma extending laterally from the spine as a left paraspinal mass *(arrows)*. (Courtesy Ian D. McLean, Davenport, Iowa.)

SP8 | Radiodense "Ivory" Vertebrae

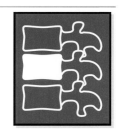

This pattern includes the appearance of radiodense ("ivory") vertebrae at one or more levels. If the entire spine is involved, the list of causes under the pattern of generalized increased bone density may be more applicable. The most common causes of an ivory vertebra are osteoblastic metastasis, Paget's disease, and lymphoma. Other less common conditions are included in the following table to provide a more comprehensive differential list of causes.

Some of the conditions listed in the table may appear as focal vertebral sclerosis instead of ivory vertebra. Conditions associated with focal vertebral sclerosis include bone islands, fractures, osteoblastic metastases, sclerosing spondylosis, lymphomas, chronic osteomyelitis, and osteoid osteomas.

DISEASE	COMMENTS
Infections	Chronic sclerosing infections seen with tuberculosis, syphilis, brucellosis, and typhoid; bone destruction and disc space narrowing is typical
Fluorosis	Chronic fluoride intoxication associated with osteophytosis and vertebral hyperostosis with calcification of the paraspinal ligaments; vertebrae have increased radiodensity; fluorosis is most marked in the innominates and lumbar spine
Fractures	Compression or healing vertebral fractures, usually appearing as a focal area of increased radiodensity, that typically do not appear uniformly dense enough to be mistaken for true ivory vertebrae
Lymphoma (FIGS. 6-54 AND 6-55) [p. 685]	Malignancy of the lymphocytes arising in the spleen, lymph nodes, and other lymphoid tissues; sclerotic vertebral lesions are more typical of Hodgkin's disease; involved vertebrae are not enlarged but may exhibit concavity of the anterior body margin secondary to erosions from enlarged prevertebral lymph nodes

Continued

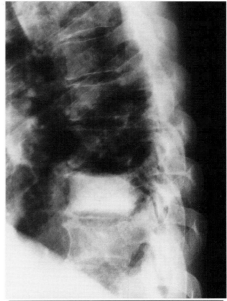

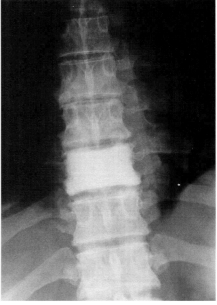

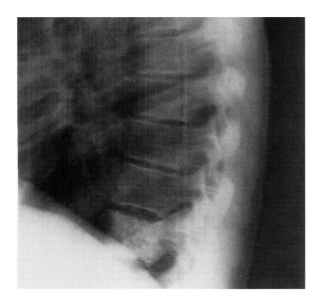

FIG. 6-54 Lymphoma causing an ivory vertebra appearance in the lower thoracic spine. (Courtesy Ian D. McLean, Davenport, Iowa.)

FIG. 6-55 Lymphoma presenting as ivory vertebra. (Courtesy Steven P. Brownstein, Springfield, NJ.)

PART TWO Bone, Joints, and Soft Tissues

DISEASE	COMMENTS
Myelofibrosis (FIG. 6-56)	Extensive and progressive bone marrow fibrosis of unknown etiology occurring in hematopoietic bones (vertebrae, pelvis, ribs, and long bones); involved areas appear osteoporotic first, later becoming patchy, then homogeneously dense; splenic enlargement also noted
Osteoblastic metastases (FIGS. 6-57, 6-58, AND 6-59) [p. 687]	Secondary to hematogenous metastases, are most commonly a result of breast or prostate primary malignancies, and exist at one or multiple levels; patients are usually over the age of 50 years; typically the size and shape of the vertebrae remain normal

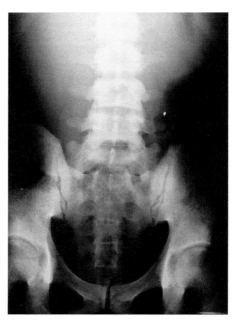

FIG. 6-56   Myelofibrosis producing radiodense vertebrae and pelvis. (Courtesy Steven P. Brownstein, Springfield, NJ.)

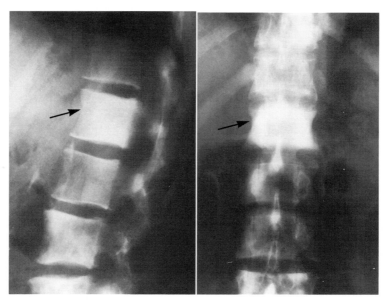

FIG. 6-57   Mixed osteolytic and osteoblastic metastasis of the lumbar spine presenting as several ivory vertebrae. The increased density of the L1 vertebrae is most notable (arrows). (Courtesy Joseph W. Howe, Sylmar, Calif.)

Osteopetrosis (Albers-Schön-berg disease) [p. 411]

Hereditary failure of calcified cartilage resorption, which interferes with the development of mature bone; the appearance is marked by sclerotic, fragile bones; vertebrae may appear "doubled" by smaller "endobones" within their bodies; well-defined transverse radiodense bands are characteristically found subjacent the endplates; multiple levels are involved

Paget's disease (FIG. 6-60) [p. 761]

Chronic skeletal disease of aberrant bone remodeling, marked by bone enlargement, softening, and (rarely) sarcomatous changes; the lumbar spine is one of the most common areas; single or multiple vertebrae may be involved, typically appearing enlarged, with thick cortices ("picture frame"); alternatively, it may present as a densely sclerotic or osteolytic lesion of the vertebrae; the disc space is uninvolved

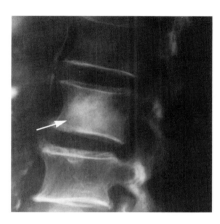

FIG. 6-58 Lateral lumbar spine demonstrating an early ivory vertebra appearance resulting from blastic metastatic bone disease affecting the L3 segment *(arrow).* (Courtesy Steven P. Brownstein, Springfield, NJ.)

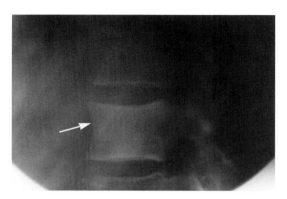

FIG. 6-59 Lateral lumbar projection demonstrating an early ivory vertebra secondary to osteoblastic metastasis *(arrow).* (Courtesy Steven P. Brownstein, Springfield, NJ.)

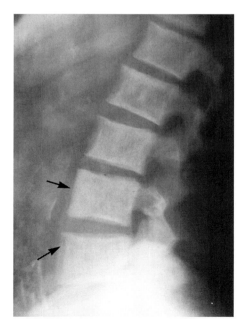

FIG. 6-60 Radiodense appearance of the lower lumbar vertebrae occurring as a result of Paget's disease. In addition, the L4 and L5 vertebrae are enlarged *(arrows).*

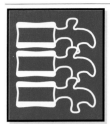

SP9 | Radiodense Vertebral Stripes

The appearance of radiodense vertebral stripes that are clearly defined and located immediately below the vertebral endplates is most closely associated with osteopetrosis. Less well-defined stripes of similar location are suggestive of hyperparathyroidism. Trauma and hypercorticism may be associated with more centrally located stripes. Other causes of dense vertebral stripes include spondylosclerosis, which has concurrent degenerative findings, and Paget's disease, which is systemic and usually has some degree of vertebral enlargement.

DISEASE	COMMENTS
Compression fractures	Fracture manifesting as decreased vertical height of the vertebra (generally less than 2 mm); recent fractures may demonstrate a horizontal radiodense zone of condensation and cortical offset "step defect" along the anterior body margin; they are often found at the L1, L2, and T12 levels
Hypercorticism	Excess levels of corticosteroids (i.e., Cushing's disease, steroid therapy); hypercorticism is associated with osteopenia, avascular necrosis, pathologic fractures; repeated microfractures of the vertebral endplate may produce horizontal, poorly defined zones of increased radiodensity in the subjacent bone
Hyperparathyroidism **(FIG. 6-61)** [p. 718]	Overproduction of parathormone, resulting from primary or secondary disorders of the parathyroid glands; the disease is marked by osteopenia, osteosclerosis, bone resorption, and soft tissue and vascular calcification; specifically, vertebrae appear osteopenic, with characteristic homogeneous radiodense bands traversing horizontally at each end of the vertebrae ("rugger-jersey" spine)
Osteopetrosis (Albers-Schön-berg disease) **(FIGS. 6-62 AND 6-63)** [p. 411]	Hereditary failure of calcified cartilage resorption, which interferes with the development of mature bone; the appearance is marked by sclerotic, fragile bones; vertebrae may appear "doubled" by smaller "endobones" within their bodies; well-defined transverse radiodense bands are characteristically found subjacent to the endplates
Paget's disease [p. 761]	Chronic skeletal disease of aberrant bone remodeling, marked by bone enlargement, softening, and rarely sarcomatous changes; the lumbar spine is one of the most common areas of involvement; the enlarged and thickened vertebral cortices appear as radiodense bands around the perimeter of the vertebra ("picture frame")
Sclerosing spondylosis	Degenerative disc disease that may produce a prominent subchondral sclerosis of the subjacent vertebra ("hemispheric spondylosclerosis") and is most common in the lower lumbar levels

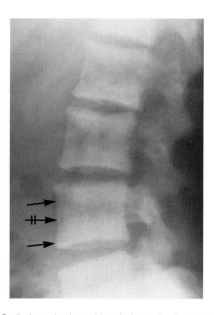

FIG. 6-61   Radiodense horizontal bands (*arrows*) adjacent to the vertebral endplates create a radiolucent horizontal band across the middle of the vertebrae (*crossed arrow*). (Courtesy Joseph W. Howe, Sylmar, Calif.)

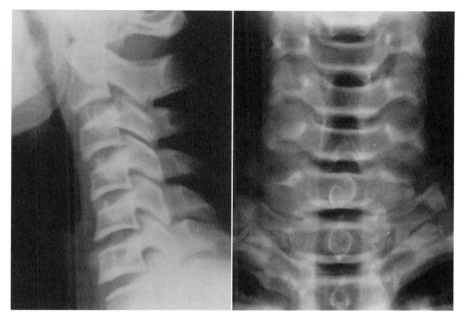

FIG. 6-62   Osteopetrosis appearing with radiodense stripes along the vertebral endplates throughout the cervical spine.

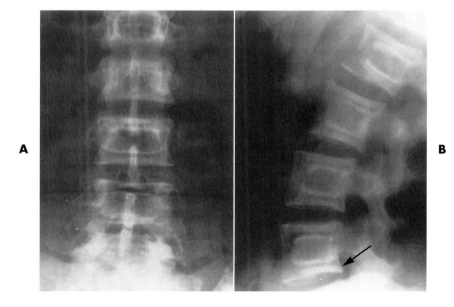

FIG. 6-63   Anteroposterior **(A)** and lateral **(B)** lumbar projections demonstrating radiodense endplate stripes *(arrow)* and bone-within-a-bone appearance of osteopetrosis. (Courtesy Joseph W. Howe, Sylmar, Calif.)

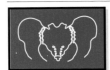

SP10 | Sacroiliac Joint Disease

The sacroiliac joint comprises a lower synovial portion and an upper ligamentous portion. Some diseases demonstrate predisposition to a specific area of the joint. For example, diffuse idiopathic skeletal hyperostosis (DISH) affects the upper portion of the joint, whereas ankylosing spondylitis affects the lower portion.

In general, sacroiliitis is initially assessed on plain film radiographs. The standard anteroposterior radiograph is most often taken. Additional radiographic projections are helpful to further assess the sacroiliac joint. The radiographic appearance of sacroiliitis is marked by osteoporosis, marginal erosions, subchondral sclerosis, loss of cortical joint margins, widened joint space with possible eventual fusion, and a return to normal bone density. Often changes are better seen on the iliac side when the lower two thirds, or synovial, portion of the sacroiliac joint is affected.

Radionuclide bone scintigraphy, computed tomography, and magnetic resonance imaging augment the plain film radiographs if infection or other serious progressive arthropathy is suspected.

DISEASE	COMMENTS		
Ankylosing spondylitis **(FIGS. 6-64, 6-65, AND 6-66)** [p. 428]	Seronegative spondyloarthropathy characterized by involvement in the sacroiliac joints and spine; the vertebrae appear square with ossification of the annulus fibrosus and paraspinal ligaments; fusion of the posterior joints are fused, and the proximal joint of the limbs are involved; distribution is bilateral symmetrical (+++)*; sacroiliitis is virtually always present; the disease has a male predominance; onset is between 15 and 35 years	Diffuse idiopathic skeletal hyperostosis (DISH) [p. 477]	Generalized articular disorder characterized by prolific hypertrophic ligamentous ossifications, especially the anterior longitudinal ligament of the spine; less commonly bilateral symmetrical (+++) distribution of sacroiliitis marked by fusion at the upper and lower margins of the joint follow more advanced spinal changes

Continued

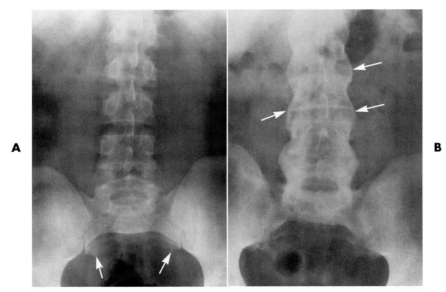

FIGS. 6-64   Ankylosing spondylitis presenting with bilateral symmetrical sacroiliitis **(A)** *(arrows)*. Ten years later, the patient's sacroiliac joint appears similar to the previous film **(B),** but the spine exhibits advanced syndesmophytes not noted on the previous film *(arrows)*. (Courtesy Joseph W. Howe, Sylmar, Calif.)

*Sacroiliac distribution: (+++), usual; (++), common; (+) rare.

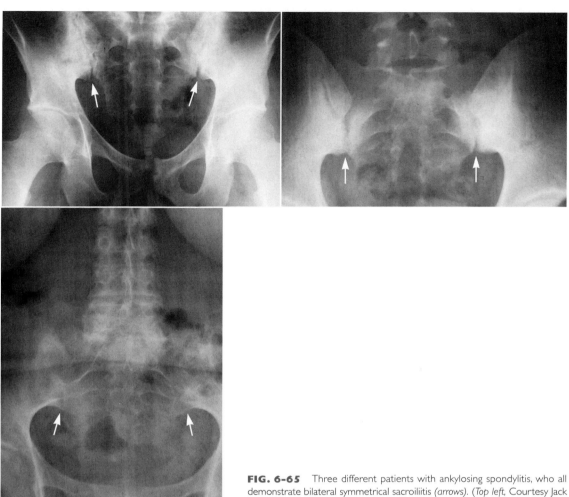

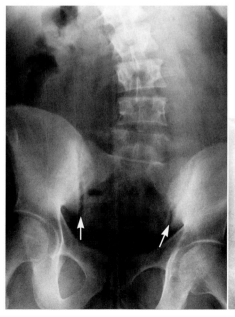

FIG. 6-65 Three different patients with ankylosing spondylitis, who all demonstrate bilateral symmetrical sacroiliitis *(arrows)*. *(Top left,* Courtesy Jack C. Avalos, Davenport, Iowa)

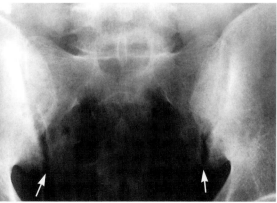

FIG. 6-66 Bilateral sacroiliitis in a patient with ankylosing spondylitis *(arrows)*.

DISEASE	COMMENTS
Gout [p. 456]	Primarily a disorder of purine metabolism that causes crystal deposits, resulting in synovial pannus, arthropathy, and large well-defined bony marginal erosions; infrequent sacroiliitis of a unilateral (++), bilateral asymmetrical (++), or bilateral symmetrical (++) distribution
Hyperparathy-roidism [p. 718]	Overproductive parathyroid glands, resulting from primary or secondary causes; the disease is marked by osteopenia, osteosclerosis, bone resorption, and soft tissue and vascular calcification; vertebrae have characteristic homogeneous radiodense bands traversing horizontally at each end of the vertebrae ("rugger-jersey" spine); less commonly, sacroiliitis with a bilateral symmetrical (++) or bilateral asymmetrical (++) distribution is noted with limited subchondral bone resorption, causing apparent widened joint space
Infections	Suppurative or tuberculosis infections of the sacroiliac joint or surrounding bone; involvement is unilateral (+++); fever and other signs of infection are helpful for differentiation when present; intravenous drug abusers are prone to *Pseudomonas* species infections, which target the "s joints" (spine, sacroiliac, symphysis pubis, and sternoclavicular)

Inflammatory bowel disease **(FIG. 6-67)**	Includes Crohn's disease, ulcerative colitis, and Whipple's disease, which are sometimes accompanied by inflammatory arthropathy, especially of the sacroiliac joints; the bilateral symmetrical (+++) distribution is indistinguishable from ankylosing spondylitis
Osteitis condensans ilii **(FIG. 6-68)**	Bilateral symmetrical (+++) triangular osteosclerosis of the iliac bones immediately adjacent to the lower, anterior portion of the sacroiliac joint; joint space appears normal; this condition represents a common variant seen among women of childbearing age
Osteoarthritis [p. 458]	Degenerative joint changes that usually develop after 40 years of age; precocious degeneration may follow biomechanical or traumatic stresses; characteristics include smooth, sclerotic joint margins with anterior osteophytes and joint space narrowing; distribution is unilateral (+++) or bilateral asymmetrical (++)
Paraplegia	Paralysis of both lower extremities and, generally, the lower trunk; sacroiliitis with a bilateral symmetrical (+++) distribution appears as joint space widening and osteoporosis

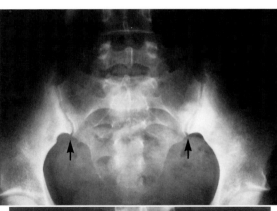

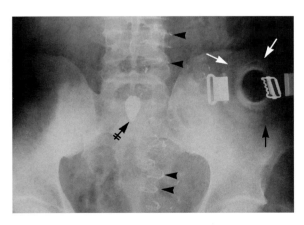

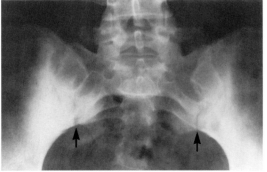

FIG. 6-67   Bilateral sacroiliitis secondary to inflammatory bowel disease. Bowel surgical staples (*arrowheads*), colostomy (*arrows*), and residual myelographic contrast (*crossed arrow*) are noted. (Courtesy Steven P. Brownstein, Springfield, NJ.)

FIG. 6-68   Two cases of osteitis condensans ilii appearing with bilateral, triangular-shaped iliac region of osteosclerosis adjacent to the low margin of the sacroiliac joint (*arrows*). (*Top,* Courtesy Joseph W. Howe, Sylmar, Calif.)

Psoriatic arthritis (FIG. 6-69) [p. 436]	Common skin disease with an associated inflammatory arthropathy; sacroiliitis is common and distribution may be unilateral (+), bilateral asymmetrical (+++), or bilateral symmetrical (++)	**Rheumatoid arthritis** [p. 442]	Systemic connective tissue disorder characterized by inflammatory arthropathy most pronounced in the hands and feet; sacroiliitis is rare, but when present it is marked by mild loss of joint space and (less commonly) erosion; distribution is bilateral asymmetrical (+++), bilateral symmetrical (++), or unilateral (+) sacroiliac
Reiter's syndrome (FIG. 6-70) [p. 440]	Encompasses triad of urethritis, conjunctivitis, and polyarthritis following sexually transmitted disease or dysentery; sacroiliitis is common and distribution may be unilateral (+), bilateral asymmetrical (+++), or bilateral symmetrical (++)		

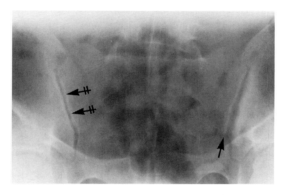

FIG. 6-69   Psoriatic sacroiliitis appearing with osteosclerosis and erosions of the left joint margins *(arrow)* and only slight osteosclerosis on the right *(crossed arrows)*. (Courtesy Joseph W. Howe, Sylmar, Calif.)

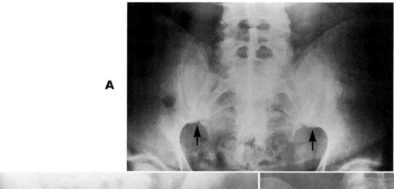

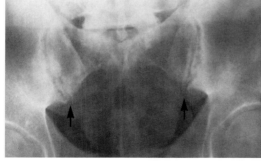

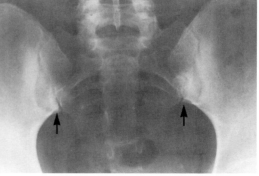

FIG. 6-70   Sacroiliitis secondary to Reiter's syndrome with bilateral asymmetrical (**A** and **B**) and nearly bilateral symmetrical (**C**) patterns *(arrows)*. (Courtesy Joseph W. Howe, Sylmar, Calif.)

PART TWO Bone, Joints, and Soft Tissues

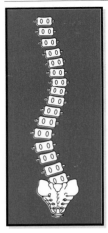

SP11 | Scoliosis

Scoliosis is a lateral curvature of the spine. The degree of curvature is quantified on a full-spine frontal projection, using the Cobb's method of assessment. Progression is assessed by periodic reevaluations. The majority of scoliosis that presents before skeletal maturity is idiopathic in nature. By contrast, those that present after skeletal maturity are typically related to degeneration, osteoporosis, or iatrogenic causes (e.g., following extensive decompressive surgery for spinal stenosis). The following table lists causes of scoliosis for all age groups.

DISEASE	COMMENTS
Chest wall abnormalities	Related to asymmetric chest wall, rib anomalies, Sprengel's deformity, or postsurgical deformities (e.g., thoracoplasty, pneumonectomy)
Congenital spinal anomaly (FIG. 6-71)	Spinal curvatures that result from structural changes of the spine representing congenital blocked vertebrae, Klippel-Feil syndrome, hemivertebrae, dysraphism, osseous bridging vertebral bars, and others; a short segment of the spine is typically involved
Congenital syndromes	Occurring with achondroplasia, cretinism, mucopolysaccharidoses, neurofibromatosis, osteogenesis imperfecta, Marfan's syndrome, homocystinuria, and others
Degenerative diseases	Most common cause of scoliosis presenting after bone maturity; scoliosis may be related to advanced degeneration of the intervertebral disc and posterior joints of the spine, particularly if asymmetrical
Iatrogenic	Typically related to extensive surgical procedures that significantly alter the spine's structural integrity (i.e., extensive decompressive laminectomy performed for spinal canal stenosis)
Idiopathic (FIG. 6-72)	Unknown—the most common type of scoliosis presenting before skeletal maturity
Infections	Examples of spinal infections: tuberculosis, pyogenic infections, brucellosis; these infections may cause focal spinal curvature secondary to bone destruction; a sharply angled kyphosis (gibbus) deformity is characteristic
Leg length deficiencies	Secondary to amputation, chiropractic subluxation, pelvic unleveling, and foot deformity
Neuromuscular disorders	Most common: poliomyelitis; others include cerebral palsy, muscular dystrophy, Friedreich ataxia, Charcot-Marie-Tooth atrophy, and syringomyelia

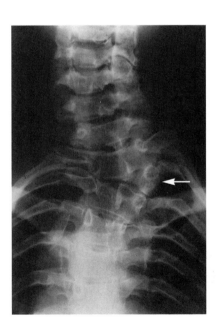

FIG. 6-71   Structural left lateral cervicothoracic scoliosis secondary to a hemivertebra interposed between the first and second thoracic segments (*arrow*). (Courtesy Joseph W. Howe, Sylmar, Calif.)

Osteoid osteoma [p. 667]	Most common neoplasm causing scoliosis; osteoid osteomas affect the vertebral arch; a painful scoliosis with sclerotic pedicle shadow on the concave side is the classic presentation; often the tumor is radiographically occult, requiring a bone scintigraphy or computed tomography to detect and confirm the diagnosis
Osteoporosis [p. 727]	Reduction in the quantity of bone that occurs most often in postmenopausal women and elderly men; sparse, thin trabeculae are present, as well as thinning (but no destruction) of cortex; smooth indentations of endplates centrally in the region of the nucleus pulposus are noted, as well as solitary or multiple level vertebral collapse; it is more typical in the lumbar and thoracic regions; severe demineralization may result in bone deformity and related scoliosis
Radiation	In a growing spine, may cause asymmetrical arrest of growth centers with resulting lateral curvature; involvement in the lumbar spine is most often in relation to treatment for Wilms' tumor and neuroblastoma; the convexity of the lateral curvature is opposite the side of irradiation
Spasms	Lateral deviation resulting from such phenomena as asymmetrical muscle spasm in response to spinal injury, retroperitoneal or abdominal abscess, hemorrhage, or ureteral or renal calculi
Trauma	Fracture or dislocation involving the spine resulting in structural deformity; in particular, fractures of the transverse processes at multiple levels are associated with scoliosis—convex to the same side

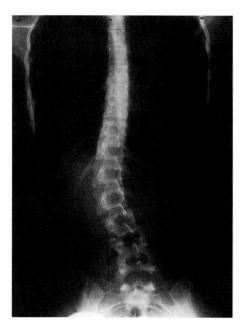

FIG. 6-72 Idiopathic right lateral lumbar scoliosis.

PART TWO Bone, Joints, and Soft Tissues

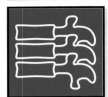

SP12 | Vertebral Collapse

Vertebral collapse is marked by a decrease of the normal vertical dimension of the vertebral body, often accompanied by an expansion of the horizontal dimension of the body. If the anterior vertebral body is more involved than the posterior margin, the appearance may resemble a "wedged" vertebra, and the differential list found in the first pattern (SP1i) of this chapter may be more helpful. Collapse secondary to fracture may lead to posterior migration and encroachment of bone fragments on the spinal canal, leading to serious neurologic complications. In addition, changes in the vertebrae's structure may have accompanying biomechanical consequences.

Most conditions known to cause a solitary vertebral collapse also cause multiple levels of vertebral collapse. Contrary to this general statement, benign bone tumors, chordomas, and traumatic ischemic necrosis virtually always involve one level, and Scheuermann's disease and sickle cell anemia typically involve multiple levels.

Advanced vertebral collapse, in which the vertebral body appears as a thin wafer disc, is termed *vertebra plana* and is characteristic of eosinophilic granuloma.

DISEASE	COMMENTS
Benign bone tumors	Giant cell bone tumors, hemangiomas, aneurysmal bone cysts, and other benign bone tumors—may present with loss of vertebral body height secondary to pathological fracture
Chordoma [p. 676]	A rare, low-grade malignancy arising from notochord remnants; only 13% arise in the spine (above the sacrum), usually at C2; appearance may include body collapse and anterior vertebral mass; tumor may cross the intervertebral disc space; there is solitary vertebral collapse
Dwarfing syndromes **(FIG. 6-73)**	Advanced flattened deformity of multiple vertebral levels—known as *platyspondyly;* associated with Morquio syndrome, spondyloepiphyseal dysplasia, thanatophoric dysplasia, and other dwarfing dysplasias
Eosinophilic granuloma **(FIG. 6-74)** [p. 747]	Proliferation of eosinophils seen most commonly in children and young adults; spine involvement in less than 10%; may appear with advanced body collapse "vertebra plana" or "coin vertebra" and involve one or multiple levels; the disease usually develops in children younger than 10 years of age

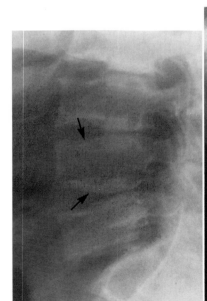
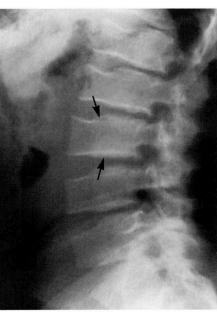

FIG. 6-73 Two cases of spondyloepiphyseal dysplasia (SED) appearing with decreased vertical body height and characteristic "heaped-up" appearance of the vertebral endplates *(arrows). (Left,* Courtesy Joseph W. Howe, Sylmar, Calif.)

Fractures	Usually involve only the anterior vertebral body height, creating a "wedged" vertebra appearance; it is more common for pathological fractures (those resulting from tumor, infection, or other causes) to also involve the posterior margin of the vertebra, which is a rare feature of fractures with purely traumatic etiologies; fractures may occur at one or several levels	**Hyperparathyroidism** [p. 718]	Overproductive parathyroid glands, resulting from primary or secondary causes; the disease is marked by osteopenia, osteosclerosis, bone resorption, and soft tissue and vascular calcification; specifically, vertebrae appear osteopenic with characteristic homogeneous radiodense bands traversing horizontally at each end of the vertebrae ("rugger-jersey" spine); solitary or multiple-level vertebral collapse occurs; the appearance may simulate osteoporosis, presenting with concave endplate deformities and marked demineralization
Hydatid (Echinococcus) cysts [p. 979]	Cysts that may be formed in bone (usually formed in the liver) by the larval stage of *Echinococcus;* such a cyst appears as a slow-growing, destructive lesion surrounded by sclerotic borders; they may cause solitary or multiple level vertebral collapse	**Infections**	Chronic sclerosing infections (e.g., tuberculosis, syphilis, brucellosis, fungus, typhus) and pyogenic infections; bone destruction and disc space narrowing is typical, distinguishing infection from metastasis and myeloma; solitary or multiple-level vertebral collapse occurs; involvement is localized to regions and not generalized; areas of cortical demineralization and destruction develop; a paraspinal mass may develop
Hypercorticism	Excess levels of corticosteroids (e.g., Cushing's disease, steroid therapy); hypercorticism is associated with osteopenia, avascular necrosis, pathologic fractures; repeated microfractures of the vertebral endplate may produce horizontal, poorly defined zones of increased radiodensity in the subjacent bone; solitary or multiple-level vertebral collapse occurs	**Ischemic necrosis (Kümmell disease)**	Controversial condition believed to represent delayed posttraumatic vertebral collapse related to ischemic necrosis of the vertebral body; presence of an intravertebral vacuum phenomena is characteristic; solitary vertebral collapse occurs

Continued

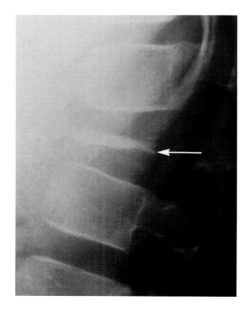

FIG. 6-74 Vertebra plana defect resulting from eosinophilic granuloma of the vertebral body (arrow).

PART TWO Bone, Joints, and Soft Tissues

DISEASE | **COMMENTS**

Lymphoma
[p. 685]

Primary and secondary (systemic non-Hodgkin's lymphoma and Hodgkin's disease) lymphoma of bone appears as permeative radiolucent lesions of the lower extremities, pelvis, and spine; less commonly the lesions appear as dense vertebral sclerosis; solitary or multiple-level vertebral collapse occurs

Metastases
(FIGS. 6-75 AND 6-76)
[p. 687]

Osteolytic metastases most commonly from primary metastases of the lung and breast; patients are usually over the age of 40 years; involvement of the pedicles and other areas of the neural arch is common and distinguishes metastasis from multiple myeloma, which does not demonstrate this tendency; solitary or multiple-level vertebral collapse occurs; the intervertebral disc space remains uninvolved, differentiating metastasis from infection

Multiple myelomas/plasmacytomas
(FIG. 6-77)
[p. 700]

Malignant proliferations of plasma cells occurring in predominately the red marrow of various bones; the skull, vertebral bodies, ribs, proximal humerus and femur are most commonly involved; osteolytic lesions simulate metastatic disease, without tendency to involve vertebral arch, which is common in metastasis; osteopenia and solitary or multiple-level vertebral collapse simulating osteoporosis occur

Neuropathic spine
[p. 483]

Primarily caused by diabetes mellitus, syringomyelia, congenital indifference to pain, and tabes dorsalisopathy; the radiographic appearance is marked by loss of intervertebral disc height, increased bone radiodensity, misalignment, fragmentation, and prominent osteophytosis; solitary or multiple-level vertebral collapse may occur

Normal variant

Mild anterior wedged configuration of vertebral body that occurs at one or several levels; the posterior vertebral body margin is not typically involved, which gives it more of a wedged appearance; it is common in the middle cervical spine and thoracolumbar junction

Osteogenesis imperfecta
[p. 409]

Inherited abnormal fragility and plasticity of bone, marked by recurring fractures following minimal trauma; other findings include ligamentous laxity, long bone deformity, blue sclerae, osteopenia, and otosclerosis; severe (congenita) and more mild forms (tarda) exist; multiple levels of wedged or completely narrowed vertebrae with biconcave endplates develop

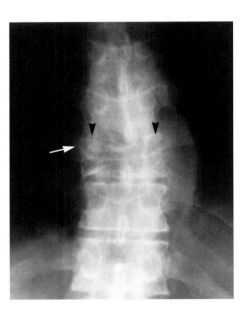

FIG. 6-75 Anteroposterior thoracic projection demonstrating vertebral collapse of T10 (arrow). The interpedicular distance is increased and the pedicles are poorly seen (arrowheads).

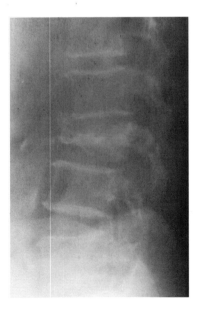

FIG. 6-76 Lateral lumbar projection revealing pathological collapse secondary to metastasis involving the L3 segment. The anterior and posterior vertebral body heights are decreased—a characteristic of pathological collapse. In addition, the anteroposterior width of the vertebra has increased, causing potential narrowing of the spinal canal. (Courtesy Joseph W. Howe, Sylmar, Calif.)

Osteomalacia
[p. 734]

Inadequate mineralization of bone, characterized by gradual softening and deformity, which develops secondary to lack of vitamin D or renal tubular dysfunction; more common in women than in men, osteomalacia often begins during pregnancy; the smooth concave deformity of the vertebral endplates simulate osteoporosis; solitary or multiple-level vertebral collapse occurs

Osteoporosis
[p. 727]

Reduction in the quantity of bone that occurs most often in postmenopausal women and elderly men; sparse, thin trabeculae, as well as thinning (but no destruction) of cortex are noted; there are smooth indentations of endplates centrally, in the region of the nucleus pulposus; solitary or multiple-level vertebral collapse occurs; the condition is more typical in the lumbar and thoracic regions

Paget's disease
[p. 761]

A generalized skeletal disease in which bone deposition and resorption are both increased, leading to abnormal thick and soft bones with disorganized, "mosaic" trabeculae; skull, pelvis, and vertebrae are common sites of involvement; vertebrae appear enlarged with thick cortices, "picture framed" vertebrae; concave endplate deformity involving one or more levels may occur but is not typical

Scheuermann's disease
[p. 413]

Posttraumatic defect in endplate maturation presenting during adolescence with multiple levels of anteriorly wedged vertebrae, narrowed anterior disc space, multiple Schmorl's nodes, and vertebral endplate irregularity; the disease usually seen in the middle and lower thoracic spine; the anteriorly wedged vertebrae produce a kyphosis; the thoracic spine is most often involved; if present, narrowing of the posterior vertebral bodies is a very prominent feature

Sickle cell anemia
(FIG. 6-78)
[p. 604]

Genetic abnormality in which red blood cells assume a sickled configuration in low oxygen tension; the sickled cells may occlude small vessels with resulting ischemia; skeletal changes include osteopenia, coarse trabeculae, dactylitis, and biconcave (more precisely, step-like or H-shaped) central endplate deformity occurring at multiple levels

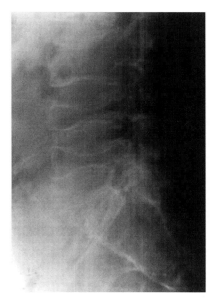

FIG. 6-77 Multiple levels of vertebral body collapse in the lumbar spine secondary to advanced multiple myeloma. The collapsed vertebrae exhibit decreased anterior and posterior vertebral body heights, a characteristic of pathological collapse. As in this case, multiple myeloma may produce decreased bone density, mimicking senile osteoporosis. (Courtesy Joseph W. Howe, Sylmar, Calif.)

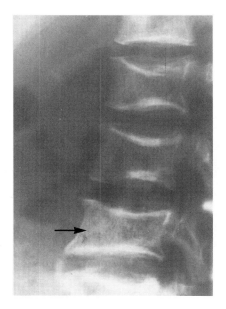

FIG. 6-78 Sickle cell anemia presenting with biconcave or H-shaped lumbar vertebrae. The L4 segment is deceased in vertical height (arrow). (Courtesy Joseph W. Howe, Sylmar, Calif.)

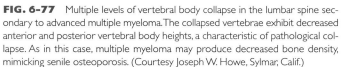

PART TWO Bone, Joints, and Soft Tissues

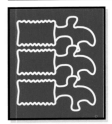

SP13 | Vertebral Endplate Alterations

Some of the more common endplate alterations include zones of increased osteosclerosis, irregularity, steplike defects, and fragmentation. One or multiple spinal levels may be involved. Often other osseous changes are present, which suggest a specific disease.

DISEASE	COMMENTS
Hyperparathyroidism [p. 718]	Overproduction of parathyroid glands, resulting from primary or secondary causes; the disease is marked by osteopenia, osteosclerosis, bone resorption, and soft tissue and vascular calcification; specifically, vertebrae appear osteopenic with characteristic homogeneous, radiodense bands traversing horizontally at each end of the vertebrae ("rugger-jersey" spine)
Limbus bone (FIG. 6-79)	Designates a small, well-corticated fragment of bone at the edge or fringe of a vertebra and develops from interosseous herniation of the nucleus pulposus between the vertebral centra and endplate, prohibiting fusion of secondary growth center to the vertebral centra; it is differentiated from fracture fragment by its well-corticated margin, lack of displacement, and absence of serious trauma history

Normal development (FIG. 6-80)	In the lateral projection, steplike defects are seen at the vertebral endplate margins (more prominent anteriorly); these defects contain the cartilage growth centers of the vertebral endplate; as ossification proceeds, a focus of bone fills the radiolucent defect (between 6 and 12 years of age), fusing to the vertebral body between 20 and 25 years of age
Nuclear impressions (notochordal persistence) (FIG. 6-81)	Nonfocal, congenital, smooth, inward deformity of all or part of the superior, inferior, or both vertebral endplates involving the entire endplate; in the frontal projection the defect has a "double-hump" or "cupid's bow" appearance

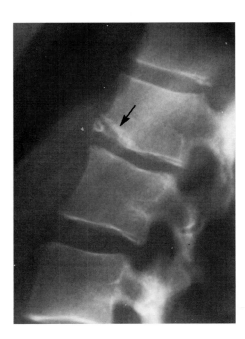

FIG. 6-79 Limbus bone with a characteristic, well-marginated appearance located at anterior inferior corner of the L2 vertebra. In contrast, a teardrop fracture is not well-marginated, does not exhibit a sclerotic band on the vertebra *(arrow)*, and is usually displaced from the vertebra.

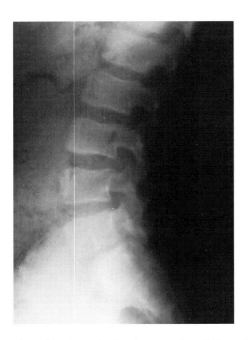

FIG. 6-80 Lateral lumbar projection demonstrating mild inward defects of the endplates with central radiodensity. This is a normal developmental appearance.

Osteopetrosis (Albers-Schön- berg disease) (FIGS. 6-82 AND 6-83) [p. 411]

Hereditary failure of calcified cartilage resorption, which interferes with the development of mature bone; the appearance is marked by sclerotic, fragile bones; vertebrae may appear "doubled" by smaller "endobones" within their bodies; well-defined, transverse, radiodense bands are characteristically found subjacent to the endplates

Osteoporosis [p. 727]

Reduction in the quantity of bone that occurs most often in postmenopausal women and elderly men; sparse, thin trabeculae, as well as thinning (but no destruction) of cortex are noted; there are smooth indentations of endplates centrally, in the region of the nucleus pulposus; bone sclerosis along endplates and solitary or multiple-level vertebral collapse occur; the disease is more typical in the lumbar and thoracic regions

Continued

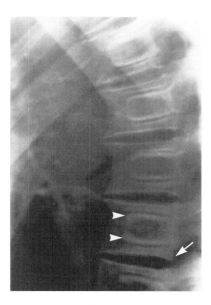

FIG. 6-82 Osteopetrosis appearing with characteristic endobone shadows in each of the thoracic vertebrae *(arrowheads)*. In addition, radiodense endplate stripes are noted *(arrow)*. The endplate stripes are not a prominent feature in this case.

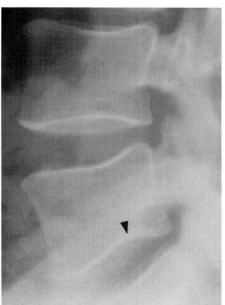

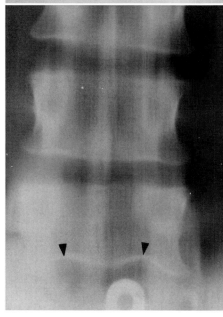

FIG. 6-81 Lateral plain film **(A)** and anteroposterior linear tomogram **(B)** radiograph demonstrating notochordal persistency *(arrowheads)*. (Courtesy Steven P. Brownstein, Springfield, NJ.)

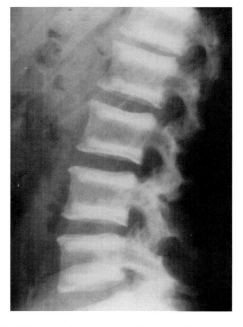

FIG. 6-83 Osteopetrosis producing radiodense stripes along the vertebral endplates throughout the lumbar spine.

DISEASE

COMMENTS

Radiation
(FIGS. 6-84 AND 6-85)

In the growing spine, may arrest the growth of the vertebra through endplate necrosis, producing short vertebrae with irregular endplates, involvement of the lumbar spine is most often in relation to treatment for Wilms' tumor and neuroblastoma; if the radiation is applied asymmetrically, scoliosis may develop with a convexity of the lateral curvature opposite the side of irradiation

Scheurmann's disease
(FIG. 6-86)
[p. 413]

Posttraumatic defect in endplate maturation presenting during adolescence with multiple levels of anteriorly wedged vertebrae, narrowed anterior disc space, multiple Schmorl's nodes, and vertebral endplate irregularity; it is usually seen in the middle and lower thoracic spine; the anteriorly wedged vertebrae produce a kyphosis; the thoracic spine is most often involved

Schmorl's nodes
(FIGS. 6-86 AND 6-87)

Prolapse of the nucleus pulposus into the vertebra producing abrupt, inward deformities of a focal area of the endplate usually with notable surrounding sclerosis; both endplates and multiple vertebrae may be involved; multiple Schmorl's nodes are encountered in Scheuermann's disease

Sickle cell anemia
(FIG. 6-88)
[p. 604]

Genetic abnormality in which red blood cells assume a sickled configuration in low oxygen tension; the sickled cells may occlude small vessels with resulting ischemia; skeletal changes include osteopenia, coarse trabeculae, biconcave (more precisely steplike or H-shaped) vertebrae, and dactylitis

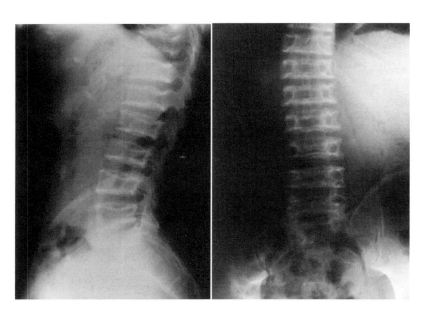

FIG. 6-84 Radiation necrosis resulting in short vertebrae and irregular endplates. (Courtesy Joseph W. Howe, Sylmar, Calif.)

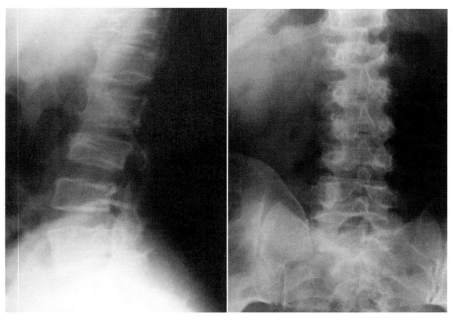

FIG. 6-85 Radiation necrosis resulting in short vertebrae and irregular endplates.

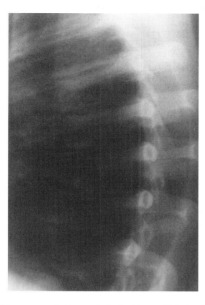

FIG. 6-86 Scheuermann's disease indicated by multiple levels of endplate irregularity and anterior vertebral wedging in the thoracic spine.

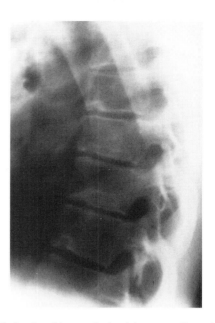

FIG. 6-87 Deformity of the vertebral endplates caused by multiple Schmorl's nodes.

FIG. 6-88 Sickle cell anemia causing biconcave deformity of the lumbar vertebrae secondary to underperfusion of the center of the vertebrae.

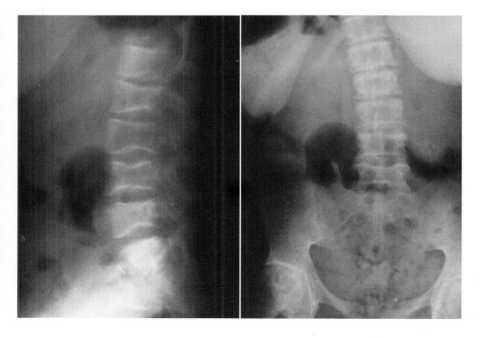

PART TWO
Bone, Joints, and Soft Tissues

Suggested Readings

Aliabadi P, Nikpoor N: Imaging evaluation of sacroiliitis, *Rheum Dis Clin North Am* 17(3):809, 1991.

Burgener FA, Kormano M: *Differential diagnosis in conventional radiology,* ed 2, New York, 1991, Thieme Medical Publishers.

Chapman S, Nakielny R: *Aids to radiological differential diagnosis,* ed 3, Philadelphia, 1995, WB Saunders.

Dahnert W: *Radiology review manual,* Baltimore, 1991, Williams and Wilkins.

Dolan KD: Cervicobasilar relationships, *Radiog Clin North Am* 15(2):155, 1977.

Eisenberg RL: *An atlas of differential diagnosis,* ed 2, Gaithersburg, 1992, Aspen.

Herman TE, McAlister WH: Inherited diseases of bone density in children, *Radiol Clin North Am* 29(1):149, 1991.

Jacobson HG: Dense bone—too much bone: radiographical considerations and differential diagnosis, *Skel Radiol* 13:1, 1985.

Jacobson HG, Edeiken J: Radiology of disorders of the sacroiliac joints, *J Am Med Assoc* 253(19): 2863, 1985.

Ravin CE, Cooper C, Leder RA: *Review of radiology,* Philadelphia, 1994, WB Saunders.

Reeder MM, Bradley WG: *Reeder and Felson's Gamuts in radiology,* ed 3, New York, 1993, Springer-Verlag.

Weinberger A, Myers AR: Intervertebral disc calcification in adults: a review, *Semin Arthritis Rheum* 8(1):69, 1978.

Weissleder R, Wittenberg J: *Primer of diagnostic imaging,* St Louis, 1994, Mosby.

Extremity Patterns

DENNIS M MARCHIORI

PART TWO
Bone, Joints, and Soft Tissues

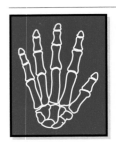

EX I | Acro-osteolysis

Acro-osteolysis represents bone resorption of the distal phalanges of the hands and feet. A wide range of congenital and acquired etiologies is responsible. Swelling or atrophy of the overlying soft tissues may also be present.

DISEASE	COMMENTS
Arteriosclerosis obliterans	Arteriosclerosis producing narrowing and occlusion of the arterial lumen; the resulting ischemia causes bone resorption
Hyperparathyroidism **(FIG. 7-1)** [p. 718]	Overproduction of parathormone resulting from primary or secondary factors affecting the parathyroid glands; the disease is marked by osteopenia, osteosclerosis, bone resorption, and soft tissue and vascular calcification; vertebrae appear osteopenic with characteristic, homogeneous, radiodense bands traversing horizontally at each end of the vertebrae ("rugger-jersey" spine); resorption of the distal tufts and radial side of the digits is characteristic
Lesch-Nyhan syndrome	Disorder characterized by hyperuricemia and uric acid urolithiasis, mental retardation, spastic cerebral palsy, and biting (self-mutilation) of fingers and lips
Neurotrophic disease **(FIG. 7-2)** [p. 483]	Bone resorption secondary to diabetes, leprosy, tabes dorsalis, syringomyelia, meningomyelocele, and congenital indifference to pain
Psoriatic arthritis **(FIG. 7-3)** [p. 436]	Arthritis occurring in fewer than 7% of patients with psoriasis; this condition involves the carpal, interphalangeal (distal interphalangeal common), and less commonly the sacroiliac joints; the digits are marked by nail pitting, swelling of the soft tissues, and less commonly erosions of the distal tufts, which relate a tapered appearance of the distal phalanges
Pyknodysostosis **(FIG. 7-4)** [p. 413]	Hereditary sclerosing dysplasia of bone, marked by short stature, dense bones (often with transverse fractures), hypoplastic angle of mandible, wormian bones, delayed closure of the fontanelles, and hypoplasia of the terminal phalanges
Raynaud's disease	Spasms of the digital arteries leading to distal tuft resorption, blanching, and pain in the hands; condition is associated with scleroderma

Continued

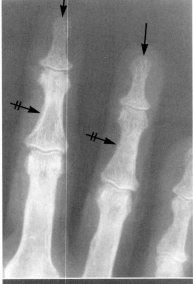

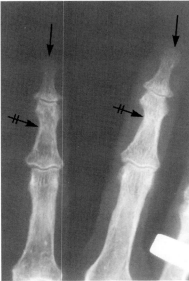

FIG. 7-1   Hyperparathyroidism with mild resorption of the distal tufts *(arrows)* and along the radial side of the middle phalanx of the second and third digits *(crossed arrows)*. (Courtesy Joseph W. Howe, Sylmar, Calif.)

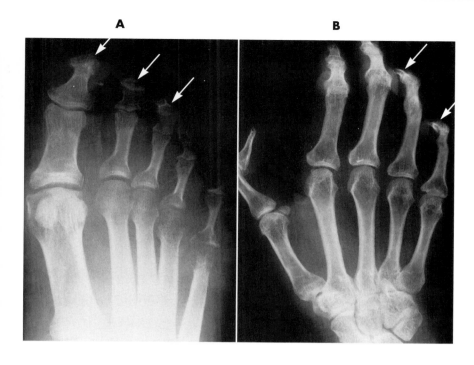

FIG. 7-2 Acro-osteolysis *(arrows)* of the feet **(A)** and hands **(B)** of different patients with leprosy. (Courtesy Steven P. Brownstein, MD, Springfield, NJ.)

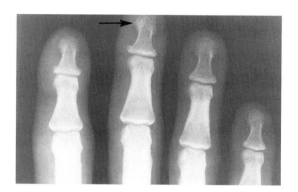

FIG. 7-3 Acro-osteolysis secondary to psoriatic arthritis *(arrow)*.

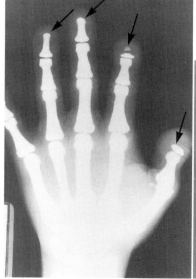

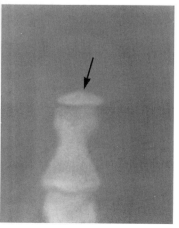

FIG. 7-4 Pyknodysostosis presenting with increased radiodensity with acro-osteolysis **(A)** and acro-osteolysis alone **(B,** *arrows)*.

DISEASE	COMMENTS
Sarcoidosis (FIG. 7-5) [p. 885]	Systemic granulomatous disease most pronounced in the lungs; less commonly the disease involves arthritis or acro-osteolysis of the hand with coarsened trabeculae and well-defined osteolytic lesions
Scleroderma (progressive systemic sclerosis) (FIG. 7-6) [p. 450]	Disease of small vessels and organ fibrosus; the soft tissues of the hands and feet undergo atrophy and calcification in addition to resorption of distal phalanges
Thermal injury (FIG. 7-7)	Resorption of the distal phalanges secondary to burns or frostbite injury; characteristically the thumb is spared in frostbite injury as the individual makes a fist around the thumb, protecting it from low temperatures
Vinyl chloride exposure	Systemic toxicant, abbreviated *VC,* that is particularly noxious to endothelium and is used for polyvinyl chloride (PVC) synthesis; occupational exposure is associated with acro-osteolysis and neuritis; the acro-osteolysis presents as transverse, bandlike radiolucent defects of the distal phalanges, usually the thumb

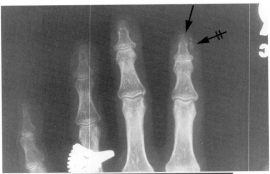

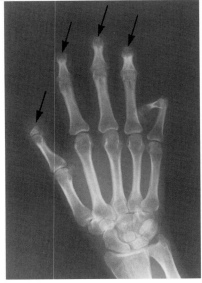

FIG. 7-6 Different patients with scleroderma with acro-osteolysis (arrows) and soft tissue calcification *(crossed arrow).* (Courtesy Joseph W. Howe, Sylmar, Calif.)

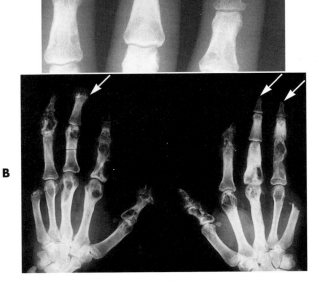

FIG. 7-5 **A** and **B,** Two cases with sarcoidosis causing acro-osteolysis *(arrows).* Sarcoidosis is an uncommon cause of acro-osteolysis. In addition, observe that several of the digits in **B** have been amputated. (A, Courtesy Joseph W. Howe, Sylmar, Calif.; B, Courtesy Steven P. Brownstein, Springfield, NJ.)

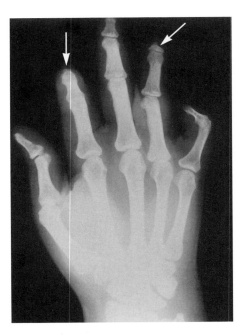

FIG. 7-7 Acro-osteolysis *(arrows)* secondary to frostbite. (Courtesy Steven P Brownstein, Springfield, NJ.)

EX2 | Calcified Intraarticular Loose Bodies

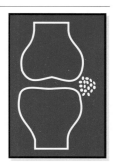

Loose intraarticular bodies are typically found in the large weight-bearing joints (e.g., knees). Degenerative disease probably represents the most common etiology. Noncalcified intraarticular bodies are not visible on plain film radiographs and necessitate specialized imaging to detect their presence. Symptoms are variable, ranging from acute joint locking to asymptomatic states.

DISEASE	COMMENTS
Degenerative joint disease [p. 458]	Very common, progressive, noninflammatory disorder involving the large weight-bearing joints and smaller joints of the hand; the radiographic appearance is characterized by joint subluxation, articular deformity, nonuniform reduction in joint space, marginal osteophytes, subchondral sclerosis, subchondral bone cysts, and intraarticular loose bodies; the knee is most commonly involved; this disease is usually seen in elderly patients
Neuropathic (Charcot) joint [p. 483]	Destructive arthropathy secondary to altered joint sensory innervation, resulting in either unchecked repetitive injury as a result of absence of pain or loss of trophic influences of innervations with local hyperemia and bone resorption; varieties are atrophic and hypertrophic; hypertrophic changes include premature and advanced degeneration marked by dislocation, destruction, intraarticular loose bodies (debris), and disorganization; the knee, hip, ankle, and lumbar spine are commonly affected
Osteochondrosis dissecans [p. 577]	Complete or incomplete separation of a portion of the joint cartilage and subjacent bone from a traumatic or osteonecrotic etiology, occurring in adolescence; the knee is usually involved, classically the lateral aspect of the medial condyle; fragments that do not reunite exist as intraarticular loose bodies
Synovial osteochondromatosis (FIGS. 7-8 AND 7-9) [p. 775]	Nonneoplastic hypertropic metaplasia of synovial tissue, producing multiple cartilage nodules, which may eventually ossify; nodules detach to become loose bodies in the joint, bursal, and tendon sheath spaces; this condition may be asymptomatic or produce acute pain with joint locking; in adults, the knee, hip, ankle, and elbow are most commonly affected
Trauma	Single or multiple loose bodies representing bone, ligament, or meniscal fragments arising from trauma; fragments may not be calcified, and therefore are not visible with plain film radiography

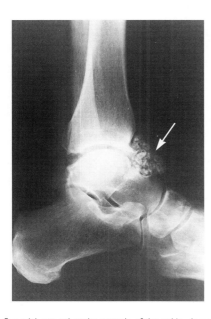

FIG. 7-8   Synovial osteochondromatosis of the ankle, demonstrating calcified loose bodies *(arrow)*. (Courtesy Joseph W. Howe, Sylmar, Calif.)

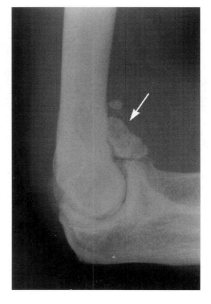

FIG. 7-9   Synovial osteochondromatosis of the elbow *(arrow)*. (Courtesy Joseph W. Howe, Sylmar, Calif.)

PART TWO
Bone, Joints, and Soft Tissues

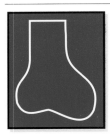

EX3 | Change in Size and Shape of Epiphyses

Alterations in the size and shape of epiphyses are related to traumatic, congenital, and metabolic disturbance of bone growth, or they may represent normal variants of bone growth and development. Joint effusion or bleeding may cause overgrowth, as is the case in juvenile rheumatoid arthritis and hemophilia. A long list of eponyms is applied to irregularity of the epiphysis associated with avascular necrosis.

DISEASE	COMMENTS
Achondroplasia [p. 385]	Congenital defect of enchondral bone formation, producing characteristic rounded lumbar "bullet-nosed" vertebrae, lumbar kyphosis, posterior scalloping of the vertebrae, increased intervertebral disc height, flattened vertebral bodies, and narrowed spinal canal; the pelvis may appear hypoplastic; epiphyses may appear "cone-shaped"; cone-shaped epiphyses are also seen with sickle cell disease, various congenital dysplasias, and as a normal variant
Avascular necrosis **(FIGS. 7-10 THROUGH 7-15)** [p. 591]	Etiologies related to vascular insufficiency (i.e., sickle cell disease, steroid therapy, trauma, alcoholism, etc.); necrosis gives the epiphyses a fragmented, radiodense, thin, and small appearance; proximal femoral epiphysis is most common; weight bearing, joint effusion, and decreased range of motion cause pain

Continued

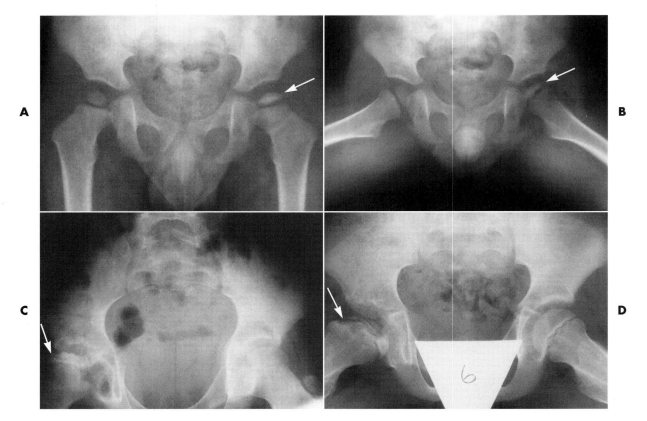

FIG. 7-10   Three cases of Legg-Calvé-Perthes (LCP) disease. Anteroposterior, **A,** and frogleg, **B,** pelvic projection of a child with a left proximal femoral epiphysis *(arrows),* which appears small and dense consistent with LCP. Second case with anteroposterior, **C,** and frogleg, **D,** projection of a different patient with similar findings of a small, fragmented, dense right epiphysis *(arrows).*   *Continued*

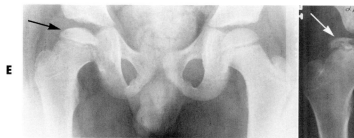
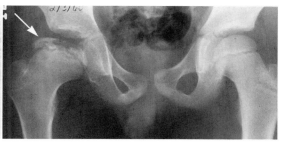

FIG. 7-10, cont'd A third case of progressive changes of fragmentation, increased density, and diminution occurring initially, **E,** and 2 years following the initial film, **F** *(arrows).* (*C* and *D,* Courtesy Jack C. Avalos, Davenport, Iowa; *E* and *F,* Courtesy Joseph W. Howe, Sylmar, Calif.)

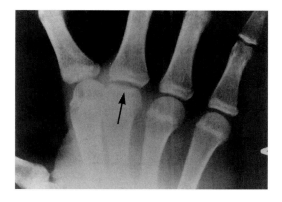

FIG. 7-11 Mauclaire's disease, presenting as avascular necrosis of the third metacarpal head *(arrow).* (Courtesy Joseph W. Howe, Sylmar, Calif.)

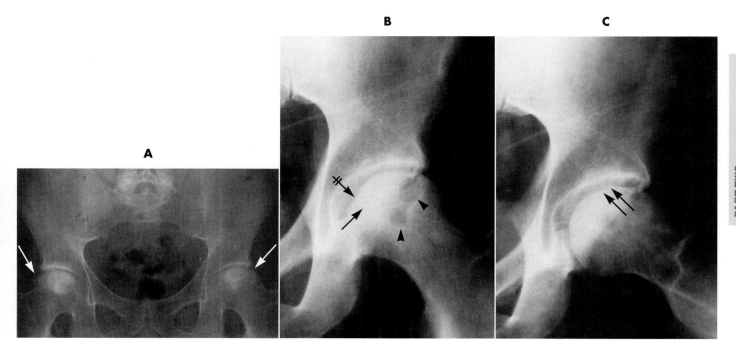

FIG. 7-12 Bilateral femoral head sclerosis and flattening of the superior articular surfaces associated with adult avascular necrosis (Chandler's disease) **A,** *(arrows).* A second patient (**B** and **C**) with sclerosis *(arrows),* cysts *(arrowheads),* cortical offset of femoral head collapse *(crossed arrow),* and subchondral lucent "crescent sign" denoting subchondral collapse *(double arrow).* (*A,* Courtesy Joseph W. Howe, Sylmar, Calif.)

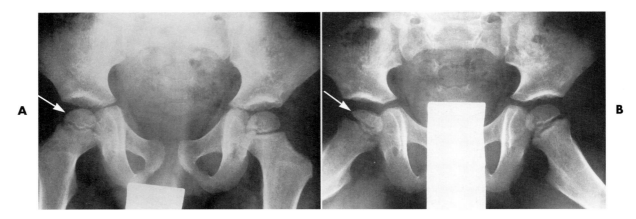

FIG. 7-13   Legg-Calvé-Perthes disease presenting with proximal femoral epiphyses that appear near normal on the anteroposterior radiography **(A)** and with loss of vertical height of the proximal femoral epiphysis on the frogleg **(B)** projection *(arrows)*. (Courtesy Robert C. Tatum, Davenport, Iowa.)

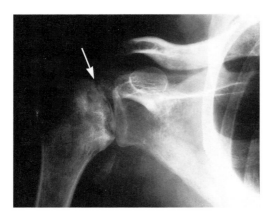

FIG. 7-14   Avascular necrosis of the humeral head (Hass's disease) *(arrow)*. (Courtesy Steven P. Brownstein, Springfield, NJ.)

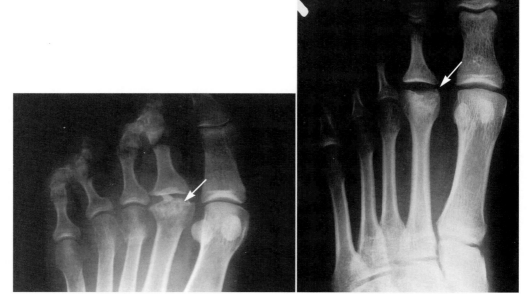

FIG. 7-15   Two patients with flattened deformity of the metatarsal head consistent with avascular necrosis (Freiberg's disease) *(arrows)*.

DISEASE

Congenital syndromes (FIG. 7-16)

Cretinism [p. 725]

COMMENTS

Chondrodysplasia punctata (Conradi's disease), multiple epiphyseal dysplasia (Fairbank-Ribbing disease), Down syndrome, and other congenital syndromes associated with irregularity, fragmentation, and stippling of multiple epiphyses

Juvenile hypothyroidism during the first year of life resulting from thymic agenesis or low maternal iodine intake during pregnancy; delayed skeletal and mental development result; epiphyses appear stippled during infancy and fragmented during childhood; cone-shaped epiphyses may develop; the proximal femoral epiphyses are most commonly involved

Hemophilia [p. 601]

Juvenile rheumatoid arthritis [p. 435]

Inherited X-linked defect of blood coagulation marked by a permanent tendency toward hemorrhages; hemarthrosis is associated with red, swollen joints, osteoporosis, precocious degeneration, and an enlargement of the epiphyses; knee, ankle, and elbow are most common; rarely, osteolytic expansile bone lesions (hemophilic pseudotumors) develop

Chronic arthritis beginning in childhood (before 16 years of age), manifesting as one of several clinical types; characteristic large, overgrown, "ballooned" epiphyses, osteoporosis, joint fusion, periostitis, and gracile long bones are secondary to hyperemia

Continued

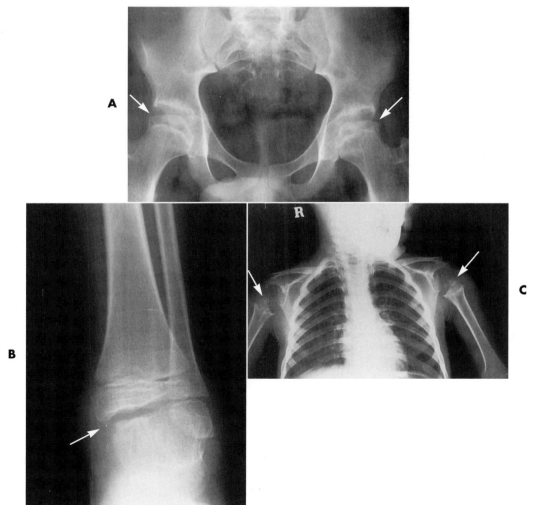

FIG. 7-16 Multiple epiphyseal dysplasia, resulting in irregular appearing epiphyses of the proximal femora **(A)** and distal tibia **(B)** *(arrows)*. **C,** Another patient with irregularity of the proximal humeri *(arrows)*. (*A* and *B*, Courtesy Jack C. Avalos, Davenport, Iowa; *C*, Courtesy Joseph W. Howe, Sylmar, Calif.)

DISEASE	**COMMENTS**
Normal variant	May be represented by symmetrical, fragmented, or irregular appearance of the epiphysis; these variants may mimic osteonecrosis
Rickets **(FIG. 7-17)** [p. 735]	Infantile or juvenile osteomalacia secondary to vitamin D deficiency, characterized clinically by irritability, listlessness, and generalized muscle weakness; an overproduction and deficient calcification of osteoid tissue results in disturbances of bone growth with resulting deformity; fractures are common; epiphyses may appear indistinct, epiphyseal plates are wide, and metaphyses appear frayed

Scurvy (Barlow's disease) **(FIG. 7-18)** [p. 738]	Defective osteogenesis secondary to abnormal collagen from vitamin C deficiency, beginning between 6 to 14 months of age; clinically marked by irritability, bleeding gums, tendency toward hemorrhage, and tenderness and weakness of lower limbs; epiphyses appear radiolucent with surrounding sclerotic rim (Wimberger's sign or ring epiphyses)
Trauma	Traumatic separation or changes in the size and shape of the epiphysis; including battered child syndrome

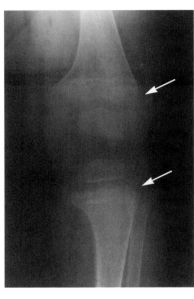

FIG. 7-17   Rickets demonstrating a widened, frayed ("paintbrush") metaphyses *(arrows)* with an indistinct epiphysis. (Courtesy Joseph W. Howe, Sylmar, Calif.)

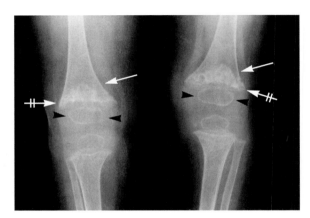

FIG. 7-18   Scurvy appearing with bilateral radiolucent epiphyses, which are outlined by a surrounding radiodense rim *(arrowheads)*. Radiolucent metaphyseal bands *(arrows)* and radiodense zone of provisional calcification *(crossed arrows)* are evident. (Courtesy Steven P. Brownstein, Springfield, NJ.)

EX4 | Cystic Lesions of Extremities and Ribs

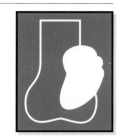

This pattern lists lesions occurring mostly in the epiphyses and metaphyses of long bones that appear as solitary or, less commonly, multiple well-defined holes in the bone. The age of presentation, host bone, presence of calcification, and symptoms are useful discriminators for the list of lesions. The infamous mnemonic *FEGNOMASHIC* includes many of this list: fibrous dysplasia, enchondroma (and eosinophilic granuloma), giant cell tumor, nonossifying fibroma, osteoblastoma, metastatic disease (and multiple myeloma/plasmacytoma), aneurysmal bone cyst, simple bone cyst, hyperparathyroidism (and hemophilic pseudotumors) infection, chondroblastoma (and chondromyxoid fibroma).

The full list may be modified if the presentation is of multiple lesions or is epiphyseal in location. A presentation of multiple lesions suggests the following etiologies: infection, fibrous dysplasia, metastasis, multiple myeloma, subchondral cysts, hyperparathyroidism, enchondromatosis, and eosinophilic granuloma. An epiphyseal location suggests infection, giant cell tumor, chondroblastoma, subchondral cyst, pigmented villonodular synovitis, and interosseous ganglion. Cystic bone lesions occurring in patients younger than 30 years of age most often result from eosinophilic granuloma, aneurysmal bone cyst, simple bone cyst, chondroblastoma, and nonossifying fibroma/fibrous cortical defect.

The mnemonic *FAME* describes cystic rib lesions: fibrous dyplasia, aneurysmal bone cyst, metastatic disease (and multiple myeloma), and enchondroma.

DISEASE	COMMENTS
Adamantinoma [p. 673]	Also known as *angioblastoma,* a rare, locally aggressive or malignant lesion composed of epithelium-like cells in dense fibrous stroma; 90% are found in the middle third of the tibia; lesions appear as central or eccentric, slightly expansile, well circumscribed, osteolytic lesions
Aneurysmal bone cyst **(FIGS. 7-19 AND 7-20)** [p. 634]	Solitary, benign, osteolytic lesion of bone, characterized by cortical expansion, usually found in patients younger than 20 years of age; this bone cyst most commonly presents as an eccentric lesion in the metaphyses of long bones; it typically causes pain

Continued

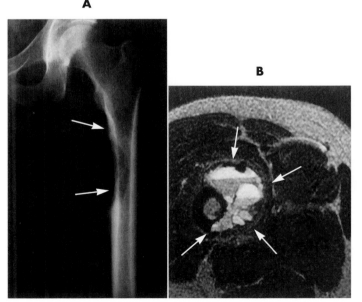

FIG. 7-19   Eccentric expansile lesion, representing an aneurysmal bone cyst of the distal tibia *(arrow).* (Courtesy Ian D. McLean, Davenport, Iowa.)

FIG. 7-20   **A,** Plain film radiograph demonstrating a seemingly aggressive expansile bone lesion in the diametaphysis of the femur *(arrows).* The T2-weighted MRI scan reveals an expanded but intact cortex surrounding the mixed signal intensity of the matrix **(B)** *(arrows).* The appearance is consistent with aneuysmal bone cyst.

PART TWO
Bone, Joints, and Soft Tissues

DISEASE	COMMENTS
Chondroblastoma [p. 641]	Rare benign bone tumor arising in the secondary growth centers of long bones; usually in patients younger than 25 years of age; 50% demonstrate matrix calcification and a rim of surrounding sclerosis
Chondromyxoid fibroma [p. 648]	Rare, benign bone tumor of mixed histology, arising most commonly in the proximal tibia and fibula; usually in patients younger than 30 years of age, they appear as noncalcified lytic lesions
Enchondroma **(FIGS. 7-21 AND 7-22)** [p. 644]	Solitary or multiple benign cystic cartilage lesion, appearing most often in the small bones of the hands and feet; stippled cartilage matrix is typically seen; no periostitis or pain is present unless fractured
Eosinophilic granuloma [p. 747]	Proliferation of eosinophils seen most commonly in children and young adults; spine involvement is present in less than 10% of patients; advanced body collapse "vertebra plana" and multiple levels may accompany the condition; long bone involvement typically occurs in the diaphysis; patients younger than 30 years of age almost exclusively represent the population affected by this disease; it may be present with solitary or multiple lesions
Fibrous cortical defect/nonossifying fibroma **(FIGS. 7-23 THROUGH 7-26)** [p. 648]	Very common, benign asymptomatic cystic bone lesions seen before the age of 30 years; marked by a thin sclerotic border without matrix calcification; common in the lower extremities, particularly around the knee

Continued

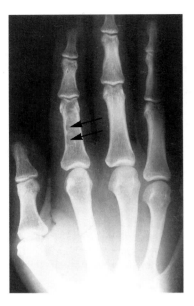

FIG. 7-21   Enchondroma of the proximal phalanx of the second digit with endosteal scalloping *(arrows)*. (Courtesy Ian D. McLean, Davenport, Iowa.)

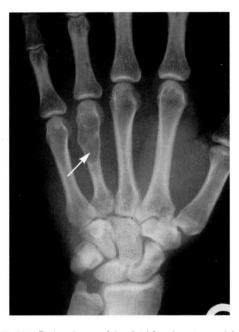

FIG. 7-22   Enchondroma of the distal fourth metacarpal *(arrow)*.

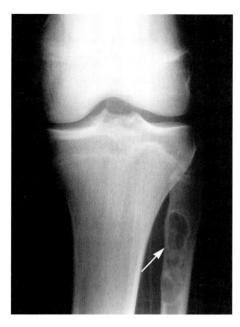

FIG. 7-23 Nonossifying fibroma of the proximal fibula *(arrow)*. (Courtesy Steven P. Brownstein, Springfield, NJ.)

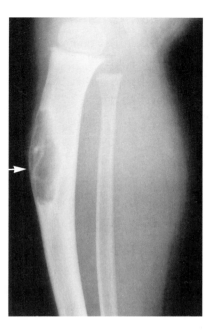

FIG. 7-24 Nonossifying fibroma of the proximal tibia *(arrow)*. (Courtesy Steven P. Brownstein, Springfield, NJ.)

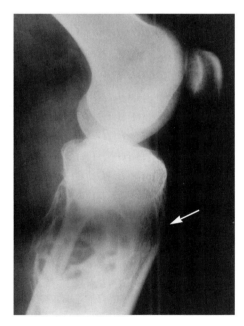

FIG. 7-25 Multiloculated, expansile lesion of the proximal tibia denoting nonossifying fibroma *(arrow)*. (Courtesy Steven P. Brownstein, Springfield, NJ.)

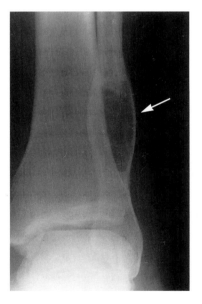

FIG. 7-26 Cystic expansile lesion of the distal fibula representing nonossifying fibroma *(arrow)*. (Courtesy Ian D. McLean, Davenport, Iowa.)

DISEASE	COMMENTS
Fibrous dysplasia **(FIGS. 7-27 THROUGH 7-29)** [p. 651]	Disturbance of bone maintenance in which bone is replaced by abnormal proliferation of fibrous tissue, possibly involving one or multiple bones; the matrix often has a characteristic "ground glass" radiodensity; lesions may be surrounded by a thick rind of bone sclerosis; most common locations are femur, ribs, tibia, craniofacial bones, and pelvis; lesion should not be painful
Giant cell tumor **(FIGS. 7-30 AND 7-31)** [p. 654]	Sometimes malignant cystic lesion of bone; subarticular, eccentric (early), sharply defined lesion appears without surrounding sclerosis; most commonly found around the knee; tumor occurs between 20 and 40 years of age

Hydatid *(Echinococcus)* cyst [p. 979]	Cyst that may be formed in bone (usually formed in the liver) by the larval stage of *Echinococcus;* it appears as a slow-growing, destructive lesion surrounded by sclerotic borders; it is primarily limited to endemic areas
Hyperparathyroidism [p. 718]	Overproduction of parathyroid glands because of primary or secondary causes; the disease is marked by osteopenia, osteosclerosis, bone resorption, and soft tissue and vascular calcification; vertebrae have characteristic homogeneous radiodense bands traversing horizontally at each endplate ("rugger-jersey" spine); subchondral bone resorption occurs, particularly at the radial aspects of the middle phalanges; lytic or sclerotic cystic bone lesion (brown tumors) may be present

Continued

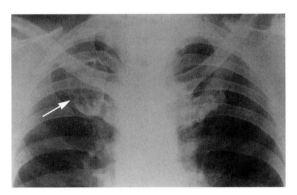

FIG. 7-27   Fibrous dyplasia causing a cystic lesion of the right first rib *(arrow).* (Courtesy Joseph W. Howe, Sylmar, Calif.)

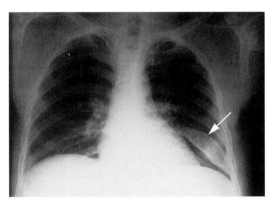

FIG. 7-28   Fibrous dyplasia, producing an expansile lesion of the posterior portion of the left eighth rib *(arrow).*

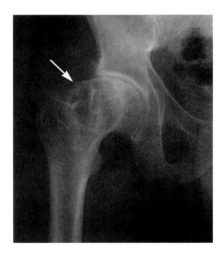

FIG. 7-29   Anteroposterior hip projection demonstrating a characteristic lesion of fibrous dysplasia of the right femoral intertochanteric region *(arrow).* (Courtesy Ian D. McLean, Davenport, Iowa.)

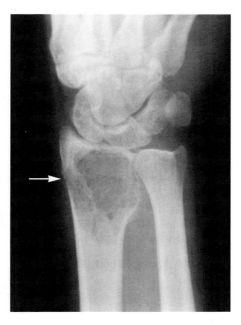

FIG. 7-30 Giant cell tumor of the distal radius. The lesion presents the characteristic osteolytic, well-defined, subarticular, and eccentric appearance *(arrow)*. (Courtesy William E. Litterer, Elizabeth, NJ.)

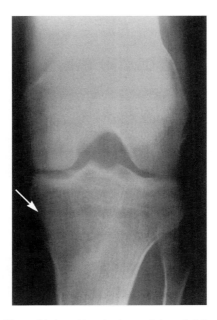

FIG. 7-31 Giant cell lesion with a classic osteolytic, well-defined, subarticular, and eccentric appearance in the proximal tibia *(arrow)*. (Courtesy Joseph W. Howe, Sylmar, Calif.)

DISEASE	COMMENTS
Infection **(FIG. 7-32)**	May occur at practically any location during any age; if found in a subarticular location, the joint is often involved with effusion; soft-tissue mass and central bone sequestrum are often present; appearance varies from cystic to sclerotic; alternatively, infections may present as aggressive bone lesions
Intraosseous lipoma **(FIG. 7-33)** [p. 661]	Intraosseous collections of fat appearing as a radiolucent lesion surrounded by a thin sclerotic rim of bone, often with a centrally located radiodense nidus; the proximal femoral and calcaneal epiphyses predominantly house the lipoma; it typically presents as an asymptomatic lesion during middle age
Metastatic disease **(FIG. 7-34)** [p. 687]	Very common cause of one or more osteolytic bone lesions in patients over the age of 40 years; atypical presentations of expansile, bubbly, solitary geographic lesions are associated with primary lesions of the thyroid and kidney; purely blastic lesions occur most often from breast, prostate, GI, bladder, and lung neoplasms
Multiple myeloma/plasmacytoma **(FIGS. 7-35 THROUGH 7-37)** [p. 700]	Malignant proliferation of plasma cells, occurring in predominately the red marrow of various bones; the skull, vertebral bodies, ribs, and proximal humerus and femurs are most commonly involved; single or multiple osteolytic lesions simulate metastatic disease, without tendency to involve vertebral arch, as is common in metastasis; osteopenia and solitary or multiple levels of vertebral collapse that together simulate osteoporosis; rarely occurs before 30 years of age
Osteoblastoma [p. 667]	Histologically similar to osteoid osteoma, but different in radiographic appearance; osteoblastomas appear as medium-sized (greater than or equal to 1.5 cm), geographic, expansile, generally nonaggressive, eccentric medullary lesions; most commonly located in the posterior elements of the spine, and less frequently in the proximal femur, tibia, talus, ribs, and hands; they usually appear before 25 years of age

Continued

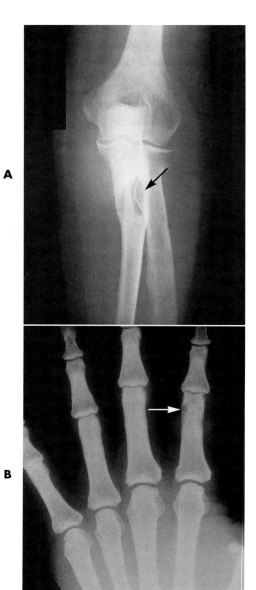

FIG. 7-32   Well-defined, seemingly relatively nonaggressive infections of the ulna, **A,** and distal portion of the proximal phalanx of the second digit, **(B)** *(arrows)*. (Courtesy Steven P. Brownstein, Springfield, NJ.)

FIG. 7-33   Interosseous lipoma appearing as a cystic lesion in the calcaneus with a central nidus of calcification *(arrow)*. (Courtesy Steven P. Brownstein, Springfield, NJ.)

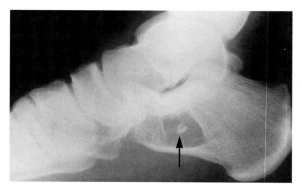

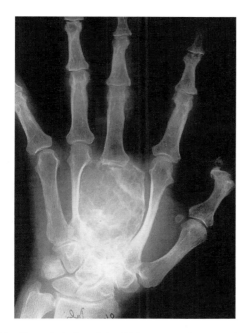

FIG. 7-34 Expansile lesion of the third metacarpal, representing metastatic bone disease secondary to primary thyroid malignancy. (Courtesy Steven P. Brownstein, Springfield, NJ.)

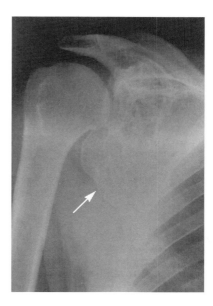

FIG. 7-35 Expansile cystic lesion of the neck of the scapula representing a plasmacytoma *(arrow).* (Courtesy Joseph W. Howe, Sylmar, Calif.)

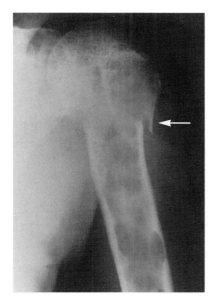

FIG. 7-36 Multiple myeloma presenting with multiple osteolytic lesions in the proximal humerus. The larger cystic lesion of the surgical neck is fractured *(arrow).* (Courtesy Joseph W. Howe, Sylmar, Calif.)

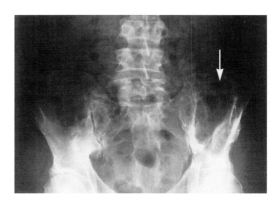

FIG. 7-37 Plasmacytoma of the left ilium, appearing as an osteolytic lesion with surrounding sclerotic margin *(arrow).* (Courtesy Steven P. Brownstein, Springfield, NJ.)

DISEASE	COMMENTS
Pigmented villo-nodular synovitis (PVNS) **(FIG. 7-38)** [p. 767]	Chronic condition marked by diffuse hyperplastic outgrowths of a joint's synovial membrane; osteolytic appearance may result from pressure erosions of bone if joint capsule is tight; usually PVNS occurs before 40 years of age, although wide age range is possible; the most common locations are the knee, hip, ankle, elbow, and shoulder
Simple (solitary) bone cyst **(FIGS. 7-39 AND 7-40)** [p. 671]	Fluid-filled cyst of uncertain etiology; the majority of cases are discovered before the age of 20 years; 90% of simple bone cysts are found in the proximal humerus and femur; bone cysts appear as mildly expansile, well-marginated, geographic lytic lesions in the metaphysis, less frequently diaphysis, or rarely epiphysis; fracture causes pain, otherwise, usually painless
Subchondral bone cyst **(FIGS. 7-41, 7-42, AND 7-43)**	Related to arthritic or synovial disorder (osteoarthritis, gout, calcium pyrophosphate deposition disease, rheumatoid arthritis, hemophilia, intraosseous ganglion, amyloidosis, and avascular necrosis); this well-defined cyst is located in the epiphysis subjacent to the articular cortex

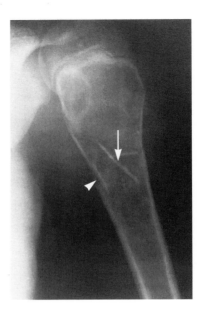

FIG. 7-39 Simple bone cyst in the proximal humerus. A fragmented septum is noted obliquely oriented and inferiorly displaced ("fallen fragment" sign) in the large radiolucent lesion *(arrow)*. Fracture of the thinned cortex is noted on the medial side of the humerus *(arrowhead)*. (Courtesy Steven P. Brownstein, Springfield, NJ.)

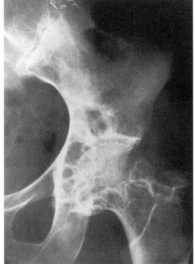

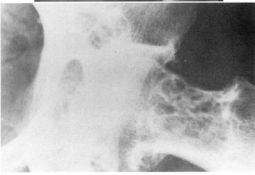

FIG. 7-38 Pigmented villonodular synovitis of the hip, causing cystic bone erosions of the femoral neck ("apple core" deformity) and the surrounding acetabulum. The bone erosions are secondary to the proliferation of the synovium. (Courtesy Joseph W. Howe, Sylmar, Calif.)

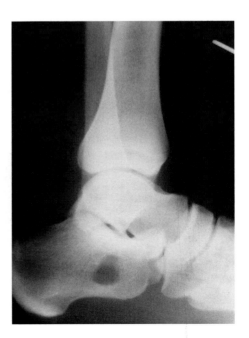

FIG. 7-40 Simple bone cyst of the calcaneus. A similar appearance may occur with interosseous lipoma or giant cell tumor. (Courtesy Steven P. Brownstein, Springfield, NJ.)

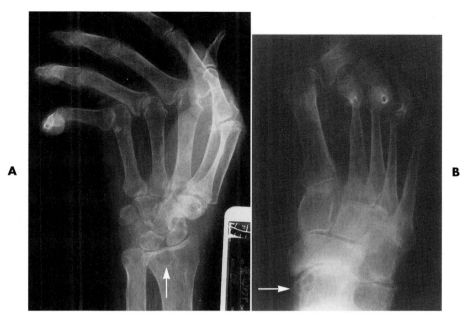

FIG. 7-41 Subchondral cysts *(arrows)* in the radius, **A,** and talus, **B,** in different patients with advanced rheumatoid arthritis. *(A,* Courtesy Jack C. Avalos, Davenport, Iowa; *B,* Courtesy Joseph W. Howe, Sylmar, Calif.)

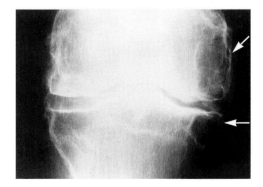

FIG. 7-42 Degenerative subchondral cysts of the tibial and femur *(arrows).* (Courtesy Joseph W. Howe, Sylmar, Calif.)

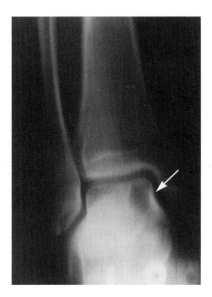

FIG. 7-43 Linear tomogram of an intraosseous ganglion of the talus *(arrow).* (Courtesy Joseph W. Howe, Sylmar, Calif.)

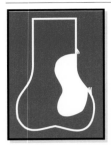

EX5 | Aggressive Osteolytic Lesions of Extremities and Ribs

The following diseases produce usually ill-defined osteolytic lesions of bone, most characteristically of the long bones. They arise from permeative or moth-eaten patterns of bone destruction, which may coalesce over time. Radiographic findings of ill-defined bone destruction suggest aggressive pathology. The majority of these patterns represent malignant bone or marrow tumors. Patients usually complain of pain and soft tissue mass over the involved bone.

Malignant bone tumors with marked periosteal reaction include Burkitt's lymphoma, Ewing's tumor, osteosarcoma, neuroblastoma metastasis, and leukemia presenting in a child. Tumors that arise in the midshaft of long bones and contain cells with round nuclei are known as *round cell lesions*. Round cell lesions are listed by the mnemonic LEMON: leukemia (and lymphoma), eosinophilic granuloma (and Ewing's tumor), multiple myeloma, osteomyelitis (mimics tumor), and neuroblastoma metastasis.

DISEASE	COMMENTS
Central chondrosarcoma **(FIG. 7-44)** [p. 673]	Aggressive malignant tumor of cartilage arising within the medullary canal of patients usually between the ages of 40 and 70 years; most are found in the pelvis, proximal femur, proximal humerus, distal femur, proximal tibia, and ribs; chondrosarcoma appears most often as metaphyseal regions of bone destruction with scattered stippled matrix calcification with endosteal cortical scalloping, but only rarely is the cortex destroyed
Eosinophilic granuloma **(FIG. 7-45)** [p. 747]	Abnormal proliferation of eosinophils seen most commonly in children and young adults; lytic skull and long bone defects mark this condition; the spine is involved in less than 10% of patients and appears as advanced body collapse "vertebra plana" possibly at multiple levels; long bone involvement typically occurs in the diaphysis appearing as solitary, or less commonly multiple osteolytic defects; almost exclusively, patients younger than 30 years of age exhibit this disease
Ewing's sarcoma **(FIG. 7-46)** [p. 676]	Highly malignant primary bone tumor occurring mostly in children and teenagers; may occur in any bone of the body, although the majority of cases present in the pelvis and long bones of the lower extremities; although a diaphyseal location is classic, the metadiaphysis is more often involved; marked by permeative lytic bone destruction, cortical erosion (saucerization), laminated or "onion skin" periosteal reaction, and large soft tissue mass

Continued

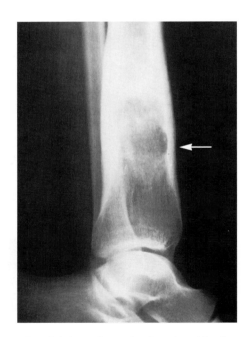

FIG. 7-44   Osteolytic bone destruction *(arrow)* resulting from chondrosarcoma in the distal tibia. (Courtesy Steven P. Brownstein, Springfield, NJ.)

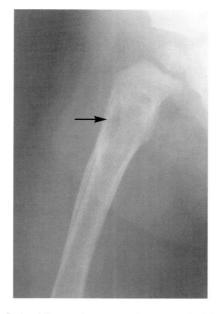

FIG. 7-45 Eosinophilic granuloma presenting as an osteolytic defect in the proximal femur *(arrow).* (Courtesy Joseph W. Howe, Sylmar, Calif.)

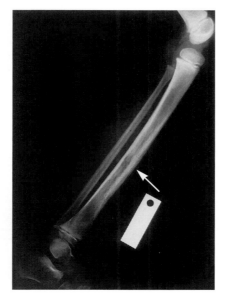

FIG. 7-46 Ewing's sarcoma representing a poorly defined osteolytic lesion of the tibial diaphysis *(arrow).* (Courtesy Ian D. McLean, Davenport, Iowa.)

DISEASE

COMMENTS

Fibrosarcoma/ malignant fibrous histiocytoma (FIGS. 7-47 AND 7-48) [p. 680]

Uncommon malignant tumors that involve fibrous tissues; most lesions are found around the knee and appear as osteolytic lesions with geographic, moth-eaten, or permeative bone destruction; typically, tumors are located in the metaphysis; cortical destruction, extraosseous mass, and aggressive periosteal reaction are often present; the tumor matrix does not exhibit calcification, although occasional bony fragments may be present

Infection (FIG. 7-49)

Infection resulting from broad spectrum causative organisms involving bone by hematogenous spread, contiguous involvement, or direct implantation; bones with rich marrow supply are frequently involved (i.e., metaphyses of long bones, spine, and ribs); bone findings begin as subtle areas of destruction; subperiosteal extension causes thick, laminated periosteal response, which encases (involucrum) the infection; disruption of the blood supply may produce osteonecrotic bone fragments (sequestrum) within the lesion

Continued

FIG. 7-47 Fibrosarcoma of the distal femur, demonstrating permeative bone destruction with no matrix calcification *(arrow)*. (Courtesy Steven P. Brownstein, Springfield, NJ.)

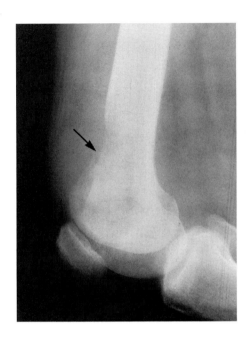

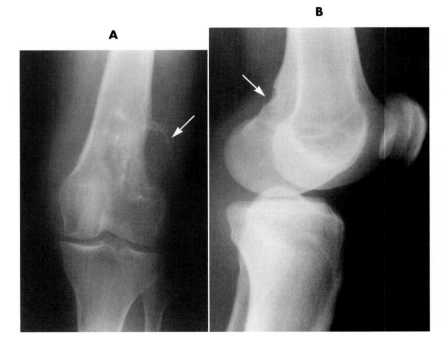

FIG. 7-48 Desmoplastic fibroma. Desmoplastic fibromas **(A)** *(arrow)* represent rare benign lesions that are histologically identical to the nontumorous alteration of the periosteum known as *juxtacortical desmoids* **(B)** *(arrow)*. As in this case, desmoplastic fibromas often appear as osteolytic lesions with prominent trabeculation. The lesions are often difficult to differentiate from fibrosarcomas. (*A,* Courtesy Joseph W. Howe, Sylmar, Calif.; *B,* Courtesy Steven P. Brownstein, Springfield, NJ.)

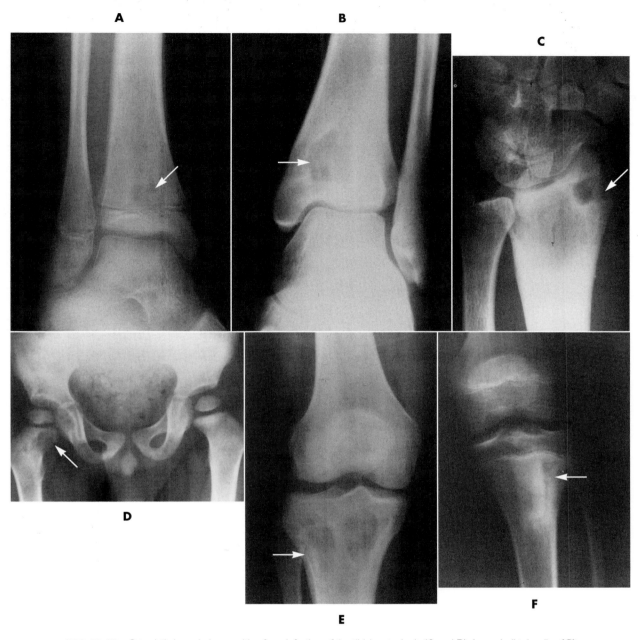

FIG. 7-49 Osteolytic bone lesion resulting from infection of the tibial metaphysis (**A** and **B**) *(arrows)*; distal radius (**C**) *(arrow)*; proximal femoral metaphysis (**D**) *(arrow)*; and the proximal tibial metaphysis (**E** and **F**) *(arrows)*.

Continued

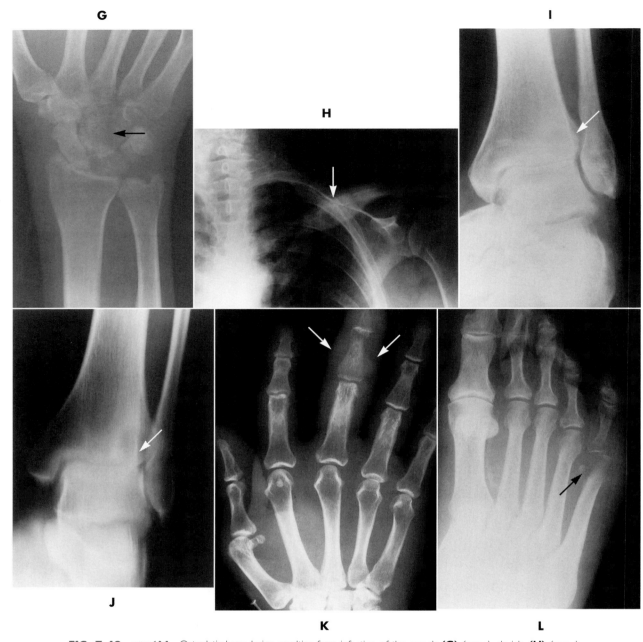

FIG. 7-49—cont'd   Osteolytic bone lesion resulting from infection of the carpals **(G)** *(arrow)*, clavicle **(H)** *(arrow)*, distal tibia **(I)** *(arrow)*, with linear tomography **(J)** *(arrow)*, and third digit of the hand **(K)** *(arrows)* and foot **(L)** *(arrow)*. *(C through J, Courtesy Joseph W. Howe, Sylmar, Calif.)*

FIG. 7-50   Primary lymphoma of bone causing permeative destruction of the ischium *(arrow)*. (Courtesy Joseph W. Howe, Sylmar, Calif.)

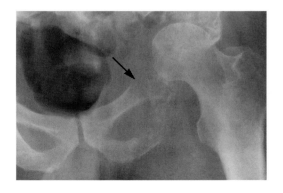

DISEASE	COMMENTS
Leukemia [p. 603]	Proliferation of abnormal leukocytes within hemopoietic tissues and other organs; variety of types is based on cell type and duration from onset to death; leukemia of bone is typically acute lymphoblastic; skeletal manifestations include diffuse demineralization, osteolytic defects, smooth periosteal reaction, and radiolucent metaphyseal bands, which become dense following chemotherapy

Lymphoma **(FIG. 7-50)** [p. 685]	Primary and secondary (systemic non-Hodgkin's lymphoma and Hodgkin's disease) lymphoma of bone, appearing as permeative radiolucent lesions of the lower extremities, pelvis, and spine; occurs over wide range of ages
Metastasis **(FIGS. 7-51** **THROUGH 7-54)** [p. 687]	Bone metastasis is common to the spine and rarely involves the skeleton distal to the elbows or knees (acral metastasis); typically appears as a polyostotic, moth-eaten pattern of osteolytic bone destruction with poorly defined zones of transition; periosteal reaction and soft tissue masses are typically small or absent; usually in patients older than age 40 years

Continued

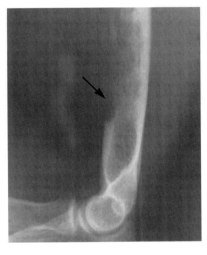

FIG. 7-51 Metastatic bone disease producing osteolytic bone destruction of the anterior, distal portion of the humerus *(arrow)*. (Courtesy Joseph W. Howe, Sylmar, Calif.)

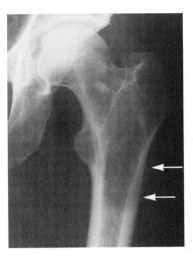

FIG. 7-53 Permeative osteolytic bone destruction of the proximal femur resulting from metastatic bone disease *(arrows)*. Lymphoma may present with a similar appearance. (Courtesy Joseph W. Howe, Sylmar, Calif.)

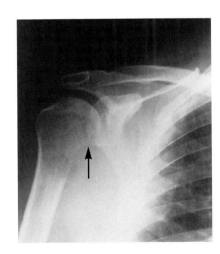

FIG. 7-52 Metastatic bone disease manifesting as poorly defined osteolytic bone destruction of the proximal humerus *(arrow)*. (Courtesy Ronnie L. Firth, East Moline, Ill.)

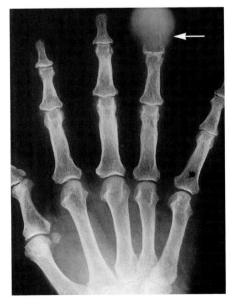

FIG. 7-54 Metastatic disease causing an aggressive lesion of the distal phalanx of the fourth digit of the left hand *(arrow)*. (Courtesy Ronnie L. Firth, East Moline, Ill.)

DISEASE	COMMENTS
Multiple myeloma/ plasma-cytoma (FIGS. 7-55 AND 7-56) [p. 700]	Malignant proliferation of plasma cells occurring in predominately the red marrow of various bones; the skull, vertebral bodies, ribs, and proximal humerus and femurs are most commonly involved; single or multiple osteolytic lesions simulate metastatic disease but typically do not involve vertebral arch, as is demonstrated by metastasis; osteopenia and solitary or multiple-level vertebral collapse may simulate osteoporosis; these diseases rarely occur before 30 years of age
Osteosarcoma (FIG. 7-57) [p. 704]	Highly aggressive, malignant tumor of bone-forming cells most commonly arising in the metaphysis of long bones, usually around the knee; people between 10 and 25 years of age primarily are affected; lesions appear as lytic or blastic areas of bone destruction with a surrounding cloudlike density of tumor matrix and aggressive periosteal reaction ("sunburst")

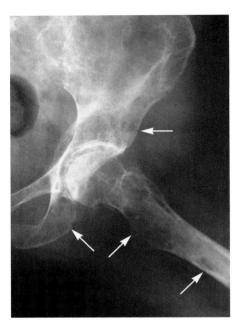

FIG. 7-56   Multiple myeloma producing multiple punched-out osteolytic lesions of the innominate and proximal femur *(arrows)*. (Courtesy Steven P. Brownstein, Springfield, NJ.)

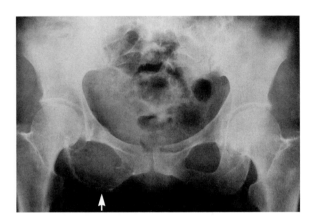

FIG. 7-55   Osteolytic destruction of the ischial tuberosity *(arrow)* secondary to multiple myeloma. (Courtesy Steven P. Brownstein, Springfield, NJ.)

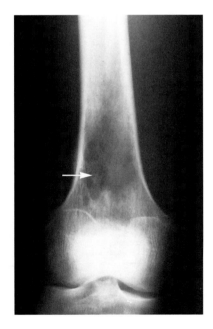

FIG. 7-57   Osteosarcoma of the distal femur, demonstrating an aggressive, purely osteolytic lesion of the distal femur *(arrow)*. No periosteal reaction is demonstrated in this single view. Approximately 25% of osteosarcomas are osteolytic, 25% osteoblastic, and 50% mixed. (Courtesy Steven P. Brownstein, Springfield, NJ.)

EX6 | Osteosclerotic Bone Lesions

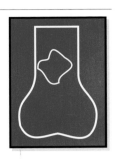

This pattern describes solitary or multiple osteosclerotic bone lesions in the extremities. Many of the diseases listed also occur in the spine, making the pattern functional for osteosclerotic spinal lesions as well. Asymptomatic, solitary osteosclerotic lesions usually represent bone islands or entities of limited consequence. In general, multiple presentations are suggestive of metastatic disease in patients over the age of 40 years.

DISEASE	COMMENTS
Bone infarct/epiphyseal avascular necrosis (FIGS. 7-58 AND 7-59) [p. 591]	Healed infarcts usually appear as serpiginous calcifications in the metadiaphysis of long bones; epiphyseal avascular necrosis (AVN) is characterized by sclerosis, cystic formations, and flattening or diminution of the involved epiphysis; both conditions most often follow trauma, irradiation, corticosteroid use, etc. *Continued*

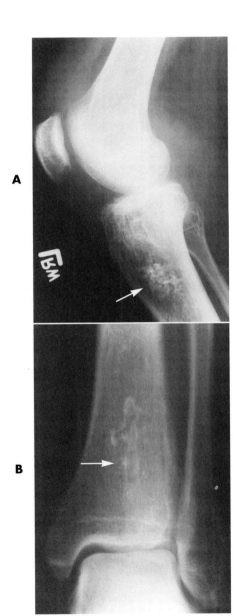

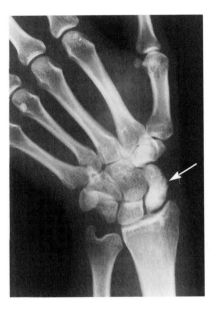

FIG. 7-59   The lunate appears osteosclerotic secondary to avascular necrosis *(arrow)*. (Courtesy Joseph W. Howe, Sylmar, Calif.)

FIG. 7-58   Different patients with stippled calcification within the medullary cavity of proximal **(A)** and distal **(B)** tibia *(arrows)*. The appearance is consistent with medullary infarct or enchondroma. (Courtesy Joseph W. Howe, Sylmar, Calif.)

PART TWO
Bone, Joints, and Soft Tissues

DISEASE	COMMENTS
Bone island/ osteopoikilosis/ osteomas (FIG. 7-60) [p. 637]	Benign, common, solitary (bone island) or less common, multiple (osteopoikilosis) foci of compact, nontrabeculated bone occurring in the extremities and less commonly the spine; similar formations in the skull and facial bones are known as *osteomas,* often occurring around the paranasal sinuses

Fibrous dysplasia [p. 651]	Nonneoplastic disturbance of bone maintenance; femur, tibia, craniofacial bones and pelvis are the most common sites; fibrous dysplasia usually appears as an osteolytic lesion with mild sclerosis within, but rarely may present as densely sclerotic lesions; it is usually solitary
Fracture	Radiodense appearance secondary to callus around healing fractures or stress fractures, which often appear in predictable locations; both are usually solitary lesions
Healing bone lesions	Osteolytic bone lesions may become sclerotic spontaneously or following treatment (i.e., radiation therapy)
Melorheostosis (FIG. 7-61) [p. 401]	Begins as a region of linear hyperostosis at the proximal end of a tubular bone and progresses distally to involve both sides of the cortex; one or more bones may be involved

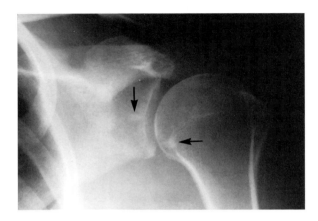

FIG. 7-60   Several bone islands in the scapula and proximal humerus *(arrows).* (Courtesy Authur W. Holmes, Foley, Ala.)

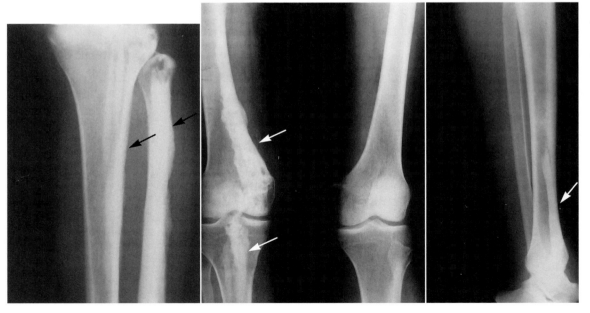

FIG. 7-61   Melorheostosis in three patients. In each patient thick endosteal osteosclerosis is noted *(arrows).* (*Left,* Courtesy Joseph W Howe, Sylmar, Calif.; *middle* and *right,* Courtesy Steven P. Brownstein, Springfield, NJ.)

Metastasis [p. 687]	Bone metastasis is common to the spine and rarely involves the skeleton distal to the elbows or knees (known as *acral metastasis*); osteosclerotic lesions are less common than osteolytic lesions, usually related to primary malignancy of the breast, prostate, GI, bladder, or lung and usually found in patients over the age of 40 years; soft tissue masses are typically small or absent; lesions may be solitary or multiple
Paget's disease **(FIG. 7-62)** [p. 761]	Chronic skeletal disease of aberrant bone remodeling, marked by bone enlargement, softening, and rarely sarcomatous changes; the pelvis, proximal femora, and lumbar spine are common areas; single or multiple osteosclerotic lesions are marked by bone enlargement, cortical thickening, and prominent trabeculae affecting the middle-aged
Primary bone tumors (benign) **(FIG. 7-63)**	Primary benign (osteoid osteoma, enchondromas, and osteochondroma) and malignant tumors (osteosarcoma, rarely multiple myeloma, and Ewing's), possibly producing osteosclerotic lesions
Sclerosing osteomyelitis	Usual related clinical symptoms; Garre's sclerosing osteomyelitis, Brodie's abscess, and chronic osteomyelitis may produce osteosclerotic bone lesions

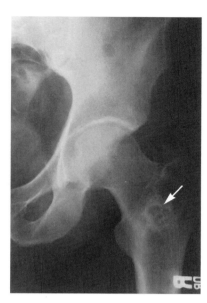

FIG. 7-63 Fibrous dysplasia presenting as a radiodense lesion of the intertrochanteric region of the left proximal femur *(arrow)*. (Courtesy Steven P. Brownstein, Springfield, NJ.)

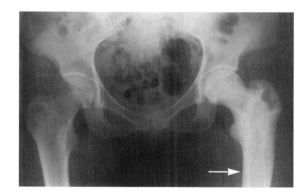

FIG. 7-62 Paget's disease. The proximal left femur appears osteosclerotic and enlarged with thick cortex *(arrow)*.

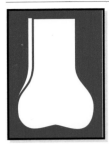

EX7 | Periosteal Reactions

Periosteal irritation occurs as a result of a wide variety of etiologies, ranging from fractures to malignant tumors. The radiographic appearance of the periosteum correlates to the aggressiveness and chronicity of the underlying lesion. Aggressive lesions (i.e., malignant bone tumors) disrupt the periosteum before bone deposition and periosteal consolidation can occur, resulting in a disrupted, spiculated, amorphous, or laminated appearance of the periosteum.

A less aggressive, benign appearance of the periosteum occurs when the underlying pathology is slowly progressive (i.e., benign bone tumors) and allows the periosteum to consolidate. Benign periosteal reaction is marked by a thick, wavy, and uniformly dense appearance. Although some benign processes may cause aggressive periosteal changes, aggressive lesions are rarely associated with a benign periosteal appearance. The periosteal reaction may be localized to a bone or appear generalized to a limb or the entire skeleton.

EX7a | Localized Periosteal Reactions

DISEASE	COMMENTS
Arthritis	Solid or laminated periosteal reaction associated with juvenile rheumatoid arthritis and Reiter's syndrome; periosteal response may appear localized or generalized
Benign bone tumor **(FIG. 7-64)**	Solid, thick (i.e., osteoid osteoma) or thin (i.e., aneurysmal bone cyst) periosteal reaction associated with benign bone lesion
Eosinophilic granuloma **(FIG. 7-65)** [p. 747]	Abnormal proliferation of histiocytes marked by osteolytic skull and long bone defects that exhibit a characteristic, beveled edge; solid or laminated periosteal reaction may be localized or generalized
Fracture	Traumatic or stress fractures; more generalized appearance occurs with battered child syndrome

Continued

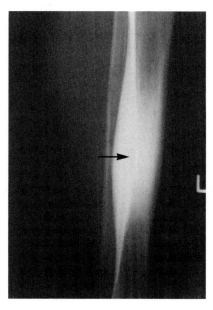

FIG. 7-64   Osteoid osteoma in the tibial diaphysis with surrounding sclerosis. New periosteal bone formation causes the localized increase in bone density. There is a subtle radiolucent nidus in the center of the sclerosis *(arrow)*. (Courtesy Joseph W. Howe, Sylmar, Calif.)

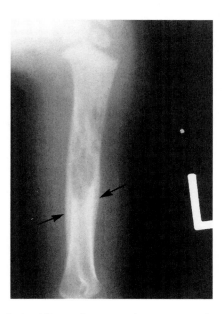

FIG. 7-65   Eosinophilic granuloma appearing as an aggressive diaphyseal lesion of the humerus with solid periosteal reaction along the medial and lateral cortices *(arrows)*.

DISEASE	**COMMENTS**
Infection (FIGS. 7-66 THROUGH 7-68)	Solid, thick, laminated periosteal reaction resulting from subperiosteal extension of infection; resulting development of involucrum surrounds central necrotic sequestrum of bone
Malignant bone tumor (FIGS. 7-69 AND 7-70)	Solid, laminated, spiculated, or amorphous appearance usually associated with either osteosarcoma or Ewing's sarcoma; multiple sites of involvement suggest leukemia or metastasis from neuroblastoma
Subperiosteal hemorrhage (FIG. 7-71)	Solid, thick, laminated periosteal reaction resulting from subperiosteal hemorrhage; it is related to trauma, hemophilia, or scurvy

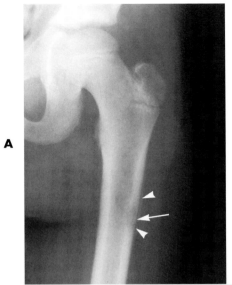

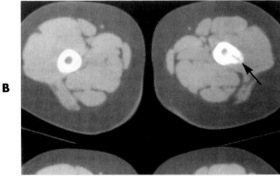

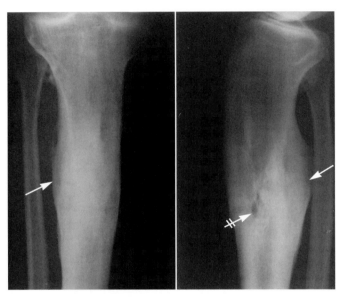

FIG. 7-66   Bone infection resulting in thick periostitis *(arrows)* and central radiolucent nidus *(crossed arrow).* (Courtesy Joseph W. Howe, Sylmar, Calif.)

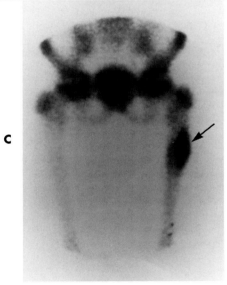

FIG. 7-67   Infection appearing with a focal region of the osteolysis **(A)** *(arrow)* with benign periosteal reaction (arrowheads). The infection demonstrates a cortical channel *(arrow)* on CT **(B)** and uptake on the radionuclide scan **(C)** *(arrows).* (Courtesy Joseph W. Howe, Sylmar, Calif.)

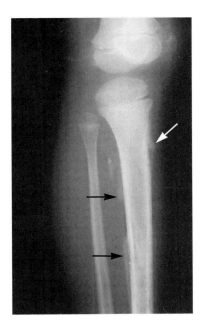

FIG. 7-68 Thick but aggressive periostitis (arrows) associated with infection or tumor in the proximal tibia.

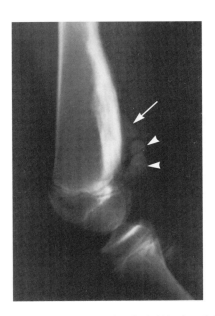

FIG. 7-69 Osteosarcoma producing localized thickening of the periosteum in the posterior distal femur (arrow). Posterior to the femur are several soft tissue masses comprising calcified osteoid material (arrowheads).

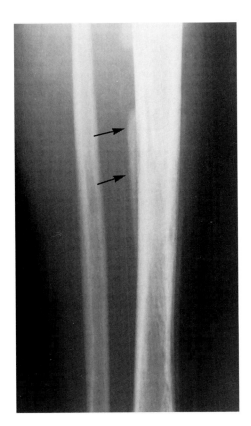

FIG. 7-70 Aggressive periostitis (arrows) associated with metastasis from neuroblastoma. (Courtesy Joseph W. Howe, Sylmar, Calif.)

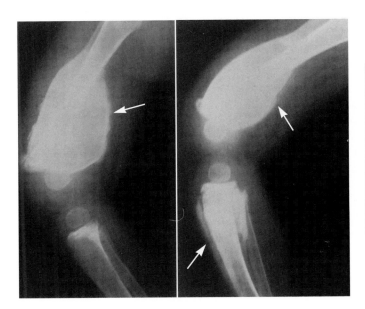

FIG. 7-71 Bilateral subperiosteal hemorrhage (arrows) in a patient with scurvy. (Courtesy Joseph W. Howe, Sylmar, Calif.)

EX7b | Generalized Periosteal Reactions

DISEASE	COMMENTS
Congenital syphilis **(FIG. 7-72)** [p. 609]	Acute or chronic infectious disease caused by *Treponema pallidum;* direct contact, usually through sexual intercourse, transmits the disease; congenital syphilis is acquired by the fetus in utero; generalized or localized diaphyseal and metaphyseal solid periosteal reaction, osteolysis, striped metaphyseal bands (radiolucent and dense), and hepatosplenomegaly are characteristic findings of congenital syphilis
Fluorosis **(FIG. 7-73)**	Chronic fluoride intoxication associated with osteophytosis, vertebral hyperostosis leading to increased radiodensity, and calcification of the paraspinal ligaments, vertebrae have increased radiodensity; fluorosis is marked in the innominates and lumbar spine; solid, symmetric periosteal reaction is most prominent in the tubular bones

Gaucher's disease [p. 744]	Genetic deficiency of glucocerebrosidase, presenting with clinical findings of hepatosplenomegaly, osteopenia, osteonecrosis, and focal osteolytic bone changes; biconcave vertebrae is a less common feature of the disease; long tubular bones may exhibit generalized solid periosteal reaction
Hypertrophic osteoarthropathy **(FIG. 7-74)** [p. 753]	Primary (e.g., pachydermoperiostosis or Touraine-Solente-Golé syndrome) or secondary (e.g., Pierre-Marie-Bamberger syndrome) disorder that presents clinically with digital clubbing, painful and swollen joints, and symmetrical undulated periosteal reaction; diaphyses of tubular bones are involved, most commonly the long bones of the arms and legs; the thickness of the periosteal reaction depends on the duration of the disease: the more chronic, the thicker the changes; secondary hypertrophic osteoarthropathy occurs in bronchogenic carcinoma (up to 10%), pulmonary abscess, pulmonary metastasis, Hodgkin's disease, cystic fibrosis, heart disease, and occasionally in other acute and chronic disorders; primary hypertrophic osteoarthropathy is less common; onset occurs during adolescence, causes thickened appearance of face and scalp, and may involve the epiphyses

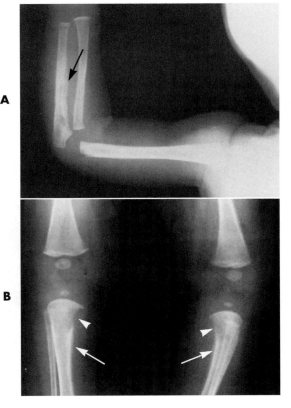

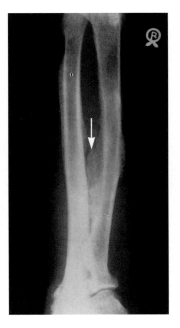

FIG. 7-72   Congenital syphilis producing a solid periosteal reaction of the ulna **(A)** *(arrow)* and tibia **(B)** *(arrows)*. Observe the characteristic bilateral destruction of the medial proximal tibia *(arrowheads)*, known as Wimberger's sign. (Courtesy Steven P. Brownstein, Springfield, NJ.)

FIG. 7-73   Thick periostitis along the diaphysis of the radius secondary to fluorosis *(arrow)*. (Courtesy Steven P. Brownstein, Springfield, NJ.)

Hypervitaminosis A [p. 731]	Condition resulting from the ingestion of an excessive amount of vitamin A; clinically alopecia, pruritus, dermatitis, and a yellow hue to the skin occur; solid periosteal reaction involves long tubular bones
Infantile cortical hyperostosis (Caffey's disease) **(FIG. 7-75)** [p. 754]	Rare disease marked by irritability, fever, swelling of the soft tissues, and palpable soft tissue masses over affected bones; periosteal new bone formation occurs over many bones, especially the mandible and clavicles and the shafts of long bones (usually ulna); although the periosteal reaction is usually generalized, a localized appearance can occur; usually present before 6 months of age, disappearing during childhood
Sickle cell disease [p. 604]	Disease characterized by altered shape and plasticity of red blood cells under low oxygen tension, causing vascular occlusion, infarct, and necrosis; predisposition to *Salmonella osteomyelitis;* generalized or localized, solid, thick, undulated periosteal reaction and osteosclerosis develop in response to diaphyseal bone infarct; dactylitis (hand-foot syndrome) occurs in children with sickle cell disease, marked by periosteal reaction and soft tissue swelling of the short tubular bones, mimicking osteomyelitis

Thyroid acropachy	Rare complication of hyperparathyroidism therapy; asymmetrical, thick, spiculated periosteal reaction occurs in the small tubular bones of the hands and, less commonly, the feet, with a predilection to the radial side; soft tissue swelling and digital clubbing occur; this can present at any age and has an equal sex incidence; patients are usually hypothyroid or euthyroid when symptoms arise
Tuberous sclerosis (Bourneville's disease)	Multisystem, neuroectodermal disorder, characterized by the triad of seizures, mental retardation, and skin nodules of the face; cerebral and retinal lesions and intracranial calcifications occur; multifocal areas of osteosclerosis are best seen in the skull and vertebrae; cortical thickening manifests in long, tubular bones; irregular solid metacarpal periosteal reaction occurs
Vascular stasis	Localized or generalized solid periosteal reaction; most often the long bones of the lower extremity are involved; vascular calcification and phleboliths may be present

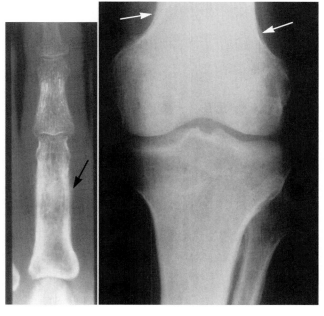

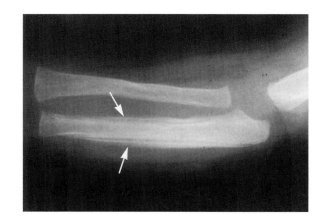

FIG. 7-74 Hypertrophic osteoarthropathy manifesting with periostitis of the small bones of the hand **(A)** *(arrow)* and in a different patient **(B)** manifesting as periostitis, seen as a thick, radiodense band parallel to the cortex in the distal femur *(arrows)*. (A, Courtesy Joseph W. Howe, Sylmar, Calif.; B, Courtesy Steven P. Brownstein, Springfield, NJ.)

FIG. 7-75 Infantile cortical hyperostosis presenting as thick periostitis along the ulna *(arrows)*. (Courtesy William E. Litterer, Elizabeth, NJ.)

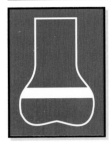

EX8 | Radiodense Metaphyseal Bands

Transverse radiodense metaphyseal bands describe zones of osteosclerosis across the metaphyses of long bones. The appearance may represent a normal variant of growth in children younger than 3 years of age. Other etiologies are described by the mnemonic *Heavy cretins shift scurrilously through rickety systems.* This mnemonic describes the following list of conditions: heavy metal poisoning, cretinism, syphilis, scurvy (congenital), rickets, and systemic illness (e.g., leukemia).

DISEASE	COMMENTS
Congenital syphilis [p. 609]	Acute or chronic infectious disease caused by *Treponema pallidum;* direct contact, usually through sexual intercourse, transmits this disease; congenital syphilis is acquired by the fetus in utero; generalized or localized diaphyseal and metaphyseal solid periosteal reaction, osteolysis, striped metaphyseal bands (dense and radiolucent), and hepatosplenomegaly are characteristic findings of congenital syphilis
Lead poisoning **(FIG. 7-76)** [p. 747]	Inhalation or ingestion of lead, causing wide metaphyses with dense transverse bands in the metaphyses of growing bones; multiple bands suggest repeat episodes of toxicity; physiologic bands may be differentiated by the involvement of other bones around the joint (i.e., fibula and tibia)
Leukemia [p. 603]	Proliferation of abnormal leukocytes within hemopoietic tissues and other organs; variety of types is based on cell type and duration from onset to death; leukemia of bone is typically acute lymphoblastic; skeletal manifestations include diffuse demineralization, osteolytic defects, smooth periosteal reaction, and radiolucent metaphyseal bands that become dense following chemotherapy
Normal variant	Dense metaphyseal band found in long bones of children younger than 3 years of age; alternatively multiple, fine, dense bands can occur, representing persistence of calcified cartilage (growth arrest lines)
Osteopetrosis (Albers-Schön-berg disease) [p. 411]	Hereditary failure of calcified cartilage resorption that interferes with the development of mature bone; the appearance is marked by sclerotic, fragile bones; vertebrae may appear "doubled" by smaller "endobones" within their bodies; well-defined transverse radiodense bands are characteristically found subjacent to the vertebral endplates and in the metaphyses of long bones
Rickets (healing) **(FIG. 7-77)** [p. 735]	Infantile or juvenile osteomalacia secondary to vitamin D deficiency, characterized clinically by irritability, listlessness, generalized muscle weakness; an overproduction and deficient calcification of osteoid tissue results in disturbances of bone growth with resulting deformity; fractures are common; epiphyses may appear indistinct with irregular and wide epiphyseal plates; with successful therapy the zone of provisional calcification is reinstated and radiographically visible as a dense metaphyseal band
Scurvy (Barlow's disease) **(FIG. 7-78)** [p. 738]	Defective osteogenesis secondary to abnormal collagen from vitamin C deficiency; onset occurs between 6 and 14 months of age; irritability, bleeding gums, tendency toward hemorrhage, and tenderness and weakness of lower limbs are clinical manifestations; epiphyses appear radiolucent with surrounding sclerotic rim (Wimberger's sign or ring epiphyses); dense metaphyseal band represents zone of provisional calcification, this zone may remain after healing
Trauma	Radiodense metaphyseal bands related to current fracture (particularly stress type), or remodeling residuum of past fracture

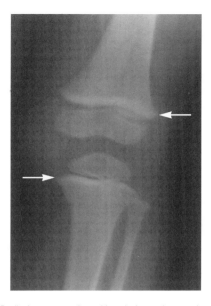

FIG. 7-76 Radiodense metaphyseal bands *(arrows)* secondary to lead intoxication. (Courtesy Joseph W. Howe, Sylmar, Calif.)

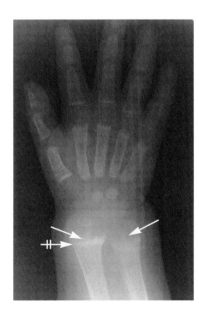

FIG. 7-77 Rickets demonstrating a widened, frayed ("paintbrush") appearance to the metaphyses *(arrows)* with indistinct epiphyses. A radiodense zone stretches across the metaphysis, indicating reconstitution of the provisional zone of calcification and the beginning stages of healing *(crossed arrow)*. (Courtesy Joseph W. Howe, Sylmar, Calif.)

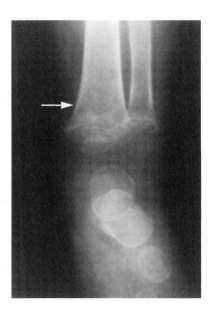

FIG. 7-78 Scurvy presenting with radiolucent metaphyseal bands *(arrow)* of the distal fibula and tibia representing disorganized osteoid material (Trümmerfeld zone). (Courtesy Joseph W. Howe, Sylmar, Calif.)

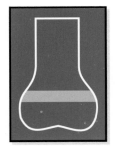

EX9 | Radiolucent Metaphyseal Bands

Radiolucent metaphyseal bands are zones of decreased bone density extending perpendicularly to the long axis of the bone. They are found at the ends of long bones. Their causes are nonspecific, representing disorganized bone growth, infection, trauma, and others.

DISEASE	COMMENTS
Congenital syphilis [p. 609]	Acute or chronic infectious disease caused by *Treponema pallidum;* direct contact, usually through sexual intercourse, transmits this disease; congenital syphilis is acquired by the fetus in utero; generalized or localized diaphyseal and metaphyseal solid periosteal reaction, osteolysis, striped metaphyseal bands (radiolucent and dense), and hepatosplenomegaly are characteristic findings of congenital syphilis
Leukemia [p. 603]	Proliferation of abnormal leukocytes within hemopoietic tissues and other organs; variety of types is based on cell type and duration from onset to death; leukemia of bone is typically acute lymphoblastic; skeletal manifestations include diffuse demineralization, osteolytic defects, smooth periosteal reaction, and radiolucent metaphyseal bands, which become dense following chemotherapy
Metastatic neuroblastoma	Highly malignant tumor of immature nerve cells arising in a retroperitoneal (usually adrenal) or mediastinal location; tumor usually develops before the age of 5 years; metastases to the liver, lungs, lymph nodes, cranial cavity, and skeleton are very common; skull metastasis are characteristic, appearing as wide sutures with bone spicules of the surrounding bone; extremity involvement resembles leukemia with radiolucent metaphyseal bands

Normal variant	Radiolucent metaphyseal bands seen as a normal variant in neonates
Scurvy (Barlow's disease) [p. 738]	Defective osteogenesis secondary to abnormal collagen from vitamin C deficiency, occuring between 6 to 14 months of age; irritability, bleeding gums, tendency toward hemorrhage, and tenderness and weakness of lower limbs are clinical manifestations; epiphyses appear radiolucent with surrounding sclerotic rim (Wimberger's sign or ring epiphyses); radiolucent metaphyseal bands (scorbutic or Trümmerfeld zone) represent disorganized osteoid
Systemic illness	Serious childhood illnesses may interfere with normal bone development and cause radiolucent metaphyseal bands
Trauma	Radiolucent metaphyseal band following traumatic fracture or battered child syndrome

Suggested Readings

Brant WE, Helms CA: *Fundamentals of diagnostic radiology,* Baltimore, 1994, Williams and Wilkins.

Burgener FA, Kormano M: *Differential diagnosis in conventional radiology,* ed 2, New York, 1991, Thieme Medical Publishers.

Chapman S and Nakielny R: *Aids to radiological differential diagnosis,* ed 3, Philadelphia, 1995, WB Saunders.

Dahnert W: *Radiology review manual,* Baltimore, 1991, Williams and Wilkins.

Eisenberg RL: *An atlas of differential diagnosis,* ed 2, Gaithersburg, 1992, Aspen.

Forrester DM, Brown JC, Nesson JW: *The radiology of joint disease,* ed 2, Philadelphia, 1978, WB Saunders.

Ravin CE, Cooper C, Leder RA: *Review of radiology,* Philadelphia, 1994, WB Saunders.

Reeder MM, Bradley WG: *Reeder and Felson's gamuts in radiology,* ed 3, New York, 1993, Springer-Verlag.

Weissleder R, Wittenberg J: *Primer of diagnostic imaging,* St Louis, 1994, Mosby.

General Skeletal Patterns

DENNIS M MARCHIORI

PART TWO Bone, Joints, and Soft Tissues

331

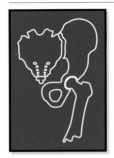

GN I | Acetabular Protrusion

Protrusio acetabuli exists if, in a frontal projection of the pelvis, the dome of the acetabulum extends medially beyond a line segment drawn from the pelvic border of the ilium to the medial border of the body of the ischium (Köhler's line). It occurs most frequently secondary to rheumatoid arthritis and Paget's disease, or as a primary anomaly (Otto pelvis).

DISEASE	COMMENTS
Bone softening **(FIG. 8-1)**	Bone deformity resulting from congenital (osteogenesis imperfecta) or acquired bone softening diseases (i.e., Paget's disease, rickets, osteomalacia, osteoporosis)
Inflammatory arthritides	Most commonly associated with advanced rheumatoid arthritis of the hip; associated findings include osteopenia, uniform loss of joint space, bilateral distribution, nonproliferative joint margins; less commonly associated with rheumatoid variants (i.e., ankylosing spondylitis, psoriatic arthritis, Reiter's syndrome, and inflammatory bowel disease)

Normal variant **(FIG. 8-2)**	May include medial protrusion of the femoral head in children
Osteoarthritis **(FIG. 8-3)** [p. 458]	Usually less-advanced degree of protrusion; patient manifests unilateral, proliferative joint changes, nonuniform reduction of joint space; this disease may be secondary to trauma, hemophilia, ochronosis, etc.
Otto pelvis **(FIG. 8-4)**	Primary protrusio acetabuli; Otto pelvis is usually bilateral and exhibits a female predominance
Miscellaneous disorders	Bone deformity resulting from posttraumatic remodeling, tumor, infection, etc.

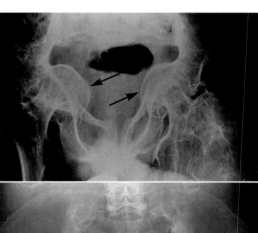

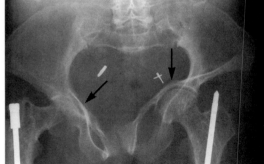

FIG. 8-1 Two cases of acetabular protrusion (*arrows*) developing in patients with osteogenesis imperfecta. (Courtesy Joseph W. Howe, Sylmar, Calif.)

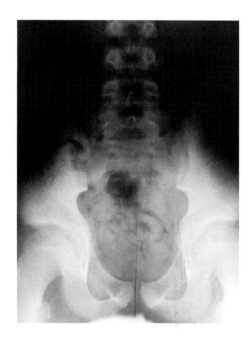

FIG. 8-2 Bilateral protrusio acetabuli presenting as a normal developmental variant. (Courtesy Lawrence J. Shell, Sandwich, Mass.)

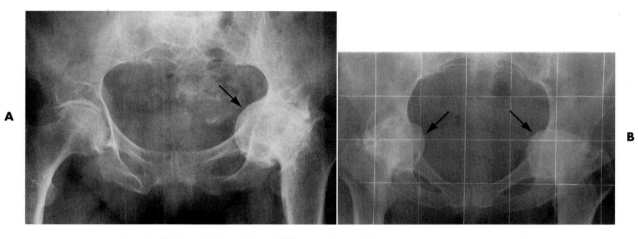

FIG. 8-3   Unilateral **(A)** and bilateral **(B)** protrusio acetabuli secondary to degeneration *(arrows)*.

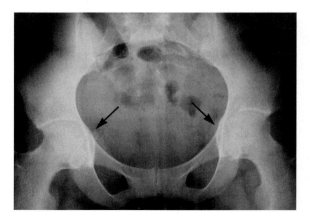

FIG. 8-4   Bilateral acetabular protrusion *(arrows)* of unknown origin (Otto pelvis).

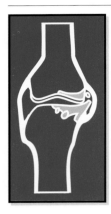

GN2 | Arthritides

Many disorders result in joint pathology. Arthritides are broadly divided into two groups: those affecting one joint and those affecting multiple joints (polyarthritis). Polyarthritis can be further divided into inflammatory, degenerative, and metabolic subcategories. Knowledge of the overall prevalence, skeletal target locations, and demography of those affected helps to narrow the long list of etiologies.

Types of arthritis occurring more commonly among men include ankylosing spondylitis, gout, hemophilia, ochronosis, and Reiter's syndrome. Common monoarticular arthritides include secondary osteoarthritis (i.e., trauma, avascular necrosis, mechanical stress), gout, and infection. Suppurative arthropathy and rheumatoid arthritis are commonly associated with surrounding osteoporosis. Behçet's syndrome, dermatomyositis, Jaccoud's arthritis, and Sjögren's syndrome characteristically produce transient arthritis, which resolves without residual bone deformity. Joint effusions are pronounced with gout, infection, hemorrhage, and rheumatoid arthritis.

DISEASE	COMMENTS
Acromegaly [p. 715]	Excess levels of growth hormone resulting from a pituitary eosinophilic adenoma that is overproducing somatotropin; this condition is marked by progressive enlargement of the hands, feet, head, jaw, and abdominal organs, in addition to enlarged vertebrae with posterior scalloping and new bone growth along the anterior body margins; arthritis is targeted to the metacarpophalangeal and hip joints
Ankylosing spondylitis **(FIG. 8-5)** [p. 428]	Seronegative spondyloarthropathy characterized by arthritis targeted to the sacroiliac joints and spine; bilateral, symmetric, thin intervertebral connections, known as *syndesmophytes,* are a prominent feature, representing ossification of the outermost lamellae of the annulus fibrosis; collectively, multiple levels produce a "bamboo spine" appearance; in addition, the anterior body margins appear straight or square

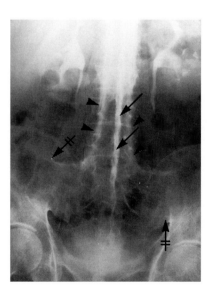

FIG. 8-5   Advanced ankylosing spondylitis presenting with fusion of the sacroiliac joints *(crossed arrows),* interspinous ligament ossification *(arrows),* and facet capsule ossification *("railroad track" sign)(arrowheads).* (Courtesy Joseph W. Howe, Sylmar, Calif.)

Chondrocal-cinosis
(FIG. 8-6)
[p. 453]

Radiographically evident cartilage calcification relating to calcium pyrophosphate dihydrate (CPPD) crystal, or other crystal, deposition disease; chondrocalcinosis is associated with arthritis targeted to the wrist, knees, elbows, hips, and shoulders

Erosive osteoarthritis
[p. 458]

Seronegative inflammatory variant of osteoarthritis particularly common in 40- to 50-year-old females; proliferative joint changes, central joint erosions, and painful, swollen joints occur; arthritis is targeted to the distal interphalangeal joints of the hands

Gout
(FIG. 8-7)
[p. 456]

Primarily a disorder of purine metabolism with crystal deposits causing synovial pannus, arthropathy, and large, well-defined, bony marginal erosions; infrequently patients demonstrate sacroiliitis and systemic dystrophic calcifications; typical sites include first metatarsophalangeal joint, insertion of the Achilles tendon, and olecranon bursa

Continued

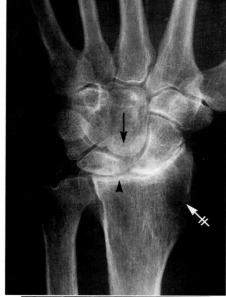

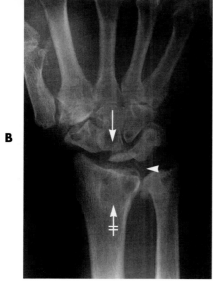

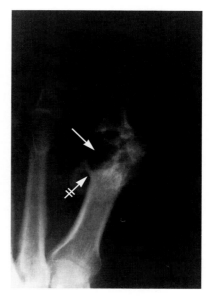

FIG. 8-7 Gout involving the first metatarsal phalangeal joints with erosions *(arrow)* and a thin, overhanging margin *(crossed arrow)*. No osteoporosis is noted. (Courtesy Joseph W. Howe, Sylmar, Calif.)

FIG. 8-6 Calcium pyrophosphate dihydrate (CPPD) deposition disease of the wrist in two different patients. Both radiographs (**A** and **B**) exhibit *ScaphoLunate* dissociation (greater than 2 to 3 mm) with *Advanced Collapse (SLAC deformity)* of the capitate toward the radius *(arrows)*, degenerative subchondral cysts *(crossed arrows)*, and chondrocalcinosis *(arrowheads)*. Additionally, **B** exhibits a radiodense appearance of the lunate consistent with lunate avascular necrosis (Keinbock's disease). (*B,* Courtesy Joseph W. Howe, Sylmar, Calif.)

DISEASE	COMMENTS		
Hemochromatosis (FIG. 8-8) [p. 600]	Disorder of iron metabolism resulting from excessive absorption of ingested or injected iron; disorder is accompanied by cirrhosis of the liver, diabetes, bronze skin pigmentation, generalized osteoporosis, and arthropathy secondary to iron deposits in synovium; the arthritis is targeted to the metacarpophalangeal and interphalangeal joints of the hands; females are protected by menstruation	**Hemophilia** [p. 601]	Inherited X-linked defect of blood coagulation, marked by a permanent tendency toward hemorrhages; hemarthrosis is associated with red, swollen joints, precocious degenerative arthritis, and an enlargement of the epiphyses; knees, ankles, and elbows are most commonly affected; rarely, expansile bone lesions (hemophilic pseudotumors) develop; arthritis is targeted to the knees, elbows, and ankles

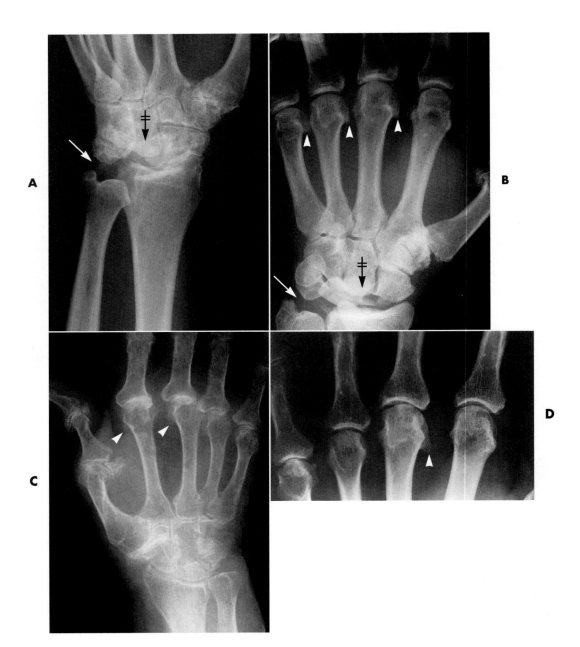

FIG. 8-8   Hemochromatosis of the hand demonstrating chondrocalcinosis of the triangular fibrocartilage (**A** and **B**) *(arrows)*, a degree of scapholunate dissociation with advance collapse (SLAC) of the capitate (**A** and **B**) *(crossed arrows)*, and prominent beaklike osteophytes from the distal metacarpals (**C** and **D**) *(arrowheads)*. (*A* and *B*, Courtesy Jack C. Avalos, Davenport, Iowa; *C*, Courtesy Robert C. Tatum, Davenport, Iowa; *D*, Courtesy Joseph W. Howe, Sylmar, Calif.)

| Infection (FIGS. 8-9 THROUGH 8-12) [p. 616] | Suppurative or tuberculosis infections marked by soft tissue swelling, juxtaarticular osteoporosis, joint space narrowing, and bone destruction; radiographic findings follow clinical presentation of pain and soft-tissue swelling by 8 to 10 days; infection may affect any joint, most commonly the hip, knee, or spine | Jaccoud's arthritis [p. 434] | Rare, nondestructive arthritis marked by reversible joint derangements, soft tissue swelling, and pain, often following episode of rheumatic fever; Jaccoud's arthritis resembles rheumatoid arthritis and affects the joints of the hands and feet |

Continued

A   **B**   **C**

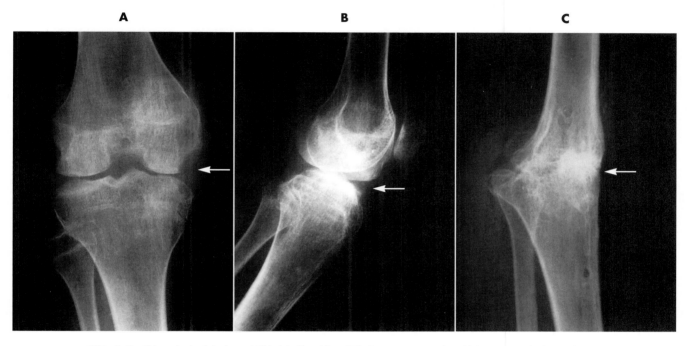

FIG. 8-9 Tuberculosis of the knee. Initial plain films (**A** and **B**) demonstrate a reduced joint space and a focus of osteolysis *(arrows)*. The lateral knee projection (**C**) taken 14 months later demonstrates ankylosis *(arrow)*. (Courtesy Steven P. Brownstein, Springfield, NJ.)

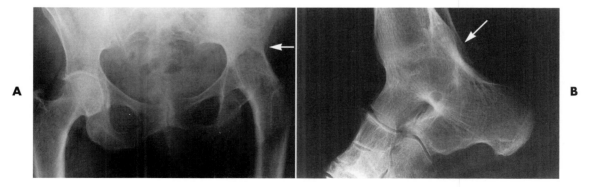

FIG. 8-10 Healed infections resulting in fusion of the left hip joint (**A**) *(arrow)* and tibiotalar joint (**B**) *(arrow)*. (Courtesy Joseph W. Howe, Sylmar, Calif.)

PART TWO Bone, Joints, and Soft Tissues

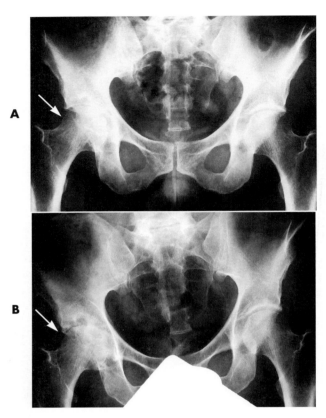

FIG. 8-11   Infection of the right hip marked by loss of joint space on the initial **(A)** and 5-month postfilm **(B)** *(arrows)*.

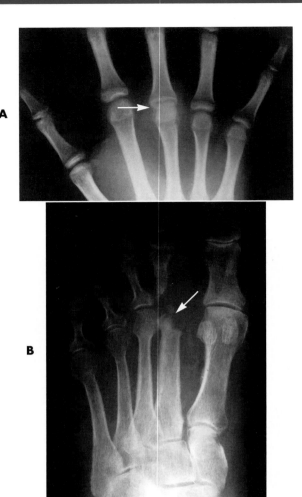

FIG. 8-12   Joint infections of the third metacarpophalangeal joint **(A)** and second metatarsophalangeal joint **(B).** All are marked by decreased joint spaces *(arrows)* and bone destruction often involving both sides of the joint. (A, Courtesy Joseph W. Howe, Sylmar, Calif.)

DISEASE	COMMENTS
Multicentric reticulohistiocytosis **(FIG. 8-13)**	Rare disorder marked by cutaneous and joint deposits of histiocytes containing glycolipids; the interphalangeal joints of the hands and feet manifest well-defined marginal erosions; shortening of the fingers often results
Neuropathic (Charcot's) joints [p. 483]	Destructive arthropathy secondary to altered joint sensory innervation, resulting in either unchecked repetitive injury resulting from absence of pain or loss of trophic influences of innervations with local hyperemia and bone resorption; atrophic and hypertrophic varieties exist; hypertrophic changes include premature and advanced degeneration, marked by dislocation, destruction, intraarticular loose bodies (debris), and disorganization; this type of arthropathy is common in the knee, hip, ankle, and lumbar spine; etiologies include diabetes, syphilis, syringomyelia, and alcoholism
Ochronosis	Inherited disorder of excessive homogentisic acid production and subsequent accumulation within connective tissues; the spine is affected by multiple levels of intervertebral disc calcification and massive osteophytosis and ankylosis, especially in the elderly; osteoporosis occurs in adjacent vertebrae; advanced degenerative joint disease may develop in the large proximal joints of the extremities (i.e., hip, knee, and shoulder)

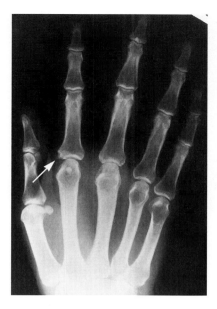

FIG. 8-13 Multicentric reticulohistiocytosis appearing with a well-defined marginal erosion of the proximal phalanges of the second digit *(arrow)*. (Courtesy Joseph W. Howe, Sylmar, Calif.)

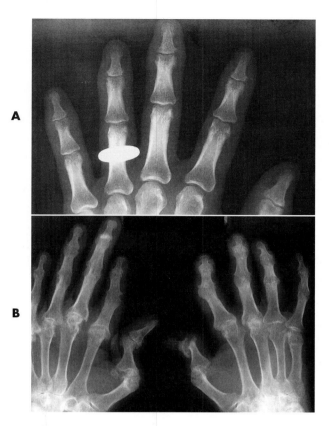

FIG. 8-14 Early **(A)** and late **(B)** psoriatic arthropathy of the hands. The changes are marked by lack of osteoporosis, soft tissue swelling, central articular erosions, proliferative marginal changes, and by a pattern of distribution that is more prominent across all joints in the same digit (ray pattern) than in the same joint across different digits. A wedding band is noted incidentally on the fourth digit **(A)**. (Courtesy Steven P. Brownstein, Springfield, NJ.)

Osteoarthritis [p. 458]	Very common, noninflammatory, degenerative joint disease with clinical presentation of pain, stiffness, crepitus; characteristic radiographic features include bilateral asymmetrical distribution, nonuniform reduction of joint space, sclerosis of subarticular bone, marginal osteophytosis, joint malalignment, subchondral cysts, and others; primary osteoarthritis is seen with increasing age and mostly affects weight-bearing joints (i.e., knee, hips, spine) and hands (i.e., distal interphalangeal, first tarsophalangeal, and first carpometacarpal joints); degeneration also occurs secondary to trauma, osteonecrosis, etc.
Pigmented villonodular synovitis (PVNS) [p. 767]	Chronic condition marked by diffuse hyperplastic outgrowths of a joint's synovial membrane; osteolytic appearance results from pressure erosion of adjoining bone; wide age range is possible, although PVNS usually occurs before 40 years of age; no juxtaarticular osteoporosis or loss of joint space exists; the most common locations are the knee, hip, ankle, elbow, and shoulder
Psoriatic arthritis (FIGS. 8-14 AND 8-15) [p. 436]	Arthritis occurring in fewer than 7% of patients with psoriasis; patients experience symptoms in the carpal, interphalangeal, and less commonly the sacroiliac joints; the digits are marked by nail pitting, swelling of the soft tissues, and erosions of the distal tufts, relating a tapered appearance of the distal phalanges

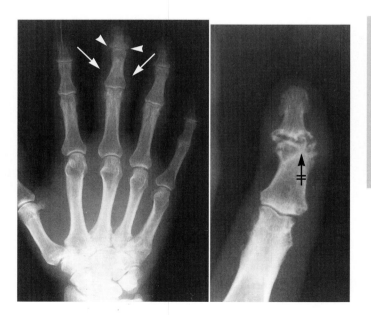

FIG. 8-15 Psoriatic arthropathy of the hands in different patients who exhibit soft tissue hypertrophy *(arrows)*, central erosions *(crossed arrow)*, and proliferative changes on the joint margins *(arrowheads)*. (Courtesy Joseph W. Howe, Sylmar, Calif.)

Continued

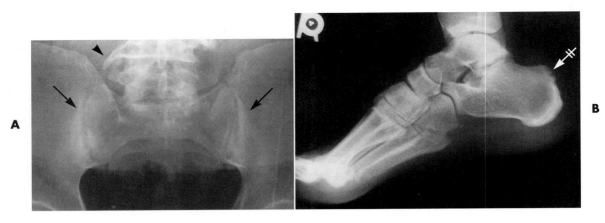

FIG. 8-16 Reiter's disease, presenting with **(A)** bilateral, slightly asymmetrical sacroiliitis *(arrows)*, syndesmophytes *(arrowhead)*, and erosions at the insertion of the calcaneal (Achilles) tendon *(crossed arrow)* in a different patient **(B).** *(A, Courtesy Joseph W. Howe, Sylmar, Calif.; B, Courtesy Arthur W. Holmes, Foley, Ala.)*

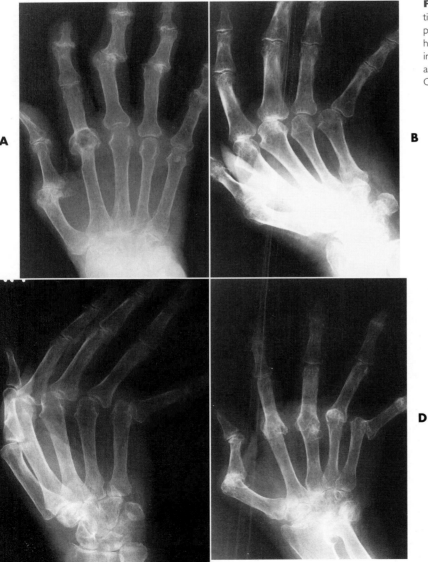

FIG. 8-17 Rheumatoid arthritis of the hand in four patients. Each patient (**A** through **D**) exhibits intercarpal, metacarpophalangeal, and interphalangeal involvement. Within each hand the distribution of the arthritis is symmetrical. The involved joint spaces are symmetrically reduced, and juxta-articular osteoporosis and misalignment are present. *(A and B, Courtesy Joseph W. Howe, Sylmar, Calif.)*

DISEASE

COMMENTS

Reiter's syndrome (FIG. 8-16) [p. 440]	Describes triad of urethritis, conjunctivitis, and polyarthritis; males, especially those between the ages of 20 and 40 years, contract this condition much more frequently than females; arthritis is targeted to the sacroiliac joints and lower extremities, especially the foot; erosions at the calcaneal insertions of the plantar and Achilles tendons are characteristic
Rheumatoid arthritis, adult (FIGS. 8-17 AND 8-18) [p. 442]	Systemic connective tissue disorder that targets synovial tissues; juxtaarticular osteoporosis, soft tissue nodules, symmetrical reduction of joint space, marginal erosions, subchondral cysts, symmetrical distribution, and rarely joint ankylosis are characteristic; most commonly the hands and feet are involved, particularly the intercarpal, metacarpophalangeal, and proximal interphalangeal joints, and counterparts in the foot; rheumatoid arthritis occurs most commonly in middle-age females
Rheumatoid arthritis, juvenile (FIG. 8-19) [p. 435]	Chronic arthritis beginning in childhood (before 16 years of age), manifesting as one of several clinical types; monoarticular distribution is more common than occurs in adult rheumatoid arthritis; target areas include cervical spine, hands, feet, and knee; joint fusion, periostitis, and growth abnormalities are characteristic
Sarcoidosis (FIG. 8-20) [p. 885]	Systemic granulomatous disease most pronounced in the lungs; less commonly the disease involves arthritis of the hand with coarsened trabeculae and well-defined osteolytic lesions

Continued

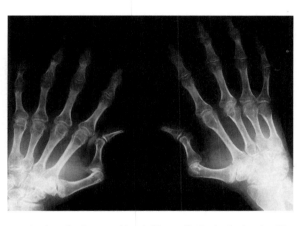

FIG. 8-19 Juvenile rheumatoid arthritis manifesting in the hands with osteoporosis, underdevelopment of the small tubular bones, and arthritis targeted to the wrist. (Courtesy Jack C. Avalos, Davenport, Iowa.)

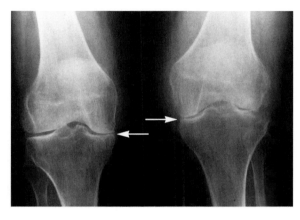

FIG. 8-18 Rheumatoid arthritis of the knees marked by nonproliferative loss of joint space *(arrows)*. (Courtesy Steven P. Brownstein, Springfield, NJ.)

FIG. 8-20 Sarcoidosis causing multiple well-defined osteolytic defects in the middle phalanx *(arrow)* with soft tissue swelling *(arrowhead)*. (Courtesy Steven P. Brownstein, Springfield, NJ.)

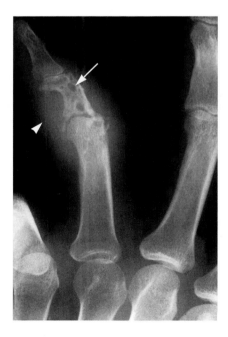

PART TWO Bone, Joints, and Soft Tissues

DISEASE	**COMMENTS**
Scleroderma (progressive systemic sclerosis) [p. 450]	Disease of small vessels and organ fibrosis; symptoms include atrophy and systemic dystrophic calcifications of the soft tissues of the hands and feet with resorption of distal phalanges; limited soft-tissue swelling, juxtaarticular osteoporosis, marginal erosions, and other similar findings to rheumatoid arthritis occurring in the hands
Systemic lupus erythematosus (FIG. 8-21) [p. 452]	Systemic inflammatory connective tissue disease marked by fever, weakness, erythematous skin lesions on the face, and arthritis most visible in the hands as reversible subluxations and dislocations of the digits, predominantly the metacarpophalangeal joints (MCPs)
Miscellaneous conditions	Transient and episodic arthritis associated with Sjögren's syndrome, dermatomyositis, relapsing polychondritis, Behçet's syndrome, etc.; patterns of involvement vary

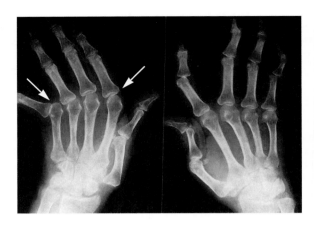

FIG. 8-21 Systemic lupus erythematosus of the hands, marked by multiple bilateral, reversible subluxations of the hands *(arrows)*. (Courtesy Steven P. Brownstein, Springfield, NJ.)

GN3 | Dwarfism

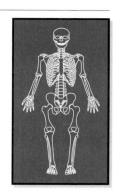

Dwarfism is the condition of being undersized. This condition may result from a variety of disorders affecting the growth and development of the tissues. Skeletal dysplasias result in dwarfism because of abnormal tissue development. Skeletal dysplasias are classified according to whether they predominantly affect the proximal or distal long bones of the limb. Rhizomelic (*rhiza-,* meaning "root" and *–melia,* meaning "limb") dysplasias affect the femur and humerus more predominantly than the tibia or radius. Mesomelic (*meso-,* meaning "middle") dysplasia describes shortening of the distal long bones (tibia, ulna, and radius), or middle of the limb in relation to the proximal limb (humerus or femur). Acromelic (*acro-,* meaning "extreme") dysplasia is a growth disturbance involving the distal portions of the limbs (hands and feet). Micromelic dysplasia involves both the proximal and distal portions of the extremity. Short spine dysplasias cause dwarfism without involving the limbs.

DISEASE	COMMENTS
Achondroplasia **(FIG. 8-22)** [p. 385]	Rhizomelic dysplasia resulting from congenital defect of enchondral bone formation; characteristics include rounded lumbar "bullet-nosed" vertebrae, lumbar kyphosis, posterior scalloping of the vertebrae, increased intervertebral disc height, flattened vertebral bodies, and narrowed spinal canal; the pelvis may appear hypoplastic; milder forms of the disease may occur
Asphyxiating thoracic dysplasia (Jeune's syndrome) **(FIG. 8-23)**	Mild micromelic dysplasia marked by small thorax; small, flared iliac bones; and shortening of the humerus, femur (rhizomelia), and distal phalanges (acromelia)

DISEASE	COMMENTS
Chondrodysplasia punctata [p. 387]	Autosomal dominant (nonrhizomelic) and recessive (rhizomelic) dysplasia; the nonrhizomelic form (Conradi-Hünermann disease) either way demonstrates tracheal underdevelopment and mild stippled epiphyses; the rarer rhizomelic form is characterized by marked limb shortening, severe punctate calcifications (stippled) epiphyses, metaphyseal splaying, and congenital cataracts

Continued

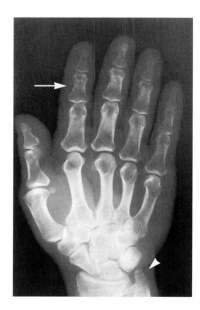

FIG. 8-22   Achondroplasia presenting as short tubular bones *(arrow)* with elongation of the ulnar styloid *(arrowhead).* (Courtesy Joseph W. Howe, Sylmar, Calif.)

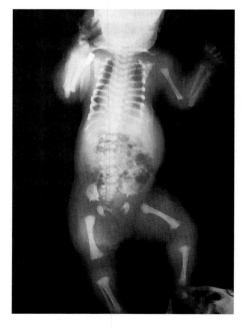

FIG. 8-23   Dwarfism related to asphyxiating thoracic dysplasia (Jeune's syndrome). (Courtesy Steven P. Brownstein, Springfield, NJ.)

DISEASE	COMMENTS
Cretinism [p. 725]	Hypothyroid dwarfism from delayed appearance and maturation of skeletal growth centers; stunted mental development occurs; disease appears during the first years of life and results from thymic agenesis or inadequate maternal intake of iodine during pregnancy; wormian bones and poorly developed sinuses are characteristic; sail-like or tonguelike vertebrae and kyphosis at the thoracolumbar junction are common; changes may regress in adulthood
Diastrophic dysplasia [p. 393]	Short spine dysplasia, characterized by scoliosis, hypoplastic first metacarpal "hitchhiker thumb," abnormal interphalangeal joints, cleft palate, and clubbed feet
Dyschondrosteosis (Leri-Weill syndrome) **(FIG. 8-24)**	Mesomelic dysplasia with long-bone shortening of the upper limbs, producing bilateral Madelung's deformities, which are marked by short radii, dorsal ulnar subluxations, and carpal wedging between the radius and ulna; elbow and distal radius dislocations result
Mucopolysaccharidosis [p. 401]	Group of lysosomal storage diseases marked by a common disorder in mucopolysaccharide metabolism, evidenced by various mucopolysaccharides excreted in the urine; these substances collect in connective tissue, resulting in bone, cartilage, and connective tissue defects; platyspondyly with dwarfism, kyphosis, and alterations in the appearance of the vertebrae are characteristic; mucopolysaccharidosis I (Hurler's syndrome) is associated with oval, posteriorly scalloped, anterior-inferiorly beaked vertebrae; mucopolysaccharidosis IV (Morquio syndrome) is associated with flattened, anterior-centrally beaked vertebrae
Osteogenesis imperfecta [p. 409]	Connective tissue disorder of immature collagen, marked by micromelic dwarfism, which is characterized by bone fragility and deformity, abnormal teeth, ligament laxity, and otosclerosis; it occurs with variable severity
Spondyloepiphyseal dysplasia	Short spine dysplasia presenting as dominant and recessive forms, marked by both platyspondyly and short trunk dwarfism
Thanatophoric dysplasia	Severe micromelic dysplasia, marked by large head with prominent frontal bone, platyspondyly, short ribs, and curved long bones with bulbous ends ("telephone receiver"-long bones).
Turner's syndrome [p. 419]	Chromosomal anomaly (XO syndrome), marked by absent secondary sex characteristics and presenting clinically with dwarfism, webbed neck, mental deficiency, valgus of elbows, pigeon chest, widely spaced nipples, infantile sexual development, and amenorrhea

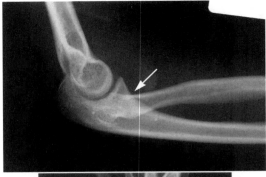
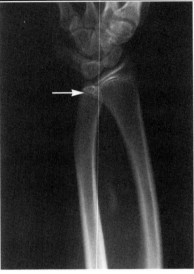

FIG. 8-24   Dyschondrosteosis exhibiting a short, bowed radius, short ulna, and dislocations (arrows). (Courtesy Joseph W. Howe, Sylmar, Calif.)

GN4 | Generalized Osteoporosis

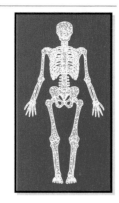

Osteoporosis is a disease of bones marked by decreased bone mass and density. The remaining bone is normal in calcification and histology. The resulting skeletal weakness increases the risk of fracture, particularly of vertebrae, wrists, and hips. Laboratory values are normal. Osteoporosis may occur as a primary, age-related phenomenon or appear secondary to an underlying condition.

Several noninvasive methods are available to evaluate bone density. These vary widely in cost, availability, and radiation dose. Dual-energy x-ray absorptiometry (DXA) offers probably the greatest reliability, safety, precision, and convenience. Standard radiographs of the spine are the most widely available measure of osteoporosis; however, they are insensitive to early changes.

DISEASE	COMMENTS
Anemia (FIG. 8-25)	Sickle cell anemia, thalassemia, spherocytosis, severe iron deficiency, all causing thin cortices secondary to bone marrow hyperplasia
Collagen disease	Osteoporosis possibly resulting from lupus erythematosus, scleroderma, dermatomyositis, rheumatoid arthritis, and ankylosing spondylitis
Congenital syndrome (FIGS. 8-26 AND 8-27)	Homocystinuria, mucopolysaccharidosis, osteogenesis imperfecta, pseudohypoparathyroidism, pseudopseudohypoparathyroidism, Ehlers-Danlos syndrome, and others
Drug-induced (iatrogenic)	Large doses of steroids, heparin, vitamin A, and various chemotherapies

Continued

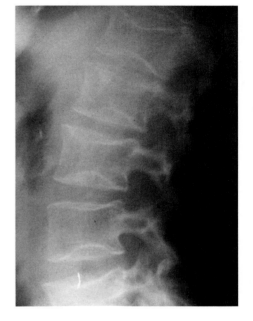

FIG. 8-26 Homocystinuria presenting with generalized osteoporosis of the lumbar spine with secondary concave endplate deformity.

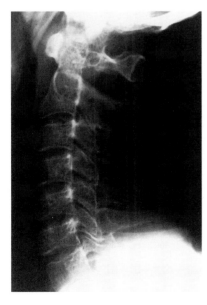

FIG. 8-25 Lateral cervical spine projection demonstrating the coarse trabecular and osteopenic pattern consistent with thalassemia (Cooley's anemia). (Courtesy Joseph W. Howe, Sylmar, Calif.)

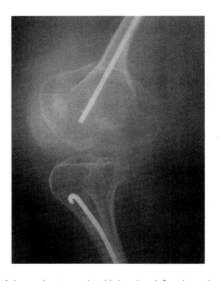

FIG. 8-27 Advanced osteopenia with bowing deformity and gracile cortices secondary to osteogenesis imperfecta. (Courtesy Joseph W. Howe, Sylmar, Calif.)

DISEASE	COMMENTS
Endocrine disorders (FIG. 8-28)	Adrenocortical abnormality (i.e., Cushing's syndrome, Addison disease), hypogonadism (i.e., menopause, oophorectomy, prepubertal castration), thyroid abnormalities (i.e., hyperthyroidism, hypothyroidism, cretinism), pancreatic abnormality (i.e., cystic fibrosis), and pituitary abnormality (i.e., acromegaly, hypopituitarism)
Hemochromatosis [p. 600]	Disorder of iron metabolism resulting from excessive absorption of ingested or injected iron; characteristics include cirrhosis of the liver, diabetes, bronze skin pigmentation, arthropathy secondary to iron deposits in synovium, and generalized osteoporosis; females are protected by menstruation
Hemophilia [p. 601]	Inherited X-linked defect of blood coagulation marked by a permanent tendency toward hemorrhages; hemarthrosis is associated with red, swollen joints, precocious degeneration, and an enlargement of the epiphyses; knees, ankles, and elbows are most commonly affected; rarely, expansile bone lesions (hemophilic pseudotumors) develop; advanced osteoporosis occurs

DISEASE	COMMENTS
Homocystinuria [p. 396]	Disorder of homocystine excretion in urine, collagen structure, ligamentous laxity, mental retardation, downward dislocation of lens, sparse blond hair, thromboembolic episodes, and osteoporosis
Idiopathic juvenile osteoporosis	Rare, usually transient, onset of osteoporosis and pain in children
Mastocytosis (systemic) [p. 754]	Abnormal proliferation of mast cells in multiple organ systems, usually seen in adults; skeletal involvement includes scattered, fairly well-defined sclerotic foci occasionally with diffuse involvement; regions of bone rarefaction are typically also present; diffuse osteopenia similar to osteoporosis is possible
Neoplastic disorders	Common manifestation of multiple myeloma, metastatic bone disease, and acute leukemia secondary to neoplastic bone marrow infiltrates
Neuromuscular diseases and dystrophies (FIG. 8-29)	Reduced muscular tone and lack of weight-bearing posture associated with cerebral palsy, spinal cord disorder, muscular dystrophy, and immobilization

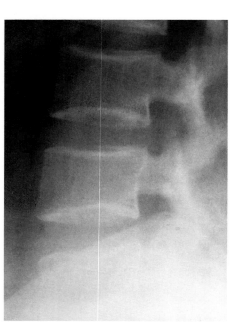

FIG. 8-28   Osteoporosis secondary to Cushing's disease.

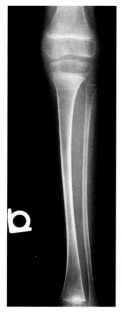

FIG. 8-29   Cerebral palsy patient with osteoporosis of the lower extremities marked by thin cortex and decreased radiopacity.

Nutritional disorders	Protein deficiency (i.e., malnutrition, nephrosis, diabetes mellitus), vitamin C deficiency (i.e., scurvy), and intestinal malabsorption (i.e., sprue, scleroderma, Crohn's disease)
Ochronosis	Inherited disorder of excessive homogentisic acid production and subsequent accumulation within connective tissues; the spine is affected by multiple levels of intervertebral disc calcification and massive osteophytosis and ankylosis, especially in the elderly; osteoporosis occurs in adjacent vertebrae; advanced degenerative joint disease may develop in the large proximal joints of the extremities (i.e., hip, knee, and shoulder)
Renal disease	Nephrosis, tubular acidosis, oxalosis, renal osteodystrophy
Senile (primary) osteoporosis (FIG. 8-30) [p. 727]	Very common age-related decrease in bone quantity; trabecular bone is resorbed more rapidly than cortical bone; the spine, proximal femur, and distal radius are the most advanced sites; complicating fractures are common causes of morbidity; women and whites are most commonly affected; rate of bone loss may be modified by therapy

Continued

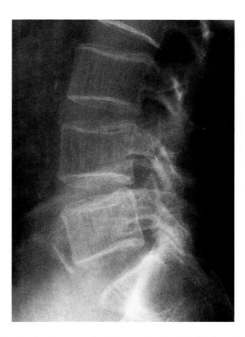

FIG. 8-30   Senile osteoporosis with prominent vertical trabecular pattern. (Courtesy Steven P. Brownstein, Springfield, NJ.)

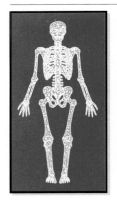

GN5 | Generalized Osteosclerosis

Generalized osteosclerosis describes skeletal-wide changes of increased bone density. Generalized osteosclerosis incorporates the causes of other patterns of increased bone density of the spine and extremities.

Disorders that more characteristically cause focal osteosclerotic lesions include bone islands, bone infarcts, avascular necrosis, enchondroma (in a long bone), fibrous dysplasia, healed fractures, healing nonossifying fibroma, osteitis condensans ilii or pubi, osteomas, osteomyelitis, osteosarcomas, and Paget's disease.

DISEASE	COMMENTS
Fibrous dysplasia (polyostotic) **(FIG. 8-31)** [p. 651]	Disturbance of bone maintenance, in which bone is replaced by abnormal proliferation of fibrous tissue; the disturbance may involve one (monostotic) or multiple (polyostotic) bones; most common locations are femur, ribs, tibia, craniofacial bones, and pelvis; lesion should not be painful, unless dysplasia is widespread with bowing deformity and pathological fractures; lesions of the medullary cavity may have radiolucent, "ground glass," or radiodense appearance
Fluorosis **(FIG. 8-32)**	Chronic fluoride intoxication associated with enthesopathies, osteophytosis, vertebral hyperostosis with calcification of the paraspinal ligaments; solid, symmetric periosteal reaction is most prominent in the tubular bones; generalized osteosclerosis is more prominent in the axial skeleton
Heavy metal intoxication **(FIG. 8-33)** [p. 747]	Osteosclerosis related to lead, phosphorus, bismuth, or cadmium poisoning; similar findings may occur following thorotrast injections (thorium dioxide in dextran)
Hyperphosphatasia **(FIG. 8-34)**	Also known as *juvenile Paget's disease;* this rare disorder of infants and children results from chronically elevated alkaline phosphatase levels; characteristics are generalized cortical thickening, bone deformity, short stature, and increased bone density
Mastocytosis (systemic) [p. 754]	Abnormal proliferation of mast cells in multiple organ systems; primarily adults are affected; skeletal involvement includes scattered, fairly well-defined sclerotic foci occasionally with diffuse involvement; regions of bone rarefaction are typically also present
Myelofibrosis	Extensive and progressive bone marrow fibrosis of unknown etiology occurring in hematopoietic bones (vertebrae, pelvis, ribs, and long bones); involved areas appear first osteoporotic, later becoming patchy, then homogeneously dense

Continued

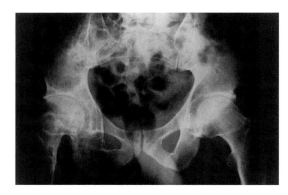

FIG. 8-31   Multiple cystic bone lesions of the pelvis resulting from polyostotic fibrous dyplasia. (Courtesy Joseph W. Howe, Sylmar, Calif.)

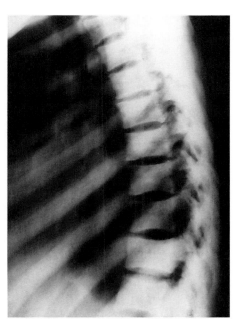

FIG. 8-32 Increased radiodense appearance of the thoracic vertebrae and ribs resulting from fluorosis. (Courtesy Steven P. Brownstein, Springfield, NJ.)

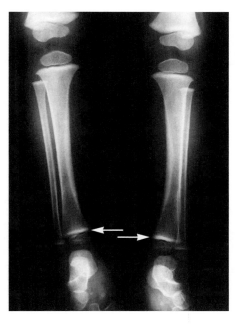

FIG. 8-33 Radiodense appearance of the tibia and fibula with metaphyseal band *(arrows)* secondary to lead intoxication. (Courtesy Steven P. Brownstein, Springfield, NJ.)

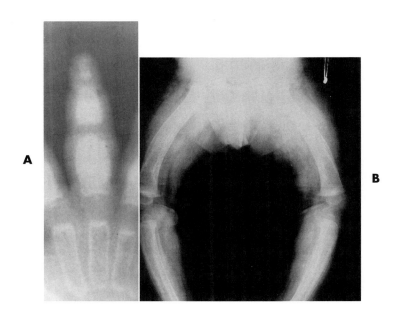

FIG. 8-34 **A,** Hyperphosphatasia causing osteosclerosis of a child's finger. **B,** A second child demonstrating increased radiodensity and thickened cortices in the lower extremities. (*A,* Courtesy Joseph W. Howe, Sylmar, Calif.; *B,* Courtesy Steven P. Brownstein, Springfield, NJ.)

DISEASE	COMMENTS
Osteoblastic metastasis (FIGS. 8-35 THROUGH 8-37) [p. 687]	Especially from breast and prostate primary lesions; typically patients are older than 40 years of age, often with a history of known malignancy; generalized osteosclerosis is less common than a presentation of multiple focal areas of osteosclerosis
Osteopetrosis (Albers-Schön-berg disease) (FIG. 8-38) [p. 411]	Hereditary failure of calcified cartilage resorption, which interferes with the development of mature bone; the appearance is marked by sclerotic, fragile bones; vertebrae may appear "doubled" by smaller "endobones" within their bodies; well-defined, transverse radiodense bands are characteristically found subjacent to the endplates
Paget's disease (FIG. 8-39) [p. 761]	Chronic skeletal disease of aberrant bone remodeling; one or more bones are affected; characteristics include bone enlargement, softening, and rarely sarcomatous changes; the lumbar spine is one of the most common areas of involvement; the enlarged and thickened vertebral cortices appear as radiodense bands around the perimeter of the vertebra (known as "picture frame"); less commonly it appears predominantly as a solitary lytic or sclerotic lesion of the vertebral body; generalized osteosclerosis may be a feature of widespread skeletal involvement

Pyknodysostosis (FIG. 8-40) [p. 413]	Hereditary sclerosing dysplasia of bone marked by short stature, dense bones (often with transverse fractures), hypoplastic angle of the mandible, wormian bones, delayed closure of the fontanelles, and hypoplasia of the terminal phalanges

Continued

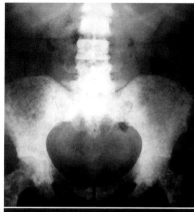

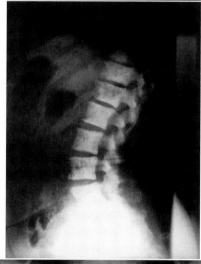

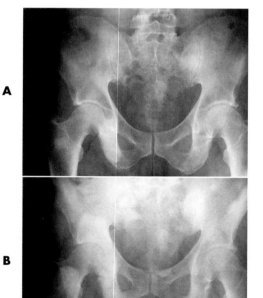

FIG. 8-35 **A,** Osteoblastic metastasis most predominantly involving the right ischium and intertrochanteric region of the femur. **B,** After approximately 1 year, increased metastasis occurs in all regions. (Courtesy Joseph W. Howe, Sylmar, Calif.)

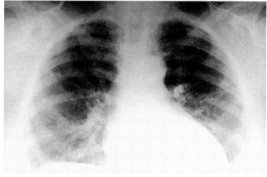

FIG. 8-36 Widely disseminated osteoblastic metastasis appearing as multiple focal radiopacities in the lumbar spine, pelvis, and chest.

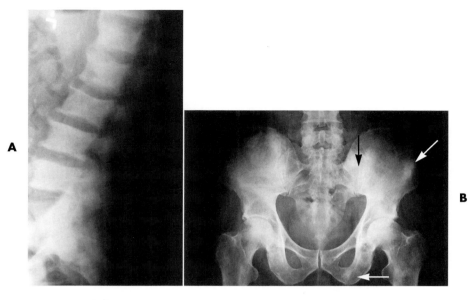

FIG. 8-37 **A,** Osteoblastic metastasis causing marked increase in vertebral density. **B,** Another patient with multiple radiodense regions of the pelvis secondary to osteoblastic metastasis *(arrows).* (Courtesy Ian D. McLean, Davenport, Iowa.)

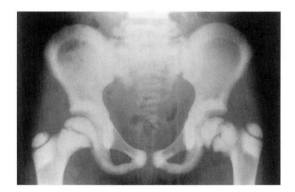

FIG. 8-38 Osteopetrosis appearing as generalized osteosclerosis of the pelvis, femora, and lumbar spine. (Courtesy Joseph W. Howe, Sylmar, Calif.)

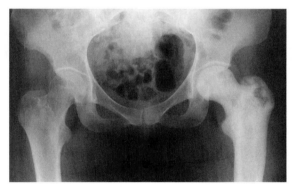

FIG. 8-39 The left femur is larger and more radiodense than the right femur secondary to Paget's disease. (Courtesy Joseph W. Howe, Sylmar, Calif.)

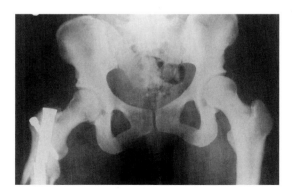

FIG. 8-40 Generalized osteosclerosis is seen in this radiograph of the pelvis of a patient with pyknodysostosis. (Courtesy Joseph W. Howe, Sylmar, Calif.)

PART TWO Bone, Joints, and Soft Tissues

DISEASE	COMMENTS
Renal osteodystrophy	Secondary to renal glomerular disease; vertebral changes occur with horizontal sclerotic bands ("rugger-jersey") and less commonly a biconcave appearance
Tuberous sclerosis (Bourneville disease) **(FIG. 8-41)**	Multisystem, neuroectodermal disorder characterized by the triad of seizures, mental retardation, and skin nodules of the face; cerebral and retinal lesions result, as well as intracranial calcifications, multifocal areas of osteosclerosis (best seen in the skull and vertebrae), cortical thickening in long, tubular bones, and irregular solid metacarpal periosteal reaction

DISEASE	COMMENTS
Sickle cell disease [p. 604]	Occurs almost exclusively in blacks, characterized by altered shape and plasticity of red blood cells under low oxygen tension, causing vascular occlusion, infarct, and necrosis; patient is predisposed to *Salmonella* osteomyelitis; generalized or localized, solid, thick, undulated periosteal reaction and osteosclerosis develop in response to diaphyseal bone infarct; dactylitis (hand-foot syndrome) occurs in children with sickle cell disease, marked by periosteal reaction and soft tissue swelling of the short tubular bones mimicking osteomyelitis

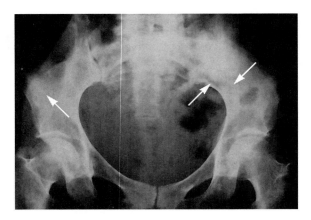

FIG. 8-41   Radiograph of a patient with tuberous sclerosis, which demonstrates multiple regions of increased bone density scattered throughout the pelvis (*arrows*).

GN6 | Polyostotic Bone Lesions

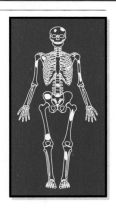

Imaging studies that indicate the presence of multiple lesions substantially narrow the differential list of conditions causing a bone lesion. The skeletal location and patient age will further narrow the list. Bone islands, fibrocytic lesions (i.e., fibrous dyplasia, fibrous cortical defect/nonossifying fibroma), and metastases represent some of the more common conditions listed in the following table.

DISEASE	COMMENTS
Anemias **(FIG. 8-42)**	Multiple osseous lesions associated with hemolytic anemias, including sickle cell disease, thalassemia, and hereditary spherocytosis
Enchondromatosis (Ollier's disease) **(FIG. 8-43)** [p. 644]	Childhood presentation of multiple benign cystic cartilage lesions most often in the small bones of the hands and feet; stippled matrix calcification is typical; 30% of cases exhibit malignant transformation; Ollier's disease with multiple soft tissue hemangiomas is termed *Maffucci's syndrome* and may have an even higher malignant transformation rate
Eosinophilic granuloma [p. 747]	Proliferation of eosinophils seen most commonly in children and young adults; spine involvement occurs in less than 10%; this condition may appear with advanced body collapse (vertebra plana) possibly at multiple levels; long bone involvement typically occurs in the diaphysis; patients are almost exclusively younger than 30 years of age; solitary or multiple lesions may occur
Fibrous cortical defect/nonossifying fibroma [p. 648]	Very common, benign, asymptomatic cystic bone lesions seen in patients younger than 30 years of age; a thin sclerotic border without matrix calcification marks this defect; the lower extremities, particularly around the knee, are commonly affected; multiple defects/fibromas are possible
Fibrous dyplasia (polyostotic) [p. 651]	Disturbance of bone maintenance in which bone is replaced by abnormal proliferation of fibrous tissue; this condition may involve one (monostotic) or multiple (polyostotic) bones; the matrix often has a characteristic "ground glass" radiodensity; lesions may be surrounded by a thick rind of bone sclerosis; most common locations are femur, ribs, tibia, craniofacial bones, and pelvis; lesion should not be painful
Fractures	Traumatic or stress fractures occurring at all ages; often seen in infants and children who are victims of battered child syndrome
Hemangiomas [p. 658]	Common congenital proliferation of vascular endothelium leading to a benign osteolytic appearance; capillary (usually in the spine) and cavernous (usually in the calvarium) types occur; multiple lesions may be present
Hemophilia [p. 601]	Inherited X-linked defect of blood coagulation, marked by a permanent tendency toward hemorrhages; hemarthrosis is associated with red, swollen joints, precocious degeneration, and an enlargement of the epiphyses; knees, ankles, and elbows are most commonly affected; rarely, expansile bone lesions (hemophilic pseudotumors) develop; advanced osteoporosis occurs

Continued

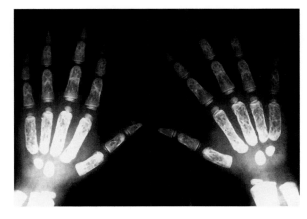

FIG. 8-42 Bilateral thin cortices and prominent coarsened trabecular pattern characteristic of thalassemia. (Courtesy Steven P. Brownstein, Springfield, NJ.)

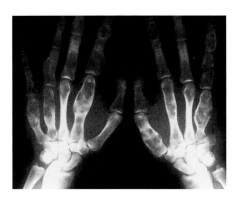

FIG. 8-43 Bilateral cystic bone lesions, characteristic of multiple enchondromatosis or Ollier's disease.

PART TWO Bone, Joints, and Soft Tissues

A   **B**   **C**

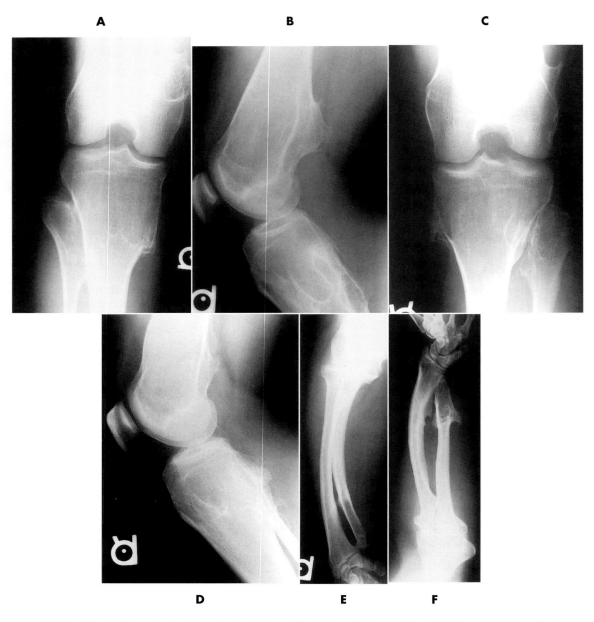

D   **E**   **F**

FIG. 8-44   Multiple osteochondromas leading to bone deformity about the knees bilaterally (**A** through **D**). This patient also exhibits the characteristic bayonet deformity of the forearms (**E** and **F**).

DISEASE	COMMENTS
Hereditary multiple exostosis (HME) **(FIG. 8-44)** [p. 663]	Describes the inherited condition of multiple osteochondromas involving growth deformity; the hips, knees, and forearms are most frequently involved; patients are typically younger than 20 years of age
Hydatid (*Echinococcus*) disease [p. 979]	Cysts that may be formed in bone (usually formed in the liver) by the larval stage of *Echinococcus;* cysts appear as slow-growing, destructive lesions surrounded by sclerotic borders; multiple lesions may appear; this occurs in endemic geographic areas
Hyperparathyroidism [p. 718]	Overproduction of parathyroid glands resulting from primary or secondary causes; the disease is marked by osteopenia, osteosclerosis, bone resorption, and soft tissue and vascular calcification; vertebrae have characteristic homogeneous radiodense bands traversing horizontally at each end of the vertebrae ("rugger-jersey" spine); subchondral bone resorption occurs, particularly at the radial aspects of the middle phalanges of the second and third digits; one or more osteolytic or sclerotic cystic bone lesions (brown tumors) may be present
Infantile cortical hyperostosis (Caffey's disease) [p. 754]	Rare disease marked by irritability, fever, swelling of the soft tissues, and palpable soft tissue masses over affected bones; periosteal new bone formation occurs over many bones, especially the mandible and clavicles and the shafts of long bones (usually the ulna); although the periosteal reaction is usually generalized, a localized appearance can occur; this condition is usually present before 6 months of age and disappears during childhood; periosteal reaction may also be localized
Infection **(FIG. 8-45)**	May occur at practically any location during any age; if found in a subarticular location, the joint is often involved with effusion; soft tissue mass and central bone sequestrum are often present; appearance varies from cystic to sclerotic; single or multiple lesions may occur
Leukemia [p. 603]	Proliferation of abnormal leukocytes within hemopoietic tissues and other organs; variety of types is based on cell type and duration from onset to death; leukemia of bone is typically acute lymphoblastic; skeletal manifestations include diffuse demineralization, osteolytic defects, smooth periosteal reaction, and radiolucent metaphyseal bands, which become dense following chemotherapy; leukemia occurs in infants and children
Lymphoma [p. 685]	Primary and secondary (systemic non-Hodgkin's lymphoma and Hodgkin's disease) lymphoma of bone, appearing as permeative radiolucent lesions of the lower extremities, pelvis, and spine; lymphoma occurs over wide range of ages
Mastocytosis (systemic) [p. 754]	Abnormal proliferation of mast cells in multiple organ systems; most patients are adult age; skeletal involvement includes scattered, fairly well-defined sclerotic foci occasionally with diffuse involvement; regions of bone rarefaction are typically also present

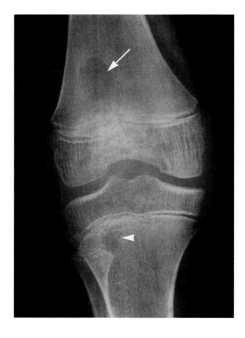

FIG. 8-45 Brodie's abscess infection noted in the distal femur *(arrow)* with a second lesion noted in the proximal tibia *(arrowhead)*. (Courtesy Steven P. Brownstein, Springfield, NJ.)

DISEASE	**COMMENTS**

Metastases (FIGS. 8-46 AND 8-47) [p. 687]

Common to the spine, rarely involves the skeleton distal to the elbows or knees (acral metastasis); metastasis typically appears as a polyostotic, moth-eaten pattern of osteolytic bone destruction with poorly defined zones of transition; it alternatively presents as predominantly mixed or purely blastic patterns; periosteal reaction and soft tissue masses are typically small or absent; this condition usually occurs in patients over the age of 40 years; neuroblastoma, retinoblastoma, rhabdomyosarcoma, and Ewing's tumor are common causes of metastasis among infants and children

Multiple myeloma (FIG. 8-48) [p. 700]

Malignant proliferation of plasma cells occurring predominantly in the red marrow of various bones; the skull, vertebral bodies, ribs, and proximal humerus and femurs are most commonly involved; single or multiple osteolytic lesions simulate metastatic disease, without tendency to involve vertebral arch, as is demonstrated by metastasis; osteopenia and solitary or multiple-level vertebral collapse simulate osteoporosis; multiple myeloma rarely occurs before 30 years of age

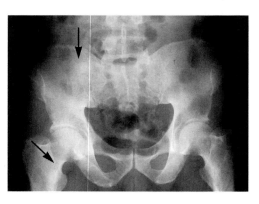

FIG. 8-46   Multiple radiodense regions of the femora, lumbar vertebrae, and pelvis secondary to osteoblastic metastasis *(arrows)*. (Courtesy Steven P. Brownstein, Springfield, NJ.)

A   **B**   **C**

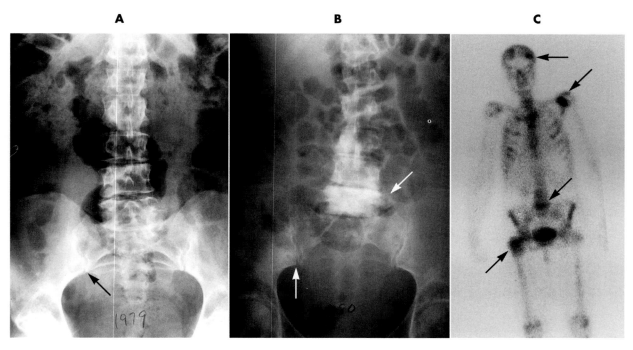

FIG. 8-47   **A,** Initial radiograph demonstrating slight osteosclerosis of the medial right ilium *(arrow)*. **B,** One year later L5 vertebral osteosclerosis is also noted *(arrows)*. **C,** Radionuclide bone scan performed around the time of the second radiograph reveals further metastatic involvement of the skull, ribs, and extremities *(arrows)*. (Courtesy Steven P. Brownstein, Springfield, NJ.)

Neurofibromatosis (von Recklinghausen's disease) [p. 755]	Congenital disturbance of mesodermal and neuroectodermal tissue development, appearing clinically with cutaneous markings, bone deformity, and neurofibromas; spinal changes include posterior vertebral scalloping, enlarged intervertebral foramina, kyphoscoliosis, and anteriorly wedged vertebrae
Osteonecrosis [p. 591]	Multiple areas of bone and marrow necrosis related to trauma, sickle cell disease, alcoholism, corticosteriods, and others; this disease appears as one or more regions of altered density and structure of bone
Paget's disease [p. 761]	Chronic skeletal disease of aberrant bone remodeling, involving one or more bones; characteristics include bone enlargement, softening, and rarely sarcomatous changes; the lumbar spine is one of the most common areas of involvement; the enlarged and thickened vertebral cortices appear as radiodense bands around the perimeter of the vertebra (similar to a picture frame); less commonly it appears as a solitary lytic or sclerotic lesion of the vertebral body; generalized osteosclerosis may be a feature of widespread skeletal involvement
Subchondral cysts	Related to arthritic or synovial disorder (osteoarthritis, gout, calcium pyrophosphate deposition disease, rheumatoid arthritis, hemophilia, intraosseous ganglion, amyloidosis, and avascular necrosis); this solitary or multiple, well-defined cyst is located in the epiphysis subjacent to the articular cortex; usually occurs in adults
Syphilis [p. 609]	Acute or chronic infectious disease caused by *Treponema pallidum;* direct contact transmits this disease, usually through sexual intercourse; congenital syphilis is acquired by the fetus *in utero;* generalized or localized diaphyseal and metaphyseal solid periosteal reaction, osteolysis, striped metaphyseal bands (lucent and dense), and hepatosplenomegaly are characteristic findings of congenital syphilis; acquired syphilis is marked by ill-defined osteolytic lesions in the skull, spine, and long bones secondary to gumma formation; both congenital and acquired types are marked by multiple foci of osteomyelitis

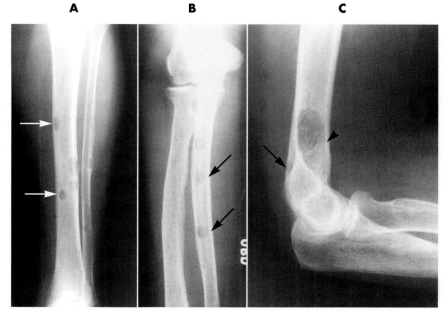

FIG. 8-48   Multiple myeloma involving the tibia **(A)**, fibula **(A)**, radius **(B)**, and humerus **(C)** with osteolytic lesions of consistent size and appearance *(arrows).* The larger and more central radiolucent defect of the distal humerus **(C,** *arrowhead)* represents the pseudocyst appearance of the epicondyle and does not represent an osteolytic bone lesion. (Courtesy Joseph W. Howe, Sylmar, Calif.).

PART TWO   Bone, Joints, and Soft Tissues

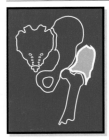

GN7 | Soft Tissue Calcification and Ossification

Soft tissue calcification describes a process in which tissue becomes hardened by deposition of calcium salts, which normally occurs only in bone and teeth. Soft tissue calcification can be classified as dystrophic, metastatic, and idiopathic.

Dystrophic calcification occurs in devitalized tissue as a result of tissue damage, degeneration, or necrosis. Associated conditions include Ehlers-Danlos syndrome, arteriosclerosis obliterans, and crystal deposition disease. Some authors describe age-related dystrophic calcification as physiologic calcification (i.e., costal cartilages).

Metastatic calcification occurs as a result of abnormal serum calcium or phosphorus levels in trophic tissues. Conditions associated with metastatic calcifications include hyperparathyroidism, selected neoplasms, milk-alkali syndrome, hypervitaminosis D, and tumoral calcinosis. Idiopathic calcinosis is unrelated to degeneration or serum calcium and phosphorus levels. Associated conditions include calcinosis universalis and calcinosis circumscripta.

Calcification is termed *ossification* if the calcified structure appears as a bone with cortex and possibly trabeculae. Nearly all disorders that cause calcification may secondarily ossify. Vascular wall calcification is a common finding in the large arteries of the abdomen and pelvis. Etiologies of vascular calcifications include arteriosclerosis, diabetes, hemangiomas, hyperparathyroidism, Mönckeberg's medial wall sclerosis, and thrombus.

Phleboliths represent dystrophic calcification of thrombi within a vein (about 0.5 cm in diameter). Phleboliths are very common, usually homogeneously dense, and particularly common in the perirectal veins of the lower pelvis.

Lymph node calcifications, usually resulting from tuberculosis or histoplasmosis infection, appear as thin curvilinear ("eggshell") segments or mottled dense nodules in characteristic locations (i.e., cervical chain, axillary).

GN7a | Calcification

DISEASE	COMMENTS
Calcific bursitis and tendinitis **(FIGS. 8-49 AND 8-50)**	Dystrophic calcification following degenerative, inflammatory, tumorous, or necrotic processes in tendons and bursae, often resulting in pain and limitation of joint motion; this condition is common in the supraspinatus tendon, subacromial and trochanteric bursa

Continued

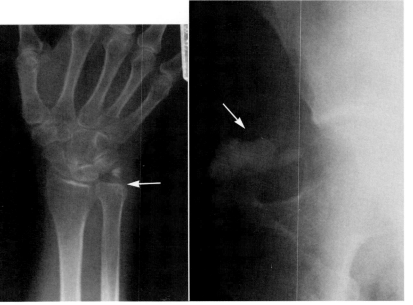

A

B

FIG. 8-49 Calcification *(arrows)* in the triangular fibrocartilage **(A)** and supratrochanteric bursae **(B).** (A, Courtesy Joseph W. Howe, Sylmar, Calif.)

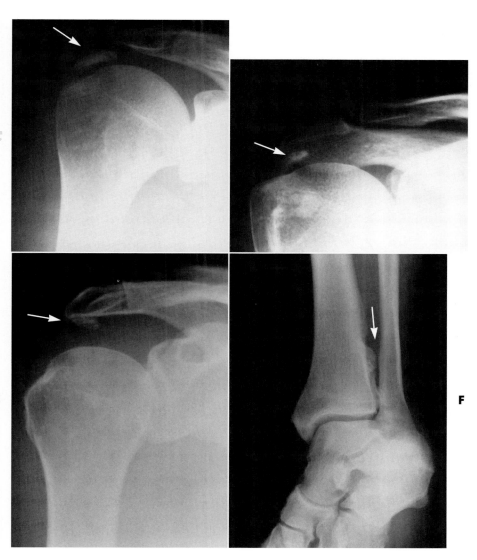

FIG. 8-49—cont'd Calcification *(arrows)* in the supraspinatus tendons (**C** through **E**) and interosseous ligament **(F).** The calcification represents postinflammatory dystrophic hydroxyapatite depositions (HADD), and signifies degeneration.

D

F

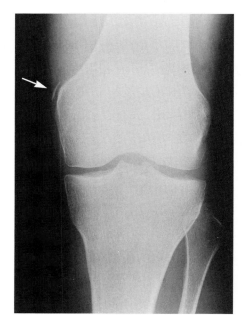

FIG. 8-50 Dystrophic calcification of the medial collateral ligament of the knee (Pellegrini-Stieda disease) *(arrow).*

DISEASE	COMMENTS
Chondrocalcinosis **(FIG. 8-51)** [p. 453]	Radiographically evident cartilage calcification relating to calcium pyrophosphate dihydrate (CPPD) or other crystal deposition disease; it may lead to symptoms of joint pain and advanced arthropathy
Dermatomyositis **(FIG. 8-52)** [p. 743]	Progressive disorder of muscular weakness and atrophy, occurring in children and adults; characteristics include linear and confluent systemic dystrophic soft tissue calcifications
Fracture	Localized dystrophic soft tissue calcifications occurring in damaged tissues and regions of hemorrhage
Gout **(FIG. 8-53)** [p. 456]	Disorder of purine metabolism with crystal deposits causing synovial pannus, arthropathy, and large, well-defined bony marginal erosions; infrequent sacroiliitis and systemic dystrophic calcifications occur; classic sites include the first metatarsophalangeal joint, insertion of the Achilles tendon, and the olecranon bursa
Hyperparathyroidism [p. 718]	Overproduction of parathyroid glands resulting from primary or secondary causes; the disease is marked by osteopenia, osteosclerosis, bone resorption, and widespread metastatic soft tissue and vascular calcification; vertebrae appear osteopenic with characteristic homogeneous, radiodense bands traversing horizontally at each end of the vertebrae ("rugger-jersey" spine); bone resorption is located predominantly at the radial aspect of the middle phalanges of the second and third digits
Hypervitaminosis D [p. 732]	Condition resulting from the ingestion of an excessive amount of vitamin D; symptoms include nausea, anorexia, drowsiness, headaches, polyuria, and polydypsia; bone deossification (parathormone-like effects) and extensive periarticular metastatic soft tissue calcification are characteristic

Continued

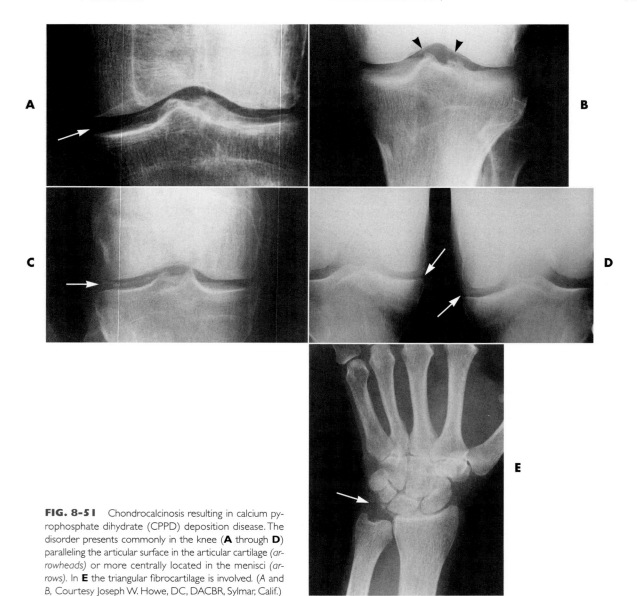

FIG. 8-51   Chondrocalcinosis resulting in calcium pyrophosphate dihydrate (CPPD) deposition disease. The disorder presents commonly in the knee (**A** through **D**) paralleling the articular surface in the articular cartilage *(arrowheads)* or more centrally located in the menisci *(arrows)*. In **E** the triangular fibrocartilage is involved. (*A* and *B*, Courtesy Joseph W. Howe, DC, DACBR, Sylmar, Calif.)

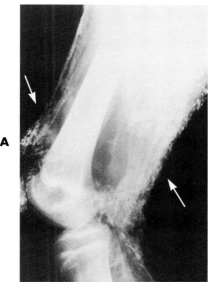

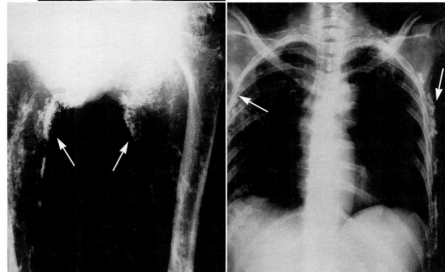

FIG. 8-52 Dermatomyositis of the knee **(A),** thighs **(B),** and chest **(C)** in different patients. All demonstrate linear cutaneous calcifications characteristic of the disease *(arrows)*. (*A,* Courtesy Joseph W. Howe, Sylmar, Calif.; *B* and *C,* Courtesy Steven P. Brownstein, Springfield, NJ.)

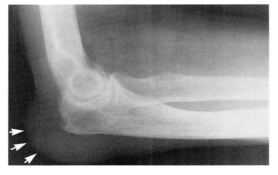

FIG. 8-53 Gout presenting with soft tissue masses about the elbow *(arrows)*. (Courtesy Joseph W. Howe, Sylmar, Calif.)

DISEASE	COMMENTS
Idiopathic	Nondystrophic, nonmetastatic etiologies
Injection granuloma	Localized postinflammatory dystrophic focus of soft tissue calcification following injection (i.e., bismuth, antibiotics, insulin, quinine) or inoculation (i.e., BCG vaccine); this disease is most commonly seen in the buttocks
Parasites (FIG. 8-54)	Systemic dystrophic calcifications of various configurations occurring secondary to parasitic infections (i.e., cysticercosis, guinea worm, trichinosis)
Scleroderma (progressive systemic sclerosis) (FIGS. 8-55 AND 8-56) [p. 450]	Disease of small vessels and organ fibrosis; atrophy and calcifications of the soft tissues of the hands and feet occur with resorption of distal phalanges
Soft tissue tumors (FIG. 8-57)	Benign (i.e., leiomyoma, lipoma, fibroma, hemangioma) and malignant (i.e., leiomyosarcoma, liposarcoma, fibrosarcoma) calcified soft tissue masses; synovial sarcomas (synoviomas) are aggressive malignant tumors of the bursa, joint capsule, or tendon
Tumoral calcinosis (FIGS. 8-58 AND 8-59)	Large, progressively enlarging, nodular, juxtaarticular soft tissue calcifications of unknown etiology, common in the hips, shoulders, wrists, and ankles; primarily otherwise healthy young individuals, age 5 to 25 years, are affected; disease is more common among blacks; this condition tends to recur following surgical removal

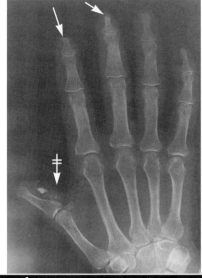

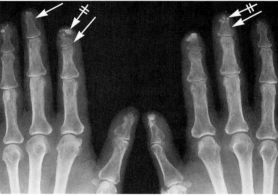

FIG. 8-55   Two cases of scleroderma with a characteristic presentation of acroosteolysis (arrows) and soft tissue calcifications (crossed arrows). (Top, Courtesy Joseph W. Howe, Sylmar, Calif.; bottom, courtesy Steven P. Brownstein, Springfield, NJ.)

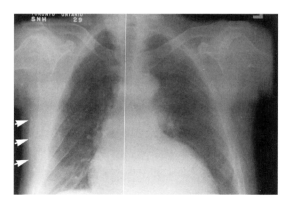

FIG. 8-54   Posteroanterior chest projection demonstrating multiple small foci of calcification in the cutaneous tissues (arrows) secondary to cysticercosis. (Courtesy Joseph W. Howe, Sylmar, Calif.)

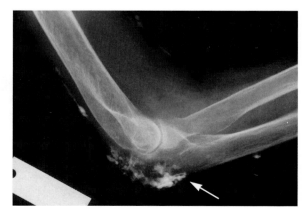

FIG. 8-56   Scleroderma with soft tissue calcification around the elbow (arrow). (Courtesy Steven P. Brownstein, Springfield, NJ.)

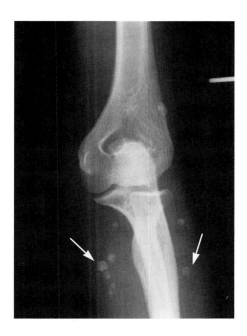

FIG. 8-57 Phleboliths *(arrows)* of a soft tissue hemangioma in the proximal forearm. (Courtesy Steven P. Brownstein, Springfield, NJ.)

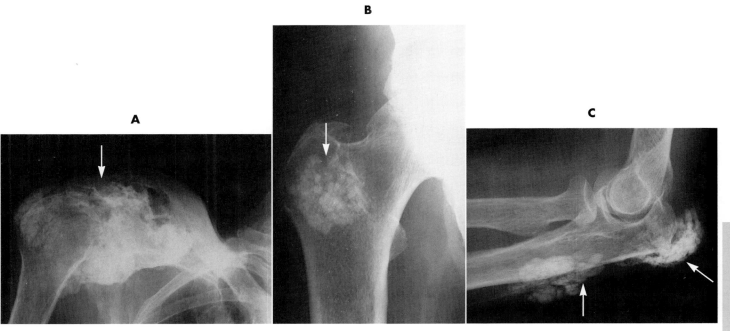

B

A

C

FIG. 8-58 Tumoral calcinosis of the shoulder **(A),** hip **(B),** and elbow **(C)** *(arrows).* (Courtesy Jack C. Avalos, Davenport, Iowa.)

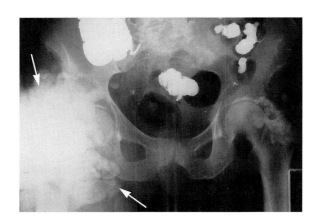

FIG. 8-59 Large, radiodense, soft tissue masses of tumoral calcinosis *(arrows).* (Courtesy Steven P. Brownstein, Springfield, NJ.)

GN7b | Ossification

DISEASE	COMMENTS
Burns	Severely burned and damaged tissue may ossify.
Degenerative	Intraarticular ossification of degenerative debris usually related to trauma
Myositis ossificans [p. 576]	Self-limiting disorder of soft tissue metaplasia to bone usually related to trauma; in early stage, it may be difficult to distinguish from primary bone tumor; a systemic, inherited, progressive form also exists
Osteosarcoma [p. 704]	Extraosseous and parosteal osteosarcomas representing aggressive primary malignancies of bone; they arise in middle-age patients, a group older than those affected with conventional osteosarcomas; lesions appear as radiodense masses
Prolonged immobilization	Paraplegia and other neuropathic conditions with development of ossification or calcifications in muscles, tendons, and ligaments
Surgical scar	Linear ossific or calcific densities in the location of past surgical sites
Synovial osteochondromatosis [p. 775]	Nonneoplastic hypertropic metaplasia of synovial tissue, producing multiple cartilage nodules; nodules detach to become loose bodies in the joint, bursal, and tendon sheath spaces and become radiographically discernible following calcification/ossification; this condition may be asymptomatic or produce acute pain with joint locking and effusion; it occurs in adults, most commonly in the knees, hips, ankles, and elbows

Suggested Readings

Bernstein ML, Neal DC: Oral lesion in a patient with calcinosis and arthritis: case report and differential diagnosis, *J Oral Pathol* 14(1):8, 1985.

Black AS, Kanat IO: A review of soft tissue calcifications, *J Foot Surg,* 24(4):243, 1985.

Brant WE: *Fundamentals of diagnostic radiology,* Baltimore, 1994, Williams and Wilkins.

Burgener FA, Kormano M: *Differential diagnosis in conventional radiology,* ed 2, New York, 1991, Thieme Medical Publishers.

Chapman S, Nakielny R: *Aids to radiological differential diagnosis,* ed 3, Philadelphia, 1995, WB Saunders.

Dahnert W: *Radiology review manual,* Baltimore, 1991, Williams and Wilkins.

Eisenberg RL: *An atlas of differential diagnosis,* ed 2, Gaithersburg, 1992, Aspen.

Forrester DM, Brown JC, Nesson JW: *The radiology of joint disease,* ed 2, Philadelphia, 1978, WB Saunders.

Ravin CE, Cooper C, Leder RA: *Review of radiology,* Philadelphia, 1994, WB Saunders.

Reeder MM, Bradley WG: *Reeder and Felson's Gamuts in radiology,* ed 3, New York, 1993, Springer-Verlag.

Weissleder R, Wittenberg J: *Primer of diagnostic imaging,* St Louis, 1994, Mosby.

chapter 9

Magnetic Resonance Imaging Patterns

IAN D MCLEAN

General Indications for MRI Examination

Magnetic resonance imaging (MRI) is the most tissue-sensitive, noninvasive imaging modality that can be used to evaluate the extraordinarily wide range of diseases affecting the neuromusculoskeletal system. It is arguably the modality of choice for the detection of osteonecrosis, occult fractures, and soft tissue neoplasms, and in the assessment of many soft tissue abnormalities. In many instances, MRI has replaced more invasive imaging techniques such as arthrography, myelography, and discography.

However, conventional radiography remains an important initial imaging tool. Plain film provides valuable information in the evaluation of common bone and joint pathologies. Conventional radiographic techniques can be more specific than MRI in the diagnosis of many bone lesions, especially bone tumors, which often produce predictable bone changes and periosteal reactions. Consequently, plain film radiographic examinations complement, and should usually precede, the MRI examination.

Critically, however, MRI has major advantages over conventional radiographic studies and even computed tomography (CT). These advantages include its ability to yield high tissue contrast, image in multiple planes, and image a large field of view, all without radiation exposure. Consequently, MRI is helpful in the evaluation of a wide range of conditions of the neuromusculoskeletal system, including traumatic muscle and tendon injuries, hematomas, infections, masses, and internal injuries to joints, including meniscal and cruciate ligament tears and brain and spinal cord pathology.

The cost of MRI is relatively high. However, an MRI examination usually yields an accurate diagnosis of the patient's condition. Furthermore, in some instances, it may preclude the need for redundant multiple examinations that may be less sensitive and specific and possibly more invasive than the MRI examination. For instance, in most clinical circumstances, MRI should be the primary imaging procedure in the evaluation of the spine, particularly in the presence of neurological symptoms. For chiropractors, therefore, MRI represents a critically needed diagnostic tool, given that diagnosis of the disorders of the spine represents a daily challenge.

The following tables illustrate some of the more common pathologies encountered in imaging the spine and extremities for musculoskeletal complaints.

MRI | Spine

DISEASE	COMMENTS
Diffuse vertebral marrow signal patterns on T1-weighted image	
Marrow appears white	Radiation
Marrow appears gray	Normal aging with fibrous marrow increased red marrow production
Marrow appears black **(FIG. 9-1)**	Increased bone formation secondary to sclerotic metastases (breast, prostate) or osteopetrosis
Infection (FIG. 9-2)	Very sensitive diagnosis of infection provided by MRI when it is used in conjunction with the clinical presentation, radiographic findings, and radionuclide studies; MRI examinations reveal joint effusions on the T2-weighted images with juxtaarticular bone marrow edema and abnormal signal within the adjacent soft tissues along with bone destruction

Intervertebral disc [p. 486]	
Annular rents	Hyperintense on T2-weighted or gradient-echo–weighted images; rents appear as high-intensity zones
Disc bulge	Diffuse contour alteration of disc space
Disc protrusion	Relatively central, broad-based—not large, sometimes described as a *subligamentous herniation*
Disc extrusion (FIG. 9-3)	Transligamentous extrusion of the disc material through the PLL
Disc sequestration	Transligamentous disc herniation without communication (migration) to the parent disc

Continued

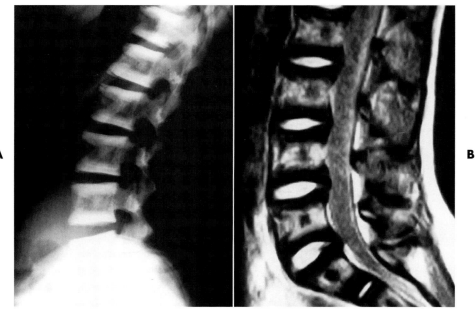

A   **B**

FIG. 9-1   Osteopetrosis on plain film **(A)** and a sagittal spin-density weighted magnetic resonance image **(B).** Densely sclerotic vertebral bands **(A)** that parallel the endplates appear markedly hypointense on the magnetic resonance image **(B).**

A **B** **C**

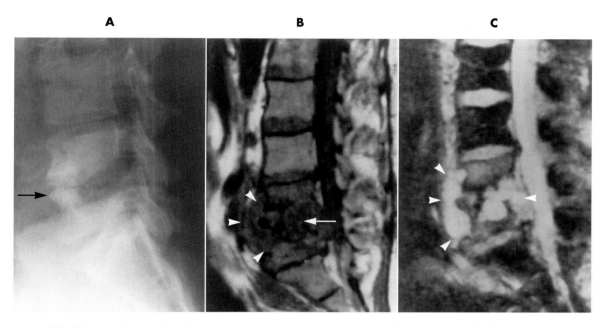

FIG. 9-2 **A,** Infection of the L4 intervertebral disc, presenting with decreased disc space on the plain film *(arrow)*. **B,** A large soft tissue mass *(arrowheads)* and hypointense signal of the infection *(arrow)* is noted on the T1-weighted MRI. **C,** These regions become hyperintense on the T2-weighted MRI *(arrowheads)*.

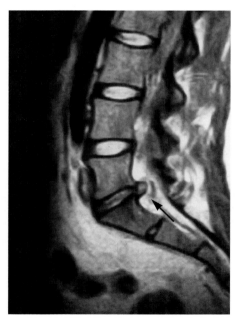

FIG. 9-3 Sagittal T2-weighted lumbar intervertebral disc extrusion at the L5 level *(arrow)*.

DISEASE

Tumors and soft tissue masses (FIG. 9-4)

COMMENTS

For normal or equivocal initial radiographs, MRI is useful for further evaluation of the presence of a serious underlying pathology such as tumor or infection; MRI are very sensitive in detecting bone abnormalities; criteria to distinguish tumor/metastasis from infection are the same as in conventional radiography, but this pattern can be recognized at a far earlier stage on an MRI; in the spine, when only a single body is involved, it is difficult to distinguish infection from tumor if the differentiation is based purely on the magnetic resonance images; the plain film criteria of endplate destruction and disc involvement are typical of infection rather than metastasis; extension of destruction into the posterior elements of a vertebra is more typical of metastatic disease; signal changes of infection are frequently equal to CSF, whereas metastatic bone disease appears more hypointense; soft tissue involvement of infection tends to be ill-defined as opposed to the soft tissue involvement of tumor, which is often more sharply defined; in general the signal changes within the vertebral bodies are nonspecific, and differentiation of benign from malignant lesions is sometimes difficult; certain masses, however, have typical MRI characteristics allowing for confident diagnosis; in general "white lesions are 'right' on T1-weighted images" and "white lesions are 'wrong' on T2-weighted images." For exam-

Tumors and soft tissue masses—cont'd

Vertebral body compression fractures [p. 536]

ple, a vertebral fat deposit that is of limited clinical significance appears as a high signal intensity on T1-weighted scans and a lower signal intensity on T2-weighted scans. By contrast, metastatic bone disease, which is highly clinically significant, will likely demonstrate a high signal intense on the T2-weighted images.

Differentiation of osteoporosis and malignant collapse may at times be difficult; old or healed fractures show preservation of the normal marrow signal, and if the fracture is chronic, a band of low signal is evident paralleling the endplate on T2-weighted images; fresh fracture creates nonhomogeneous bone marrow changes, reflective of hemorrhage; by contrast tumor replacement of marrow tends to create homogeneous signal changes within the vertebral bodies; multiple levels of vertebral body marrow abnormalities with fracture are typical for metastatic disease; CT findings of an osteoporotic vertebral body fracture can be applied to MRI and include cortical fractures without bone destruction retropulsion of bone fragments, intravertebral vacuum phenomenon, and thin, diffuse paraspinal soft tissue mass; CT findings of collapse secondary to malignancy include destruction of the anterolateral or posterior cortical bone of the vertebral body; characteristics include destruction of the vertebral body, destruction of a pedicle, and focal soft tissue mass or epidural mass

Continued

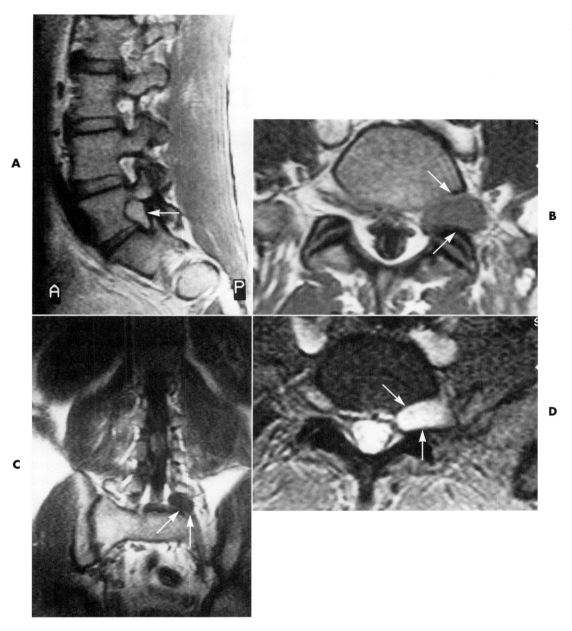

FIG. 9-4 Neurofibroma presenting as a mass in the intervertebral foramen *(arrows)* on sagittal **(A)**, axial **(B)** and coronal **(C)** MRIs. **D,** The mass becomes hyperintense on the T2-weighted images *(arrows)*.

DISEASE

Vertebral (modic)
endplate changes
[p. 468]

Type I
(FIG. 9-5)

COMMENTS

Represents edema/granulation tissue and appears hypointense on the T1-weighted images and hyperintense on the T2-weighted images

Type II
(FIG. 9-6)

Represents fat tissue phase and appears hyperintense on the T1-weighted images and mildly hyperintense on the T2-weighted images

Type III

Represents bone sclerosis and appears hypointense on the T1- and T2-weighted images

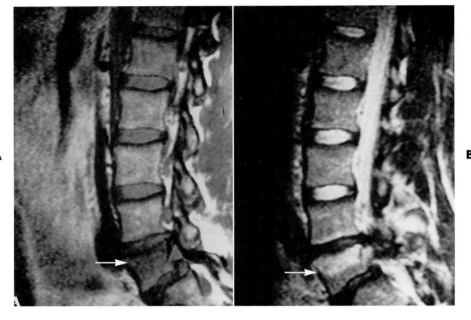

A   **B**

FIG. 9-5   Modic type I endplate changes consistent with inflammatory vertebral marrow alterations. Notably the hypointense regions *(arrow)* on the T1-weighted image **(A)** appear hyperintense *(arrow)* on the T2-weighted image **(B).**

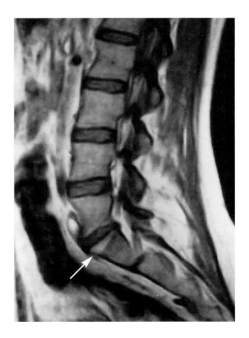

FIG. 9-6   Modic type II endplate changes consistent with fat marrow changes. The imaging findings denote focal signal hyperintensity on the sagittal T1-weighted MR lumbar scan *(arrow)*.

<table>
<tr><td>

Miscellaneous conditions (FIGS. 9-7 THROUGH 9-11)

</td><td>

MRI excellent for imaging of the spinal canal; abnormalities such as dural ectasia, multiple sclerosis, tethered cord syndrome, ligamentum flavum calcification, and syringomyelia are readily noted

Continued

</td></tr>
</table>

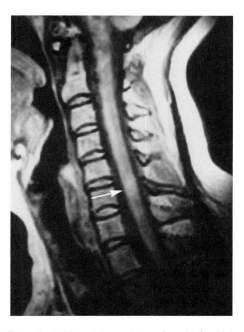

FIG. 9-8 Demyelinated, hyperintense plaques *(arrow)* of multiple sclerosis on this sagittal T1-weighted cervical MRI without contrast.

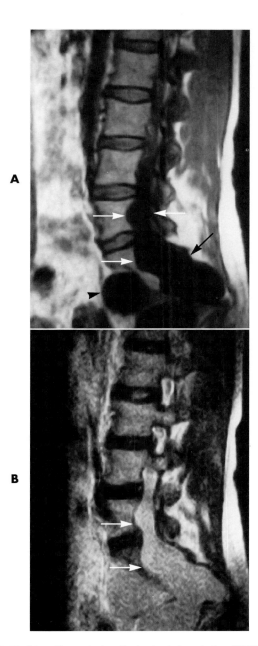

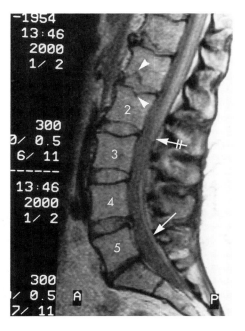

FIG. 9-7 Neurofibromatosis with dural ectasia noted as CSF-filled saccular redundancy of the dura *(arrows)* with ventral meningocele *(arrowhead)* appearing **(A)** hypointense on the T1-weighted image and **(B)** hyperintense on the T2-weighted images *(arrows)*.

FIG. 9-9 Tethered cord syndrome. Sagittal T1-weighted MRI demonstrating fat infiltrate of the filum terminale *(arrow)*. The spinal cord termination is at the L2/L3 intervertebral disc space *(crossed arrow)*, which is lower than the normal L1-L2 level of termination. Schmorl's nodes *(arrowheads)* of the upper lumbar spine and advanced degenerative disc disease at the L4 and L5 levels are also noted.

PART TWO Bone, Joints, and Soft Tissues

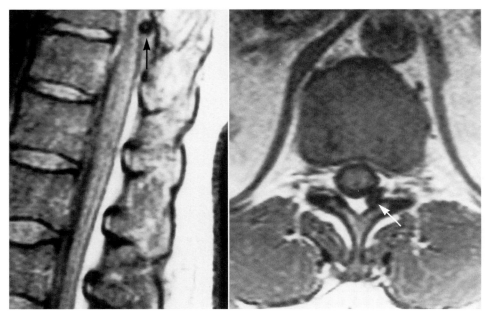

FIG. 9-10   Ligamentum flavum calcification *(arrows)* appearing as focal hypointensity in the vertebral canal at the thoracolumbar junction.

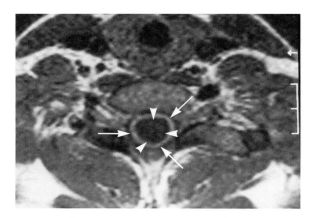

FIG. 9-11   Syringomyelia presenting as a cavity in the center of the hyperintense spinal cord *(arrows)* filled with hypointense CSF *(arrowheads)* on this axial T1-weighted image.

MR2 | Joints

Most causes of joint pain are poorly portrayed with conventional radiography. Tissue contrast with MRI is high, and early changes in marrow, subchondral bone, and cartilage can be evaluated, including arthritis, trauma, infection, and neoplasia. MRI should be considered when a need exists to evaluate internal joint derangement and juxtaarticular pathology or if a poor response occurs to conservative management.

MR2a | Shoulder

DISEASE	COMMENTS
Biceps tendon abnormalities **(FIG. 9-12)**	Rupture or dislocation possible when biceps tendon is not visible in its expected location; fluid may also be observed within the biceps tendon sheath

DISEASE	COMMENTS
Glenoid labral tears **(FIG. 9-13)** [p. 543]	Sequelae of anterior shoulder dislocation with involvement of the anterior labrum (Bankart lesion); osseous fractures of the underlying glenoid margin may accompany labral tear

Continued

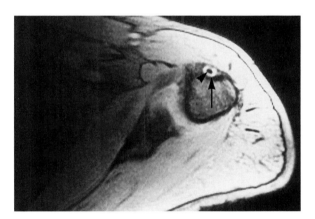

FIG. 9-12 Bicipital tendinitis noted by a hyperintense effusion *(arrow)* surrounding the central hypointense biceps tendon *(arrowhead)* within the bicipital groove on this T2-weighted axial MRI.

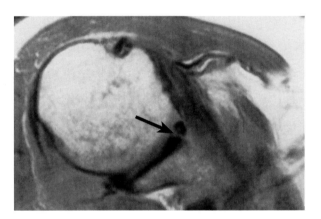

FIG. 9-13 Bucket-handle tear of the glenoid labrum. Larger bucket-handle–type tears can be seen as areas of linear high signal intensity within the labrum on multiple images *(arrow).* (From Stark DD, Gradley WG: *Magnetic resonance imaging,* ed 2, St. Louis, 1992, Mosby.)

PART TWO Bone, Joints, and Soft Tissues

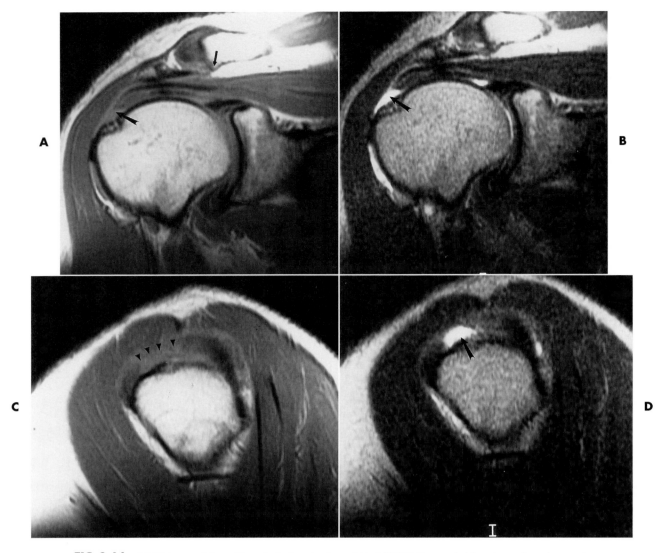

FIG. 9-14   Full-thickness rotator cuff tear. **A,** Proton-density–weighted (2500/14) coronal oblique image. A gap is present in the supraspinatus tendon near its insertion site *(arrow)*. Some proliferative changes affect the acromioclavicular joint, including a small, downward-pointing spur *(small arrow)*. **B,** T2-weighted (2500/70) coronal oblique image. The tendon gap is very bright *(arrow)* and is most likely filled with fluid. No intact tendon exists above or below the abnormal area. **C,** Proton-density-weighted (2500/70) sagittal oblique image. Anterosuperiorly the normal dark band of the rotator cuff is interrupted by a fuzzy area of relatively increased signal *(arrowheads)*. **D,** T2-weighted (2500/70) sagittal oblique image. The anterior part of this area becomes very bright *(arrow)*. The remainder brightens only slightly. Often a tear is adjacent to or surrounded by an area of tendonopathy. (From Haaga JR: *Computed tomography and magnetic resonance imaging of the whole body,* St Louis, 1994, Mosby.)

DISEASE

Rotator cuff tear
(FIGS. 9-14 AND 9-15)
[p. 544]

COMMENTS

Complete tear revealing a T2-weighted signal hyperintensity extending through the rotator cuff; the supraspinatus musculotendinous junction retracts, and fluid accumulates in the subacromial bursa; secondary signs include loss of the subdeltoid fat, atrophy of the supraspinatus muscle, cystic changes of the humeral head, principally at the site of the supraspinatus tendon insertion

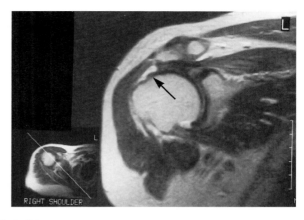

FIG. 9-15 Full-thickness tear of the supraspinatus with the tendon gap filled with fluid on this T1-weighted coronal magnetic resonance image *(arrow)*.

MR2b | Wrist

The multiplanar imaging potential of MRI is advantageous in evaluating the complex anatomy of the wrist, an area that is often difficult to visualize with conventional imaging techniques.

DISEASE	COMMENTS		
Carpal tunnel syndrome (FIG. 9-16) [p. 556]	Compression of the median nerve with flattening, swelling, and increased signal intensity; palmar bowing of the transverse ligament occurs	**Osteonecrosis of the scaphoid (FIG. 9-17)** [pp. 551 and 591]	Typically low signal intensity within the bone marrow on T1-weighted images with regions of increased signal intensity on the T2-weighted images; the T2-weighted appearance is thought to represent hemorrhage or edema

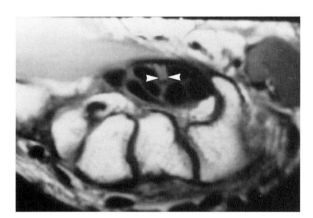

FIG. 9-16 Axial T1-weighted MR scan of the wrist, demonstrating alteration of the normally oval median nerve width *(arrowheads)*, suggesting compression within the carpal tunnel.

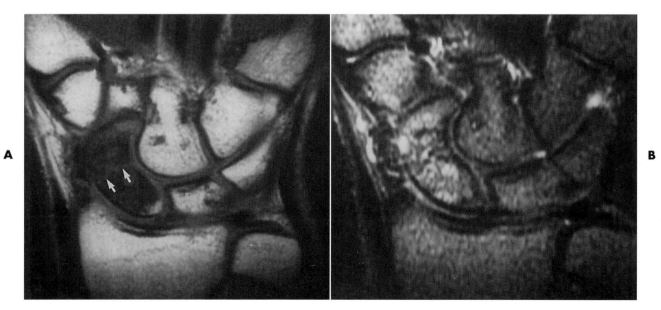

FIG. 9-17 Avascular necrosis of the scaphoid. Coronal sections through the wrist were obtained with TR/TE of 500/20 **(A)** and TR/TE of 200/80 **(B)**. A fracture of the scaphoid is present (**A,** *arrows*). A diffuse loss of the normally high signal intensity of the marrow is seen on the T1-weighted image, and mottled high and low signal intensity is seen on the T2-weighted image. (From Stark DD, Gradley WG: *Magnetic resonance imaging,* ed 2, St Louis, 1992, Mosby.)

MR2c Hip

DISEASE	COMMENTS
Legg-Calvé-Perthes disease [p. 592]	Idiopathic osteonecrosis of the femoral head in children, usually between 4 and 8 years of age; characteristic radiographic findings include increase in density of the femoral head, subchondral collapse, flattening, and diffuse sclerosis of an irregularly ossified femoral capital epiphysis
Osteonecrosis **(FIGS. 9-18 AND 9-19)** [p. 591]	Condition that results from ischemic death of the cellular aspects of bone marrow and bone; MRI is optimal for use with patients with normal or equivocal conventional radiographs following clinical complaint of the hip; radiography is comparatively insensitive in the early diagnosis of osteonecrosis; when stages of bone repair or collapse become evident, the classic radiographic findings become obvious; radionuclide bone scintigraphy is sensitive but lacks specificity; consequently, MRI detects early osteonecrosis and differentiates osteonecrosis from other bone pathology; char-
Osteonecrosis—cont'd	acteristic features of osteonecrosis of the hip include a circumscribed ovoid- or crescent-shaped rim of low signal circumscribed ovoid- or crescent-shaped rim of low signal on T1-weighted scans occurring - in a subchondral location and corresponding to the interface of repair between ischemic and the normal bone ("double-line" sign); joint effusions along with the presence of a diffuse signal abnormality of the head and neck are also observed
Transient osteoporosis of the hip	Condition of unknown etiology; may be related to regional migratory osteoporosis and reflex sympathetic dystrophy; conventional radiographs are often normal; MRI reveals a diffuse loss of normal marrow fat signal on T1-weighted images with hyperintense signal on the T2-weighted images representing bone marrow edema; condition tends to resolve spontaneously in 6 to 12 months

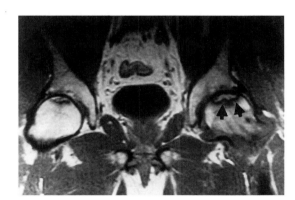

FIG. 9-18 T1-weighted coronal section demonstrating bilateral femoral head avascular necrosis, more advanced on the patient's left (arrows).

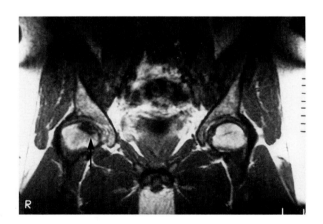

FIG. 9-19 T1-weighted coronal section demonstrating a hypointense focus in the right femoral head, consistent with avascular necrosis (arrow).

PART TWO Bone, Joints, and Soft Tissues

MR2d | Knee

DISEASE

Anterior cruciate injuries

(FIG. 9-20)
[p. 564]

COMMENTS

Midsubstance discontinuity, abnormal angulation of the course of the anterior cruciate, abnormal cruciate buckling, increased curvature of the posterior cruciate ligament, anterior tibial subluxation, thinning of the fibers of the ACL hematomas about the intact fibers of the ACL, increased signal intensity within the ACL but with intact fibers

Posterior cruciate ligament injuries

(FIG. 9-21)
[p. 565]

Midsubstance discontinuity of the ligament with avulsion occurring at the tibial insertion; isolated posterior cruciate ligament (PCL) tears are uncommon, and associated injuries to the anterior cruciate ligament or the menisci should be sought

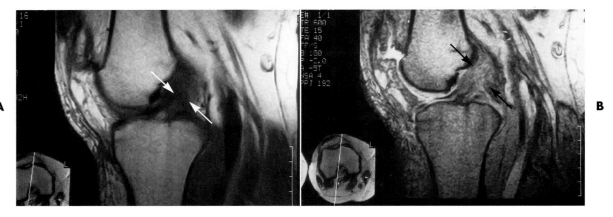

FIG. 9-20   Anterior cruciate ligament tear noted by the interruption of the normally hypointense ligament band with surrounding hemorrhage and edema present on the sagittal T1-weighted MRI **(A)** and T2-weighted **(B)** MRIs *(arrows)*.

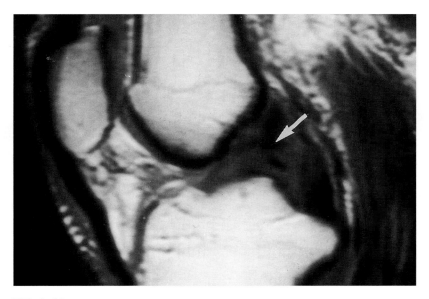

FIG. 9-21   Posterior cruciate ligament tear. Sagittal T1-weighted image shows no identifiable PCL configuration. Hemorrhage and edema replace the region of a complete tear *(arrow)*. (From Haaga JR: *Computed tomography and magnetic resonance imaging of the whole body*, St Louis, 1994, Mosby.)

Chondromalacia patellae	MRI studies showing early cartilage thinning or erosion of the cartilaginous surface along with focal regions of edema and later marked hypointensity (sclerosis) on T1- and T2-weighted images of the subchondral bone	**Patellar subluxation**	Triad of patellar bone bruise, femoral bone bruise, and associated tearing of the medial retinacular attachments; patellar subluxation may involve a large effusion; this condition is associated with hypoplastic lateral femoral condyle, genu valgum, abnormal lateral insertion of the patellar tendon and patella alta
Collateral ligament injuries (FIG. 9-22) [p. 566]	T2-weighted images demonstrating edema and hemorrhage surrounding the usually low signal intensity fibers of the ligament; complete tears are seen as a loss of continuity of the ligament fibers		
Meniscal tears (FIGS. 9-23 AND 9-24) [p. 566]	Three grades of abnormal signal intensity associated with abnormal menisci: grade 1 represents globular foci of abnormal signal correlating with mucinous degeneration (the signal does not extend to the meniscal articular surface); grade 2 represents a linear, horizontal region of increased signal intensity that does not extend to the articular surface; grades 1 and 2 are arthroscopically normal; grade 3 represents an abnormal signal intensity (often linear) that extends to an articular surface		
Osteochondritis dissecans [p. 577]	Low signal intensity, subchondral foci involving the non–weight-bearing lateral surface of the medial femoral condyle on both T1 and T2; *in situ* bone and cartilage fragment with or without evidence of displacement or migration		

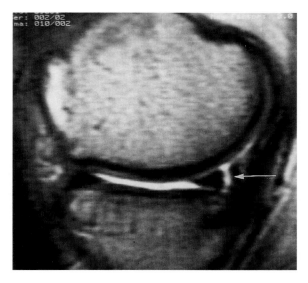

FIG. 9-23 Peripheral meniscal tear. Sagittal T2-weighted image shows high signal intensity at the periphery of the posterior horn of the medial meniscus *(arrow)*. A joint effusion is present. (From Haaga JR: *Computed tomography and magnetic resonance imaging of the whole body,* St Louis, 1994, Mosby.)

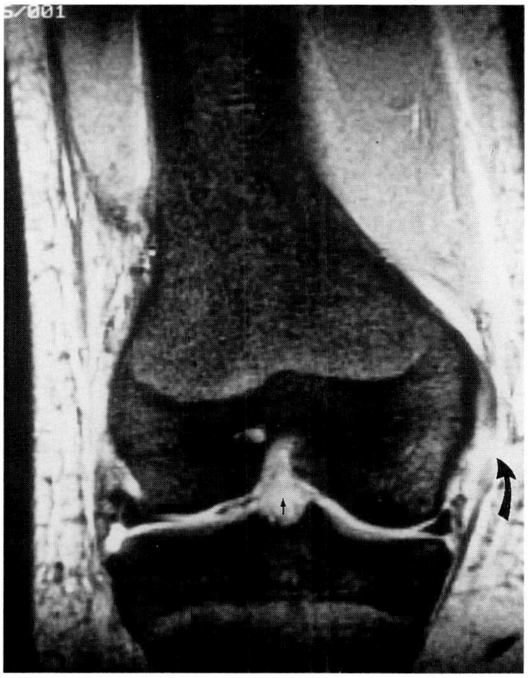

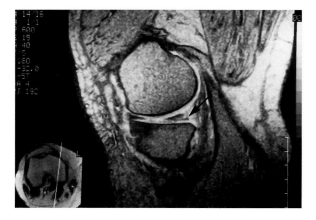

FIG. 9-22 Medial collateral ligament tear, grade 3. Coronal gradient echo image shows complete disruption of the medial collateral ligament *(curved arrow)*. In addition, a normal ACL is not seen at the intercondylar region and is therefore torn *(small arrow)*. (From Haaga JR: *Computed tomography and magnetic resonance imaging of the whole body,* St Louis, 1994, Mosby.)

FIG. 9-24 Hyperintense tear of the posterior horn of the lateral meniscus (arrow).

MR2e | Ankle

DISEASE	COMMENTS
Tendon ruptures	Most commonly affecting the Achilles and tibialis posterior; the peroneus brevis and longus are also frequently affected
Transchondral injuries	Including osteochondral fractures, osteochondritis dessicans, and talar dome fractures, which are usually found to involve either the medial or lateral talar dome with extension into both the articular cartilage and subchondral bone; characteristics include associated focal cartilaginous signal alteration and joint effusion

MR3 | General Skeletal

DISEASE	COMMENTS
Bone bruises	Seen as ill-defined low and high signal intensity changes within the bone marrow on the T1-weighted and T2-weighted images, respectively; in the knee these are associated with anterior and posterior cruciate ligament injuries and medial collateral ligament injuries
Bone marrow disorders (FIGS. 9-25 AND 9-26)	Healthy bone marrow of adults is composed predominantly of fat with characteristic high signal intensity on T1-weighted images; disease processes that replace bone marrow, including fluid, blood, pus, or calcification, cause an abnormal MRI bone marrow signal; consequently, MRI is exquisitely sensitive to such diseases as osteonecrosis, primary and secondary tumors, infection, systemic bone marrow diseases, and trauma; the signal characteristics of the medullary space also depend on the age of the patient and the quantity of cancellous bone and the ratios of red and yellow marrow; in children and young adults, high signal intensity of yellow marrow is observed in the femoral epiphyses in contrast with the intermediate signal intensity of the hematopoietic marrow in the metaphysis and the pelvis; with aging, fatty marrow gradually replaces hematopoietic marrow and the MRI signal changes to the characteristic high signal intensity on the T1-weighted images; MRI provides critical diagnostic information on bone marrow disorders; bone marrow processes include age-related marrow conversion and reconversion, hematologic disorders, neoplasia processes, ischemic disorders, infection, and metabolic bone disorders

Continued

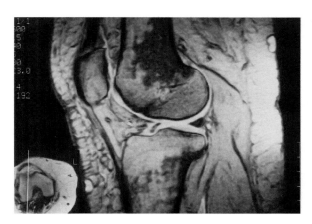

FIG. 9-25 Conspicuous red marrow reconversion in a long-term smoker. Most notable are the focal regions of hypointense hemopoietic marrow within the normal hyperintense adult yellow marrow, yielding a heterogeneous marrow signal pattern.

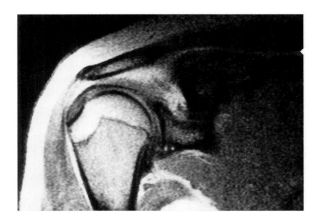

FIG. 9-26 Coronal T1-weighted MR scan of the proximal humerus, denoting normal bone marrow contrast of the epiphyses and the signal hypointense hemopoietic metaphysis in a young patient.

PART TWO Bone, Joints, and Soft Tissues

DISEASE	COMMENTS
Fractures (FIG. 9-27)	MRI is very sensitive in the diagnosis of acute and stress fractures and should be used when conventional radiographs show no abnormalities or only questionable findings; the typical findings of fatigue fractures include linear regions of decreased signal intensity on the T1-weighted images with associated edematous changes within the marrow of low signal intensity on T1-weighted images and high signal intensity on T2-weighted images; importantly, stress fractures may be bilateral
Joint effusions (FIG. 9-28)	Low signal intensity on T1-weighted and high signal intensity on T2-weighted scans; a characteristic saddlebag appearance appears on the coronal images within the suprapatellar bursa
Osteoarthritis [p. 458]	Characteristic features including osteophytes, loss of joint space, and subchondral cysts
Pigmented villonodular synovitis (PVNS) [p. 767]	Monoarticular synovial proliferative disorder presenting as soft tissue masses about the joint; MRI findings consist of mixed signal intensity changes, with the T2-weighted images showing foci of decreased signal intensity consistent with hemosiderin deposition, in addition to areas of increased signal intensity in the adjacent synovial fluid
Rheumatoid arthritis [p. 442]	Multicompartmental disease with subchondral and marginal erosions with diffuse loss of cartilage; moderate joint effusions with popliteal cysts about the knee are common, best demonstrated on the T2-weighted images; thickening of the synovium is a relatively consistent feature of inflammatory joint diseases; MRI examination of rheumatoid joints also helps to exclude osteonecrosis as a complication of steroid therapy
Synovial osteochondromatosis [p. 775]	Joint effusions and multiple filling effect shown on MRI within the effusions, which represent osteocartilaginous loose bodies; calcified cartilaginous bodies may be seen on conventional radiographs; however, in approximately one third of the cases, calcification is not apparent

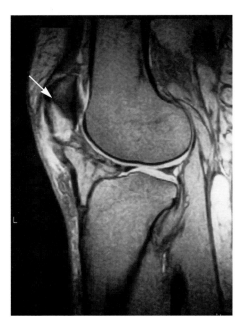

FIG. 9-27   Fracture of the patella, producing altered signal pattern appearing as hypointense signal in the upper pole and hyperintense signal in the lower pole *(arrow)*.

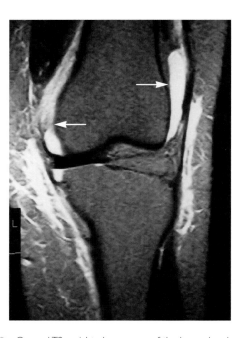

FIG. 9-28   Coronal T2-weighted sequence of the knee, showing a homogeneous posttraumatic collection of fluid-producing joint effusion *(arrows)*.

Suggested Readings

Gosfield E, Alavi A, Kneeland B: Comparison of radionuclide bone scans and magnetic resonance imaging in detecting spinal metastases, *J Nucl Med* 34:2191, 1993.

Grundy CR, Fritts HM: Magnetic resonance imaging of the musculoskeletal system, *Clin Orthop Rel Res* 338:275,

Haaga JR: *Computed tomography and magnetic resonance imaging of the whole body,* ed 3, St Louis, 1994, Mosby.

Kneeland JB: Magnetic resonance imaging of the musculoskeletal system. I. Fundamental principles, *Clin Orthop Rel Res* 321:274, 1995.

Mitchell DG et al: Femoral head avascular necrosis: correlation with MR imaging, radiographic staging, radionuclide imaging, and clinical features, *Radiol* 162:709, 1987.

Pomeranz SJ: *Pitfalls and variations in neuro-orthopedics,* MRI-EFI publications. Cincinnati, 1995.

Runge VM: *Magnetic resonance imaging of the spine,* Philadelphia, 1995, JB Lippincott.

chapter 10

Congenital Diseases

TIMOTHY J MICK

Achondroplasia

BACKGROUND

Classic, heterozygous, autosomal dominant achondroplasia is the most common dwarfing skeletal dysplasia and is typically evident at birth. Recently, achondroplasia has been mapped to the 2.5 Mb locus of chromosome 4p16.3.[74] The name (*a-*, meaning "not," *chondroplasia,* meaning "formation of cartilage") seems to imply that a complete lack of normal cartilage formation exists. This is not the case, although the hallmark of the condition is hypochondrogenesis, with a decreased rate of formation of essentially normal cartilage.

Achondroplasia is generally compatible with a normal life expectancy. Therefore this condition occurs at any age. Achondroplasia is easily recognized clinically and is readily differentiated from other dwarfing dysplasias.

IMAGING FINDINGS

General. Imaging findings in achondroplasia reflect gross anatomical changes, especially regarding the craniofacial region. The ilii are broad and squared, with constricted sciatic notches. The pelvic inlet has a "champagne glass" configuration. The sacrum is horizontal and deeply seated in the pelvis. The ribs are broad and short, resulting in a diminished anteroposterior dimension of the thorax. The sternum is short and broad. As noted, typically a "bullet-shaped" vertebra with central beak exists at the thoracolumbar junction resulting from underdevelopment of the primary ossification center for the vertebral body (Fig. 10-1). The long and tubular bones are shortened and the developing metaphyses flared, somewhat resembling the characteristics of rickets. Limb shortening is more profound proximally than distally (rhizomelic micromelia).

Epiphyses. Epiphyseal changes may resemble a variety of epiphyseal dysplasias. Broad, short proximal phalanges and short middle phalanges of the feet and, more classically, the hands, may occur and result in a clinically apparent trident-shaped hand in infants. (The trident is a three-pronged spear wielded by the fish-god of classical mythology.)

Limb length. As limb-lengthening procedures pioneered by the Russian physician Ilizarov become more widely utilized, clinicians may encounter achondroplasts with atypical postoperative long bone changes.[29,53] One case series from Germany demonstrated average limb lengthening of approximately 8 cm at a rate of about 1 cm every 50 days using the Ilizarov apparatus.[75] A U.S. study demonstrates gains in limb length averaging 10 cm (32%) for the femur and 11 cm (40%) for the humerus.[5] Workers at the University of Milan achieved total increases in limb length of 18 to 23 cm in each of six children studied.[194]

Studies in growth hormone therapy for achondroplasia are not extensive, although subjects receiving growth hormone demonstrate sustained increases in rate of growth for 4 to 6 years. Because the treatment is investigational, patients receiving this therapy are unlikely to seek treatment from a practitioner who is not part of the study.[30,109,179,293]

Spine. Plain films highlight most of the characteristic spinal abnormalities; however, advanced imaging is necessary to directly identify compression of neural elements. Posterior vertebral body scalloping results from dysplasia and dural ectasia. Platyspondyly is typical, although it may not be remarkable. The pedicles are short and the interpediculate distance decreases in a cephalocaudal direction in the lumbar spine, which is opposite of what normally occurs. Spinal canal stenosis results, and a typical trefoil configuration is noted on axial images from advanced imaging.

Degenerative disc disease and facet arthrosis are common in older adult patients because of biomechanical and gross anatomical factors. Vertebral osteophytes may contribute significantly to central canal and nerve root canal stenosis, complications that any health care provider working with achondroplasts should recognize. The surgical approach to treatment may range from single-level laminectomy to complete craniospinal decompression from brainstem to cauda equina. This reportedly (but incredibly) does not produce spinal instability.[273]

CLINICAL COMMENTS

Achondroplastic dwarfs have macrocephaly; a broad, flat nasal bridge; and prominence of the frontal bone and frontal sinuses, sometimes described as "frontal bossing." Achondroplastic adults are obviously short, ranging in height from 112 to 145 cm. However, these are not the shortest of the dwarfs. Patients with spondy-

385

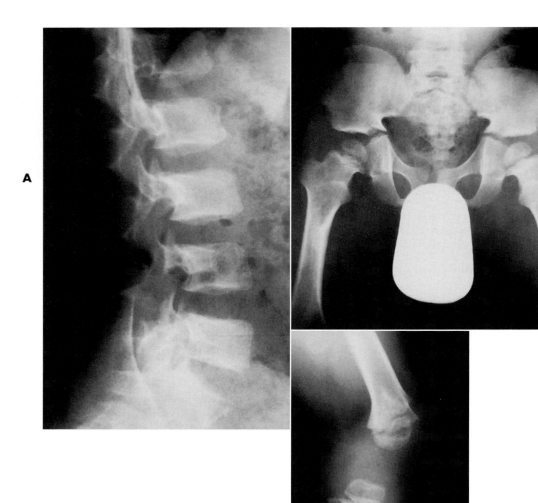

FIG. 10-1 Achondroplasia in a 5-month-old girl. **A,** Platyspondyly, posterior scalloping. **B,** Broad, square ilia, hemispheric capital femoral epiphyses, short femoral necks. **C,** Exaggerated tibial tubercle apophysis, fibulae overgrowth. (From Taybi H, Lachman RS: *Radiology of syndromes, metabolic disorders, and skeletal dysplasias,* ed 4, St Louis, 1996, Mosby.)

loepiphyseal dysplasia (SED) or spondylometaepiphyseal dysplasia range from 94 to 132 cm and have much more apparent trunkal shortening than they do extremity shortening.[102]

Clinically and radiographically apparent thoracolumbar angular kyphosis, with a classic "bullet-shaped" vertebra at the thoracolumbar junction, is a hallmark of the condition and is present at birth, whereas lumbar hyperlordosis tends to develop secondarily in children and adult achondroplasts.[140]

Achondroplasia is a prototypical cause of developmental spinal canal stenosis, often causing spinal cord, cauda equina, and nerve root compression. Stenosis of the foramen magnum may lead to brainstem, cerebellar, or upper cervical cord compression, angulation, or displacement in addition to hydrocephalus, which is commonly diagnosed in infancy or early childhood. This may produce neurological complications, including ataxia, incontinence, and depression of respiratory function, which is occasionally lethal.[191,225,278] Advanced diagnostic imaging has been valuable in identifying infants at risk for these complications and associated abnormalities, such as Chiari malformation.[54] Abnormalities on polysomnography, as well as clinical findings of hyperreflexia and clonus, have also been considered to be indications for surgical decompression of the cervicomedullary junction. About 10% of infants will fit this clinical picture. It is important to universally screen achondroplastic babies for these findings.[192]

Achondroplasts often have a waddling gait because of hip joint involvement, frequently leading to advanced osteoarthritis early in life. Femoral epiphyseal changes may resemble those of Legg-Calvé-Perthes disease.

KEY CONCEPTS

- *Achondroplasia is a common dwarfing dysplasia typified by the circus dwarf.*
- *A normal or near normal trunk and marked rhizomelic micromelia are characteristic.*
- *A number of classic radiographic changes affect the entire axial and appendicular skeleton.*
- *Anomalies involving the skull and spine are particularly important because of their potential association with neurological complications.*
- *Achondroplasia is a prototypical cause of developmental spinal canal stenosis, often causing spinal cord, cauda equina, and nerve root compression.*
- *In the peripheral skeleton, in addition to the obvious limb shortening, early, severe, and sometimes debilitating osteoarthritis may develop.*

Chondrodysplasia Punctata

BACKGROUND

Chondrodysplasia punctata is a rare familial disorder characterized by punctate or "stippled" calcification of developing epiphyses. As with other dysplasias, chondrodysplasia punctata is actually a heterogeneous group of disorders rather than a single disease entity, with at least four distinct forms reported.[143,253]

IMAGING FINDINGS

Radiographs illustrate marked shortening of tubular bones and expanded metaphyses, with marked rhizomelic shortening of long tubular bones (Fig. 10-2). Epiphyseal ossification is delayed and irregular, with characteristic "stippling" bilaterally and symmetri-

cally. This diminishes over time in infants who survive. Generalized bone density also decreases over time. Similar stippled calcification occurs in the spine and pelvis, as well as in the ribs, laryngeal and tracheal cartilages, tarsal and carpal regions, and the patellae.

Radiographic changes reflect histological and gross anatomical changes resulting from altered development and alignment of chondrocytes.[85] Poznanski[202] has emphasized the fact that finding punctate or "stippled" epiphyses represents a radiographic sign, not a specific disease entity. In fact, the differential diagnosis for stippled epiphyses is rather extensive. The conditions most closely resembling chondrodysplasia punctata radiographically are Zellweger syndrome and warfarin or alcohol-related embryopathy. The presence of brain lesions distinguishes Zellweger syndrome from chondrodysplasia punctata. A history of warfarin (coumadin) treatment or alcoholism in the mother of an infant who is affected is a red flag for warfarin or alcohol-related embryopathy.[143,202] Evidence exists that warfarin-induced changes may result from the same deficiency of a novel sulfatase enzyme seen in chondrodysplasia punctata.[73]

Chondrodysplasia punctata, along with Kniest syndrome, metatropic dwarfism, and some forms of osteopetrosis, may demonstrate a coronal cleft in the vertebral bodies in utero. This cleft is generally obliterated prior to birth. Dysplasia of vertebral bodies may result in kyphoscoliosis or other spinal deformity. Rare manifestations of chondrodysplasia have been reported, including asymmetrical or unilateral involvement, which may overlap with a so-called "CHILD" syndrome, comprising congenital hemidysplasia, ichthyosiform erythroderma, and limb defects.[96] Reported characteristics include a long bone, cone-shaped phalanges and metacarpal bones, brachydactyly, and bowing of the long bones.[143]

CLINICAL COMMENTS

The most readily identifiable form of chondrodysplasia punctata is an autosomal recessive form characterized by rhizomelic shortening of the extremities, microcephaly, a depressed nasal bridge, developmental delays, congenital cataracts, and joint contracture. Clinical features are usually apparent in infancy and the condition is typically lethal. A milder, autosomal dominant form (Conradi-Hünermann syndrome) demonstrates similar but less severe changes, with patients more often experiencing a normal lifespan and no significant neurological deficit.[44,238,241] An X-linked dominant form and a mild sporadic form (Sheffield type) have also been identified.[143,157] In addition to characteristic epiphyseal changes seen radiographically, an icthyosiform (resembling fish scales) dermatitis exists.[143] Otherwise, a relative lack of associated classical clinical features is evident.

KEY CONCEPTS

- *Many clinicians are unlikely to encounter patients with any of the forms of chondrodysplasia punctata.*
- *The classic radiographic feature of "stippled" epiphyses may also be seen in other conditions, such as warfarin or alcohol-induced embryopathy and are therefore not pathognomonic for this condition.*
- *Other radiographic findings, including dysplasia of long bones and vertebrae, are variable and nonspecific.*
- *Likewise, clinical findings are not distinctive, with considerable overlap with other conditions.*

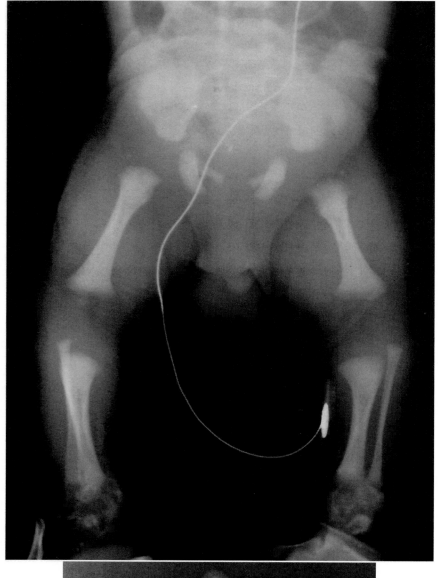

A,

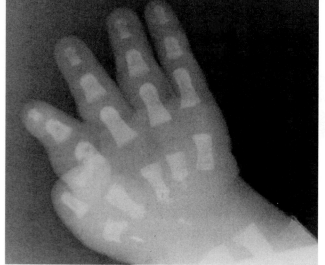

B,

FIG. 10-2   Chondrodysplasia punctata, tibial-metacarpal type in the neonate. **A,** Diffuse areas of stippling in hips, ankles, and sacrum; short femurs, long fibulae with very short tibiae. **B,** Generalized brachydactyly with special shortening of the first, third, and fourth metacarpals and the proximal phalanx of the second digit combined with stippling in these areas and the carpus.

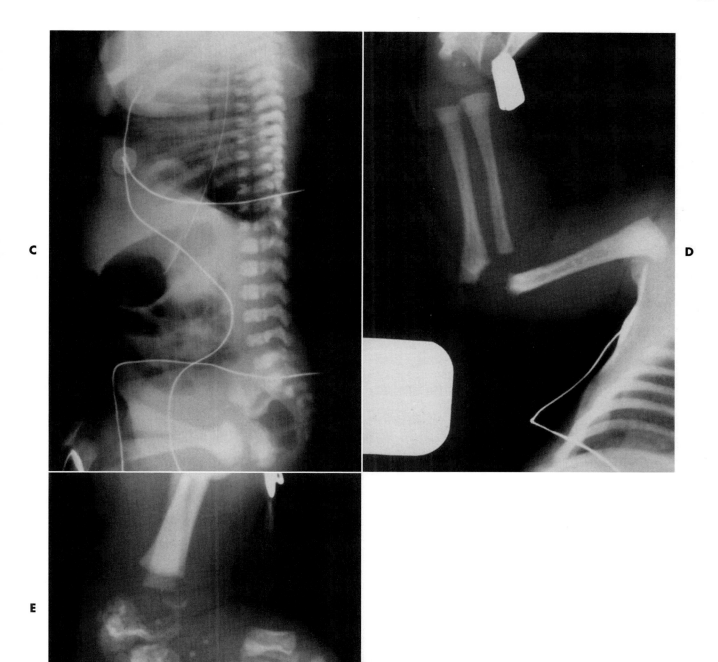

FIG. 10-2—cont'd   C, Coronal cleft vertebrae and sacrococcygeal stippling. **D,** Mild upper extremity shortening with epiphyseal area stippling. **E,** Severe stippling in the tarsal region. (From Taybi H, Lachman RS: *Radiology of syndromes, metabolic disorders, and skeletal dysplasias,* ed 4, St Louis, 1996, Mosby.)

Chondroectodermal Dysplasia

BACKGROUND

Chondroectodermal dysplasia (Ellis-van Creveld syndrome) is an autosomal recessive, short-limbed, dwarfing dysplasia associated with polydactyly, congenital heart anomalies, and ectodermal dysplasia, which are evident at birth. The condition, classified as a short-ribbed polydactyly syndrome (SRPS), is linked to consanguineous relationships. Previously, this was particularly common among the old order Amish community, but an awareness of this problem has prompted the Amish to encourage young adults to move away and seek a spouse from another Amish community.

IMAGING FINDINGS

Radiographic changes resemble those of Jeune's asphyxiating thoracic dysplasia. Ribs are short and broad anteriorly, with an increased anteroposterior dimension but constriction of the thorax. The ilia are hypoplastic. Alterations include variation in shape, size, and number of the tubular bones of the hands and feet. Characteristics include polydactyly, with or without syndactyly, polycarpy, carpal coalition across carpal rows, and cone-shaped epiphyses. Hexadactyly (six digits on each hand and foot) always occurs with this condition. Congenital radial head dislocation and marked widening of the distal radial and proximal ulnar metaphyses occur, with metaphyseal flaring producing a so-called drumstick appearance. More generalized alteration of bone formation in the epimetaphyseal region may be seen. Genu valgum resulting from a hypoplastic medial tibial plateau may resemble Blount's disease. Tibiotalar slant and bony excrescences at the medial aspect of the proximal tibia are also commonly seen. The axial skeleton is largely spared, with generally normal skull and spine.[47,166] Coronal vertebral clefts may be seen.[283]

CLINICAL COMMENTS

Patients are short, with greater limb shortening distally. Skeletal anomalies of size, shape, and number, along with congenital synostoses, may be suspected clinically, but they are best assessed radiographically. Nails and teeth are agenetic or markedly dysplas-

tic. Cardiopulmonary complications often lead to death in early childhood, although some individuals survive into adulthood. Dandy-Walker malformation has been reported, but it is unclear whether this is directly related or a coincidental occurrence.[303]

KEY CONCEPTS

- *The classic patient with Ellis-van Creveld disease presents in infancy or childhood with hexadactyly, marked phalangeal and nail hypoplasia, congenital heart anomaly, typical thoracic anomalies, and genu varum.*
- *Radiologic changes reflect these clinical phenomena and reveal findings that may not be readily detected on physical examination. These include developmental metaphyseal alterations and congenital synostosis, especially carpal coalition.*

Cleidocranial Dysplasia

BACKGROUND

Despite a name that implies a process limited to the clavicle (*cleido*, meaning "clavicle") and calvarium, cleidocranial dysplasia is actually a generalized autosomal dominant dysplasia combining developmental midline spinal defects, delayed skeletal maturity, dental anomalies, and the more widely recognized skull and clavicle abnormalities. This rather rare condition was first described in 1898, but the autosomal dominant genetic abnormality has only recently been localized to the short arm of chromosome 6p.[66,81] This refutes an earlier report that the chromosomal abnormality involved was the 8q locus.[32] One third of cases represent new mutations.

As with most skeletal dysplasias, identification of specific genetic markers has vastly enhanced the ability to distinguish between conditions that share many clinical and radiographic features. This led to identification of newly described dysplasias that would otherwise have been lumped together with another more familiar or more common syndrome.[242,296] As a result, it may seem the study of skeletal dysplasias has advanced from an esoteric and uncertain exercise undertaken by a small, erudite group of pediatric and bone radiologists to a more certain (perhaps still esoteric) exercise carried out by a small (perhaps still erudite) group of geneticists. A report of cleidocranial dysplasia occurring in three consecutive genera-

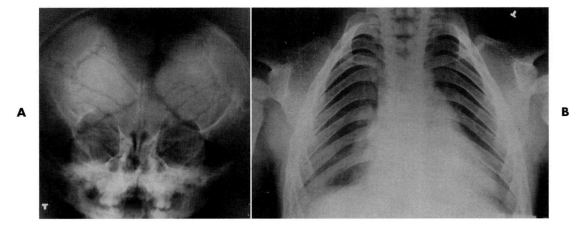

FIG. 10-3   Cleidocranial dysplasia in a 5-year-old boy with "soft shoulders," large head, prominent anterior fontanelle open down through forehead, and poor teeth. **A,** Widely open sutures and fontanelle, and wormian bones. **B,** Partial aplasia of clavicles, droopy shoulders, small scapulae, spina bifida, wide ribs. (From Taybi H, Lachman RS: *Radiology of syndromes, metabolic disorders, and skeletal dysplasias,* ed 4, St Louis, 1996, Mosby.)

tions but previously unrecognized in the first two has prompted recommendation of assessment of family members in every case of what may appear to be a sporadic occurrence of the disorder.[37]

IMAGING FINDINGS

Skull. Cleiodocranial dysplasia is characterized by multiple wormian (intrasutural) bones, especially within the lambdoid suture, frontal bossing of the calvarium, and variable hypoplasia and dysplasia of the clavicles (Fig. 10-3). Examination of the development of the cranium in neonates with this condition has revealed a marked delay in skeletal maturity over the first 6 months of life. Also, normal mineralization of the calvarium is typically grossly reduced. Calvarial size may be relatively normal, taking into account marked postpartum deformity secondary to the poor mineralization. Widening of the skull has been reported in some cases. About 60% of patients have an inverted "pear-shaped" calvarium and a persistent anterior fontanelle, one of the midline defects so typical of this disorder. The portion of the skull base formed through enchondral ossification is narrowed and shows delayed ossification. Also apparent is craniad displacement of the clivus and sella turcica, with anteriorly facing foramen magnum, often accompanied by basilar invagination. The sphenooccipital synchondrosis is widened.[117,119]

Clavicles. Fewer than 10% of patients show complete agenesis of the clavicles.[32] Other clavicular anomalies involving hypoplasia and dysplasia are consistent and specific enough that the diagnosis may be at least suspected in utero; this may aid decision making prenatally.[95]

Face and sinuses. Consistent with abnormality predominating in bones formed through intramembranous ossification, the paranasal sinuses are characteristically absent or hypoplastic. The sella turcica is often hypoplastic and the dorsum sellae is often bulbous. Nasal bones are almost always hypoplastic or agenetic. Likewise, the zygomatic arches are hypoplastic or absent.[119] All craniofacial regions are affected in cleidocranial dysplasia.[117] Even the hyoid bone may demonstrate decreased ossification.[210] The height and width of the mandible and maxilla are decreased, with anterior inclination of the mandible.[117] The coronoid process of the mandible is slender and obliquely oriented in a posterosuperior direction. Persistence of a midline suture at the mandibular symphysis is classic for cleidocranial dysplasia.[65] Facial abnormalities appear to progress with increasing age and may not be readily apparent in younger children.[119,120]

Other anomalies. Other anomalies include incompletely descended, hypoplastic scapulae, with shallow glenoid fossae. The iliac wings are hypoplastic and ossification of the pubic bones and obturator rings is delayed and deficient. Pubic diastasis is characteristic and resembles changes associated with exstrophy of the bladder (Fig. 10-4). Either coxa vara or valga may occur; the latter is more common. Long bones may be overtubulated. Fibular agenesis or congenital pseudoarthrosis of the femur may occur. In the spine, the predominant finding is spina bifida occulta, most commonly in the cervicothoracic region. Another potential anomaly is structural scoliosis resulting from vertebral segmentation anomalies. The hands may demonstrate hypoplasia of carpal bones and distal phalanges, with relative hyperplasia of the epiphyses, especially of the distal phalanges.[211] The second and fifth metacarpals are typically long and the second and fifth middle phalanges short. Supernumerary ossification centers may be apparent.

CLINICAL COMMENTS

The clinical manifestations of cleidocranial dysplasia are highly variable. Affected individuals may be somewhat below average in height. The head is large but brachycephalic, with frontal bossing

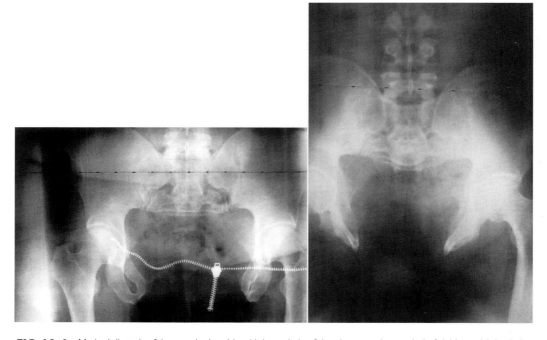

FIG. 10-4 Marked diastasis of the symphysis pubis, with hypoplasia of the obturator rings, typical of cleidocranial dysplasia, but often indistinguishable from the pelvic anomaly associated with exstrophy of the bladder. In left illustration, note zipper artifact and artifact from trifold 14-inch × 36-inch film.

and a small face. The shoulders may appear drooped and demonstrate an increased range of motion. Genu valgum and brachydactyly may also be seen. Respiratory dysfunction may result from a developmentally narrow thorax.[211]

Unlike other conditions involving midline defects and spinal dysraphism, cleidocranial dysplasia is not classically associated with neurological deficit. When present, neurological abnormality should prompt assessment for other abnormalities of the central nervous system, such as neoplasm, syringomyelia, or other developmental anomaly.[58,190] Supernumerary and other anomalous teeth are typical in cleidocranial dysplasia, previously necessitating a long and often difficult regimen of surgical and orthodontic intervention, frequently with limited success. However, a strategy has been devised to successfully predict the development of supernumerary teeth before the permanent teeth are fully developed. This allows extraction of the supernumerary teeth and, when indicated, of the primary teeth and overlying bone, which improves eruption of the remaining permanent teeth.[118,213]

■ KEY CONCEPTS

- *Although neonatal respiratory distress may result from dysplasia of the thoracic cage, individuals with cleidocranial dysplasia may be remarkably normal clinically, despite rather diffuse skeletal anomalies.*
- *The most classic anomalies include midline skeletal defects, especially mild spinal dysraphism (spina bifida occulta) and clavicular anomalies, usually in the form of hypoplasia or partial agenesis.*

Congenital Insensitivity to Pain

BACKGROUND

Congenital insensitivity to pain is sometimes described as "indifference to pain." This, however, is somewhat misleading and implies that pain is perceived but ignored. Instead, a basic lack of or marked diminution in pain perception exists, whereas all other sensory findings are normal. The condition, first described in 1932, may spare sensation of light touch and deep tendon reflexes may be normal.

IMAGING FINDINGS

The radiographic findings of congenital insensitivity to pain are those in common with other neuropathic conditions and summarized as the classic *6 D's* of neuroarthropathy, or "degenerative joint disease with a vengeance." These include joint destruction, disorganization, diminished joint space, intraarticular debris (detritus), joint distention, and reactive subchondral sclerosis (density). Because of its presence from infancy, congenital insensitivity to pain typically leads to disruption of the physes, essentially representing insufficiency fracture through the growth plate. This also may be evident in children with spinal dysraphism. Extensive subperiosteal hemorrhage may also occur, which, along with periarticular disintegration and fragmentation, has been mistaken for child abuse.[252] In the spine, radiographic changes are similar to the changes seen in neuroarthropathy resulting from syphilis or diabetic neuropathy.[198]

In addition to neuroarthropathy, patients with congenital insensitivity to pain may have complicating infections, of both the soft tissues and skeleton. This results from a chronic open wound resulting from an abrasion, burn, or other superficial injury.[188] Such infections may necessitate amputation. Other complications that may necessitate extensive orthopedic or neurosurgical intervention include pathologic fracture, dislocation, autoamputation, and rapidly progressing scoliosis.[90,99]

CLINICAL COMMENTS

Generally, the abnormality is manifested in infancy or early childhood as a marked absence of reaction to pain stimuli, frequently with cutaneous manifestations of scars and burns, unnoticed by the child. Self-mutilation and aggressive behavior may occur, especially in conjunction with Lesch-Nyhan syndrome or familial dysautonomia (Riley-Day syndrome). Patients with these and related hereditary sensory neuropathies (HSN) or dysautonomic conditions may also suffer from mental retardation, anhidrosis (inability to sweat), and resultant alteration of thermoregulation.[57,185]

A distinct form of congenital insensitivity to pain with anhidrosis (CIPA) has been identified, also known as *hereditary sensory and autonomic neuropathy type IV.* Nearly 20% of patients with this disorder die within the first 3 years of life because of hyperpyrexia.[220] At least five variants of HSN exist and in some cases, a precise distinction of one disorder from another may not be possible without prolonged follow-up and nerve biopsy. Reports detail patients initially diagnosed with congenital insensitivity to pain, who were later determined to have a hereditary sensory and autonomic neuropathy.[141] Nerve biopsies reveal loss of nonmyelinated and small myelinated fibers.[220]

Recently, abnormalities of muscle have also been reported in patients with congenital insensitivity to pain. Clinically, muscle weakness and hyporeflexia or areflexia may be evident. Histologically and anatomically, the involved muscle demonstrates marked variation in fiber size, some small fibers having central nuclei and a few small angulated fibers.[261]

■ KEY CONCEPTS

- *The classic patient with congenital insensitivity to pain is an infant or young child with traumas involving burns, abrasions, and other wounds initially unnoticed by the patient and parents.*
- *Repeated traumas to joints and surrounding structures, resulting from a lack of protective proprioceptive feedback, lead to an appearance of "degenerative joint disease with a vengeance."*
- *Developing physes are vulnerable to insufficiency fractures, with significant fragmentation and other architectural distortion.*
- *A loose periosteum in infants and children and subperiosteal hemorrhage may lead to remarkable periosteal reaction.*
- *Severe burns may be associated with joint contractures.*

Developmental Dysplasia of the Hip

BACKGROUND

Developmental dysplasia of the hip (DDH) is lateral displacement of the hip with varying degrees of acetabular dysplasia. In the past, the condition was termed *congenital hip dysplasia.* However, more recent literature suggests a developmental and not congenital etiology.

IMAGING FINDINGS

The hip may be partially or completely dislocated. Displacement is difficult to detect at the time of birth because of the incomplete mineralization of the hip and pelvis. Classic imaging findings are summarized in Putti's triad, which describes lateral displacement of the femur, a small or absent femoral capital epiphysis, and increased acetabular angulation (Fig. 10-5). Roentgenometrics are useful tools to assess the acetabular angle and to determine whether lateral superior displacement of the hip has occurred. The acetabular center-edge angle and acetabular index are useful measures of the acetabular angle. Shenton's line and the iliofemoral line are helpful to

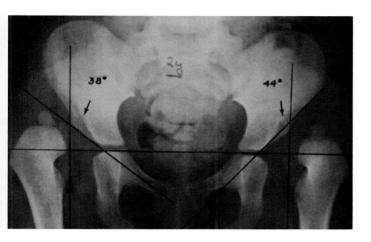

FIG. 10-5   Bilateral developmental dysplasia of the hip (DDH) in a girl 2 years of age. Putti's triad is present on both sides; the right acetabular angle is enlarged to 38 degrees, the left to 44 degrees. The arrow point to bilateral false acetabula. (From Silverman FN, Kuhn JP: *Caffey's pediatric x-ray diagnosis: an integrated imaging approach*, ed 9, St. Louis, 1993, Mosby.)

assess for displacement. These roentgenometrics are presented in Chapter 3. Ultrasonography, arthrography, and computer tomography are useful to further delineate the anatomy of the hip and acetabulum. In particular, these modalities are useful to locate the position of the acetabular labrum, which affects clinical outcome.

CLINICAL COMMENTS

Detection of displacement is accomplished largely through the application of appropriate imaging. Ortolani's and Barlow's orthopedic maneuvers are helpful and suggestive of the condition. Early detection is paramount. Management is most effective when the condition is detected early, preferably in the neonatal period. Mild cases can be successfully treated by keeping the hips in a position of flexion and abduction. This may be accomplished by double or triple diapering the infant. In more advanced cases, a Pavlik harness is used to maintain hip flexion and abduction. When conservative treatment fails, surgery may be indicated to achieve reduction.

Successful reduction is largely dependent on the location of the acetabular labrum. If the labrum is displaced lateral to the femoral head, reduction is achieved with good outcome. However, if the labrum becomes inverted into the acetabulum during lateral displacement of the hip, successful reduction is more difficult.

KEY CONCEPTS

- *Developmental hip dysplasia describes lateral displacement of the proximal femur with related dysplasia of the acetabulum.*
- *Classic imaging findings are summarized in Putti's triad, which describes the lateral displacement of the femur, a small or absent femoral capital epiphysis, and increased acetabular angulation.*
- *Ultrasonography, arthography, and computed tomography are useful modalities to demonstrate the position of the acetabular labrum, the location of which affects clinical outcome.*
- *Management is most effective when the condition is detected early.*

Diastrophic Dysplasia

BACKGROUND

This autosomal recessive dwarfing dysplasia derives its name from the twisted appearance of the spine and extremities resulting from

scoliosis, which may be progressive, as well as deformities, contractures, subluxations, and dislocations of the extremities. The condition is particularly common in Finland, although the reason is not clear. A study from the University of Helsinki demonstrated ankle and foot anomalies in 93% of cases, with the most common deformity involving combined metatarsal valgus and metatarsus adductus or equinovarus.[226]

IMAGING FINDINGS

General. Radiographic changes are consistent with the dwarfing and diffuse skeletal deformities seen clinically (Fig. 10-6). Severe peripheral deformities typically lead to early, advanced degenerative joint disease, which may necessitate arthroplasty.[193] Tubular bones are markedly shortened and metaphyses are widened, which does not help much in distinguishing this from other dwarfing conditions.

Hands. The first metacarpal is characteristically more severely affected and may be oval in shape. The carpal bones may demonstrate multiple accessory ossification centers, premature ossification, and deformity.

Epiphyses. The appearance of epiphyseal ossification centers is delayed, and other epiphyseal changes, which tend to be most marked at the proximal femora, resemble those of severe Legg-Calvè-Perthes disease. Developmental joint space narrowing may occur, and equinovarus deformity is common.[211]

Spine. Severe cervical kyphosis resulting from dysplastic vertebrae occurs in about one third of patients and may reach 180 degrees, with the spine literally folded upon itself. Unlike extremity deformities, which typically increase as the child ages, some of these kyphoses will completely resolve by adulthood. Others may lead to myelopathy or even death.[15] Scoliosis occurs in about one third of all patients, but it is more common in females, seen in about 50%. Although they typically develop at a much younger age than idiopathic scolioses (usually apparent by 2 to 4 years of age), fewer than 15% of these curves will progress to beyond 50 degrees.[201] Diastrophic dysplasia represents a rare cause of atlantoaxial subluxation.[212] Congenital central spinal canal stenosis often occurs, with a narrowed interpediculate distance, although this is not as marked nor as consistent as in achondroplasia.

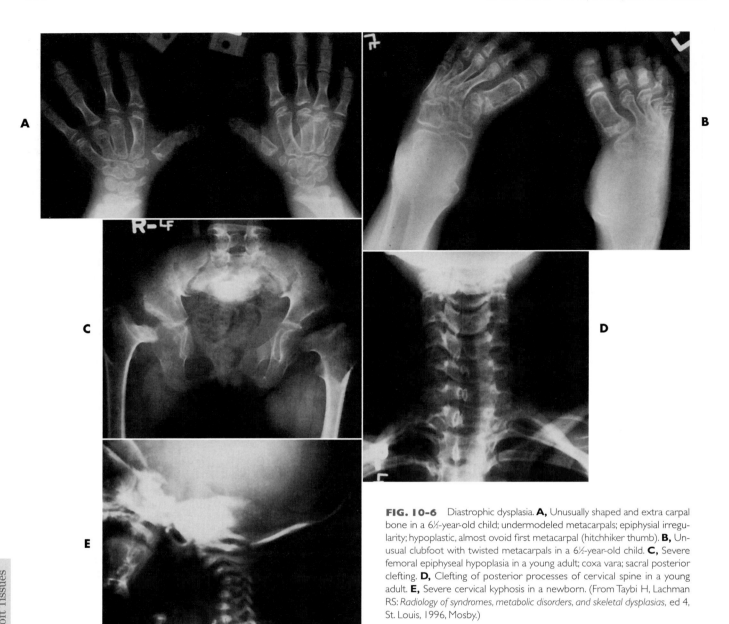

FIG. 10-6   Diastrophic dysplasia. **A,** Unusually shaped and extra carpal bone in a 6½-year-old child; undermodeled metacarpals; epiphysial irregularity; hypoplastic, almost ovoid first metacarpal (hitchhiker thumb). **B,** Unusual clubfoot with twisted metacarpals in a 6½-year-old child. **C,** Severe femoral epiphyseal hypoplasia in a young adult; coxa vara; sacral posterior clefting. **D,** Clefting of posterior processes of cervical spine in a young adult. **E,** Severe cervical kyphosis in a newborn. (From Taybi H, Lachman RS: *Radiology of syndromes, metabolic disorders, and skeletal dysplasias,* ed 4, St. Louis, 1996, Mosby.)

CLINICAL COMMENTS

Clubfoot deformity has frequently been reported in the literature, although a true clubfoot (talipes equinovarus) is actually not seen. Hands and feet are short and broad, demonstrating a characteristic abduction or "hitchhiker" deformity of the thumbs and great toes. Peculiar cystic masses develop on the external ears, resulting in clinically apparent deformity. Cleft palate is seen in about 75% of cases, although only about half of these are open and clinically obvious.[214]

Expression is variable, with some patients attaining a normal lifespan and others dying in infancy from respiratory complications. A milder form of diastrophic dysplasia has been referred to, probably inappropriately, as "diastrophic variant."[110,137] Conversely, particularly severe cases with cervical spine dislocations and congenital heart anomalies have previously been considered by some to represent a unique lethal form of the condition.[91]

KEY CONCEPTS

- *The most classic features in diastrophic dysplasia include a progressive kyphoscoliosis and narrowed interpediculate distance in the spine, especially in the lumbar region.*
- *The hands and feet demonstrate supernumerary, delta-shaped epiphyses; the typical deformity of the thumb is described as a "hitchhiker's thumb."*
- *Severe kyphoscoliosis, which may demonstrate remarkable improvement over time, is common.*

Down Syndrome

BACKGROUND

Down syndrome was first described in 1959 in individuals with ocular abnormality, dystonia, mental and developmental retardation, brachycephaly, and macroglossia. Although most affected individuals abnormally demonstrate 47 chromosomes, this "trisomy 21" configuration is absent in 5% to 10% of individuals with the typical phenotype. Such cases exhibit translocation and mosaicism.[289] A well-known relationship exists between advancing maternal age and an increased incidence of trisomy 21. Women over 35 years of age are typically offered prenatal testing. Maternal serum markers have more recently been used, typically to detect unborn babies in the second trimester at risk for Down syndrome. The first of these serum markers to be used was maternal serum alpha-fetoprotein (MSAFP), but unconjugated estriol (uE3) and human chorionic gonadotropin (hCG) are also being used. None of these is infallible and there remains some controversy regarding which is the best method of detection in utero. Combining measurement of MSAFP and free-beta HCG with maternal age reportedly results in an 80% detection rate and a 5% false-positive rate. This would still leave mothers with a 1 chance in 20 of choosing to abort a normal baby in response to a positive test and a 1 chance in 5 of having a baby with Down syndrome, despite a negative test.[150]

IMAGING FINDINGS

Atlantoaxial instability. The single most important articulation to evaluate in a patient with Down syndrome is the anterior atlantoaxial articulation, which is subluxated or unstable in 20% of affected individuals.[170] The most critical ligamentous structure to assess is the transverse ligament. The most crucial plain film study is a lateral cervical film with head nod or flexion to evaluate for anterior atlantoaxial subluxation or the far less commonly atlantooccipital instability. This is essential, especially with patients in whom activity, anticipated therapy (especially spinal manipulation), or past atlantoaxial surgical fusion may place the upper cervical complex or craniovertebral junction at risk.[221]

The relationship between Down syndrome and congenital laxity of the transverse portion of the cruciate ligament of C1 is well known and is generally considered to be the primary etiology for most cases of atlantoaxial instability and subluxation. However, other factors such as odontoid hypoplasia and dysplasia, along with upper respiratory infections and trauma, are believed to contribute.[159,270] The atlantoaxial relationship in Down syndrome does not tend to change significantly over time, at least in asymptomatic individuals. Unless a clinical indication exists, serial lateral and flexion lateral cervical radiographs should not be necessary.[205]

Atlas hypoplasia. A lesser-known, associated anomaly is a developmentally short posterior arch of C1, seen in just over one quarter of patients in one study.[160] This could present a sort of "double jeopardy" in the presence of atlantoaxial instability. This anomaly is readily detected on lateral cervical radiographs and appears as an anterior displacement of the spinolaminar junction line of C1 relative to that of C2. When anterior atlantoaxial subluxation is present resulting from abnormality of the transverse ligament, it is difficult to estimate the potential contribution to spinal canal stenosis by a short posterior arch. Down syndrome patients also have an increased incidence of occipitoatlantal hypermobility and instability. Anteroposterior translation of the occiput between the neutral and fully flexed neck posture averages about 0.6 mm in normal individuals. A measurement of more than 1 mm in an adult implies instability. A study of 38 children with Down syndrome demonstrated an average of 2.3 mm, with a range from 0 to 6.4 mm. However, only one of these patients had symptoms that might be attributed to occipitoatlantal instability. The clinical implications are not entirely clear, but caution is indicated and craniovertebral junction instability is possible, even in the presence of an apparently stable atlantoaxial articulation.[162]

Cervical spine. Other abnormalities of the cervical spine identified on plain film radiographs include an unusually high incidence of degenerative joint changes in the mid to upper cervical spine, congenital synostosis, and developmental platyspondyly. A relationship is reported between Down syndrome and small separate ossicles in the upper cervical region, thought to represent avulsions of the distal aspect of the dens rather than associated anomalies.[76] Partial or complete hypopneumatization of the sphenoid sinus may also be noted on the lateral cervical neutral view, although typically without clinical relevance.[170,265] Other abnormalities associated with Down syndrome include inconsequential but classic findings, such as a prominent conoid tubercle of the clavicle.[280]

Organ systems. A variety of other anomalies have been reported in individuals with Down syndrome, affecting virtually all organ systems. Plain film radiography may be used to identify infants with duodenal atresia, the most common gastrointestinal anomaly, or thoracic anomalies such as diaphragmatic hernia. Angiography may demonstrate anomaly of the radial, anterior interosseous, ulnar, subclavian, or vertebral artery.[149,209]

Other anomalies. Milder skeletal changes include rib anomalies, especially agenesis of the twelfth ribs, microcephaly with hypopneumatized sinuses and clinodactyly and brachydactyly, with hypoplasia of the middle phalanx of the fifth digit, seen in about 60% of patients. Characteristics may include a short, arched hard palate, a small posterior fossa, and calcification of the basilar ganglia, best demonstrated on CT.[113,215] Accessory epiphyses and supernumerary ossification centers of the manubrium may be seen in as many as 90% of patients.[46,215] Knee pain and dysfunction should prompt an evaluation for patellofemoral dislocation, which may be present in about 4% to 8% of individuals with Down syndrome but is rarely disabling.[60] Infants with Down syndrome demonstrate flared iliac wings and flat acetabular roofs. In ambulatory adult patients, this may contribute to hip instability and frequently early, advanced osteoarthritis.[112]

SPECIALIZED IMAGING

Computed tomography (CT) and magnetic resonance imaging (MRI) have demonstrated a variety of intracranial abnormalities, including abnormally large sylvian fissures, mega cisterna magna, and cerebellar hypoplasia. Hippocampal and neocortical structures are smaller, whereas the parahippocampal gyrus is larger in Down patients. CT may demonstrate intracranial calcification in as many as 85% of patients, most of which are not directly associated with clinical findings. These calcifications affect the basal ganglia, choroid plexus, and pineal gland. However, some overlap is likely with normal physiologic calcification, because a high percentage of normal individuals will demonstrate similar calcifications.[3] It does not appear that these calcifications are related to the increased incidence of seizure disorders in patients with Down syndrome.[254]

Older adult Down patients experience greater ventricular dilatation, peripheral atrophy, and deep white matter lesions when compared with the normal aging population. Vascular studies demonstrate decreasing cerebral perfusion, presumably related to altered blood-brain barrier permeability. Dynamic MRI shows a fluctuating cortical CSF volume in aging Down patients, similar to otherwise normal elderly individuals with shunted hydrocephalus. This finding, first reported in 1995, suggests a relationship between aging in Down syndrome and edematous states of the brain.[64]

CLINICAL COMMENTS

Leukemia. One of the most serious complications of Down syndrome is leukemia, with about 50% of cases representing acute megakaryoblastic leukemia (AMKL). This form typically occurs by age 4 years. It is preceded by a transient leukemia (TL), involving a megakaryoblastosis that clears by 3 months of age. Between 20% and 30% of infants with TL will, however, develop AMKL.[306] Transient leukemoid reactions, myelofibrosis, and leukemia may all result from an increased sensitivity of cells to interferon in patients with Down syndrome. This results in aberrant antigen expression, which leads to autoimmune disease. In the bone marrow, this may manifest itself as premature egress of blast cells as in TL inflammation, incomplete repair as in myelofibrosis, and binding of autoantibodies to cell nuclei, resulting in malignant transformation and leukemia.[305]

Atlantoaxial instability. A second potentially life-threatening complication commonly encountered is atlantoaxial subluxation and instability. In otherwise neurologically intact individuals, the only clinical finding that may have some predictive value for the presence of this condition is gait disturbance, but in 180 children with Down syndrome, the sensitivity of this finding was only 50%, with a specificity of 81%.[234] This study failed to identify any reliable clinical indicators of atlantoaxial subluxation or instability. This study also concluded that x-rays, like clinical indicators, were not reliable for detecting this complication, although other studies concluded differently. Measurement of the anterior atlantodental interspace on neutral and flexion lateral cervical radiographs is still typically performed to identify at-risk individuals.[170,221,265] This includes those being considered for spinal manipulation, those participating in contact sports, and preoperatively in patients being anesthetized, especially for otolaryngeal surgery.[97,171]

OTHER FINDINGS

In addition to the features described in the original syndrome, gastrointestinal anomalies, especially duodenal atresia, are typical.[246] Cardiac anomalies and pulmonary hypertension are frequent, with congenital heart disease found in some 40% to 50% of patients. Atrioventricular and ventriculoseptal defects and tetralogy of Fallot are among the most common, whereas certain other anomalies, including situs inversus and transposition of the great vessels are distinctly uncommon.[158] In about a dozen reports, Down syndrome has been associated with moyamoya disease, an intracranial vascular anomaly.[14] About 40% of patients have developmental dysplasia of the hips.[142,215] Tracheal, anorectal, and esophageal anomalies are also seen.[271,282] A characteristic form of subpleural cystic pulmonary disease has been reported, which is typically difficult to appreciate on plain films and may require high-resolution CT of the chest.[92]

Down syndrome is associated with celiac disease. Because of other common abdominal complaints, considerable delay may frequently occur in diagnosing celiac disease in Down patients, when compared with otherwise normal patients. The length of time between initial symptoms and diagnosis averages 2.5 years in Down patients versus 8 months in non-Down patients.[104] This condition should be suspected in any child showing failure to thrive, especially when accompanied by chronic diarrhea.[104]

An increased incidence of a variety of autoimmune diseases occurs in Down syndrome, including thyroid disease. Although hypothyroidism is most common, reports exist of hyperthyroidism in the form of classic Graves' disease.[264]

In addition to gastrointestinal and autoimmune diseases, males with Down syndrome seem to have an increased risk for testicular cancer.[72]

KEY CONCEPTS

- *Down syndrome, or trisomy 21, produces classic clinical features and is typically diagnosed or at least suspected prior to radiography.*
- *Plain film radiographs and other diagnostic imaging studies are typically obtained to assess for the multitude of associated anomalies seen in this condition.*
- *These anomalies affect most organ systems, including the gastrointestinal tract, cardiovascular system, and skeletal system.*
- *Potentially life-threatening atlantoaxial subluxation and instability are special concerns even after other serious internal organ system anomalies have been ruled out in the prenatal and neonatal period.*

Homocystinuria

BACKGROUND

Homocystinuria is actually a group of three related genetic abnormalities resulting in a deficiency of cystathionine synthetase, the enzyme that metabolizes methionine. The autosomal recessive condition was first described in the early 1960s as a variant of Marfan's syndrome and is most common in individuals of northern European descent.[35,83,84,168,245]

According to common belief, homocystinuria results in abnormal aldehyde cross-linkages and defective collagen synthesis, similar to the pathogenesis of Ehlers-Danlos syndrome, Marfan's syndrome, and osteogenesis imperfecta. It should be no surprise, therefore, that these conditions share features, especially radiographically. However, homocystinuria has actually been classified with alkaptonuria (ochronosis), Menke's syndrome, and pseudoxanthoma elasticum because it secondarily affects the fibrous components of connective tissues.[123,167]

IMAGING FINDINGS

Osteopenia. The imaging findings in homocystinuria may be nonspecific and are not present at birth. Osteopenia is a typical finding and is believed to result from deficiency of collagen cross-linking rather than a gross deficiency in collagen itself.[152] The presence of osteoporosis, often with multiple compression fractures, helps to distinguish homocystinuria from Marfan's syndrome.

Skeleton. Skeletal abnormalities occur in up to 60% of patients. They closely resemble Marfan's syndrome. Extremities are long and thin and patients are usually above average in height. Arachnodactyly is typically seen. Multiple growth resumption lines may be present. Scoliosis, pectus excavatum, and generalized joint laxity may appear to be identical to Marfan's syndrome. Joint contractures may occur in the knees, elbows, and digits, whereas such contractures are usually limited to the fifth digits in Marfan's syndrome. Ligamentous laxity may result in genu valgum, patella alta, and repeated subluxations. Infants and children may demonstrate metaphyseal flaring and irregularity of epiphyseal ossification centers.

Other reports include a variety of other less common or less classic imaging findings diffusely affecting the skeleton, in addition to vascular calcification and medullary sponge kidney.[28,31,45,168]

Skull and facial changes in homocystinuria include sinus expansion, a widened diploic space, prognathism, and dural calcification.[168,245] The spine may show early advanced degenerative disc disease, and posterior vertebral body scalloping may be present.

This appears to be a primary developmental abnormality rather than a pressure-related change, as occurs in dural ectasia.[28,245]

The radiographic changes of homocystinuria may be distinguished from Marfan's syndrome primarily by osteoporosis, flared metaphyses, and joint contractures, which are absent in Marfan's syndrome.[28,245]

CLINICAL COMMENTS

Homocystinuria is generally asymptomatic in infants and very young children, although urinary levels of homocystine are increased. Skin lesions begin to develop, including a malar flush, striae over the extremities and buttocks, and "cigarette paper" scars. The palate is high and arched and dentition is poor. Hair is usually thin and sparse.[168]

Homocystinuria affects primarily the central nervous system, eye, skeleton, and cardiovascular system. Increased homocystine levels are strongly correlated to atherosclerotic, coronary artery, and thromboembolic disease. Cardiopulmonary diseases are the most common causes of death.[49] Although cystic medial necrosis occurs, as in Marfan's syndrome, aortic dissection, a common cause of premature death in Marfan's syndrome, is not generally seen in homocystinuria. Accumulation of homocystine may adversely affect platelets, clotting factors, and vascular endothelial cells.

It is believed that individuals with deficiencies of vitamin B_6, B_{12}, or folic acid or who are heterozygous for cystathionine synthetase deficiency are at increased risk for occlusive vascular disease and that supplementation may lower the plasma homocystine levels in some affected individuals.[31,163,217] Diets low in methionine and supplementation with betaine or its precursor choline may be beneficial in management of homocystinuria.[248,287] Decision making, especially when considering elective surgery, must reflect the fact that surgeries increase the risk for vascular catastrophies.[28]

The most characteristic ocular lesion is dislocation of the lens, also seen in Marfan's syndrome. Lens dislocation may be detected in infancy in homocystinuria, but not in Marfan's syndrome.[28] Other optic anomalies may also occur, including congenital cataracts and glaucoma.

Unlike Marfan's syndrome, central nervous system involvement leading to mental deficit and seizures is seen in about 30% of patients, although the pathogenesis has not been clearly delineated. CNS complications may be modified by therapy.[245]

KEY CONCEPTS
- *Homocystine and methionine accumulate in the tissues as a result of an autosomal recessive deficiency of cystathionine synthetase.*
- *The accumulation of homocystine and methionine leads to mental deficit in 60% of patients and marfanoid features, including tall, thin stature, and arachnodactyly, as well as scoliosis, pectus excavatum or carinatum, and genu valgum.*
- *Vascular changes are similar to those of Marfan's syndrome, with medial degeneration of arteries.*
- *Lens subluxation, common to both conditions, is typically inferior in homocystinuria and superior in Marfan's syndrome.*
- *Osteoporosis is a distinctive feature of homocystinuria, as is the presence of flared metaphyses and diffuse joint contractures.*

Klippel-Feil Syndrome

BACKGROUND

As with so many other syndromes bearing the name of long-dead scholars who cannot defend or explain themselves, the Klippel-Feil syndrome has gradually evolved from a concise clinical triad to a confusing collection of loosely related vertebral anomalies. Purists still apply the term to only the same triad first described in 1912 by Klippel and Feil without benefit of radiographs. They described patients with a short neck, low hairline, and restricted cervical range of motion, although these features were not carefully quantified. They also described anomalies of the skull base and thoracic cage, which have received little attention over the years.[131,132] It has subsequently been discovered that such patients typically demonstrate vertebral segmentation anomalies, primarily in the form of congenital nonsegmentation ("block vertebrae").

Today, whether proper or improper, the term has been expanded to include any situation with nonsegmentation of even a single vertebral motion unit. In the context of this broadened definition, fewer than 50% of individuals with the requisite segmentation anomalies demonstrate the complete clinical triad. A diagnosis that was once dictated by clinical findings is now made primarily on the basis of radiographic changes.

IMAGING FINDINGS

Congenital nonsegmentation most commonly affects vertebral level C2-C3. About two thirds of cases involving C2-C3 nonsegmentation also involve assimilation of C1 to occiput ("occipitalization" of C1). Nonsegmentation varies from minimal to extensive and may be continuous or intermittent, with intervening normal disc levels (Figs. 10-7, 10-8, and 10-9). The anomaly may extend caudally to the mid to upper thoracic spine, and some cases may involve similar nonsegmentation in the lower thoracic and lumbar regions. At some levels, incomplete or abbreviated forms of congenital nonsegmentation may occur. Associated anomalies may exist, especially spina bifida occulta and hemivertebrae, which are seen in about 20% of cases and may be associated with structural scoliosis and kyphosis. Intraspinal anomalies such as syringomyelia and diastematomyelia may occur.[78]

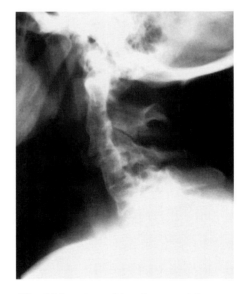

FIG. 10-7 Klippel-Feil syndrome. Note the congenital nonsegmentation and dysplasia of C2 through C4 and C5-C6, with only two functional disc spaces in the cervical spine. Assimilation of the C1 posterior arch to occiput and marked hypoplasia of the dens are also noted. The neck appears to be short, which would be more obvious clinically, along with a low hairline and diminished range of motion. Similar vertebral segmentation anomalies may also be seen as an isolated finding or in other syndromes, including neurofibromatosis.

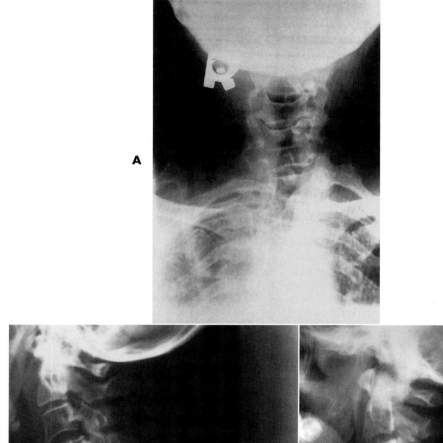

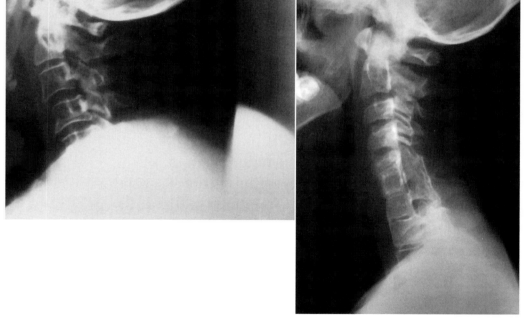

FIG. 10-8　Klippel-Feil syndrome with classic clinical and radiographic findings. **A,** 62-year-old female with multiple vertebral segmentation anomalies and rib anomalies at the cervicothoracic junction. Sprengel's anomaly represents failure of descent of the right scapula. **B,** On the lateral view marked cervicothoracic kyphosis is obvious, with soft tissue prominence resembling the "buffalo hump" of Cushing's syndrome or the "dowager's hump" of osteoporosis. The vertebral anomalies themselves would go unnoticed, without a swimmer's view. **C,** Younger female with classic segmentation anomalies in the cervicothoracic region.

Other skeletal anomalies commonly accompany the vertebral segmentation anomalies. Failure of descent (often improperly described as "elevation") of one or both scapulae is seen in about 25% of cases and is more common in patients with extensive and upper cervical involvement. This deformity may be surgically corrected.[36,181] Between 30% and 40% of Sprengel's deformity will be associated with an omovertebral "bone," an osseous, fibrous, or cartilaginous structure extending from the scapula (*omo-*, meaning "scapula") to the posterior vertebral elements, most often in the mid to lower cervical region. Solid fusion or an accessory articulation may exist at both the scapular and vertebral junctions.[181] Similar bones have been reported extending from the upper ribs or clavicles

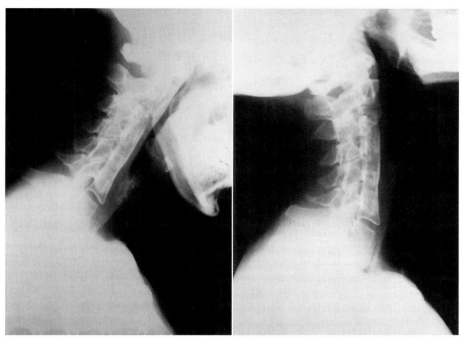

FIG. 10-9 Extensive congenital nonsegmentation of C3 through C6. The more normal C2-C3 and C6-C7 motion units at the cephalic and caudal ends of the nonsegmentation are prone to hypermobility/instability and subsequent premature degenerative disc disease and facet arthrosis.

to the vertebrae, although these are rare.[88] Cervical ribs, Srb's anomaly, and a variety of rib anomalies, including agenesis or synostosis, are common in Klippel-Feil syndrome.

Craniovertebral junction anomalies may accompany Klippel-Feil syndrome. Basilar impression is common, with or without assimilation of C1 to occiput. Diagnosis of basilar impression is based upon observance of the tip of the dens projecting significantly above McGregor's line on a well-positioned lateral skull or lateral cervical neutral view. Chiari type I malformation may also occur, in which the cerebellar tonsils project significantly below the foramen magnum and herniate into the region typically occupied by the upper cervical cord. Dens anomalies may also be seen. Imaging of the thorax, abdomen, and pelvis may be ordered based upon clinical findings and may demonstrate common anomalies such as cardiac anomalies (especially septal defects), enteric cysts, accessory lobes of the lung, and anomalies of the urinary tract.[101]

CLINICAL COMMENTS

Klippel-Feil syndrome affects males and females equally. The prevalence of congenital nonsegmentation of at least one spinal motion segment has been estimated to be as high as 0.5% in the general population.[236] In Klippel-Feil syndrome, the segmentation defects tend to be more extensive and may be associated with neurological deficit, most often seen with marked upper cervical and craniovertebral junction anomalies. Many patients, however, are relatively asymptomatic. Cosmetic concerns, including associated spinal curvatures, scapular elevation, or pterygium colli (webbed neck), may first drive the patient to seek clinical attention.

Lateral flexion and rotation motion are most markedly restricted, with lesser decrease in sagittal plane rotation (flexion-extension). The head may appear to be resting on the shoulders. Patients may present with acute torticollis. Other signs and symptoms range from

neck pain to paresis and paralysis. Hyperreflexia and pathologic reflexes may occur, such as upward-going toes on Babinski testing, signifying an upper motor neuron lesion. Neurological deficit may be gradual in onset or may appear acutely, secondary to often trivial trauma. Cranial nerve dysfunction may also occur, including oculomotor disturbance. Some patients may demonstrate cardiopulmonary, gastroenteric, or genitourinary tract anomalies.

KEY CONCEPTS

- *As most frequently defined today, the Klippel-Feil syndrome is a classic clinical triad of short neck, low hairline, and diminished cervical range of motion, associated with radiographic evidence of multiple vertebral segmentation anomalies.*
- *Commonly, one or more possibly occult underlying anomalies of the internal organ systems occur, especially of the genitourinary tract.*
- *A wide variety of other clinically or radiographically apparent findings have been described in this heterogeneous syndrome.*

Marfan's Syndrome

BACKGROUND

Marfan's syndrome is an autosomal dominant disorder of connective tissues primarily affecting the ocular, cardiovascular, and musculoskeletal systems. As many as 30% of cases may be due to sporadic mutations. The condition bears the name of Antonin Marfan, who first described the phenotype in 1896. Marfan's syndrome is estimated to affect between 4 and 6 people per 100,000.[154,304] Several famous characters from history were, at one time or another, believed to have had Marfan's syndrome. This includes Mary, Queen of Scots, and musicians and composers Niccolo Paganini and Rachmaninov.[33,156,298] Despite significant investigation and impressive advances in understanding this condition, Marfan's syndrome remains, in many ways, an enigma. Numerous questions have gone unanswered regarding the precise etiology of the ligamentous laxity, muscular hypotonia, and skeletal changes that characterize this disorder.[154]

IMAGING FINDINGS

In addition to clinically apparent scoliosis and other postural changes, protrusio acetabulum has been reported in nearly half of a study group of 22 patients.[136] This was bilateral in 50% of cases. When the protrusio was unilateral, it occurred on the side of a scoliotic convexity 90% of the time. Presumably, the inherent abnormality of formation of connective tissues in combination with altered stresses associated with scoliosis leads to protrusio acetabulum in Marfan's syndrome.[136]

Another associated abnormality emphasizing the generalized effects of Marfan's syndrome on connective tissues is dural ectasia, which may first be suspected on the basis of pedicle thinning, posterior body scalloping, or erosion and widening of the interpediculate distance on plain films (Fig. 10-10). Although the condition may be asymptomatic and found incidentally, follow-up MRI is indicated to exclude other more serious space-occupying lesions of the central spinal canal associated with similar pedicle or central canal changes on plain films.[197,255] Multiple meningeal cysts have also been reported in Marfan's syndrome and may result in similar gradual pressure erosion of the neural arch or posterior vertebral body margin.[216,218] Also, bones may appear long and thin (dolichostenomelia) (see Fig. 10-10).

CLINICAL COMMENTS

The clinical features overlap considerably in several related disorders characterized by dolichostenomelia (abnormally long limbs) and arachnodactyly (spiderlike digits). Patients may demonstrate Marfanoid habitus, with tall stature and arachnodactyly, yet not truly have Marfan's syndrome. A biomolecular assay is valuable in firmly establishing the diagnosis. In as many as 50% of cases, patients initially diagnosed as having Marfan's syndrome may be reclassified.[276] In some instances, patients may demonstrate an incomplete Marfanoid phenotype, whereas other family members have unequivocal Marfan's syndrome.

Initially, the most noticeable clinical features include tall stature, exceeding the 95th percentile for age, race, and sex in most cases. The condition is more common in blacks. Long, gracile limbs and digits are also readily apparent, as well as hyperextendable joints (especially genu recurvatum), frequently with history of subluxation, secondary to generalized ligamentous laxity. Scoliosis, an akyphotic thoracic spine, and pectus excavatum are also typical. Subcutaneous fat and muscular atrophy exaggerate the skeletal changes. The arm span may equal or exceed the height. The ratio of the upper body segment (from vertex of skull to symphysis pubis) versus the lower body segment (from symphysis pubis to the floor) is often greatly reduced, but this is variable, significantly affected by scoliosis. This clinical feature is not diagnostic, although suggestive of the diagnosis. The maximally apposed thumb overlaps the ulnar aspect of the hand ("thumb sign"), and when one hand grasps the opposite wrist, the first and fifth distal phalanges overlap ("wrist sign"). These latter signs are also not definitive and may be seen in some normal individuals.[154]

From 50% to 80% of patients have cephalic lens dislocation in the eye. This is usually bilateral and typically present at birth. The zonules remain intact and the eye accommodates normally. In contrast, homocystinuria, which resembles Marfan's in various ways, demonstrates caudal lens dislocation, with zonular disintegration and lack of accommodation. Myopia and retinal detachment are frequent complications of Marfan's syndrome because of increased axial length of the globe. This, along with flattening of the corneas, contributes to impaired visual acuity.[43]

The cardiovascular complications of Marfan's syndrome are more serious and well known. These include mitral valve prolapse, mitral regurgitation, aortic root dilatation, aortic regurgitation, and proximal aortic dissection, which is the most immediately life-threatening complication commonly occurring in Marfan's syndrome. Sudden onset of severe chest pain should prompt consider-

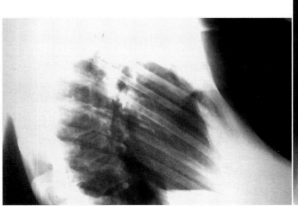
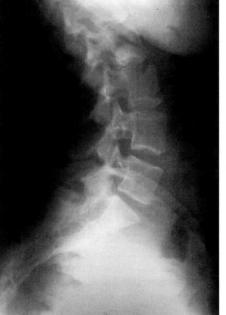

FIG. 10-10 Marfan's syndrome in a young adult black female not previously diagnosed. **A,** Note "tall" lumbar vertebrae and gracile ribs along with pectus excavatum. **B,** The sacrum is also remarkably thin and elongated—a "tall" sacrum.

ation of either aortic dissection or spontaneous pneumothorax, another complication of Marfan's syndrome Mitral valve prolapse and aortic root dilatation are the most common cardiovascular complications, with one or both present in at least 80% of patients. Although mitral prolapse is frequently associated with dyspnea, chest pain, palpitations, and lightheadedness, aortic root dilatation is usually asymptomatic, unless accompanied by aortic regurgitation or aortic dissection. Auscultation reveals most cases of regurgitation or nonejection systolic clicks.[106]

A rare complication of Marfan's syndrome reported in a father and his two sons is spontaneous bilateral pneumothorax. The precise etiology is uncertain.[297] Another rare complication is retroperitoneal fibrosis, apparently secondary to abnormality of the abdominal aorta. This may lead to hydronephrosis or other nephropathy.[38]

KEY CONCEPTS

- *Marfan's syndrome is an autosomal dominant connective tissue disorder, in which affected individuals are tall and thin, with gracile limbs and generalized joint laxity.*
- *Scoliosis and other postural alterations are common, seen in more than half of all patients, along with pectus excavatum or carinatum.*
- *Superior versus inferior lens dislocation and lack of osteoporosis help to distinguish Marfan's syndrome from homocystinuria.*
- *Dilatation and aneurysms of the ascending thoracic aorta are common, frequently with sudden onset and dissection, which is fatal in about 90% of cases; aneurysms of other vessels are less frequent.*

Melorheostosis

BACKGROUND

Melorheostosis was first described by Leri and Joanny in France in 1922 and has also been referred to as *Leri-Joanny syndrome*. To date, the precise etiology of this unusual syndrome is unknown, but theories include vascular insufficiency, inflammation or degeneration of connective tissues, and developmental abnormality of innervation.[211]

IMAGING FINDINGS

The classic radiographic appearance of melorheostosis is that of linear and curvilinear hyperostoses extending varying distances along the endosteal and periosteal surfaces, particularly of long and short tubular bones. These may demonstrate a wavy or irregular margin, resembling candle wax flowing along the bone, from which the condition derives its name. The hyperostosis may predominate on the radial side of the upper extremity. Spinal, pelvic, and craniofacial involvement may occur less frequently.[288] In the extremities, the hyperostosis follows a single sclerotome in about two thirds of the cases, a feature first described in 1979. In the remaining cases, multiple sclerotomes appear affected, leading to the theory that melorheostosis is a late result of a segmental sensory nerve lesion. An association with paraarticular ossification in some cases raises the question of involvement of the corresponding myotome.[55,175]

Melorheostosis is typically first discovered on plain films, but radiologists should also be familiar with its scintigraphic appearance. A bone scan demonstrates asymmetrical cortical uptake of radionuclide, which may extend across joints to affect contiguous bones.[48] The MR image features of melorheostosis and its associated soft tissue masses have been described. MRI is the optimal imaging study for assessing the extent of soft tissue involvement.[301]

The occurrence of melorheostosis in combination with radiographic changes of osteopoikilosis and osteopathia striata has been termed *mixed sclerosing bone dystrophy (MSBD)*. These patients may demonstrate diffuse sclerosis of the axial skeleton.[285] Although most cases of MSBD involve both upper and lower extremities, single limb involvement has been reported.[184] Isolated reports of regression of melorheostosis have appeared, and osteosarcoma arising in an affected femur has also been reported.[19,124] These features appear to be exceptional.

CLINICAL COMMENTS

Melorheostosis varies in its clinical presentation and may be asymptomatic or may be associated with pain along its typically sclerotomal distribution. Joint contractures, growth disturbances, other gross postural or biomechanical alterations, and linear scleroderma may occur.[175,240] Other changes in the overlying soft tissues may include tight, shiny, erythematous skin, discoloration, induration, and fibrosis. Such changes, which may be present at birth, may precede obvious osseous abnormality. Paraspinal soft tissue mass lesions and intrathecal lipoma were found in several patients with axial melorheostosis and linear cutaneous vascular malformation in one other patient with peripheral involvement; this emphasizes the fact that the disease affects mesenchymal tissue generally, rather than being confined to bone.[79,87,208] Single case reports exist of melorheostosis with hypophosphatemic rickets, minimal change nephrotic syndrome with mesenteric fibromatosis and capillary hemangioma, or renal artery stenosis.[114,145,219]

Although melorheostosis may not be discovered until adulthood, lesions are known to become apparent in children. Typical clinical findings include soft tissue contractures, joint pain and stiffness, and anisomelia, generally resistant to surgical correction.[204] Pain is uncommon in children and, when present, is mild. In one study of melorheostosis in children, the average delay between onset of clinical findings and diagnosis was 6 years.[299] Case reports of carpal tunnel syndrome secondary to melorheostosis exist, including one apparently congenital case in an infant.[9,18,19] In adults, pain may be severe and debilitating. Nifedipine and a disodium salt of diphosphonic acid have both been used successfully for pain control.[126,235]

KEY CONCEPTS

- *Melorheostosis is characterized radiographically by thick, wavy periosteal new bone formation, usually following a spinal sclerotome, myotome or, less frequently, a dermatome and sometimes crossing a joint space.*
- *Although axial involvement may occur, the extremities are more typically affected.*
- *Variable changes of the overlying soft tissues and adjacent joints may be seen in this painful, sometimes deforming idiopathic condition.*

Mucopolysaccharidoses

BACKGROUND

The mucopolysaccharidoses (MPSs) represent a heterogeneous group of conditions sharing the common feature of an abnormal sulfatase enzyme, leading to intralysosomal accumulation of partially degraded mucopolysaccharides. The first such condition was described in 1952 in individuals with physical features of gargoylism (coarse facies resembling the mythical gargoyle) and dwarfism. Histologic studies revealed collagen tissues and organs laden with water-soluble material also identified in the urine as mucopolysaccharide, in the form of glycosaminoglycans (GAGs).

Subsequently, at least eight different MPSs and a number of mucolipidoses (MLs), which result in similar clinical and radiographic changes, have been recognized.[26,59] Several of these also have been divided into subtypes, which demonstrate considerable variation in clinical and radiographic changes. Other storage disorders that may show some resemblance to MPS include aspartylglycosaminuria, fucosidosis, gangliosidosis, and mannosidosis.[211]

Differentiation of the various MPSs is based upon examination of the pattern of inheritance and the urinary excretion of a particular acid mucopolysaccharide (GAGs). The originally reported screening urinalysis based upon the color reaction of GAGs with dimethylmethylene blue was modified to reduce protein interference and may also be used to determine GAGs in other body fluids.[50] The better known MPSs are Morquio (Brailsford) syndrome (MPS IV) (Fig. 10-11), Hurler syndrome (MPS IH), Hunter syndrome (MPS II), and San Filippo syndrome (MPS III).

IMAGING FINDINGS

General. The skeletal changes common to the MPSs and MLs have been described as *dysostosis multiplex*. They include macrocephaly and dolichocephaly, related to premature closure of the sagittal suture and a characteristic J-shaped sella turcica and pituitary fossa. Widening of the diploic space and hypopneumatized sinuses are typically seen.

Intracranial. In patients with mental retardation, MRI has been used to demonstrate such abnormalities as deficient myelination, enlarged ventricles resulting from hydrocephalus, and widened fissures and sulci.[122,174,279] MRI has also been used to identify characteristic "cribriform" (multicystic, or sievelike) changes in the peri- and supraventricular parietal white matter, corpus callosum, and basal ganglia. These changes were most severe in Hunter and Hurler syndrome and were inversely related to the amount of atrophy, ventricular dilatation, and white matter abnormality. There appears to be a progression from cribriform changes to white matter changes and, finally, atrophy.[146] As for cardiac complications, bone marrow transplantation has shown promise in limiting central nervous system complications, when performed early, prior to demonstrable atrophy.[237]

Spine. The developing vertebrae are initially oval, with a beaklike appearance anteriorly, resulting from a combination of developmental deficiency, hypotonia, and anterior herniation of the nucleus pulposus. The beak is most frequently seen in Morquio's syndrome, in which it is centrally located (see Fig. 10-11). In Hurler's syndrome, as well as other congenital syndromes including Down syndrome and congenital hypothyroidism (cretinism), the beak is inferior. Beaked or hook-shaped vertebrae contribute to angular kyphosis or gibbus deformity, most typical in the thoracolumbar junction. In ambulatory patients, increasing kyphosis increases the altered stress on developing abnormal vertebrae and perpetuates the deformity. Developmental platyspondyly may result, typically not obvious until later childhood and resembling the changes of spondyloepiphyseal dysplasia.

Advanced imaging may reveal dural ectasia, which may result in spinal cord or thecal sac compression.[251] Reported atlantoaxial subluxation and instability is due to odontoid hypoplasia, os odontoideum, and other anomalies of the atlantoaxial articulation.[199,268]

Thorax. In the thorax, mucopolysaccharide deposition in the wall of the trachea may lead to luminal narrowing, which may be visible on plain films. In one series, 9 out of 56 patients demonstrated this finding, which is not necessarily symptomatic.[196] Ribs are widened generally, but with marked narrowing near their articulation with the spine, resulting in an oarlike appearance. The clavicles are also typically short and wide. Pectus carinatum may result from premature fusion of the sternal ossification centers.

Pelvis. The pelvis shows an increase in the acetabular angles and a widened appearance to the acetabular roofs. Characteristics include delayed ossification and dysplasia of the femoral heads.

Extremities. The long bones show delayed ossification of the epiphyses and cortical thinning with osteopenia. These changes are greater in the upper extremities. Initial undertubulation of metaphyses and diaphyses and valgus deformity may give way to overtubulation (overconstriction) and varus deformity, especially at the proximal humeri and femora. Other changes of the proximal femora resemble those of Legg-Calvè-Perthes disease. Premature osteoarthritis may be present.

The distal ulnae and radius are tapered, decreasing the carpal angle. The tubular bones of the hands and, to a lesser extent, the feet, may be affected. The metacarpal and metatarsal bones are proximally tapered, with relative sparing of the first. The distal phalanges are hypoplastic and the remaining phalanges are wide and short. In addition, dysplasia and hypoplasia of the carpal bones may also occur.

CLINICAL COMMENTS

The conditions share many features, such as macroglossia, adenoidal hyperplasia, and abnormal dentition. Patients may be short or average in height.

Cardiomegaly and associated cardiac abnormality may occur, as well as hepatosplenomegaly. Cardiopulmonary complications, when severe, may lead to death in infancy or childhood. Pneumonia, upper airway obstruction, and aortic regurgitation are among the complications that frequently lead to death. Bone marrow transplantation has been shown to diminish or at least limit the progression of cardiac complications in about two thirds of patients.[80] In one study of 45 patients, chronic otitis media was reported in more than 70% of the cases. More than half of all the patients in that study required some type of operative management by an otolaryngologist, with seven undergoing tracheostomy to relieve upper airway obstruction.[27] Congenital umbilical and inguinal hernias are common. Joint stiffness and contractures occur in some individuals, whereas other individuals may demonstrate joint laxity. Joint deformities, including genu valgum, may be apparent clinically as well as radiographically.

Carpal tunnel syndrome appears to be an unusually common complication of mucopolysaccharidosis or mucolipidosis and was reported in 17 of 18 patients in one case series.[292] In that study, the only patient without nerve conduction abnormality indicative of carpal tunnel syndrome was a 6-month-old infant.[292] Optic nerve head swelling and secondary optic atrophy have been reported as common complications of several of the mucopolysaccharidoses.[41]

Mental deficit in these syndromes is highly variable both within and between the various disorders, ranging from absent to profound. Morquio's syndrome is generally associated with normal mentation. Behavior problems occur at high rates, especially among children with San Filippo and Hunter syndromes. These include destructiveness, restlessness, and aggressiveness, as well as sleep disturbance in about two thirds of patients.[10]

KEY CONCEPTS

- *Mucopolysaccharidoses have been classified along with the mucolipidoses and oligosaccharidoses as conditions of "dysostosis multiplex."*
- *Accordingly, a given mucopolysaccharidosis may demonstrate varying degrees of alteration of bone texture; widening or undertubulation of the diaphyses; dysplasias of the distal radius and ulna (Madelung's deformity); tapered metacarpal bases; macrocephaly and thickening of the calvarium, with a J-shaped sella turcica; and an anterior beak of a vertebral body at the thoracolumbar junction.*
- *Beyond the consistent, radiographically apparent skeletal anomalies, a variety of other system-wide anomalies may be seen, depending upon the type and severity of the disorder from among this heterogenous group of dysplasias.*

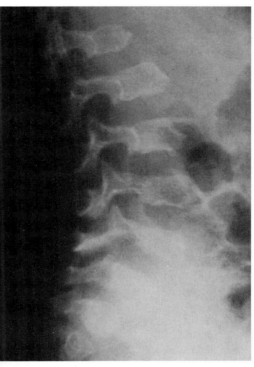

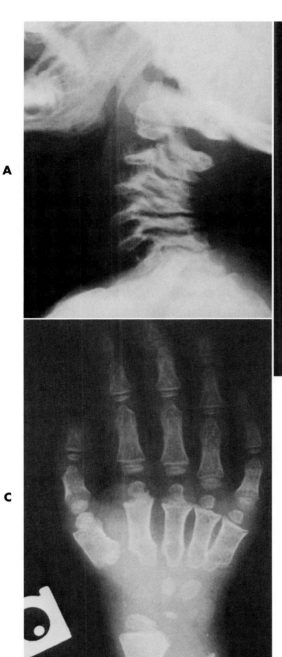

FIG. 10-11 Mucopolysaccharidosis IV A in a 3-year-old girl. **A,** Platyspondyly of the cervical vertebrae, underdevelopment of the odontoid process of the axis, and atlantoaxial subluxation in the extension position. **B,** Universal platyspondyly of the lumbar vertebrae and a central beak protruding from the vertebral bodies. **C,** Marked irregularity of the distal metaphysis of the radius and ulna, pointed proximal end of the second through fifth metacarpals, short metacarpals, and pointed distal end of the middle and distal phalanges. (From Taybi H, Lachman RS: *Radiology of syndromes, metabolic disorders, and skeletal dysplasias,* ed 4, St Louis, 1996, Mosby.)

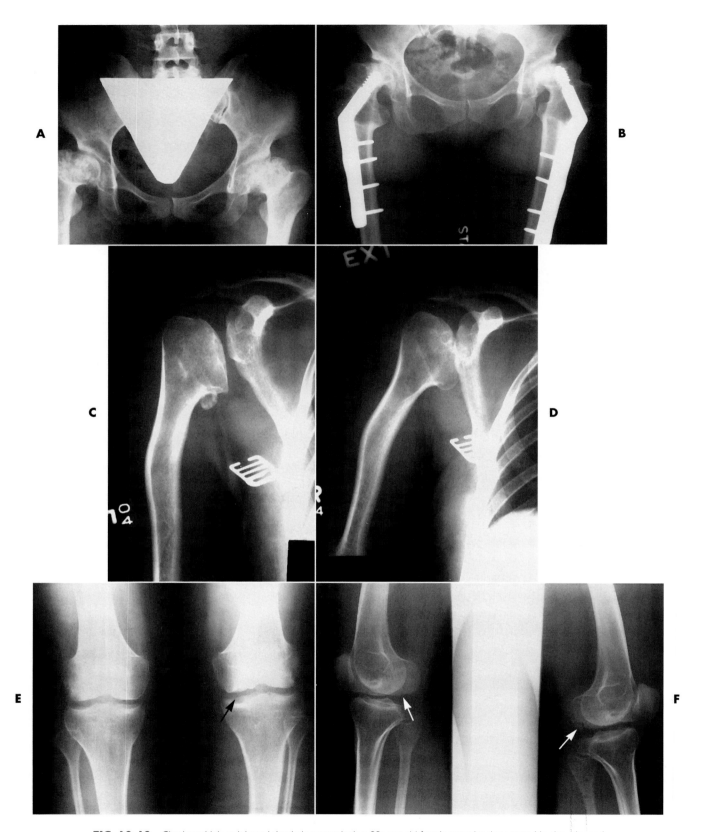

FIG. 10-12 Classic multiple epiphyseal dysplasia congenita in a 39-year-old female experiencing severe hip, shoulder, and knee involvement. **A,** Initial hip films at age 25 years resembled severe bilateral Legg-Calvè-Perthes disease but with more significant acetabular involvement. Note the oversized triangular gonadal shield obscuring the lumbosacral region. **B,** Osteotomy and instrumentation was performed at age 31 years in an attempt to alter weightbearing stresses on the femoral heads. **C** and **D,** The glenoid fossae are markedly hypoplastic and shallow with chronic subluxation of the "hatched head" proximal humeri. **E** and **F,** The knees are only mildly affected, with changes resembling osteochondritis dissecans (arrows). Dwarfing has resulted from rhizomelic shortening, most prominent at the humeri.

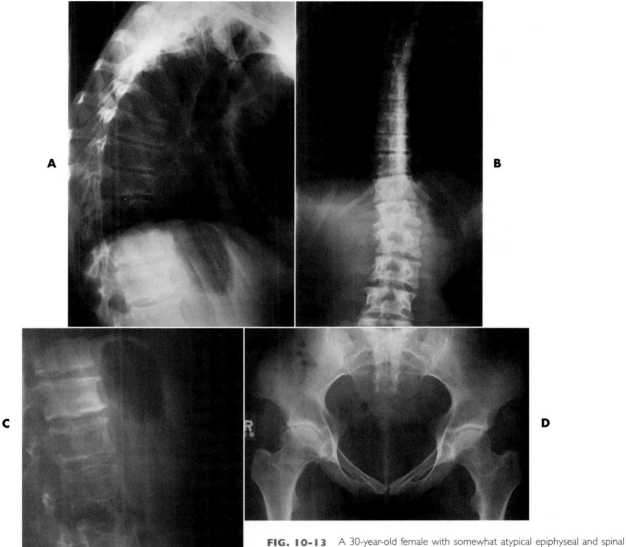

FIG. 10-13 A 30-year-old female with somewhat atypical epiphyseal and spinal dysplasia diagnosed previously as a form of MED ("Fairbanks disease"). Note unusually marked thoracic spine (**A** and **B**) changes more reminiscent of SED but with few classic changes in the lumbar (**C**) and cervical regions. The hips (**D**) and shoulders were only mildly affected, with the most apparent changes at the right hip, where moderate painful osteoarthritis had developed. One might question the diagnosis of MED tarda and suggest the possibility that this represents one of the rare autosomal dominant variants of SED.

Multiple Epiphyseal Dysplasia (MED)

BACKGROUND

This autosomal dominant condition is characterized by dwarfism, brachydactyly, and altered appearance and development of epiphyseal ossification centers, which commonly leads to early, severe osteoarthritis.[189]

The condition typically is apparent clinically by ages 5 to 14 and may necessitate bilateral total joint arthroplasties by early to middle adulthood (Fig. 10-12). Second only to the hips, other weight-bearing joints and the wrists are the most frequently and most severely affected. Unlike spondyloepiphyseal dysplasia, the spine is usually normal or only minimally affected (Fig. 10-13).

IMAGING FINDINGS

Two distinct subtypes based on degree of abnormality of the developing hips have been described; this classification may assist in prognosis and treatment planning. Type I is associated with more severe changes, including fragmented and flattened ossification centers and acetabular dysplasia. Markedly deformed femoral heads at skeletal maturity almost invariably lead to premature severe osteoarthritis. Type II hips show no gross femoral head deformity at skeletal maturity and are less likely to demonstrate severe osteoarthritis.[272]

Similarly, a study of shoulders in 50 patients with MED demonstrated two distinct clinical and radiological subtypes.[115] The first group with minor epiphyseal changes developed painful osteoarthritis in middle age but retained shoulder movement until the osteoarthritis was severe radiographically. The other group demonstrated more severe deformity, described as a "hatchet head" epiphysis. These patients had markedly restricted glenohumeral motion early but, like the other group, did not experience pain until in their 40s or 50s.[115]

A limited focal epiphyseal dysplasia isolated to the femoral heads is termed *dysplasia epiphysealis capitis femoris* or *Meyer's dysplasia.* This is bilateral in about 50% of cases and five times more common in males. Most cases are symptomatic, but a waddling gait sometimes occurs. Radiographs show a hypoplastic proximal femoral epiphysis, with a delayed appearance of single or multiple ossification centers. This improves with age and by 6 years the separate ossification centers consolidate and develop a nearly normal appearance. The only residual finding is a slightly diminished cephalocaudal dimension to the femoral head.[127]

CLINICAL COMMENTS

The person with MED has normal intelligence. Joint pain and gait disturbance are among the most notable clinical manifestations. Urine and blood laboratory indices are within normal limits.

KEY CONCEPTS

- *Multiple epiphyseal dysplasia is a familial disorder that may show delayed and abnormal appearance and development of the epiphyseal ossification centers, although generally with a normal time of fusion.*
- *The result is early, often severe, and disabling osteoarthritis; short, stubby digits; and dwarfing that is milder than spondyloepiphyseal dysplasia because of lack of significant spinal involvement.*

Os Odontoideum

BACKGROUND

Os odontoideum describes a condition in which a variable portion of the ossification center for the odontoid process of C2 is separate from the body and is often associated with atlantoaxial subluxation and instability (Fig. 10-14). In the past, prior to advanced diagnostic imaging, os odontoideum may have been misdiagnosed as agenesis or hypoplasia of the dens, because the separate ossicle may be obscured by superimposed osseous structures on plain films. It was long taught that the dens represents the embryological derivative of the atlas body, but it is now known that it is, instead, merely a bony projection arising from the C2 body.

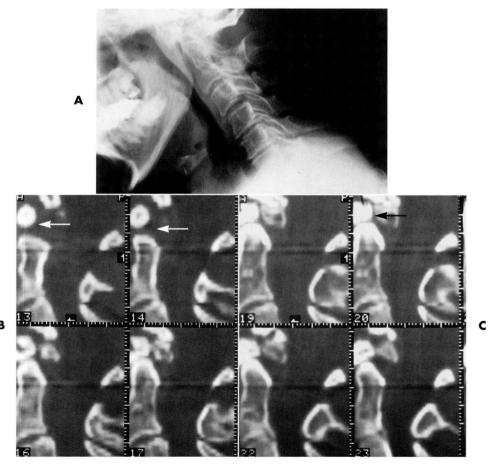

FIG. 10-14   Os odontoideum. **A,** The flexion lateral cervical projection does not show signs of instability assessed by the normal relationship maintained between the spinolaminar junction lines of C1 and C2. A congenital nonsegmentation exists at C2-C3. **B** and **C,** Reformatted sagittal CT images demonstrate the separated dens to better advantage (*arrows*).

Abnormal motion, sometimes in the form of a specific acute trauma, appears to be essential to the development of the os odontoideum. This increased motion may also be in conjunction with a syndrome such as Down syndrome or Morquio's syndrome.[42,256] The first clear evidence that os odontoideum could be produced from a single traumatic event was found in a case report in 1991.[231] Prior to that, the lesion was considered to be congenital.

IMAGING FINDINGS

Rarely would an os odontoideum be an anticipated finding on plain film radiographs. In fact, even to those familiar with plain film radiography of the spine, the os odontoideum may be overlooked or confused with a recent dens fracture. Plain films demonstrate a separate ossicle of varying conspicuity, frequently largely obscured on an anteroposterior open-mouth view. On the lateral view, a helpful finding is hypertrophy and sclerosis of the anterior tubercle of the atlas. This finding, which may also be seen in other long-standing upper cervical abnormalities such as spina bifida occulta or rheumatoid arthritis, is due to abnormal stresses concentrated on the anterior tubercle and may be quite helpful in distinguishing the os odontoideum from an acute dens fracture, posttraumatically.[108]

Carefully positioned flexion lateral views typically reveal atlantoaxial subluxation and instability (Figs. 10-15 through 10-17). The spinolaminar junction line of C1 is displaced anteriorly to that of C2 on flexion, yet the anterior atlantodental interspace (ADI) is normal, a very important sign of either os odontoideum or dens fracture. In instability resulting from disruption of the transverse ligament, both the ADI and the relationship of the spinolaminar junction lines at C1-C2 are altered. In the neutral posture, the upper cervical relationship may be normal or altered and an extension lateral view illustrates typical posterior subluxation, with the spinolaminar junction line of C1 now lying posterior to that of C2.

Another helpful plain film finding is a smooth, well-corticated margin at the inferior aspect of the separate odontoid and at the base of the dens. This does not, of course, definitively distinguish a long-standing ununited dens fracture from an os odontoideum, but it will help to exclude a recent dens fracture when this might otherwise be in question.

Additionally, the posterior articular margin of the anterior tubercle of C1 is often remodeled, demonstrating a posteriorly directed, V-shaped configuration representing a "molding" defect. The anterior tubercle may also be fused to the separate dens (Fig. 10-18).

In addition to plain films, other diagnostic imaging techniques that either diagnose or gain additional information regarding os odontoideum include plain film and computerized tomography, myelography, and magnetic resonance imaging. Today, the preferred diagnostic procedure beyond plain film radiographs is typically MRI, which will generally answer the clinical questions most likely to arise with os odontoideum, particularly whether or not there is evidence of cord compression. It is possible that dynamic MRI or at least a conventional MRI with the head and neck in flex-

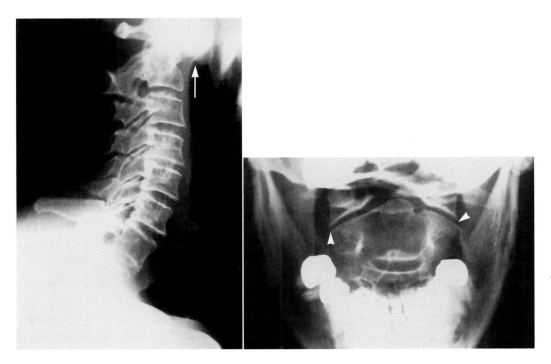

FIG. 10-15   Os odontoideum with anterior *(arrow)* and lateral *(arrowheads)* subluxation. Note marked decrease in the space available for the cord, measuring only 1 cm. A more typical measurement would be 2 cm. Despite the narrowing, this 68-year-old male had only mild neck pain and stiffness, without clinical evidence of cord compression and myelopathy. Gradual onset of the upper cervical spinal stenosis and presumed compensatory changes of the cord help to explain his lack of symptoms. Additionally, compressible, loose areolar connective tissue occupies as much as one third of the central canal dimension; the other two thirds is occupied by cord and dens. The same degree of subluxation or dislocation occurring rapidly would likely be much more devastating.

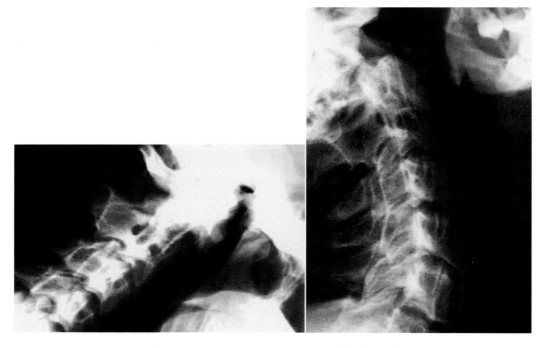

FIG. 10-16   Atypical unstable os odontoideum with adjacent C2-C3 congenital nonsegmentation.

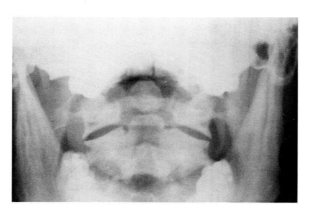

FIG. 10-17   Os odontoideum with history of multiple traumas over the past 3 years.

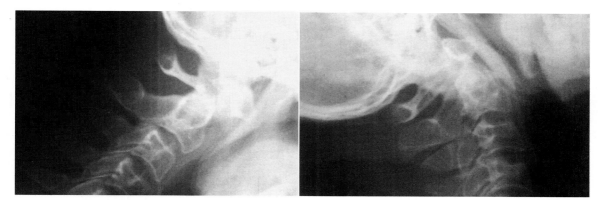

FIG. 10-18 Unstable os odontoideum on flexion-extension lateral views. Note typical angular configuration at the posterior margin of the anterior tubercle of C1, known as a "molding" defect. This defect represents a classic associated developmental anomaly and helps to distinguish os odontoideum from dens fracture following trauma.

ion may provide the most information by maximally stressing the upper cervical complex. As with functional radiographs, this type of imaging requires careful monitoring to ensure safety of the patient and prevent additional neurological injury.[295]

CLINICAL COMMENTS

The clinical presentation of patients with os odontoideum varies considerably. The abnormality is sometimes discovered as an incidental finding on plain films of patients who are either asymptomatic or whose symptoms are apparently unrelated. Other symptoms include headaches or upper cervical or suboccipital pain of varying severity. Still others are discovered in previously asymptomatic patients who experience trauma, in which case the findings may include significant neurological deficit.

Given the previously mentioned role of abnormal motion or specific trauma in the development of os odontoideum, most authorities today probably favor an acquired etiology for the os odontoideum. However, compelling evidence still exists that at least some os odontoidea are congenital, including a report of identical twins with os odontoideum and a known association between os odontoideum and Down syndrome.[71,129] A case report from 1989 indicates that at least some cases may be familial and associated with syndromes involving spinal anomalies, such as Klippel-Feil syndrome.[173]

In some instances, it is unclear whether the os odontoideum is congenital or acquired, especially when relatively minor trauma has occurred.[103] Os odontoideum is probably sometimes congenital and sometimes acquired. Clements et al[40] state that the question of primary importance is not whether a given case of os odontoideum is congenital or traumatic but rather how the condition should best be managed once discovered to ensure the best outcome for the patient. Of course, among academicians and lawyers, the question of traumatic or congenital may still hold significant weight and the debates continue.[40]

Surgical management for os odontoideum has included interlaminar wiring alone and posterior screw fixation, with or without bone graft or combined bone-wire fixation. Procedures that do not involve sublaminar passage of wire are associated with a lesser risk for neural injury.[257] Some have advocated the use of cineradiography to help determine the most appropriate means of surgical fixation.[111]

In addition to the obvious potential for upper cervical cord compression, a less widely recognized complication of the unstable os odontoideum is compromise of the vertebral artery, which may lead to brainstem, cerebellar, or cerebral infarction. This may be associated with neurological deficit that ranges from permanent and profound to partially or completely reversible.[16,128,172,262]

KEY CONCEPTS

- *Whether posttraumatic, developmental, or congenital, the os odontoideum represents a relatively uncommon but important abnormality of the upper cervical complex.*
- *Its presence may compromise the stability of the atlantoaxial articulation, which may be catastrophic, especially when a previously asymptomatic and seemingly normal individual experiences hyperflexion or other trauma to the upper cervical complex.*
- *The os odontoideum may be seen alone or in conjunction with other anomalies of the cervical spine and craniovertebral junction.*

Osteogenesis Imperfecta

BACKGROUND

Osteogenesis imperfecta (OI), also known as *Lobstein's disease, Ekman syndrome,* and *osteopsathyrosis,* encompasses a heterogenous group of genetic disorders that are marked by abnormal collagen type I formation. Osteogenesis imperfecta may be inherited as a dominant or recessive defect, or it may arise from a mutation. At least four distinct types exist, ranging in clinical presentation from mild osteopenia with normal stature to dwarfism with multiple fractures occurring in utero. In the past, the disease was dichotomized into congenita and tarda forms; however, this is no longer thought to be valid.[266]

Type I is the most common form, marked by easily fractured bones, blue sclera, abnormal dentition, normal stature, joint hypermobility, and a tendency toward spinal curvatures.

IMAGING FINDINGS

The radiographic studies may demonstrate osteopenia, one or more fractures, hypoplastic dentition, dwarfism, and kyphoscoliosis (Fig. 10-19). The bone cortices may be thin, most apparent in the long bones, which may also demonstrate bowing deformity. The skull may be large, exhibiting delayed ossification and wormian bones.

CLINICAL COMMENTS

Severe types of the disease are lethal. Milder forms of the disease are characterized by weakened, easily fractured bones. Patients may exhibit blue sclera, translucent skin, and deafness.

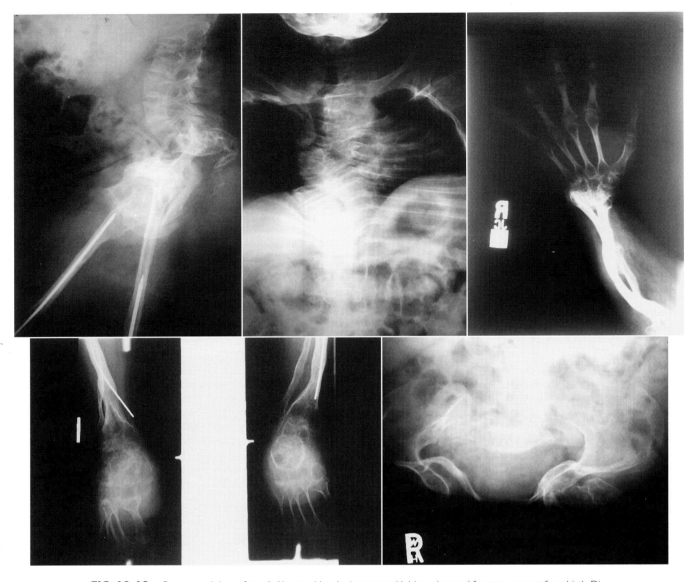

FIG. 10-19   Osteogenesis imperfecta. A 41-year-old male drummer with blue sclera and fractures present from birth. Diagnosis was first made at 7 months and patient had experienced more than 200 fractures before age 20. As is typical, the rate of new fracture decreased markedly after puberty. Note gracile, overtubulated long bones with multiple healed fractures and severe osteopenia. Marked protrusio acetabulum, multiple vertebral compression fractures, and sacral and rib fractures are present. Lifelong wheelchair confinement has contributed to deformity of the trunk, with scoliosis and short stature noted.

At present, no cure exists for osteogenesis imperfecta. Treatment is directed toward limiting deformity and injury. Conservatively, this may entail limiting physical activity. More aggressive approaches involve surgically inserting rods to prevent long bone deformity and fracture.

KEY CONCEPTS

- *Osteogenesis is a heterogenous group of genetic disorders that are marked by abnormal collagen.*
- *The severity of the clinical presentation varies.*
- *Radiographic examination may reveal osteoporosis, fractures, abnormal dentition, dwarfism, kyphoscoliosis, thin cortices, delayed calvarium ossification, and wormian bones.*
- *Treatment is directed toward limiting deformity and injury.*

Osteopetrosis

BACKGROUND

Rather than a single disease, osteopetrosis syndromes include at least four distinct entities, with varying clinical and radiographic features. These are grouped with a larger collection of diseases known as the *sclerosing bone dysplasias,* sharing a common feature of increased density of bone.

A severe and intermediate autosomal recessive form of osteopetrosis exists. A third autosomal recessive form is associated with tubular acidosis and was recognized as a unique syndrome in 1972. It has been referred to as "marble brain disease," owing to the typical intracranial calcifications, especially in the basal ganglia and cerebral hemispheres.

Finally, a mild, autosomal dominant form exists, most likely to be discovered incidentally in patients x-rayed for other reasons. This condition has been named *Albers-Schönberg disease* after the radiologist who first reported it. Osteopetrosis has previously been separated grossly into benign and aggressive or "malignant" forms. This simplistic classification system is invalid because of the heterogeneity within the various forms.

IMAGING FINDINGS

Radiographic findings vary widely, both between and within the various forms of osteopetrosis, but the typical changes are a result of deficient osteoclastic activity. Although the number of osteoclasts is generally normal, most of the population is dysfunctional. As expected, this condition involves a lack of proper remodeling of bones, especially the most metabolically active portions, the ends of long bones. Undertubulation, with a widened appearance of the metaphyses and metadiaphyseal regions is described as an "Erlenmeyer flask" deformity. A loss of distinction may occur between cortical and medullary bone and, in the most severe cases, completely obliterate the medullary spaces.

A "bone-within-a-bone" appearance, or "endobone," is due to persistence of infantile bone matrix within the medullary cavity and is often most striking in the spine (Fig. 10-20). In the skull, changes predominate in the enchondral bone of the skull base. Paranasal sinuses are underdeveloped. Acute and insufficiency type stress fractures may be seen. Other characteristics of osteopetrosis include an especially high incidence of lumbar spondylolysis and spondylolisthesis. Dental anomalies may also be seen, including supernumerary teeth, retention of infantile teeth, and impaction of permanent teeth.

Although all forms of osteopetrosis may show at least minimal improvement of radiographic changes, this feature is most characteristic of the recessive form associated with renal tubular acidosis. The intracranial calcifications in this form of osteopetrosis are also unique and are most readily demonstrated on computed tomography, predominating in the basal ganglia.[182,243,244] A relationship may exist between osteopetrosis and calcific tendinitis, although this remains uncertain.[206]

CLINICAL COMMENTS

The severe autosomal recessive form of osteopetrosis is often, although not invariably, lethal in infancy. Frequently osteopetrosis is marked by hydrocephalus and macrocephaly, failure to thrive, hepatosplenomegaly, and cranial nerve dysfunction, resulting from stenosis of skull foramina. Death is typically due to severe anemia resulting from stenosis of the medullary, hematopoietic regions of bone. Thrombocytopenia, including leukocytopenia, predisposes to infections, which may also be fatal.

The intermediate recessive form is associated with hepatomegaly, anemia, below-average height, and pathological fractures.[12,130] The intermediate recessive form with renal acidosis may be associated with mental deficit. Symptoms may include failure to thrive, muscle weakness, hypotonia, and other clinical findings of renal acidosis.[182, 243,244]

Although many with the autosomal dominant form (Albers-Schönberg) of the disease remain asymptomatic, some experience anemia, cranial nerve dysfunction, and pathological fractures, which may first bring the condition to a clinician's attention.[105,121,247]

KEY CONCEPTS

- *Osteopetrosis is actually a combination of several related conditions formerly divided simply into benign and malignant forms, all with an underlying decrease in osteoclastic activity, resulting in lack of normal bone resorption.*
- *Those with the more severe autosomal recessive form die within the first decade from complications of severe anemia.*
- *An autosomal recessive form with renal tubular acidosis tends to improve radiographically, and bone density may appear to be relatively normal by later childhood; intracranial calcifications are invariably seen, which distinguishes this form from the others.*
- *The autosomal dominant tarda form is the one most likely to be encountered by the typical clinician and may be found incidentally on radiographs performed for another reason, such as the evaluation of back pain.*
- *Those with the autosomal dominant tarda form may experience mild anemia, cranial nerve compromise, pathologic acute and stress fractures, and osteomyelitis resulting from dental extraction, although most who are affected remain asymptomatic throughout their life.*

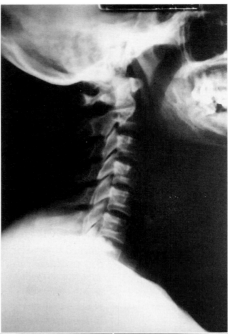

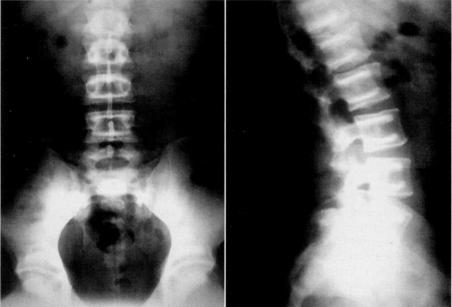

FIG. 10-20 Mild form of osteopetrosis with typical "bone within a bone" appearance resulting from defective osteoclastic activity, which fails to fully remove the immature vertebral body anlage. Note also spondylolisthesis of L5 secondary to ununited stress fractures of the pars interarticulares. This is extremely common in osteopetrosis and attests to the fact that the bones are more prone to fracture than normal bones, despite the increased radiographic density. The vertebrae, sometimes described as "sandwich" vertebrae, might be confused with the "rugger jersey" appearance of renal osteodystrophy. In this condition (also known as *secondary hyperparathyroidism*) the bands of sclerosis are reactive, a response to resorption of bone at the discovertebral junction. They are therefore immediately adjacent to the endplates, as opposed to several millimeters away from the endplates as seen here in osteopetrosis.

Pyknodysostosis (Pycnodysostosis)

BACKGROUND

Pyknodysostosis is a rare autosomal recessive syndrome comprising diffuse osteosclerosis; below-average height; skull changes; broad; short hands; hypoplasia of the mandible; acro-osteolysis; hypoplastic nails; and abnormal dentition. Although some have considered this to be a variant of osteopetrosis, it appears to be a distinct entity, first described by Maritoux and Lamy in 1962. Toulouse-Lautrec probably suffered from this condition.

IMAGING FINDINGS

Changes of the skull are most striking, with frontal and occipital bossing, a small face, and micrognathia (Fig. 10-21). The mandible is hypoplastic and the mandibular angle increased. Closure of skull

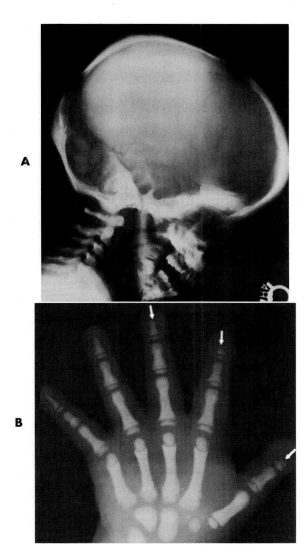

FIG. 10-21   Pyknodysostosis in a 5-year-old girl. **A,** Dense bones, widely open cranial sutures, prognathism obtuse angle of mandible, lack of normal development of mastoids and paranasal sinuses. **B,** Generalized osteosclerosis, partial absence of ossification of distal phalanx of thumb and middle and index fingers *(arrows)*. (From Taybi H, Lachman RS: *Radiology of syndromes, metabolic disorders, and skeletal dysplasias,* ed 4, St Louis, 1996, Mosby.)

sutures is delayed. The anterior fontanelle often persists into adulthood, and multiple wormian bones are common. As in osteopetrosis, the skull base is particularly sclerotic and dentition is abnormal. Unlike osteopetrosis, portions of the calvarium may actually be thinned and osteopenic and normal diploic markings are generally absent. Short tubular bones of the hands and feet are hypoplastic, and the distal phalangeal tufts are often marked by resorption or hypoplasia (Fig. 10-20, *B*). In addition to sclerosis of the spine, segmentation anomalies, especially of the upper cervical spine, are common.

In contrast to osteopetrosis, in which skeletal changes remain static or may even improve over time, skeletal changes tend to progress in pyknodysostosis. As in osteopetrosis, characteristics of pyknodysostosis may include pathological fractures and insufficiency fractures, including cervical and lumbar pars interarticularis defects (spondylolysis).[45,63,300] Fracture complications arise most frequently in the second decade of life. Another associated complication is osteomyelitis of the mandible, which appears to be related to a combination of hypovascularity and abnormal dentition.[45,153]

CLINICAL COMMENTS

Although affected individuals often have a normal lifespan, hyperplasia of the uvula may lead to hypoventilation and subsequent cardiac or hepatic failure.[4,300]

KEY CONCEPTS

- This autosomal recessive disorder demonstrates generalized sclerosis of bone and short stature, without true dwarfism, along with dysplasia of the terminal tufts of the phalanges.
- Cranial, facial, spinal, and clavicular anomalies are common.

Scheuermann's Disease

BACKGROUND

History. In 1921 Scheuermann published the first reports of the common spinal condition that bears his name, introducing the term *kyphosis dorsalis juvenilis* and the characteristic morphological changes of the discovertebral junctions resembling those of Legg-Calvè-Perthes disease of the proximal femur.[230] It seems that no other developmental spinal condition, with the possible exception of spondylolytic spondylolisthesis, has engendered as much confusion and controversy as Scheuermann's disease. In fact, the pathogenesis, epidemiology, and clinical relevance of these two conditions share some common features.

Both Scheuermann's disease and lumbar spondylolysis were first reported decades ago and have given rise to a perplexing array of etiological hypotheses and revisions. Both are considered to be related in some measure to repetitive altered stresses on what may be inherently vulnerable developing structures in adolescents, the pars interarticularis for spondylolisthesis and the osteocartilaginous endplate junction in Scheuermann's disease. Although both conditions seem to have some genetic component, lumbar spondylolysis should be considered to represent stress fracture of the pars interarticularis and is essentially never congenital.[93] Scheuermann's disease is best classified as a stress-related apophysitis, rather than a congenital process. Both conditions may be asymptomatic, and the severity of symptoms is often unrelated to the degree of abnormality demonstrated on diagnostic imaging and clinical examination. In both, more severe symptoms are often a result of associated or secondary abnormalities, such as intervertebral disc herniations, which are much more common in patients with these conditions than in the general population. Interestingly, an increased incidence is reported in lumbar spondylolysis in Scheuermann's disease, occurring in 32% to 50% of patients, as compared with about 7% in the general population.[89,183]

Terminology. Even the naming of Scheuermann's disease has led to confusion over the years. Scheuermann's disease has been variably referred to as *vertebral epiphysitis, osteochondrosis juvenilis dorsi, adolescent kyphosis, osteochondrosis juvenilis Scheuermann, juvenile kyphosis, spinal osteochondrosis,* and *osteochondritis.*[7,23,94,165,258] In fact, in some instances, the same author has published different articles using arbitrarily several different names for the same condition.[7]

Diagnosis. The diagnosis of Scheuermann's disease is typically established on the basis of plain film radiographs, in conjunction with clinical findings of increasing kyphosis and variable back pain. Schmorl's nodes, resulting from intravertebral disc protrusions through natural fissures (i.e., vascular channels) in the developing cartilaginous endplate, are an essential feature, along with more generalized endplate irregularity, anterior vertebral body wedging, and diminished disc height. Involvement is usually multilevel, typically of the lower thoracic or thoracolumbar region.

Although Scheuermann did allow for the diagnosis in cases of isolated changes at one disc level, some experts feel that the term *Scheuermann's disease* is only appropriate for classic cases with three or more affected vertebral levels, each with at least 5 degrees of anterior vertebral body wedging, leading to hyperkyphosis.[211] It should not be used to describe minimal Schmorl's node formation even at more than one level if it is not accompanied by increasing kyphosis. Because developmental and traumatic endplate changes

occur on a continuum, some of these cases may be considered to be formes fruste of Scheuermann's disease.

As with idiopathic scoliosis, attention has been focused upon an alteration in biosynthesis of collagen and other ground substances as a fundamental abnormality leading to the typical gross anatomical and radiographic features of Scheuermann's disease.[7] Other authors have theorized that inadequate nutrition, structural weakness, or a combination of these lead to Scheuermann's-like changes in the thoracolumbar region and premature degenerative disc disease of the lower lumbar spine. This constellation of findings has been described as "juvenile discogenic disease."[100] Studies demonstrating similar spinal changes in identical twins, sibling recurrence, and transmission over three generations lend credence to a fundamental genetic abnormality, with disease severity influenced by biomechanical stresses.[165,274] One researcher demonstrated disorganized enchondral ossification resembling the changes of Blount's disease of the tibia and thought to be secondary to increased axial loading of the developing anterior vertebral body margin.[232]

Over the years, other theories regarding the cause or causes of Scheuermann's disease have included idiopathic osteochondrosis or avascular necrosis, hamstring tightness, a nonspecific myopathy, or even emotional stress.[67,70,164]

Prevalence. It is impossible to calculate a precise estimate of the prevalence of Scheuermann's disease, because a specific figure demands a well-defined entity. A conservative definition yielded an estimate as low as 0.4% in adolescents between the ages of 11 and 13 years who were tracked for 3 years through their pubertal period.[180] As previously noted, one study calculated an incidence of 13%.[98] An-

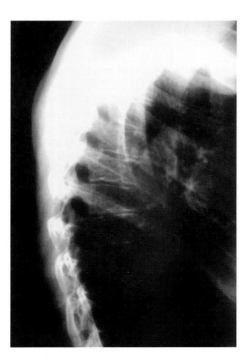

FIG. 10-22　Residuals of Scheuermann's disease. Note the focally more marked anterior vertebral body wedging at T7. Following trauma, this type of finding is frequently mistaken for a compression fracture. Also, observe the moderate disc space narrowing focally at T7-T8, associated with an especially prominent Schmorl's node formation.

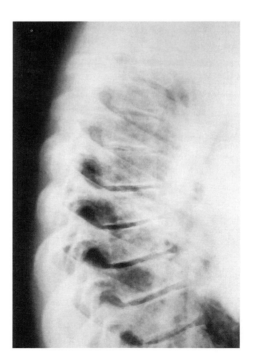

FIG. 10-23　Residuals of Scheuermann's disease in a 25-year-old male. Note the marked platyspondyly and increased kyphosis with less apparent endplate irregularities and Schmorl's node formation, as well as mild disc space narrowing.

other paper reported MRI changes of Scheuermann's disease in 38% of 90 asymptomatic subjects.[290] Still another article, basing the diagnosis on a lateral plain film of the thoracic and lumbar spine, along with a questionnaire and assessment of passive stretch of the hamstrings, reported a prevalence of 60% of males and 23% of females from among 96 students ages 17 to 18 years.[68] A later study by these same authors using a larger sample size of 500 subjects showed an incidence of 56.3% in males and 30.3% in females aged 17 to 18 years. Risk factors identified in this study included above-average height, greater than 2 weeks spent in bed because of illness or injury, and hamstring tightness, which had been previously found in 85% of individuals with Scheuermann's disease.[67,69]

IMAGING FINDINGS

Plain film radiographs are the initial diagnostic imaging modality used in most cases, but Scheuermann's disease has been widely studied using CT, MRI, and even planar bone scintigraphy and SPECT scanning (Figs. 10-22 through 10-27). These advanced imaging techniques may be indicated in atypical presentations of Scheuermann's disease that might mimic other more serious conditions such as disc space infection or when there is suspicion for intervertebral disc herniation or other complications.[6,155]

Conversely, nonspecific studies such as scintigraphy, ordered for further evaluation of back pain unresponsive to conservative management, may be negative or show abnormal findings indistinguishable from other processes such as disc space infection.[6,222] This fact, along with the similar sensitivity and greater specificity of MRI versus bone scan, makes MRI the diagnostic imaging procedure of choice in virtually all cases requiring further investigation beyond plain films, particularly when symptoms are localized.

CLINICAL COMMENTS

General. Scheuermann described a condition of increased thoracic kyphosis in adolescents demonstrating unique multilevel thoracic endplate irregularities and Schmorl's nodes, along with anterior vertebral body wedging. Milder cases and abbreviated forms of Scheuermann's disease may be clinically occult and asymptomatic, with radiographic changes noted incidentally. Severe cases may lead to progressive deformity, pain, disability, and, infrequently, acute neurological deficit secondary to angular kyphosis, with or without disc herniation.[224,294]

Patients with Scheuermann's disease may have associated musculoskeletal abnormality, such as lumbar or cervical hyperlordosis and muscular imbalance and hypertonicity, although a clear cause-and-effect relationship has not been established.[250]

As with idiopathic scoliosis, no clear predictive factors have been delineated to assist in determining which cases are likely to progress and which are likely to halt. Reports conflict regarding the clinical significance of Scheuermann's-related endplate changes, especially chronic or residual changes in adults. A recent 25-year prospective cohort study of 640 school children failed to demonstrate a positive correlation between thoracolumbar changes of Scheuermann's disease and back pain, either in adolescence or adulthood. Thirteen percent of these children had radiographic evidence of Scheuermann's disease. Interestingly, these authors did find a strong correlation between adolescent back pain combined

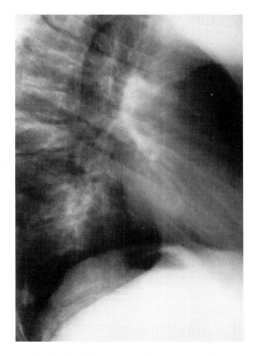

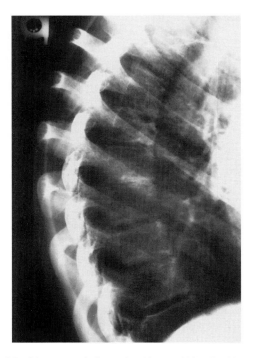

FIG. 10-24 Residuals of Scheuermann's disease in a 19-year-old male. The patient experienced severe focal sternal and rib pain with mild back pain following a fall while skiing. Platyspondyly in the midthoracic spine should not be mistaken for compression fracture. Patients with hyperkyphosis may be at increased risk for sternal fracture or stress fracture. This is especially true with kyphosis related to postmenopausal osteoporosis in females. Advanced imaging should be considered, because sternal fracture may be difficult to diagnosis on plain films.

FIG. 10-25 Scheuermann's disease in a 14-year-old female with moderate to severe progressive thoracic kyphosis. A markedly wedged midthoracic segment could be mistaken for a compression fracture, but no trauma occurred and symptoms were not focally more pronounced.

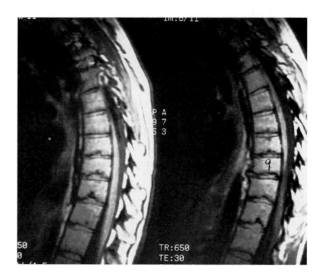

FIG. 10-26   With the exception of hyperkyphosis, the changes of Scheuermann's disease and its complications are generally much better seen on MRI than on plain films. Schmorl's node formation may appear to be minimal on plain films but substantial on MRI. Note the anterior disc protrusion at T9-T10. A marked increase exists in the incidence of disc bulge and herniation in Scheuermann's patients versus a normal population.

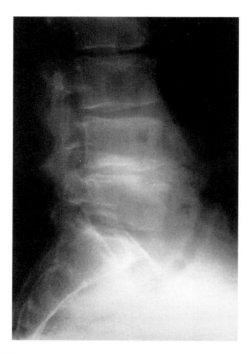

FIG. 10-27   Anteroposterior expansion of the L3 through L5 vertebral bodies secondary to prominent Schmorl's node formation, as seen occasionally in Scheuermann's disease or, a related condition, juvenile discogenic disease.

with a familial occurrence of back pain and pain in the same adolescents into adulthood, regardless of the presence or absence of radiographic abnormality.[98]

Activity. Historically Scheuermann's disease has been linked to activities that increase axial loading of the spine in adolescents, such as diving, gymnastics, weightlifting, or heavy lifting at work; however, this relationship has not been universally confirmed.[69,267] Although such activities have not been clearly demonstrated to cause the radiographic changes of Scheuermann's disease, the onset of symptoms in patients with this condition is often temporally linked to such activities.[89]

Scoliosis. Some authors have examined the relationship between Scheuermann's disease and idiopathic scoliosis and have concluded that they may share a common pathogenesis. One study found that 70% of patients with Scheuermann's disease had scoliosis, averaging 15 degrees. Just less than one third of these had an apex at the same level as the Scheuermann's kyphosis. The number of right convexities equalled that of left convexities. Also present was an equal distribution among males and females, unlike scoliosis unrelated to Scheuermann's disease, which is far more common in females and results in a right convexity in about 90% of cases. The remaining lumbar curves, most commonly below the Scheuermann's kyphosis, averaged 16 degrees but were still felt to be compensatory. These curves did show the more typical right-sided thoracic convexity and higher female prevalence that are characteristic of idiopathic scoliosis.[52]

Osteoporosis. An apparent relationship has been noted between Scheuermann's disease and osteoporosis developing in adolescence.[22,25] Osteoporosis limited to the axial skeleton, primarily the affected thoracic spine, could be explained by a combination of hyperemia and disuse. However, it has been subsequently shown that the osteoporosis is generalized, involving the appendicular skeleton as well and to roughly the same degree.[151] Another study found abnormal levels of serum alkaline phosphatase and urine hydroxyproline as well as deficient dietary calcium intake in 12 adolescents with Scheuermann's disease and osteopenia.[22,25] In keeping with the controversial nature of Scheuermann's disease, yet another study found no evidence of a relationship between this condition and osteoporosis, even in the axial skeleton. However, the disparity may be explained by different inclusion criteria for defining Scheuermann's disease.[86]

Intervertebral disc disease. Thoracic disc herniation resulting in cord or nerve root compression is one of the more clinically significant lesions secondary to Scheuermann's disease, resulting in focal back and radicular intercostal pain as well as occasional neurological deficit such as gait disturbance or bowel and bladder dysfunction.[17] Individuals with Scheuermann's disease demonstrate MRI changes of thoracolumbar degenerative disc disease by their early twenties in about 55% of the cases, as compared with about 10% in asymptomatic controls.[186] Another study also found that plain film changes of Scheuermann's disease, with associated disc space narrowing, were always associated with MRI evidence of degenerative disc disease.[187] This study did not, however, unearth a similar relationship between Scheuermann's disease and spondylolisthesis. A relationship has been noted between Scheuermann's disease and central spinal stenosis secondary to severe osteochondral changes, which may not be evident on plain films. Although these authors identified stenosis using myelogram, it is reasonable to conclude that either MRI or CT would typically be more suitable alternatives to myelography.[263]

Treatment. Treatment of Scheuermann's disease depends largely upon the clinical findings. Although watchful monitoring is all that may be necessary in most cases, progressive deformity, intractable moderate to severe pain, or development of neurological deficit would warrant more aggressive treatment. This ranges from bracing and application of orthoses to surgery, although the efficacy of nonsurgical treatments has not been established and the complications of surgery should limit its application to debilitating pain, neurological deficit, or spinal cord compression.[21,24,302]

KEY CONCEPTS

- *Scheuermann's disease and its abbreviated forms represent common developmental spinal abnormalities that may be asymptomatic or may lead to significant back pain and deformity.*
- *Physicians in a setting in which they will encounter adolescents with back complaints will certainly see many patients with this disorder and should be familiar with the clinical and diagnostic imaging findings (endplate irregularity, narrowed disc spaces, multiple Schmorl's nodes, and decreased anterior vertebral body height).*
- *Patients with more severe pain should be considered for advanced imaging, specifically MRI, to assess for the common complication of thoracic disc herniation, which is otherwise comparatively uncommon.*
- *Patients with more severe kyphosis may require bracing or, in a few cases, surgery to arrest or partially correct the deformity.*

Spondyloepiphyseal Dysplasia (SED)

BACKGROUND

Spondyloepiphyseal dysplasia (SED) congenita is an autosomal dominant dwarfing chondrodysplasia that is evident at birth and demonstrates a short trunk, generalized platyspondyly, and epiphyseal dysplasia. This has been linked to the gene locus COL2AI for type II collagen production.[2,239]

The more familiar SED tarda was first described by Maroteaux, Lamy, and Bernhard in 1957 in 20 patients from 3 families, although reports as early as 1937 describe what may have been SED tarda.[125] This is an X-linked recessive disorder characterized by epiphyseal and spinal apophyseal dysplasia, with spinal changes predominating. The condition is usually first suspected in young males from 5 to 10 years of age who demonstrate impaired spinal growth.[139] Chest expansion may occur, along with typical trunk shortening. A Danish study of more than 450,000 people demonstrated a prevalence of SED tarda of 7 per million, as compared with 40 per million for MED tarda.[1]

Rare variants of SED tarda have been reported in the last decade. These include a presumably autosomal recessive form occurring in females with mild to moderate mental retardation.[133] Another paper reported a case of localized spondyloepiphyseal dysplasia apparently affecting only the proximal femora and thoracolumbar junction. This case was discovered incidentally at 11 months and was therefore classified as SED congenita.[107] One case series from a family with several affected members involved autosomal dominant transmission and, in some instances, hearing deficit. The precise cause for the auditory complication was not indicated.[228] In another family, five patients in three generations demonstrated autosomal dominant SED tarda, associated with congenital hypotrichosis.[284]

In 1990 a report of a new form of SED tarda was published. This probably autosomal dominant condition, termed *spondyloepiphyseal dysplasia of Maroteaux,* demonstrated generalized platyspondyly as in Morquio syndrome but without anterior vertebral body beaks. Also unlike Morquio syndrome, no increase was noted in excretion of keratosulfate or corneal opacities. Patients were of normal intelligence and skeletal changes were not apparent at birth, features shared with Morquio syndrome.[56] An interesting variant of SED has been reported in 19 white South Africans of German descent, with mild to moderate dysplasia, progressive infantile kyphoscoliosis, altered trabecular pattern, and generalized joint laxity.[134]

IMAGING FINDINGS

Spinal changes predominate in the lumbar region but may affect the entire spine. Characteristics include generalized endplate irregularity and platyspondyly, which may resemble changes of severe Scheuermann's disease. A characteristic "heaped up" appearance of the vertebral "endplates," especially superiorly, helps to distinguish SED tarda from other conditions, although a similar appearance may infrequently result from isolated Schmorl's node formation (Fig. 10-28).

Degenerative disc space narrowing is asymmetrical, affecting the posterior aspect of the disc to a greater extent and sometimes leading to false impression of a widened anterior disc space. In the pelvis, the innominate and femoral neck may be hypoplastic. The epiphyses of the larger joints (shoulders and hips) may be slightly flattened, and early, advanced osteoarthritis, especially of the hips, may occur.[134,135,200] The epiphyseal changes are much milder and the spinal changes considerably more pronounced than in multiple epiphyseal dysplasia (MED).

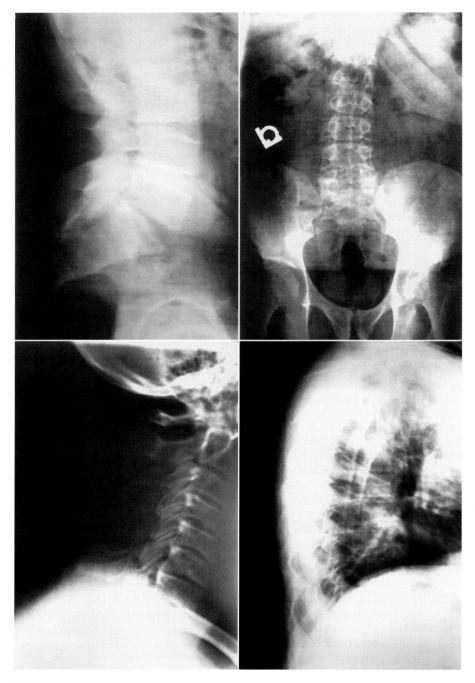

FIG. 10-28   Spondyloepiphyseal dysplasia tarda. Note generalized platyspondyly, premature degenerative disc disease, prominent nuclear impressions, and typical "heaped up" appearance to the posterior aspect of the superior endplates, more apparent in the thoracic and lumbar spine.

CLINICAL COMMENTS

In addition to a short trunk, generalized playspondyly, and epiphyseal dysplasia, patients with spondyloepiphyseal dysplasia congenita demonstrate other clinical findings, which include myopia, hypertelorism, frequent retinal detachment, short neck, mild thoracic kyphoscoliosis, and an expanded anteroposterior thoracic dimension. One case involved a dysplastic and unstable cervical spine, requiring surgical management.[144]

Individuals affected with the tarda form of SED often complain of back and hip pain, especially in early adulthood. Early, advanced degenerative disc disease begins in later adolescence and may be severe by ages 25 to 30 years.

A case series involving three boys with SED tarda and growth failure suggested an association with the nephrotic syndrome. Two of these patients showed focal and segmental glomerulosclerosis on renal biopsy.[62] Yet another report has appeared of three siblings with an autosomal recessive form of SED tarda, leading to severe, progressive arthropathy mimicking juvenile rheumatoid arthritis.[216]

KEY CONCEPTS

- *With some rather isolated exceptions, spondyloepiphyseal dysplasia may be seen as an autosomal recessive (spondyloepiphyseal dysplasia congenita) form or as an autosomal dominant (spondyloepiphyseal dysplasia tarda) form, the latter being more common.*
- *Generalized platyspondly with endplate irregularities and classic "heaped up" endplates is expected and is associated with significant short-trunk dwarfism.*
- *Epiphyseal regions are more mildly affected, especially when compared with multiple epiphyseal dysplasia.*

Turner's Syndrome

BACKGROUND

The phenotype of females with infantile secondary sexual characteristics, webbed neck (pterygium colli), and cubitus valgus was first described by Henry Turner more than 50 years ago. Shortly thereafter, gonadal dysgenesis was recognized as an integral part of the syndrome. It was not until about 20 years later, however, that Otto Ullrich identified the typical chromosomal abnormality, 45,XO, along with recognizing additional cases of mosaicism. Ullrich's name is sometimes attributed to the syndrome as well.[286]

IMAGING FINDINGS

The most widely recognized skeletal abnormality associated with Turner's syndrome is osteoporosis, which may be detectable prior to puberty. Turner's patients show below-average bone density, relative to bone age, chronological age, and body mass index (BMI) but normal density for height age. Adolescents with Turner's syndrome show a predilection to fractures of the distal radius, although it is not clear that these are related to alteration of bone density.[223] Turner's patients receiving growth hormone replacement in adolescence do not demonstrate osteoporosis. Thus it appears that growth hormone therapy has the double benefit of preventing markedly shortened stature and delayed skeletal maturity, as well as preventing osteoporosis.[138,178]

Isolated reports of skeletal changes resembling spondyloepiphyseal dysplasia (SED) have appeared. These include platyspondly and marked endplate irregularity, short femoral necks, coxa valga, coxa magna, and acetabular hypoplasia.[161,176] Anomalies of the sternum have been reported in Turner's syndrome. In addition to pectus excavatum, characteristics include shortening of the sternum, premature fusion of the manubriosternal joint or manubrium, and double manubrial ossification centers. These types of anomalies do not appear to be more common in patients with congenital heart disease.[169]

Radiographs of the hands may provide clues to the diagnosis. A classic, but by no means pathognomonic, radiographic finding in Turner's syndrome is shortening of one or more metacarpal bones, seen in about 50% of patients. The fourth metacarpal bone is the most commonly affected, although the third and fifth may also be involved. Other possible characteristics include carpal coalition; and, as in other syndromes producing coalition, the synostosis tends to be across rather than along carpal rows. Cubitus valgus, which is generally readily apparent clinically and seen in about 70% of patients, may be confirmed and accurately quantified radiographically, allowing planning for orthopedic intervention when necessary. The incidence of Madelung's deformity of the forearm is increased. The lower extremities may experience pes cavus and hyperplasia of the medial tibial plateau, with or without a small exostosis arising inferomedial to the tibial plateau.

CLINICAL COMMENTS

Turner's syndrome occurs in 1/2000 to 1/5000 live female births. The diagnosis is typically suspected early on the basis of overt clinical findings, although some patients may show nothing more than markedly diminished height. Analysis of chromatin bodies in buccal smears was hoped to represent a helpful screening tool in this population, but this has not proven to be true.[51] Individuals with Turner's syndrome have a decreased life expectancy of about 10 to 12 years below average. This is primarily a result of increased mortality from cardiovascular complications of congenital heart disease and aortic dissections.[203]

Cardiovascular anomalies are present in about 20% of affected patients, 70% of which are aortic coarctation. Echocardiography may show an asymptomatic aortic root dilatation. Besides aortic coarctation, congenital cardiovascular anomalies include partial anomalous pulmonary venous return, bicuspid aortic valve, mitral valve prolapse, aortic sinus aneurysm, and hypoplastic left heart (HLH) syndrome.[177,260,275]

Hypertension is also frequently seen, present in childhood in about one quarter of patients and with at least episodic hypertension in nearly 50% of adults. Estrogen replacement therapy may initiate or exacerbate the hypertension.[277] Aortic dissection is typically related to cystic medial necrosis. This underlying abnormality, similar to that seen in Marfan's syndrome, may play an important role in the development of other cardiovascular complications.[260] Patients with Turner's syndrome and their families should be made aware of these potential complications and prophylaxis should be considered, to include methods of preventing bacterial endocarditis and monitoring and control of blood pressure. The onset of aortic dissection may be characterized by unexplained, often severe chest pain, dyspnea, or sudden hypotension.[147]

Renal anomalies are seen in about one third of patients and are typically screened for using ultrasonography. The most common anomalies are horseshoe kidneys and duplication of the collecting system, accounting for somewhat less than half of all urinary tract anomalies (Fig. 10-29). Less often, renal agenesis, crossed ectopia, or pelvic kidney may occur. These anomalies may lead to urinary tract obstruction and may play a role in the development of hypertension.[148] An association may also exist between renal anomalies and altered renal vitamin D metabolism. This may be an important factor in the development of osteoporosis, particularly because osteoblastic function has not been found to be impaired.[227] Turner's patients may have insulin-resistant diabetes mellitus. This appears

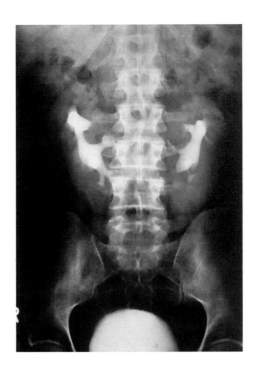

FIG. 10-29 Horseshoe kidney. Intravenous urogram optimally demonstrates typical renal morphology that would be better seen than on plain films. These and other renal anomalies may be seen in a variety of syndromes involving vertebral anomalies, including a distinctive "VATER syndrome," which includes vertebral anomalies, anal atresia, tracheoesophageal fistula, and renal anomalies.

to be related to abnormality at the muscular receptor site and may be partially overcome by increasing the insulin dose.[34,259]

Webbing of the neck (pterygium colli) is a frequent finding in Turner's syndrome, resembling some cases of Klippel-Feil syndrome. This may be corrected surgically, both for functional and cosmetic reasons.[269] Turner's syndrome patients typically have a broad chest, with widely spaced nipples and mild pectus excavatum. A high incidence of chronic otitis media (about 80%) is noted, frequently with associated sensorineural hearing loss (about 35%), and routine otological and audiological assessment has been advocated.[233]

Turner's syndrome is related to other diseases. The incidence of autoimmune diseases is increased among Turner's patients, although a relationship between specific diseases such as juvenile rheumatoid arthritis and Turner's syndrome has not been firmly established.[8] A frequent association exists between Turner's syndrome and congenital lymphedema, which typically resolves in the first year of life. Persistence of lymphedema may signal congenital lymphangiectasia, which was not described until 1986.[195] Turner's syndrome is also reportedly associated with pedal angioma.[281] Some of the associated disorders seen in Turner's syndrome may be related to treatment rather than to the disease itself. For example, an increased incidence of some types of uterine adenomyomas results from estrogen therapy.[39]

The variety of abnormalities reported in Turner's syndrome may result in complications being overlooked or receiving little attention. This may be true of central nervous system dysfunction, which may result from intrinsic anomaly or may be secondary to a cerebral vascular anomaly. This may lead to cognitive abnormalities and seizure disorders. Turner's patients experience an increased incidence of malignant transformation of the dysgenetic ovary, prompting questions regarding the role of prophylactic oophorectomy.[249] Turner's is also accompanied by an increased incidence of melanocytic nevi. Particularly in patients with multiple nevi and those on growth hormone therapy (which has been shown to increase the rate of growth of nevi), periodic skin examinations and restriction of unprotected sun exposure are prudent to minimize the risk of malignant transformation to malignant melanoma.[11,20]

KEY CONCEPTS

- *Turner's syndrome is an inherited disorder of XO chromosomal pattern, associated with short stature, delayed skeletal maturity, osteoporosis, and varying multisystem anomalies.*
- *Approximately 10% of patients have a mental deficit.*
  Classically associated anomalies of the various organ systems include aortic coarctation, ovarian dysgenesis, and horseshoe kidney.
- *The skeleton may demonstrate, among other things, scoliosis, kyphosis, cubitus valgus, pes cavus, Madelung's deformity, and enlargement of the medial tibial plateau.*
- *The most familiar anomaly of the skeleton is probably a short fourth metacarpal, although this is seen in only about half of all cases and may also be seen in a variety of other clinical settings, including as a normal variant.*

van Buchem's Disease

BACKGROUND

van Buchem's disease is a sclerosing bone dysplasia first described in 1955. Until fairly recently, the eponym was used to describe what are now considered to be several separate and distinct entities.[116] Classic van Buchem's disease, an autosomal recessive condition, is characterized by the same endosteal hyperostosis as its autosomal dominant counterpart, Worth's syndrome, and another autosomal recessive form known as *sclerosteosis*. In both conditions, the underlying histological abnormality appears to be a defect in the endochondral modulatory step regulating transformation of osteoclasts to osteoblasts.[61]

The latter may be fatal in infancy or early childhood.[291] Sclerosteosis is more common among South African Afrikaners than in other regions of the world and is less common in Holland.[13] Although Worth's syndrome becomes apparent clinically by early childhood, van Buchem's disease may not become apparent until puberty and demonstrates more severe skeletal changes, especially involving the mandible and skull. Frontal bossing and a broad nasal bridge are typical. Laboratory examination may be normal, or the serum alkaline phosphatase level may rise. Worth's syndrome, on the other hand, invariably demonstrates normal alkaline phosphatase levels. Symptoms associated with the bony changes are typically mild, and the condition may be found incidentally.

Skull changes may result in headache and cranial nerve palsies, with the facial and auditory nerves most frequently affected. Cranial nerve compression resulting from sclerosis and thickening of bone around the foramina may occur in early infancy, even before sclerosis and thickening of the skull is apparent radiographically.[77] Basal foraminal encroachment is another feature absent in Worth's syndrome and this may also assist in distinguishing between these two very similar conditions.[82]

IMAGING FINDINGS

Characteristic imaging changes involve diffuse, symmetrical sclerosis and cortical thickening, affecting both the axial and appendicular skeleton. The calvarium is thick and sclerotic, the mandible is enlarged, and a torus palatinum may exist. Unlike other syndromes affecting mandibular morphology, dental occlusion is unaltered.[229] Peculiar bony excrescences may be seen at the ends of long bones, a finding not seen with Worth's syndrome. Sclerosis and expansion of bone is often most prominent at the clavicles and ribs. Although the differences are minimal, bony expansion and lack of abnormalities of bone remodeling may also help to distinguish between van Buchem's disease and Worth's syndrome.[61,116]

KEY CONCEPTS

- *van Buchem's disease is a sclerosing bone dysplasia involving cranial and endosteal hyperostosis.*
- *It may closely resemble other sclerosing bone dysplasias, especially Worth's syndrome and sclerosteosis.*
- *It may be confused with other uncommon disorders, such as familial hyperphosphatasia, osteopetrosis, and diaphyseal dysplasia (Camurati-Engelmann disease).*

References

1. Andersen PE Jr et al: Bilateral femoral head dysplasia and osteochondritis. Multiple epiphyseal dysplasia tarda, spondylo-epiphyseal dysplasia tarda, and bilateral Legg-Perthes disease, *Acta Radiol* 29:705, 1988.
2. Anderson IJ et al: Spondyloepiphyseal dysplasia congenita: genetic linkage to type II collagen (COL2AI), *Am J Hum Genet* 46:896, 1990.
3. Arai Y et al: Brain CT studies in 26 cases of aged patients with Down syndrome, *Brain & Develop* 27:17, 1995.
4. Aronson DC et al: Cor pulmonale and acute liver necrosis, due to upper airway obstruction as part of pycknodysostosis, *Eur J Pediatr* 141:251, 1984.
5. Atar D et al: New method of limb deformities correction in children, *Bull NY Acad Med* 68:447, 1992.
6. Atkinson RN et al: Bone scintigraphy in discitis and related disorders in children, *Aust N Z J Surg* 48:374, 1978.
7. Aufdermauer M, Spycher M: Pathogenesis of osteochondrosis juvenilis Scheuermann, *J Orthop Res* 4:452, 1986.
8. Balestrazzi P et al: Juvenile rheumatoid arthritis in Turner's syndrome, *Clin Exp Rheumatol* 4:61, 1986.
9. Barfred T, Ipsen T: Congenital carpal tunnel syndrome, *J Hand Surg* 10A:246, 1985.
10. Bax MC, Colville GA: Behaviour in mucopolysaccharide disorders, *Arch Dis Child* 73:77, 1995.
11. Becker B et al: Melanocytic nevi in Turner syndrome, *Pediatr Dermatol* 11:120, 1994.
12. Beighton P et al: Osteopetrosis in South Africa. The benign, lethal and intermediate forms, *S Afr Med J* 55:659, 1979.
13. Beighton P et al: The syndromic status of sclerosteosis and van Buchem disease, *Clin Genet* 25:175, 1984.
14. Berg JM, Armstrong D: On the association of moyamoya disease with Down syndrome, *J Ment Defic Res* 35:398, 1991.
15. Bethen D et al: Disorders of the spine in diastrophic dwarfism, *J Bone Joint Surg Am* 62:529, 1980.
16. Bhatnagar M et al: Pediatric atlantoaxial instability presenting as cerebral and cerebellar infarcts, *J Pediatr Orthop* 11:103, 1991.
17. Bhojraj SY, Dandawate AV: Progressive cord compression secondary to thoracic disc lesions in Scheuermann's kyphosis managed by posterolateral decompression, interbody fusion and pedicular fixation. A new approach to the management of a rare clinical entity, *Eur Spine J* 3:66, 1994.
18. Bostman OM, Bakalim GE: Carpal tunnel syndrome in a melorheostotic limb, *J Hand Surg* 10B:101, 1985.
19. Bostman OM et al: Osteosarcoma arising in a melorheostotic femur: a case report, *J Bone Joint Surg Am* 69:1232, 1987.
20. Bourguignon JP et al: Effects of human growth hormone therapy on melanocytic naevi, *Lancet* 341:1505, 1993.
21. Bradford DS: Juvenile kyphosis, *Clin Orthop* 128:45, 1977.
22. Bradford DS et al: Scheuermann's kyphosis: a form of osteoporosis?, *Clin Orthop* 118:10, 1976.
23. Bradford DS et al: Scheuermann's kyphosis and roundback deformity. Results of Milwaukee brace treatment, *J Bone Joint Surg Am* 56:740, 1974.
24. Bradford DS et al: Scheuermann's kyphosis. Results of surgical treatment by posterior spine arthrodesis in twenty-two patients, *J Bone Joint Surg Am* 57:439, 1975.
25. Bradford DS, Moe JH: Scheuermann's juvenile kyphosis. A histologic study, *Clin* 110:45, 1975.
26. Brante G: Gargoylism: a mucopolysaccharidosis, *Scand J Clin Lab Invest* 4:43, 1952.
27. Bredenkamp JK et al: Otolaryngologic manifestations of the mucopolysaccharidoses, *Ann Otol Rhinol Laryngol* 101:472, 1992.
28. Brenton DP, Dow CJ: Homocystinuria and Marfan's syndrome. A comparison, *J Bone Joint Surg Br* 54:277, 1972.
29. Bridgeman SA et al: Leg lengthening, *J R Coll Surg Edinb* 38:101, 1993.
30. Bridges NA, Brook CG: Progress report: growth hormone in skeletal dysplasia, *Hormone Res* 42:231, 1994.
31. Brill PW et al: Homocystinuria due to cystathionine synthetase deficiency: clinical roentgenologic correlation, *AJR* 121:45, 1974.
32. Brueton LA et al: Apparent cleidocranial dysplasia associated with abnormalities of 8q22 in three individuals, *Am J Med Genet* 43:612, 1992.
33. Buchanan WW: The arthritis of Mary Queen of Scots: due to Marfan's syndrome?, *Clin Rheumatol* 5:419, 1986.
34. Caprio S et al: Insulin resistance: an early metabolic defect of Turner's syndrome, *J Clin Endocrinol Metab* 72:832, 1991.
35. Carson NAJ et al: Homocystinuria: clinical and pathological review of ten cases, *J Pediatr* 66:565, 1965.
36. Carson WG et al: Congenital elevation of the scapula. Surgical correction by the Woodward procedure, *J Bone Joint Surg Am* 63:1199, 1981.
37. Chitayat D et al: Intrafamilial variability in cleidocranial dysplasia: a three generation family, *Am J Med Genet* 42:298, 1992.
38. Chong WK, al-Kutoubi MA: Retroperitoneal fibrosis in Marfan's syndrome, *Clin Radiol* 44:386, 1991.

39. Clement PB, Young RH: Atypical polypoid adenomyoma of the uterus associated with Turner's syndrome. A report of three cases, including a review of "estrogen-associated" endometrial neoplasms and neoplasms associated with Turner's syndrome, *Int J Gynecol Pathol* 6:104, 1987.

40. Clements WD et al: Os odontoideum - congenital or acquired? That's not the question, *Injury* 26:640, 1995.

41. Collins ML et al: Optic nerve head swelling and optic atrophy in the systemic mucopolysaccharidoses, *Ophthalmology* 97:1445, 1990.

42. Crockard HA, Stevens JM: Craniovertebral junction anomalies in inherited disorders: part of the syndrome or caused by the disorder, *Eur J Pediatr* 154:504, 1995.

43. Cross HE, Jensen AD: Ocular manifestations in the Marfan syndrome: a heritable disorder of connective tissue, *Am J Ophthalmol* 75:405, 1973.

44. Curless RG: Dominant chondrodysplasia punctata with neurological symptoms, *Neurology* 33:1095, 1983.

45. Currarino G: Primary spondylolysis of the axis vertebra (C2) in three children, including one with pyknodysostosis, *Pediatr Radiol* 19:535, 1989.

46. Currarino G, Swanson GE: A developmental variant of ossificaion in manubrium sterni in mongolism, *Radiol* 82:916, 1964.

47. da Silva EO et al: Ellis-van Creveld syndrome: report of 15 cases in an inbred kindred, *J Med Genet* 17:349, 1980.

48. Davis DC et al: Melorheostosis on three-phase bone scintigraphy. Case report, *Clin Nucl Med* 17:561, 1992.

49. Davis JW et al: Amino acids and collagen-induced platelet aggregation. Lack of effect of three amino acids that are elevated in homocystinuria, *Am J Dis Child* 129:1020, 1975.

50. de Jong JG et al: Measuring urinary glycosaminoglycans in the presence of protein: an improved screening procedure for mucoplysaccharidoses based on dimethylmethylene blue, *Clin Chem* 38:803, 1992.

51. de Mel T et al: Screening for Turner syndrome: how useful is the buccal smear test?, *Ceylon Med J* 37:83, 1992.

52. Deacon P et al: Combined idiopathic kyphosis and scoliosis. An analysis of the lateral spinal curvatures associated with Scheuermann's disease, *J Bone Joint Surg Br* 67:189, 1985.

53. D'iachkova GV: X-ray diagnosis of the state of soft tissues in patients with achondroplasia in limb lengthening using Ilizarov technique, *Vestn Rentgenol Radiol* 2:46, 1995.

54. DiMario FJ et al: Brain morphometric analysis in achondroplasia, *Neurology* 45:519, 1995.

55. Dissing I, Zafirovski G: Para-articular ossifications associated with melorheostosis Leri, *Acta Orthop Scand* 50:717, 1979.

56. Doman AN et al: Spondyloepiphyseal dysplasia of Maroteaux, *J Bone Joint Surg Am* 72:1364, 1990.

57. Domingues JC et al: Congenital sensory neuropathy with anhidrosis, *Pediatr Dermatol* 11:231, 1994.

58. Dore DD et al: Cleiodcranial dysostosis and syringomyelia. Review of the literature and case report, *Clin Orthop* 214:229, 1987.

59. Dorfman A, Lorincz AE: Occurrence of urinary acid mucopolysacharides in the Hurler syndrome, *Proc Natl Acad Sci U S A* 43:443, 1957.

60. Dugdale TW, Renshaw TS: Instability of the patellofemoral joint in Down syndrome, *J Bone Joint Surg Am* 68:405, 1986.

61. Eastman JR, Bixler D: Generalized cortical hyperostosis (van Buchem disease): nosological considerations, *Radiology* 125:297, 1977.

62. Ehrich JH et al: Association of spondylo-epiphyseal dysplasia with nephrotic syndrome, *Pediatr Nephrol* 4:117, 1990.

63. Elmore SM: Pycnodysostosis. A review, *J Bone Joint Surg Am* 49:153, 1967.

64. Emerson JF et al: Magnetic resonance imaging of the aging brain in Down syndrome, *Progr Clin Biol Res* 393:123, 1995.

65. Eppley BL et al: Developmental significance of delayed closure of the mandibular symphsis, *J Oral Maxillofac Surg* 50:677, 1992.

66. Feldman GJ et al: A gene for cleidocranial dysplasia maps to the short arm of chromosome 6, *Am J Hum Genet* 56:938, 1995.

67. Fisk JW, Baigent ML: Hamstring tightness and Scheuermann's disease: a pilot study, *Am J Phys Med Rehabil* 60:122, 1981.

68. Fisk JW et al: Incidence of Scheuermann's disease. Preliminary report, *Am J Phys Med Rehabil* 61:32, 1982.

69. Fisk JW et al: Scheuermann's disease. Clinical and radiological survey of 17 and 18 year olds, *Am J Phys Med Rehabil* 63:18, 1984.

70. Fitzsimons RB: Idiopathic scoliosis, Scheuermann's disease and myopathy: two case reports, *Clin Exp Neurol* 16:303, 1979.

71. Forlin E et al: Understanding the os odontoideum, *Orthop Rev* 21:1441, 1992.

72. Fountzilas G et al: Extragonadal choriocarcinoma in a patient with Down syndrome, *Am J Clin Oncol* 17:452, 1994.

73. Franco B et al: A cluster of sulfatase genes on Xp22.3: mutations in chondrodysplasia punctata (CDPX) and implications for warfarin embryopathy, *Cell* 81:15, 1995.

74. Francomano CA et al: Localization of the achondroplasia gene to the distal 2.5 Mb of human chromosome 4p, *Hum Molec Genet* 3:787, 1994.

75. Franke J et al: Ilizarov-Techniken zur Beinverlangerung. Probleme und Ergebnisse, *Orthopade* 21:197, 1992.

76. French HG et al: Upper cervical ossicles in Down syndrome, *J Pediatr Orthop* 7:69, 1987.

77. Fryns JP, Van den Bergh H: Facial paralysis at the age of 2 months as a first clinical sign of van Buchem disease, *Eur J Pediatr* 147:99, 1988.

78. Gardner WJ, Collins JS: The Klippel-Feil syndrome. Syringomyelia, diastematamyelia and myelomeningocele - one disease?, *Arch Surg* 83:638, 1961.

79. Garver P et al: Melorheostosis of the axial skeleton with associated fibrolipomatous lesions, *Skeletal Radiol* 9:41, 1982.

80. Gatzoulis MA et al: Cardiac involvement in mucoplysaccharidoses: effects of allogenic bone marrow transplantation, *Arch Dis Child* 73:259, 1995.

81. Gelb BD et al: Genetic mapping of the cleidocranial dysplasia (CCD) locus on chromosome band 6p21 to include a microdeletion, *Am J Med Genet* 58:200, 1995.

82. Gelman MI: Autosomal dominant osteosclerosis, *Radiology* 125:289, 1977.

83. Gerrittsen T, Waisman HA: Homocystinuria, an error in metabolism of methionine, *Pediatrics* 33:413, 1964.

84. Gibson JB et al: Pathological findings in homocystinuria, *J Clin Pathol* 17:427, 1964.

85. Gilbert EF et al: Chondrodysplasia punctata - rhizomelic form, *Eur J Pediatr* 123:89, 1976.

86. Gilsanz V et al: Vertebral bone density in Scheuermann disease, *J Bone Joint Surg Am* 71:894, 1989.

87. Goldman AB et al: Case report 778. Melorheostosis presenting as two soft tissue masses with osseous changes limited to the axial skeleton, *Skeletal Radiol* 22:206, 1993.

88. Goodwin CB et al: Cervical vertebral-costal process (costovertebral bone)—a previously unreported anomaly. A case report, *J Bone Joint Surg Am* 66:1477, 1984.

89. Greene TL et al: Back pain and vertebral changes simulating Scheuermann's disease, *J Pediatr Orthop* 5:1, 1985.

90. Guidera KJ et al: Orthopaedic manifestations in congenitally insensate patients, *J Pediatr Orthop* 10:514, 1990.

91. Gustavson KH et al: Lethal and non-lethal diastrophic dysplasia. A study of 14 Swedish cases, *Clin Genet* 28:321, 1985.

92. Gyves-Ray K et al: Cystic lung disease in Down syndrome, *Pediatr Radiol* 24:137, 1994.

93. Halal F et al: Dominant inheritance of Scheuermann's juvenile kyphosis, *Am J Dis Child* 132:1105, 1978.

94. Hall GS: A continution to the study of melorheostosis: unusual bone changes associated with tuberous sclerosis, *Q J Med* 12:77, 1943.

95. Hamner LH et al: Prenatal diagnosis of cleidocranial dysplasia, *Obstet Gynecol* 83:856, 1994.

96. Happle R et al: The CHILD surndrome: congenital hemidysplasia with ichthyosiform erythroderma and limb defects, *Eur J Pediatr* 134:27, 1980.

97. Harley EH, Collins MD: Neurological sequelae secondary to atlantoaxial instability in Down syndrome. Implications in otolaryngologic surgery, *Arch Otolaryngol Head Neck Surg* 120:159, 1994.

98. Harreby M et al: Are radiologic changes in the thoracic and lumbar spine of adolescents risk factors for low back pain in adults? A 25-year prospective cohort study of 640 school children, *Spine* 20:2298, 1995.

99. Heggeness MH: Charcot arthropathy of the spine with resulting paraparesis developing during in a patient with congenital insensitivity to pain. A case report, *Spine* 19:95, 1994.

100. Heithoff KB et al: Juvenile discogenic disease, *Spine* 19:335, 1994.

101. Hensinger RN et al: Klippel-Feil syndrome. A constellation of associated anomalies, *J Bone Joint Surg Am* 56:1246, 1974.

102. Hertel NT, Muller J: Anthropometry in skeletal dysplasia, *J Pediatr Endocrinol* 7:155, 1994.

103. Heselson NG, Marus G: Chronic atlanto-axial dislocation with spontaneous bony fusion, *Clin Radiol* 39:555, 1988.

104. Hilhorst MI et al: Down syndrome and coeliac disease: five new cases with a review of the literature, *Eur J Pediatr* 152:884, 1993.

105. Hinkle CO, Beilard D: Osteopetrosis, *AJR* 74:46, 1955.

106. Hirata K et al: The Marfan syndrome: cardiovascular physical findings and diagnostic correlates, *Am Heart J* 123:743, 1992.

107. Hoeffel JC et al: Localized form of spondylo-epiphyseal dysplasia congenita, *Rontgen-Blatter* 41:20, 1988.

108. Holt RG et al: Hypertrophy of C1 anterior arch: useful sign to distinguish os odontoideum from acute dens fracture, *Radiology* 173:207, 1989.

109. Horton WA et al: Growth hormone therapy in achondroplasia, *Am J Med Genet* 42:667, 1992.

110. Horton WA et al: The phenotypic variability of diastrophic dysplasia, *J Pediatr* 93:609, 1978.

111. Hosono N et al: Cineradiographic motion analysis of atlantoaxial instability in os odontoideum, *Spine* 16:S480, 1991.

112. Hresko MT et al: Hip disease in adults with Down syndrome, *J Bone Joint Surg Br* 75:604, 1993.

113. Ieshima A et al: A morphometric CT study of Down syndrome showing small posterior fossa and calcification of basal ganglia, *Neuroradiology* 26:493, 1984.

114. Iglesias JH et al: Renal artery stenosis associated with melorheostosis, *Pediatr Nephrol* 8:441, 1994.

115. Ingram RR: The shoulder in multiple epiphyseal dysplasia, *J Bone Joint Surg Br* 73:277, 1991.

116. Jacobs P: van Buchem's disease, *Postgrad Med* 53:479, 1977.

117. Jensen BL: Cleidocranial dysplasia: craniofacial morphology in adult patients, *J Craniofac Genet Dev Biol* 14:163, 1994.

118. Jensen BL, Kreiborg S: Dental treatment strategies in cleidocranial dysplasia, *Br Dent J* 172:243, 1992.

119. Jensen BL, Kreiborg S: Development of the skull in infants with cleidocranial dysplasia, *J Craniofac Genet Dev Biol* 13:89, 1993.

120. Jensen BL, Kreiborg S: Craniofacial growth in cleidocranial dysplasia —a roentgencephalometric study, *J Craniofac Genet Dev Biol* 15:35, 1995.

121. Johnson CC et al: Osteopetrosis. A clinical, genetic, metabolic and morphologic study of the dominantly inherited benign type, *Medicine* 47:149, 1968.

122. Johnson MA et al: Magnetic resonance imaging of the brain in Hurler's syndrome, *Am J Neuroradiol* 5:816, 1984.

123. Kang AH, Trelstad RL: A collagen defect in homocystinuria, *J Clin Invest* 52:2571, 1973.

124. Kanis JA, Thomson JG: Mixed sclerosing bone dystrophy with regression of melorheostosis, *Br J Radiol* 48:400, 1975.

125. Katona K et al: Spondyloepiphyseal dysplasia tarda, *Rontgen-Blatter* 38:397, 1985.

126. Kawabata H et al: Melorheostosis of the upper limb: a report of two cases, *J Hand Surg* 9:871, 1984.

127. Khermosh O, Wientroub S: Dysplasia epiphysealis capitis femoris. Meyer's dysplasia, *J Bone Joint Surg Br* 73:621, 1991.

128. Kikuchi K et al: Bilateral vertebral artery occlusion secondary to atlantoaxial dislocation with os odontoideum: implication for prophylactic cervical stabilization by fusion—case report, *Neurol Med Chir* 33:769, 1993.

129. Kirlew KA et al: Os odontoideum in identical twins: perspective on etiology, *Skeletal Radiol* 22:525, 1993.

130. Kivara N et al: Intermediate form of osteopetrosis, with recessive inheritance, *Skeletal Radiol* 9:47, 1982.

131. Klippel M, Feil A: Absence de colonne cervicale. Cage thoracique remontant jusqu'à la base du crane, *Presse Med* 20:411, 1912.

132. Klippel M, Feil A: Anomalie de la colonne vertebrale par absence des vertebres cervicales; cage thoracique remontant jusqu'à la base du crane, *Bull Mem Soc Anat Paris* 87:185, 1912.

133. Kohn G et al: Spondyloepiphyseal dysplasia tarda: a new autosomal recessive variant with mental retardation, *J Med Genet* 24:366, 1987.

134. Kozlowski K, Beighton P: Radiographic features of spondyloepiphyseal dysplasia with joint laxity and progressive kyphoscoliosis. Review of 19 cases, *Rofo Fortschr Rontgenstr Neuen Bildgeb Verfahr* 141:337, 1984.

135. Kozlowski K, Masel J: Spondyloepiphysial dysplasia tarda (report of 7 cases), *Australas Radiol* 27:285, 1983.

136. Kuhlman JE et al: Acetabular protrusion in the Marfan syndrome, *Radiology* 164:415, 1987.

137. Lachman R et al: Diastrophic dysplasia: the death of a variant, *Radiology* 140:79, 1981.

138. Lanes R et al: Bone mineral density of prepubertal age girls with Turner's syndrome while on growth hormone therapy, *Horm Res* 44:168, 1995.

139. Langer LO: Spondyloepiphyseal dysplasia tarda. Hereditary chondrodysplasia with characteristic vertebral configuration in the adult, *Radiology* 82:833, 1964.

140. Langer LO et al: Achondroplasia, *AJR* 100:12, 1967.

141. Larner AJ et al: Congenital insensitivity to pain: a 20 year follow up, *J Neurol Neurosurg Psychiatry* 57:973, 1994.

142. Laughlin GM et al: Sleep apnea as a possible cause of pulmonary hypertension in Down syndrome, *J Pediatr* 98:435, 1981.

143. Lawrence JJ et al: Unusual radiographic manifestations of chondrodysplasia punctata, *Skeletal Radiol* 18(1):15, 1989.

144. LeDoux MS et al: Stabilization of the cervical spine in spondyloepiphyseal dysplasia congenita, *Neurosurgery* 28:580, 1991.

145. Lee SH, Sanderson J: Hypophosphataemic rickets and melorheostosis, *Clin Radiol* 40:209, 1989.

146. Lee C et al: The mucopolysaccharidoses: characterization by cranial MR imaging, *Am J Neuroradiol* 14:1285,1993.

147. Lin AE et al: Aortic dilation, dissection and rupture in patients with Turner's syndrome, *J Pediatr* 109(5):820, 1986.

148. Lippe B et al: Renal malformations in patients with Turner syndrome: imaging in 141 patients, *Pediatrics* 82:852, 1988.

149. Lo RN et al: Abnormal radial artery in Down syndrome, *Arch Dis Child* 61:885, 1986.

150. Loncar J et al: Advent of maternal serum markers for Down syndrome screening, *Obstet Gynecol* 50:316, 1995.

151. Lopez RA et al: Osteoporosis in Scheuermann's disease, *Spine* 13:1099, 1988.

152. Lubec B et al: Evidence for McKusick's hypothesis of deficient collagen cross-linking in patients with homocystinuria, *Biochimic Biophys Acta* 1315:159, 1996.

153. Lyritis G et al: Orthopaedic problems in patients with pycnodysostosis, *Prog Clin Biol Res* 104:199, 1982.

154. Magid D et al: Musculoskeletal manifestations of the Marfan syndrome: radiologic features, *AJR* 155:99, 1990.

155. Mandell GA et al: Bone scintigraphy in patients wih atypical lumbar Scheuermann disease, *J Pediatr Orthop* 13:622, 1993.

156. Mantero R: The Marfan hands of Niccolo Paganini, *Ann Chir Main Memb Super* 7:335, 1988.

157. Manzke H et al: Dominant sex-linked inherited chondrodysplasia punctata. A distinct type of chondrodysplasia punctata, *Clin Genet* 17:97, 1980.

158. Marino B: Congenital heart disease in patients with Down syndrome: anatomical and genetic aspects, *Biomed Pharmacother* 47:197, 1993.

159. Martel W, Tishler JM: Observations on the spine in mongoloidism, *AJR* 97:630, 1966.

160. Martich V et al: Hypoplastic posterior arch of C1 in children with Down syndrome: a double jeopardy, *Radiology* 183:125, 1992.

161. Massa G, Vanderschueren-Lodeweyckx M: Spondyloepiphyseal dysplasia tarda in Turner syndrome, *Acta Paediatr Scand* 78:971, 1989.

162. Matsuda Y et al: Atlanto-occipital hypermobility in subjects with Down syndrome, *Spine* 20:2283, 1995.

163. Mayer EL et al: Homocysteine and coronary atheroclerosis, *J Am Coll Cardiol* 27:517, 1996.

164. McCallum MJ: Scheuermann's disease the result of emotional stress? *Med J Austr* 140:184, 1984.

165. McKenzie L, Sillence D: Familial Scheuermann disease: a genetic and linkage study, *J Med Genet* 29:41, 1992.

166. McKusick VA et al: Dwarfism in the Amish. The Ellis-Van Creveld syndrome, *Bull Johns Hopkins Hosp* 115:306, 1964.

167. McKusick VA: The classification of hereditable disorders of connective tissue, *Birth Defects* 11:1, 1975.

168. McKusick VA: *Hereditable disorders of connective tissues,* ed 4, St Louis, 1972, Mosby.

169. Mehta AV et al: Radiologic abnormalities of the sternum in Turner's syndrome, *Chest* 104:1795, 1993.

170. Miller JD et al: Changes at the skull and cevical spine in Down syndrome, *Can Assoc Radiol J* 37:85, 1986.

171. Mitchell V et al: Down syndrome and anaesthesia, *Pediatric Anaesthesia* 5:379, 1995.

172. Miyata I et al: Pediatric cerebellar infarction caused by atlantoaxial subluxation—case report, *Neurol Med Chir* 34:241, 1994.

173. Morgan MK et al: Familial os odontoideum. Case report, *J Neurosurg* 70:636, 1989.

174. Murata R et al: MR imaging of the brain in patients with mucoplysaccharidosis, *Am J Neuroradiol* 10:1165, 1989.

175. Murray RO, McCredie J: Melorheostosis and the sclerotomes: a radiological correlation, *Skeletal Radiol* 4:57, 1979.

176. Nakashima N et al: Two cases of Turner's syndrome with spondyloepiphyseal dysplasia like bone appearance, *Fukuoka Igaku Zasshi* 81:384, 1990.

177. Natowicz M, Kelley RI: Association of Turner syndrome with hypoplastic left heart-syndrome, *Am J Dis Child* 141:218, 1987.

178. Neely EK et al: Turner syndrome adolescents receiving growth hormone are not osteopenic, *J Clin Endocrinol Metab* 76:861, 1993.

179. Nishi Y et al: Growth hormone therapy in achondroplasia, *Acta Endocrinologica* 128:394, 1993.

180. Nissinen M: Spinal posture during pubertal growth, *Acta Paediatr* 84:308,1995.

181. Ogden JA et al: Sprengel's deformity. Radiology of the pathologic deformation, *Skeletal Radiol* 4:(2)204, 1979.

182. Ohlsson A et al: Marble brain disease: recessive osteopetrosis, renal tubular acidosis and cerebral calcification in three Saudi Arabian families, *Dev Med Child Neurol* 22:72, 1980.

183. Olgilvie JW, Sherman J: Spondylolysis in Scheuermann's disease, *Spine* 12:251, 1987.

184. Ostrowski DM, Gilula LA: Mixed sclerosing bone dystrophy presenting with upper extremity deformities. A case report and review of the literature, *Br J Hand Surg* 17:108, 1992.

185. Ozbarlas N et al: Congenital insensitivity to pain with anhidrosis, *Cutis* 51:373, 1993.

186. Paajanen H et al: Disc degeneration in Scheuermann disease, *Skeletal Radiol* 18:523, 1989.

187. Paajanen H et al: Magnetic resonance study of disc degeneration in young low-back pain patients, *Spine* 14:982, 1989.

188. Parker RD, Froimson AI: Neurogenic arthropathy of the hand and wrist, *J Hand Surg* 11A:706, 1986.

189. Patrone NA, Kredich DW: Arthritis in children with multiple epiphyseal dysplasia, *J Rhematol* 12:145, 1985.

190. Pattisapu J et al: Cleidocranial dysostosis and schwannoma, *Neurosurgery* 18:827, 1986.

191. Pauli RM et al: Apnea and sudden unexpected death in infants with achondroplasia, *J Pediatr* 104:342, 1984.

192. Pauli RM et al: Prospective assessment of risks for cervicomedullary junction compression in infants with achondroplasia, *Am J Hum Genet* 56:732, 1995.

193. Peltonen JI et al: Cementless hip arthroplasty in diastrophic dysplasia, *J Arthroplasty* 7 suppl:369, 1992.

194. Peretti G et al: Staged lengthening in the prevention of dwarfism in achondroplastic children: a preliminary report, *J Pediatr Orthop* 4:58, 1995.

195. Perry HD, Cossari AJ: Chronic lymphangiectasis in Turner's syndrome, *Br J Ophthalmol* 70:396, 1986.

196. Peters ME et al: Narrow trachea in mucopolysaccharidoses, *Pediatr Radiol* 15:225, 1985.

197. Peyritz RE et al: Dural ectasia is a common feature of the Marfan syndrome, *Am J Hum Genet* 43:726, 1988.

198. Piazza MR et al: Neuropathic spinal arthropathy in congenital insensitivity to pain, *Clin Orthop* 236:175, 1988.

199. Pizzutillo PD et al: Atlantoaxial instability in mucopolysaccharidosis type VII, *J Pediatr Orthop* 9:76, 1989.

200. Poker N et al: Spondyloepiphyseal dysplasia tarda. Four cases in childhood and adolescence, and some considerations regarding platyspondyly, *Radiol* 85:474, 1965.

201. Poussa M et al: The spine in diastrophic dysplasia, *Spine* 16:881, 1991.

202. Poznanski AK: Punctate epiphyses: a radiological sign not a disease, *Pediatr Radiol* 24:418, 1994.

203. Price WH et al: Mortality ratios, life expectancy, and causes of death in patients with Turner's syndrome, *J Epidemiol Community Health* 40:97, 1986.

204. Pruitt DL, Manske PR: Soft tissue contractures from melortheostosis involving the upper extremity, *J Hand Surg* 17A:90, 1992.

205. Pueschel SM et al: A longitudinal study of atlanto-dens relationships in asymptomatic individuals with Down syndrome, *Pediatrics* 89:1194, 1992.

206. Quinn SF, Dyer R: Osteopetrosis with calcifying tendinitis, *South Med J* 77:400, 1984.

207. Qureshi F et al: Skeletal histopathology in fetuses with chondroectodermal dysplasia (Ellis-Van Creveld syndrome), *Am J Med Genet* 45:471, 1993.

208. Raby N, Vivian G: Case report 478: melorheostosis of the axial skeleton with associated intrathecal lipoma, *Skeletal Radiol* 17:216, 1988.

209. Rathore MH, Sreenivasan VV: Vertebral and right subclavian artery abnormalities in the Down syndrome, *Am J Cardiol* 63:1528, 1989.

210. Reed MH, Houston CS: Abnormal ossification of the hyoid bone in cleidocranial dysplasia, *Can Assoc Radiol J* 44:277, 1993.

211. Resnick D: Diagnosis of bone and joint disorders, ed 3, Philadelphia, 1995, WB Saunders.

212. Richards BS: Atlanto-axial instability in diastrophic dysplasia. A case report, *J Bone Joint Surg Am* 73:614, 1991.

213. Richardson A, Deussen FF: Facial and dental anomalies in cleidocranial dysplasia: a study of 17 cases, *Internat J Paediatr Dent* 4:225, 1994.

214. Rintala A et al: Cleft palate in diastrophic dysplasia. Morphology, results of treatment and complications, *Scand J Plast Reconstr Surg Hand Surg* 20:45, 1986.

215. Roberts GM et al: Radiology of the pelvis and hips in adults with Down syndrome, *Clin Radiol* 31:475, 1980.

216. Robinson D et al: Spondyloepiphyseal dysplasia associated with progressive arthropathy. An unusual disorder mimicking juvenile rheumatoid arthritis, *Arch Orthop Trauma Surg* 108:397, 1989.

217. Robinson K et al: Homocysteine and coronary artery disease, *Cleveland Clin J Med* 61:438, 1994.

218. Robinson L et al: Multiple meningeal cysts in Marfan syndrome, *Am J Neuroradiol* 10:1275, 1989.

219. Roger D et al: Melorheostosis with associated minimal change nephrotic syndrome, mesenteric fibromatosis and capillary hemangiomas, *Dermatology* 188:166, 1994.

220. Rosemberg S et al: Congenital insensitivity to pain with anhidrosis hereditary sensory and autonomic neuropathy type IV, *Pediatr Neurol* 11:50, 1994.

221. Rosenbaum DM et al: Atlanto-occipital instability in Down syndrome, *AJR* 146:1269, 1986.

222. Rosenshtein A, Negrin JA: Increased Tc-99MDP in multiple lumbar intervertebral disk spaces in Scheuermann disease without concomitant radiographic calcification or discitis, *Clin Nucl Med* 19:863, 1994.

223. Ross JL et al: Normal bone density of the wrist and spine and increased wrist fractures in girls with Turner's syndrome, *J Clin Endocrinol Metab* 73:355, 1991.

224. Ryan MD, Taylor TK: Acute spinal cord compression in Scheuermann's disease, *J Bone Joint Surg* 64B:409, 1982.

225. Ryken TC, Menezes AH: Cervicomedullary compression in achondroplasia, *J Neurosurg* 81:43, 1994.

226. Ryoppy S et al: Foot deformities in diastrophic dysplasia. An analysis of 102 patients, *J Bone Joint Surg* Br 74:441, 1992.

227. Saggese G et al: Mineral metabolism in Turner's syndrome: Evidence for impaired renal vitamin D metabolism and normal osteoblast function, *J Clin Endocrinol Metab* 75:998, 1992.

228. Schantz K et al: Spondyloepiphyseal dysplasia tarda. Report of a family with autosomal dominant transmission, *Acta Orthop Scand* 59:716, 1988.

229. Schendel SA: van Buchem disease: surgical treatment of the mandible, *Ann Plast Surg* 20:462, 1988.

230. Scheuermann HW: Kyphosis dorsalis juvenilis, *Z Orthop Chir* 41:305, 1921.

231. Schuler TC et al: Natural history of os odontoideum, *J Pediatr Orthop* 11:222, 1991.

232. Scoles PV et al: Vertebral alterations in Scheuermann's kyphosis, *Spine* 16:509, 1991.

233. Sculerati N et al: Otitis media and hearing loss in Turner syndrome, *Arch Otolaryngol* 116:704, 1990.

234. Selby KA et al: Clinical predictors and radiological reliability in atlanto-axial subluxation in Down syndrome, *Arch Dis Child* 66:876, 1991.

235. Sembel EL et al: Successful symptomatic treatment of melorheostosis with nifedipine, *Clin Exp Rheumatol* 4:277, 1986.

236. Shands AR, Jr., Bunden WD: Congenital deformities of the spine. An analysis of the roentgenograms of 700 children, *Bull Hosp Jt Dis* 17:110, 1956.

237. Shapiro EG et al: Neuropsychological outcomes of several storage diseases with and without bone marrow transplantation, *J Inherit Metab Dis* 18:413, 1995.

238. Sheffield LJ et al: Chondrodysplasia punctata - 23 cases of a mild and relatively common variety, *J Pediatr* 89:916, 1976.

239. Sher C et al: Mild spondyloepiphyseal dysplasia (Namaqualand type): genetic linkage to the type II collagen gene COL2AI, *Am J Hum Genet* 48:518, 1991.

240. Siegel A, Williams H: Linear scleroderma and melorheostosis, *Br J Radiol* 65:266, 1992.

241. Silengo MC et al: Clinical and genetic aspects of Conradi-Hunermann disease, *J Pediatr* 97:911, 1980.

242. Silverman FN, Reiley MA: Spondylo-megaepiphyseal-metaphyseal dysplasia: a new bone dysplasia resembling cleidocranial dysplasia, *Radiology* 156:365, 1985.

243. Sly WS et al: Recessive osteopetrosis, a new clinical phenotype, *Am J Hum Genet* 24:34, 1972.

244. Sly WS et al: Carbonic anhydrase II deficiency in twelve families with autosomal recessive syndrome of osteopetrosis and renal tubular acidosis and cerebral calcifications, *N Engl J Med* 313:139, 1985.

245. Smith GV, Teele RL: Delayed diagnosis of duodenal obstruction in Down syndrome, *AJR* 134:937, 1980.

246. Smith SW: Roentgen findings in homocystinuria, *AJR* 100:147, 1967.

247. Smith NH: Albers-Schönberg disease (osteopetrosis). Report of a case and review of the literature, *Oral Surg Oral Med Oral Patho Oral Radiol Endodl*, 22:6, 699, 1966

248. Smolin LA et al: The use of betaine for treatment of homocystinuria, *J Pediatr* 99:467, 1981.

249. Soh LT et al: Embryonal carcinoma arising in Turner's syndrome, *Ann Acad Med Singapore* 21:386, 1992.

250. Somhegyi A, Ratko I: Hamstring tightness and Scheuermann's disease, *Am J Phys Med Rehabil* 72:44, 1993.

251. Sostrin RD et al: Myelographic features in mucopolysaccharidosis—a new sign, *Radiology* 125:421, 1977.

252. Spencer JA, Grieve DK: Congenital indifference to pain mistaken for non-accidental injury, *Br J Radiol* 63:308, 1990.

253. Spranger JW et al: Heterogeneity of chondrodysplasia punctata, *Hum Genet* 11:190, 1971.

254. Stafstrom CE: Epilepsy in Down syndrome: clinical aspects and possible mechanisms, *Am J Ment Retard* 98(suppl):12, 1993.

255. Stern WE: Dural ectasia and the Marfan syndrome, *J Neurosurg* 69:221, 1988.

256. Stevens JM et al: A new appraisal of abnormalities of the odontoid process associated with atlanto-axial subluxation and neurological disability, *Brain* 117:133, 1994.

257. Stillerman CB, Wilson JA: Atlanto-axial stabilization with posterior transarticular screw fixation: technical description and report of 22 cases, *Neurosurgery* 32:948, 1993.

258. Stoddard A, Osborn JF: Scheuermann's disease or spinal osteochondrosis: its frequency and relationship with spondylosis, *J Bone Joint Surg* 61B:56, 1979.

259. Stoppoloni G et al: Characteristics of insulin resistance in Turner syndrome, *Diabetes Metab* 16:267, 1990.

260. Subramaniam PN: Turner's syndrome and cardiovascular anomalies: a case report and review of the literature, *Am J Med Sci* 297:260, 1989.

261. Tachi N et al: Muscle involvement in congenital insensitivity to pain with anhidrosis, *Pediatr Neurol* 12:264, 1995.

262. Takakuwa T et al: Os odontoideum with vertebral artery occlusion, *Spine* 19:460, 1994.

263. Tallroth K, Schlenzka D: Spinal stenosis subsequent to juvenile lumbar osteochondrosis, *Skeletal Radiol* 19:203, 1990.

264. Tambyah PA, Cheah JS: Hyperthyroidism and Down syndrome, *Ann Acad Med Singapore* 22:603, 1993.

265. Tangerud A et al: Degenerative changes in the cervical spine in Down syndrome, *J Ment Defic Res* 34:179, 1990.

266. Taybi H: *Radiology of syndromes, metabolic disorders, and skeletal dysplasias,* ed 4, St Louis, 1996, Mosby.

267. Tertti M et al: Disc degeneration in young gymnasts. A magnetic resonance imaging study, *Am J Sports Med* 18:206, 1990.

268. Thomas SL et al: Hypoplasia of the odontoid with atlanto-axial subluxation in Hurler's syndrome, *Pediatr Radiol* 15:353, 1985.

269. Thomson SJ et al: Web neck deformity; anatomical considerations and options in surgical management, *Br J Plast Surg* 43:94, 1990.

270. Tishler JM, Martel W: Dislocation of the atlas in mongoloidism. A preliminary report, *Radiology* 84:904, 1965.

271. Torfs CP et al: Anorectal and esophageal anomalies with Down syndrome, *Am J Med Genet* 44:847, 1992.

272. Treble NJ et al: Development of the hip in multiple epiphyseal dysplasia. Natural history and susceptibility to premature osteoarthritis, *J Bone Joint Surg* 72B:1061, 1990.

273. Uematsu S et al: Total craniospinal decompression in achondroplastic stenosis, *Neurosurg* 35:250, 1994.

274. van Linhoudt D, Revel M: Similar radiologic lesions of localized Scheuermann's disease of the lumbar spine in twin sisters, *Spine* 19:987, 1994.

275. van Wassenaer AG et al: Partial anomalous pulmonary venous return in Turner syndrome, *Eur J Pediatr* 148:101, 1988.

276. Viljoen D, Beighton P: Marfan syndrome: a diagnostic dilemma, *Clin Genet* 37:417, 1990.

277. Virdis R et al: Blood pressure behaviour and control in Turner syndrome, *Clin Exp Hypertens* 8:787, 1986.

278. Waters KA et al: Breathing abnormalities in sleep in achondroplasia, *Arch Dis Child* 69:191, 1993.

279. Watts RWE et al: Computed tomography studies on patients with mucopolysaccharidosis, *Neuroradiology* 21:9, 1981.

280. Weinberg B et al: The prominent conoid process of the clavicle: a new radiographic sign in Down syndrome, *AJR* 160:591, 1993.

281. Weiss SW: Pedal hemangioma (venous malformation) occurring in Turner's syndrome: an additional manifestation of the syndrome, *Hum Pathol* 19:1015, 1988.

282. Wells TR et al: Association of Down syndrome and segmental tracheal stenosis with ring tracheal cartilages: a review of nine cases, *Pediatr Pathol* 12:673:1992.

283. Wells TR et al: Studies of vertebral coronal cleft in rhizomelic chondrodysplasia punctata, *Pediatr Pathol* 13:123, 1993.

284. Whyte MP et al: Hypotrichosis with spondyloepimetaphyseal dysplasia in three generations: a new autosomal dominant syndrome, *Am J Med Genet* 36:288, 1990.

285. Whyte MP et al: Mixed sclerosing bone dystrophy: report of a case and review of the literature, *Skeletal Radiol* 6:95, 1981.

286. Wiedemann HR: Otto Ullrich and his syndromes, *Am J Med Genet* 41:128, 1991.

287. Wilcken DEL et al: Homocystinuria—the effects of betaine in treatment of patients not responsive to pyridoxine, *N Engl J Med* 309:448, 1983.

288. Williams JW et al: Craniofacial melorheostosis: case report and review of the literature, *Br J Radiol* 64:60, 1991.

289. Willich E et al: Skeletal manifestations in Down syndrome. Correlation between roentgenologic and cytogenetic findings, *Ann Radiol* 18:355, 1975.

290. Wood KB et al: Magnetic resonance imaging of the thoracic spine. Evaluation of asymptomatic individuals, *J Bone Joint Surg Am* 77:1631, 1995.

291. Worth HM, Wollin DG: Hyperostosis corticalis generalisata congenita, *J Can Assoc Radiol* 17:69, 1966.

292. Wraith JE, Alani SM: Carpal tunnel syndrome in the mucopolysaccharidoses and related disorders, *Arch Dis Child* 65:962, 1990.

293. Yablon JS et al: Thoracic cord compression in Scheuermann's disease, *Spine* 13:896, 1988.

294. Yamashita Y et al: Atlantoaxial subluxation. Radiography and magnetic resonance imaging correlated to myelopathy, *Acta Radiol* 30:135, 1989.

295. Yamate T et al: Growth hormone (GH) treatment in achondroplasia, *J Ped Endocrinol* 6:45, 1993.

296. Yang SS et al: Two lethal chondrodysplasias with giant chondrocytes, *Am J Med Genet* 15:615, 1983.

297. Yellin A et al: Familial multiple bilateral pneumothorax associated with Marfan syndrome, *Chest* 100:577, 1991.

298. Young DA: Rachmaninov and Marfan's syndrome, *BMJ* 299:1624, 1986.

299. Younge D et al: Melorheostosis in children. Clinical features and natural history, *J Bone Joint Surg* 61B:415, 1979.

300. Yousefzadeh DK et al: Radiographic studies of upper airway obstruction with cor pulmonale in a patient with pycnodysostosis, *Pediatr Radiol* 8:45, 1979.

301. Yu JS et al: Melorheostosis with an ossified soft tissue mass: MR features, *Skeletal Radiol* 24:367, 1995.

302. Yucel M et al: Treatment of florid dorsal Scheuermann's disease with two new breathable plaster-of-paris casts and their biomechnical principles of action, *Z Orthop Ihre Grenzgeb* 119:292, 1981.

303. Zangwill KM et al: Dandy-Walker malformation in Ellis-van Creveld syndrome, *Am J Med Genet* 31:123, 1988.

304. Zettergvist P et al: The man behind the syndrome: Antonin Marfan, *Lakartidningen* 86:2205, 1989.

305. Zihni L: Downs' syndrome, interferon sensitivity and the development of leukaemia, *Leuk Res* 18:1, 1994.

306. Zipursky A et al: Leukemia in Down syndrome: a review, *Pediatr Hematol Oncol* 9:139, 1992.

chapter 11

Arthritides

Inflammatory Arthritides

TAWNIA ADAMS AND DEBORAH M FORRESTER

Metabolic and Deposition Arthritides

TAWNIA ADAMS AND DEBORAH M FORRESTER

Degenerative Arthritides and Related Conditions

DENNIS M MARCHIORI AND DEBORAH M FORRESTER

Background

Arthritis is the most common self-reported chronic condition among whites, the second most common among Native Americans and Hispanics, the third most common among blacks, and the fourth most common condition among Asians. For all groups, arthritis is a more prevalent chronic condition than heart disease, hearing impairments, chronic bronchitis, asthma, and diabetes.[65] Arthritis and its related conditions have a significant impact on activities of daily living, such as housekeeping, sleeping, driving, and working. Early recognition and appropriate management of arthritis are important to limit its progression and related disabilities.

Imaging

Plain film radiography is still the most useful imaging modality for evaluating arthropathy.[338] It adequately demonstrates bone erosions, osteophytes, alterations of joint space, joint swelling, and misalignment. Because plain film radiographs are relatively inexpensive and rapidly obtained, serial radiography can be used to provide important information about the progression of the disease. The addition of intraarticular injections of air or contrast allows limited demonstrations of the internal components of joints.

Computed tomography (CT) provides excellent anatomical detail and images in an axial plane. Magnetic resonance imaging (MRI) is used to evaluate the cartilaginous and ligamentous joint structures and the marrow of the adjacent bone. Scintigraphy provides a useful method of gathering functional information to aid in morphological assessments provided by other imaging modalities. Ultrasonography has the capability to define joint effusions and identify edematous connective tissues.

Classification

In general, arthritis can be grouped into three major categories: inflammatory (e.g., rheumatoid), degenerative (e.g., osteoarthritis), and metabolic deposition (e.g., gout). Inflammatory arthritides are subdivided into rheumatoid types (seropositive) and rheumatoid variants (seronegative) based on the serological presence of the rheumatoid factor.

Arthritis may be monoarticular or polyarticular. All types of arthritis may be monoarticular early in their pathological course. Joint abnormalities that are caused by trauma or infections usually remain monoarticular. Arthritides are differentiated on the basis of clinical data and imaging studies (Table 11-1). The most useful information about them comes from plain film radiographs coupled with clinical data that relates to skeletal distribution, patient age, patient gender, joint swelling, joint stiffness, joint range of motion, symptom response to physical activity, and laboratory tests (e.g., erythrocyte sedimentation rate [ESR], antinuclear antibodies [ANA], human leukocyte antigen [HLA] typing).

TABLE 11-1
Relationship of Selected Arthritides to Age, Gender, and Skeletal Regions

Arthritide	Age of onset (years)	Relationship to gender*	Skeletal region typically affected
Ankylosing spondylitis	15-35	1-10:1	Axial
CPPD	>40	1:1	Knee, wrist
DISH	>50	More men affected	Axial
Enteropathic arthritides	Adolescent†	1:1	Axial
Gout	40-50	20:1	Foot (first MTP)
Osteoarthritis	>40	Varies according to region affected	Axial, knee
Psoriatic arthritides	30-50	1:1	SI, hand
Reiter's syndrome	15-35	5:1	SI, foot
Rheumatoid arthritis			
Adult	20-50	1:2-3	MCP, wrist
Juvenile	<16	1:1	Cervical, wrist
Scleroderma	20-50	1:3	Hand
SLE	20-40	1:9	Hand

*Ratios—male:female.
†Wide variation in age of onset, depending on the underlying condition.

Inflammatory Arthritides

Ankylosing Spondylitis

BACKGROUND

Ankylosing spondylitis, also referred to as *Bechterew's disease* or *Marie-Strümpell disease,* is the most common of the seronegative spondyloarthropathies, affecting approximately 0.1% to 0.2% of white North Americans.[190] It is a chronic, progressive, inflammatory condition involving predominantly the synovial and cartilaginous joints of the axial skeleton and often the large, proximal appendicular joints. Alterations at *entheses,* the sites where ligaments and tendons attach to bone, are also a prominent feature.

The disease is more common and severe in men, with ratios of 1:1 to 10:1 reported.[91,105,113,185,402] The onset is usually between 15 and 35 years of age. Although the etiology remains unknown, the high prevalence (greater than 90%) of the genetic marker HLA-B27 in white patients with ankylosing spondylitis as compared with unaffected white patients (6% to 8%) suggests the disease may have a genetic etiology.[50,190,275]

IMAGING FINDINGS

Regardless of location the radiographic findings reflect the underlying inflammatory condition, which is characterized by erosions, osseous proliferation, and bony ankylosis. Joint involvement in the axial and appendicular skeleton is typically bilateral and symmetrical, although this may vary early in the disease process.

Sacroiliac joint. The sacroiliac joints are the classic sites to be initially involved in ankylosing spondylitis, with the ensuing changes predominantly affecting the middle and lower two thirds of the sacroiliac joints and affecting the iliac surface to a greater degree than the sacral surface because of the thinner iliac cartilage.[45] The early stages are characterized by subtle periarticular osteoporosis and loss of cortical bone definition. More obvious erosions then develop, leading to irregular joint margins and joint space

widening. Patchy and ill-defined reactive sclerosis accompanies the erosions and becomes more diffuse and uniform as the disease advances (Fig. 11-1). Bony bridges form across the joint, leading to eventual fusion or ankylosis, which appears radiographically as obliteration of the sacroiliac articulations. After ankylosis occurs, the reactive sclerosis is resorbed, and generalized osteoporosis becomes a prominent feature (Fig. 11-2). Approximately 50% of patients will progress to sacroiliac fusion, whereas in the other 50% the disease will arrest short of complete ankylosis.

Spine. Spondylitis occurs in about 50% of patients and as a rule develops after sacroiliac disease, with the thoracolumbar and lumbosacral junctions being the most common initial target sites.[98] The disease process typically ascends the spine contiguously without skip lesions and progresses bilaterally and symmetrically. The most characteristic spinal finding occurs at the discovertebral junction, but the inflammatory process may also affect the apophyseal joints, posterior ligamentous attachments, costovertebral joints, and atlantoaxial joint.

Discovertebral junction. The classic spinal findings associated with ankylosing spondylitis are thin, vertical ossifications or syndesmophytes that bridge adjacent vertebrae and cause ankylosis of multiple segments. As the disease progresses, complete ankylosis occurs, resulting in a distinctive, undulating spinal outline that radiographically resembles a piece of bamboo. The classic "bamboo spine" occurs in a minority of patients and takes an average of 10 years to develop (Fig. 11-3).

A syndesmophyte begins as a focal osteitis or erosion with surrounding sclerosis at the anterior vertebral body margins. The small corner erosions, or *Romanus lesions,* lead to a loss of the normal anterior vertebral body concavity and cause "squaring," which is most apparent in the lumbar spine. This early finding is often overlooked, but new techniques are being designed to evaluate this sub-

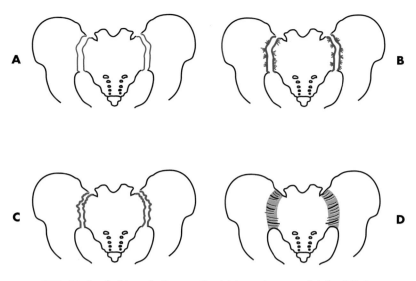

FIG. 11-1 **A,** Normally the sacroiliac joint margins are well-defined. **B,** Inflammation may initially appear hazy with loss of cortical definition. Progression leads to joint space widening, erosions **(C),** and fusion **(D).**

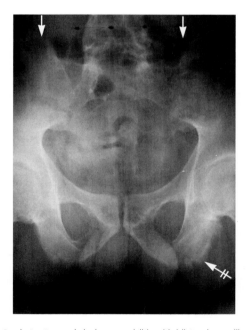

FIG. 11-2 Late stage ankylosing spondylitis with bilateral sacroiliac fusion *(arrows).* The pubic symphysis is irregular and sclerotic. Periostitis is present along the ischial rami *(crossed arrow).*

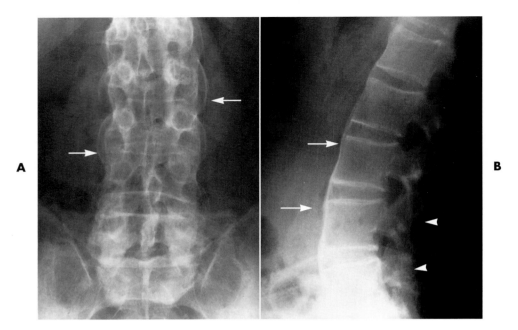

FIG. 11-3   The AP **(A)** and lateral **(B)** lumbar radiographs demonstrate the classic spinal finding associated with ankylosing spondylitis—ossification of the outer annulus fibrosis. These thin, vertical bridging ossifications are called *syndesmophytes (arrows).* A "bamboo spine" appearance results when ankylosis develops in several segments **(A).** Posterior fusion of the apophyseal joints **(B)** is also evident *(arrowheads).*

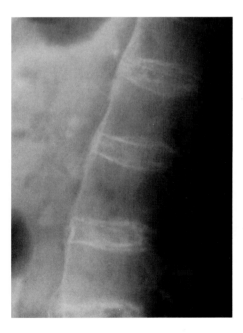

FIG. 11-4   On this lateral lumbar radiograph of a patient with AS, note the radiopacity of the intervertebral discs relative to the vertebral bodies and adjacent soft tissue. Calcification can be seen in the disc, whereas the vertebrae have become osteoporotic.

tle change in an attempt to aid early radiological diagnosis and assess spinal progression.[327] The radiographic brightness of reactive sclerosis is intensified by the accompanying vertebral body osteoporosis and is appropriately called the *shiny corner sign.* Ossification then develops in the outer annular fibers and results in thin, marginal syndesmophytes that are predominantly found on the anterolateral aspects of the spine but can arise posteriorly and may cause symptomatic spinal stenosis.[154]

Other abnormalities occurring at the discovertebral junction include discal calcification (Fig. 11-4), which is common to many conditions of spinal hypomobility; discal ballooning, which is found in the later stages of spinal ankylosis as osteoporosis causes the endplates to weaken and become biconcave, causing the disc to take on a ballooned, or biconvex, appearance; and Andersson lesions, which are caused by a localized erosive or destructive process involving the central and/or peripheral aspect of the discovertebral junction, whose theorized etiology ranges from posttraumatic pseudoarthrosis to infection.

Apophyseal joints and posterior ligaments. Ankylosis of the apophyseal joints is secondary to an underlying erosive process that leads to osseous fusion and capsular ossification. This process is considered a prerequisite for the postural changes of reduced lumbar and cervical lordosis and increased thoracic kyphosis associated with patients in the later stages of the disease (Fig. 11-5). Radiographically, bilateral apophyseal fusion resembles two thick, vertically oriented linear radiopacities, which are known as the *railroad track sign,* on the anteroposterior (AP) radiograph. If this appearance is present in combination with ossification of the interspinous and supraspinous ligaments, the resulting three vertical stripes are referred to as the *trolley track sign.* If found alone, the single vertical stripe caused by ossification of only the supraspinous and interspinous ligaments is called the *dagger sign* (Fig. 11-6).

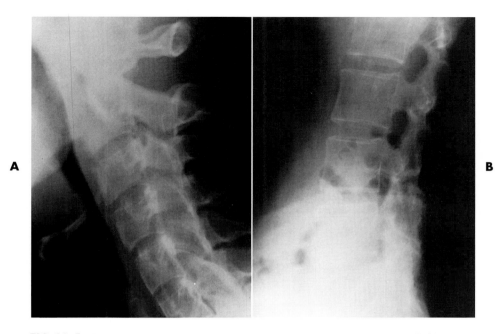

FIG. 11-5 Posterior joint fusion on the lateral cervical **(A)** and lumbar **(B)** radiographs of a 23-year-old male with AS. Both films were taken weight-bearing and in a neutral position. Notice the reduced lordosis in both regions and the anterior weight-bearing posture of the cervical spine.

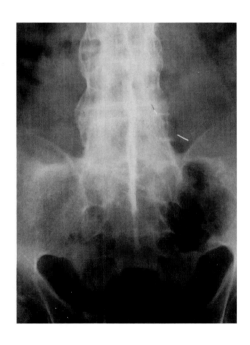

FIG. 11-6 AP view showing changes associated with advanced stages of ankylosing spondylitis: generalized osteoporosis, sacroiliac fusion, syndesmophyte formation, apophyseal joint fusion, and supraspinous and interspinous ligament ossification.

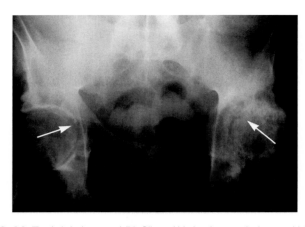

FIG. 11-7 Ankylosing spondylitis. Bilateral hip involvement is shown, which includes features that are consistent with many inflammatory arthritides (e.g., axial migration of femur heads [*arrows*], mild erosions). Hyperostosis is also shown, a finding more commonly associated with the seronegative spondyloarthropathies. Osseous bridging of the pubic symphysis is apparent.

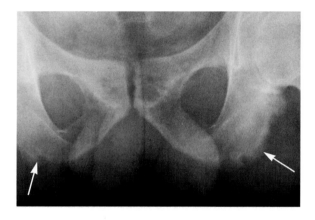

FIG. 11-8 Clearly visible periostotic "whiskering" of the ischial tuberosities on the radiograph of a man with ankylosing spondylitis (*arrows*).

Costovertebral joints. Osseous fusion of the costovertebral joints is responsible for the limited chest expansion associated with ankylosing spondylitis. It is difficult to visualize on plain film and may require specialized imaging such as radionuclide scintigraphy or CT.

Atlantoaxial. Although less frequent and severe, atlantoaxial involvement mimics the changes seen in patients with rheumatoid arthritis. Inflammatory changes of the synovium and adjacent ligamentous and osseous structures may lead to atlantoaxial subluxation, cranial settling, odontoid erosions, or complete destruction of the dens.

Appendicular skeleton. Ankylosing spondylitis has an affinity for the large proximal joints (rhizomelic spondylitis), primarily the hip, which it affects in up to 50% of patients. The associated radiographic findings are consistent with any inflammatory disorder, and include concentric joint space narrowing, mild erosions, and possibly protrusio acetabuli. Bony proliferation may occur as femoral osteophytosis, forming a circumferential ring around the femoral neck (Fig. 11-7).

The glenohumeral joint is the second most common peripheral joint affected, with erosive and proliferative changes mirroring those in the hip. Chronic involvement may lead to rotator cuff disruption, which appears on the radiograph as elevation of the humeral head relative to the glenoid cavity.

Enthesopathy. Bony erosions and osseous proliferation at entheses are common, most notably affecting the pelvis, calcaneus, and patella. This reactive new bone is termed *periostotic whiskering,* which describes its frayed radiographic appearance (Fig. 11-8).

CLINICAL COMMENTS

Diagnosis. Early diagnosis of patients with ankylosing spondylitis may be delayed because of its mild and vague clinical presentation, nonspecific laboratory findings, and subtle radiographic changes. The initial complaint usually includes an insidious onset of low back pain and morning stiffness, which is relieved with activity and aggravated by resting in the supine position. In the early stages, pain is intermittent, becoming constant as the disease progresses and diminishing or disappearing as the paraspinal ligaments and apophyseal joints ossify.[220] Recurrence of pain after diminution may signal a superimposed complication such as a fracture.[299,337] On rare occasions, acute iritis is the initial complaint.

Additional early physical findings may include limited range of motion, limited chest expansion, postural changes (to ease back pain), fever, fatigue, anorexia, weight loss, and anemia. Neurological signs and symptoms may include radiating leg pain that does not extend below the knee, cauda equina syndrome, and myelopathic changes caused by stenosis or a fracture.[113,151,255]

Spinal, or "carrot stick," fractures are not uncommon and are usually a result of trivial trauma to bone that has become severely osteoporotic due to disease-related ankylosis or surgical fusion.[261] Extraskeletal manifestations include heart disease (especially aortic insufficiency), upper lobe pulmonary fibrosis, and inflammatory bowel disease.

Diagnosis is confirmed by radiographic examination. Currently, plain film radiography is considered to be the primary and most important imaging modality for diagnosis and assessment, but MRI and other imaging techniques are playing expanding roles, with the potential to help with early diagnosis and provide a better understanding of treatment response.[14,57,328,329]

Assessment. Assessment and progression of the disease course may eventually be carried out in the office without costly or invasive tests. Investigators are finding relationships between specific radiographic findings and physical signs and symptoms, such as pain, stiffness and reduced range of motion.[389,410] If plain films are negative for ankylosing spondylitis, laboratory studies may be helpful but are not specific for ankylosing spondylitis and must be considered only when significant clinical suspicion exists. HLA-B27, probably the most well-known laboratory finding associated with ankylosing spondylitis, may be found in all patients with seronegative spondyloarthropathies and in a small percent of the unaffected patients (6% to 8%). The ESR is also nonspecific and may be increased in patients with any inflammatory or necrotic conditions. Tests for rheumatoid factor and ANA are characteristically negative and are more useful for excluding seropositive disorders than diagnosing ankylosing spondylitis.

Treatment. Treatment should focus on pain relief and a long-range plan to prevent, decrease, or delay joint and postural deformities. A rehabilitation and exercise regimen is needed to maintain proper joint motion and function and promote proper posture by strengthening muscle groups that oppose the direction of the ensuing deformity. If joints are inflamed and painful, nonsteroidal antiinflammatory drugs (NSAIDs) may be used to suppress pain, inflammation, and spasms in an effort to facilitate exercise. Although the prognosis varies, the majority of patients will experience periods of mild to moderate exacerbation that alternate with periods of no symptoms and with proper treatment will have minimal to no disability. Occasionally the disease course is severe and progressive, leading to significant deformities and incapacitation.

KEY CONCEPTS

- *Ankylosing spondylitis is the most common seronegative spondyloarthropathy.*
- *It primarily involves the synovial and cartilaginous joints of the axial skeleton*
- *Males are predisposed to developing the condition (1:1 to 10:1), with usual onset from 15 to 35 years of age.*
- *The radiographic findings are characterized by erosions, osseous proliferation, and bony ankylosis.*
- *Involvement is bilateral symmetrical and targeted to the spine, hips, shoulders, and particularly the sacroiliac joints.*
- *The condition causes decreased cervical and lumbar lordosis and increased thoracic kyphosis.*
- *Ankylosing spondylitis also causes sacroiliac joint widening, sclerosis, and fusion.*
- *It is associated with vertebral changes such as body squaring, Romanus lesions, shiny corner sign, syndesmophytes, and posterior joint fusion.*
- *Clinical characteristics include pain, limited range of motion, limited chest expansion, fever, fatigue, and weight loss.*
- *Diagnosis is made by radiographic appearance, negative test for rheumatoid factor, positive test for HLA-B27 antigen marker, and an elevated ESR.*
- *Treatment includes pain relief, with a long-range plan to decrease or delay joint and postural deformities.*

Enteropathic Arthritis

BACKGROUND

Enteropathic arthritis, or arthropathy, encompasses the resultant articular alterations that are associated with a group of gut abnormalities, predominantly inflammatory bowel disorders. The condition is most frequently associated with ulcerative colitis and regional enteritis (Crohn's disease), but Whipple's disease; enteritis caused by *Salmonella, Shigella,* or *Yersinia* organisms; cirrhosis; hepatitis; pancreatic disease; and intestinal bypass surgery are all conditions that somehow can induce joint disease. The suspected mechanisms include simultaneous joint and bowel infections or bowel infections that subsequently reach the synovial tissue, an immune response of antibodies against a common bowel and joint antigen, and genetic factors related to the increased proportion of HLA-B27 in affected individuals compared with unaffected individuals.[275]

The axial and appendicular skeletons may be separately or simultaneously involved. Peripheral arthritis is seen in 15% to 20% of patients with inflammatory bowel disease, is most common in the lower extremities, and develops after the onset of bowel disease; arthritic flares correlate with the underlying disease activity.[147] Axial involvement is noted in 3% to 18% of patients with inflammatory bowel disease, may precede or follow onset of bowel disease, and shows no strong association with disease activity.[147] No particular associations with gender have been noted.

IMAGING FINDINGS

Radiographic alterations reflect the underlying inflammatory disease process, showing peripheral joint involvement similar to rheumatoid arthritis and axial changes identical to ankylosing spondylitis.

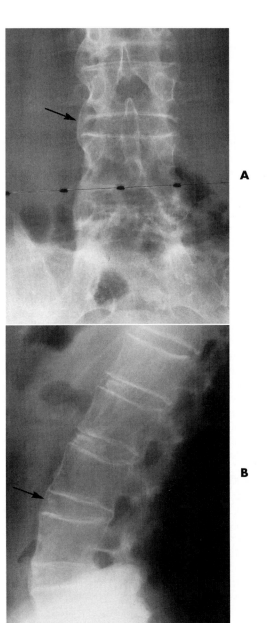

FIG. 11-9 AP **(A)** and lateral **(B)** lumbar radiographs of a patient with an inflammatory bowel disease show spinal features that are identical to ankylosing spondylitis. Note the bridging syndesmophyte formation *(arrows)* and posterior joint involvement.

Axial skeleton. Bilateral and symmetrical sacroiliac erosions and sclerosis, joint space narrowing, and possible subsequent fusion occurs in combination with spinal changes or as isolated asymptomatic sacroiliitis in 4% to 18% of patients.[147] The spondylitis that occurs in 3% to 6% of patients begins as a marginal vertebral body osteitis, progressing to the characteristic syndesmophyte bridging adjacent vertebrae, and resulting in intersegmental fusion (Fig. 11-9).

Appendicular skeleton. Initially, the peripheral joint involvement associated with inflammatory bowel disease was thought to be rheumatoid arthritis caused by similar inflammatory episodes. However, enteropathic arthritis is usually nondestructive and asymmetrical, consisting primarily of soft tissue swelling and periarticular osteopenia. In rare cases, osseous and cartilaginous destructive changes occur. The arthropathy is usually self-limiting but tends to recur with a flare-up of bowel disease. The most commonly affected joint is the knee, followed by the ankle, shoulder, wrist, elbow, and joints of the hand and feet respectively.[29]

CLINICAL COMMENTS

Not only do the radiographic features mimic ankylosing spondylitis, but so can the clinical manifestations (e.g., in a young patient with low back pain). Obviously, patients may complain of symptoms associated with inflammatory bowel disease, such as abdominal pain, malaise, weight loss, diarrhea, or constipation. However, the arthropathy can precede the onset of symptoms from the bowel disease, or the actual bowel disease itself. An ileocolonic study may be useful if inflammatory bowel disease is a possibility in a patient with unusual peripheral arthropathy or radiographic features consistent with ankylosing spondylitis.[224]

Laboratory test findings will typically reflect those of other seronegative spondyloarthropathies. The percentage of positive HLA-B27 patients varies with the underlying gut abnormality and arthritic distribution. For example, the antigen is present in approximately 75% of patients with ulcerative colitis or Crohn's disease who develop axial involvement but is not an associated genetic marker in patients with peripheral arthritis.[275] Tests for the rheumatoid factor is typically negative, and the ESR may be elevated.

Treatment involves control of the intestinal inflammation, which may incorporate the use of NSAIDs, as well as conservative management of the arthralgia. Surgical removal of the diseased portion of the colon can result in improvement of the peripheral arthropathy but does not seem to affect the progression of axial involvement.[105]

KEY CONCEPTS

- *Enteropathic arthritis is a seronegative spondyloarthropathy associated with disorders of the gut and most commonly related to inflammatory bowel disease.*
- *The radiographic features of the axial skeleton mimic ankylosing spondylitis.*
- *The radiographic features of the appendicular skeleton mimic rheumatoid arthritis but are typically not erosive.*
- *Enteropathic arthritis has laboratory findings that are typical of other seronegative arthropathies*

Jaccoud's Arthropathy

BACKGROUND

Jaccoud's arthritis, or arthropathy or syndrome, is a nonerosive, relatively asymptomatic deforming arthropathy of the hands and feet. It was initially described in 1867 (and for some time thereafter) as a rare complication of rheumatic fever (i.e., "postrheumatic fever arthritis").[181,366] Jaccoud's arthropathy has since been reported in patients without a previous history of rheumatic fever as well as in association with multiple connective tissue disorders, such as systemic lupus scleroderma, dermatomyositis, psoriatic arthritis, sarcoidosis, and in lung disease patients.*

Although the etiology is unclear, biopsy studies reveal no evidence of synovial pathology and do not indicate the presence of an inflammatory condition. Jaccoud's arthropathy is characterized by capsular fibrosis and in certain cases secondary degenerative changes, which are presumably caused by long-standing joint deformities.[142,398]

IMAGING FINDINGS

The hallmark of Jaccoud's arthropathy is a nonerosive, reversible joint deformity. The joint deformities cannot be actively corrected by the patient but can be corrected by an examiner if the patient relaxes the joint. Radiographic examination of the hands may reveal this passive reducibility; when the cassette puts pressure on the hand during the posteroanterior (PA) view, the hand is restored to nearly normal alignment, but it is not restored during the oblique radiography procedure. The most common deformities are ulnar deviation and metacarpophalangeal (MCP) joint flexion, which is most marked in the fourth and fifth digits, and flexion and fibular deviation of the metatarsophalangeal (MTP) articulations (Fig. 11-10).[274] Swan-neck and boutonnière deformities of the digits are also noted.[197] The bone density may be normal or exhibit periarticular osteoporosis. Joint space is preserved until late in the disease, when mechanical stress of the accompanying subluxation may cause secondary degeneration. Osseous erosions are rare, but when they occur they appear as "hook lesions" on the radial and palmar aspect of the metacarpal heads.[300]

CLINICAL COMMENTS

Jaccoud's arthropathy is no longer considered a rare condition and should be mentioned in the differential diagnosis of chronic arthritis.[274] The pattern of joint involvement mimics that of rheumatoid arthritis and systemic lupus and may therefore be misdiagnosed. Laboratory tests may help establish the correct diagnosis because patients with Jaccoud's arthropathy typically have negative tests for the rheumatoid factor and ANA. Clinically, patients with Jaccoud's arthropathy (despite its striking deformities) usually have no pain and good functional capabilities. In fact, the arthropathy may not be the reason the patient is seeking care.

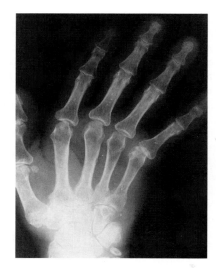

FIG. 11-10 Jaccoud's arthritis with ulnar deviation of the digits and advanced degeneration and radial subluxation of the first metacarpal. (Courtesy Joseph W. Howe, Sylmar, Calif.)

---

*References 15, 47, 48, 175, 186, 236, 244, 249, 298, 368, 382, 386, 394.

Juvenile Rheumatoid Arthritis

BACKGROUND

Juvenile rheumatoid arthritis (JRA) is the most common disease in a group of related diseases called *juvenile chronic arthritis* that develop during childhood (i.e., before 16 years of age).[420] In one review the prevalence of JRA in the general population ranged from between 12 and 113 cases per 100,000 people.[370] Within its major classification, JRA can be subdivided according to the presence or absence of rheumatoid factor, systemic symptoms within the first 6 months of onset, and the number of joints involved.

Juvenile onset adult rheumatoid arthritis, or seropositive chronic arthritis, typically develops in teenage girls, has a frequency of 5% to 10% among the juvenile chronic arthritides, and is similar clinically and radiographically to adult rheumatoid arthritis.[9,350] Juvenile patients may present with subcutaneous nodules, although this symptom occurs less frequently in juveniles than adults. The joints most commonly affected are the hands, wrists, knees, feet, and cervical spine.

Seronegative chronic arthritis, or Still's disease, encompasses approximately 70% of juvenile chronic arthritides and includes three subsets of children with systemic and/or articular manifestations who test negative for the rheumatoid factor:

(1) The classic systemic disease occurs in children under 5 years of age; affects males and females equally; and presents with spiking fevers and a characteristic rash, hepatosplenomegaly, adenopathy, leukocytosis, and mild polyarthritis.

(2) Pauciarticular disease is found in young children under 5 years of age and involves fewer than five joints, generally affecting large joints (i.e., knees, ankles, elbows, wrists). This form is frequently accompanied by iridocyclitis.

(3) The polyarticular form involves more than five joints, has a preponderance among females, and is distributed bilaterally and symmetrically, which is similar to the distribution of adult rheumatoid arthritis.

IMAGING FINDINGS

The radiographic presentation of JRA is similar to adult rheumatoid arthritis with few exceptions (Table 11-2), and although features within each subset of JRA can differ, those features common to all subsets include fusiform periarticular soft tissue swelling, juxtaarticular osteopenia that may become diffuse, joint space narrowing, osseous erosions, bony ankylosis (Figs. 11-11 and 11-12), and joint contractures.

Distinct features of JRA include periostitis and growth abnormalities, which are the result of the disease process combined with skeletal immaturity. Periostitis commonly involves the diaphysis of the metacarpals, metatarsals, and proximal phalanges and may be an early and prominent finding that is likely explained by the exposure of loosely attached periosteum to an inflammatory and hyperemic process. Growth abnormalities result from hyperemia to the epiphysis and growth plates causing an overgrown or "ballooned" epiphysis and/or premature growth plate fusion, leading to shortening of limbs or limb length discrepancies.

Overall joint involvement mimics that of adult rheumatoid arthritis; however, some distinctive findings at specific joints are as follows.

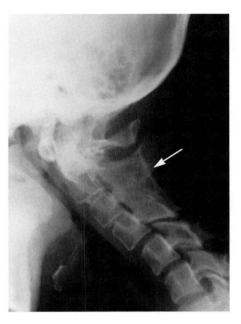

FIG. 11-11 Juvenile rheumatoid arthritis with vertebral hypoplasia and fusion of the posterior joints *(arrow)* in the cervical spine. Although inflammation may affect the posterior facets in both adult and juvenile forms of rheumatoid arthritis, resultant apophyseal fusion is common in the child and unlikely in the adult. Vertebral body and disc hypoplasia are also prominent features in juvenile rheumatoid arthritis. (Courtesy Jack C. Avalos, Davenport, Iowa.)

TABLE 11-2
Radiographic Findings Associated with Juvenile and Adult Rheumatoid Arthritis

Radiographic finding	Juvenile rheumatoid	Adult rheumatoid
Joint space narrowing	Common in late stages of disease	Common in early stages of disease
Marginal bony erosions	Common in late stages of disease	Common in early stages of disease
Intraarticular fusion	Common	Uncommon
Growth abnormalities	Common	Absent
Periostitis	Common	Absent

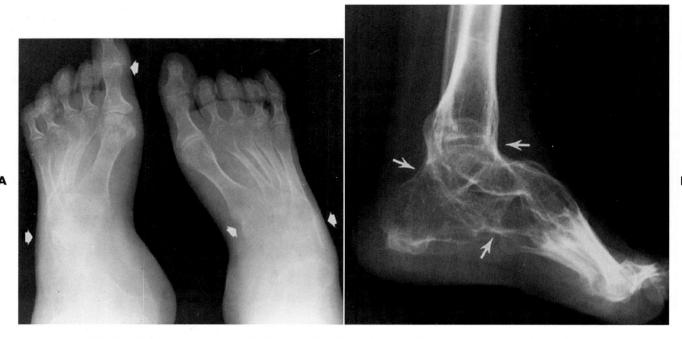

FIG. 11-12   Juvenile chronic arthritis. **A,** Symmetric findings include generalized osteopenia, diaphyseal overtubulation, widespread joint space narrowing, evolving ankylosis *(arrows)*, and diffuse muscle wasting. **B,** Another patient exhibits widespread ankylosis *(arrows)* in the hindfoot and midfoot with a cavus deformity secondary to the disease and stabilizing surgery. Osteopenia and muscle atrophy are also evident. Differential diagnosis should include consideration of other causes of disuse beginning in childhood, as well as certain congenital foot deformities. (From Sartoris DJ: *Musculoskeletal imaging: the requisites,* St Louis, 1996, Mosby.)

Hand and wrist. Early findings include soft tissue swelling and juxtaarticular osteoporosis of the carpals, MCPs, and proximal interphalangeals (PIPs); preservation of joint space; lack of erosions; and periostitis. Carpal and carpometacarpal ankylosis may be prominent, and boutonnière and swan-neck deformities may be present.

Knee. Effusion; enlargement, or "ballooning," of the metaphysis and epiphysis; widening of the intercondylar notch; and patellar squaring are the most distinctive findings associated with JRA in the knee.

Hip. JRA may be indicated by femoral head enlargement, early growth plate closure, coxa valga deformity, and acetabular protrusion. Osteonecrosis may also develop as a complication of the disease or treatment (ie, corticosteroids).

Cervical spine. Atlantoaxial subluxation and odontoid erosions occur but not as frequently as they do in adult patients with rheumatoid arthritis. Posterior joint ankylosis is a common occurrence following facet erosions in the upper and mid cervical spine (Fig. 11-11). The ankylosis is thought to cause vertebral body and disc hypoplasia.

CLINICAL COMMENTS

The approach to therapy is similar to that for adult rheumatoid arthritis and varies depending on the course of the disease. Aspirin and NSAIDs are usually given to help with inflammation, whereas the use of systemic corticosteroids is initially avoided because growth retardation is a major complication. Active exercise, maintaining joint range of motion, and physical therapy may aid in preserving or restoring joint space and leading to clinical improvements.[301] Ophthalmological examinations should be given semiannually to detect asymptomatic iridocyclitis.

> ### KEY CONCEPTS
> - *Juvenile rheumatoid arthritis is the most common juvenile chronic arthritide, which all affect children before they reach 16 years.*
> - *Seronegative (Still's disease) and seropositive (juvenile onset of adult rheumatoid arthritis) varieties exist.*
> - *Although joint involvement mimics that of adult rheumatoid arthritis, intraarticular fusion is much more common and periostitis and growth abnormalities are noted only in the juvenile type.*
> - *Hands, wrists, knees, hips, and the cervical spine are commonly affected.*
> - *Therapy is similar to that used for adult rheumatoid arthritis.*

Psoriatic Arthritis

BACKGROUND

Psoriatic arthritis is an inflammatory arthritide that affects approximately 5% to 7% of patients with psoriasis and usually follows the onset of the skin disease.[83,310] Although the etiology remains unclear, the pathogenesis of both skin and joint diseases is believed to be mediated by the immune system, as well as environmental and genetic factors.[20,82,83,297,408]

The age of onset is usually between 30 and 50 years of age; there is no significant correlation between being male or female and developing the condition.[82,105] The main target areas are the distal joints of the hands and to a lesser degree the feet. Because axial involvement occurs in 20% to 40% of patients, psoriatic arthritis is classified as a seronegative spondyloarthropathy.[105]

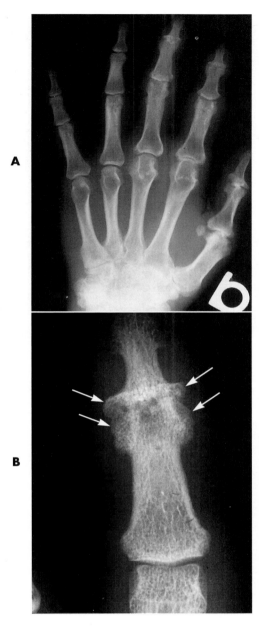

FIG. 11-13 Psoriatic arthritis. **A,** PA hand radiograph reveals soft tissue swelling of the first, second, and third digits. Small erosions and accompanying periostitis is present at the DIP, PIP, and MCP joints of these digits. The fourth and fifth digits have been spared. Overall bone density appears normal. **B,** Detail of DIP, second digit, demonstrates the proliferative new bone formation in a configuration referred to as "mouse ear" periostitis *(arrows).*

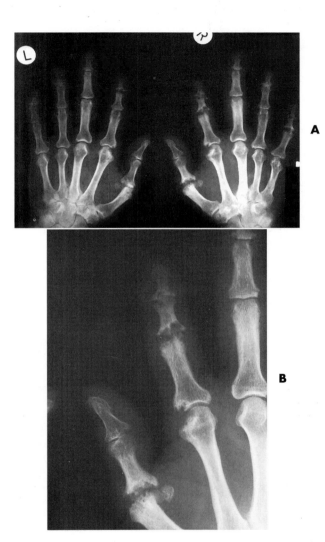

FIG. 11-14 Psoriatic arthritis. **A,** Bilateral hand radiograph reveals swelling of entire digits (sausage digits) and central and peripheral erosions affecting multiple articulations; the most severely affected joints are the IP joints of the index finger bilaterally and fifth digit of the right hand and the MCP joints of the thumb and index finger of the right hand. **B,** PIP joint of the index finger of the right hand reveals a pencil-in-cup deformity, which is characteristic of psoriatic arthritis.

PART TWO Bone, Joints, and Soft Tissues

IMAGING FINDINGS

Although the radiographic changes in the appendicular and axial skeleton are similar to the changes associated with of rheumatoid arthritis and ankylosing spondylitis, there are some distinct differences.

Hands and wrist. Patients with psoriatic arthritis typically have asymmetrical small joint involvement, with erosions predominantly involving the distal interphalangeal joints. Erosions may be marginal, involving the bare area and accompanied by fluffy new

bone formation ("mouse ears") (Fig. 11-13), or central, possibly forming a "pencil-and-cup deformity"(Fig. 11-14), and may be followed by intraarticular fusion (Fig. 11-15).[312] The pattern formed by involvement of all joints of a digit is referred to as a *ray pattern.* Tuft resorption or acroosteolysis may also develop.[228] Although uncommon, the course of the disease may progress to a debilitating form known as *arthritis mutilans* (Fig. 11-16). Wrist abnormalities usually follow distal interphalangeal (DIP) involvement and may occur within any compartment (Fig. 11-17).

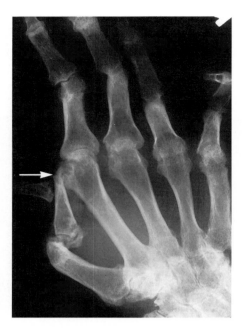

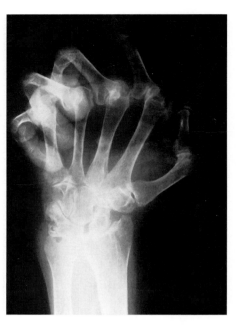

FIG. 11-15   PA view of the right hand of a 59-year-old male showing fusion of the PIP joints of the third and fourth digits. A pencil-in-cup deformity of the interphalangeal joint of the thumb is present *(arrow)*, in addition to a hitchhiker's deformity. The swan-neck deformity of the fifth digit is similar to that in patients with rheumatoid arthritis.

FIG. 11-16   Psoriatic arthritis of the hand resulting in severe subluxation and subsequent arthritis mutilans. A similar condition may be found in patients with rheumatoid arthritis but is less common.

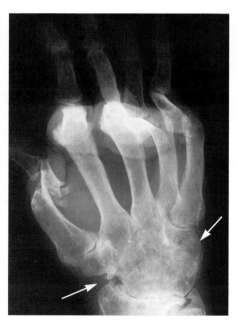

FIG. 11-17   Pancompartmental inflammatory changes in the wrist resulting in complete carpal fusion *(arrows)*.

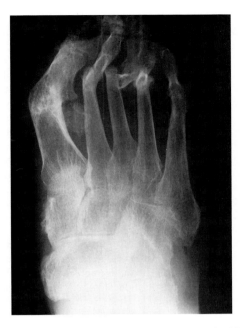

FIG. 11-18 Significantly affected MTP joints with fusion of multiple joints.

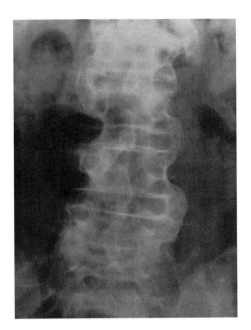

FIG. 11-19 Nonmarginal syndesmophytes. In contrast to ankylosing spondylitis, the syndesmophytes associated with psoriatic arthritis are typically thicker and nonmarginal and skip segments. (Courtesy Trevor Ireland, Anchorage, Alaska.)

Feet. Changes in the feet caused by psoriatic arthritis are similar to those of the hand. The interphalangeal joint of the great toe is commonly affected, as well as the distal interphalangeal articulations of all digits (Fig. 11-18). An ivory phalanx may result from osseous proliferation and sclerosis. Erosive and subsequent proliferative changes may take place at the calcaneal entheses, leading to findings similar to those associated with other seronegative spondyloarthropathies.

Sacroiliac joints. In patients with psoriatic arthritis, erosions, joint space widening, sclerosis, and possible fusion are usually bilateral and symmetrical, but the bilateral and symmetric nature is less frequent than in patients with ankylosing spondylitis.

Spine. Spinal involvement is usually but not always associated with sacroiliitis. In contrast to patients with ankylosing spondylitis, the spinal lesions in patients with psoriatic arthritis are typically bulky, asymmetrical, nonmarginal, paravertebral ossifications (i.e., nonmarginal syndesmophytes), which most commonly develop at the lateral aspects of the vertebral bodies in the thoracolumbar junction and tend to skip segments (Fig. 11-19).[312] Radiological differentiation between the spondylitis caused by psoriatic arthritis and spondylitis caused by Reiter's syndrome is impossible, although the latter may be less severe.[302]

CLINICAL COMMENTS

Although the majority of patients with psoriatic arthritis will be aware of the psoriasis, some may not. They may have a single, hidden lesion and be unaware they have the condition, or the patient may fail to mention the skin disorder after it has cleared, assuming it is not related to their joint pain. Therefore, if psoriatic arthritis is a diagnostic consideration, a prudent cutaneous search is needed, and the patient's history should be directly questioned. Although the onset of arthritis usually follows the development

of the skin lesions, up to 20% of patients may develop arthritis before psoriasis.

Physical examination of patients with psoriatic arthritis may reveal skin lesions, soft tissue swelling of an entire digit ("sausage digit"), and nail pitting, the latter of which seems to best correlate with the arthritis.[105] Low back, hand, and foot pain may be initial presenting complaints. Laboratory tests will usually reveal an increased sedimentation rate, be negative for rheumatoid factor, and possibly be positive for HLA-B27 (in 25% to 60% of patients).[50]

Treatment is directed at controlling the joint inflammation. NSAIDs, or in more resistant cases methotrexate, may be useful. Cyclosporine has recently been noted as the drug of choice because it aids in treating both the skin and joint conditions.[345] High doses of vitamin D may also be beneficial.[170] Recently the clinical symptoms and syndromes considered to be associated with psoriatic arthritis have significantly increased in scope.[345]

KEY CONCEPTS

- *Psoriatic arthritis is a seronegative spondyloarthropathy that develops in 5% to 7% of patients with psoriasis.*
- *The age of onset is between 30 and 50 years of age and does not develop more often in a particular gender.*
- *The changes in the axial skeleton mimic the changes in patients with ankylosing spondylitis, but the patients may have unilateral or asymmetrical sacroiliac involvement. Syndesmophyte formation may be thick and asymmetrical with skip lesions.*
- *The effects on the hands are similar to those caused by rheumatoid arthritis, but the DIPs are usually affected first. Erosions may be central and more severe.*
- *Physical examination of the hands may reveal nail pitting, skin lesions, and soft tissue swelling of a digit.*

Reiter's Syndrome

BACKGROUND

Reiter's syndrome, a seronegative spondyloarthropathy, is an asymmetrical polyarthritis that targets the large joints of the lower extremities and small joints of the feet. Only a minority of patients have the classic triad of symptoms (arthritis, urethritis, and conjunctivitis) that originally characterized the syndrome introduced by Hans Reiter in 1916.[307]

Considered a form of reactive arthritis, probable immune-mediated, sterile inflammatory process, occurring distant to the primary focus of infection, generally in the genitourinary or gastrointestinal tracts), its etiology appears to be linked to genetic factor(s) and infection, given the high incidence of HLA-B27 (80%), and frequent occurrence after an infectious episode.[195,325] Most cases follow sexually transmitted infections from *Chlamydia* organisms; however, *Shigella, Yersinia,* and *Salmonella* species are common pathogens associated with Reiter's syndrome after enteric bacterial infections. Males are affected five times more frequently than females, with the average age of onset from 15 to 35 years.[118]

IMAGING FINDINGS

Reiter's syndrome and psoriatic arthritis may be radiographically indistinguishable. However, the propensity for patients with Reiter's syndrome to have lower extremity involvement and patients with psoriatic arthritis to have upper extremity involvement has been noted. Differential diagnosis is accomplished through clinical distinction (e.g., presence of balanitis circinata and keratoderma blennorrhagicum in patients with Reiter's syndrome or nail pitting and psoriasis in patients with psoriatic arthritis), not radiological appearance.[128,196]

Feet. The feet are the most common site of Reiter's syndrome involvement, with the calcaneus and the metatarsophalangeal articulations being specifically affected (Figs. 11-20 and 11-21). Erosion followed by fluffy periosteal new bone formation occurs at the insertion of the plantar fascia and Achilles tendon (enthesopathies).[367] These inflammatory heel spurs are present in approximately 59% of patients and suggest Reiter's syndrome.[365] The erosive changes involving the MTPs are similar to those that occur in patients with rheumatoid arthritis; these patients also have periostitis and sausage digits and relatively little osteopenia.

Tendons. Tenosynovitis is striking in patients with Reiter's syndrome, particularly in the tendons of the feet. MRI is useful to demonstrate the distended tendon sheath.

Large joints of lower extremities. The knee and ankle are frequently affected in patients with Reiter's syndrome, whereas the hip is rarely affected. The radiographic findings are consistent with other inflammatory arthritides: loss of joint space and erosions. In addition, mild productive changes are usually seen, and osteopenia typically does not develop. Severe joint destruction is uncommon.[241,365]

Sacroiliac joints. Sacroiliitis is often asymmetrical or unilateral, with changes mirroring those of the other seronegative spondyloarthropathies. Progression to complete joint fusion in patients with Reiter's syndrome is much less common than in patients with ankylosing spondylitis.[365]

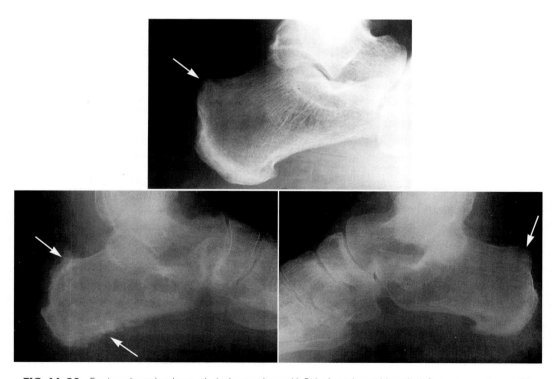

FIG. 11-20 Erosive calcaneal enthesopathy in three patients with Reiter's syndrome. Note the inflammatory enthesopathic changes in each patient, which commonly involve the calcaneus and may develop at the insertion of the plantar fascia and/or Achilles tendon (*arrows*). (Courtesy Steven P. Brownstein, Springfield, NJ.)

Spine. The thoracolumbar junction is the most common spinal site affected.[307] Thick, nonmarginal syndesmophytes, identical to those associated with psoriatic arthritis, bridge the spine and commonly skip segments (Fig. 11-22).

CLINICAL COMMENTS

Reiter's syndrome typically develops within days or weeks following sexual exposure to the disease-causing bacteria or dysentery. The patient generally experiences lower extremity polyarthritis for at least 1 month in addition to one or more of the following: ure-thritis; conjunctivitis (less commonly uveitis); mucocutaneous lesions; nail changes; dysentery; heel pain; or radiographic signs of sacroiliitis, periostitis, or heel spurs. The initial disorder is usually self-limiting, but most patients have recurrent episodes of active arthritis.[325]

Reiter's syndrome may produce two characteristic cutaneous lesions. Balanitis circinata is present in about 25% of post-Shigella and post–Chlamydia-infected patients and is characterized by small, painless ulcers on the glans penis and urethral meatus. Keratoderma blennorrhagica, which develops in 12% to 14% of patients, is char-

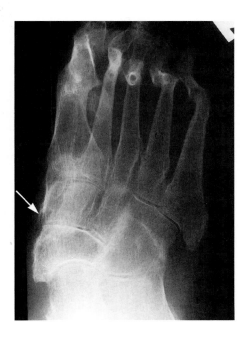

FIG. 11-21 Erosive changes and multiple subluxations affecting predominantly the MTP articulations. Mild periostitis can be seen along the medial aspect of the tarsals *(arrow)*. Bone density is usually relatively well preserved in Reiter's syndrome; however, in this patient, pain has caused disuse and resulting osteoporosis.

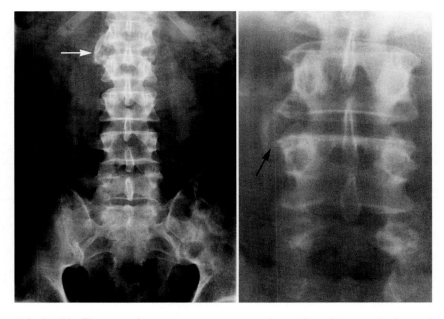

FIG. 11-22 Two cases of asymmetric paravertebral ossification *(arrows)* characterize the spinal changes associated with Reiter's syndrome. These syndesmophytes are radiographically indistinguishable from those caused by psoriatic arthritis. (*Left,* Courtesy Steven P. Brownstein, Springfield, NJ; *Right,* Courtesy Arthur W. Holmes, Foley, Ala.)

acterized by hyperkeratotic skin lesions that are usually on the plantar surface of the feet, toes, penis, and trunk.

Tetracycline or erythromycin is the usual treatment for sexually transmitted chlamydial infections. Until recently, similar antibiotic therapy for the treatment of Reiter's syndrome was unsuccessful[325]; however, more current studies have yielded favorable results.[18,19,219,295] It has been suggested that prophylactic antibiotics may eventually benefit individuals who are at risk for developing Reiter's syndrome.[19] At the onset, arthritic flare-ups usually respond to NSAIDs, but local steroid injections may be required if they are severe.

KEY CONCEPTS

- *Reiter's syndrome is a seronegative spondyloarthropathy that predominately affects the large joints of the lower extremities and small joints of the feet.*
- *Five times more men than women develop the syndrome. The average age of onset is between 15 and 35 years.*
- *The radiographic changes of the axial skeleton (sacroilitis and spondylitis) may be identical to the changes seen in psoriatic arthritis.*
- *Inflammatory changes in the feet are similar to those associated with rheumatoid arthritis. Calcaneal enthesopathies (erosive and proliferative) are characteristic.*
- *Only a minority of patients develop the classic triad of arthritis, urethritis, and conjunctivitis that is associated with Reiter's syndrome.*
- *It is associated with venereal disease and enteric bacterial infections.*

Rheumatoid Arthritis

BACKGROUND

Rheumatoid arthritis is the most common inflammatory arthritide, affecting approximately 1% of the general population and 2% of the population over the age of 60.[155,374,378] This systemic connective tissue disorder primarily affects the synovial lined joints.

Rheumatoid arthritis is characterized by an inflammatory, hyperplastic synovitis (pannus), resulting in cartilage and bone destruction and consequent loss of function. Although it is known that genetic and immunological factors play a role in its pathogenesis, the underlying etiology remains uncertain.[296,330] Proposed etiological theories revolve around genetic, hormonal, and environmental possibilities.[17,84,422]

Joint involvement is typically bilateral and symmetrical, with the small joints of the hands and feet, the wrists, knees, elbows, hips and shoulders being particularly affected.[56] The peak occurrence of disease onset is between 20 and 50 years of age. Women are affected more often than men; although some studies have shown a ratio as high as 7:1, it is generally accepted that women are affected two to three times more frequently.[42,84,247,378] If the disease onset occurs at a more advanced age (over 60 years), this ratio approaches 1:1.[404]

IMAGING FINDINGS

Plain film radiography is used not only to aid in the diagnosis of rheumatoid arthritis but also to follow its progression and the effectiveness of treatment.[362] MRI has been shown to detect many of the initial subtle joint changes much earlier but because of the high cost is not routinely used; therefore this section will focus on plain film findings.[78,108,311]

The general radiographic findings of rheumatoid arthritis may involve any synovial joint and reflect the underlying pathological change of chronic synovial joint inflammation with associated hyperemia, edema, and pannus formation. The first feature, which is usually the sole finding for the first few months, is fusiform periarticular soft tissue swelling arising from capsular distention caused by excessive fluid accumulation. Increased blood flow to the synovium leads to juxtaarticular osteoporosis, which later becomes more generalized because of inactivity.[188,231]

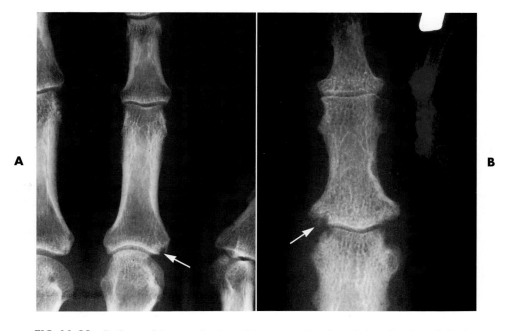

FIG. 11-23   Fusiform soft tissue swelling, loss of joint space, and small marginal erosions *(arrows)* affecting the MCP articulation of the index finger **(A)** and the PIP articulation of the third digit **(B)** on two patients with rheumatoid arthritis.

Joint spaces eventually narrow uniformly as the cartilage is destroyed by the enzymatic nature of pannus. Osseous erosions usually become apparent within the first 2 years of the disease, first occurring at the unprotected bone margins (bare area) (Fig. 11-23), where the pannus has direct contact, and later in the subchondral bone. Subchondral cysts or geodes typically develop and may communicate with the synovium.[242,401]

Later stages of the disease give rise to joint deformities resulting from tendon and ligament laxity, ruptures, and contractures. During periods of prolonged remission, radiographic signs of secondary osteoarthritis may develop and, on rare occasions, ankylosis may occur.

Hands and feet. The earliest clinical and radiographic changes are characteristically found in the hands and feet.[401] Most evaluation methods of rheumatoid arthritis utilize radiographs of the hands, but the feet may show osseous erosions first and to a greater extent.[54,179,400] The initial involvement is of the head of the fifth metatarsal, with erosion and narrowing of the fifth MTP joint.

The classic joint distribution of rheumatoid arthritis in the hands is bilateral and symmetrical involvement of the MCP and PIP articulations (Fig. 11-24). Some or all of the general radiographic features may be seen, with the earliest osseous erosions occurring at the radial aspect of the metacarpal heads (Fig. 11-25). Characteristic joint deformities include the swan-neck deformity, the boutonnière deformity, and the hitchhiker's thumb. The swan-neck deformity results from hyperextension of the PIP and hyperflexion of the DIP (Fig. 11-26), while the boutonnière deformity represents the opposite configuration of hyperflexion of the PIP and hyperextension of the DIP. The hitchhiker's thumb is secondary to MCP flexion and interphalangeal (IP) extension (Fig. 11-27). Ulnar deviation at the MCPs combined with radial deviation in the radiocarpal articulations is also common (Fig. 11-28).

Changes in the feet tend to parallel those of the hands, with the MTP articulations commonly becoming affected first and other deformities, including lateral deviation at the MTPs, flexion of the DIPs (hammer toes), and extension of the MTPs eventually devel-

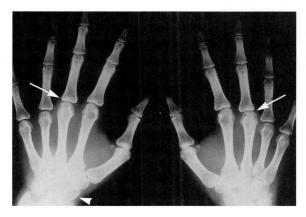

FIG. 11-24   Rheumatoid arthritis classically involves joints bilaterally and symmetrically. Juxtaarticular osteoporosis is present in this patient, in addition to small erosions at the base of the proximal phalanges (arrows). A large subchondral cyst can be seen in the scaphoid of the left wrist (arrowhead).

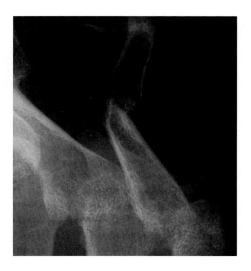

FIG. 11-26   Oblique spot view of the fifth digit of a 62-year-old woman showing a swan-neck deformity.

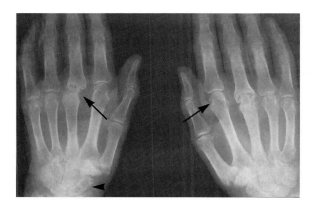

FIG. 11-25   Some of the early osseous changes of a rheumatoid hand are erosions at the second and third MCP articulations (arrows) as seen in this patient with bilateral metacarpal head erosions of the third digit, bilateral erosions at the base of the first metacarpals, and a subchondral cyst on the scaphoid (arrowhead).

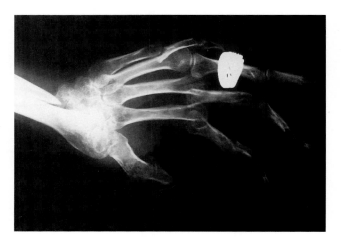

FIG. 11-27   Features associated with advanced stages of rheumatoid arthritis in the hand: diffuse osteoporosis, complete erosion of the distal ulna, and subluxation in the MCP and PIP joints that has resulted in a hitchhiker's deformity in the thumb. Note the ring on the fourth digit.

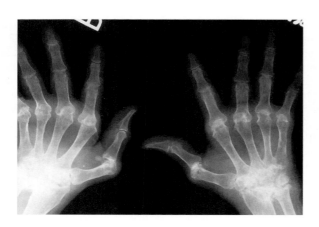

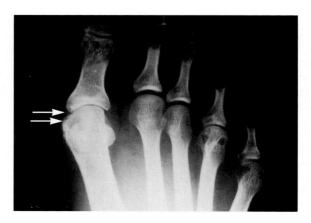

FIG. 11-28 Advanced rheumatoid arthritis with diffuse osteoporosis. Severe erosions and subluxations are present in the MCP joints and carpus bilaterally. The distal and proximal interphalangeal joints have been relatively spared. Ulnar deviation at the MCPs is noted.

FIG. 11-29 Small rat-bite erosions (arrows) and loss of joint space at the MTP articulation of the great toe. Loss of joint space is also apparent at the fourth MTP articulation.

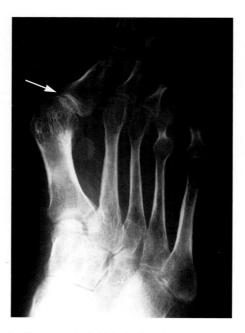

FIG. 11-30 Rheumatoid arthritis in the foot. Fibular deviation at the MTP articulations (arrow) is the most prominent feature in this man with rheumatoid arthritis.

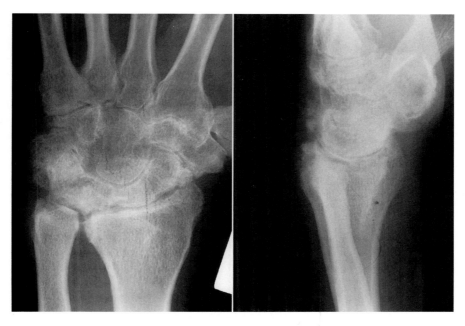

FIG. 11-31 Rheumatoid arthritis in the wrist. Inflammation is most notable in the proximal row of carpals, radiocarpal compartment, and distal ulna. Mild osseous proliferation is noted, suggesting clinical quiescence.

oping (Figs. 11-29 and 11-30). In the heel, retrocalcaneal bursitis, Achilles tendonitis, or Achilles tendon rupture may occur.

Wrist. Pancompartmental involvement is typical in the wrist, with the earliest erosions usually involving the radial and ulnar styloid processes; distal radioulnar joint; and waist of the scaphoid, triquetrum, and pisiform (Fig. 11-31). Ligamentous instability results in patterns that parallel posttraumatic lesions, such as scapholunate dissociation, distal radioulnar dissociation, and dorsiflexion/volar flexion instability.

Elbows. Joint effusion is recognized by a positive fat pad sign (Fig. 11-32). Osseous erosions may be noted at each of the articulating surfaces.

Shoulders. The glenohumeral and acromioclavicular joints may be affected. Resorption of the distal clavicle, in addition to erosions at the coracoclavicular ligament insertion on the undersurface of the clavicle, is not uncommon. Erosion may be observed on the medial aspect of the humeral neck as it abuts the glenoid process from elevation of the humerus, which is caused by a rotator cuff tear secondary to a chronically inflamed supraspinatus tendon.

Hips. Axial migration of the femoral head and acetabular protrusion are common findings that accompany the other general features of rheumatoid arthritis (Fig. 11-33).[86]

Knees. Tricompartmental involvement is typical (Fig. 11-34). A genu valgus deformity is more likely to develop than a varus joint deformity. Soft tissue swelling may be present in the form of suprapatellar effusion or a large popliteal, or Baker's, cyst.

Cervical spine. Rheumatoid arthritis involvement is rare in other regions of the axial skeleton but affects the cervical spine in over half the patients within the first 10 years of disease onset.[401] Atlantoaxial subluxation is the most common radiographic abnormality encountered in the cervical spine, with the prevalence varying from 19% to 70% depending on the patient selection.[193] Move-

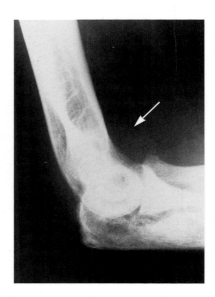

FIG. 11-32 Rheumatoid arthritis in the elbow. Elevation of the anterior fat pad is consistent with joint effusion *(arrow)*. (Courtesy Joseph W. Howe, Sylmar, Calif.)

ment may occur in several directions (listed in order of decreasing frequency): anterior (most frequent—9.5% to 36%), lateral, vertical, or posterior.[35,66] Movement is usually the result of odontoid erosions or transverse ligament laxity, although the alar and apical ligaments may also be involved (Figs. 11-35, 11-36, and 11-37).

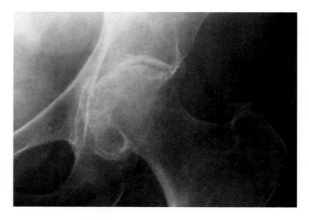

FIG. 11-33   Early rheumatoid arthritis of the hip shown by concentric loss of joint space, small erosions of the femoral head and acetabulum, and osteopenia. Note the lack of osteophytosis and eburnation.

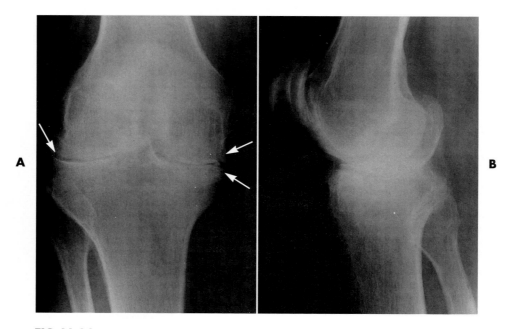

FIG. 11-34   AP **(A)** and lateral **(B)** radiographs showing changes typically associated with rheumatoid arthritis of the knee. The most striking finding is tricompartmental loss of joint space and joint effusion. Small marginal osteophytes indicate secondary osteoarthritis *(arrows)*.

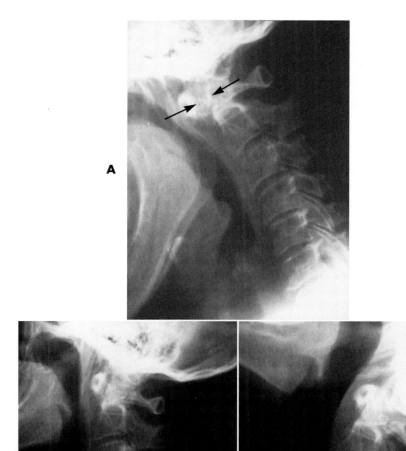

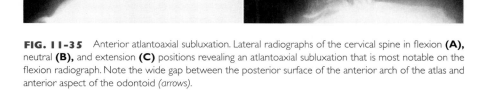

FIG. 11-35 Anterior atlantoaxial subluxation. Lateral radiographs of the cervical spine in flexion **(A),** neutral **(B),** and extension **(C)** positions revealing an atlantoaxial subluxation that is most notable on the flexion radiograph. Note the wide gap between the posterior surface of the anterior arch of the atlas and anterior aspect of the odontoid *(arrows).*

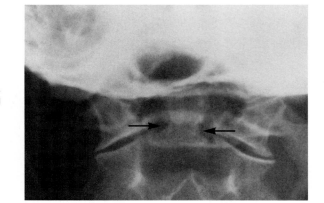

FIG. 11-36   Odontoid erosions. AP open-mouth radiograph of patient in Fig. 11-35 revealing erosions at the base of the odontoid process *(arrows)*. The lateral atlantoaxial joints appear unaffected.

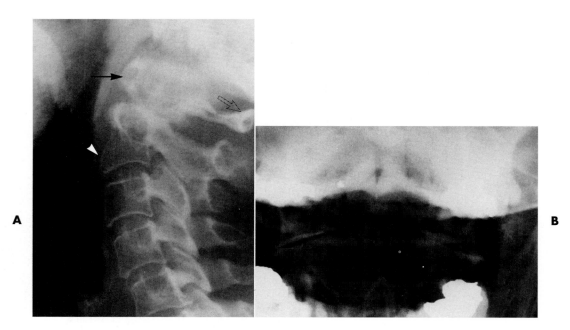

FIG. 11-37   Posterior atlantoaxial subluxation. **A,** Neutral lateral cervical radiograph demonstrating posterior displacement of the anterior arch of C1 *(arrow)* relative to the C2 body *(arrowhead)*. The spinolaminar line of the atlas *(open arrow)* is also posterior with respect to the remaining cervical vertebrae. **B,** Open-mouth radiograph revealing lateral subluxation of the dens with erosions and reduced joint space and subluxation of the lateral atlantoaxial articulations.

The degree of anterior subluxation shown on conventional radiography correlates poorly with neurological signs and the presence of cord compression, which is in part a result of the unknown thickness of the synovial pannus not visible (Fig. 11-38).[34,333] The standard method for determining anterior atlantoaxial subluxation has been an anterior atlantodental interval* (ADI) of greater than 3 mm,

but it has been shown that a posterior atlantodental interval† (PADI) of 14 mm or less may be a more reliable predictor for neural compression and necessitate an MRI for evaluation of true cord space.[34]

Subaxial subluxations are less common than upper cervical spine subluxations, with an estimated occurrence rate of 7% to 27%, but are potentially more important neurologically because of

---

*The ADI is the distance between the posterior-inferior aspect of the anterior arch of the atlas and the most anterior point of the odontoid process. Measurements of greater than 3 cm is considered abnormal. The measurement should be obtained from a lateral flexion radiograph.

†The PADI is measured from the posterior wall of the dens to the anterior aspect of the C1 lamina.

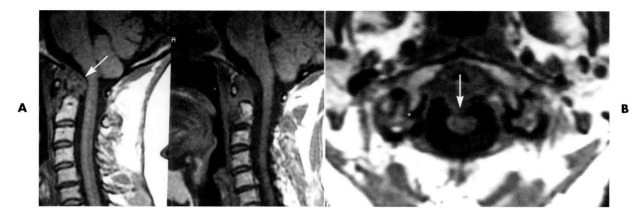

FIG. 11-38 Sagittal T1-weighted gradient echo **(A)** and axial gradient echo **(B)** MRI images revealing prominent synovial inflammation (pannus) in the posterior median atlantoaxial joint *(arrows)* with apparent destruction of the dens and mild compression of the spinal cord *(arrows)*.

the smaller spinal canal dimensions (Fig. 11-39).[34,66] A canal measurement may be taken from the lateral radiograph in a similar way the PADI is taken. If the subaxial canal diameter measures less than 14 mm, MRI is advised.[34]

Erosions of the vertebral endplates, facet joints, and spinous processes are other less severe signs of rheumatoid involvement. These signs are often subtle and difficult to diagnose on plain film radiographs.

CLINICAL COMMENTS

Diagnosis. The criteria for the diagnosis of rheumatoid arthritis, which was originally designed to aid in research consistency, have been revised and are now easier for the clinician to use.[12] The diagnosis can be made if the patient meets at least four of the following criteria established by the American College of Rheumatology. The first four must be present for at least 6 weeks.

1. Stiffness in the morning that lasts at least 1 hour
2. Swelling of at least three joints
3. Swelling of the wrist, MCP, or PIP joints
4. Symmetrical swelling
5. Rheumatoid nodules
6. Positive rheumatoid factor test
7. Radiographic changes consistent with rheumatoid arthritis

Laboratory tests aid in establishing the diagnosis and assessing disease activity. The test for the presence of rheumatoid factor will be positive in approximately 70% to 80% of patients with rheumatoid arthritis but will also be positive in approximately 5% of individuals who do not have rheumatoid arthritis, as well as in patients with other nonrheumatoid diseases.[226,426] Therefore a positive or negative rheumatoid factor test must be correlated closely with other clinical features. A complete blood count, ESR, and ANA assay may also be performed to initially evaluate and follow up with patients with rheumatoid arthritis.[426]

Although the main sites affected by rheumatoid arthritis are the joints, extraarticular manifestations are common. Rheumatoid nodules are the classic extraarticular lesions. These subcutaneous lesions are found in approximately 25% to 40% of patients and are typically located on the extensor surfaces at sites subject to trauma.[247,378] These nodules can also be present in visceral organs. Pulmonary and cardiovascular systems are often affected in patients

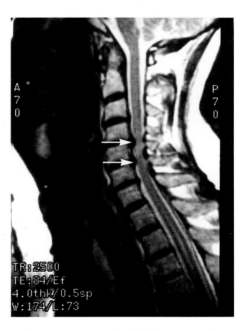

FIG. 11-39 Subaxial subluxations. Sagittal T2-weighted MRI image of patient in Figure 11-35 revealing marrow changes of the odontoid process, synovial inflammation, and multiple subaxial subluxations in the mid and lower regions of the cervical spine with disc protusions *(arrows)* and resulting cord compression.

with rheumatoid arthritis. Pleural involvement (e.g., pleurisy, pleural effusion) is the most common lung manifestation and is usually asymptomatic.[7] Other pulmonary manifestations include interstitial and airway disease. Two syndromes associated with rheumatoid arthritis are Felty's (a combination of rheumatoid arthritis, splenomegaly, and neutropenia) and Sjögren's (marked by rheumatoid arthritis and dry eyes and mouth).

Patients with rheumatoid arthritis tend to have reduced life expectancies and decreases in their ability to perform activities of daily living and work.[278,309] The disease course is variable, ranging

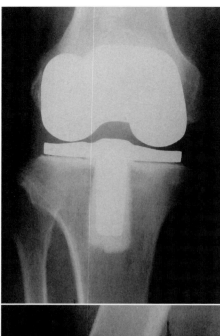

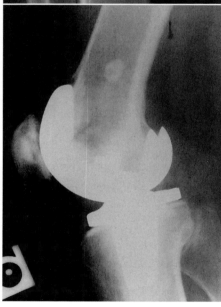

FIG. 11-40   Total resurfacing knee arthroplasty of patient in Fig. 11-34 because of advanced rheumatoid arthritis.

from mild with periods of remission to severe and quickly progressive. The highest rate of joint damage and progression occurs early in the disease; therefore treatment should begin immediately after the diagnosis is made so that irreversible joint damage is prevented.[401] Known risk factors may increase the possibility of developing the severe stages of the disease and early mortality, so these patients may need a more aggressive treatment.[308,309,404,406]

Treatment. Treatment is multifaceted and must address both pain and disability. Conservative therapy includes patient education and emotional support; rest; application of heat or cold; dietary changes or supplementation; and resistance training, exercise, and joint mobilization to improve joint range of motion, strengthen muscles, and minimize joint deformity.* Pharmacological treatment includes NSAIDs as well as more aggressive second-line of defense drugs (corticosteroids, antimalarial drugs, gold salts, penicillamine, immunosuppressive drugs).[43,378] Surgical intervention may also be indicated to replace joints (Fig. 11-40) or treat neurological compromise.[137]

KEY CONCEPTS

- *Rheumatoid arthritis is the most common inflammatory arthritide.*
- *Females are more likely to develop the disease (two or three times more likely, less in older populations), with peak incidence occurring between 20 and 50 years of age.*
- *The primary sites affected are the synovial tissues of the hands, feet, wrists, hips, knees, elbows, and shoulders. Affected MCP and PIP joints of the hand and atlantoaxial subluxation of the cervical spine are most characteristic.*
- *The arthritide is marked by a bilateral symmetrical distribution; periarticular soft tissue swelling; initial juxtaarticular osteoporosis progressing to generalized, uniform loss of joint space; marginal erosions (bare areas) progressing to subchondral erosions; subchondral cysts; and joint deformities.*
- *Hip involvement leads to acetabular protrusion.*
- *Subluxations and joint deformities, including swan-neck, boutonnière, and hitchhiker's thumb, are characteristic.*
- *Treatment is directed toward limiting pain and disability and may include surgery for joint replacement or to address neurological complications.*

Scleroderma

BACKGROUND

Scleroderma—or progressive systemic sclerosis (PSS), a term that more appropriately describes the entire disease process—is a connective tissue disorder characterized by small vessel disease and fibrosis that affects the skin (scleroderma), musculoskeletal system, and internal organs.

Although the etiology is unknown, the immune system and environmental agents are believed to play important roles in the pathogenesis.† The annual incidence rate in the United States has been reported to be approximately 17 per million population. It is unclear whether this rate is stable or increasing.[250,257] Women are affected three times more frequently than men, especially during the childbearing years, with the diagnosis usually made between 20 and 50 years of age.[379,380] Although there is no overall significant racial predisposition, young black women are stricken most often and most severely.[257]

Scleroderma has been divided into different classifications depending on the existence and extent of systemic involvement and

*References 2, 92, 97, 160, 326, 423.
†References 13, 27, 63, 189, 256, 257.

the rapidity of disease progression. Several syndromes are associated with scleroderma or scleroderma-like features, the classic one being the CREST syndrome (*Calcinosis, Raynaud's phenomenon, Esophageal abnormalities, Sclerodactyly,* and *Telangiectasia*).

IMAGING FINDINGS

The major abnormalities found by plain film radiography that are associated with PSS are noted in the hands and include soft tissue atrophy, osseous resorption, and subcutaneous calcification. Gastrointestinal contrast studies may reveal characteristic findings in the esophagus, small intestine, and large bowel that are mainly caused by fibrosis and atrophy.

Hands. Atrophy of the soft tissues at the fingertips (acral tapering) is a very common feature, the incidence of which increases if the patient has accompanying Raynaud's phenomenon.[21] Bone resorption or erosion is also frequently noted, involving primarily the distal tufts (acro-osteolysis) (Fig. 11-41) and (to a much lesser degree) the distal and proximal interphalangeal articulations.[100] The presence of subcutaneous calcinosis is prominent in the hands but also develops around other joints and over bony eminences (Fig. 11-42).[100,117,414]

Chest. The two major pulmonary manifestations associated with scleroderma are pulmonary hypertension and interstitial lung disease (inflammation and fibrosis). If the fibrosis is extensive enough to be visible on a chest radiograph, the reticular pattern predominates in the lower lungs.

Gastrointestinal tract. Smooth muscle dysfunction causes esophageal aperistalsis and reduced lower esophageal sphincter pressure resulting in gastro-esophageal reflux and an increased incidence of peptic stricture and Barrett's esophagus. The esophageal changes lead to dysmotility and may be reflected on plain film as air or air-fluid levels within the esophagus.[288] Barium studies may initially re-

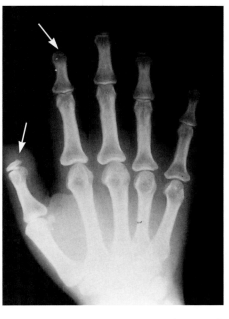

FIG. 11-41 Scleroderma causing acro-osteolysis of the hand *(arrows)*. (Courtesy Joseph W. Howe, Sylmar, Calif.)

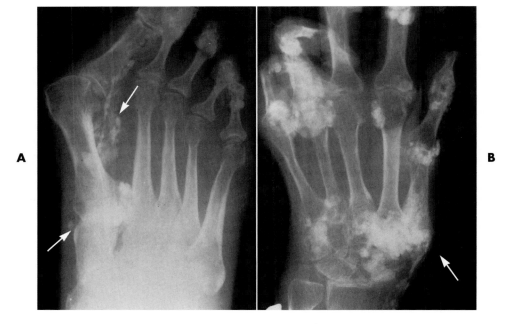

FIG. 11-42 Different patients with scleroderma exhibiting subcutaneous and periarticular soft tissue calcification *(arrows)* of the foot **(A)** and hand **(B)**. Although fibular subluxations of the phalanges at the MTP articulations are evident, no signs of significant erosions are present.

veal rapid transit; esophageal reflux; dilatation of the esophagus and small bowel; and large-mouthed sacculations or pseudodiverticula in the colon, jejunum, and ileum. Over time, barium studies reveal decreased motility and possibly obstruction.

CLINICAL COMMENTS

Changes in the skin's appearance (thickness and fibrosis, tightening, shininess, atrophy), Raynaud's phenomenon, and polyarthralgia may be the first signs of systemic sclerosis, although visceral involvement may have already occurred.[95,176,387] The gastrointestinal tract is the most common internal site affected, with complications including dysphagia, gastroesophageal reflux, Barrett's esophagus, small bowel bacterial overgrowth, malnutrition, and intestinal pseudo-obstruction.[136,371] Periodontal membrane thickening causes loose teeth, which further complicates maintaining a good nutritional status. The heart, lungs, and kidneys may also become involved; pulmonary disease causes higher mortality than kidney failure.[69,95,158,222] A thorough, multisystem evaluation is needed to detect serious problems that may exist in a seemingly asymptomatic patient.[222]

Laboratory tests may reveal an elevated ESR, the presence of rheumatoid factor in approximately 30% of patients, and the presence of serum ANAs in more than 90% of cases. A variety of disease-specific autoantibodies have been discovered that provide markers for certain clinical features.[13]

Treatment includes patient education, dietary modification, drug therapy, and surgery and is directed toward the varied systemic manifestations of the disease.[258,273,283,371] No generalized therapy for progressive systemic sclerosis has been proven to be effective; however, the continuous accumulation of information about pathogenesis of scleroderma and the numerous therapies that are being studied provide hope for the development of a successful treatment.[283,349,396]

KEY CONCEPTS

- *Scleroderma is a connective tissue disorder that affects the skin, musculoskeletal system, and internal organs.*
- *Women are three times more likely to develop the condition than men.*
- *The disorder typically develops between 20 and 50 years of age.*
- *The hands develop distal tuft resorption (acro-osteolysis), acral tapering caused by soft tissue atrophy, and subcutaneous calcinosis.*
- *Major pulmonary manifestations include hypertension and interstitial fibrosis.*
- *Gastrointestinal manifestations include esophageal dysmotility and large-mouthed bowel sacculations.*
- *Laboratory tests may reveal an elevated ESR, the presence of rheumatoid factor in 30% of patients, and the presence of serum ANAs in 90% of patients.*

Systemic Lupus Erythematosus

BACKGROUND

Systemic lupus erythematosus (SLE) is an inflammatory connective tissue disorder characterized by excessive immunoreactivity. The resulting production of autoantibodies affects multiple organ systems.[281,332] Although the factor that activates this immune response is unclear, a major element of the underlying pathogenesis is widespread vasculitis, which may be secondary to local deposition of immune complexes.[24] The clinical manifestations reflect the capillary damage to the affected structures. Virtually any tissue can be damaged, but the joints, skin, kidneys, and serosal membranes are most frequently affected.[48,111,214]

SLE follows an irregular course of flare-ups and remissions. The majority of SLE cases develop between 20 and 40 years of age. Women are affected up to nine times more often than men, with the most significant ratio variance occurring during childbearing years. Pregnancy may increase the disease's morbidity.[306] It is generally reported that blacks are affected more often than whites. However, in one reported study, in the United States, women who develop the disease are more likely to be white, whereas all racial groups of men are equally likely to develop the disease.[126] A familial link has also been documented.

IMAGING FINDINGS

Although up to 90% of patients complain of articular problems, prominent and severe radiographic changes are not commonly seen.[213] The most frequently affected joints are the hands, feet, wrists, and knees. Soft tissue swelling and minimal periarticular osteoporosis are the earliest radiographic manifestations and usually present bilaterally and symmetrically. In later stages, joint deformities may ensue. Subcutaneous calcifications, particularly those involving the legs, may be present but are not commonly seen.[418]

Hands. SLE often affects the hands and has a joint distribution similar to that of rheumatoid arthritis (i.e., in the MCPs and PIPs).[280,334] Chronic joint inflammation and effusion may lead to ligamentous laxity and result in joint deformities, the most common of which include ulnar deviation at the MCPs, flexion and extension deformities of the IP articulations resembling swan-neck and boutonnière deformities, and malalignment of the first carpometacarpal joint. These deformities are nonerosive and reducible and are therefore more visible on an oblique or lateral view of a hand radiograph as compared to a PA view, where the pressure of the cassette may make the subluxations less pronounced. These nonerosive, flexible deformities are considered pathognomonic and are present in less than half of patients with SLE who have articular abnormalities. Although rarely, these deformities may eventually become permanent or fixed.

Axial skeleton. Although spinal changes are uncommon, atlantoaxial subluxation has been reported in 8.5% of patients with SLE; it is wise to obtain a lateral cervical flexion radiograph because this abnormality may be present but not apparent on a neutral lateral radiograph.[16]

Sacroiliitis, which has radiographic features that are similar to those associated with the seronegative spondyloarthropathies, has been reported as an uncommon manifestation of SLE.[210]

Osteonecrosis. Avascular necrosis is a common complication in patients with SLE. The radiographic features are identical to those associated with osteonecrosis caused by factors other than SLE. The femoral condyles and humeral and femoral heads are the most common sites affected, with the femoral heads being affected more than the humeral heads or femoral condyles. Other common sites include the distal femur and proximal and distal tibia. Although high doses of corticosteroids can significantly increase the risk of osteonecrosis, some treatment regimens may reduce this risk.[260] Regardless, the disease process seems to increase risk for developing osteonecrosis, because those patients not receiving steroids have developed the condition.[209]

CLINICAL COMMENTS

The clinical presentation varies according to the distribution of lesions and the extent of systemic involvement. Many patients initially present with constitutional signs and symptoms (malaise, fever, weight loss), polyarthritis, or a skin rash. The classic malar "butterfly" erythema may be noted but is only one of several cutaneous lesions that may present intermittently during the course of the disease.[214] The renal system is involved, but the extent differs widely from one patient to the next.[11] Manifestations in any organ system (e.g., respiratory, cardiac, gastrointestinal, central nervous) may eventually appear.[355]

The screening test for SLE detects the presence of ANAs, which are present in virtually all patients with SLE. Although this test is sensitive for SLE, it is not specific so it may also be positive in other nonlupus conditions. However, the presence of antibodies to native (double-stranded [ds]) DNA strongly suggests SLE. Lupus erythematosus cells* may also be observed. Rheumatoid factor is found in a minority of patients, which may indicate an overlap syndrome other than true SLE.

The diagnosis of idiopathic lupus should be made only after ruling out the possibility of a drug-induced condition, which can be concluded if discontinuing use of a suspected drug alleviates all signs and symptoms.[165] Treatment depends on the location and

---

*ANAs react with nuclei of damaged cells, which disrupts the cells' chromatin structures and transforms them into lupus erythematosus bodies. These bodies undergo phagocytosis by neutrophils to form lupus erythematosus cells.

severity of the disease. In mild cases it may involve counseling, exercise, and NSAIDs, whereas in more severe disease immediate corticosteroid or other immunosuppressive drug therapy may be required.[85,232] Unfortunately, the use of immunosuppressive drugs increases the risk of infection, which is currently a major cause of morbidity and mortality in these patients.[178] New drug therapies are being tested that may reduce disease activity.[167,395] Because of their immunomodulatory properties, sex hormones are also being investigated as potential therapeutic agents.[405]

KEY CONCEPTS

- *SLE is an inflammatory connective tissue disorder that affects many organs.*
- *Women develop the disease nine times more often than men, with the majority of cases developing between 20 and 40 years of age.*
- *The MCP and PIP joints of the hands are affected, and nonerosive, flexible deformities develop.*
- *A serious complication includes possible atlantoaxial subluxation.*
- *The clinical presentation is marked by arthralgia, a "butterfly" rash, and constitutional signs and symptoms.*
- *Laboratory tests include a test for the presence of ANAs, lupus erythematosus cells, and rheumatoid factor.*

Metabolic and Deposition Arthritides

Calcium Pyrophosphate Dihydrate Crystal Deposition Disease

BACKGROUND

The deposition of calcium pyrophosphate dihydrate crystals in and around joints results in an arthropathy with protean manifestations. The nomenclature relating to this process and disease is often confusing and incorrectly used. For the purposes of simplification, the text will focus on the following three major presentations of the calcium pyrophosphate deposition disease (CPPD):

1. *Chondrocalcinosis.* The classic presentation of CPPD is radiographic evidence of calcified articular cartilage (chondrocalcinosis) involving characteristic sites, which include the knee, wrist, MCPs, and symphysis pubis. Less commonly, crystals may also be deposited and radiographically visible in the synovium, joint capsules, tendons, and ligaments.

   The term *chondrocalcinosis* is often used as a synonym for CPPD. Although calcium pyrophosphate is the most common crystal to cause chondrocalcinosis, the terms *CPPD* and *chondrocalcinosis* are not truly interchangeable because crystals other than calcium pyrophosphates can be deposited, and factors other than crystal deposition can lead to cartilage calcification.

2. *Pyrophosphate arthropathy.* The intraarticular deposition of crystals may degrade the cartilage and lead to a second manifestation of CPPD that radiographically mimics severe joint degeneration, a condition called *pyrophosphate arthropathy.* The radiographic image may be difficult to distinguish from primary osteoarthritis or secondary osteoarthritis following trauma, although pyrophosphate arthropathy typically develops in a location that is not characteristic for primary osteoarthritis (OA), and no history of trauma is documented.

3. *Pseudogout.* The clinical presentation of CPPD varies; a patient can be completely asymptomatic or have an acutely painful and inflamed joint that is similar to the joints associated with gout. The latter presentation has been appropriately referred to as *pseudogout.*

The underlying cause of this CPPD is unknown, but its frequent association with other conditions such as gout, hyperparathyroidism, hemochromatosis, diabetes mellitus, and neurotrophic osteoarthropathy suggests that it may be secondary to metabolic or degenerative changes in the cartilage. It has also been proposed that the simultaneous occurrence of pseudogout and the mentioned conditions is purely coincidental.

It is generally accepted that the prevalence of chondrocalcinosis increases with age but that no particular gender develops the condition more often.[107,122,424] A recent study suggests this increased prevalence with age and lack of association with a certain gender may correlate with the affected tissues.[430] The study, which focused on structures of the knee, concluded that the prevalence of hyaline cartilage calcification increases with age but is not related to gender, whereas meniscal calcification is significantly more prevalent in men but is not related to age.

IMAGING FINDINGS

General radiographic features of CPPD can consist of a characteristic solitary finding such as chondrocalcinosis or a combination of features, including other intraarticular and periarticular calcifications, soft tissue swelling, and progressive structural joint damage that may mimic degenerative joint disease (DJD) or, if severe, neurotrophic arthropathy.

Chondrocalcinosis. Cartilage calcification may involve hyaline or fibrocartilage. Fibrocartilage calcification is most common in the menisci of the knees (Fig. 11-43), triangular cartilage

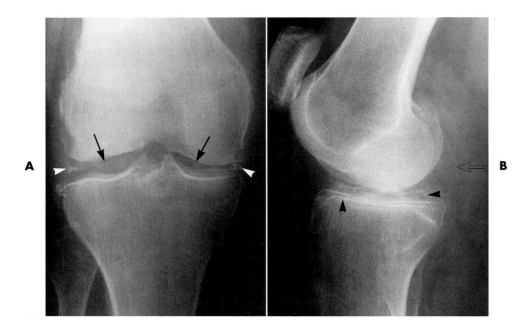

FIG. 11-43 **(A)** AP and **(B)** lateral radiographs of the knee showing calcification of the hyaline *(arrows)* and fibrocartilage *(arrowheads)* and involvement of the capsule *(open arrow)*. The retropatellar compartment appears mildly reduced, a finding characteristic of CPPD.

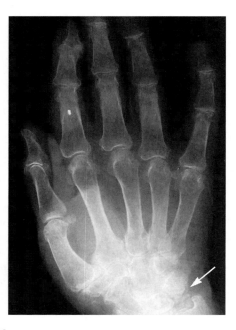

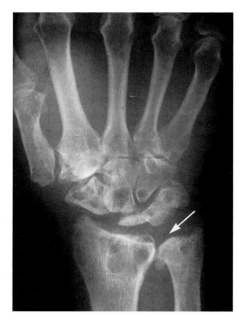

FIG. 11-44 PA hand radiograph of a patient with CPPD revealing thick calcification in the region of the triangular fibrocartilage *(arrow)* and thin linear calcification within the MCP articulations.

FIG. 11-45 PA hand radiograph of a patient with CPPD showing calcification of the triangular fibrocartilage *(arrow)*, multiple subchondral cysts, avascular necrosis of the lunate, and proximal collapse of the capitate.

complex of the wrist (Figs. 11-44 and 11-45), symphysis pubis, and acetabular labrum. The calcification presents radiographically as a thick, irregular radiopaque focus within the affected structure. Hyaline cartilage calcification is also most common in the knee (see Fig. 11-43), wrist, and hip (Fig. 11-46), as well as the MCPs (see Fig. 11-44), elbows, and shoulders. On a radiograph it appears as a thin, linear radiopacity that parallels the articular surface of bone.

Pyrophosphate arthropathy. Chronic pyrophosphate crystal deposition within hyaline cartilage may lead to intraarticular damage that simulates DJD. These changes tend to be progressive and severe, with advanced joint space narrowing, prominent bony proliferation, and often dramatic cyst formation (Fig. 11-46). The articular and intra-articular (or compartmental) distribution classically differs from that of primary osteoarthritis and should aid in the diagnosis. Non–weight-bearing joints such as the shoulder, elbow, wrist, and patellofemoral joint, are involved, as well as weight-bearing articulations such as the knee and hip. In a patient with no history of trauma, a DJD pattern in the mentioned non–weight-bearing joints suggests pyrophosphate arthropathy. Isolated involvement of the patellofemoral compartment (Fig. 11-47), advanced tricompartmental disease of the knee, and selective radiocarpal or trapezioscaphoid joint degeneration are also unusual for nontraumatic DJD and suggests the possibility of an underlying crystal deposition.

CLINICAL COMMENTS

The varied clinical presentations of CPPD can cause a diagnostic dilemma. CPPD, may masquerade as DJD (chronic progressive joint pain, crepitus, and limited range of motion), manifest as an acute inflammatory disorder such as rheumatoid arthritis or gout (with intermittent attacks of painful, red, swollen joints), or have no clinical symptoms in a patient with a concomitant disorder.

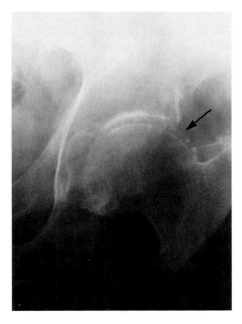

FIG. 11-46 AP hip radiograph revealing calcification that parallels the lateral aspect of the femoral head *(arrow)*.

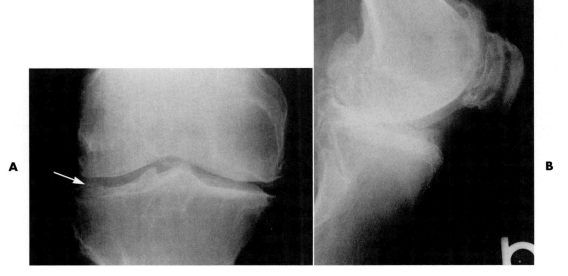

FIG. 11-47 Pyrophosphate arthropathy. AP **(A)** and lateral **(B)** knee radiographs revealing characteristic features of pyrophosphate arthropathy. Advanced femoropatellar compartment degenerative changes are present; the medial and lateral compartments of the knee are relatively spared. Meniscal calcification is also apparent *(arrow)*. Primary osteoarthritis has an affinity for the medial femorotibial compartment and tends to spare the lateral and retropatellar compartments.

The diagnostic possibilities narrow if the clinical signs and symptoms are combined with radiographic evidence of chondrocalcinosis. This combination indicates that the patient probably has CPPD, and survey radiographs (such as an AP view of the knees, a PA view of the hands and wrists, and an AP view of the symphysis) may need to be taken. The clinician must keep in mind that chondrocalcinosis may not develop and as mentioned is not the only characteristic radiographic finding. If the clinician seriously suspects the patient has CPPD, a diagnosis can be confirmed by synovial aspiration and consequent microscopic identification of calcium pyrophosphate crystals. Other laboratory findings are not diagnostic but may reveal additional diseases such as diabetes, gout, hyperparathyroidism, or hemochromatosis.

The treatment and prognosis for CPPD vary because they depend on the clinical presentation, radiographic findings, and the presence of any underlying or associated disorders. The clinician must be aware that the patient may have an additional disease to make an appropriate investigation and provide the necessary treatment. The prognosis of CPPD with no additional diseases is usually excellent but in some cases may be poor (e.g., severe joint damage), requiring administration of colchicine intravenously or NSAIDs to control inflammatory episodes and possibly colchicine orally to prevent acute attacks.

Although immobilization may help reduce overt inflammation, it may have a more adverse affect on the articular cartilage than the inflammation itself; therefore, joint mobility should be maintained to the patient's tolerance.[117] A balance of exercise and rest is necessary to preserve the articular cartilage and control pain from active inflammation.

KEY CONCEPTS

- *CPPD is a disease in which calcium pyrophosphate dihydrate crystals are deposited in and around joints; the disease has three common presentations.*
  1. The first presentation is marked by calcification of hyaline and fibrocartilage in and around joints (chondrocalcinosis).
  2. The second clinical presentation involves progressive joint degeneration (pseudoosteoarthritis, pyrophosphate arthropathy).
  3. The third clinical presentation is characterized by acutely painful, swollen joints and simulates the clinical presentation of gout (pseudogout).
- *The sites commonly affected by CPPD are the knees, wrists, hips, and MCPs.*
- *CPPD is often associated with another underlying disorder (e.g., hemosiderosis, hyperparathyroidism, gout, amyloidosis).*

Gout

BACKGROUND

Gout is a clinical disorder associated with monosodium urate crystal deposits in the connective tissues, including articular cartilage. Gout is classified into two forms based on etiology: (1) an idiopathic or primary form and (2) a much less common secondary form that is associated with a host of preexisting enzymatic, hereditary, hematological, endocrine, and renal disorders.[44] The first attack of gout is most common among individuals between 40 and 50 years of age and is 20 times more common in men.[146] In general, women who develop gout tend to be older than men. The disorder is characterized by recurrent, acute, or chronic joint pain and swelling (arthritic gout), large soft tissue accumulations (tophaceous gout), and impaired renal function (gouty nephropathy).

Uric acid is the normal by-product of purine catabolism in patients with aberrant purine metabolic pathways. *Hyperuricemia,* which is defined as serum urate concentrations of more than 7 mg/dL in men and 6 mg/dL in women, develops in these patients, and the excess urate crystallizes as monosodium salt, mainly in the oversaturated tissues of the joints. The needle-shaped monosodium crystals may act as mechanical irritants to the joint, producing an arthropathy. However, the exact mechanism by which monosodium urate crystals cause inflammation and arthropathy is not well understood.[377]

Only a minority of patients (about 20%) with hyperuricemia ever develop gout. Gout development depends on multiple factors. Hyperuricemia is requisite but by itself does not always lead to gout.

Four phases of gout are recognized: asymptomatic gout, acute gouty arthritis, intercritical gout, and chronic tophaceous gout. The first phase is hyperuricemia, which as stated previously may not lead to gout. Patients experiencing their first attack of acute gout have had sustained hyperuricemia for 20 to 30 years. The second phase involves acute inflammatory arthritis, usually involving the first MTP joint of the first toe. The ankle, tarsals, and knee are also commonly involved. Early attacks tend to subside without treatment in a period of 7 to 10 days. The third, or intercritical, phase is the period between acute attacks. The fourth, or chronic tophaceous gout stage is marked by the development of radiographically evident subcutaneous monosodium urate crystal tophi in the synovium, subchondral bone, olecranon bursae, extensor surface of forearm, infrapatellar and calcaneal tendons, and helix of the ear. Often, patients in the chronic phase of gout may not exhibit tophi for 10 to 12 years.

IMAGING FINDINGS

Gout tends to affect lower extremities, particularly the feet. During the course of the disease, 90% of patients will exhibit changes in the MTP joint of the first toe. Changes are more pronounced on the dor-

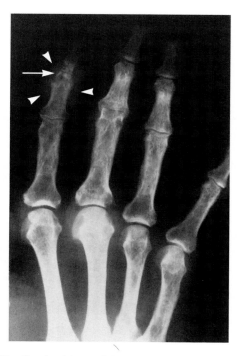

FIG. 11-48   Gout involving the DIP joint of the second digit. Soft tissue density *(arrowheads)* and mechanical joint erosions *(arrow)* are noted. (Courtesy Joseph W. Howe, Sylmar, Calif.)

sal and medial aspects of the this joint. Swelling over the dorsum of the foot results from involvement of the tarsometatarsal articulations.

Asymmetrical joint changes may be noted in the wrists and hands, particularly the carpometacarpal joints. The medial aspect of the knee and prepatellar bursa may be involved. The axial skeleton is only rarely involved.

It is difficult for radiography to detect the early phases of gout. Soft tissue swelling and capsular distention are usually present around the involved joint but are difficult to recognize radiographically. In patients with chronic gout, tophaceous deposits cause intraarticular or periarticular bone erosions, which are seen on the radiograph as thin, "overhanging edge" margins of bone that cover a portion of the tophaceous deposit (Fig. 11-48). The margins of these bone erosions are sclerotic, which is characteristic of their mechanically erosive etiology. Large tophaceous deposits (Fig. 11-49) are often seen on the dorsum of the feet and near the olecranon (Fig. 11-50). Osteoporosis is not characteristic of gout, but severe pain can cause disuse atrophy and lead to this condition. The joint space is preserved until late in the disease.

CLINICAL COMMENTS

Serum urate levels may be high or low and are therefore often misleading. A definitive diagnosis depends on confirming the presence of monosodium urate crystals. Fluid samples are ordinarily drawn

from the first MTP joint. Following diagnosis, treatment is directed toward limiting pain and joint destruction and preventing the renal stones that often develop. Medical treatment usually entails the administration of NSAIDs, corticosteriods, and colchicine. With the advent of modern treatment, chronic tophaceous gout is an uncommon condition.

KEY CONCEPTS

- *Gout is an idiopathic or secondary disorder of purine metabolism that results in monosodium urate crystal deposition in the connective tissues.*
- *Four gout phases are recognized: asymptomatic gout, acute arthritic gout, intercritical gout, and chronic tophaceous gout.*
- *The lower extremities are most commonly affected, and the first MTP joint is eventually affected in 90% of gout patients.*
- *Radiographic features that develop in the early stages of gout include soft tissue swelling and capsular distentions.*
- *Radiographic features that develop in the late stages of gout include eccentric nodular soft tissue prominences, which often develop over the dorsum of the foot or olecranon; preservation of the joint space until the later stages of the disease; and intraarticular or periarticular bony erosions with an "overhanging edge" produced by tophaceous deposits.*
- *The calcium density in patients with tophaceous gout is the feature that distinguishes gouty deposits from deposits associated with amyloidosis and multicentric reticulohistiocytosis.*

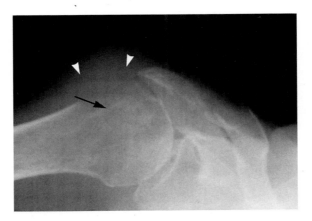

FIG. 11-49 Gout. Large tophaceous deposits (*arrowheads*) and osseous erosions of the lateral portion of the humeral head (*arrows*).

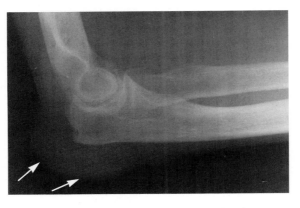

FIG. 11-50 Gout. Large tophaceous deposits on the olecranon process (*arrows*).

Degenerative Arthritides and Related Conditions

Degenerative Joint Disease

BACKGROUND

DJD (also referred to as *osteoarthritis* or *osteoarthrosis [OA]* is the most common type of arthropathy. It is slowly progressive, primarily affects joint cartilage, and is the first or second (following cardiovascular disease) most common cause of disability in adults.[234,259,432] Although the term *DJD* implies that a synovial joint is affected, similar changes occur in cartilaginous joints (e.g., acromioclavicular, intervertebral disc [IVD]).

Etiology. Degeneration can be caused by multiple factors that include a heterogenous collection of processes that affect the joints and periarticular tissues. Degeneration is classically divided into primary (or idiopathic) and secondary forms based on the identification of an underlying condition or traumatic event. Primary degeneration has no identified causative factors. Secondary degeneration is caused by a preexisting abnormality and is the most common type of degeneration. The overall validity of the primary classification has been questioned by some because they assert that some type of mechanical deviation always precedes degeneration.[340]

Secondary degeneration most commonly develops when a patient has had a trauma (acute or repetitive) or has avascular necrosis, diabetes mellitus, Paget's disease, a slipped capital femoral epiphysis, chondrocalcinosis, neuropathy, acromegaly, ochronosis, hereditary collagen disorders, or a variety of other conditions.

There are several theories explaining the cause of degeneration, including repetitive trauma, changes in the synovium, or changes in the subchondral bone.[31,102,143,235] The most widely held theory is that changes in the joint cartilage microenvironment play a significant role in degeneration.[60,153] Chondrocytes facilitate the production of extracellular proteolytic enzymes that degrade the upper layers of the articular cartilage. Repair processes begin, but they are unable to surpass the rate of degradation. Cartilage degradation eventually leads to similar degenerative changes of the synovium and subchondral bone because they are all interdependent.

Risk factors. Many factors that increase the risk for developing degeneration have been identified; they are often categorized as either systemic or local. Age is a systemic factor, and it has the strongest and most consistent correlation with degeneration.[88] Heredity, hormones, gender, and diet are other systemic influences.[348] Mechanical influences including trauma are the most important local influences, resulting in site-specific degeneration.[88] The significance of risk factors varies in all people and their joints, so individual variations are common.

Bone density. Studies have shown a decrease in the incidence of degeneration among individuals with osteoporosis. It has been postulated osteoporotic bone may be a better shock absorber than normal bone and protect joints from trauma. However, this concept is not universally accepted. Other studies have found an inverse relationship between bone density and the incidence of degeneration.[276] The influence of bone density on the incidence of degeneration remains unclear.

Age. Increasing age is highly correlated with development and progression of degeneration.[259,403] One study found all patients over the age of 65 years had DJD in either the hands, feet, knees, hips, or spine.[221] Other studies indicated that radiographic evidence of degeneration could be found in 63% to 85% of Americans over the age of 65 years, 35% to 50% of whom have associated pain.[68,348,432] Although increased age is a major risk factor, degeneration is not necessarily a consequence of aging, shown by the fact that degenerated cartilage in elderly patients differs structurally and biochemically from normal cartilage found in elderly patients.[234,276,322,384,397] Therefore degeneration is age related but not age dependent (Fig. 11-51).[152]

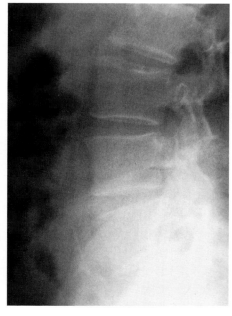

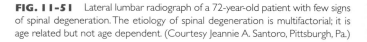

FIG. 11-51   Lateral lumbar radiograph of a 72-year-old patient with few signs of spinal degeneration. The etiology of spinal degeneration is multifactorial; it is age related but not age dependent. (Courtesy Jeannie A. Santoro, Pittsburgh, Pa.)

Gender. Gender plays a role in certain aspects of joint degeneration. Women are at greater risk than men for developing DJD in the knees, hands, and feet.[372] Heredity has also been linked to the development of DJD in the hands of women, whereas the influence of inheritance is less obvious in men.

Obesity. Obesity increases the risk of developing DJD in the knees, hips, and possibly hands.[124] Obesity appears to increase the risk more in females.[374] Weight loss reduces the risk of developing symptomatic DJD in the knees.[68,123]

Physical activity. Exercise and occupation influence the distribution of the disease, with athletes and construction workers developing characteristic patterns more frequently than individuals in other occupations.[4,77,138,173] For example, DJD often develops in the feet of ballet dancers, ankles of soccer players, knees of football players, shoulders of baseball pitchers, hands of boxers, and elbows of pneumatic drill operators.[52,324,411]

Research suggests that normal joints tolerate prolonged vigorous low-impact exercise without accelerated development of degeneration.[168,215,216] However, the risk of developing degeneration appears to increase with high-impact activities, biomechanical alterations, sports played at the professional or elite levels, activities with torsional loading, and among individuals who continue exercise programs while injured.[168,216,217] It is important not to discourage patients with osteoarthritis from exercising. Evidence suggests that stretching, muscle strengthening, and aerobic conditioning can improve deficits in these patients.[433]

Trauma. Trauma is probably the single most important local factor in predisposing a joint toward developing DJD.[230] Normal, daily wear and tear explains many of the manifestations of DJD, but it does not account for all of the biochemical changes found in degenerative cartilage.

In the clinical setting, obtaining a simple history about the patient's previous traumas and making an assessment may not be sufficient to elicit the appropriate information. For example, in one study, 700 subjects were asked to rate the severity of pain, lifestyle disability, and past trauma associated with any current neck complaint.[237] An association between the amount of cervical spine degeneration and reported history of past trauma was not found, which was probably a result of the overly simplistic dichotomous (yes or no) design of the trauma question on the intake form. A more detailed assessment of the patients' past traumas would likely have demonstrated a relationship between degeneration and certain types of trauma.

IMAGING FINDINGS

The radiographic features of DJD are characterized by nonuniform reduction of the joint spaces, osteophytes, subchondral sclerosis, subchondral cysts, intraarticular loose bodies, and joint misalignment and deformity (Fig. 11-52) (Table 11-3). Narrowing of the joint spaces is the criterion variable most often used to assess the development of DJD in research trials.[331] Some of the radiographic features are more prominent in specific regions of the skeleton.

Although weight-bearing joints are most often affected, there is no consistent relationship between weight-bearing joints and the development of DJD because the ankles are rarely affected.[322] Nontraumatic osteoarthritis in the shoulder, elbows, wrists, or middle of the foot can indicate the presence of an underlying disease such as calcium pyrophosphate arthropathy or hemochromatosis.[259] Some of the more common locations of joint degeneration follow.

Spine. Degeneration of the spine may affect the posterior joints (facets), IVDs, uncovertebral joints, costovertebral joints, and costotransverse joints. Degeneration of the IVDs can be easily seen on radiographs. Because the disc is not a synovial joint, the use of the terms *DJD* or *osteoarthritis* is inappropriate to describe IVD degeneration. Instead the terms *spondylosis* or *degenerative disc disease (DDD)* are used.

Because the disc and facets are closely related anatomically and physiologically, degeneration affecting one will eventually affect the other.[38] Although determining a causal relationship between degeneration in discs and facets is difficult, limited evidence suggests

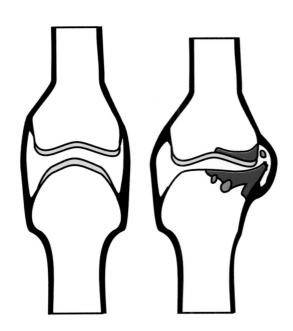

FIG. 11-52 Normal and degenerating joints. Degenerative joint disease is marked by nonuniform reduction of joint space, osteophytes, subchondral sclerosis, subchondral cysts, intraarticular loose bodies, joint misalignment, and deformity.

Text continued on p. 467

PART TWO Bone, Joints, and Soft Tissues

TABLE 11-3
Physiopathology of Radiographic Features Associated with Degeneration

Feature	Physiopathology
Reduced joint space	Widely used criteria for radiographically assessing degeneration; this feature develops secondary to degenerative thinning of the articular cartilage or IVD.

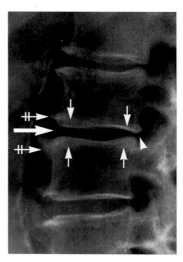

Degenerative disc disease of the lumbar spine with reduced disc spaces *(large arrow)*, osteophytes *(crossed arrows)*, retrolisthesis *(arrowhead)*, and endplate sclerosis *(small arrows)*.

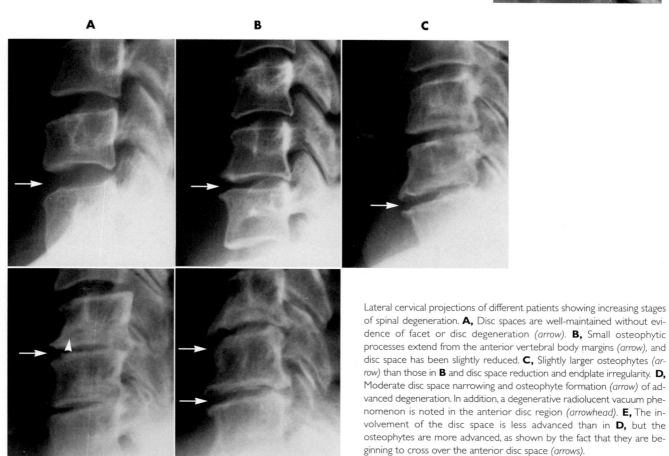

Lateral cervical projections of different patients showing increasing stages of spinal degeneration. **A,** Disc spaces are well-maintained without evidence of facet or disc degeneration *(arrow)*. **B,** Small osteophytic processes extend from the anterior vertebral body margins *(arrow)*, and disc space has been slightly reduced. **C,** Slightly larger osteophytes *(arrow)* than those in **B** and disc space reduction and endplate irregularity. **D,** Moderate disc space narrowing and osteophyte formation *(arrow)* of advanced degeneration. In addition, a degenerative radiolucent vacuum phenomenon is noted in the anterior disc region *(arrowhead)*. **E,** The involvement of the disc space is less advanced than in **D,** but the osteophytes are more advanced, as shown by the fact that they are beginning to cross over the anterior disc space *(arrows)*.

TABLE 11-3
Physiopathology of Radiographic Features Associated with Degeneration—cont'd

Feature	Physiopathology
Osteophyte	Outgrowth that develops as part of the reparative and stabilization process of a degenerative joint; enchondral bone formation produces internal (central) and external (marginal) osteophytes; periosteal osteophytes (buttressing) result from intramembranous bone growth; capsular osteophytes resulting from capsular tension[318]; spinal osteophytes result from traction forces on the Sharpey's fiber insertions of the outer annulus into the compact bone of the outer vertebral rim[339]; dividing spinal osteophytes into curved "claw" and horizontal "traction" types based on appearance is problematic and should be avoided; it has been postulated that osteophytes tend to develop in a marginal location in an attempt to stabilize and reduce the range of joint motion[324] or increase the surface area of the articular surface, thereby reducing joint load, whereas some postulate that the marginal location of osteophytes is merely the default growth pattern occurring in the direction of least resistance[3,140,157,240]; similar marginal bony outgrowths occur secondary to traction forces applied to the insertion of ligaments and tendons into bone (enthesis); osteophytes should be distinguished from the thinner syndesmophytes that develop in patients with inflammatory arthropathies (e.g., ankylosing spondylitis, rheumatoid arthritis) or thick syndesmophytes that develop in patients with Reiter's syndrome and psoriatic arthropathy

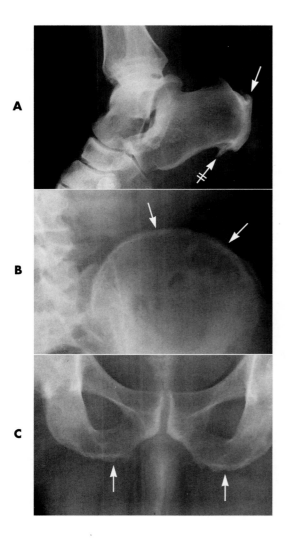

A, Degenerative osteophytes at the insertions (entheses) of the calcaneal (Achilles) tendon *(arrow)* and plantar aponeurosis *(crossed arrow)*. In different patients, similar enthesopathy *(arrows)* is noted at the iliac crest **(B)** and ischial tuberosities **(C).**

TABLE 11-3
Physiopathology of Radiographic Features Associated with Degeneration—cont'd

Feature	Physiopathology

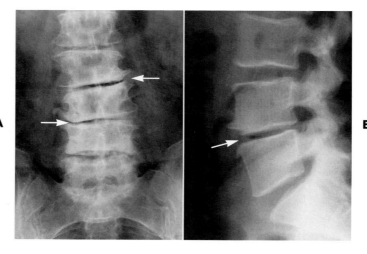

Anteroposterior **(A)** and lateral **(B)** lumbar radiographs on different patients with advanced **(A)** and moderately advanced **(B)** intervertebral disc degeneration and vacuum phenomena *(arrows)*.

Vacuum phenomena*

Knuttson's sign—radiolucent defects indicating the presence of nitrogen gas accumulations in annular and nuclear degenerative fissures; the nitrogen gas is thought to arise from the extracellular spaces; because the gas accumulates in areas of lower pressure, it is often seen in fissures of the anterior disc on extension radiographs; the presence of a vacuum phenomenon virtually excludes the possibility of an infection causing a narrow IVD (except in the rare cases in which a patient has a gas-forming infection); vacuum phenomena are normal in synovial joints under slight distraction[135] (i.e., vacuum is often seen in the anteroposterior projection of the glenohumeral joint because of the weight of the arm slightly distracting the joint)

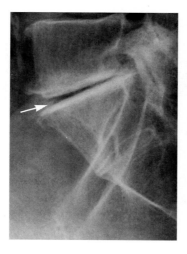

Degenerative vacuum phenomena in the L5 disc *(arrow)*.

* Characteristics of degenerative disc disease (DDD) only.

TABLE 11-3
Physiopathology of Radiographic Features Associated with Degeneration—cont'd

Feature	Physiopathology

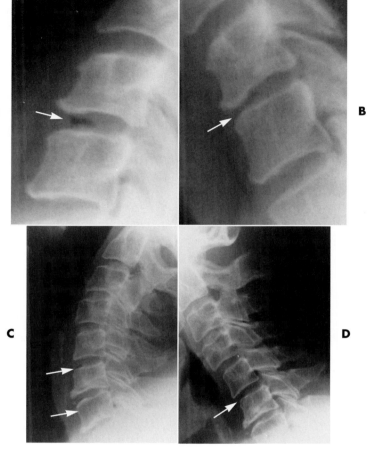

Lateral cervical radiographs with the patients in extension (**A** and **C**) revealing intradiscal vacuum phenomena *(arrows)* that disappear during flexion (**B** and **D**). The extension movement decreases the intradiscal pressure, which makes vacuum phenomena more easily seen. (*Bottom,* Courtesy Joseph W. Howe, Sylmar, Calif.)

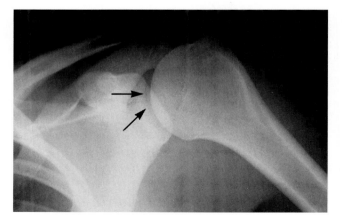

Intraarticular vacuum phenomena (arrows) are normal when found in distracted extremity joints. They are not normal when found in the IVD.

Continued

TABLE 11-3
Physiopathology of Radiographic Features Associated with Degeneration—cont'd

Feature	Physiopathology
Cartilaginous (Schmorl's) nodes*	Abupt, focal, radiolucent intravertebral IVD displacements; Schmorl's nodes are usually normal variants that develop in weakened areas of the vertebral endplate where a blood vessel or the chordal dorsalis has regressed from the cartilaginous endplate and usually develop in young patients; the more clinically significant Schmorl's nodes, which typically develop in a patient's 30s or 40s, are related to intervertebral osteochondrosis or are the result of an endplate fracture (and are called *traumatic Schmorl's nodes)*

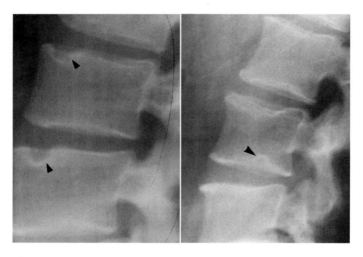

Schmorl's node herniations seen in a lateral lumbar projection as abrupt focal intravertebral endplate intrusions on two patients *(arrowheads)*. (*Left,* Courtesy Steven P. Brownstein, Springfield, NJ.)

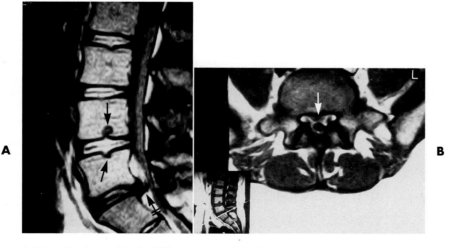

A, T2-weighted sagittal lumbar MRI scan demonstrating Schmorl's node herniations at the superior endplate of L5 and inferior endplate of L4 *(arrows)*. In addition, an L5 disc herniation is present *(crossed arrow)*. **B,** T1-weighted axial lumbar MRI scan at the lower L5 disc level demonstrating the central location of the disc herniation *(arrow)*.

*Characteristics of degenerative disc disease (DDD) only.

TABLE 11-3

Physiopathology of Radiographic Features Associated with Degeneration—cont'd

Feature	Physiopathology
Subchondral sclerosis	Also known as eburnation; represents infraction, compression, and necrosis of stressed subchondral bone trabeculae[62,159]; at times subcondral vertebral sclerosis may appear exaggerated (hemispheric spondylosclerosis), mimicking an infection; absence of bone destruction, paravertebral mass, and historical indicators assist the exclusion of an infection

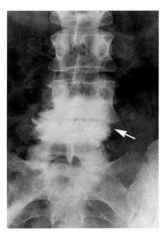

Anteroposterior lumbar projection showing advanced IVD degeneration of L4 marked by reduced L4 disc space by surrounding osteophytes from the vertebral margins and dense radiopacity of the subchondral bone in response to the degeneration *(arrow)*. Because of the advanced degeneration and subsequent joint laxity, laterolisthesis of L4 on L5 developed. (Courtesy Joseph W. Howe, Sylmar, Calif.)

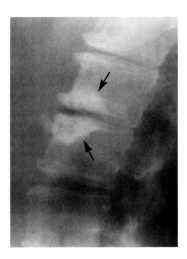

Marked vertebral body sclerosis surrounding the narrowed degenerative disc *(arrows)* with vacuum phenomena. Vertebral sclerosis may be visually confused with an infection. However, the presence of vacuum phenomena virtually excludes non–gas-producing infection as a cause for the vertebral sclerosis. The theory is that an infection would replace the air-filled vacuum with pus and edema, eliminating the air density on the radiograph. (Courtesy Ronnie L. Firth, East Moline, Ill.)

Subchondral cysts (see Figs. 11-63 and 11-65)	Also known as *geodes*—regions in which synovial fluid has been forced through degenerative cartilaginous fissures in the subchondral bone
Joint misalignment (see previous table section on Subchondral Sclerosis and Fig. 11-63)	Misalignment of articular surfaces occurring secondary to reduced joint space and laxity of surrounding ligaments; in the spine, advanced facet arthrosis may lead to anterior displacement of the vertebral body (degenerative spondylolisthesis); degenerative spondylolisthesis is common in the "three Fs"—*females* over *forty* at the *fourth* lumbar level, and the degree of displacement partially depends on the severity of concurrent IVD and facet degeneration; another example of joint misalignment occurs as muscle tension laterally displacing the first metacarpal secondary to joint laxity associated with advanced first carpometacarpal joint degeneration
Joint deformity (see Fig. 11-63)	Redistribution of forces across the joint surfaces and secondary bone remodeling that can be caused by advanced degeneration.
Intraarticular fragments (see Fig. 11-64)	Also referred to as *loose bodies* or *joint mice*—intraarticular postdegenerative fragments of bone, cartilage, meniscus, and synovium

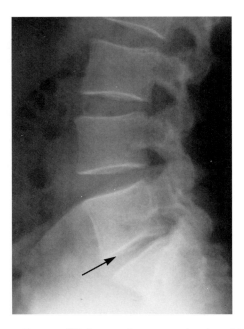

FIG. 11-53 Decreased L5 disc space. Because no other signs of degeneration are present (e.g., osteophytes, vacuum phenomena), the narrowing of the L5 disc *(arrow)* is probably not degenerative, especially in young patients. Disc hypoplasia is a common cause of a narrow disc space.

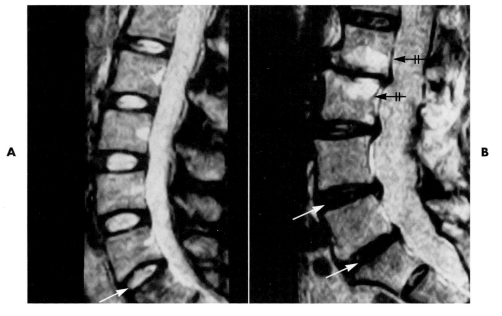

FIG. 11-54 Sagittal T2-weighted MRI scans of different patients. **A,** Bright nuclear signal intensities at the L1 to L4 levels and a slight decrease in intensity at the L5 level *(arrow)*. High signal intensity indicates that the water content is high and the inner disc is healthy. **B,** Low signal intensity indicating loss of water and degeneration of the inner disc *(arrows)*. High signal intensity is noted in the region of the vertebral body marrow subjacent to the endplates surrounding the L2 disc *(crossed arrows)*. Bright signal intensity corresponds to vascularized tissue formed in response to degeneration (Modic type I). On the T1-weighted scans *(not shown)* the region of the vertebra was less intense.

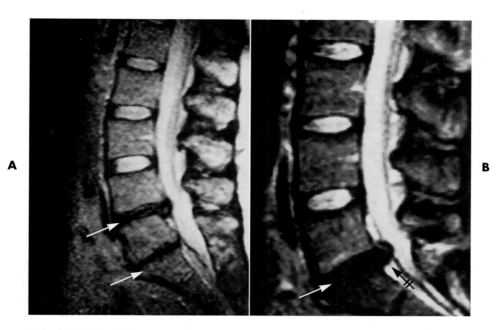

FIG. 11-55 Sagittal lumbar MRI scans of two different patients exhibiting decreased nuclear signal intensity, which indicates disc degeneration. **(A),** Degeneration involving the L4 and L5 levels *(arrows)*. **(B),** Degeneration of only the L5 level *(arrow)*. A large disc herniation is noted at the L5 disc level *(crossed arrow)*.

that degeneration may first appear in the IVD and progress to the facets.[59] The hypothesis is that loss of disc height leads to increased force loading and subsequent degeneration of the facet joints.

Intervertebral disc. Spondylosis, or DDD, presents with a narrowed disc space, osteophytes, misalignment, and eburnation—findings that are all similar to those in patients with DJD. However, DDD also presents with vacuum phenomena and Schmorl's nodes, which are both unique to degeneration of IVDs (see Table 11-3). Only in rare cases that are usually very advanced are all of the radiographic features present concurrently. Marginal osteophytes and IVD narrowing are the most common and reliable degenerative radiographic findings. Osteophytes are less pronounced on the left side throughout the middle to lower levels of the thoracic spine because of the pulsations of the adjacent descending aorta.[360] Narrowing of the posterior lumbosacral disc height to less than 5.5 mm on plain film is associated with degeneration.[71] However, because the fifth lumbar disc space is often developmentally narrow (Fig. 11-53), it is important not to interpret a narrow fifth lumbar disc space with no associated osteophytes or other concurrent signs of degeneration as indicative of degeneration.

For description purposes, spondylosis can be divided into two loci of degeneration that are often parallel. Degeneration of the outer portion of the annulus fibrosis, which is identified by marginal osteophytes, is called *spondylosis deformans.*[238,339] Degeneration of the innermost portion of the annulus fibrosus, combined with dehydration of the nucleus pulposus and breakdown of the cartilaginous endplate, is referred to as *intervertebral chondrosis.* The term *intervertebral osteochondrosis* is used if the adjacent vertebrae appear to be involved, which is suggested by vertebral endplate sclerosis (also known as *eburnation*). Degeneration of the inner disc is demonstrated radiographically by reduction of the IVD height and central intradiscal vacuum phenomena.[238,339]

MRI is particularly helpful in visualizing IVDs. The normally well-hydrated nucleus pulposus has a high signal intensity on the sagittal T2-weighted spin echo MRI sequence. Loss of nuclear signal intensity indicates dehydration and alterations in the macromolecule content and distribution in the nucleus pulposus.[266,353] These changes are the result of senescence and degeneration (Figs. 11-54 and 11-55).*

In addition to delineating the IVD anatomy directly, MRI reveals characteristic vertebral body changes that occur in response to IVD degeneration. These changes have been categorized into three types based on the vertebral appearance on a spin echo MRI sequence.[10,94,245,264] (Table 11-4). Any relationship between these marrow changes and patient symptoms remains unclear.

Uncovertebral joints. The bilateral posterolateral uncinate processes of the third through seventh cervical vertebrae articulate with the corresponding vertebral grooves above to form cartilaginous uncovertebral joints, which also called *joints of Luschka* or *neurocentral joints.* Uncovertebral degeneration presents as pointed or bulbous osteophytes extending from the uncinate processes, which may encroach on the intervertebral foramina, possibly causing radiculopathy (Fig. 11-56).[225,425] Hypertrophic uncinate processes may compromise the vertebral artery blood flow.[76,363]

Degeneration is most common in the middle and lower cervical levels. Uncinate degeneration is readily demonstrated on frontal or oblique radiographic projections. In the lateral radiographic projection, uncinate process hypertrophy may give the appearance of a radiolucent fracture line (pseudofracture) extending horizontally

*References 32, 139, 166, 183, 223, 262, 263, 264, 266, 290, 294, 304, 351, 353, 359, 429.

TABLE 11-4
Classification of the MRI Appearance of Vertebral Body Marrow Patterns Resulting from
Degenerative Disc Disease

Classification (Modic)	Appearance on MRI	Histology and significance
Type I	Decreased signal intensity (causing darkness) on T1-weighted images and increased signal intensity (causing brightness) and T2-weighted images	Highly vascularized fibrous tissue in the vertebral body corresponding to acute stages of disc degeneration

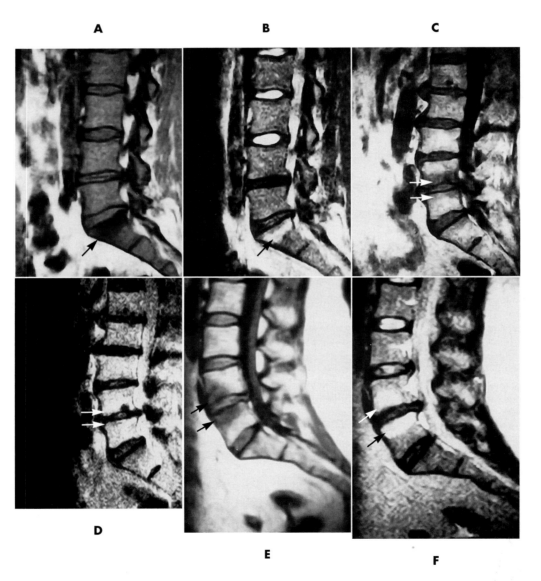

Modic Type I vertebral changes. Three patients who all exhibit decreased vertebral marrow signal intensity *(arrows)* on the T1-weighted studies (**A, C,** and **E**) that increased on the corresponding T2-weighted images (**B, D,** and **F**), indicating the presence of highly vascularized fibrous tissue.

TABLE 11-4

Classification of the MRI Appearance of Vertebral Body Marrow Patterns Resulting from Degenerative Disc Disease—cont'd

Classification (Modic)	Appearance on MRI	Histology and significance
Type II	Increased signal intensity (causing brightness) on T1-weighted images and equal to slightly increased signal intensity (medium) on T2-weighted images	Continuation of type I vertebral changes in which vascularized fibrous tissue is replaced by yellow bone marrow
Type III	Decreased signal intensity (causing darkness) on both T1-weighted and T2-weighted images	Extensive body sclerosis that is associated with long-standing degeneration and correlates with radiographic evidence of vertebral sclerosis

A   **B**

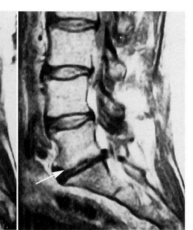

Modic Type II vertebral changes. Vertebral bands of increased signal intensity *(arrow)* on the T1-weighted image **(A)** remain increased on the T2-weighted image **(B),** indicating the presence of yellow bone marrow.

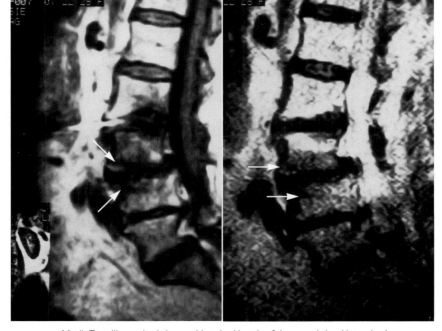

Modic Type III vertebral changes. Vertebral bands of decreased signal intensity *(arrows)* on the T1-weighted image **(A)** remain decreased on the T2-weighted image **(B),** indicating bone sclerosis.

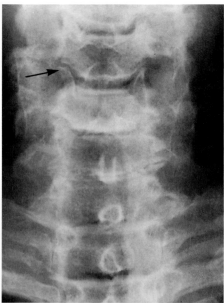

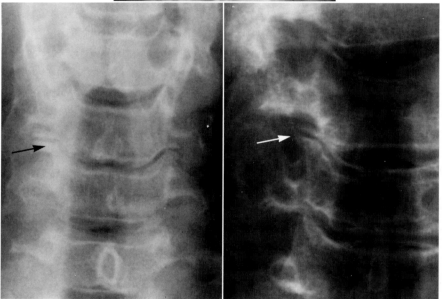

FIG. 11-56 AP projections of the middle cervical region of different patients showing degenerative changes of the uncinate processes *(arrows)*. (Courtesy Arthur W. Holmes, Foley, Ala.)

across the lower cervical body at the level above the degeneration (Fig. 11-57).[344] CT may help further delineate clinically relevant levels.

Zygapophyseal joints. The zygapophyseal (apophyseal, facet, posterior) joints are synovial articulations formed between the paired superior and inferior articular processes of adjacent vertebrae from C2-S1. Radiographically, degeneration is most often observed in the middle cervical, upper and middle thoracic, and lower lumbar regions.[207,239] It is characterized by joint irregularity, increased sclerosis, vertebral anterolisthesis (degenerative spondylolisthesis), and osteophytosis. The oblique projection best demonstrates the zygapophyseal joints. The axial images provided by CT and MRI are particularly helpful in assessing degenerative changes and existing soft tissue complications (Fig. 11-58).

Factors influencing zygapophyseal degeneration are similar to those affecting other joints. In particular, alterations in the stress across the articulations, which occurs in patients with kyphosis, scoliosis, and probably facet tropism, increase the incidence of zygapophyseal degeneration.[34,390]

Costovertebral joints. The costovertebral joints are the articulations between the rib heads and transverse processes. The costotransverse joints (Fig. 11-59) are the articulations between the rib tubercles and the transverse processes. Both joints are synovial and exhibit osteophytosis, sclerosis, and irregularity when they degenerate. Degeneration most often affects costovertebral joints at the lower thoracic levels.

Sacroiliac joints. Degeneration of the sacroiliac joints is characterized by increased sclerosis and irregularity of the joint margins (Fig. 11-60). In patients who are in the advanced stages of

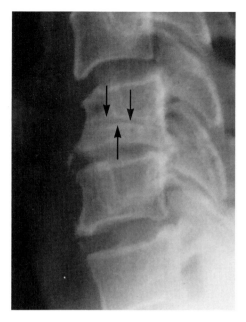

FIG. 11-57 Partial view of a lateral cervical radiograph. The pseudofracture appearance created by uncinate degeneration causes a radiolucent appearance above the bulbous uncinate process (arrows).

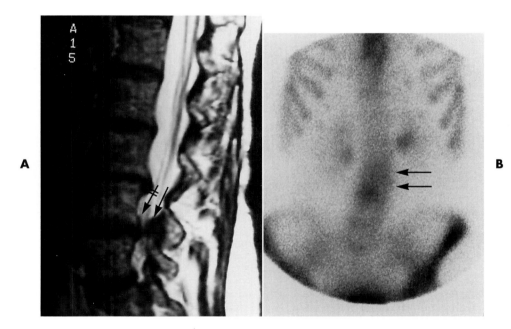

A

B

FIG. 11-58 Sagittal lumbar MRI scans. **(A),** Posterior joint arthrosis (arrow) and disc bulge (crossed arrow) narrow the sagittal dimension of the spinal canal. **(B),** The posterior joint arthrosis causes increased radionuclide uptake on the bone scan (arrows).

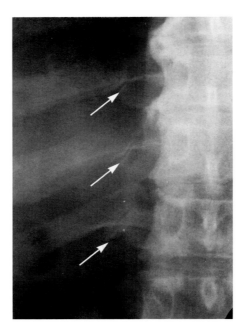

FIG. 11-59 Degeneration of the costotransverse joints *(arrows).*

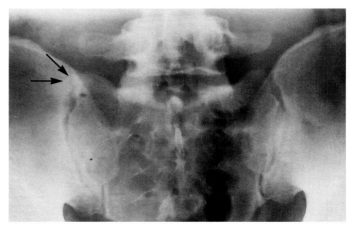

FIG. 11-60 Degeneration of the upper portion of the right sacroiliac joint *(arrows)* indicated by marginal sclerosis and osteophytes. (Courtesy Joseph W. Howe, Sylmar, Calif.)

degeneration, portions of the joint space may not be clearly seen because of bridging osteophytes. Intraobserver and interobserver error limit the reliability of correct interpretation of degeneration in such an irregularly shaped joint on radiographs.[342]

Shoulders. The acromioclavicular joint is more commonly involved than the glenohumeral joint (Fig. 11-61). Large osteophytes may project from the inferior margin of the acromioclavicular joint, producing rotator cuff tendonopathy, which usually develops in the supraspinatus tendon. Inflammation and compromise of the tendon leads to superior migration of the humeral head because of the unopposed action of the deltoid, with consequential narrowing of the acromiohumeral space (shoulder impingement syndrome). Advanced degeneration of the glenohumeral joint often results from complete rupture of the supraspinatus tendon, disruption of the joint capsule, and loss of synovial fluid. MRI is particularly valuable in evaluating the integrity of the supraspinatus tendon. Radiographic evidence of dystrophic calcification or hydroxyapatite deposition

disease (HADD) can usually be seen in the supraspinatus tendon just proximal to its insertion on the greater tuberosity.

Hands. The interphalangeal joints are commonly involved. Characteristic nodes of the degenerative distal (Heberden's nodes) or proximal (Bouchard's nodes) interphalangeal joints are seen (Kellgren's arthritis).

A distinct variant of DJD is found in middle-aged females and is known as *erosive DJD.* Erosive DJD is differentiated from typical, secondary DJD by its bilateral symmetrical pattern of distribution and its greater tendency to be painful.[23] As the name implies, the diagnosis of erosive DJD depends on the presence of central joint erosions, or "gull wing" sign (Fig. 11-62, *A-C*).[23,343] Whether erosive DJD is a type of DJD or a separate disease is not clear.[70] As a general rule, erosive DJD is distinguished from rheumatoid arthritis in that it affects the interphalangeal joints initially, whereas rheumatoid arthritis affects the MCP joints (Fig. 11-62, *D*) before progressing distally. Erosive DJD is distinguished from psoriatic

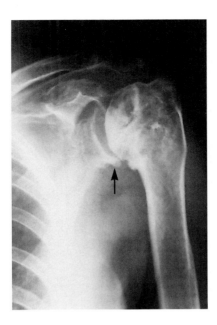

FIG. 11-61 Degeneration of the glenohumeral joint. The degeneration followed mechanical alterations secondary to avascular necrosis of the humeral head. The degeneration is indicated by osteophytes at the lower margins of the articular surfaces *(arrow)*. (Courtesy Joseph W. Howe, Sylmar, Calif.)

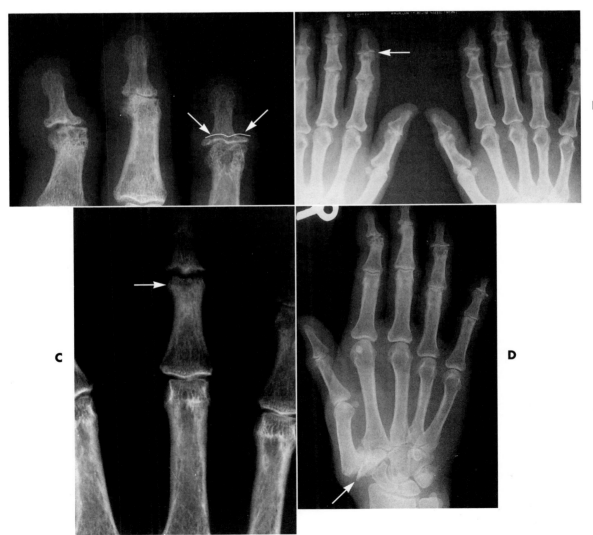

FIG. 11-62 **A-C,** Three patients with primary osteoarthritis shown by the characteristic gull wing deformity of the DIP joints of the hands *(arrows)*. **D,** The patient in **A** also has degenerative changes in the first carpometacarpal articulation *(arrow)*. *(Top left and bottom right,* Courtesy Jack C. Avalos, Davenport, Iowa; *Bottom left,* Courtesy Joseph W. Howe, Sylmar, Calif.)*

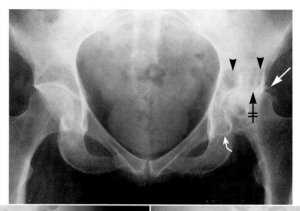

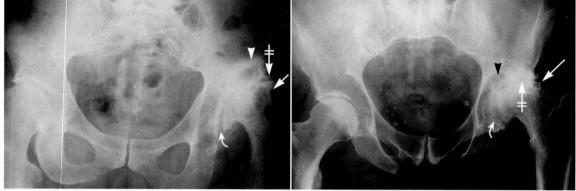

FIG. 11-63   Three patients with advanced hip degeneration secondary to avascular necrosis. Degeneration is noted by the marginal osteophytes *(arrows)*, reduced joint space *(crossed arrows)*, subchondral degenerative cysts *(arrowheads)*, and joint deformity with lateral displacement of the femoral head from the teardrop of the pelvis *(curved arrows)*.

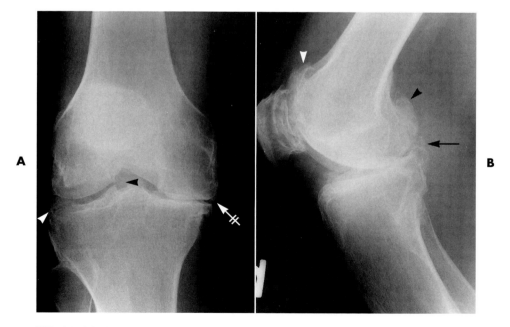

FIG. 11-64   Anteroposterior **(A)** and lateral **(B)** projections with reduced medial joint space *(crossed arrow)*, marginal osteophytes *(arrowheads)*, and interarticular debris *(arrow)* consistent with degenerative joint disease of the knee.

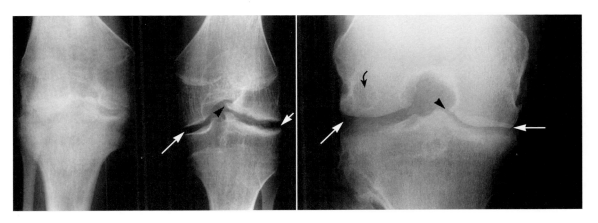

FIG. 11-65 Degenerative joint disease in two patients. Degeneration is noted by asymmetrical joint loss *(arrows)*, osteophytes *(arrowheads)*, subchondral degenerative cysts *(curved arrow)*, and subchondral sclerosis.

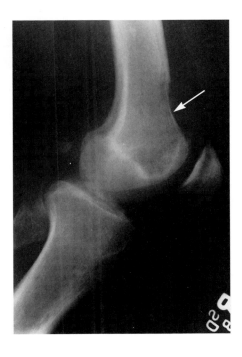

FIG. 11-66 CPPD of the knee leading to secondary degeneration of the patellofemoral joint. A pressure erosion is noted on the anterior distal portion of the femur *(arrow)* caused by contact with the suprapatellar osteophyte. (Courtesy Joseph W. Howe, Sylmar, Calif.)

arthritis, which has a propensity for DIP involvement, by the central erosions of the proximal articular surface; marginal erosions of the distal articular surface ("mouse ears") are associated with psoriatic arthritis. Also, erosive DJD is symmetrical in distribution, and psoriatic tends to be asymmetrical.

Hips. Asymmetrical reduction in the joint space with subsequent superior, axial, or medial migration of the femoral head is the earliest sign of degeneration of the hip (Fig. 11-63). Superior migration is by far the most common pattern and accompanies an increased distance between the medial margin of the femoral head and the lateral margin of the acetabulum (Waldenström's sign). Axial migration indicates concentric loss of joint space that is more typical of an inflammatory arthropathy (e.g., rheumatoid arthritis). Medial migration occurs in less than 20% of cases and may be accompanied by a mild degree of acetabular protrusion.[204] Periosteal osteophytes accumulation, or buttressing, is noted on the medial and (less commonly) lateral side of the femoral neck.[318]

Knees. The knee is one of the most common joints to degenerate. Of the three compartments in the knee, the medial femorotibial joint compartment is most often affected (Fig. 11-64). Internal or central osteophytes may be seen extending from the tibial eminence (Fig. 11-65).[1,317] Osteophytes arising from the proximal pole of the patella may cause an erosive defect in the anterior distal femur (Fig. 11-66). Occasionally in the tangential projection, tiny, bony proliferative projections may appear to be extending from the external proximal surface of the patella near the insertion of the patellar tendon (the "patellar tooth" sign).

Isolated DJD in the patellofemoral compartment is unusual. If this situation develops, the presence of underlying conditions (e.g., CPPD, hemochromatosis, chondromalacial patella, previous trauma) should also be considered. In comparison to DJD in other joints, DJD in the knees is less likely to exhibit subchondral sclerosis and cysts and more likely to exhibit intraarticular loose bodies.[289]

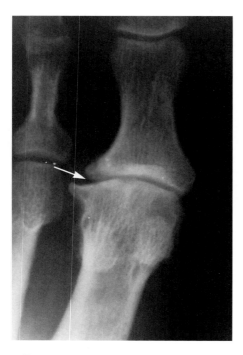

FIG. 11-67   Degenerative osteophytes extending from the medial aspect of the MTP joint with accompanying decrease in the joint space *(arrow)*. (Courtesy Joseph W. Howe, Sylmar, Calif.)

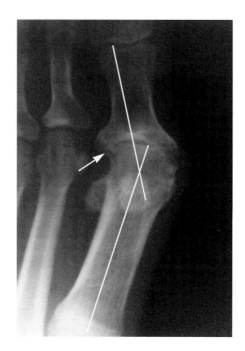

FIG. 11-68   Selected view of an AP radiograph showing hallux valgus deformity *(lines)*, marginal osteophytes, reduced joint space, joint erosions, and joint misalignment associated with degeneration of the first MTP joint *(arrow)*. (Courtesy Joseph W. Howe, Sylmar, Calif.)

TABLE 11-5
Treatment Options for Degenerative Joint Disease

Treatment	Uses
Chiropractic adjustments; improvement of muscle strength, range of motion, and balance and flexibility	Used to restore function
Pharmacology	Used to decrease inflammation (aspirin, NSAIDs) and pain (acetaminophen)
Surgery	Used for joint replacement, joint fusion, osteotomy, arthroscopic debridement, and joint space wash
Social support	Used to encourage social interaction, improve coping skills, manage stress, and coordinate support services
Reduction of body weight, modification of activities, use of walkers or canes, use of orthotics to shift weight	Used to protect joint
Physiotherapy (ice, heat [paraffin baths, diathermy], hydrotherapy)	Used to alter circulation and as palliative relief

Feet. DJD in the first MTP joint is extremely common (Figs. 11-67 and 11-68). Often it is accompanied with clinical symptoms of pain and stiffness caused by the hypertrophic changes, a condition referred to as *hallux rigidus*. First metatarsal varus hallux valgus joint misalignment is often present.

Advanced imaging methods. Plain film radiography is the most widely used modality to assess the presence and progression of an arthropathy; however, the need to visualize the soft tissues limits the use of this procedure. MRI is a valuable adjunct because it provides superior imaging of the cartilage and detects the presence of synovitis as well as the reaction of the bone to the arthropathy.[41] MRI has the advantage of providing true multiplanar imaging, superior soft tissue contrast, and being noninvasive.[30,125]

Radionuclide bone scintigraphy, CT, arthrography, and arthroscopy represent some of the other methods that can be used for joint assessment. Each has advantages and disadvantages depending on the application and clinical situation.

CLINICAL COMMENTS

DJD is associated with joint pain, which is usually related to activity. Because cartilage has no nerve endings, symptoms arise from other joint components.[5] Multiple mechanisms have been proposed to explain the production of pain, including distention of joint capsule, joint inflammation, muscle spasm, contracture of joint capsule, periosteal elevation, or direct pressure on subchondral bone caused by loss of articular cartilage.

The pain limits activity, leading to loss of muscle strength (deconditioning), reduced range of motion (contracture), limited function (disability), crepitus, occasional joint effusion, and localized inflammation. The pain worsens with activity in early stages of the disease but increases with rest in later stages of the disease.[276] Not all degenerating joints are painful or disabling. Disability is more likely to result if concurrent psychological disorders such as depression or anxiety are present or in patients who have insufficient social supports.[381,383]

Treatment is aimed at limiting pain, maintaining function and independence, and preventing complications. Treatment plans are individualized and directed toward multiple areas (Table 11-5). Treatment is often directed at the maintenance of joint motion. Cartilage does not have a blood supply and depends on joint motion to provide nutrition and eliminate toxins.[31]

Pain control is crucial if the patient is to maintain activity and motion. However, little evidence supports the long-term use of NSAIDs, which may interfere with normal repair mechanisms.[68,251] In addition, chronic ingestion of NSAIDs is linked to systemic complications, including gastric ulceration, one third of which are asymptomatic. NSAIDs should be administered only when inflammation is present.[49,131] If the pain and disability are severe, joint replacement surgery may be a necessary treatment. In fact, more than 70% of total hip and knee replacements are for osteoarthritis.[124]

Clinicians must keep in mind that it is very difficult to correlate the patient's clinical complaint to the degree of spondylosis and facet degeneration present on radiographs.* However, the chronicity of the patient's complaint is associated with the degree of spondylosis.[239] Limited evidence has suggested that in women, spondylosis is associated with changes in lifestyle activities; further study is needed.[239]

---

*References 106, 129, 130, 144, 145, 161, 239.

Spondylotic radiculopathy usually responds to conservative management. Spondylotic myelopathy, the most serious complication of spondylosis, is more complex and difficult to resolve with a conservative approach to treatment. Surgical intervention is warranted in patients with progressive neurological deficits.[254] Although results of laboratory tests are usually within normal limits, they can help identify the presence or absence of other diseases.[276]

KEY CONCEPTS

- *DJD (osteoarthritis/osteoarthrosis [OA]) is the most common of the arthropathies.*
- *The disease has a multifactorial etiology that is influenced by local and systemic factors: trauma, aging, obesity, genetics, activity, gender, bone density, and nutritional status.*
- *The spine, hips, knees, first metatarsal, and phalanges are most commonly involved.*
- *The classic radiographic findings include narrowing of the joint spaces, osteophytosis, subchondral bone sclerosis, subchondral cysts, intraarticular loose bodies, and joint misalignment or deformity.*
- *The radiographic findings for IVD degeneration (spondylosis, DDD) also include vacuum phenomena and Schmorl's nodes.*
- *Erosive DJD is a variant of DJD that affects middle-aged women and is characterized by central joint erosions (the gull wing sign).*
- *MRI is a valuable adjunct to plain film radiography because it offers superior imaging of the cartilage and detects the presence of synovitis and the bone's reaction to the arthropathy.*
- *The axial images provided by CT and MRI are helpful in assessing intricate joints of the regions such as the spine, ankle, and wrist.*
- *Pain is a common clinical complaint, although the severity of pain does not correlate well with the radiographic appearance.*
- *Pain limits activity, leading to loss of muscle strength (deconditioning), reduced range of motion (contracture), limited function (disability), crepitus, occasional joint effusion, and localized inflammation.*
- *Treatment is aimed at limiting pain, maintaining function, continuing independence, and preventing complications. Pain control is crucial to the continuance of activity and motion.*
- *Results of laboratory tests are usually within normal limits, but they can still help identify the presence or absence of comorbid diseases.*

Diffuse Idiopathic Skeletal Hyperostosis

BACKGROUND

Diffuse idiopathic skeletal hyperostosis (DISH), also referred to as *ankylosing hyperostosis of the spine* and *Forestier disease*, is a common rheumatological abnormality characterized by exuberant proliferation of bone at osseous sites of ligamentous and tendinous attachments throughout the body. Both spinal and extraspinal sites are affected, but the most notable development of this disease occurs in the anterior longitudinal ligament (ALL) of the spine.

A high prevalence (13% to 49%) of the disease is noted among diabetics and in the general population (8.5% to 20%).[127,356,409] The incidence of DISH increases with age, being most common in the middle-aged and elderly, and develops more frequently in men.[127] The etiology of this bone-forming disorder remains unknown despite several avenues of investigation: growth hormone, insulin, and vitamin A or retinoid derivatives and associated metabolic syndromes.[89,388,409]

Initial studies evaluating levels of growth hormone in patients with DISH revealed little useful information, but more recent investigations support the hypothesis that growth hormone (GH) may indeed act as a bone-growth promoting factor in patients with DISH just as it promotes tissue growth in patients with acromegaly.[6,93]

It has been suggested that insulin may also play a role in the new bone formation associated with DISH because it may act as a growth factor. Elevated insulin levels and marked hyperinsulinemia following a glucose challenge have been reported.[93,227] Although it has been reported that a high percentage of patients with DISH also have diabetes (as cited previously), a more recent study revealed that no difference in the percentage of diabetics exists between patients with DISH and a control group.[87]

IMAGING FINDINGS

Spine. The diagnosis of spinal involvement is based on the following three strict radiographic criteria, which aid in distinguishing DISH from spondylosis deformans (degeneration) and ankylosing spondylitis (Figs. 11-69 and 11-70)[336]:

1. Flowing ossification of the anterolateral aspect of at least four contiguous vertebral bodies
2. Relative preservation of disc height in the involved segments and absence of radiographic changes associated with DDD (vacuum sign or discogenic sclerosis)
3. Absence of sacroiliitis and facet ankylosis

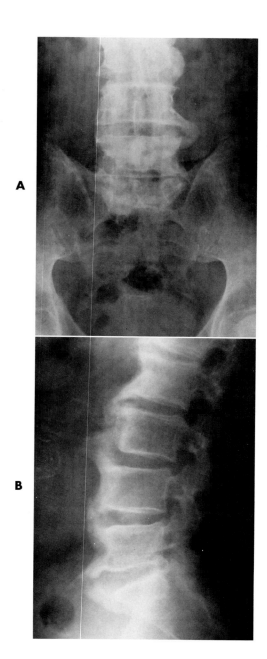

FIG. 11-69 DISH. AP lumbopelvic **(A)** and lateral **(B)** lumbar radiographs reveal large flowing ossification over several contiguous segments. The disc heights are relatively well preserved. There is no sacroiliac or posterior joint fusion.

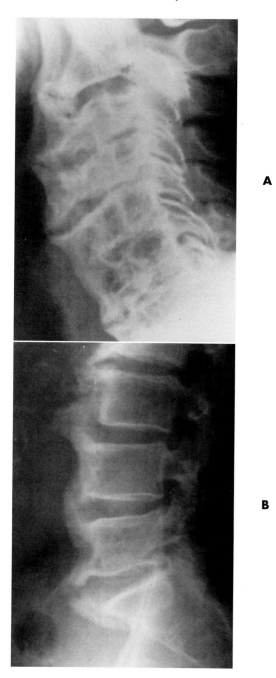

FIG. 11-70 DISH of the cervical **(A)** and lumbar **(B)** spine in different patients. Both cases show flowing exostosis and preservation of the disc heights and have no posterior joint involvement. (**A,** Courtesy Joseph W. Howe, Sylmar, Calif.)

The anterior ossification can be subtle or very dramatic depending on its thickness and contour. The hyperostotic outline may be smooth or bumpy, continuous or interrupted, and range from 1 or 2 mm to more than 20 mm in thickness. There may be lucent defects through the ossification anterior to the disc space that represent discal extrusions, not fractures, through the new bone formation (Fig. 11-71).

The most common site of involvement is the mid to lower thoracic spine where the new anterolateral bone formation is more of-ten on the right, apparently because of the pulsating descending thoracic aorta on the left. Upper lumbar hyperostosis is noted almost as frequently as in the lower thoracic segments, with the ossification occurring bilaterally and predominantly on the anterior aspect. Lower cervical spine abnormalities are also common and include posterior alterations (e.g., posterior spinal osteophytes, ossification within the nuchal ligament and the posterior longitudinal ligament) in addition to the more common anterior bone deposition.

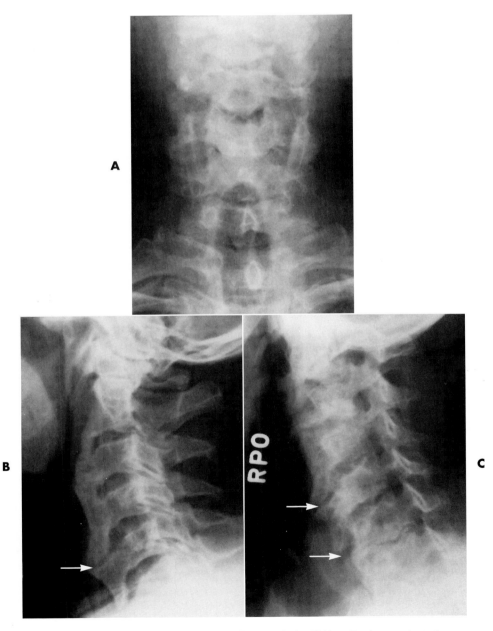

FIG. 11-71 AP **(A)**, lateral **(B)**, and oblique **(C)**, cervical spine. Thick ossification anterior to the vertebral bodies is noted in this 57-year-old male with DISH. A lucent defect is seen running through this bone formation (arrows), which indicates discal extensions.

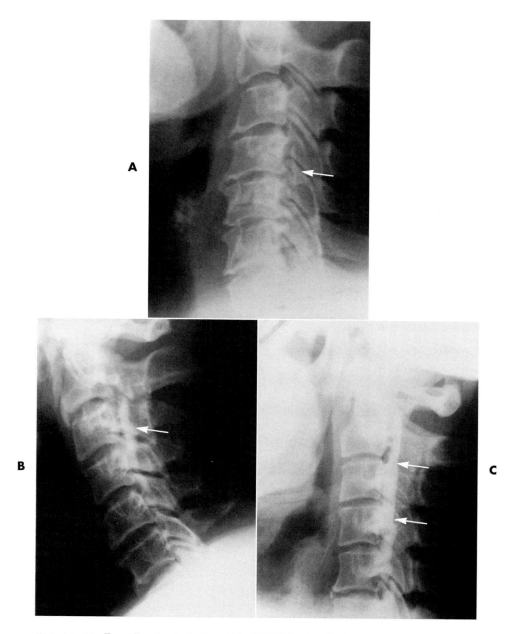

FIG. 11-72 Two different patients **(A** and **B)** with DISH and ossification of the posterior longitudinal ligament (OPLL) *(arrows)* in the cervical spine. A third patient **(C)** demonstrates OPLL *(arrows)* without stigmata of DISH. *(Bottom right,* Courtesy Joseph W. Howe, Sylmar, Calif.)

Ossification of the posterior longitudinal ligament (OPLL), formerly known as the "Japanese disease" because of its frequent development in members of the Asian race, is a condition that may develop alone or in conjunction with DISH. One study found that 50% of patients with DISH who were radiographed revealed evidence of calcification or OPLL, and other studies found that DISH was present in approximately 40% of patients with OPLL.[335]

If visible on a plain film radiograph, OPLL is best seen on the lateral view, appearing as a thin, linear calcification that runs parallel and posterior to the vertebral bodies (Fig. 11-72). A lucent cleft may be sandwiched between the dense ligament and vertebral bodies. The cervical spine is most commonly involved; in rare cases the thoracic and lumbar spine are involved (Fig. 11-73). OPLL may not be identified on a plain film radiograph because of overlying anatomy; if OPLL is suspected or the clinician would like to determine the extent of ossification and possible cord compression, CT is the recommended procedure (Figs. 11-74 and 11-75).[252,277,285,436]

Sacroiliac joints. The synovial portion, or lower two thirds, of the sacroiliac joint is not commonly affected; however, the upper third may become blurred or indistinct. The superior and inferior portions of the joints also are often bridged by paraarticular ligamentous calcification.

Extraspinal enthesopathy. The typical sites of involvement include the pelvis (see Table 11-3), calcaneus (Fig. 11-76), and patella. The enthesopathic changes that ensue are purely productive; there are no erosive components. This is initially visualized radiographically by roughening, or fraying, of the bone and later by extensive proliferation.

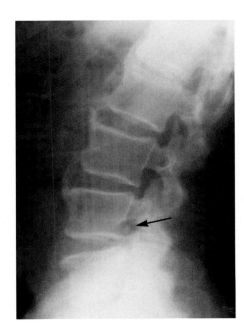

FIG. 11-73 DISH and ossification of the posterior longitudinal ligament *(arrow)* in the lumbar spine.

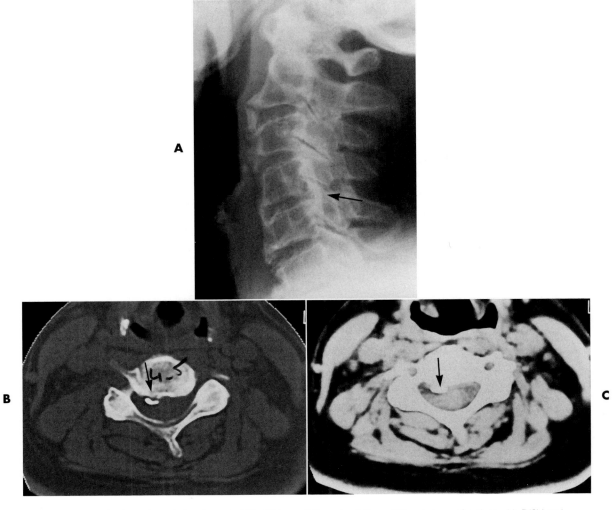

FIG. 11-74 Lateral cervical radiograph **(A),** CT bone **(B),** and soft tissue **(C),** windows of patient with DISH and OPLL *(arrows).* CT may be used to evaluate the presence of possible cord compression.

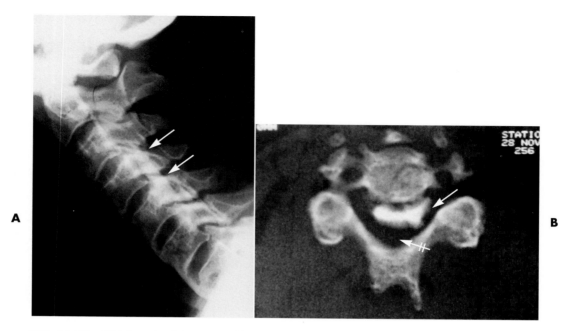

FIG. 11-75   OPLL *(arrows)* well demonstrated in the lateral cervical projection **(A)** and on CT **(B)** *(arrow).* The CT scan reveals very little space for the cord to pass *(crossed arrow).* (Courtesy Steven P. Brownstein, Springfield, NJ.)

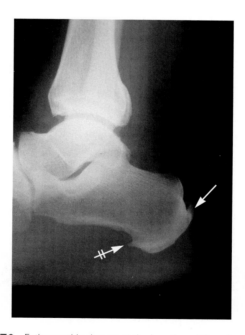

FIG. 11-76   Enthesopathic changes at the insertion of the calcaneal tendon *(arrow)* and plantar aponeurosis *(crossed arrow).* Differential diagnosis includes idiopathic degeneration, DISH, acromegaly, hypoparathyroidism, fluorosis, and vitamin D resistant osteomalacia.

CLINICAL COMMENTS

The clinical complaints of mild pain and stiffness that are associated with the majority of patients with DISH are much less remarkable than the extensive radiographic changes suggest. Although these findings are uncommon, patients may develop dyspnea and hoarseness dysphagia, aspiration pneumonia, myelopathies, peripheral nerve entrapment, or tendinitis.[192, 218,253,415,427] These complications may result from direct compression that requires surgical intervention or may manifest because of associated tissue inflammation.[253] Given the lack of clinical relevance associated with spinal and extraspinal hyperostosis, other causes should be investigated before DISH is assumed to be responsible for the patient's complaints.[26,352]

Spinal fractures in patients with DISH are rarely reported but can occur in patients with spinal ankylosis who sustain even trivial traumas.[58,61,163,292,320] These patients should be carefully evaluated to avoid a delay in diagnosing the patient and to minimize possible complications, including pseudoarthrosis, neurologic injury, and death.[58,163,292,320]

KEY CONCEPTS

- *DISH is a variant of degenerative disease marked by exuberant proliferation of bone at osseous sites of ligament and tendon attachments.*
- *DISH develops more frequently in men and usually presents near 40 years of age; incidence increases with age.*
- *Radiographic characteristics usually include ossification of the ALL, with relative maintenance of the disc height and absence of posterior joint fusion or sacroiliac joint involvement.*
- *The disease is associated with OPLL and possibly diabetes mellitus.*
- *Dysphagia and dysphasia may develop.*

Neuropathic Arthropathy

BACKGROUND

Neuropathic, or neurotrophic or neurogenic, arthritis is a destructive arthropathy caused by impaired pain perception and/or proprioception (position sense).[358] The joints lose their normal protective reflexes and muscle tone, leading to a cycle of repeated, unrecognized episodes of trauma and resultant joint damage. Distribution is usually monarticular and depends on the underlying etiology of the arthropathy.

The epidemiology is also etiology dependent. Today, diabetes and syringomyelia are the two most common causes respectively of neuropathic arthropathy. Tabes dorsalis resulting from syphilis is no longer a leading cause; however, when it was discovered that tabes dorsalis was associated with joint destruction, its resulting arthropathy was given the eponym *Charcot's joints.* Charcot's joint is now used interchangeably to refer to all joints affected with neuropathic arthropathy, regardless of the underlying disease.

IMAGING FINDINGS

Radiographic findings can be divided into two major categories. The hypertrophic, or bone-forming, variety is likely to occur in weight-bearing joints such as the spine and lower extremities, whereas the atrophic, or resorptive, form develops more often in the non–weight-bearing joints of the upper extremities. These two forms may occur independently or together (Figs. 11-77 and 11-78).[55]

Hypertrophic. The hypertrophic radiographic features manifest as a severely aggressive osteoarthritis. These proliferative joint changes are often referred to as the *6 D's* (*D*ense subchondral bone, joint *D*istension, *D*ebris or loose bodies, joint *D*isorganization, *D*islocation, and *D*estruction of articular cortex) or, in an abbreviated

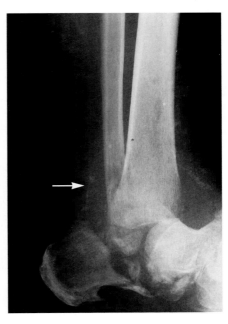

FIG. 11-77 A 52-year-old woman with diabetes developed a neurotrophic ankle joint. Destruction of the joint and bony debris are evident; vascular calcification *(arrow)* is also apparent. Diabetes is the most common cause of a neurotrophic arthropathy.

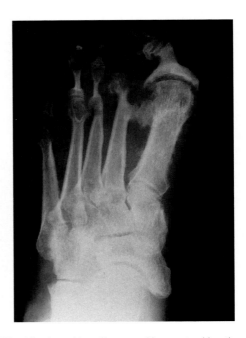

FIG. 11-78 Mixed atrophic and hypertrophic neurotrophic arthropathy of the foot in a patient with diabetes. (Courtesy Steven P. Brownstein, Springfield, NJ.)

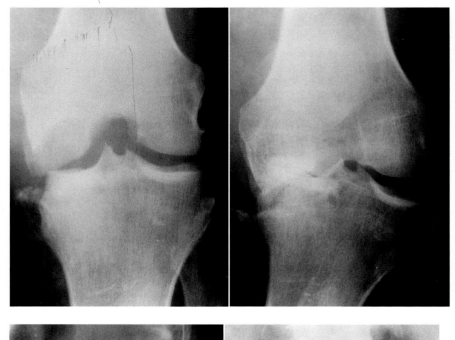

FIG. 11-79 Sequential films (taken 4 months apart) of a 65-year-old woman with neurosyphilis showing features consistent with a Charcot joint: destruction of the articulating bone ends, joint disorganization and subluxation, bony debris, and joint distension.

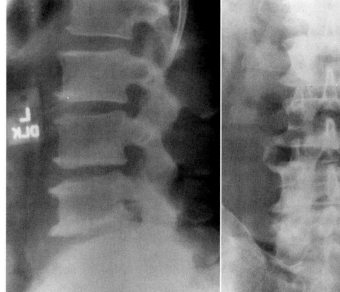

A

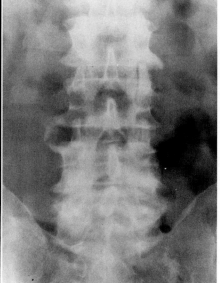

B

FIG. 11-80 Hypertrophic neurotrophic disease of the spine before (**A** and **B**) and after (**C** and **D**) the changes have occurred. The neuropathies are secondary to syphilis. (Courtesy Joseph W. Howe, Sylmar, Calif.)

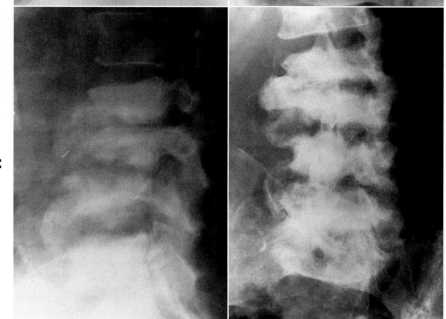

C

D

version, as *distension in 3D* (D*islocation*, D*estruction*, and D*egeneration*).[358] Patients with diabetes, syphilis, and spinal cord trauma are prone to developing this form of neurotrophic arthropathy in the feet, knees (Fig. 11-79), and spine (Fig. 11-80) respectively.

Atrophic. The atrophic radiographic features may be visualized as an osteolytic process that (1) completely resorbs the articulating bone end, leaving a sharp transverse demarcation at the meta-

diaphysis similar to that caused by surgical amputation, or (2) tapers the bone end to a sharp "pencil point." The former is most frequently seen in patients with syringomyelia, with osteolysis affecting the proximal humerus (Figs. 11-81 and 11-82). The latter reflects findings that often involve the metatarsals and phalanges of diabetic patients (Fig. 11-83).

CLINICAL COMMENTS

Obviously, the diagnosis of Charcot's joint should be suspected in a patient with an associated neurological disorder who develops a painless, swollen joint and has radiographic signs of bony destruction. Consideration must also be given to the fact that one third of patients affected with Charcot's joint may have no demonstrable neurological deficit,[358] one third may experience pain, and the osseous radiographic findings may initially be unremarkable or resemble early osteoarthritis.

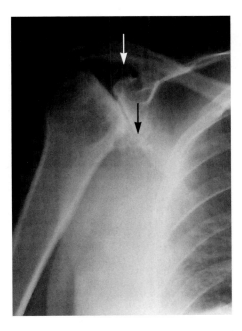

FIG. 11-81 A 47-year-old female with syringomyelia developed an extremely swollen and mildly uncomfortable shoulder joint. AP shoulder radiograph reveals joint destruction, debris *(arrows)*, and subluxation of the humeral head.

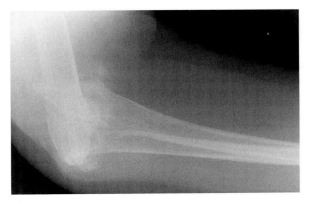

FIG. 11-82 Mostly atrophic changes of the elbow secondary to syringomyelia. (Courtesy Joseph W. Howe, Sylmar, Calif.)

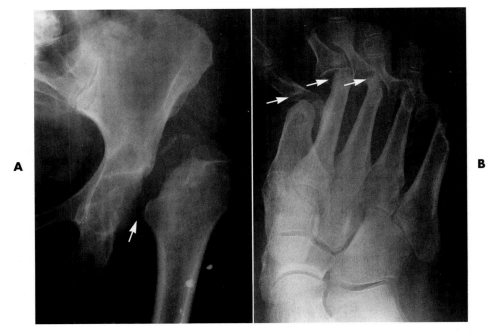

FIG. 11-83 Atrophic neurotrophic arthropathy *(arrows)* of the hip **(A)** and foot **(B)** secondary to syphilis. (Courtesy Joseph W. Howe, Sylmar, Calif.)

PART TWO Bone, Joints, and Soft Tissues

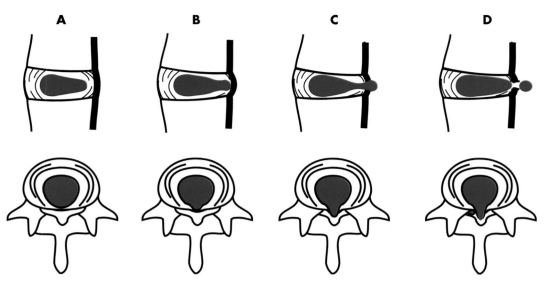

FIG. 11-84   Disc herniation. **A,** Bulge. **B,** Protrusion. **C,** Extrusion. **D,** Sequestration.

Joint infection and a crystal deposition diseases such as CPPD may have the clinical and radiographic features of a neuropathic joint, presenting a possible diagnostic dilemma. Joint sepsis may also be a complication of Charcot's joint.

Treatment is directed toward the underlying disease in an attempt to slow or reverse the destructive arthropathy; in addition, antiinflammatories, splints, braces, and other devices to prevent further weight-bearing trauma may aid in limiting joint damage.

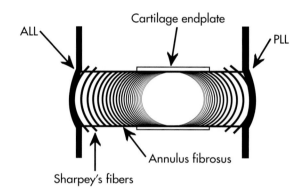

FIG. 11-85   The IVD comprises a central nucleus pulposus, surrounding annulus fibrosus, and cartilaginous endplates above and below.

KEY CONCEPTS

- *Neuropathic arthropathy is a destructive arthropathy resulting from impaired pain perception and/or proprioception.*
- *Diabetes (foot and ankle) and syringomyelia (upper extremity) are the most common causes.*
- *Radiographic features may be classified as hypertrophic or atrophic, although some joints can have characteristics of both categories.*
- *Hypertrophic changes (the 6 D's—Dense subchondral bone, joint Distension, Debris or loose bodies, joint Disorganization, Dislocation, and Destruction of articular cortex) commonly occur in the weight-bearing joints.*
- *Atrophic changes (pseudoamputation, tapered bone ends) occur more often in the non–weight-bearing joints of the upper extremity.*

Intervertebral Disc Herniation

BACKGROUND

An IVD herniation is the extension of nucleus pulposus through the annulus fibrosus and beyond adjacent vertebral margins.[141] Fragments from the annulus fibrosus and cartilaginous endplate may occur in addition to the displaced nucleus pulposus.

Disc herniations are more common among males, smokers, the obese, and those exposed to vehicular vibration.[132-134,198] Any relationship of heredity is less certain.[132-134] Herniations rarely develop before 20 and after 65 years of age; they most commonly develop in 25- to 45-year olds.[198] Although many risk factors have been identified, it is difficult to assess which cause disc herniations and which merely aggravate its symptoms.[341]

Classification.   The continuum of IVD herniations ranges from very small focal protrusions to large sequestered fragments (Fig. 11-84) (Table 11-6). This continuum is usually divided into subtypes based on the extent of nuclear displacement: protrusions

(contained herniations), extrusions (herniations that are not contained), or sequestrations (free fragments). An IVD bulge is not a herniation. An IVD bulge is a broad-based extension of the annulus fibrosus with no nuclear displacement. No system of classification is universally accepted. Often the individual interpreting the imaging studies and the clinician who reads the radiology report use different definitions of the same terms. Confusion can be avoided by emphasizing the use of accurate anatomical descriptions of the imaging findings and not relying too heavily on the use of categorical descriptions.

Anatomy.   An IVD herniation is one manifestation of the ongoing process of IVD degeneration.[164] Because herniated discs are degenerative, this discussion continues and expands on the previous discussion (Intervertebral Disc Degeneration) under the heading Degenerative Joint Disease in this chapter. An understanding of the structure and cellular metabolism of the intervertebral components provides a more complete picture of the physiopathology of IVD herniations.

IVDs unite adjacent vertebrae from C2 through S1. Each disc is named for the vertebra immediately above it. The IVD is composed of a central nucleus pulposus, the surrounding annulus fibrosus, and the cartilaginous endplate above and below the majority of the IVD (Fig. 11-85). The cross-sectional anatomy of the spinal canal is visualized with CT (11-86) and MRI (Fig. 11-87).

Text continued on p. 493

Classification	Description
Normal	The nucleus has a high signal intensity; the annulus is intact and has only a small outward posterior bulge *(arrow)*.
Diffuse bulge	Broad-based, concentric outward bulge of the annulus fibrosus beyond the margins of the vertebral endplate that usually occurs in all directions symmetrically; diffuse bulges are common among individuals over the age of 40 years.
Protrusion Prolapse Contained herniation	Focal displacement of nuclear, annular, or endplate material beyond the peripheral margin of the IVD that is defined by the osseous boundaries of the adjacent vertebral body endplates; the protruded material remains under or contained by some portion of intact outer annulus
Extrusion Herniation Noncontained herniation	Same as previous entry, except that the protruding material extends beyond a section of the annulus; if a central disc herniation does not extend past the posterior longitudinal ligament (PLL), the term *subligamentous herniation* is appropriate, whereas if the herniation passes through the PLL, the term *transligamentous herniation* is used; *contained* and *noncontained* refer to the annulus fibrosus, not the PLL (although some sources disagree, contending that distinction between the annulus and PLL is not possible on available imaging systems and that the term *extrusion* implies extension beyond the PLL).

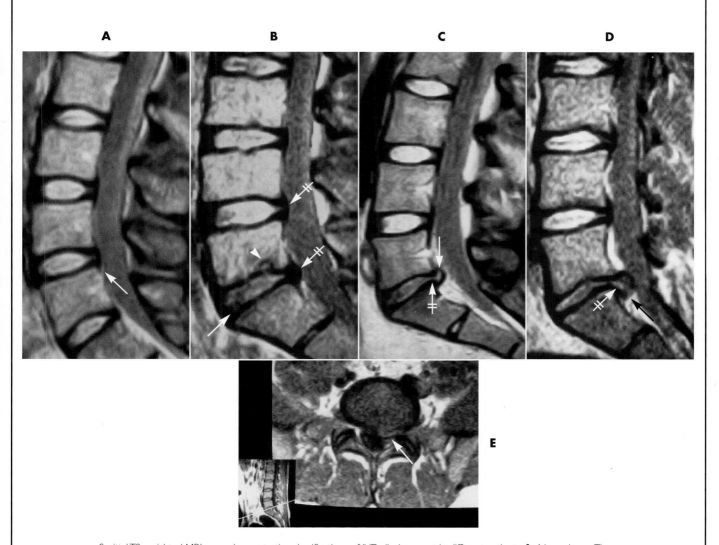

Sagittal T2-weighted MRI scans demonstrating classifications of IVD displacement in different patients. **A,** Normal scan. The nucleus has a high signal intensity. The annulus is intact and has a normal configuration *(arrow)*. **B,** Disc bulges at the L4 and L5 level *(crossed arrows)*. In addition, decreased nuclear signal intensity *(arrow)* and a Schmorl's node at L5 *(arrowhead)* are noted. **C,** L5 disc protrusion is indicated by the thinned but intact annulus *(arrow)* and posteriorly displaced nuclear material *(crossed arrow)*. Although the nucleus is posteriorly displaced, it is still contained by the thinned annulus and is therefore alternatively referred to as a *contained disc herniation*. **D,** L5 disc extrusion is indicated by the disrupted posterior annulus *(arrow)* and posteriorly displaced nucleus *(crossed arrow)*, which is no longer contained by the annulus (a noncontained herniation). **E,** T1-weighted axial MRI scan of the same patient in **D.** The herniation effaces the thecal sac as it projects left of the midline *(arrow)*.

Continued

TABLE 11-6
MRI Classification of Intervertebral Disc Displacement[149,164]—cont'd

Classification	Description
Sequestration	Migration of a "free fragment" of herniated material that has no connection to the IVD; fragments (in decreasing order of frequency) migrate laterally, superiorly, or inferiorly; stay in the midline; or disperse in multiple directions.[149]

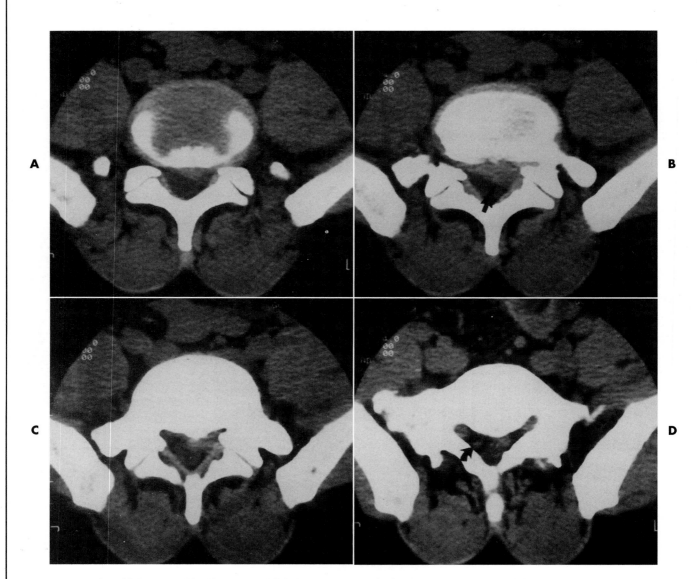

An L4-5 herniated disk with extension inferiorly and migration of a free fragment affecting the left S1 descending nerve root. **A** and **B,** Axial CT slices show large herniations with a major component on the left (*arrow* in **B**). **C,** An axial slice through the upper part of the L5 pedicle shows extension inferiorly on the left side. Note the obliteration of epidural fat anteriorly and anterolaterally on the left. **D,** Axial slice 8 mm below **C,** through the lower portion of the L5 pedicles. The arrow points to the normal right descending S1 nerve root. A small migrated free fragment is present on the left, engulfing the left S1 descending root. There was no abnormality 4 mm above this level indicating detachment of the fragment (visible in **D**) from the extended herniated disk (visible in **C**). (From Firooznia H et al: *MRI and CT of the musculoskeletal system,* St Louis, 1992, Mosby).

TABLE 11-6

MRI Classification of Intervertebral Disc Displacement[149,164]—cont'd

Classification	Description

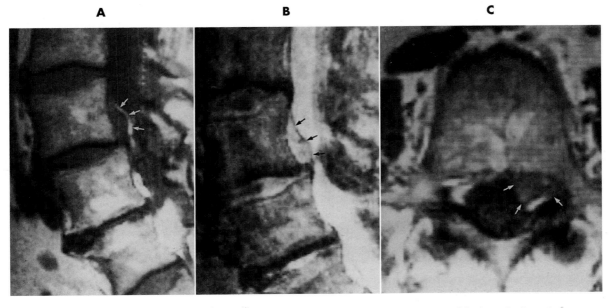

Migrated free fragment from the L4-L5 disk. **A,** Sagittal T1-weighted (500/17) spin-echo image of the lower lumbar spine showing narrowing of the L4-5 and L5-S1 disk spaces with type II vertebral body changes at the latter level. A soft tissue density fragment is seen posterior to the inferior aspect of L3 *(arrows).* The high signal intensity surrounding is probably epidural fat. Surgery revealed that the fragment was posterior to the vertebral body but anterior to the posterior longitudinal ligament. **B** and **C,** Sagittal T2-weighted (2000/90) spin echo and axial T1-weighted (500/17) spin echo images. The migrated fragment is indicated by the small arrows. (From Modic M et al: *Magnetic resonance imaging of the spine,* ed 2, St Louis, 1994, Mosby.)

Ruptured disc	Complete tear through the annulus; a herniation may or may not be present, whereas patients with disc herniations always have disc ruptures.
Hard disc	Colloquialism used to describe the presence of osteophytosis from the posterior margin of the vertebral endplate or uncinate process, which mimics the clinical presentation of a herniation or "soft disc."

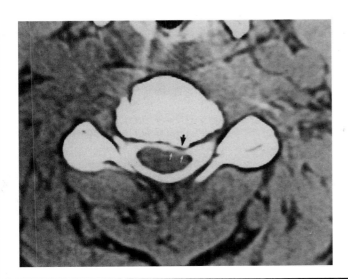

Hard disk. CT-myelography demonstrating a small left-sided osteophytic ridge *(black arrow).* Note the mild flattening on the left side of the anterior cord *(white arrows).* (From Firooznia H et al: *MRI and CT of the musculoskeletal system,* St Louis, 1992, Mosby.)

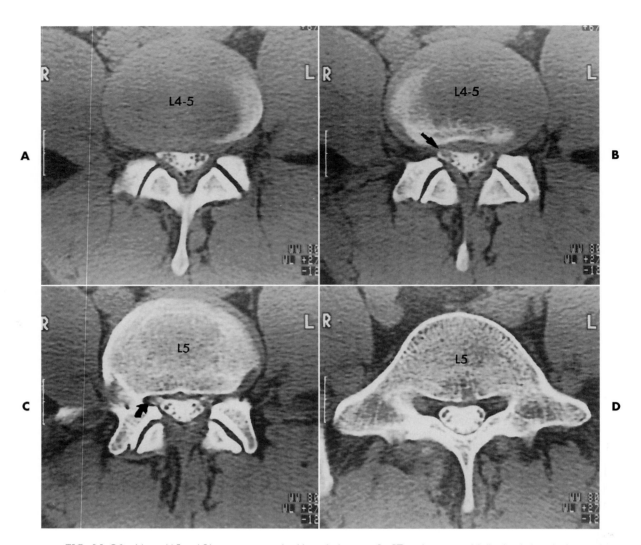

FIG. 11–86 Normal L5 and S1 nerve roots and exiting spinal nerves. **A,** CT-myelogram—axial slice just below the inferior endplate of L4. Descending roots are found in the dural sac anterolaterally; however, the L5 roots have not separated from the sac yet. **B,** Axial slice at the superior endplate of L5. The L5 descending roots are just budding. The arrow points to the right L5 root. **C,** Four mm below **B.** The descending lumbar roots are completely separated from the dural sac and are within the sleeves. The arrow points to the right L5 root. **D,** A slice that is distal to the end of the L5 dural sleeve. The descending L5 roots are visible in the lateral recess of L5. The descending sacral roots are close to the anterolateral corners of the dural sac.

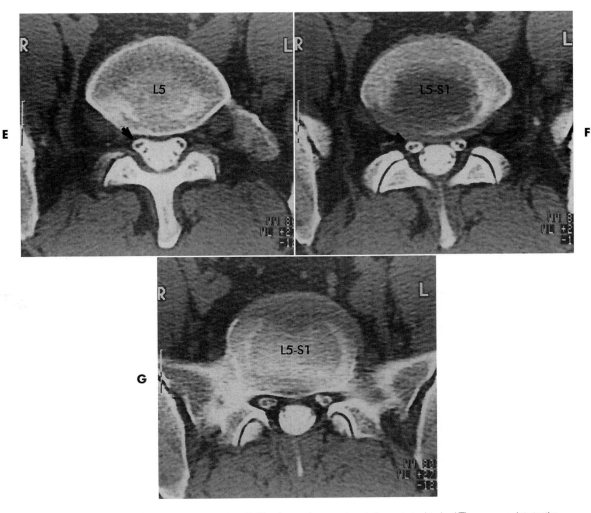

FIG. 11-86—cont'd **E,** Eight mm below **D.** The descending sacral roots have started to bud. The arrow points to the right S1 root. **F,** Four mm below **E.** The sacral roots are in the anterior epidural space posterior to the L5-S1 disc. **G,** Eight mm below **F.** The descending sacral roots can be seen in the lateral recess of S1. (From Firooznia H et al: *MRI and CT of the musculoskeletal system,* St Louis, 1992, Mosby.)

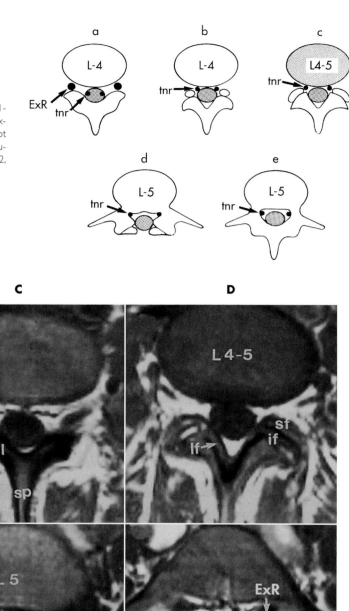

FIG. 11-87 **A,** Axial plane of the lumbar spine. **B-G,** Schematic of the T1-weighted MRI image (500/17) through L4-5. *TNR,* Traversing nerve root; *ExR,* exiting nerve root; *p,* pedicle; *lr,* lateral recess; *tp,* transverse process; *drg,* dorsal root ganglion; *l,* lamina; *sp,* spinous process; *lf,* ligamentum flavum; *if,* inferior facet; *sf,* superior facet. (From Modic M et al: *Magnetic resonance imaging of the spine,* ed 2, St Louis, 1994, Mosby.)

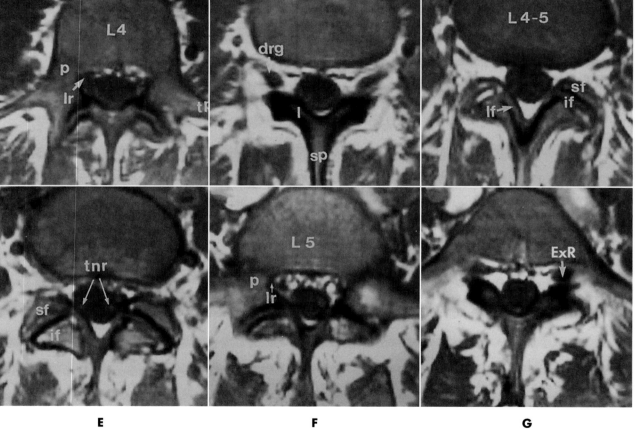

Nucleus pulposus. The semifluid nucleus pulposus is composed of a loose network of cells of notochordal origin that are interspersed within a collagen and proteoglycan matrix. Nuclear proteoglycans have a strong affinity for water, giving the nucleus a positive swelling pressure, or turgor.[391] The nucleus lacks nerve or blood supply.

Annulus fibrosus. The annulus fibrosus consists of about 20 concentric lamellae that surround the nucleus. Each lamella is composed of obliquely oriented bundles of collagen fibers. The direction of the bundles' obliquity alternates with each successive lamella. The inner third of the lamellae are anchored into the cartilaginous endplates, forming a retaining envelope around the nucleus. The outer two thirds of the lamellae are functionally and histologically more similar to ligaments and are firmly attached to the vertebrae.[172] The outer lamellae are innervated posteriorly by the sinuvertebral nerve, posterolaterally by ventral rami, and anteriorly by grey rami communicants.[37] Blood vessels are found in the outermost lamellae.[391]

Cartilage endplates. The cartilage endplates and the unossified epiphyses are homologous; they cover each end of the vertebrae.[391] The endplates are encircled by the ossified ring apophysis of the vertebrae. Endplates are about 1 mm thick and facilitate fluid exchange between the vertebrae and IVDs.[116] Although a blood supply is present during early phases of development, it subsequently regresses, leaving the cartilaginous endplates completely avascular by adulthood.[391] No neural elements are present.

Pathophysiology

Function. In the healthy state the disc is remarkably resilient to injury. The annulus fibrosus and nucleus pulposus work together to prevent spinal loading. Forces applied to the nucleus become attenuated when dispersed peripherally to the surrounding annulus. In addition, the central and well-hydrated nucleus pulposus retains the shape and function of the annulus fibrosus.

Maintaining the function of the IVD depends largely on the ability of cells to maintain the stability of their matrices. Mechanical, chemical, or nutritional factors may affect the viability of these cells[169]; cellular death and matrix alterations create more stressors, and a vicious cycle of degeneration develops. As with degeneration in other joints, many of these changes are age related and slowly progressive. However, in some individuals degeneration can progress rapidly, resulting in spinal pain and disability. As a result of degeneration, altered function, and impaired metabolism, the IVDs become susceptible to injury from axial, shear, and rotational forces.

Injury to the annulus fibrosus. Injury to the annulus fibrosus progressively decreases its effectiveness to prevent spinal loading. Circumferential, radial, and transverse fissures develop significant annular breakdown.[119,120] The cleft of a circumferential tear is oriented in the same direction as the lamellae, extending in an arc around the center of the IVD. Radial tears disrupt adjacent annular lamellae, with the cleft of the tear oriented perpendicular to the fibers of the lamellae. Transverse tears are found at the rim of the disc at the interface of the outer annulus and vertebral ring apophysis.[164]

The posterior and posterolateral portions of the annulus are particularly susceptible to tearing for two reasons: (1) they are thin, and (2) the posteriorly concave design of the lumbar disc places the posterolateral fibers at a mechanical disadvantage.[121] The latter is particularly true if a combined flexion and rotation posture is assumed.[303]

As portions of the annulus begin to tear and fragment, a greater load is placed on the remaining healthy annulus, leading to further breakdown. The resulting large radial fissures that develop provide a pathway for displacement of the nucleus pulposus into the spinal canal.

Injury to the nucleus pulposus. The evolution of a herniated disc is more complicated than the development of a radial fissure that allows displacement of the nucleus pulposus.[313] If a pathway resembling a radial fissure is experimentally cut into the annulus and the spinal segment is loaded, a posterior disc herniation will not develop.[51,303,412] Some authors attribute this phenomenon to the lack of concurrent breakdown of the nucleus pulposus.[36,40,399] They contend that a healthy nucleus pulposus exhibits natural cohesive properties that prevent herniation. They further propose that these cohesive properties become less effective as a consequence of vertebral endplate fractures. Endplate fractures expose the avascular and immunologically unfamiliar nucleus to the ample blood supply in the vertebral body. The ensuing autoimmune reaction destroys the cohesiveness, permitting herniation of the nucleus through existing annular defects.

Alternatively, if the nucleus pulposus breaks down in the absence of an annular defect, the inner IVD becomes disrupted but herniation will not occur.[81] Internal disc disruption is marked by narrowing of the disc height and a slight annular bulge but not herniation. See the References[36,40] for sources describing a more complete discussion of this model.

Distribution of herniations. Disc herniations are most common in the lumbar spine; they are uncommon in the thoracic spine. Ninety percent of lumbar herniations occur at the L4 and L5 levels, 5% to 7% occur at the L3 level, and only in rare cases do they occur at the L1 or L2 levels.[171,305] Most herniations are directed posterolaterally, whereas only 5% directed posterocentrally.

Thoracic disc herniations that are large enough to encroach on the thecal sac are rare. When they do develop, they are typically posterocentral and much more likely to cause myelopathy than radiculopathy.

Ninety percent of cervical disc herniations occur at the C5 and C6 levels, with the remainder occurring mostly in the lower cervical spine. The herniations are usually directed posterolaterally (similar to those in the lumbar spine). Because the epidural space is less capacious than that of the lower lumbar spine, a small herniation in the cervical spine is more apt to cause symptoms. Because less substantial nucleus pulposus exists, large herniations like those found in the lumbar spine are not seen. Most cervical disc herniations result in radiculopathy, although myelopathy develops much more often in the cervical spine than in the upper lumbar spine.

IMAGING FINDINGS

The appearance of IVD herniation depends on the imaging modality employed, level of involvement, presence of concurrent degeneration, and chronicity of the lesion.

Plain film radiography. Because the IVD is not visualized directly, disc herniations are not seen on plain film radiographs.[305] Disc bulging accompanies degeneration and can be indicated by extensive marginal osteophytosis and disk height narrowing. In rare cases a calcified sequestration, visualized as a radiopaque ossicle in the spinal canal, can be seen.

Myelography. Myelography depends on the introduction of a water-based (e.g., metrizamide, iohexol [Omnipaque] or iopamidol [Isovue]) or oil-based (iophendylate [Pantopaque]) contrast agent into the subarachnoid space.[22] If a herniation is present and of sufficient size, the column of contrast will demonstrate a slight indentation and possibly amputation of the nerve root sleeve.[200,201] Herniations at the L5 level may not be noticed or sufficiently visualized because of the large epidural space (Fig. 11-88).

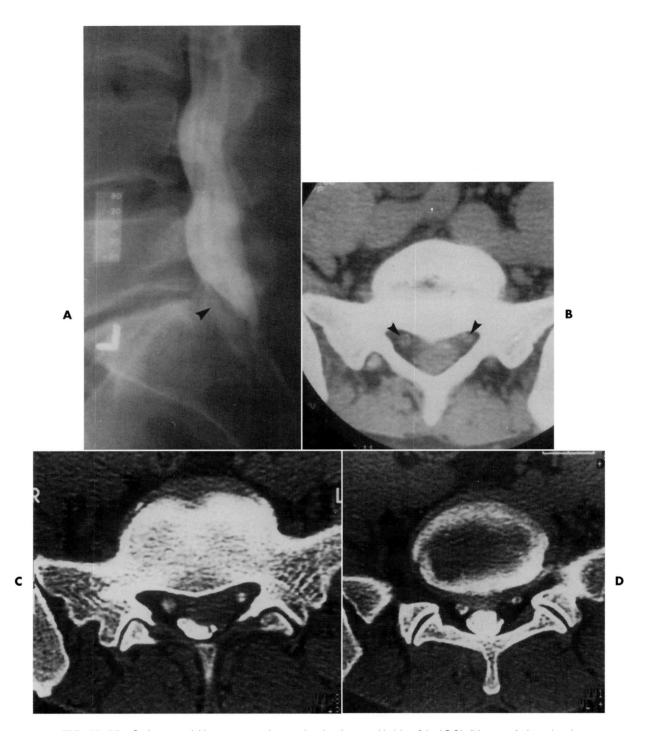

FIG. 11-88   A, A water-soluble contrast myelogram showing decreased height of the L5-S1 disk space. A short thecal sac can be seen, and an insensitive ventral epidural space is also present *(arrowhead).* **B,** A CT slice without intrathecal contrast obtained at the vertebral endplate level of S1 shows the descending roots in the lateral S1 recesses *(arrowheads).* The thecal sac is present centrally and appears unremarkable. A small fleck of calcification is visible to the left of midline anteriorly within the thecal sac. **C,** A postmyelographic CT scan at the same level reveals a large epidural defect indicative of an extruded herniated disk situated anterolaterally to the left of midline and displacing the left S1 root laterally. It compresses the thecal sac focally (especially to the left of midline). **D,** Another postmyelographic CT slice, this time through the disk space of L5-S1, demonstrates a mild focal epidural defect centrally without distortion of the thecal sac or the right S1 root sleeve. The left S1 root sleeve is displaced laterally. (From Firooznia H et al: *MRI and CT of the musculoskeletal system,* St Louis, 1992, Mosby.)

Although myelography was the procedure of choice to identify and define discal pathology for many years, it is currently inferior to CT and MRI. Myelography combined with CT provides anatomical detail that is superior to detail provided by either study used independently. It is most often performed in the cervical and thoracic regions.

Myelography is advantageous because it provides a large field of study and allows for provocation of patients with spinal stenosis. It is used in place of CT and MRI to study patients who are too large to fit in the scanners or patients who have large, metallic constructs that may cause numerous artifacts in the images.[164]

Discography. Discography entails injecting radiopaque contrast into the nucleus pulposus and imaging the morphology of the dye with plain films or CT (Fig. 11-89). The injected dye disperses throughout the nucleus pulposus and into the annular fissures that communicate with the nucleus. If a disc herniation is present, the injected dye will enter the spinal canal and an annular fissure will be clearly delineated by the trail of contrast extending to the spinal canal. For the most part, discography has been superseded by CT and MRI. It is only commonly used before chemonucleolysis or a percutaneous nucleotomy.

In addition to its application in imaging, discography is the only provocative method that can be used to determine whether a disc is causing a patient's pain.[72,73,74,112,115] Contrast injected into the nucleus pulposus distends the annulus; a reproduction or amplification of the patient's pattern of pain is evidence of a discogenic pathogenesis. Discography may be helpful in determining the symptomatic level of disc herniation if multiple herniation levels are demonstrated by CT or MRI.

Computed tomography. It is advantageous to use CT to evaluate patients with suspected herniations for several reasons: it is available in most hospitals, offers an axial plane of imaging, is quick, and yields excellent visualization of the bony anatomy and good visualization of possible disc herniations (Fig. 11-90).

The disadvantages of CT are that radiation is used, true multiplanar imaging is not possible, only a limited region can be examined, and it does not visualize components of the intervertebral disc or contents of the thecal sac—these structures can be seen only if contrast is introduced.

Advantages of CT over MRI include its shorter examination times, higher resolution of cortical bone, and usual capacity to visualize thinner sections than MRI. The latter is particularly advantageous when imaging the cervical spine.

Magnetic resonance imaging. The quality of MRI images 15 years ago was poor, but in recent years substantial improvements have occurred. At present, most would agree MRI has become the primary imaging modality for investigating the spine and spinal canal.* In some spinal imaging circumstances (e.g., in which visualization of osseous detail is paramount), MRI remains inferior to CT. Some examiners prefer CT myelography to MRI for imaging the intricate detail of the cervical spine and canal. However, as advances continue, the application and superiority of MRI will most likely broaden and become more certain.

---

*References 22, 149, 233, 265, 268, 373.

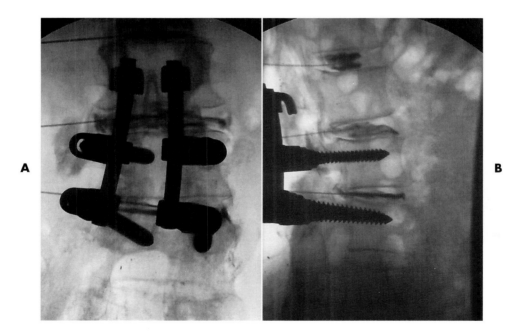

FIG. 11-89 AP **(A)** and lateral **(B)** discography projection demonstrating a normal internal disc at the L1 level and disc herniation at the L2 and L3 levels. Stabilization hardware is also noted.

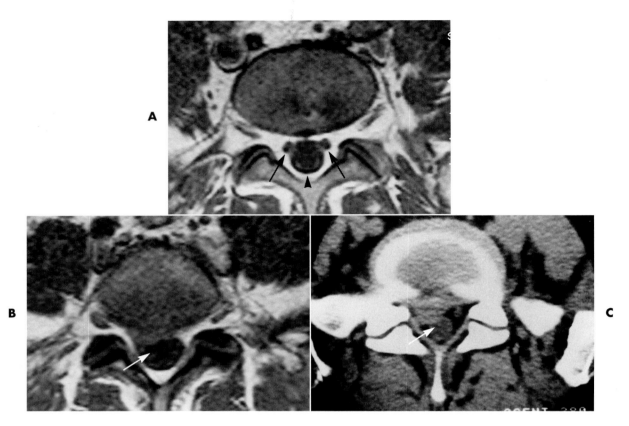

FIG. 11-90   Disc herniation in axial plane. **A,** T1-weighted axial MRI slice exhibiting the normal configuration of the the-cal sac *(arrowhead)* and branching nerve roots *(arrows)*. Notice the hyperintense epidural fat interposed between the thecal sac and the vertebra. **B,** T1-weighted axial MRI slice in a different patient reveals a large disc herniation to the right of mid-line projecting into the thecal sac *(arrow)* with loss of the interposed epidural fat. **C,** CT scan soft tissue window of a third patient with a large right-sided L5 disc herniation *(arrow)*. The right nerve root is not visualized. *(Bottom right,* Courtesy Steven P. Brownstein, Springfield, NJ.)

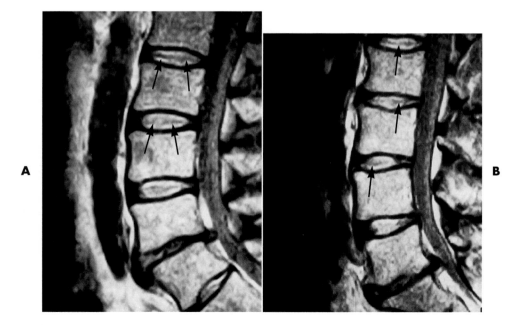

FIG. 11-91   Sagittal T2-weighted lumbar MRI scans of two patients. **A,** An L4 disc herniation with anterior and poste-rior displacement *(arrows)*. **B,** A posterior L5 herniation is noted. Both patients demonstrate high nuclear signal intensity, with dark horizontal bands indicating intranuclear clefts created by fibrous tissue invaginations *(arrows)*.

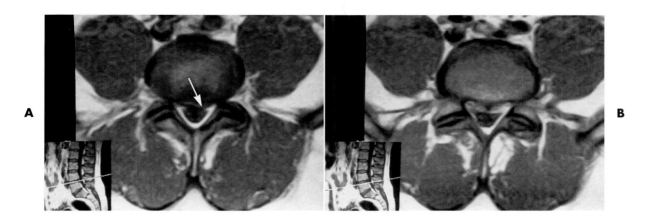

FIG. 11-92   T1-weighted (TR 750, TE 25) axial MRI scans denoting left parasagittal disc protrusion at the L4 level **(A)** *(arrow)*. One slice below does not reveal the abnormality **(B)**.

The advantages of MRI are that it is noninvasive, provides true three-dimensional imaging, has a field of examination extending from the conus to the sacrum, and visualizes the bone marrow and intrathecal contents. Disadvantage are its long examination times, unavailability in some areas, expense, and low resolution of cortical bone.

Both CT and MRI are excellent at showing the morphological changes associated with an intervertebral disc herniation (see Fig. 11-90). However, only MRI provides information on the physio-chemical changes within the disc. On T2-weighted MRI images, the high signal intensity (brightness) of the nucleus pulposus and inner annulus can be differentiated from the low signal intensity (darkness) of the outer annulus.[435] In healthy individuals over 30 years of age, it is common to see a dark horizontal band, which is an intranuclear cleft in the middle of the nucleus (Fig. 11-91). This cleft is caused by an ingrowth of fibrous tissue, which is thought to be a natural consequence of aging. The nuclear signal intensity on the T2-weighted image depends on the hydration and macromolecular composition of the nucleus.[417] The signal intensity or brightness of the nucleus inversely correlates to aging and degeneration.*

Annular tears. Transverse and radial annular tears have been visualized by MRI[435] as small foci of increased signal intensity on the T2-weighted image. They are best seen when hydrated nuclear material fills the cleft of the tear. If neovascularity is adequate, annular tears may become brightly enhanced on the T1-weighted image after administration of an intravenous contrast agent (e.g., gadolinium diethylenetriamine pentaacetic acid, Gd-DTPA). The ability to observe annular tears is highly dependent on their orientation.

Intervertebral disc herniations. Examination of the sagittal proton density image is probably the most helpful means of assessing the integrity of the annulus fibrosus and posterior longitudinal ligament.[202] Axial images provide the best information regarding the direction of the herniation and resulting thecal (neural) sac effacement and nerve root encroachment (Figs. 11-92, 11-93, 11-94, and 11-95).

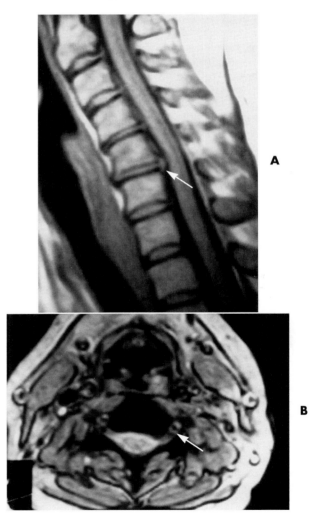

FIG. 11-93   Cervical disc herniation. Sagittal T1-weighted **(A)** and axial **(B)** MRI scan of a patient with focal disc herniation at the C5 *(arrows)*. The axial images demonstrate an uncinate osteophyte encroaching on the left intervertebral foramen.

*References 32, 139, 166, 183, 223, 262-264, 266, 290, 294, 306, 351, 353, 359, 429.

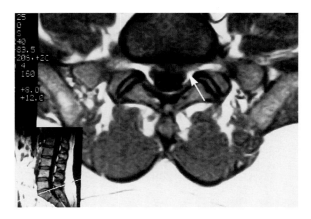

FIG. 11-94   Axial T1-weighted MRI image of a left-sided L5 disc herniation that posteriorly displaces the budding nerve root from the thecal sac *(arrow)*.

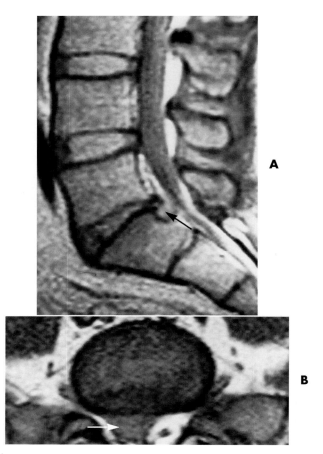

FIG. 11-95   Sagittal **(A)** and axial **(B)** T2-weighted images of a large right-sided disc herniation *(arrows)*.

Disc extrusions and sequestered fragments may exhibit high signal intensity on the T2-weighted images.[246] It is not clear whether these lesions represent acute herniations that have not desiccated completely or the high signal intensity has something to do with neovascularity or inflammation of the disc pathology.

MRI is helpful with differentiating recurrent disc herniations from surgical scars or tumors in the same location. When compared with the surrounding epidural fat, postoperative scars typically have lower signal intensity on T1-weighted images and higher signal intensity on T2-weighted images. Their appearance is difficult to differentiate from that of recurrent disc herniation. However, distinction is easier following the administration of intravenous contrast (e.g., gadolinium diethylenetriamine pentaacetic acid, Gd-DTPA). After use of contrast, postoperative scars and tumors exhibit diffuse enhancement on T1-weighted images, whereas recurrent herniations enhance only peripherally (Fig. 11-96).

CLINICAL COMMENTS

Clinical complaint.   The most common clinical complaint of a patient with a disc herniation is severe low back pain and possibly leg pain; however, only 5% of patients with a complaint of low back pain actually have this pain as a result of a disc herniation.[28] The pain typically occurs immediately after or within a few hours of an injury. The pain is typically increased by flexion, sneezing, bowel movements, and sitting.

Pain types.   Pain may be local, referred, or radicular. Local pain is limited to the area of the lesion and can only develop in innervated areas. Referred (sclerotomal) pain is limited to anatomical regions of similar embryological origin. Referred pain is usually described as deep, dull, and poorly localized and does not extend beyond the knee or elbows.[413] Radicular (dermatomal) pain is located along dermatomal nerve root distributions and may be accompanied by predictable sensory or motor deficits (Table 11-7). It is usually described as superficial, sharp, and well-defined.

Radicular pain is thought to be related to nerve root inflammation.[385] Loss of muscle strength and muscle atrophy is typically attributed to nerve root pressure. Local and referred spinal pain patterns may arise from irritation of the spinal dura, paravertebral muscles, ligaments, and joints (e.g., IVD, facet, sacroiliac).[39,80] It is difficult to pinpoint the affected tissue.

A displaced disc typically affects the nerve root exiting at the same level in the cervical spine and one segment below in the lum-

FIG. 11-96   Scar formation mimicking disc herniation. **A,** Lateral lumbar spot projection showing a narrowed L5 disc space and small osteophyte extending from the posterior aspect of L5 *(arrow)*. **B,** T1-weighted (TR 700, TE 25) sagittal lumbar MRI scan demonstrating two levels of disc herniations *(arrows)*. **C,** The preconstrast T1-weighted axial image demonstrates a midline L4 disc herniation that appears to contact but not flatten the thecal sac *(arrow)*. **D,** Following administration of gadopentetate dimeglumine contrast the mass becomes enhanced along its periphery *(arrows)*, indicating L4 disc herniation. **E,** At the L5 level a larger mass extending from the disc spaces is noted to the left of midline effacing the thecal sac *(arrow)*. **F,** Following the gadopentetate dimeglumine contrast administration the suspected disc herniation becomes diffusely enhanced *(arrows)*. This pattern of enhancement is associated with the highly vascular nature of scar formation, not disc herniation, which tends to become only peripherally enhanced. In addition, enhancement of a surgical scar from a previous laminectomy is noted in the region of the posterior arch of L5 *(curved arrows)*. (Courtesy Ian D. McLean, Davenport, Iowa.)

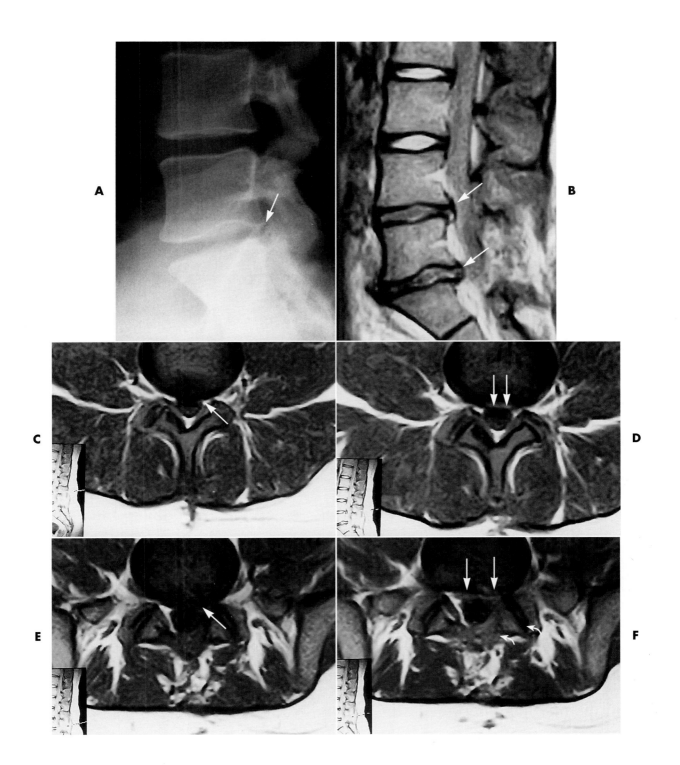

bar spine (see Table 11-7). For example, an L4 disc herniation will affect the L5 nerve root, but it will not affect the L4 nerve root unless it is a far lateral herniation or laterally migrated sequestration.

Myelopathy. IVD displacement in the cervical, thoracic, and upper lumbar spine may produce long tract deficits secondary to cord pressure (myelopathy). Symptoms include complaints of bilateral numbness, muscle weakness, and spasticity. The pain and numbness do not follow dermatomal patterns, which differentiates it from radiculopathy.

Asymptomatic herniations. Not all patients with disc herniations are symptomatic.[33,75,393] In one study, cervical disc herniations were found in 5 (10%) of 40 asymptomatic patients who were under 40 years of age and in 1 (5%) of 23 patients who were over 40 years of age.[33] In another study of 98 asymptomatic individuals with a mean age of 48, a lumbar disc bulge was found in 58%, protrusion in 27%, and extrusion in 1% of subjects.[184] Annular tears were noted in 14%.[184] The prevalence of disc herniations determined by MRI, CT, and myelographic studies is estimated to be between 20% and 35% in asymptomatic subjects.[164]

The size of the spinal canal and presence of concurrent facet joint arthrosis or ligamentum flavum hypertrophy are important features in determining who will experience symptoms, but currently it is not clear why some herniations are painful and others are not.[287] Prospective data are needed to determine the long-term consequences of disc herniations.

Physical examination. Abdominal and erector spinal muscle spasm is commonly found in the physical examination. Patients are usually apprehensive during palpation and experience tenderness that is typically more pronounced on one side of the body. A functional scoliosis is common.[413] A positive straight-leg raising orthopedic test is positive in 95% of patients with disc herniations.[96] A positive straight-leg raising test of the asymptomatic leg (contralateral straight-leg raising test) is less often positive but more accurate for disc herniation when the test is positive.[96]

Clinical course. Patients with IVD herniations usually have a good prognosis.[347] Cauda equina syndrome is one of the most serious complications of an IVD herniation and is marked by altered bowel and bladder function, impotence, progressive muscle atro-

---

TABLE 11-7
Clinical Findings Associated with Disc Herniations[8,419]

Disc level	Nerve root	Reflex affected	Muscle affected	Location of sensation
C4-5	C5	Biceps	Deltoid, biceps	Lateral arm
C5-6	C6	Brachioradialis	Wrist extensors, biceps	Lateral forearm
C6-7	C7	Triceps	Wrist flexors, triceps	Middle finger
C7-T1	C8	None reliable	Finger flexors	Medial forearm
L1-2	L2	None reliable	Iliopsoas	Anterior thigh, groin
L2-3	L3	Patellar	Quadriceps	Anterior and lateral thigh
L3-4	L4	Patellar	Anterior tibialis	Medial leg and foot
L4-5	L5	None reliable	Extensor hallucis	Lateral leg and foot
L5-S1	S1	Achilles	Peroneus longus	Lateral foot and fifth toe

TABLE 11-8
Management of Intervertebral Disc Herniations

Type of management	Comments
Chiropractic	Judicious application of side posture and flexion distraction adjustments for lumbar discs and other approaches for cervical herniations; chiropractic care is beneficial for many patients with confirmed disc herniations.
Other conservative measures	NSAIDs and other analgesics, muscle relaxants, epidural steroid injections, oral steroids, traction, ice biofeedback, limited bed rest, braces, acupuncture.
Chemonucleolysis	Injection of the enzyme chymopapain into the nucleus puplosus; indiscrimite destruction of the disc often results in poor outcome; generally, surgery is preferrable for patients who do not respond to conservative care.
Surgery	Options: removing the offending disc through a needle without the aid of an incision (percutaneous discectomy), using a small incision to make a hemilaminotomy and removing the offending disc material (microdiscectomy), removing a larger portion of the lamina (laminectomy) and possibly removing a portion of the disc (discectomy—most common approach), performing central or lateral decompression, spinal fusion; these surgical techniques are directed toward alleviating nerve root or cord pressure or stabilizing the vertebral segments.

phy, and saddle paresthesia. It is uncommon, occurring among 1% to 16% of patients.[141] This syndrome it is widely regarded as a surgical emergency because nerve pressure must be alleviated and function restored.

The use of serial imaging studies to assess the impact of treatments on disc lesion size is complicated by the natural evolution of disc herniations. Over time, herniations undergo cicatrization and retraction as part of their normal healing process.[177,346,392] Moreover, it is theorized that exposure of material extruded from disc herniations to the epidural blood supply facilitates phagocytosis of the material—the larger the lesion, the greater the resorption.[248] Extrusions demonstrate greater resorption than prolapses (contained herniations).[180] The degree of sequestration resorption is positively associated with its distance of migration.[203]

Management. Generally, imaging studies of the IVD or spinal canal during the initial 4 to 6 weeks after onset of symptoms that suggest disc herniation are unnecessary.[164] Exceptions to this generalization include patients with suspected cauda equina syndrome; progressive neurological deficit; intractable pain; and constitutional signs and symptoms suggesting tumor, fracture, infection or other aggressive pathology.[416] If the patient is not responsive to conservative therapy, imaging studies are usually warranted to determine whether the management plan should be altered.[164] Management approaches are listed in Table 11-8.

Conservative management. The management paradigm should begin with conservative measures, typically for at least 2 or 3 months.[229,316] If agreed on by the patient, slow recoveries can be managed even longer.[229] However, the use of muscle relaxants, analgesics, and bed rest for more than 2 weeks may further deteriorate the patient's status.[141] Activities that exacerbate back pain, such as heavy lifting and repetitive axial rotation or flexion should be avoided.[96,413] Often psychological counseling is helpful.[413] Chiropractic care has been observed to be beneficial by numerous investigators,* and a few experimental studies have confirmed these observations.[64,286] Serious complications caused by the judicious application of chiropractic care are rare.[64,79,357]

Surgery. Immediate surgery may be indicated if intractable pain, a significant or progressive neurological deficit, and loss of bowel and bladder function (e.g., cauda equina syndrome) develop.[229] The decision about whether to perform surgery is usually based on patients' symptoms, not their neurological deficits. This accounts for the wide variation in the number of surgeries performed.[133]

Surgery may provide immediate and dramatic relief of symptoms, but the symptoms often return[316] and may be worse than they were originally. Only about 5% to 10% of patients with radicular pain require surgery.[141]

The mere presence of a disc herniation is not an absolute indication of surgery. Appropriate patient selection is the key to surgical success.[270] The failure of a few selective conservative management measures is not an appropriate criterion for determining whether to use surgical intervention.[347] Surgery is most successful on patients who have exhausted all other options.[385,413]

---

*References 64, 79, 150, 205, 212, 286, 323, 364.

KEY CONCEPTS

- An IVD herniation describes the extension of nuclear, annular, or endplate substance through the annulus fibrosus.
- IVD herniations are more common among males, smokers, the obese, those exposed to vehicular vibration, and those between the ages of 25 and 45 years.
- Herniations exist along a continuum and may be categorized into protrusions (contained herniations), extrusions (uncontained herniations), and sequestrations (free fragments).
- Bulges are not herniations, instead, they are broad-based extensions of the annulus fibrosus with no associated focal displacement of nuclear substance.
- Herniations are most common in the lumbar region of the spine, followed by the cervical and then thoracic regions, respectively; 90% of lumbar herniations occur at the L4 and L5 levels, and 90% of cervical herniations occur at the C5 and C6 levels.
- Plain films do not visualize disc herniations.
- Myelography is considered antiquated and is only used in specific circumstances.
- A discography is performed before chemonucleolysis and is a provocative test for suspected discogenic pain syndromes.
- The advantages of CT are that it provides axial images, has shorter examination times, provides excellent osseous detail, and has the capability of visualizing very thin sections. It may be combined with myelography to visualize the thecal sac.
- MRI is widely regarded as the best imaging modality for the spine and canal contents. It is noninvasive; provides true three-dimensional imaging; allows the region from the conus to the sacrum to be examined; and provides excellent visualization of the IVD, bone marrow, and intrathecal contents.
- Symptoms associated with disc herniations are usually described as severe low back pain and possibly leg pain that are exaggerated by flexion, sneezing, bowel movement, and sitting.
- Many disc herniations produce no symptoms; the prevalence of disc herniations that are found by MRI, CT, and myelographic studies is estimated to be between 20% and 35% in asymptomatic subjects.
- The size of the spinal canal and presence of concurrent facet joint arthrosis or ligamentum flavum hypertrophy are important features in determining who will experience symptoms.
- The ipsilateral straight-leg raiser test is positive in 95% of patients with disc herniation; the contralateral straight-leg raiser test is positive less often but is more accurate.
- Cauda equina syndrome is one of the most serious complications of an IVD herniation and is characterized by altered bowel and bladder function, impotence, progressive muscle atrophy, and saddle paresthesia.
- The use of serial imaging studies to assess the impact of treatments on disc lesion size is complicated by the fact that disc herniations naturally resorb over time.
- The management paradigm should begin with conservative measures, typically for at least 2 or 3 months.
- Use of muscle relaxants, analgesics, and bed rest for more than 2 weeks may further compromise the patient's status.
- Chiropractic care has been reported to be beneficial; complications are rare.
- Immediate surgery may be indicated if intractable pain, a significant or progressive neurological deficit, and loss of bowel and bladder function develop.
- Appropriate patient selection is the key to surgical success. Surgery is most successful on patients who have exhausted all other options.

Spinal Stenosis

BACKGROUND

Spinal stenosis refers to narrowing of the spinal canal or intervertebral foramen (IVF), or neuroforamen, secondary to adjacent soft tissue or bone enlargement.[99,109,291] Stenosis may involve one or more levels.[271]

Demographics. Spinal stenosis appears to affect more men than women,[291,361] except for the cases involving degenerative spondylolisthesis, which are more common in women. Stenosis is more common among middle-aged (e.g., 40 to 50 years of age) individuals.[67,361] No clear relationship has been found between spinal stenosis and occupation or body size. Valid incidence and prevalence data are difficult to obtain because of the lack of specific diagnostic criteria for spinal stenosis.[243,431] Stenosis occurs most commonly in the cervical and lumbar regions of the spine; central lumbar stenosis is most common at the L4 level.

Classification system. Stenosis is typically divided into two types that are based on etiology: (1) congenital (e.g., achondroplasia, Morquio's and Down syndromes) and (2) acquired (e.g., IVD herniation, zygapophyseal arthrosis, postsurgical) (Table 11-9) (Fig. 11-97). Another classification system divides spinal stenosis into three types based on the anatomical region involved: (1) central

(narrowing of the spinal canal), (2) neuroforaminal (narrowing of the IVF), and (3) lateral recess (narrowing of the lateral zone—the distance between the thecal sac and the IVF).[99] Combined narrowing of the lateral recess and neuroforamen is termed *peripheral stenosis.*

IMAGING FINDINGS

Plain film radiographs. Plain film radiographs are of limited value in the diagnosis of spinal stenosis.[314,315] Because of gender, race, and age differences, radiographic measures of the spinal canal or neuroforamina lack specificity.[103,104,151,162,187] Variations of the shape of the canal appear to be more important than size variations of the canal.[354]

Projectional distortion may alter the appearance of the canal or neuroforamina, which may lead to spurious conclusions. This is a particularly common pitfall when observing the neuroforamina on the lateral lumbar radiograph. The lower lumbar neuroforamina are directed anterolaterally, and they appear to be more narrow than their actual anteroposterior dimensions (Fig. 11-98).

Plain film radiographs are very helpful in excluding conditions often associated with spinal stenosis (e.g., achondroplasia, Paget's disease, spondylosis, spondylolisthesis).

TABLE 11-9
Conditions Related to Spinal Stenosis

Condition	Description
Congenital stenosis	
Achondroplasia	Narrowing of interpeduncular distance and all components of the spinal canal secondary to aberrant enchondral bone formation; the condition is most severe in the lumbar spine.[272,319]
Idiopathic stenosis	Usually characterized by uniform narrowing of the lumbar spinal canal and neuroforamina of congenital origin (usually) but not associated with a congenital syndrome[45]; symptoms are most common in middle-aged patients.
Morquio's mucopolysaccharoidosis	Metabolic disease associated with spinal stenosis secondary to altered vertebral shape, posterior segmental displacements, and thoracolumbar kyphosis.[25]
Acquired stenosis	
Calcification or ossification of ligamentum flavum or posterior longitudinal ligament	Condition that may lead to spinal canal stenosis; ossification of the posterior longitudinal ligament is more common among Japanese men[279] and is a characteristic complication of DISH[335]; calcification or ossification of the ligamentum flavum is less common and is usually secondary to CPPD or degeneration.[191,194]
Spondylolisthesis	Degenerative (nonspondylolitic) spondylolisthesis results from zygophohyseal joint degeneration and up to 33% forward displacement of the vertebra; degenerative spondylolistheses most commonly occur among middle-aged women at the L4 level[282]; by contrast, because of the pars defect, spondylolytic spondylolisthesis is rarely associated with spinal stenosis; because of the pars defect, the zygophyseal joints maintain normal alignment and the vertebrae slips forward, effectively enlarging the spinal canal, although advanced forward displacement may encroach on the thecal sac from the segment above.[428]
Spondylosis (see Fig. 11-58)	Degeneration of the IVD, zygopophyseal joints, and uncovertebral joints of the cervical spine; it is marked by proliferative osteophytic changes, decreased joint space, segmental misalignment, disc bulging, and associated hypertrophy and forward buckling of the ligamentum flavum,[314-316] which narrows the spinal canal; neuroforamina are most affected by degeneration of the uncovertebral and zygopophyseal joints.
Postsurgical	Spinal stenosis following laminectomy, fusion, or chemonucleolysis that occurs in 30% to 40% of cases[53,321,174]; chemonucleolysis narrows the IVD space and projects the superior articular facet into the neuroforamina.[90]
Metabolic/endocrine/other	Acromegaly: associated with spinal stenosis secondary to advanced osteophytosis[110]; CPPD: affects the spinal ligaments, particularly the ligamentum flavum[194]; the bone overgrowth associated with Paget's disease narrows the spinal canal[421] and neuroforamen; a deformity caused by trauma may lead to spinal stenosis.

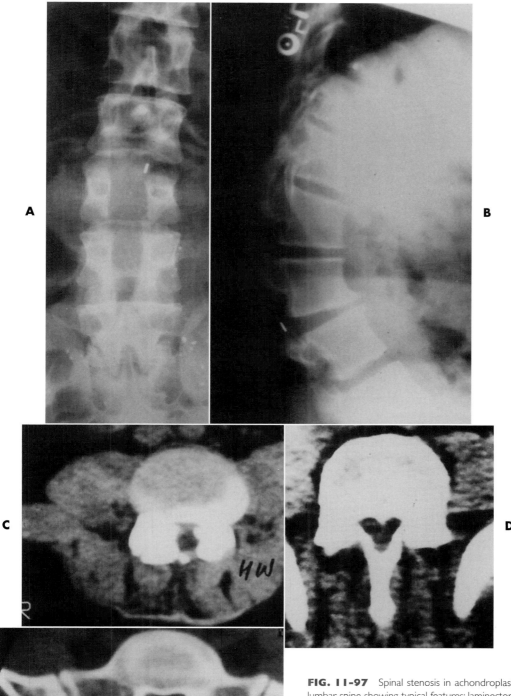

FIG. 11-97 Spinal stenosis in achondroplasia. **A,** Frontal projection of the lumbar spine showing typical features; laminectomy has been performed. **B,** Lateral projection of the thoracolumbar region showing the exaggerated concavity of the posterior vertebral surfaces. **C,** Axial CT at L3-4. Note the marked stenosis of the canal following the laminectomy. Superimposed degenerative disease of the facet joints is also present, which has contributed to the stenosis. **D** and **E,** Note the triangular configuration of the spinal canal **(D)** and the degenerative disease of the facet joints at S1 **(E).** The protruding hypertrophied facets have caused further distortion and stenosis of the canal. (From Firooznia H et al: *MRI and CT of the musculoskeletal system,* St Louis, 1992, Mosby.)

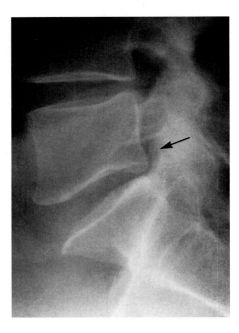

FIG. 11-98   Lateral lumbosacral spot projection demonstrating a narrow L5-S1 IVF *(arrow)*. In the lower lumbar spine the IVF is directed anterolaterally; therefore a lateral projection underestimates the anteroposterior dimension of the foramen.

Advanced imaging.   CT and MRI are the most helpful procedures used to assess spinal stenosis and have essentially eliminated the use of myelography. Both CT and MRI yield axial images that allow assessment of the size and shape of the spinal canal and neuroforamen (Figs. 11-99, 11-100, and 11-101). CT seems to have an advantage over MRI for diagnosing spondylolysis; contrast-enhanced CT is preferred by some clinicians for evaluating cervical spine stenosis.[182] MRI is a better method to use for assessing the thecal sac and contents. The cerebrospinal fluid of the thecal sac contrasts well with the epidural fat on T2-weighted images, so these are the best types of images to use when assessing for the presence of spinal canal (central) stenosis. Epidural fat is best seen on T1-weighted images, so these are the best types of images to use when evaluating for the presence of peripheral stenosis.

CLINICAL COMMENTS

Clinical symptoms.   Spinal stenosis results in compression of the nerves, arteries, capillaries, and veins.[206,208] It is theorized that pain results from arterial obstruction, venous hypertension, and pressure on the primary rami and recurrent meningeal nerves (sinuvertebral nerves).[101,211,269]

The patient's pain patterns are related to the region in which the stenosis has developed. Neuroforaminal stenosis is associated with well-defined pain patterns that correspond to the level of stenosis. Conversely, spinal stenosis typically produces vague, poorly defined pain patterns. Both patterns are usually preceded by a long history of intermittent spinal complaints.[151]

Spinal region.   The symptoms associated with stenosis of the cervical region of the spine differ from those associated with the lumbar region of the spine. Many patients with stenosis in the cervical region may have long tract and radicular signs and symptoms[99,156,291,407] and usually have headaches and neck pain.[291] Lumbar stenosis is associated with radicular signs and symptoms, not headaches or long tract findings. Flexion of the cervical region of the spine often causes sudden electric-like shocks to extend down the spine and extremities (Lhermitte's sign). Stenosis in the cervical region may mimic the clinical presentation of multiple sclerosis, syringomyelia, and amyotrophic lateral sclerosis.[407] Concurrent stenosis in the cervical and lumbar regions produces a perplexing clinical presentation marked by gait disturbance and mixed- and multiple-level myelopathy and radiculopathy that closely resemble symptoms associated with amyotrophic lateral sclerosis or another motor neuron disease.[111]

Neurogenic claudication.   Neurogenic claudication (pseudoclaudication) may occur in patients with lumbar spinal canal stenosis.[151] It is characterized by poorly defined leg pain accompanied by limb numbness and muscle weakness. The pain is exacerbated by standing and alleviated by flexing the trunk.[99,151,206,291,376] Patients often assume a Simian stance—a posture of trunk, hip, and knee flexion.[369] Although vascular claudication has symptoms that are similar to those of neurogenic claudication, symptom-aggravating movements can be used to differentiate them clinically. Vascular claudication is worsened by exercise and improved by standing and lying down. Neurogenic claudication is exacerbated by standing and spinal extension but is not dramatically changed by exercise.

Differentiating disc herniation.   Differentiating spinal stenosis pain from discogenic pain is difficult because the two conditions often coexist.[99,428] Disc herniation is a common cause of stenosis. Symptom-aggravating movements may provide a basis for differentiation between the two conditions. Sitting, bending, lifting, and Valsalva maneuvers aggravate discogenic back pain but have no affect on pain caused by spinal stenosis.[99,206,291] Conversely, walking may aggravate spinal stenosis complaints and alleviate discogenic pain.[99,206,291] Symptoms of spinal stenosis are more chronic than those associated with IVD herniation.[291]

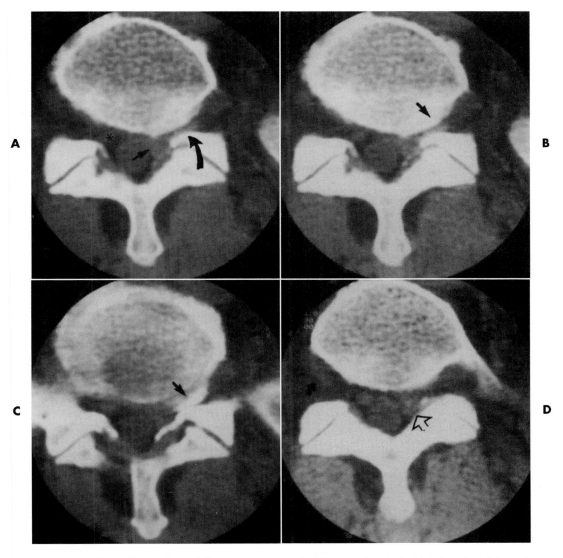

FIG. 11-99 Neural foraminal stenosis. Two window settings of a CT examination obtained just above the inferior endplate of L5. There are hypertrophic changes of the posterolateral border of L5 on the left, which have caused stenosis of the lower portion of the L5-S1 foramen. The curved arrow in **A** denotes the stenotic foramen. The normal descending right S1 nerve root *(asterisk)* has already separated from the dural sac. A soft tissue density *(straight arrow)* in the epidural space occupies the anterolateral portion of the spinal canal on the left; it is a migrated fragment of herniated disk. The left descending S1 nerve root is obscured by the herniated disk. **B,** Hypertrophic changes on the posterolateral border of L5 *(arrow)*. **C,** An axial slice obtained 4 mm below **A** and **B** showing the hypertrophic changes and a calcified ridge *(arrow)*. A soft tissue density, which is herniated disk material, obscuring the left anterior epidural fat and extending laterally, also obscuring the left descending S1 nerve root and lateral recess. **D,** An axial slice just below the L5 pedicle showing the neural foramen to be normal at this level. The dorsal root ganglion also is normal *(curved arrow)*. The fragment of herniated disk obscures the descending left S1 nerve root *(hollow arrow)*. This patient has marked stenosis in the lower portion of the neural foramen but no evidence of compression of the L5 dorsal root ganglion in the upper part of the foramen. The exiting L5 spinal nerve is more anterior and lateral to the site of the stenosis and is not involved. (From Firooznia H et al: *MRI and CT of the musculoskeletal system,* St Louis, 1992, Mosby.)

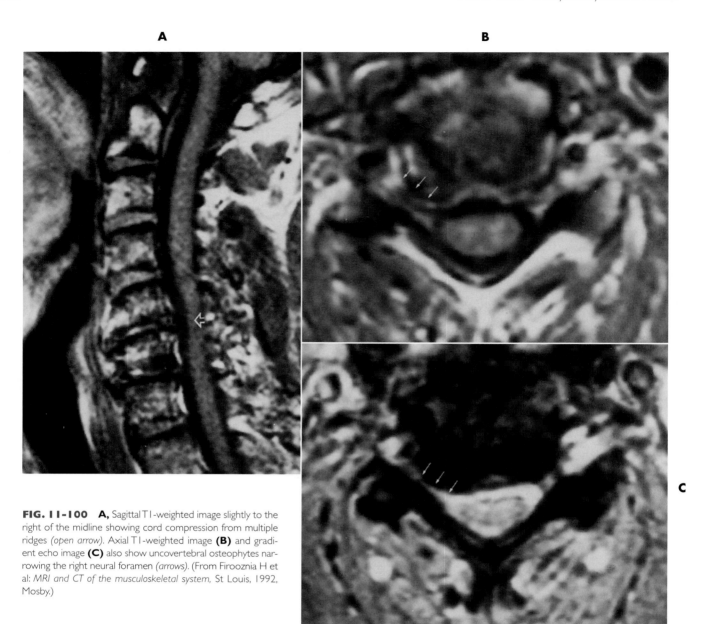

A

B

C

FIG. 11-100 **A,** Sagittal T1-weighted image slightly to the right of the midline showing cord compression from multiple ridges *(open arrow)*. Axial T1-weighted image **(B)** and gradient echo image **(C)** also show uncovertebral osteophytes narrowing the right neural foramen *(arrows)*. (From Firooznia H et al: *MRI and CT of the musculoskeletal system,* St Louis, 1992, Mosby.)

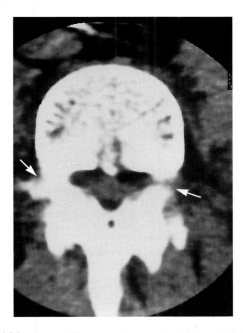

FIG. 11-101 Lumbar CT scan revealing a narrowed intervertebral canal secondary to short, thick pedicles *(arrows)*. (Courtesy Steven P. Brownstein, Springfield, NJ.)

Management. The type of treatment for spinal stenosis is usually based on the types of symptoms being experienced by the patient. Most patients with intermittent or mild symptoms can be managed nonsurgically.[293,437] If the patient does not respond to nonsurgical methods, surgical decompression and possibly fusion is an option.[67]

■ KEY CONCEPTS

- *Spinal stenosis is narrowing of the spinal canal or IVF (neuroforamen) secondary to adjacent soft tissue or bone enlargement.*
- *Overall stenosis is more common in men and middle-aged (40 to 50 years of age) individuals.*
- *Spinal stenosis is more common in the cervical and lumbar regions of the spine than in the thoracic region.*
- *Spinal stenosis can be divided by etiology: (1) congenital (e.g., achondroplasia, Morquio's and Down syndromes) and (2) acquired (e.g., IVD herniation, zygapophyseal arthrosis, postsurgical).*
- *Spinal stenosis can also be categorized by location: (1) central (spinal canal), (2) neuroforaminal (IVF), and (3) lateral recess (lateral zone—the distance between the thecal sac and the IVF).*
- *Plain film radiographs are the most helpful to evaluate related conditions (e.g., spondylolisthesis, Paget's disease, achondroplasia).*
- *CT and MRI provide axial images and allow evaluation of thecal sac deformities.*
- *Neuroforaminal stenosis is associated with a well-defined pain pattern. Spinal stenosis produces vague, poorly defined pain patterns.*
- *Patients with spinal stenosis usually relate a chronic history of complaints related to the spine; patients with disc herniations more often do not.*
- *Stenosis in the cervical region of the spine is commonly associated with myelopathy and diffuse symptoms.*
- *Neurogenic claudication (pseudoclaudication) is common in patients with lumbar spinal canal stenosis. It is characterized by poorly defined leg pain accompanied by limb numbness and muscle weakness that tend to resolve on trunk flexion.*

References

1. Abrahim-Zadeh R, Yu JS, Resnick D: Central (interior) osteophytes of the distal femur. Imaging and pathologic findings, *Invest Radiol* 29:1001, 1994.
2. Adam O: Nutrition as adjuvant therapy in chronic polyarthritis, *Z Rheumatol* 52:275, 1993.
3. Alexander CJ: Osteoarthritis: a review of old myths and current concepts, *Skeletal Radiol* 19:327, 1990.
4. Alexander CJ: Relationship between utilization profile of individual joints and their susceptibility to primary osteoarthritis, *Skeletal Radiol* 18:199, 1989.
5. Altman RD et al: Future therapeutic trends in osteoarthritis, *Scand J Rheumatol Suppl* 77:37, 1988.
6. Altomonte L et al: Growth hormone secretion in diffuse idiopathic skeletal hyperostosis, *Ann Ital Med Int* 7(1):30, 1992.
7. Anaya JM, Diethelm L, Ortiz LA: Pulmonary involvement in rheumatoid arthritis, *Semin Arthritis Rheum* 24:242, 1995 (review).
8. Andersson GBJ, Deyo RA: History and physical examination in patients with herniated lumbar discs, *Spine* 21(suppl 24):10, 1996.
9. Ansell BM: Joint manifestations in children with juvenile chronic polyarthritis, *Arthritis Rheum* 20:204, 1977.
10. Aoki J et al: Endplate of the discovertebral joint: degenerative change in the elderly adult, *Radiology* 164:411, 1987.
11. Appel GB, Valeri A: The course and treatment of lupus nephritis, *Annu Rev Med* 45:525, 1994.
12. Arnett FC et al: The American Rheumatism Association 1987 revised criteria for the classification of rheumatoid arthritis, *Arthritis Rheum* 31:315, 1988.
13. Arnett FC: HLA and autoimmunity in scleroderma (systemic sclerosis), *Int Rev Immunol* 12:107, 1995.
14. Azouz EM, Duffy CM: Juvenile spondyloarthropathies: clinical manifestations and medical imaging, *Skeletal Radiol* 24:399, 1995.
15. Babini SM et al: Tendinous laxity and Jaccoud's syndrome in patients with systemic lupus erythematosus. Possible role of secondary hyperparathyroidism, *J Rheumatol* 16:494, 1989.
16. Babini SM et al: Atlantoaxial subluxation in systemic lupus erythematosus: further evidence of tendinous alterations, *J Rheumatol* 17:173, 1990.
17. Baker GHB, Brewerton DA: Rheumatoid arthritis: a psychiatric assessment, *Br Med J* 282:2014, 1981.
18. Bardin T, Enel C, Lathrop GM: Treatment of tetracycline and erythromycin of urethritides allows significant prevention of postvenereal arthritic flares in Reiter's syndrome patients, *Arthritis Rheum* 33(suppl):26, 1990 (abstract).
19. Bardin T, Lathrop GM: Postvenereal Reiter's syndrome in Greenland, *Rheum Dis Clin North Am* 18:81, 1992.
20. Barker JN: The immunopathology of psoriasis, *Baillieres Clin Rheumatol* 8:429, 1994 (review).
21. Basset L et al: Skeletal findings in progressive systemic sclerosis (scleroderma), *AJR* 136:1121, 1981.
22. Bates D, Ruggeri P: Imaging modalities for evaluation of the spine, *Radiol Clin North Am* 29:675, 1991.
23. Belhorn LR, Hess EV: Erosive osteoarthritis, *Semin Arthritis Rheum* 22:298, 1993.
24. Belmont HM, Abramson SB, Lie JT: Pathology and pathogenesis of vascular injury in systemic lupus erythematosus, *Arthritis Rheum* 39:9, 1996.
25. Bethem D et al: Spinal disorders of dwarfism, *J Bone Joint Surg Am* 63:1412, 1981.
26. Beyeler C et al: Diffuse idiopathic hyperostosis (DISH) of the elbow: a cause of elbow pain? A controlled study, *Br J Rheumatol* 31:319, 1992.
27. Bezrodnyhk AA, Karelin AP: Systemic lupus erythematosus and systemic scleroderma in patients from the aboriginal people and the newcomers of Yakutia under the extreme conditions of the far north, *Alaska Med* 36:102, 1994.
28. Bigos SJ et al: The new thinking on low back pain, *Patient Care* 29:140, 1995.

29. Bjorkengren AG, Resnick D, Sartoris DJ: Enteropathic arthropathies, *Radiol Clin North Am* 25:189, 1987.

30. Blackburn WD, Chivers S, Bernreuter W: Cartilage imaging in osteoarthritis, *Semin Arthritis Rheum* 25:273, 1996.

31. Bland JH: The reversibility of osteoarthritis: a review, *Am J Med* 74:16, 1983.

32. Bobest M et al: Hydrogen nuclear magnetic resonance study of intervertebral discs: a preliminary report, *Spine* 11:709, 1986.

33. Boden SD et al: Abnormal magnetic resonance scans of the cervical spine in asymptomatic subjects, *J Bone Joint Surg Am* 72:1178, 1990.

34. Boden SD et al: Orientation of the lumbar facet joints: association with degenerative disc disease, *J Bone Joint Surg Am* 78:403, 1996.

35. Boden SD: Rheumatoid arthritis of the cervical spine. Surgical decision making based on predictors of paralysis and recovery, *Spine* 19:2275, 1994.

36. Bogduk N, Twomey LT: *Clinical anatomy of the lumbar spine,* ed 2, Melbourne, 1991, Churchill Livingstone.

37. Bogduk N, Tynan W, Wilson AS: The nerve supply to the human lumbar intervertebral discs, *J Anat* 132:39, 1981.

38. Bogduk N: Pathology of lumbar disc pain, *J Manual Med* 5:72, 1990.

39. Bogduk N: The anatomical basis for spinal pain syndromes, *J Manipulative Physiol Ther* 18: 603, 1995.

40. Bogduk N: The lumbar disc and low back pain, *Neurosurg Clin N Am* 2:791, 1991.

41. Bohndorf K, Schalm J: Diagnostic radiography in rheumatoid arthritis: benefits and limitations, *Baillieres Clin Rheumatol* 10:399, 1996.

42. Boki DA et al: Examination of HLA-DR4 as a severity marker for rheumatoid arthritis in Greek patients, *Ann Rheum Dis* 52:517, 1993.

43. Borenstein DG, Silver G, Jenkins E: Approach to initial medical treatment of rheumatoid arthritis, *Arch Fam Med* 2:545, 1993.

44. Boss GR, Seegmiller JE: Hyperuricemia and gout. Classification, complications and management, *N Engl J Med* 300:1459, 1979.

45. Bowen V, Cassidy JD: Macroscopic and microscopic anatomy of the sacroiliac joint from embryonic life until the eighth decade, *Spine* 6:620, 1981.

46. Bowen V, Shannon R, Kirkaldy-Willis WH: Lumbar spinal stenosis: a review article, *Childs Brain* 4:257, 1978.

47. Bradley JD: Jaccoud's arthropathy in adult dermatomyositis, *Clin Exp Rheumatol* 4:273, 1986.

48. Bradley JD, Pinals RS: Jaccoud's arthropathy in scleroderma, *Clin Exp Rheumatol* 2:337, 1984.

49. Brandt KD: Nonsurgical management of osteoarthritis, with an emphasis on nonpharmacologic measures, *Arch Fam Med* 4:1057, 1995.

50. Brewerton DA et al: HL-A 27 and the arthropathies associated with ulcerative colitis and psoriasis, *Lancet* 1:956, 1974.

51. Brinckmann P: Injury of the annulus fibrosus and disc protrusions: an in vitro investigation on human lumbar discs, *Spine* 11:149, 1986.

52. Brodelius A: Osteoarthrosis of the talar joints in footballers and ballet dancers, *Acta Orthop Scand* 30:309, 1960.

53. Brodsky AE: Post-laminectomy and post-fusion stenosis of the spine, *Clin Orthop* 15:130, 1976.

54. Brook A, Corbett M: Radiographic changes in early RA, *Ann Rheum Dis* 36:71, 1977.

55. Brower A, Allman R: Pathogenesis of the neurotrophic joint: neurotraumatic vs neurovascular, *Radiology* 139:349, 1981.

56. Brown JH, Deluca SA: The radiology of rheumatoid arthritis, *Am Fam Physician* 52:1372, 1995.

57. Burgos-Vargas R, Pineda C: New clinical and radiographic features of the seronegative spondyloarthropathies, *Curr Opin Rheumatol* 3:562, 1991.

58. Burkus JK, Denis F: Hyperextension injuries of the thoracic spine in diffuse idiopathic hyperostosis. Report of four cases, *J Bone Joint Surg Am* 76:237, 1994.

59. Butler D et al: Discs degenerate before facets, *Spine* 15:111, 1990.

60. Byers PD, Contepomi CA, Farkas TA: Post-mortem study of the hip joint. Part III, Correlations between observations, *Ann Rheum Dis* 35:122, 1976.

61. Callahan EP, Aguillera H: Complications following minor trauma in a patient with diffuse idiopathic skeletal hyperostosis, *Ann Emerg Med* 22:1067, 1993.

62. Cameron HU, Fornasier VL: Trabecular stress fractures, *Clin Orthop* 11:266, 1975.

63. Casciola-Rosen L, Wigley F, Rosen A: Scleroderma autoantigens are uniquely fragmented by metal-catalyzed oxidation reactions: implications for pathogenesis, *J Exp Med* 185:71, 1997.

64. Cassidy JD, Thiel HW, Kirkaldy-Willis WH: Side posture manipulation for lumbar intervertebral disk herniation, *J Manipulative Physiol Ther* 16:96, 1993.

65. Centers for Disease Control: Prevalance leisure-time physical activity among persons with arthrithis and other rheumatic conditions, *MMWR* 9:18, 1997.

66. Chang DJ, Paget SA: Neurologic complications of rheumatoid arthritis, *Rheum Dis Clin North Am* 19(4):955, 1993.

67. Chase JA: Spinal stenosis. When arthritis is more than arthritis, *Nurs Clin North Am* 26:53, 1991.

68. Cicuttini FM, Spector TD: Osteoarthritis in the aged. Epidemiological issues and optimal management, *Drugs Aging* 6:409, 1995.

69. Clements P: Clinical aspects of localized and systemic sclerosis, *Curr Opin Rheumatol* 4:843, 1992.

70. Cobby M et al: Erosive osteoarthritis: is it a separate disease entity? *Clin Radiol* 42:258, 1990.

71. Cohn EL et al: Plain film evaluation of degenerative disk disease at the lumbosacral junction, *Skeletal Radiol* 26:161, 1997.

72. Colhoun E et al: Provocation discography as a guide to planning operations on the spine, *J Bone Joint Surg Br* 70:267, 1988.

73. Collins HR: An evaluation of cervical and lumbar discography, *Clin Orthop* 107:133, 1975.

74. Collins JS, Gardner WJ: Lumbar discography—an analysis of 1,000 cases, *J Neurosurg* 19:452, 1962.

75. Connell MD, Wiesel SW: Natural history and pathogenesis of cervical disk disease, *Orthop Clin North Am* 23:369, 1992.

76. Constantin P, Lucretia C: Relations between the cervical spine and the vertebral arteries, *Acta Radiol* 11:91, 1971.

77. Cooper C: Occupational activity and the risk of osteoarthritis, *J Rheumatol Suppl* 43:10, 1995.

78. Corvetta A et al: MR imaging of rheumatoid hand lesions: comparison with conventional radiology in 31 patients, *Clin Exp Rheumatol* 10:217, 1992.

79. Cox JM, Feller J, Cox-Cid J: Distraction chiropractic adjusting: clinical application and outcome of 1,000 cases, *Top Clin Chiro* 3:45, 1996.

80. Cramer GD, Darby SA: Clinical pathoanatomy related to low back pain, *Top Clin Chiro* 3:1, 1996.

81. Crock HV: Internal disc disruption: a challenge to disc prolapse 50 years on, *Spine* 11:650, 1986.

82. Cuellar ML, Espinoza LR: Psoriatic arthritis. Current developments, *J Fla Med Assoc* 82:338, 1995.

83. Cuellar ML, Silveira LH, Espinoza LR: Recent developments in psoriatic arthritis, *Curr Opin Rheumatol* 6:378, 1994.

84. Da Silva JA, Spector TD: The role of pregnancy in the course and aetiology of rheumatoid arthritis, *Clin Rheumatol* 11:189, 1992.

85. Daltroy LH et al: Effectiveness of minimally supervised home aerobic training in patients with systemic rheumatic disease, *Br J Rheumatol* 34:1064, 1995.

86. Damron TA, Heiner JP: Rapidly progressive protrusio acetabuli in patients with rheumatoid arthritis, *Clin Orthop* 289:186, 1993.

87. Daragon A et al: Vertebral hyperostosis and diabetes mellitus: a case-control study, *Ann Rheum Dis* 54:375, 1995.

88. Davis MA: Epidemiology of osteoarthritis, *Clin Geriatr Med* 4:241, 1988.

89. De Bandt M et al: Ossifcation of the posterior longitudinal ligament, diffuse idiopathic skeletal hyperostosis, abnormal retinol and retinol binding protein: a familial observation, *J Rheumatol* 22:1395, 1995.

90. Deburge A, Rocolle J, Benoist M: Surgical findings and results of surgery after failure of chemonucleolysis, *Spine* 10:812, 1985.

91. Deesomchok U, Tumrasvin T: Clinical comparison of patients with ankylosing spondylitis, Reiter's syndrome, and psoriatic arthritis, *J Med Assoc Thai* 76:61, 1993.

92. Denisov LN et al: Therapeutic nutrition and sparing diet therapy in the combined treatment of rheumatoid arthritis, *Klin Med (Mosk)* 71:46, 1993.

93. Denko CW, Boja B, Moskowitz RW: Growth promoting peptides in osteoarthritis and diffuse idiopathic skeletal hyperostosis—insulin, insulin-like growth factor-I, growth hormone, *J Rheumatol* 21:1725, 1994.

94. deRoos A et al: MR imaging of marrow changes adjacent to endplates in degenerative lumbar disk disease, *AJR* 149:531, 1987.

95. Desai Y et al: Renal involvement in scleroderma, *J Assoc Physicians India* 38:768, 1990.

96. Deyo RA, Loeser JD, Bigos SJ: Herniated lumbar intervertebral disk, *Ann Intern Med* 112:598, 1990.

97. Diethelm U: Nutrition and chronic polyarthritis, *Schweiz Rundsc Med Prax* 82:359, 1993.

98. Dihlmann W: Current radiodiagnostic concept of ankylosing spondylitis, *Skeletal Radiol* 4:179, 1979.

99. Dorwart RH, Vogler JB, Helms CA: Spinal stenosis, *Radiol Clin North Am* 21:301, 1983.

100. Doyle T et al: The radiographic changes of scleroderma in the hands, *Australas Radiol* 34:53, 1990.

101. Edgar MA, Ghadially JA: Innervation of the lumbar spine, *Clin Orthop* 115:35, 1976.

102. Ehrlich MG: Degradative enzyme systems in osteoarthritic cartilage, *J Orthop Res* 3:170, 1985.

103. Eisenstein S: Measurement of the lumbar spinal canal in 2 racial groups, *Clin Orthop* 115:42, 1976.

104. Eisenstein S: The morphometry and pathological anatomy of the lumbar spine in South African negroes and caucasoids with specific reference to spinal stenosis, *J Bone Joint Surg Br* 59:173, 1977.

105. El-Khoury GY, Kathol MH, Brandser EA: Seronegative spondyloarthropathies, *Rad Clin North Am* 34:343, 1996.

106. Elias F: Roentgen findings in the asymptomatic cervical spine, *N Y State J Med* 58:3300, 1958.

107. Ellman MH, Brown NL, Levin B: Prevalence of knee chondrocalcinosis in hospital and clinic patients aged 50 and older, *J Am Geriatr Soc* 29:189, 1981.

108. Eng BJ et al: Use of MRI with 3-dimensional reconstruction to measure changes in the synovium and joints in rheumatoid arthritis, *Arthritis Rheum* 35(suppl):196, 1992.

109. Epstein BS, Epstein JA, Jones MD: Lumbar spinal stenosis, *Radiol Clin North Am* 15:227, 1977.

110. Epstein H, Whelan M, Benjamin V: Acromegaly and spinal stenosis, *J Neurosurg* 56:145, 1982.

111. Epstein NE et al: Coexisting cervical and lumbar spinal stenosis: diagnosis and management, *Neurosurgery* 15:489, 1984.

112. Errico TJ: The role of diskography in the 1980s, *Radiology* 162:285, 1987.

113. Escalante A: Ankylosing spondylitis. A common cause of low back pain, *Postgrad Med* 94:153, 1993.

114. Eustace S, Coughlan RJ, McCarthy C: Ankylosing spondylitis. A comparison of clinical and radiographic features in men and women, *Ir Med J* 86:120, 1993.

115. Executive Committee of the North American Spine Society: Position statement on discography, *Spine* 13:1343, 1988.

116. Eyring EJ: The biochemistry and physiology of the intervertebral disc, *Clin Orthop* 67:16, 1969.

117. Fam AG, Pritzker KP: Acute calcific periarthritis in scleroderma, *J Rheumatol* 19:1580, 1992.

118. Fan PT, Yu DTY: Reiter's syndrome. In Schumacher HR Jr, Klippel JH, Koopman WJ, editors: *Primer on rheumatic disease,* ed 10, Atlanta, 1993, Arthritis Foundation.

119. Farfan HF et al: The effects of torsion on the lumbar intervertebral joints: the role of torsion in the production of disc degeneration, *J Bone Joint Surg Am* 52:468, 1970.

120. Farfan HF, Gracovetsky S: The nature of instability, *Spine* 9:174, 1984.

121. Farfan HF: A reorientation in the surgical approach to degenerative lumbar intervertebral joint disease, *Orthop Clin North Am* 8:9, 1977.

122. Felson DT et al: The prevalence of chondrocalcinosis in the elderly and its association with knee osteoarthritis: the Framingham study, *J Rheumatol* 16:1241, 1989.

123. Felson DT et al: Weight loss reduces the risk for symptomatic knee osteoarthritis in women: the Framingham study, *Ann Intern Med* 116:535, 1992.

124. Felson DT: Weight and osteoarthritis, *Am J Clin Nutr* 63(suppl 3):4305, 1996.

125. Fernandez-Madrid F et al: MR features of osteoarthritis of the knee, *Magn Reson Imaging* 12:703, 1994.

126. Fessel JW: Systematic lupus erythematosus in the community, *Arch Intern Med* 134:1027, 1974.

127. Forgacs SS: Diabetes mellitus and rheumatic disease, *Clin Rheum Dis* 12:279, 1986.

128. Fox R et al: The chronicity of symptoms and disability in Reiter's syndrome, *Ann Intern Med* 91:190, 1979.

129. Friedenberg AH, Miller WF: Degenerative disc disease of the cervical spine, *J Bone Joint Surg Am* 45:1171, 1963.

130. Friedenberg ZB et al: Degenerative disc disease of the cervical spine: clinical and roentgenographic study, *JAMA* 174:375, 1960.

131. Fries JF et al: Nonsteroidal anti-inflammatory drug-associated gastropathy: incidence and risk factor models, *Am J Med* 91:213, 1991.

132. Frymoyer JW: Can low back pain disability be prevented? *Baillieres Clin Rheumatol* 6:595, 1992.

133. Frymoyer JW: Lumbar disk disease: epidemiology, *Instr Course Lect* 41:217, 1992.

134. Frymoyer JW: Predicting disability from low back pain, *Clin Orthop* 279:101, 1992.

135. Fuiks DM, Grayson CE: Vacuum pneumarthrography and the spontaneous occurance of gas in the joint spaces, *J Bone Joint Surg Am* 32:933, 1950.

136. Fulp SR, Castell DO: Scleroderma esophagus, *Dysphagia* 5:204, 1990.

137. Garfin SR, Ahlgren BD: Current management of cervical spine instability, *Curr Opin Rheumatol* 7:114, 1995.

138. Genti G: Occupation and osteoarthritis, *Baillieres Clin Rheumatol* 3:193, 1989.

139. Gibson MJ et al: Magnetic resonance imaging and discography in the diagnosis of disc degeneration, *J Bone Joint Surg* 68B:369, 1986.

140. Gilbertson EMM: Development of peri-articular osteophytes in experimentally induced osteoarthritis in the dog, *Ann Rheum Dis* 34:12, 1975.

141. Gilmer HS, Papadopoulos SM, Tuite GF: Lumbar disk disease: pathophysiology, management and prevention, *Amer Fam Physician* 47(5):1141, 1993.

142. Girgis FL, Popple AW, Bruckner FE: Jaccoud's arthropathy. A case report and necropsy study, *Ann Rheum Dis* 37(6):561, 1978.

143. Glynn LE: Primary lesion in osteoarthrosis, *Lancet* 1(8011):574, 1977.

144. Gore DR, Sepic SB, Gardner GF: Roentgenographic findings of the cervical spine in asymptomatic people, *Spine* 11:521, 1986.

145. Gore DR et al: Neck pain: A long-term follow-up of 205 patients, *Spine* 12:1, 1987.

PART TWO Bone, Joints, and Soft Tissues

146. Grahame R, Scott JT: Clinical survey of 354 patients with gout, *Ann Rheum Dis* 29:461, 1970.

147. Gravallese EM, Kantrowitz FG: Arthritic manifestations of inflammatory bowel disease, *Am J Gastroenterol* 83(7):703, 1988.

148. Grishman E, Venkatasehan VS: Vascular lesions in lupus nephritis, *Mod Pathol* 1:235-241, 1988.

149. Hackney DB: Degenerative disk disease, *Top Magn Reson Imaging* 4(2):12, 1992.

150. Hadler NM et al: A benefit of spinal manipulation and adjunctive therapy for acute low back pain: a stratified controlled trial, *Spine* 12(7):703, 1987.

151. Hall S et al: Lumbar spinal stenosis: clinical features, diagnostic procedures, and results of surgical treatment in 68 patients, *Ann Intern Med* 103:271, 1985.

152. Hamerman D: Current leads in research on the osteoarthritic joint, *J Am Geriatr Soc* 31:299, 1983.

153. Hamerman D: The biology of osteoarthritis, *N Engl J Med* 320:1322, 1989.

154. Hammoudeh M, Rahim Siam A, Khanjar I: Spinal stenosis due to posterior syndesmophytes in a patient with seronegative spondyloarthropathy, *Clin Rheumatol* 14:464, 1995.

155. Harris EDJ: Rheumatoid arthritis: pathophysiology and implications for therapy, *N Engl J Med* 322:1277, 1990.

156. Harris P: Cervical spine stenosis, *Paraplegia* 15:125, 1977.

157. Harrison MHM, Schajowicz F, Trueta J: Osteoarthritis of the hip: study of the nature and evolution of the disease, *J Bone Joint Surg Br* 35:598, 1953.

158. Harrison NK et al: Insulin-like growth factor-I is partially responsible for fibroblast proliferation induced by bronchoalveolar lavage fluid from patients with systemic sclerosis, *Clin Sci (Colch)* 86:141, 1994.

159. Havdrup T, Huth A, Telhag H: The subchondral bone in osteoarthritis and rheumatoid arthritis of the knee: a histologic and microradiographical study, *Acta Orthop Scan* 47:345, 1976.

160. Hayes KW: Heat and cold in the management of rheumatoid arthritis, *Arthritis Care Res* 6:156, 1993.

161. Heller CA et al: Value of x-ray examinations of the cervical spine, *BMJ* 287:1276, 1983.

162. Helms CA: CT of the lumbar spine—stenosis and arthrosis, *Comput Radiol* 6:359, 1982.

163. Hendrix RW et al: Fracture of the spine in patients with ankylosis due to diffuse skeletal hyperostosis: clinical and imaging findings, *AJR* 162:899, 1994.

164. Herzog RJ: The radiologic assessment for a lumbar disc herniation, *Spine* 21(suppl 24):19, 1996.

165. Hess EV, Mongey AB: Drug-related lupus, *Bull Rheum Dis* 40:1, 1991.

166. Hickey DS et al: Analysis of magnetic resonance images from normal and degenerated lumbar intervertebral discs, *Spine* 11:702, 1986.

167. Hirohata S, Ohnishi K, Sagawa A: Treatment of systemic lupus erythematosus with lobenzarit: an open clinical trial, *Clin Exp Rheumatol* 12:261, 1994.

168. Hoffman DF: Arthritis and exercise, *Primary Care* 20:895, 1993.

169. Holm S: Pathophysiology of disc degeneration, *Acta Orthop Scand* 64(suppl 251):13, 1993.

170. Huckins D, Felson DT, Holick M: Treatment of psoriatic arthritis with oral 1,25-dihydroxyvitamin D3: a pilot study, *Arthritis Rheum* 33:1723, 1990.

171. Hudgins WR: The predictive value of myelography in the diagnosis of ruptured lumbar disks, *J Neurosurg* 32:152, 1970.

172. Humzah MD, Soames RW: Human intervertebral disc: structure and function, *Anat Rec* 220:337, 1988.

173. Hunter D, McLaughlin AIG, Perry KMA: Clinical effects of the use of pneumatic tools, *Br J Intern Med* 2:10, 1945.

174. Hutter CG: Spinal stenosis and posterior lumbar interbody fusion, *Clin Orthop* 193:103, 1985.

175. Ignaczak T et al: Jaccoud arthritis, *Ann Intern Med* 135:577, 1975.

176. Ihn H et al: Ultrasound measurement of skin thickness in systemic sclerosis, *Br J Rheumatol* 34:535, 1995.

177. Ikeda T et al: Pathomechanism of spontaneous regression of the herniated lumbar disc: histologic and immunohistochemical study, *J Spinal Disord* 9:136, 1996.

178. Iliopoulos AG, Tsokos GC: Immunopathogenesis and spectrum of infections in systemic lupus erythematosus, *Semin Arthritis Rheum* 25:318, 1996.

179. Isomaki HA, Kaarela K, Martio J: Are hand radiographs the most suitable for the diagnosis of rheumatoid arthritis? *Arthritis Rheum* 31:1452, 1988.

180. Ito T, Yamada M, Ikuta F: Histologic evidence of absorption of sequestration-type herniated disc, *Spine* 21:230, 1996.

181. Jaccoud S: Vingt-troisieme leçon, sur une forme de rhumatisme chronique. Leçons de Clinique Medicale faites á l'Hôpital de la Charité, ed 1, Paris, 1867, Adrien Delahaye.

182. Jahnke RW, Hart BL: Cervical stenosis, spondylosis, and herniation disc disease, *Radiol Clin North Am* 29:777, 1991.

183. Jenkins JPR et al: MR imaging of the intervertebral disc: a quantitative study, *J Bone Joint Surg Br* 58:705, 1985.

184. Jensen MC et al: Magnetic resonance imaging of the lumbar spine in people without back pain, *N Engl J Med* 331:69, 1994.

185. Jimenez-Balderas FJ, Mintz G: Ankylosing spondylitis: clinical course in women and men, *J Rheumatol* 20:2069, 1993.

186. Johnson JJ, Leonard-Segal A, Nashel DJ: Jaccoud's-type arthropathy: an association with malignancy, *J Rheumatol* 16:1278, 1989.

187. Jones RAC, Thomson JLG: The narrow lumbar canal: a clinical and radiological review, *J Bone Joint Surg Br* 50:595, 1968.

188. Jones SM, Bhalla AK: Osteoporosis in rheumatoid arthritis, *Clin Exp Rheumatol* 11:557, 1993.

189. Kahaleh B: Immunologic aspects of scleroderma, *Curr Opin Rheumatol* 5:760, 1993.

190. Kahn MS: Pathogenesis of ankylosing spondylitis, *J Rheumatol* 20:1273, 1993.

191. Kamakura K et al: Cervical radiculomyelopathy due to calcified ligamenta flava, *Ann Neurol* 5:193, 1979.

192. Karlins NL, Yagan R: Dyspnea and hoarseness. A complication of diffuse idiopathic skeletal hyperostosis, *Spine* 16:235, 1991.

193. Kauppi M et al: Pathogenetic mechanism and prevalence of the stable atlantoaxial subluxation in rheumatoid arthritis, *J Rheumatol* 23:831, 1996.

194. Kawano N, Yoshida S, Ohwada T: Cervical radiculomyelopathy caused by deposition of calcium pyrophosphate dihydrate crystals in the ligamenta flava, *J Neurosurg* 52:279, 1980.

195. Keat A, Thomas BJ, Taylor-Robinson D: Chlamydial infection in the aetiology of arthritis, *Br Med Bull* 39:168, 1983.

196. Keat A: Reiter's syndrome and reactive arthritis in perspective, *N Engl J Med* 309:1606, 1983.

197. Kelly WL: *Textbook of rheumatology*, Philadelphia, 1997, WB Saunders.

198. Kelsey JL, Golden AL, Mundt DJ: Low back pain/prolapsed lumbar intervertebral disc, *Rheum Dis Clin North Am* 16:699, 1990.

199. Khan MA, van der Linden SM: Ankylosing spondylitis and other spondyloarthropathies, *Rheum Dis Clin North Am* 16:551, 1990.

200. Kieffer SA, Cacayorin ED, Sherry RG: The radiological diagnosis of herniated lumbar intervertebral disc: a current controversy, *JAMA* 251:1192, 1984.

201. Kieffer SA et al: Bulging lumbar intervertebral disc: myelographic differentiation from herniated disc with nerve root compression, *AJR* 138:709, 1982.

202. Kim KY et al: MRI classification of lumbar herniated intervertebral disc, *Orthopedics* 15:493, 1992.

203. Kimori H et al: The natural history of herniated nucleus pulposus with radiculopathy, *Spine* 21:225, 1996.

204. Kindyns P et al: Osteophytes of the knee. Anatomic, radiologic, and pathologic investigation, *Radiology* 174:841, 1990.

205. Kirkaldy-Willis WH, Cassidy JD: Spinal manipulation in the treatment of low-back pain, *Can Fam Physician* 31:535, 1975.

206. Kirkaldy-Willis WH et al: Lumbar spinal stenosis, *Clin Orthop* 99:30, 1974.

207. Kirkaldy-Willis WH et al: Pathology and pathogenesis of lumbar spondylosis and stenosis, *Spine* 3:319, 1978.

208. Kirkaldy-Willis WH: The relationship of structural pathology to the nerve root, *Spine* 9:49, 1984.

209. Klipper AR et al: Ischemic necrosis of bone in systemic lupus erythematosus, *Medicine* 55:251, 1976.

210. Kohli M, Bennett RM: Sacroiliitis in systemic lupus erythematosus, *J Rheumatol* 21:170, 1994.

211. Kubota M, Baba I, Sumida T: Myelopathy due to ossification of the ligamentum flavum of the cervical spine. A report of two cases, *Spine* 6:553, 1981.

212. Kuo P, Loh Z: Treatment of lumbar intervertebral disc protrusion by manipulation, *Clin Orthop* 215:47, 1987.

213. Labowitz R, Schumacher HR Jr: Articular manifestations of systemic lupus erythematosus, *Ann Intern Med* 74:911, 1971.

214. Laman SD, Provost TT: Cutaneous manifestations of lupus erythematosus, *Rheum Dis Clin North Am* 20:195, 1994.

215. Lane NE et al: Long-distance running, bone density, and osteoarthritis, *JAMA* 255:1147, 1986.

216. Lane NE: Exercise: a cause of osteoarthritis, *J Rheumatol Suppl* 43:3, 1995.

217. Lane NE: Physical activity at leisure and risk of osteoarthritis, *Ann Rheum Dis* 55:682, 1996.

218. Laroche M et al: Lumbar and cervical stenosis. Frequency of the association, role of the ankylosing hyperostosis, *Clin Rheumatol* 11:533, 1992.

219. Lauhio A et al: Double-blind, placebo-controlled study of three-month treatment with lymecycline in reactive arthritis, with special reference to chlamydia arthritis, *Arthritis Rheum* 34:6, 1991.

220. Laurent-Haupt L, Westmark KD: Long-standing ankylosing spondylitis with back pain, *Rheum Dis Clin North Am* 17:813, 1991.

221. Lawrence JS, Bremner JM, Bier F: Osteoarthrosis: prevalence in the population and relationship between symptoms and x-ray changes, *Ann Rheum Dis* 25:1, 1966.

222. Lee P: Clinical aspects of systemic and localized sclerosis, *Curr Opin Rheumatol* 5:785, 1993.

223. Lee SH, Coleman PE, Hahn FL: Magnetic resonance imaging of degenerative disc disease of the spine, *Radiol Clin of North Am* 26:949, 1988.

224. Leirisalo-Repo M: Enteropathic arthritis, Whipple's disease, juvenile spondyloarthropathy, and uveitis, *Curr Opin Rheumatol* 6:385, 1994.

225. Lestini WF, Wiesel SW: The pathogenesis of cervical spondylosis, *Clin Orthop* 239:69, 1989.

226. Lisse JR: Does rheumatoid factor always mean arthritis? *Postgrad Med* 94:133, 1993.

227. Littlejohn GO, Smythe HA: Marked hyperinsulinemia after glucose challenge in patients with diffuse idiopathic skeletal hyperostosis, *J Rheumatol* 8:965, 1981.

228. Loebl DH et al: Psoriatic arthritis, *JAMA* 42:2447, 1979.

229. Long DM: Decision making in lumbar disc disease, *Clin Neurosurg* 39:36, 1992.

230. Lukoschek M et al: Synovial membrane and cartilage changes in experimental osteoarthritis, *J Orthop Res* 6:475, 1988.

231. Magaro M et al: Generalized osteoporosis in non-steroid treated rheumatoid arthritis, *Rheumatol Int* 11:73, 1991.

232. Maisiak R et al: The effect of person-centered counseling on the psychological status of persons with systemic lupus erythematosus or rheumatoid arthritis: a randomized, controlled trial, *Arthritis Care Res* 9:60, 1996.

233. Manelfe C: Imaging of degenerative processes of the spine, *Curr Opin Radiol* 4:63, 1992.

234. Mankin HJ, Brandt KD, Shulman LE: Workshop on etiopathogenesis of osteoarthritis, *J Rheumtol* 13:1130, 1986.

235. Mankin HJ, Treadwell BV: Osteoarthritis: a 1987 update, *Bull Rheum Dis* 36:1, 1986.

236. Manthorpe R et al: Jaccoud's syndrome. A nosographic entity associated with systemic lupus erythematosus, *J Rheumatol* 7:169, 1980.

237. Marchiori DM, Henderson CNR: A cross-sectional study correlating cervical radiographic degenerative findings to pain and disability, *Spine* 21:2747, 1996.

238. Marchiori DM et al: A comparison of radiographic signs of degeneration to corresponding MRI signal intensities in the lumbar spine, *J Manipulative Physiol Ther* 17:238, 1994.

239. Marchiori DM: A survey of radiographic impressions on a selected chiropractic patient population, *J Manipulative Physiol Ther* 19:109, 1996.

240. Marshall JL: Periarticular osteophytes, *Clin Orthop* 62:37, 1969.

241. Martel W et al: Radiologic features of Reiter's disease, *Radiology* 132:1, 1979.

242. Martel W, Hayes JT, Diff IF: The pattern of bone erosion in the hand and wrist in rheumatoid arthritis, *Radiology* 84:206, 1965.

243. Martinelli TA, Wiesel SW: Epidemiology of spinal stenosis, *Instr Course Lect* 41:179, 1992.

244. Martini A et al: Systemic lupus erythematosus with Jaccoud's arthropathy mimicking juvenile rheumatoid arthritis, *Arthritis Rheum* 30:1062, 1987.

245. Masaryk TJ et al: Effects of chemonucleolysis demonstrated by MR imaging, *J Comput Assist Tomogr* 10:917, 1986.

246. Masaryk TJ et al: High-resolution MR imaging of sequestered lumbar intervertebral disks, *AJNR* 150:1155, 1988.

247. Massardo L et al: Clinical expression of rheumatoid arthritis in Chilean patients, *Semin Arthritis Rheum* 25:203, 1995.

248. Matsubara Y et al: Serial changes on MRI in lumbar disc herniations treated conservatively, *Neuroradiology* 37:378, 1995.

249. Mavrikakis M et al: Optic neuritis and Jaccoud's syndrome in a patient with systemic lupus erythematosus, *Scand J Rheum* 12:367, 1983.

250. Mayes MD et al: Epidemiology of scleroderma in Detroit tricounty area 1989-1991: prevalence, incidence, and survival rates. Proceedings of the American College of Rheumatology meeting, Orlando, Florida, 1996.

251. Mazzuca SA et al: Therapeutic strategies distinguish community based primary care physicians from rheumatologists in the management of osteoarthritis, *Br J Rheumatol* 20:80, 1993.

252. McAfee PC, Regan JJ, Bohlman HH: Cervical cord compression from ossification of the posterior longitudinal ligament in non-orientals, *J Bone Joint Surg Br* 89:569, 1987.

253. McCafferty RR et al: Ossification of the anterior longitudinal ligament and Forestier's disease: an analysis of seven cases, *J Neurosurg* 83:13, 1995.

254. McCormack BM, Weinstein PR: Cervical spondylosis. An update, *West J Med* 165:43, 1996.

255. McFadden JW: The stress lumbar discogram, *Spine* 13:931, 1988.

256. McHugh NJ et al: Anti-topoisomerase I in silica-associated systemic sclerosis. A model for autoimmunity, *Arthritis Rheum* 37:1198, 1994.

257. Medsger TA Jr: Epidemiology of systemic sclerosis, *Clin Dermatol* 12:207, 1994.

258. Medsger TA Jr: Treatment of systemic sclerosis, *Ann Rheum Dis* 50:877, 1991.

259. Michet CJ: Osteoarthritis, *Arthritis* 20:815, 1993.

260. Migliaresi S et al: Avascular osteonecrosis in patients with SLE: relation to corticosteroid therapy and anticardiolipin antibodies, *Lupus* 3:37, 1994.

261. Miller FH, Roger LF: Fractures of the dens complicating ankylosing spondylitis with atlantooccipital fusion, *J Rheumatol* 18:771, 1991.

262. Miller JAA, Schmatz C, Schultz AB: Lumbar disc degeneration: correlation with age, sex, and spine level in 600 autopsy specimens, *Spine* 13:173, 1988.

263. Modic MT, Herfkens RJ: Intervertebral disk: normal age-related changes in MR signal intensity, *Radiology* 177:332, 1990.

264. Modic MT et al: Imaging of degenerative disk disease, *Radiology* 168:177, 1988.

265. Modic MT et al: Lumbar herniated disk disease and canal stenosis: prospective evaluation by surface coil MR, CT, and myelography, *AJNR* 7:709, 1986.

266. Modic MT et al: Magnetic resonance imaging of intervertebral disc disease, *Radiology* 152:103, 1984.

267. Modic MT et al: Degenerative disk disease: assessment of changes in vertebral body marrow with MR imaging, *Radiology* 166:193, 1988.

268. Modic MT et al: Nuclear magnetic resonance imaging of the spine, *Radiology* 148:757, 1983.

269. Mooney V, Robertson J: The facet syndrome, *Clin Orthop* 115:149, 1976.

270. Mooney V: When is surgery appropriate for patients with low back pain? *J Musculoskeletal Med* 7:61, 1990.

271. Moreland LW, Lopez-Mendez A, Alarcon GS: Spinal stenosis: a comprehensive review of the literature, *Semin Arthritis Rheum* 19:127, 1989.

272. Morgan DF, Young RF: Spinal neurological complications of achondroplasia. Results of surgical treatment, *J Neurosurg* 52:463, 1980.

273. Morita A et al: Successful treatment of systemic sclerosis with topical PUVA, *J Rheumatol* 22:2361, 1995.

274. Moro C et al: Jaccoud's arthropathy in patients with chronic rheumatic valvular heart disease, *Eur J Cardiol* 6:459, 1978.

275. Morris R et al: HL-A-B27 a useful discriminator in the arthropathies of inflammatory bowel disease, *N Engl J Med* 290:1117, 1974.

276. Moskowitz RW: Primary osteoarthritis: epidemiology, clinical aspects, and general management, *Am J Med* 83:5, 1987.

277. Murakami J et al: Computed tomography of posterior longitudinal ligament ossification: its appearance and diagnostic value with special reference to thoracic lesions, *J Comput Tomogr* 6:41, 1982.

278. Myllykangas-Luosujarvi RA, Aho K, Isomaki A: Mortality in rheumatoid arthritis, *Semin Arthritis Rheum* 25:193, 1995.

279. Nakanishi T et al: Symptomatic ossification of the posterior longitudinal ligament of the cervical spine, *Neurology* 24:1139, 1974.

280. Nalebuff EA: Surgery of systemic lupus erythematosus arthritis of the hand, *Hand Clin* 12:591, 1996.

281. Naparstek Y, Plotz PH: The role of autoantibodies in autoimmune disease, *Annu Rev Immunol* 11:79, 1993.

282. Newman PH: Stenosis of the lumbar spine in spondylolisthesis, *Clin Orthop* 115:116, 1976.

283. Ng SC, Clements PJ, Paulus HE: Management of systemic sclerosis—a review, *Singapore Med J* 31:269, 1990.

284. Niepel GA, Sitaj S: Enthesopathy, *Clin Rheum Dis* 5:857, 1979.

285. Nose T et al: Ossification of the posterior longitudinal ligament: a clinio-radiological study of 74 cases, *J Neurol Neurosurg Psych* 50:321, 1987.

286. Nwuga VCB: Relative therapeutic efficacy of vertebral manipulation and conventional treatment in back pain management, *Am J Phys Med* 61:273, 1982.

287. O'Donnell JL, O'Donnell AL: Prostaglandin E₂ content in herniated lumbar disc disease, *Spine* 21:1653, 1996.

288. Olive A et al: Air in the oesophagus: a sign of oesophageal involvement in systemic sclerosis, *Clin Rheumatol* 14:319, 1995.

289. Ostlere SJ, Seeger LL, Eckhardt JJ: Subchondral cysts of the tibia secondary to osteoarthritis of the knee, *Skeletal Radiol* 19:287, 1990.

290. Paajanen H et al: Magnetic resonance study of disc degeneration in young low back pain patients, *Spine* 14:982, 1989.

291. Paine KWE: Clinical features of lumbar spinal stenosis, *Clin Orthop* 29:315, 1976.

292. Paley D et al: Fractures of the spine in diffuse idiopathic skeletal hyperostosis, *Clin Orthop* 267:22, 1991.

293. Palumbo MA, Lucas P, Akelman E: Lumbar spinal stenosis: a review, *Rhode Island Med* 78:321, 1995.

294. Panangiotacopulos ND et al: Water content in human intervertebral discs, *Spine* 12:912, 1987.

295. Panayi GS, Clark B: Minocycline in the treatment of patients with Reiter's syndrome, *Clin Exp Rheumatol* 7:100, 1989.

296. Panayi GS: The pathogenesis of rheumatoid arthritis and the development of therapeutic strategies for the clinical investigation of biologics, *Agents Actions Suppl* 47:1, 1995.

297. Panayi GS: Immunology of psoriasis and psoriatic arthritis, *Baillieres Clin Rheumatol* 8:419, 1994.

298. Panichewa S, Chitrabamrung S, Vatanasuk M: Hand deformities in a patient with chronic lung disease: Jaccoud's arthropathy, *Clin Rheumatol* 2:65, 1983.

299. Park WM et al: The detection of spinal pseudoarthrosis in ankylosing spondylitis, *Br J Radiol* 54:467, 1981.

300. Pastershank SP, Resnick D: "Hook" erosions in Jaccoud's arthropathy, *J Can Assoc Radiol* 31:174, 1980.

301. Patriquin HB, Camerlain M, Trias A: Late sequelae of juvenile rheumatoid arthritis of the hip: a follow-up study into adulthood, *Pediatr Radiol* 14:151, 1984.

302. Patton JT: Differential diagnosis of inflammatory spondylitis, *Skeletal Radiol* 1:77, 1976.

303. Pearcy MJ: Inferred strains in the intervertebral discs during physiological movements, *J Manual Med* 5:68, 1990.

304. Pech P, Haughton VM: Lumbar intervertebral disk: correlative MR and anatomic study, *Radiology* 156:699, 1985.

305. Peterson HO, Kieffer SA: Radiology of intervertebral disk disease, *Semin Roentgenol* 7:260, 1972.

306. Petri M: Systemic lupus erythematosus and pregnancy, *Rheum Dis Clin North Am* 20:87, 1994.

307. Pinals RS: Polyarthritis and fever, *N Eng J Med* 330:769, 1994.

308. Pincus T, Callahan LF: What is the natural history of rheumatoid arthritis? *Rheum Dis Clin North Am* 19:123, 1993.

309. Pincus T: Long-term outcomes in rheumatoid arthritis, *Br J Rheumatol* 34:59, 1995.

310. Pitzalis C et al: Cutaneous lymphocyte antigen-positive T lymphocytes preferentially migrate to the skin but not to the joint in psoriatic arthritis, *Arthritis Rheum* 39:137, 1996.

311. Poleksic L et al: Magnetic resonance imaging of bone destruction in rheumatoid arthritis: comparison with radiography, *Skeletal Radiol* 22:577, 1993.

312. Porter GG: Psoriatic arthritis. Plain radiology and other imaging techniques, *Baillieres Clin Rheumatol* 8:465, 1994.

313. Porter RW: Pathology of symptomatic lumbar disc protrusion, *J R Coll Surg Edinb* 40:200, 1995.

314. Postacchini F et al: Ligamenta flava in lumbar disc herniation and spinal stenosis, *Spine* 19:917, 1994.

315. Postacchini F: Lumbar spinal stenosis and pseudostenosis, definition, and classification of pathology, *Ital J Orthop Traumatol* 9:339, 1983.

316. Postacchini F: Results of surgery compared with conservative management for lumbar disc herniations, *Spine* 21:1383, 1996.

317. Pottenger LA, Phillips FM, Draganich LF: The effect of marginal osteophytes on reduction of varus-valgus instability in osteoarthritic knee, *Arthritis Rheum* 30:853, 1990.

318. Preidler KW, Resnick D: Imaging of osteoarthritis, *Radiol Clin North Am* 34:259, 1996.

319. Pyeritz RE, Sack GLH, Udvarhely GB: Genetics clinics of the Johns Hopkins Hospital. Surgical intervention in achondroplasia. Cervical and lumbar laminectomy for spinal stenosis in achondroplasia, *Johns Hopkins Med J* 146:203, 1980.

320. Quagliano PV, Hayes CW, Palmer WE: Vertebral pseudoarthrosis associated with diffuse idiopathic skeletal hyperostosis, *Skeletal Radiol* 23:353, 1994.

321. Quencer RM et al: Postoperative bone stenosis of the lumbar spinal canal: evaluation of 164 symptomatic patients with axial radiography, *AJR* 131:1059, 1978.

322. Quinet RJ: Osteoarthritis: increasing mobility and reducing disability, *Geriatrics* 41:36, 1986.

323. Quon JA et al: Lumbar intervertebral disc herniation: treatment by rotational manipulation, *J Manipulative Physiol Ther* 12:220, 1989.

324. Radin EL, Paul IL, Rose RM: Role of mechanical factors in pathogenesis of primary osteoarthritis, *Lancet* 1:519, 1972.

325. Rahman MU, Hudson AP, Schumacher HR: Chlamydia and Reiter's syndrome (reactive arthritis), *Rheum Dis Clin North Am* 18:67, 1992.

326. Rall LC et al: The effect of progressive resistance training in rheumatoid arthritis, *Arthritis Rheum* 39:415, 1996.

327. Ralston SH et al: A new method for the radiological assessment of vertebral squaring in ankylosing spondylitis, *Ann Rheum Dis* 51:330, 1992.

328. Ramos-Remus C, Russell AS: Clinical features and management of ankylosing spondylitis, *Curr Opin Rheumatol* 5:408, 1993.

329. Ramos-Remus C, Russell AS: New clinical and radiographic features of ankylosing spondylitis, *Curr Opin Rheumatol* 4:463, 1992.

330. Rankin JA: Pathophysiology of the rheumatoid joint, *Orthop Nurs* 14:39, 1995.

331. Ravaud P: Quantitative radiography in osteoarthritis: plain radiographs, *Baillieres Clin Rheumatol* 10:409, 1996.

332. Reichlin M: Systemic lupus erythematosus. Antibodies to ribonuclear proteins, *Rheum Dis Clin North Am* 20:29, 1994.

333. Reijnierse M et al: The cervical spine in rheumatoid arthritis: relationship between neurologic signs and morphology on MR imaging and radiographs, *Skeletal Radiol* 25:113, 1996.

334. Reilly PA et al: Arthropathy of hands and feet in systemic lupus erythematosus, *J Rheumatol* 17:777, 1990.

335. Resnick D et al: Association of diffuse idiopathic skeletal hyperostosis (DISH) and calcification and ossification of the posterior longitudinal ligament, *AJR* 131:1049, 1978.

336. Resnick D, Niwayama G: Radiographic and pathologic features of spinal involvement in diffuse idiopathic skeletal hyperostosis (DISH), *Radiology* 119:559, 1976.

337. Resnick D, Williamson S, Alazraki N: Focal spinal abnormalities on bone scans in ankylosing spondylitis, *Clin Nucl Med* 6:213, 1981.

338. Resnick D: Common disorders of synovium-lined joints: pathogenesis, imaging abnormalities, and complications, *AJR* 151:1079, 1988.

339. Resnick D: Degenerative diseases of the vertebral column, *Radiology* 156:3, 1985.

340. Resnick D: *Diagnosis of bone and joint disorders,* ed 3, Philadelphia, 1995, WB Saunders.

341. Riihimaki H: Low-back pain: its origin and risk indicators, *Scand J Work Environ Health* 17:81, 1991.

342. Rothschild BM et al: Inflammatory sacroiliac joint pathology: evaluation of radiologic assessment techniques, *Clin Exp Rheumatol* 12:267, 1994.

343. Rovetta G, Bianchi G, Monteforte P: Joint failure in erosive osteoarthritis of the hands, *Int J Tissue React* 17:33, 1995.

344. Rowe LJ: The split vertebral body: a pseudofracture, *J Austral Chiro Assoc* 29:5, 1990.

345. Ruzicka T: Psoriatic arthritis. New types, new treatments, *Arch Dermatol* 132:215, 1996.

346. Saal JA, Saal JS, Herzog RJ: The natural history of lumbar intervertebral disc extrusions treated non-operatively, *Spine* 15:683, 1990.

347. Saal JA: Natural history and nonoperative treatment of lumbar disc herniations, *Spine* 21(suppl 24):2, 1996.

348. Sack KE: Osteoarthritis. A continuing challenge, *West J Med* 163:579, 1995.

349. Sattar MA, Guindi RT, Sugathan TN: Penicillamine in systemic sclerosis: a reappraisal, *Clin Rheumatol* 9:517, 1990.

350. Schaller JG: Chronic arthritis in children. Juvenile rheumatoid arthritis, *Clin Orthop* 182:79, 1984.

351. Schiebler ML et al: Normal and degenerated intervertebral disk: in vivo and in vitro MR imaging with histopathologic correlation, *AJR* 157:93, 1991.

352. Schlapbach P et al: Diffuse idiopathic skeletal hyperostosis of the spine: a cause of back pain? *Br J Rheumatol* 28:299, 1989.

353. Schneiderman G et al: Magnetic resonance imaging in the diagnosis of disc degeneration: correlation with discography, *Spine* 12:276, 1987.

354. Schonstrom NS, Bolender NF, Spengler DM: The pathomorphology of spinal stenosis as seen on CT scans of the lumbar spine, *Spine* 10:806, 1985.

355. Schwab EP et al: Pulmonary alveolar hemorrhage in systemic lupus erythematosus, *Semin Arthritis Rheum* 23:8, 1993.

356. Scutellari PN, Orzincolo C, Castaldi G: Association between diffuse idiopathic skeletal hyperostosis and multiple myeloma, *Skeletal Radiol* 24:489, 1995.

357. Senstad O, Leboeuf-Yde C, Borchgrevink C: Frequency and characteristics of side effects of spinal manipulative therapy, *Spine* 22:435, 1997.

358. Sequeira W: The neuropathic joint, *Clin Exp Rheumatol* 12:325, 1994.

359. Sether LA, Yu S, Haughton VM: Intervertebral disk: normal age-related changes in MR signal intensity, *Radiology* 177:385, 1990.

360. Shapiro R, Balt H: Unilateral thoracic spondylosis, *AJR* 83:660, 1960.

361. Sharma S et al: Spinal stenosis: diagnosis and management—a clinical and radiological study, *Int Surg* 67:565, 1982.

362. Sharp JT: Radiologic assessment as an outcome measure in rheumatoid arthritis, *Arthritis Rheum* 32:221, 1989.

363. Sheehan S, Bauer R, Meyer J: Vertebral artery compression in cervical spondylosis, *Neurology* 10:968, 1960.

364. Shekelle P, et al: Spinal manipulation for low back pain, *BMJ* 117:590, 1992.

365. Sholkoff SD, Glickman MG, Steinbach HL: Roentgenology of Reiter's syndrome, *Radiology* 97:497, 1970.

366. Short CL, Bauer W, Reynolds WE: Rheumatoid arthritis, Cambridge, Mass, 1957, Harvard University Press.

367. Shumacher TM et al: HLA-B27 associated arthropathies, *Radiology* 126:289, 1978.

368. Siam AR, Hammoudeh M: Jaccoud's arthropathy of the shoulders in systemic lupus erythematosus, *J Rheumatol* 19:980, 1992.

369. Simkin PA: Simian stance: a sign of spinal stenosis, *Lancet* 2:652, 1982.

370. Singsen BH: Rheumatic diseases of childhood, *Rheum Dis Clin North Am* 16:581, 1990.

371. Sjogren RW: Gastrointestinal motility disorders in scleroderma, *Arthritis Rheum* 37:1265, 1994.

372. Slemenda CW: The epidemiology of osteoarthritis of the knee, *Curr Opin Rheumatol* 4:546, 1992.

373. Smoker WRK et al: The role of MR imaging in evaluating metastatic spinal disease, *AJNR* 8:901, 1987.

374. Spector TD: The fat on the joint. Osteoarthritis and obesity, *J Rheumatol* 17:284, 1990.

375. Spector TD: Rheumatoid arthritis, *Rheum Dis Clin North Am* 16:513, 1990.

376. Spengler DM: Degenerative stenosis of the lumbar spine, *J Bone Joint Surg Am* 69:305, 1987.

377. Spilberg I: Current concepts of the mechanism of acute inflammation in gouty arthritis, *Arthritis Rheum* 18:129, 1975.

378. Starz TW, Miller EB: Diagnosis and treatment of rheumatoid arthritis, *Primary Care* 20:827, 1993.

379. Steen VD et al: Twenty-year incidence survey of systemic sclerosis, *Arthritis Rheum* 31(suppl):57, 1988.

380. Steen VD: Systemic sclerosis, *Rheum Dis Clin North Am* 16:641, 1990.

381. Stewart AL et al: Functional status and well-being of patients with chronic conditions. Results from the Medical Outcomes Study, *JAMA* 262:907, 1989.

382. Sukenik S et al: Jaccoud's-type arthropathy: an association with sarcoidosis, *J Rheumatol* 18:915, 1991.

383. Summers MN et al: Radiographic assessment and psychologic variables as predictors of pain and functional impairment in osteoarthritis of the knee or hip, *Arthritis Rheum* 31:204, 1988.

384. Swedberg JA, Steinbauer JR: Osteoarthritis, *Am Fam Physician* 45:557, 1992.

385. Swezey RL: Pathophysiology and treatment of intervertebral disk disease, *Rheum Dis Clin North Am* 19:741, 1993.

386. Szczepanski L, Targonska B, Piotrowski M: Deforming arthropathy and Jaccoud's syndrome in patients with systemic lupus erythematosus, *Scand J Rheumatol* 21:308, 1992.

387. Takehara K, Soma Y, Ishibashi Y: Early detection of scleroderma spectrum disorders in patients with Raynaud's phenomenon, *Dermatologica* 183:164, 1991.

388. Tangrea JA et al: Skeletal hyperostosis in patients receiving chronic, very low-dose isotretinoin, *Arch Dermatol* 128:921, 1992.

389. Taylor HG et al: The relationship of clinical and laboratory measurements to radiological change in ankylosing spondylitis, *Br J Rheumatol* 30:330, 1991.

390. Taylor JR, Twomey LT: Age changes in lumbar zygopophyseal joints. Observations on structure and function, *Spine* 11:739, 1986.

391. Taylor JR: The development and adult structure of lumbar intervertebral discs, *J Manual Med* 5:43, 1990.

392. Teplick JG, Haskin ME: Spontaneous regression of herniated nucleus pulposus, *AJR* 145:371, 1985.

393. Teresi LM et al: Asymptomatic degenerative disc disease and spondylosis of the cervical spine: MR imaging, *Radiology* 164:83, 1987.

394. Tishler M, Yaron M: Jaccoud's arthropathy and psoriatis arthritis, *Clin Exp Rheumatol* 11:663, 1993.

395. Tokuda M et al: Effect of low-dose cyclosporin A on systemic lupus erythematosus disease activity, *Arthritis Rheum* 37:551, 1994.

396. Torres MA, Furst DE: Treatment of generalized systemic sclerosis, *Rheum Dis Clin North Am* 16:2217, 1990.

397. Tsang IK: Update on osteoarthritis, *Can Fam Physician* 36:539, 1990.

398. Twigg HL, Smith BF: Jaccoud's arthritis, *Radiology* 80:417, 1963.

399. Twomey L, Taylor TR: Structural and mechanical disc changes with age, *J Manual Med* 5:58, 1990.

400. van der Heijde DMFM et al: Biannual radiographic assessments of hands and feet in a three-year prospective follow-up of patients with early rheumatoid arthritis, *Arthritis Rheum* 35:26, 1992.

401. van der Heijde DMFM: Joint erosions and patients with early rheumatoid arthritis, *Br J Rheumatol* 34:74, 1995.

402. van der Linden SF et al: The risk of developing ankylosing spondylitis in HLA-B27 positive individuals, *Arthritis Rheum* 27:241, 1984.

403. Van Saase JL et al: Epidemiology of osteoarthritis: Zoetermeer survey. Comparison of radiological osteoarthritis in a Dutch population with that of 10 other populations, *Ann Rheum Dis* 48:271, 1989.

404. Van Schaardenburg D, Breedveld FC: Elderly-onset rheumatoid arthritis, *Semin Arthritis Rheum* 23:367, 1994.

405. Van Vollenhoven RF, McGuire JL: Estrogen, progesterone, and testosterone: can they be used to treat autoimmune diseases? *Cleve Clin J Med* 61:276, 1994.

406. van Zeben D, Breedveld FC: Prognostic factors in rheumatoid arthritis, *J Rheumatol* 23:31, 1996.

407. Veidlinger OF et al: Cervical myelopathy and its relationship to cervical stenosis, *Spine* 6:551, 1981.

408. Veys EM, Mielants H: Current concepts in psoriatic arthritis, *Dermatology* 189:35, 1994.

409. Vezyroglow G et al: A metabolic syndrome in diffuse idiopathic skeletal hyperostosis. A controlled study, *J Rheumatol* 23:672, 1996.

410. Viitanen JV et al: Correlation between mobility restrictions and radiologic changes in ankylosing spondylitis, *Spine* 20:492, 1995.

411. Vincelette P, Laurin CA, Levesque HP: The footballer's ankle and foot, *Can Med Assoc* 107:872, 1972.

412. Virgin WJ: Experimental investigations into the physical properties of the intervertebral disc, *J Bone Joint Surg Br* 33:607, 1951.

413. Vlok GJ, Hendrix MR: The lumbar disc: evaluating the causes of pain, *Orthopedics* 14:419, 1991.

414. Walden CA et al: Case report 620. Progressive systemic sclerosis (PSS) with paraspinous and intraspinous calcifications, *Skeletal Radiol* 19:377, 1990.

415. Warnick C, Sherman MS, Lesser RW: Aspiration pneumonia due to diffuse cervical hyperostosis, *Chest* 98:763, 1990.

416. Weber H: The natural history of disc herniation and the influence of intervention, *Spine* 19:2234, 1994.

417. Weidenbaum M et al: Correlating magnetic resonance imaging with the biochemical content of the normal human intervertebral disc, *J Orthop* 10:552, 1992.

418. Weinberger A, Kaplan JG, Myers AR: Extensive soft tissue calcification (calcinosis universalis) in systemic lupus erythematosus, *Ann Rheum Dis* 38:384, 1979.

419. Weinstein JN, Rydevik BL, Sonntag VKH: *Essentials of the spine,* New York, 1995, Raven Press.

420. Weissman BN: Juvenile rheumatoid arthritis. In Feldman F, editor: Radiology, pathology, and immunology of bones and joints: a review of current concepts, New York, 1978, Appleton-Century-Croft.

421. Weisz GM: Lumbar spinal canal stenosis in Paget's disease, *Spine* 8:192, 1983.

422. Weyand CM, Goronzy JJ: Inherited and noninherited risk factors in rheumatoid arthritis, *Curr Opin Rheumatol* 7:206, 1995.

423. Wilhelmi G: Potential influence of nutrition with supplements on healthy and arthritic joints, *J Rheumatol* 52:191, 1993.

424. Wilkin E et al: Osteoarthritis and articular chondrocalcinosis in the elderly, *Ann Rheum Dis* 42:280, 1983.

425. Wilkinson HA, LeMay ML, Ferris EJ: Roentgenographic correlations in cervical spondylosis, *AJR* 105:370, 1969.

426. Williams RC: Rheumatoid arthritis: using laboratory tests in diagnosis and follow-up, *J Musculoskel Med* 13:14, 1996.

427. Wilson FM, Jaspan T: Thoracic spinal cord compression caused by diffuse idiopathic skeletal hyperostosis (DISH), *Clin Radiol* 42:133, 1990.

428. Wiltse LL, Kirkaldy-Willis WH, Melvor GWD: The treatment of spinal stenosis, *Clin Orthop* 115:83, 1976.

429. Wiltse LL: The effect of the common anomalies of the lumbar spine upon disc degeneration and low back pain, *Orthop Clin North Am* 2:569, 1971.

430. Yang BY et al: Calcium pyrophosphate dihydrate crystal deposition disease: frequency of tendon calcification about the knee, *J Rheumatol* 23:883, 1996.

431. Yates DAH: Spinal stenosis, *J R Soc Med* 74:334, 1981.

432. Yelin E: Impact of musculoskeletal conditions on the elderly, *Geriatr Med Today* 8:103, 1989.

433. Ytterberg SR, Mahowald ML, Krug HE: Exercise for arthritis, *Baillieres Clin Rheumatol* 8:161, 1994.

434. Yu S et al: Progressive and regressive changes in the nucleus pulposus, *Radiology* 169:93, 1988.

435. Yu S et al: Tears of the annulus fibrosus: correlation between MR and pathologic findings in cadavers, *AJNR* 9:367, 1988.

436. Yusof ZB, Pratap RC: Cervical cord compression due to ossified posterior longitudinal ligament associated with difuse idiopathic skeletal hyperostosis, *Aust N Z J Med* 29:697, 1990.

437. Zdeblick TA: The treatment of degenerative lumbar disorders, *Spine* 20(suppl 24):126S, 1995.

chapter 12

Trauma

DENNIS M MARCHIORI
*with content expertise from Ian D McLean**

Imaging
Battered Child Syndrome
Bone, Joint, and Soft Tissue Trauma

Myositis Ossificans
Osteochondritis Dissecans

Slipped Capital Femoral Epiphysis
Spondylolisthesis

This chapter reviews trauma to the skeleton, particularly bone and joint trauma. Most of the tables list fractures and soft tissue injuries categorized by body region. Also presented are other topics related to trauma, such as battered child syndrome, spondylolisthesis, and osteochondritis dissecans.

Imaging

Imaging of skeletal trauma is dominated by plain film radiology. However, magnetic resonance imaging (MRI) is indicated if any of the following situations occur: a significant soft tissue component is suspected, visualization of bone marrow is needed, or neurological findings are present. In addition, computed tomography (CT) is beneficial for exhibiting complex anatomy of the head and spine. CT provides imaging in an axial plane and is particularly adept at demonstrating cortical bone.

Like CT, MRI provides axial imaging, but in addition, it offers true multidimensional imaging in other planes (i.e., frontal, sagittal). Additional benefits are that MRI is noninvasive and can evaluate a wide range of both intraarticular and extraarticular anatomy. The greatest impact of articular musculoskeletal MRI has been in the evaluation of the knee. In many circumstances, MRI has replaced knee arthrography. It is probably the preferred examination method for patients with symptoms severe enough to warrant arthroscopy.[142] MRI is very accurate in the evaluation of meniscal tears; the diagnostic certainty is approximately 95%, and the likelihood of MRI failing to detect a clinically significant meniscal tear is quite low.[32]

Battered Child Syndrome

BACKGROUND

Battered child syndrome is the result of nonaccidental trauma to children, representing a major cause of morbidity and mortality of children.[54] The abuse is usually inflicted by acquaintances of the parents, stepparents, babysitters, and others responsible for the child's care. The children most frequently abused are stepchildren and handicapped and first-born children. Most victims are younger than 2 years of age,[129] with a reported average age of 16 months.[97]

IMAGING FINDINGS

Although uncommon,[97] the presence of multiple fractures in different stages of healing is a classic radiographic presentation of battered child syndrome. Fractures of the skull, spinous processes, scapula, posterior ribs, and sternum strongly indicate abuse. Metaphyseal fractures are particularly indicative of abuse. Metaphyseal fractures occur as avulsions secondary to twisting action of the distal limb. Two varieties are identified: corner fractures represent small fragments of avulsed immature metaphysis, and bucket-handle fractures represent separation of a circumferential segment of immature metaphysis (Fig. 12-1).[88]

Extreme periosteal reaction is often present. Radionuclide bone scans or skeletal surveys are useful to detect other sites of injury.[78,87,159] Osteogenesis imperfecta, scurvy, syphilis, and other diseases that may mimic the radiographic findings of battered child syndrome are usually differentiated by clinical data and specific radiographic findings.[37]

CLINICAL COMMENTS

Often the reported patient history of trauma is inadequate to explain the presenting injuries. Concurrent burns, bruises, retinal damage, subdural hemorrhages, and other soft tissue injuries may accompany the osseous injuries.

KEY CONCEPTS

- *Classic representation of battered child syndrome is multiple fractures in various stages of healing.*
- *Abused children may have corner and bucket-handle metaphyseal fractures.*
- *Most victims of child abuse are under the age of 2 years.*

Bone, Joint, and Soft Tissue Trauma

BACKGROUND

Bone injuries. Traumatic lesions of the skeleton are common to all ages and patient populations. Traumatic bone insult may be fairly innocuous, manifesting with little more than a bone bruise, or may be severe enough to break the bone, producing a fracture. A fracture is a break in the structural continuity of bone, manifesting

*Special thanks to Ian D. McLean for writing most of the soft tissue entries in the tables. I would also like to thank Murray Solomon for providing editorial comments related to the chapter design.

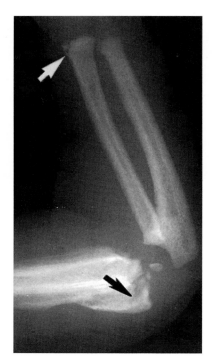

FIG. 12-1   Metaphyseal corner fractures *(arrows)* of differing ages in battered child syndrome. Similar findings may occur in Menkes' syndrome (also called *kinky-hair syndrome*) and in scurvy. (From Sartoris DJ: *Musculoskeletal imaging: the requisites,* St Louis, 1993, Mosby.)

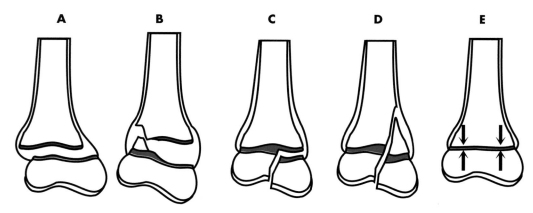

FIG. 12-2   Salter-Harris classification of epiphyseal injuries. **A,** Fracture through the physis. **B,** Fracture through the physis and metaphysis. **C,** Fracture through the physis and epiphysis. **D,** Fracture through the physis, metaphysis, and epiphysis. **E,** Compression injury of the epiphyseal plate.

as minor cracks, crumpling, splintering, or complete disruption of the cortex. If the overlying skin remains intact, the fracture is considered closed (or simple); if the skin is disrupted, the fracture is considered open (or compound).

Fractures develop from a single application of stress outside of the normal range (traumatic, acute, or strain fracture), from repetitive application of stress within the normal range (fatigue or stress fracture) (see Table 12-1, pp. 517-518), or from the single (pathological) or repeated (insufficiency) application of stress within the normal range applied to bone that has been weakened by pathology (e.g., Paget's disease and metastatic bone disease).

Fractures are oriented transverse or oblique to the long axis of the bone. Spiral fractures result from rotational stresses and have an oblique fracture plane that encircles the long axis of the bone. Complete fractures extend through the bone and produce at least two fragments. Those with more than two fragments are termed *comminuted fractures.* Because of the pliability of long bones in children, a fracture may not extend through the entire bone. If one side of

the periosteum remains intact, the fracture is considered incomplete. Incomplete fractures of long bones present with either distraction (greenstick) or impaction (buckle or torus) of the completely fractured cortical side of the bone (see Table 12-2, pp. 519-524).

Reports of a fracture should include the following information: identity of injured bone, location of fracture within the bone, fragment apposition (shift), alignment (tilt), rotation (twist), distraction (separation), and any resulting alteration in limb length. Individual fractures are listed by region in Tables 12-3 through 12-6 (pp. 525-572).

Epiphyseal injuries. Approximately 6% to 15% of long bone fractures occurring in children under 16 years of age involve the epiphysis.[121,138,152] Because the epiphysis is responsible for longitudinal bone growth, this area is particularly susceptible to injury. The distal tibia, fibula, ulna, and radius are the most common sites affected. Several variations of epiphyseal injury have been identified. The Salter-Harris classification is the most widely used system used to describe these injuries (see Table 12-2 and Fig. 12-2).[143]

Text continued on p. 573

TABLE 12-1
Common Stress Fractures[133]

Skeletal location	Related activities or conditions
Calcaneus	Jumping, parachuting, prolonged standing, being recently immobilized

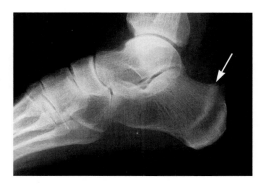

Radiodense line traversing the posterior portion of the calcaneus, representing a stress fracture (arrow).

Cervical and thoracic vertebrae (spinous processes)	Shoveling clay or coal
Femur (shaft and neck)	Ballet dancing, long distance running, marching, performing gymnastics

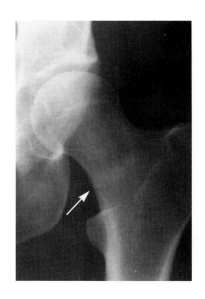

Radiodense line indicating stress fracture oriented parallel to the intertrochanteric line/crest (arrow). (Courtesy Joseph W. Howe, Sylmar, Calif.)

Fibula (shaft)	Long distance running, jumping, parachuting
Hamate (hook)	Golfing, playing racquet sports, swinging a baseball bat
Humerus (distal shaft)	Throwing a ball, using a pitchfork, propelling self in wheelchair
Lumbar vertebrae (pars interarticularis)	Ballet dancing, lifting, scrubbing floors
Metatarsal shaft	Marching, prolonged standing, ballet dancing
Navicular	Marching, long distance running
Patella	Hurdling
Pelvis (obturator ring)	Stooping, bowling, performing gymnastics

Continued

TABLE 12-1
Common Stress Fractures[133]—cont'd

Skeletal location	Related activities or conditions
Ribs	Carrying a heavy pack, golfing, coughing

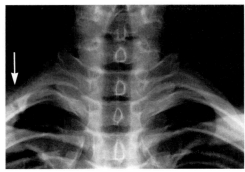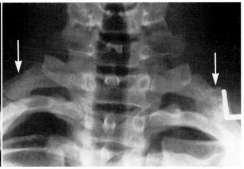

A, Stress fracture of the right first rib *(arrow).* **B,** Bilateral first rib stress fractures *(arrows)* in an elite powerlifter secondary to repetitive trauma related to the squatting lift (front squats).

Skeletal location	Related activities or conditions
Scapulae (coracoid process)	Trapshooting
Sesamoid bones	Prolonged standing
Tibia (shaft)	Long distance running

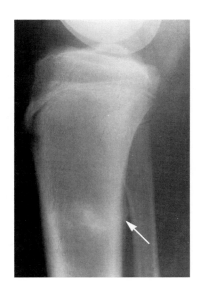

Radiodense line indicating stress fracture extending into the posterior aspect of the proximal tibia *(arrow).* (Courtesy Joseph W. Howe, Sylmar, Calif.)

Skeletal location	Related activities or conditions
Ulna (coronoid process)	Throwing a ball, using a pitchfork, propelling a wheelchair by person in the wheelchair

TABLE 12-2
Fractures: Descriptive Terminology

Type of fracture or related condition	Comments
Avulsion fracture	Fracture in which ligament or tendon is pulled from the bone at the attachment, taking a small bone fragment with it; the fragments are often highly serrated

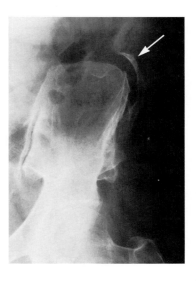

Old avulsion fracture of the iliac crest with fingerlike appearance of avulsed fragment *(arrow)*. (Courtesy Steven P. Brownstein, Springfield, NJ.)

Closed (simple) fracture	Fracture that does not penetrate the skin
Comminuted fracture	Fracture that has more than two fragments; a butterfly fragment describes a triangular-shaped bone fragment split from one of the main fragments

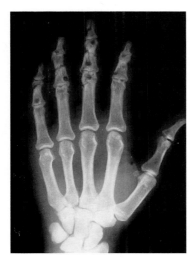

Multiple comminuted fractures of the phalanges secondary to a crush injury from a steel press. (Courtesy Steven P. Brownstein, Springfield, NJ.)

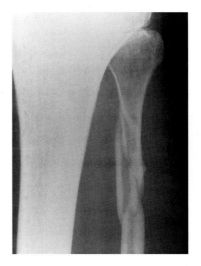

Comminuted fracture of the proximal fibula. (Courtesy Joseph W. Howe, Sylmar, Calif.)

Continued

TABLE 12-2
Fractures: Descriptive Terminology—cont'd

Type of fracture or related condition	Comments
Complicated fracture	Fracture that is accompanied by such complications as damage to nerves, vessels, and viscera
Corner (chip) fracture	Fracture in which the fragment originates from articular margin

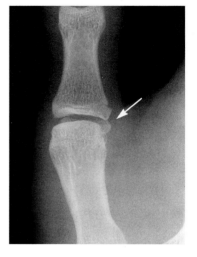

Small corner fracture of the proximal phalanx of the first digit *(arrow)*.

Diastatic fracture	Fracture that is a separation injury of synarthrodial joints (i.e., pubic symphysis, proximal and distal tibiofibular joints)
Epiphyseal (Salter-Harris) fracture	Fracture that involves the epiphyses of long bones
Type I	Fracture that involves separation of the entire growth plate and epiphysis from the metaphysis
Type II	Fracture that involves separation of the entire growth plate and epiphysis with the additional separation of a small fragment of the metaphysis (Thurston-Holland fragment), which remains in contact with the epiphyseal plate

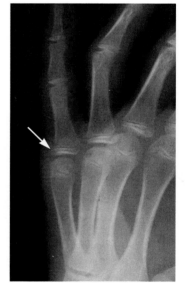

Type II Salter-Harris injury to the proximal epiphyseal plate of the proximal phalanx of the fifth digit *(arrow)*. Note the metaphyseal fragment that remains in contact with the growth plate. (Courtesy Steven P. Brownstein, Springfield, NJ.)

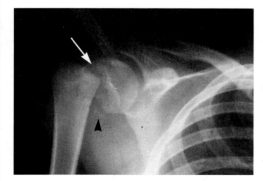

Type II Salter-Harris injury to the proximal humerus *(arrow)*. Note the metaphyseal fragment that remains in contact with the growth plate *(arrowhead)*.

TABLE 12-2

Fractures: Descriptive Terminology—cont'd

Type of fracture or related condition	Comments
Type III	Fracture that involves separation of a portion of the growth plate and epiphysis
Type IV	Fracture that involves separation of a portion of the growth plate, epiphysis, and metaphysis
Type V	Fracture that involves impaction of the epiphysis onto the metaphysis, crushing the growth plate, possibly causing growth retardation of involved bone; prognosis is poor; the fracture is practically impossible to see with plain film radiography
Impacted (crush) fracture	Fracture that occurs when bone fragment is driven or telescoped into the cancellous portion of the remaining bone from which the fragment originated
Depression fracture	Fracture that occurs when one bone is driven into the adjacent bone, as occurs with the femur forced into the softer tibia

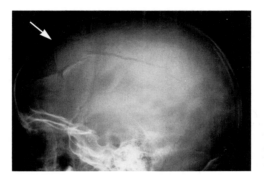

Depression and linear *(arrow)* fractures of the skull.

Compression fracture	Fracture that occurs when articular surfaces of a bone approximate one another, as occurs with vertebrae
Incomplete fracture	Fracture line that appears to traverse or penetrate the entire bone (periosteum may be intact); this fracture occurs most commonly in children, in whom the bones are soft and pliable

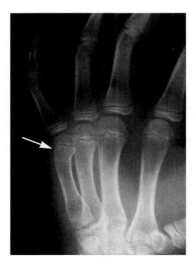

Incomplete fracture of the fifth metacarpal denoting cortical disruption without clear fracture through the entire bone *(arrow)*. (Courtesy Steven P. Brownstein, Springfield, NJ.)

Continued

TABLE 12-2
Fractures: Descriptive Terminology—cont'd

Type of fracture or related condition	Comments
Incomplete fracture—cont'd *Greenstick fracture*	Incomplete fracture of long bones seen in children; one cortex of the bone is impacted with an occult fracture line and the opposite cortex is distracted with an obvious fracture line

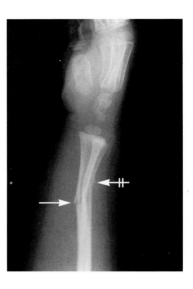

Child with a greenstick fracture of the distal radius *(crossed arrow)* and torus fracture of the distal ulna *(arrow).* Both bones are posteriorly angulated without evidence that each fracture extends through the entire bone. (Courtesy Steven P. Brownstein, Springfield, NJ.)

Torus (buckle) fracture	Nondistracted greenstick fracture common in the distal radius of children

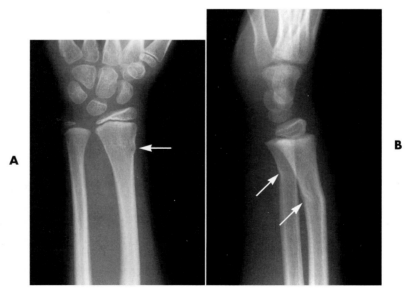

Different patients demonstrating torus fractures of the radius (**A** and **B**) and ulna (**B**) denoting an incomplete fracture with cortical bulge *(arrows).* (A, Courtesy Robert C. Tatum, Davenport, Iowa; B, Courtesy Joseph W. Howe, Sylmar, Calif.)

TABLE 12-2

Fractures: Descriptive Terminology—cont'd

Type of fracture or related condition	Comments
Insufficiency fracture	Stress fracture of diseased bone
Intraarticular fracture	Fracture that extends into the articular surface of a joint
Oblique fracture	Fracture line oriented oblique to the long axis of the bone, but does not exhibit a spiral path
Occult fracture	Clinical, but not radiographic, evidence of fracture; radiographic evidence usually develops within several weeks
Open (compound) fracture	Fracture that penetrates the skin
Pathological fracture	Fracture occurring in bone that has been weakened by disease; the disease may be localized (infection, tumor, disuse, etc.) or more generalized (osteogenesis imperfecta, osteoporosis, rickets, osteomalacia, etc.); pathological fractures are often oriented transverse to the long axis of the bone

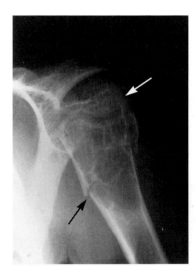

Pathological fracture through simple bone cyst in proximal humerus (*arrows*). (Courtesy Joseph W. Howe, Sylmar, Calif.)

A

B

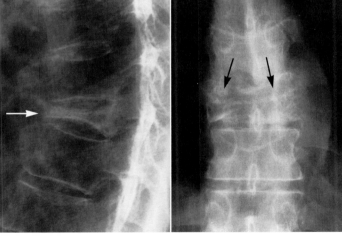

Lateral **(A)** and anteroposterior **(B)** lumbar radiograph demonstrating pathological compression fractures. Both the anterior (*arrow*) and posterior body height is decreased **(A).** Further, the interpeduncular distance is widened **(B,** *arrows*).

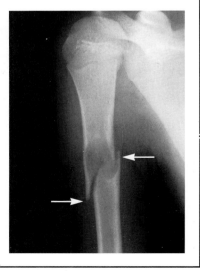

Pathological fracture through a simple bone cyst in the proximal diaphysis of the humerus (*arrows*). (Courtesy Steven P. Brownstein, Springfield, NJ.)

Continued

TABLE 12-2
Fractures: Descriptive Terminology—cont'd

Type of fracture or related condition	Comments
Pseudoarthrosis	Articulation that develops between bone fragments following nonunion
Spiral fracture	Oblique fracture line that coils around the long axis of the bone
Stress fracture	Fractures caused by repeated stresses on bones; there are two types—fatigue and insufficiency; fatigue fractures result from repeated applications of abnormal stresses on bones of normal elastic resistance; insufficiency fractures result from repeated application of normal stresses on bones of abnormal elastic resistance; common stress fractures are listed in Table 12-7

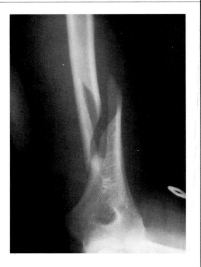

Spiral fracture of the distal humerus.

A   **B**   **C**

Serial studies of stress fractures in one patient. **A,** One stress fracture of the second metatarsal's shaft (arrow). **B,** 19 days later a second stress fracture is noted in the shaft of the third metatarsal (arrows). **C,** 40 days following the second film, a third radiograph demonstrates a third stress fracture in the fourth metatarsal (arrows). (Courtesy Steven P. Brownstein, Springfield, NJ.)

Transverse fracture	Fracture line oriented perpendicular to the long axis of the bone; fractures of transverse orientation suggest underlying osseous pathology (e.g., Paget's disease, metastatic bone disease, etc.)
Unstable/stable fracture	Unstable: fracture that tends to displace once the fracture has been reduced and immobilized; stable: fracture that tends not to displace once the fracture has been immobilized

TABLE 12-3

Fractures and Soft Tissue Injuries of the Skull and Face

Injury	Comments
Basilar skull fracture	Result of blow to the front of the skull; basilar skull fracture is difficult to detect with plain film radiography; most often CT is needed to demonstrate the fracture line; air-fluid level or opacification of sphenoid sinus is the most reliable sign of basilar skull fractures[135]
Depression fracture (see Depression Fracture, p. 521)	Impact injury to cranial vault, causing depression of fragments; this type of fracture represents 15% of all skull fractures; fracture usually occurs in the frontoparietal area; 33% are associated with dural tears, which are suspected when fragments are depressed beyond 5 mm of skull surface or beyond inner table,[162] indicated by depressed fragments beyond 5 mm of skull surface; the plasticity of a child's skull allows depression without obvious fracture, known as a *ping-pong fracture*
Diastatic fracture	Trauma causing widening of the cranial sutures, accounting for 5% of skull fractures,[65] most commonly lambdoid and sagittal sutures; diastatic fractures are often associated with, or are extensions of, linear fractures
LeFort fracture	Occurs along three planes of weakness in the facial skeleton; all types are unstable and bilateral, involve the pterygoid processes, and separate a large fragment of bone from the face; LeFort type I is a transverse fracture through the maxilla separating the upper dentition (floating palate)[40]; LeFort type II is an oblique fracture through the maxilla, separating a pyramidal shaped segment of the midface[39]; LeFort type III is a nearly vertical fracture through the nasal bones and septum, maxilla, and orbits, completely separating the face from the skull[39]

A   **B**

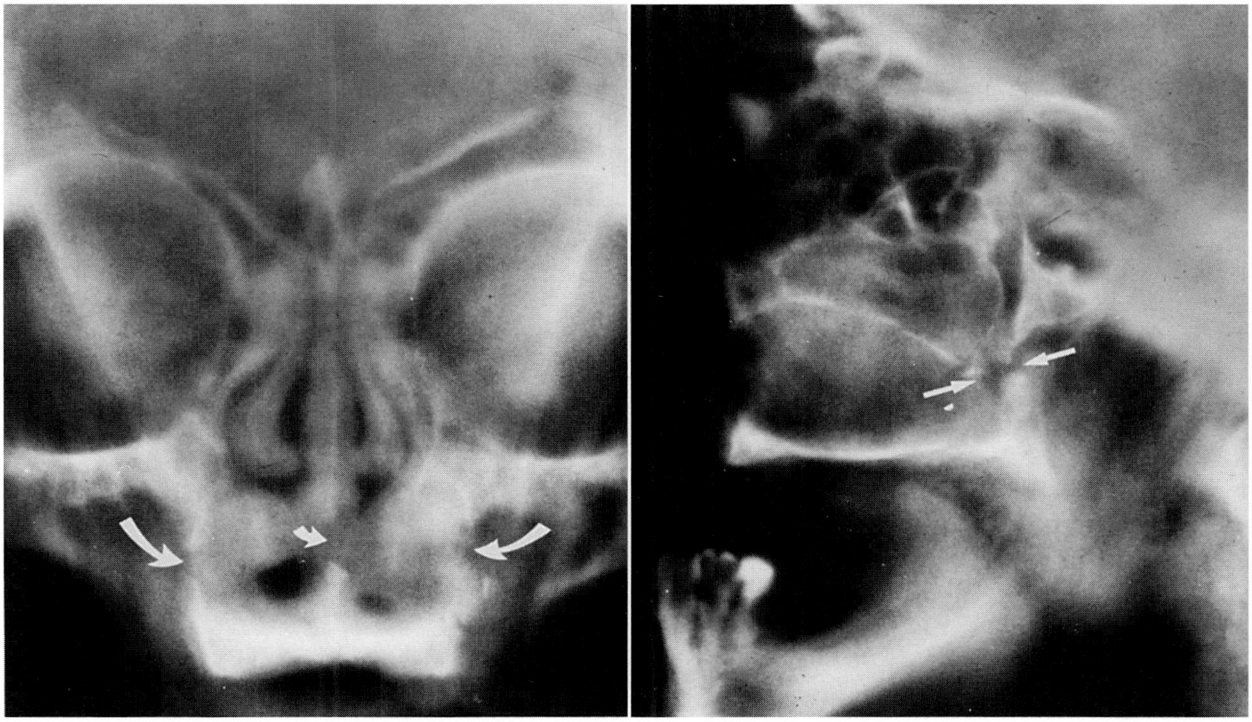

A, Coronal multidirectional tomogram shows a LeFort type I fracture *(arrows).* **B,** Lateral multidirectional tomogram shows a Le Fort type I fracture. The extension of the fracture through the pterygoid plates is seen *(arrows).* (From Som PM, Curtin HD: *Head and neck imaging,* ed 3, St Louis, 1996, Mosby.)

Leptomeningeal cyst	Fracture complication resulting from arachnoid mater extending through a tear in the dura mater, into a skull fracture; the pulsatility of the CSF may inhibit fracture healing and, at times, erode the perimeter of the fracture appearing as a ("growing" fracture)

Continued

TABLE 12-3

Fractures and Soft Tissue Injuries of the Skull and Face—cont'd

Injury	Comments
Linear fracture (see Depression Fracture, p. 521)	Lucent line of several centimeters, representing 80% of all skull fractures; the bone affected is usually the parietal or temporal bone; it may cross sutures and vascular grooves and does not exhibit a branching pattern[139]

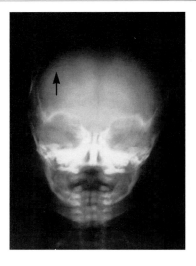

Linear fracture of the skull *(arrow)*. (Courtesy Tim Mick, St. Paul, Minn.)

Mandibular fracture	Third most common facial fracture (after nasal and maxilla); most fractures occur at the body (40%) and the angle (30%) of the mandible[104]; fractures are often bilateral[111,166] and multiple; assault and automobile accidents account for 80% of mandibular fractures[11,104]
Nasal bone fracture	Frequent facial fractures: typically transverse orientation[80,148]; fragments are usually depressed and displaced; nasofrontal suture or longitudinal groove are often mistaken for fractures

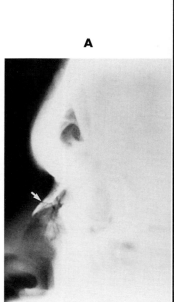
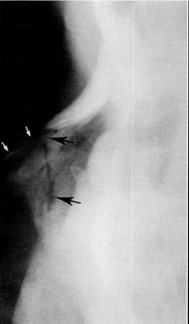
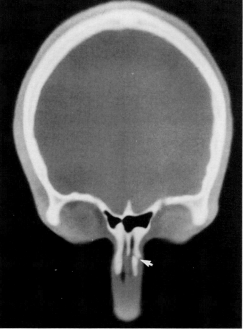

Lateral view of a nasal bone fracture. **A,** Nondisplaced fracture *(arrow)* is seen extending from the midline nasal bones laterally. **B,** Lateral view shows comminuted nasal bone fracture *(small arrows)* with extension of the fracture into the lateral nasal bones and frontal processes of the maxilla *(large arrows)*. **C,** Coronal CT scan shows an isolated, minimally depressed left nasal fracture *(arrow)*. (From Som PM, Curtin HD: *Head and neck imaging,* ed 3, St Louis, 1996, Mosby.)

TABLE 12-3
Fractures and Soft Tissue Injuries of the Skull and Face—cont'd

Injury	Comments

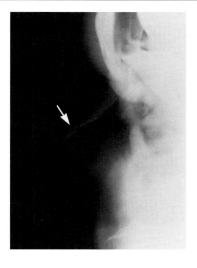

Fracture of the nasal bone *(arrow)*. (Courtesy Tim Mick, St. Paul, Minn.)

Orbital fracture	Occurs as isolated fracture to the rim or walls of the orbit or as components of more complex tripod or LeFort fractures; fractures of the infraorbital wall (blowout fractures) may be complicated by entrapment of the inferior rectus and inferior oblique muscles; medial wall fractures may be complicated by entrapment of the medial rectus

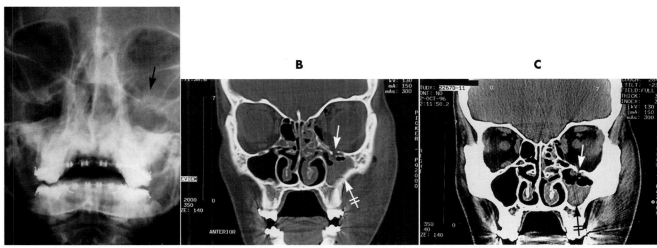

Fracture of the orbital floor *(arrow)* seen on plain film **(A)**, bone **(B)**, and soft tissue **(C)** CT windows. The patient's left maxillary sinus is opacified secondary to accumulations of blood and edema *(crossed arrows)*. (Courtesy Jack C. Avalos, Davenport, Iowa.)

Tripod (trimalar) fracture	Sometimes reported as the most common fracture of the face[139] or second most common fracture of the face[80,148] following nasal bones; termed *tripod* because three limbs of the zygoma are fractured, separating the zygoma from its frontal, temporal, and maxillary attachments by direct blow to the malar prominence[93]; isolated, usually comminuted, fractures of the zygomatic arch are common following direct blows to the side of the face
Pneumocephalus	Fracture complication resulting from air in the subarachnoid space; trauma to the walls of the air-filled paranasal sinus or mastoid air cells permits dissection of air into the subarachnoid space; other causes include infection, neoplasm, and surgery

TABLE 12-4

Fractures, Dislocations, and Soft Tissue Injuries of the Spine and Thorax

Injury	Comments
Atlantooccipital dislocation	Rare, secondary to cervical hyperextension injury; anterior direction is most common
Atlas posterior arch fracture	Bilateral vertical fracture secondary to cervical hyperextension injury; minimal risk of neurological deficit exists; this is the most common fracture of the atlas[151]

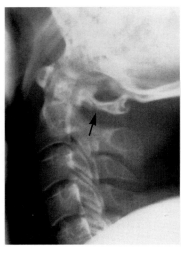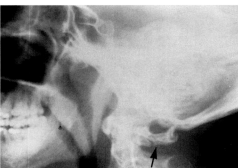

Two cases of linear fracture of the posterior arch of atlas *(arrows)*. (Courtesy Tim Mick, St. Paul, Minn.)

Jefferson fracture	Bursting fracture of the atlas involving both the posterior and anterior arches secondary to an axial force; this type of fracture is indicated by the lateral offset of lateral masses on their C2 articulations in the frontal projection; offset of more than 7 mm may indicate rupture of the transverse atlantal ligament and resulting instability[139]

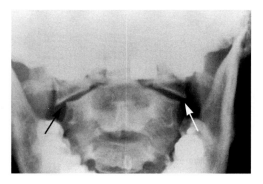

Anteroposterior open mouth projection demonstrating a Jefferson fracture noted by lateral overhanging of the lateral mass beyond the lateral margins of the C2 superior articular processes *(arrows)*. (Courtesy Steven P. Brownstein, Springfield, NJ.)

Atlantoaxial dislocation	Acquired or congenital damage of the transverse atlantal ligament resulting in anterior translation of the atlas, producing a guillotine effect on the cord

TABLE 12-4

Fractures, Dislocations, and Soft Tissue Injuries of the Spine and Thorax—cont'd

Injury	Comments	
Hangman's fracture (traumatic spondylolisthesis of axis)	Bilateral fracture of the pedicles or pars interarticularis of C2, usually related to cervical hyperextension, representing about 25% of C2 fractures[139]; this is difficult to detect in the frontal projection	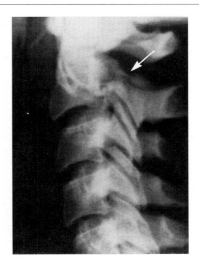
	Bilateral fracture through the pars interarticularis region of axis (traumatic spondylolisthesis or hangman's fracture) *(arrow)*.	
Axis odontoid process fractures	Represent about 50% of all C2 fractures[139] and are divided into three types based on location: type I is avulsion of the tip of the odontoid process; type II is a transverse fracture at the base of the odontoid process and is the most common type; type III is a fracture of the C2 body, below the base of the odontoid process	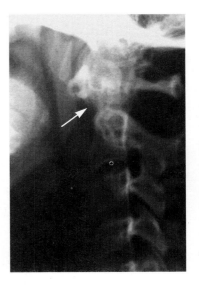
	Type II odontoid fracture *(arrow)*. Note the anterior displacement of the atlas, potentiating myelopathy. (Courtesy Joseph W. Howe, Sylmar, Calif.)	

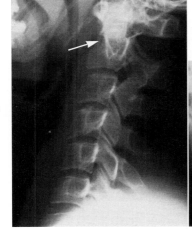

Lateral **(A)** and anteroposterior open mouth **(B)** projection of the cervical spine demonstrating fracture below the base of the odontoid (type III) *(arrows)*. (Courtesy Steven P. Brownstein, Springfield, NJ.)

Continued

PART TWO Bone, Joints, and Soft Tissues

TABLE 12-4
Fractures, Dislocations, and Soft Tissue Injuries of the Spine and Thorax—cont'd

Injury	Comments

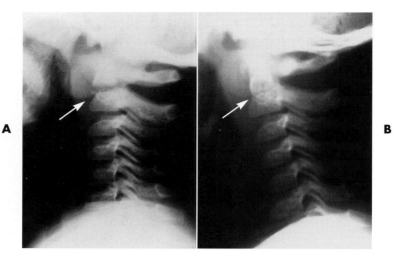

A, Initial film demonstrating a type II odontoid fracture *(arrow).* **B,** The fracture line is less prominent one month later *(arrow).* (Courtesy Jack C. Avalos, Davenport, Iowa.)

Burst fracture

Special type of compression fracture in which axial loads drive portions of the intervertebral disc into the adjacent vertebra, producing a comminuted fracture marked by posterior displacement of fracture fragments into the vertebral canal, that may produce neurological deficits[5]; fractures usually have a sagittal component[86] and often demonstrate an increased interpeduncular distance in frontal projection[5]; nearly 50% occur at the L1 level[5]

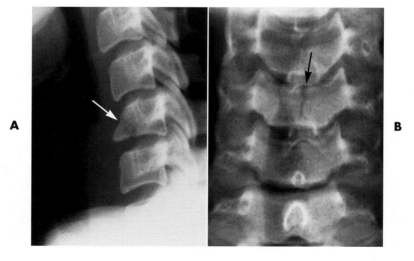

A, Lateral cervical projection demonstrating kyphosis and burst fracture of C5 marked by a radiolucent fracture extending through the anterior lower margin of the vertebrae *(arrow).* **B,** In the frontal projection, the lucent fracture line extends vertically through the vertebra *(arrow).*

TABLE 12-4

Fractures, Dislocations, and Soft Tissue Injuries of the Spine and Thorax—cont'd

Injury	Comments	
Teardrop fracture	Most common at C2; teardrop fractures are produced from hyperflexion or hyperextension injuries compressing or avulsing a small, usually triangular segment of the inferior, less commonly superior, vertebral body[12]; although both are serious injuries often associated with neurological deficits, the flexion teardrop fracture is more severe, because it represents disruption of the posterior ligamentous system and results in acute anterior cord syndrome in almost 90% of cases[67]	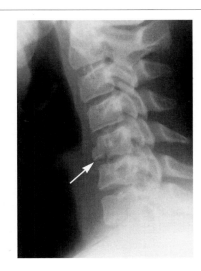

Teardrop fracture of the anterior-inferior margin of the C5 vertebral body *(arrow)*. (Courtesy Steven P. Brownstein, Springfield, NJ.)

A   **B**

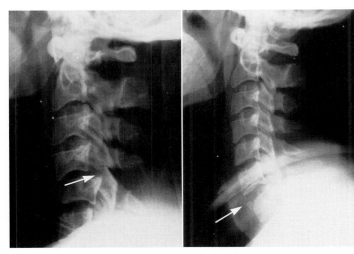

Unilateral facet dislocation. **A,** One of the inferior facets of C4 *(arrow)* is located anterior to the superior facets of C5. **B,** This patient underwent traction for her injuries and the dislocation reduced. However, on this 3 months' follow-up film, the increased field of view allowed a teardrop fracture of C7 to be recognized *(arrow)*. (Courtesy Robert C. Tatum, Davenport, Iowa.)

Cervical articular pillar fractures	Hyperextension and rotation injury, most common at the C6 and C7 levels; in the lateral projection the articular pillar may appear as a double shadow ("double outline" sign)

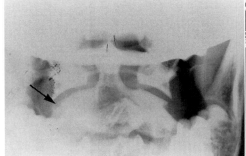
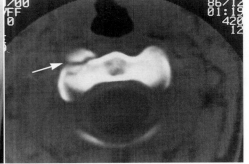

A   **B**

C2 pillar fracture demonstrated by plain film **(A)** and CT **(B,** *arrows)*. (Courtesy Tim Mick, St. Paul, Minn.)

Continued

TABLE 12-4
Fractures, Dislocations, and Soft Tissue Injuries of the Spine and Thorax—cont'd

Injury	Comments
Cervical facet dislocation (see Teardrop Fracture [lower figure])	Unilateral facet dislocation is a usually stable lesion because of a flexion rotation injury; it occurs most often at a C4 to C7 level; the dislocated inferior articular process appears "locked" or "perched" anterior to the superior articular process of the segment below; the dislocated facet simulates a "bow-tie" appearance in the lateral and oblique projection and "fanning" spinous processes in the lateral projection, accompanying fractures[12] and radicular symptoms may be present[179]; bilateral facet dislocation is a usually unstable lesion resulting from a flexion injury, occurring most often at the C4 to C7 level, in the lateral projection "fanning" spinous processes, narrowed disc space, and anterolisthesis are usually evident, cord damage is common[67] and bilateral facet dislocation is at least as common as unilateral facet dislocations[57]

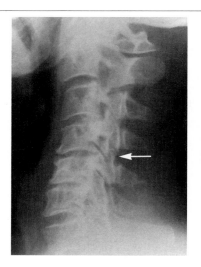

Unilateral facet subluxation indicated by gross misalignment of the articulating facets *(arrow).* The radiographic findings do not demonstrate facet dislocation nor complete misalignment of articulating facets. (Courtesy Tim Mick, St. Paul, Minn.)

Injury	Comments
Clay shoveler's (coal shoveler's)	Flexion injury resulting in an oblique avulsion fracture of the spinous process at the level of C6-T1; best seen in the lateral projection, it appears as "double-spinous" sign in the AP projection; irregularity and distraction of the fragment differentiates the fracture from nonunion of secondary growth center of the spinous process

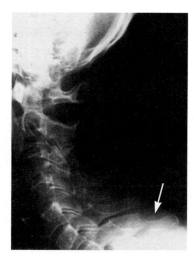

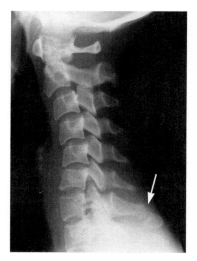

Fracture of the C7 spinous process (clay shoveler's fracture) denoted by disruption of the cortices with inferior displacement of the fragment *(arrow).* Occasionally, a radiolucent line is noted traversing the spinous process, but in the absence of irregularity, history of trauma, or inferior displacement, an isolated radiolucent line most likely represents nonunion of the secondary growth center of the spinous process and not fracture.

Fracture and inferior displacement of the C7 spinous process (clay shoveler's fracture) *(arrow).* Prominent kyphosis is also noted. (Courtesy Steven P. Brownstein, Springfield, NJ.)

TABLE 12-4

Fractures, Dislocations, and Soft Tissue Injuries of the Spine and Thorax—cont'd

Injury	Comments	
Lumbar chance (seatbelt, fulcrum)	Transverse fracture through the spinous process, neural arch, into and possibly through the vertebral body; typically this fracture results from automobile accidents in which flexion forces are applied to the spine while the patient is held down by a lap seatbelt, which acts as a fulcrum; in the frontal projection a radiolucent region ("empty" or "ghost" vertebra) is seen at the region of fracture	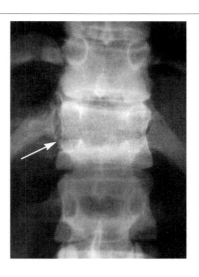

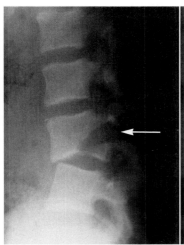 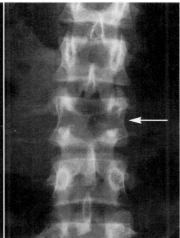

Chance (seatbelt) fracture of L3 noted by the split vertebral arch and posterior vertebral body (arrow). (Courtesy Steven P. Brownstein, Springfield, NJ.)

Horizontal zone of radiolucency transecting the pedicle shadows on this anteroposterior lumbar radiograph (arrows). These fractures are also referred to as chance or seatbelt fractures.

Injury	Comments	
Lumbar pars interarticularis fracture	Best seen in the oblique projection; acute fractures are uncommon and develop from hyperextension injuries	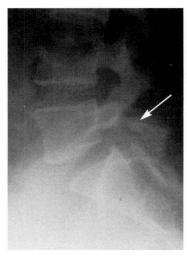

Fracture of the pars interarticularis (arrow) with resulting spondylolisthesis. (Courtesy Tim Mick, St. Paul, Minn.)

Continued

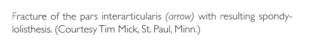

TABLE 12-4
Fractures, Dislocations, and Soft Tissue Injuries of the Spine and Thorax—cont'd

Injury	Comments
Transverse process fracture	Common, often multiple, fracture usually in the upper lumbar spine; this occurs as a vertical or oblique fracture; irregularity of the fracture line and distraction of the fragment differentiates it from nonunion of the transverse process

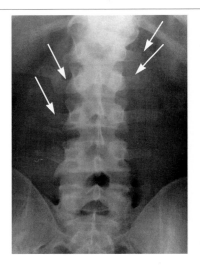

Multiple levels of transverse process fractures *(arrows)*. (Courtesy Tim Mick, St. Paul, Minn.)

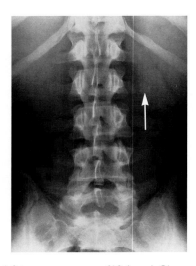

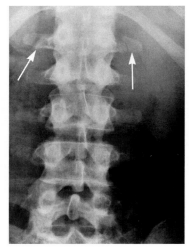

Fracture of the left transverse process of L2 *(arrow)*. Observe the rough medial margin of the distracted fragment.

Bilateral nonunion of the terminal growth center of the transverse process (arrows). The margins of the bone fragments are smooth and nondisplaced, mitigating against fracture.

Flail chest fracture	Multiple fractures of the same ribs, isolating a segment of one or more ribs that are now free to move inward and outward in response to respiration; the movement of the fractured segment is paradoxical to normal rib movement during the respiratory cycle
Golfer's fracture	Lateral rib fracture occurring when a golf club strikes the ground before striking the ball

TABLE 12-4

Fractures, Dislocations, and Soft Tissue Injuries of the Spine and Thorax—cont'd

Injury	Comments
Rib fracture	Most commonly affects the sixth, seventh, and eighth ribs; this type of fracture is more frequent in the posterior and middle two thirds; the risk of pulmonary complications is more significant than the fractures themselves; fracture of the upper ribs indicates the patient has experienced severe trauma[126,134]

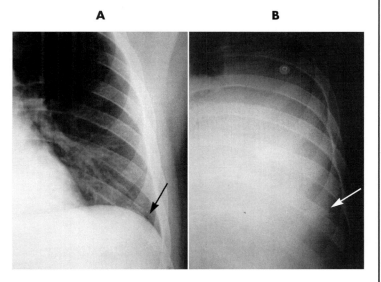

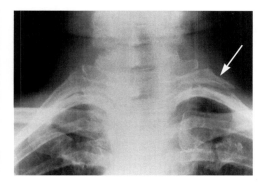

Fracture of the first rib (arrow).

A, Rib fracture with a subtle appearance (arrow) on the PA chest film. **B,** It is more apparent on the lateral decubitus projection (arrow). (Courtesy Robert C. Tatum, Davenport, Iowa.)

Sternal fractures	Common result of direct frontal forces (e.g., steering wheel during automobile accident), causing a transverse fracture of the sternal body; hyperflexion injuries of the spine often result in a posterior dislocation of manubrium at the manubriosternal joint; 40% of sternal fractures occur with associated spinal fracture[79]; 25% to 45% mortality results from cardiac and other associated injuries

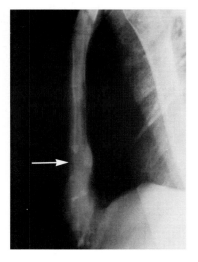

Lateral thoracic projection showing a sternal fracture (arrow).

Continued

TABLE 12-4

Fractures, Dislocations, and Soft Tissue Injuries of the Spine and Thorax—cont'd

Injury	Comments
Vertebral compression fractures	Most frequent at the L1, L2, and T12 levels; vertebral compression fractures appear as a loss of anterior body height (generally, 2 mm less than posterior except at the T11-L1 level, where normal trapezoidal variants are common) and/or depression of the vertebral endplate secondary to forces of forward rotation and axial loading; in those people older than 40 years of age, pathological compression fractures resulting from such conditions as metastatic bone disease and multiple myeloma need to be excluded from fractures caused by osteoporosis or acute injury alone; differentiation is aided by a history of malignancy, past radiographs, other sites of involvement (e.g., pedicles), cortical bone destruction, associated soft tissue mass, collapse of posterior body margin, specialized imaging, and occasionally laboratory work (e.g., multiple myeloma); the presence of a horizontal radiopaque zone of condensation and cortical offset "step defect" along the anterior body margin indicates the fracture is recent (within 2 months prior to the radiograph)[180]

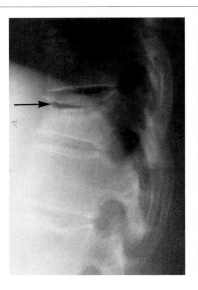

Compression fracture with intravertebral vacuum phenomena (*arrow*). (Courtesy Joseph W. Howe, Sylmar, Calif.)

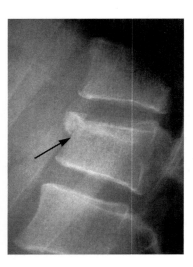

Vertebral compression fracture denoting a horizontal zone of condensation and offset of the anterior cortex ("step defect") (*arrow*). Both the line of condensation and step defect suggest the fracture is less than 2 months old.

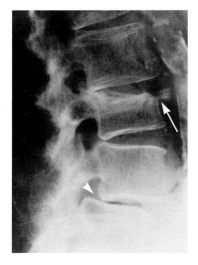

Compression fracture of L3 with anterior displacement of the traumatic fragment (*arrow*). The posterior body height is maintained. Also seen is advanced degenerative disc disease of L4 with degenerative spondylolisthesis (*arrowhead*) and vascular calcification of the abdominal aorta, although the vessel does not appear dilated. (Courtesy Joseph W. Howe, Sylmar, Calif.)

TABLE 12-4
Fractures, Dislocations, and Soft Tissue Injuries of the Spine and Thorax—cont'd

Injury	Comments

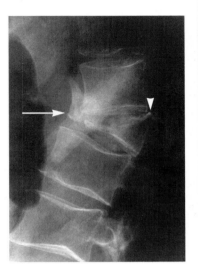

Compression fracture of T12 with displacement of anterior fragment *(arrow)*. The posterior body height is maintained, but slight retropulsion is noted *(arrowhead)*. (Courtesy Joseph W. Howe, Sylmar, Calif.)

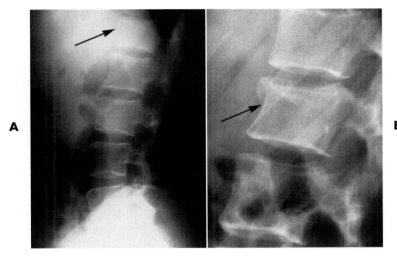

A, Lateral lumbar projection demonstrating a subtle fracture of L1 *(arrow)*. **B,** By limiting beam distortion, motion, and scatter, recumbent spot radiography of the region yields a much improved image *(arrow)*. The fracture exhibits a thin horizontal zone of condensation and offset of the anterior cortex ("step defect"). Both the line of condensation and step defect suggest the fracture is less than 2 months old.

"Whiplash" syndrome

Medicolegal term describing a hyperextension-hyperflexion mechanism of injury; radiographic findings that suggest cervical spine injury include the following: widened retropharyngeal space, widened retrotracheal space, displacement of the prevertebral fat stripe, tracheal deviation and laryngeal dislocation, soft tissue emphysema, loss or reversal of lordosis, widened interspinous space, acute angular kyphosis, altered intersegmental motion, and vertebral body rotation[180]

TABLE 12-5
Fractures, Dislocations, and Soft Tissue Injuries of the Upper Extremities

Injury	Comments

Shoulder
Fracture sites
Clavicle

Most common bone fractured during birth and childhood[180]; 80% of fractures occur in the middle, 15% in the lateral, and 5% in the medial third; hypertrophic callus formation may impinge upon the neurovascular bundle exiting the root of the neck (thoracic outlet syndrome); the distal clavicle may undergo focal osteolysis following acute injury or repetitive stress, as in weightlifting

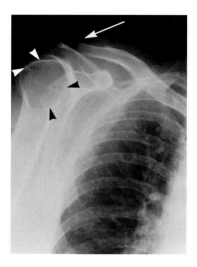

Fracture of the distal clavicle *(arrow)*. Also note the pseudocyst appearance of the greater tuberosity when projected en face *(arrowheads)*. (Courtesy Steven P. Brownstein, Springfield, NJ.)

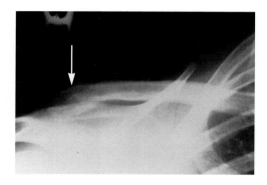

Fracture of the distal third of the clavicle with inferior angulation of the distal fragment *(arrow)*.

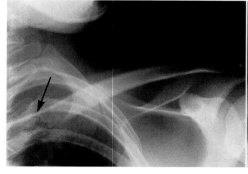
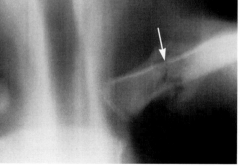

Anteroposterior plain film **(A)** and linear tomogram **(B)** of a fracture of the medial end of the left clavicle *(arrows)*.

TABLE 12-5

Fractures, Dislocations, and Soft Tissue Injuries of the Upper Extremities—cont'd

Injury	Comments

Shoulder—cont'd
Fracture sites—cont'd

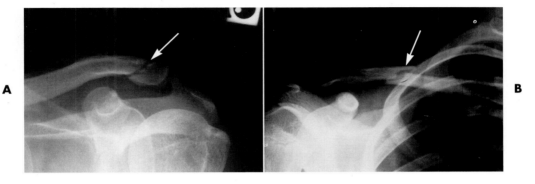

Clavicle fractures through the distal **(A)** and middle **(B)** third of the clavicle in different patients *(arrows)*. (Courtesy Steven P. Brownstein, Springfield, NJ.)

Proximal humerus

Most proximal humerus fractures occur at the surgical neck (distal to tuberosities); avulsion of the greater tuberosity ("flap" fracture) and impaction of the posterolateral surface on the inferior glenoid tubercle (Hill-Sachs fracture or "hatchet" defect) are associated with anterior dislocations of the humerus

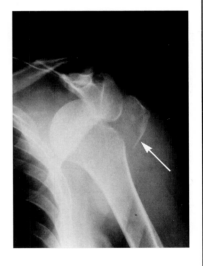

Fracture of the posterior aspect of the humeral head with lateral displacement of the fragment *(arrow)* and anterior dislocation of the humerus.

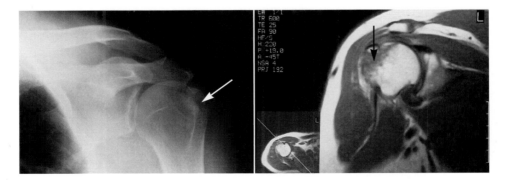

Anteroposterior shoulder projection demonstrating fracture of posterior humeral head with a subtle presentation on the radiograph, but it is easily seen through loss of normal marrow signal on the T1-weighted MRI scan *(arrows)*. This case also demonstrates Ian McLean's lack of dexterity on skis. (Courtesy Ian D McLean, Davenport, Iowa.)

Continued

TABLE 12-5
Fractures, Dislocations, and Soft Tissue Injuries of the Upper Extremities—cont'd

Injury	Comments

Shoulder—cont'd
Fracture sites—cont'd
Scapula

Usually fractures of the body and neck of scapula, rarely as isolated fractures; these fractures are often overlooked because attention is focused on more severe accompanying injuries[68]; avulsion of the inferior glenoid rim (Bankart fracture) is related to anterior dislocation of the humerus

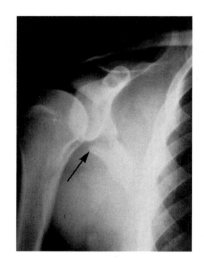

Fracture through the lateral border of the scapula *(arrow)*. (Courtesy Steven P. Brownstein, Springfield, NJ.)

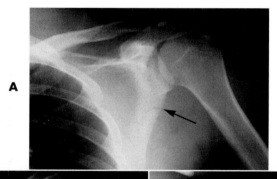

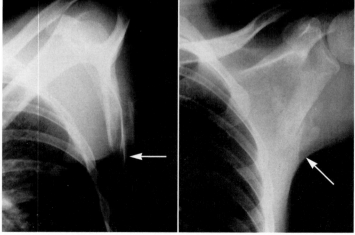

Fracture through the lateral border **(A)** and body **(B** and **C)** of the scapula *(arrows)*. (Courtesy Steven P. Brownstein, Springfield, NJ.)

TABLE 12-5
Fractures, Dislocations, and Soft Tissue Injuries of the Upper Extremities—cont'd

Injury	Comments
Shoulder—cont'd	
Dislocations	
Acromioclavicular joint	Three grades or stages of acromioclavicular injury: grade I is a ligamentous sprain with no radiographic evidence of injury; grade II is rupture of the joint capsule and acromioclavicular ligaments, with radiographic evidence of joint space widening and elevation; grade III is a tear of the coracoclavicular ligaments, resulting in increased coracoclavicular distance (greater than 1.3 cm or 40% asymmetry from side to side); the separation of the joint may be detected only when a 5- to 10- lb weight is held in the hand or tied to the wrist of the involved side

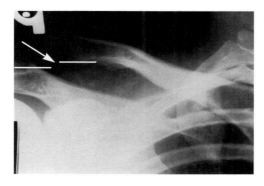

Disruption of the acromioclavicular joint with elevation of the inferior margin of the clavicle above the superior surface of the acromion process, denoting a grade III separation *(arrow)*.

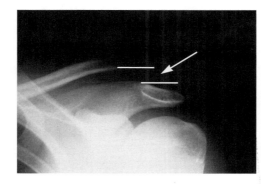

Grade III dislocation *(arrow)* of the acromioclavicular joint noted by the superior migration of the inferior margin of the clavicle above the acromion process of the scapula *(lines)*. (Courtesy Steven P. Brownstein, Springfield, NJ.)

Old grade II acromioclavicular joint separation with bone callus *(arrow)*. (Courtesy Tim Mick, St. Paul, Minn.)

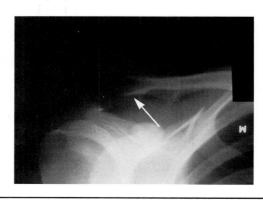

Continued

PART TWO
Bone, Joints, and Soft Tissues

TABLE 12-5

Fractures, Dislocations, and Soft Tissue Injuries of the Upper Extremities—cont'd

Injury	Comments

Shoulder—cont'd

Dislocations—cont'd

Glenohumeral

95% Anterior, 60% of which are associated with impaction fractures of the posterolateral surface of the humeral head (Hill-Sachs fracture), 15% with avulsion of the greater tuberosity (flap fracture), and less commonly a fracture of the infraglenoid tubercle (Bankart fracture); the radiographic appearance of an anterior humeral dislocation is marked by an intrathoracic (between ribs), subclavicular, subcoracoid (most common), or subglenoid position of the humeral head; posterior dislocations are less common (occur in 5% of patients) and anecdotally associated with epileptic or electric shock convulsions; posterior humeral dislocations are marked by joint widening between the humeral head and anterior glenoid rim (greater than 6 mm, "rim" sign), an impaction of the medial humeral head may be seen ("trough line")[26]; rarely the humeral head becomes inferiorly displaced under the glenoid process (luxatio erecta) most often related to extreme hyperabduction injury

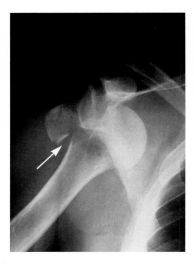

Anterior humeral dislocation in subcoracoid location with impaction of the posterolateral surface of the humeral head on the inferior portion of the glenoid rim causing a Hill-Sachs fracture (hatchet defect) with lateral displacement of the fragment (arrow). (Courtesy Steven P. Brownstein, Springfield, NJ.)

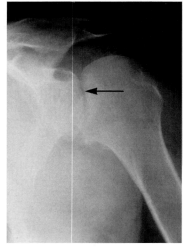

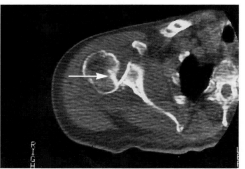

Plain film **(A)** and CT scan **(B)** of a posterior dislocation of the humerus with impaction fracture of the medial humeral head on the posterior aspect of the glenoid rim (arrows). (Courtesy Steven P. Brownstein, Springfield, NJ.)

Sternoclavicular joint

Usually results from a blow to the posterior shoulder; medial end of the clavicle typically dislocates anteriorly; direct anterior blow will dislocate medial end of the clavicle posteriorly, which is potentially lethal if it encroaches on the great vessels; in those younger than 25 years of age, many seemingly identical lesions represent separation of the growth plate and not true dislocations[139]

TABLE 12-5
Fractures, Dislocations, and Soft Tissue Injuries of the Upper Extremities—cont'd

Injury	Comments

Shoulder—cont'd

Soft tissue injuries (ligaments and cartilage)

Biceps tendon injuries   Tendon of the long head of the biceps usually appearing as a round, low-signal intensity structure within the intertubercular groove on the axial images of the shoulder; when not seen within its expected location, rupture and dislocation are considerations; fluid may also be observed within the biceps tendon sheath

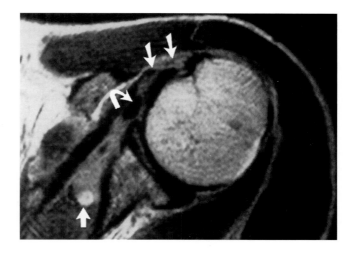

Dislocated biceps tendon, left shoulder. Axial proton density (1800/30) image. The long head of the biceps tendon *(curved arrow)* is displaced out of the bicipital groove and into the glenohumeral joint through the torn transverse ligament and subscapularis tendon *(slanted arrows)*. A high-signal loose body is visible in the distended subscapularis bursa *(straight arrow)*. (From Firooznia H et al: *MRI and CT of the musculoskeletal system,* St Louis, 1992, Mosby.)

Glenoid labral tears   Usually a sequelae of anterior shoulder dislocations when the anterior glenoid labrum is torn (Bankart lesion) with separation of the anterior capsule from the glenoid rim; the glenoid margin itself may be fractured (Bankart fracture) along with a fracture of the humeral head as impaction occurs against the inferior glenoid rim

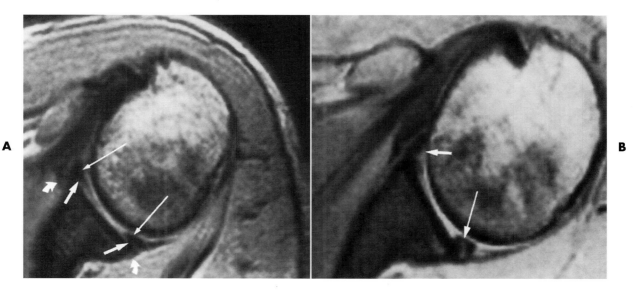

Normal glenoid labrum morphology and MR patterns of glenoid labral tears. **A,** Axial gradient echo sequence (400/191/65 degrees). The anterior and posterior glenoid labrum is visualized as a signal void structure *(long arrows)*. The medium-signal hyaline glenoid articular cartilage extends beneath the labrum to the glenoid margin *(short arrows)*. Note the smooth contour of the capsule and the clearly visualized anterior and posterior glenoid insertions *(curved arrows)*. **B,** Axial gradient echo sequence (400/19/65 degrees). Tearing of the anterior labrum is evidenced by contour abnormality *(short arrow)*. A linear tear of the posterior labrum is manifested by a band of medium signal through the labral substance *(long arrow)*. (From Firooznia H et al: *MRI and CT of the musculoskeletal system,* St Louis, 1992, Mosby.)

Continued

TABLE 12-5
Fractures, Dislocations, and Soft Tissue Injuries of the Upper Extremities—cont'd

Injury	Comments

Shoulder—cont'd

Soft tissue injuries (ligaments and cartilage)—cont'd

Rotator cuff tears — MRI—best method to diagnose tears and is almost 90% accurate in diagnosing full thickness tears of the rotator cuff; the principal finding of a rotator cuff tear is a hyperintense signal on the T2-weighted image, extending through the rotator cuff with discontinuity of the tendon and communicating with the subacromial or subdeltoid space; retraction of the musculotendinous junction of the supraspinatus muscle can also be seen along with significant fluid accumulation in the subacromial bursa; secondary signs include loss of the subdeltoid fat, atrophy of the supraspinatus muscle, cystic changes of the humeral head principally at the site of the supraspinatus tendon insertion; the tears are often classified by a three grade system: grade I represents a tendinitis demonstrating normal morphology with high signal intensity on T1-weighted images and normal low signal intensity on T2-weighted images; grade II represents partial-thickness tears on either the articular or bursal surface of the tendon and are seen as high-signal intensity lesions on T2-weighted images; grade III represents full-thickness tears that show a high signal intensity gap in the tendon on T2-weighted images

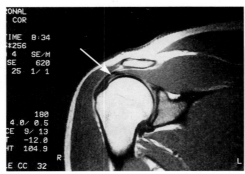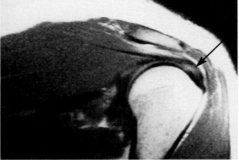

Rotator cuff tendonopathy indicated by the increased signal intensity *(arrows)* in the normally hypointense (dark) supraspinatus tendon in these coronal T1-weighted MR images of different patients.

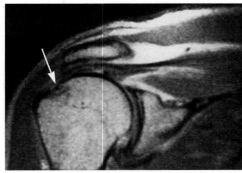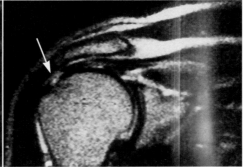

A   **B**

Supraspinatus tear indicated by increased signal intensity *(arrows)* on the T1-weighted **(A)** and T2-weighted **(B)** coronal images.

TABLE 12-5
Fractures, Dislocations, and Soft Tissue Injuries of the Upper Extremities—cont'd

Injury	Comments

Shoulder—cont'd
Soft tissue injuries (ligaments and cartilage)—cont'd

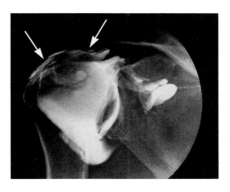

Arthrogram demonstrating migration of injected contrast from the glenohumeral joint to the subacromial space *(arrows),* which implies a tear in the supraspinatus tendon. (Courtesy Tim Mick, St. Paul, Minn.)

Shoulder impingement syndrome	May be secondary to the narrowing of the subacromial space, which includes changes in the shape and slope of the acromion process, subacromial osteophytes, and degenerative joint disease of the acromioclavicular articulation; these changes create chronic effacement of the rotator cuff tendon and are often a precursor to rotator cuff tears; in older patients the combination of repetitive overhead activity along with a congenitally narrowed subacromial space is a common cause of osteophytes on the undersurface of the acromion; in younger patients, however, involvement with sports that require high-velocity overhand throwing can be an additional cause of instability

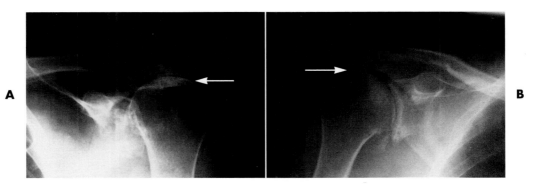

Shoulder impingement syndrome, **A** and **B.** Incompetence of the rotator cuff allows superior elevation of the humerus resulting from the unopposed muscle tension of the deltoid. The acromiohumeral space is narrowed *(arrows)* and evidence of arthrosis, marked by bone sclerosis, may be present.

Continued

TABLE 12-5
Fractures, Dislocations, and Soft Tissue Injuries of the Upper Extremities—cont'd

Injury	Comments

Elbow
Fractures
Distal humerus

Most commonly supracondylar fractures in children[30,48]; comminuted intracondylar fractures of a T or Y configuration are common in adults[89,111]; a small osteochondral flake fractured off the convex surface of the capitellum is termed *Kocher's fracture;* in children the appearance of normal secondary ossification centers may mistakenly be interpreted as fractures; the acronym *CRITOE* describes the order of appearance of the secondary ossification centers about the elbow: capitellum, radial head, internal epicondyle, trochlea, olecranon, and external epicondyle; hence the presence of a trochlea requires the presence of an internal epicondyle

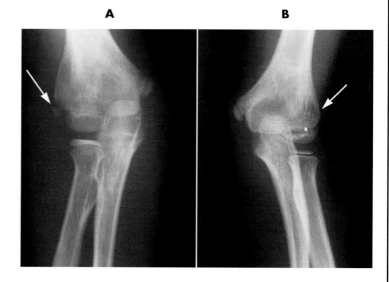

A   **B**

A, Avulsion fracture of the lateral epicondyle of the distal humerus *(arrow).* On occasion, normal growth centers can be misinterpreted as fractures. As in this case, the fracture fragment is typically irregular and distracted from its parent bone. **B,** Radiograph of the contralateral elbow; it exhibits the normal configuration *(arrow).* (Courtesy Steven P. Brownstein, Springfield, NJ.)

Little leaguer's elbow[18]
Olecranon

Avulsion of the medial epicondyle resulting from traction forces of the flexor-pronator tendons[25]
Second most common elbow fracture after those of the proximal radius[139]; fracture line is usually oriented transversely[72] and easily noted in the lateral projection

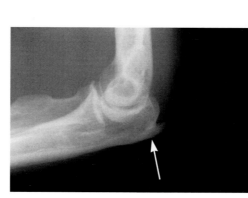
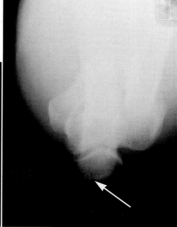

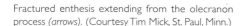
Fractured enthesis extending from the olecranon process *(arrows).* (Courtesy Tim Mick, St. Paul, Minn.)

TABLE 12-5

Fractures, Dislocations, and Soft Tissue Injuries of the Upper Extremities—cont'd

Injury	Comments

Elbow—cont'd

Fractures—cont'd

Radial head

Most common elbow fractures in the adult[139]; these are difficult to detect on radiographs; a radial head fracture oriented with the long axis of the bone is termed *chisel fracture;* thin fat pads are located between the synovial and fibrous layers of the joint capsule of the elbow; in the lateral flexed elbow position, an injury with resulting joint effusion may cause elevation of the normally visible anterior fat pad and visibility of the normally invisible posterior fat pad (fat pad sign)[13,90]

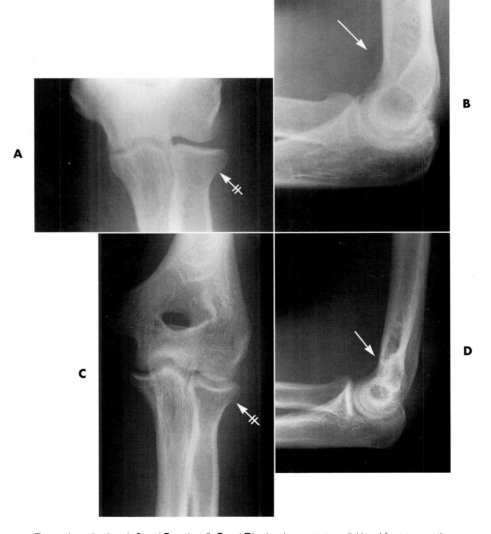

Two patients (patient 1, **A** and **B**; patient 2, **C** and **D**) who demonstrate radial head fractures on the anteroposterior elbow projections (**A** and **C**) *(crossed arrows)*. In the lateral projections (**B** and **D**), the anterior fat pads are visible *(arrows)*. (Courtesy Joseph W. Howe, Sylmar, Calif.)

Continued

TABLE 12-5

Fractures, Dislocations, and Soft Tissue Injuries of the Upper Extremities—cont'd

Injury	Comments

Elbow—cont'd
Fractures—cont'd

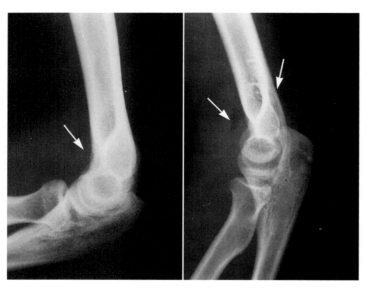

Two patients who demonstrate elevation of the humeral fat pads *(arrows)* consistent with elbow injury; however no evidence of fracture is noted in either patient. (Right, Courtesy Steven P. Brownstein, Springfield, NJ.)

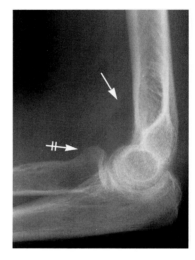

An elevated anterior fat pad *(arrow)* and subtle radial head fracture *(crossed arrow)*.

Dislocations
Elbow dislocations

Third most common dislocation in adults, following shoulder and interphalangeal dislocations; most common dislocation in children[4]; overall these are more common in children than in adults; the direction of dislocations of both the radius and ulna is usually posterior (90% of the time)[128]; concurrent fractures occur at a high rate; on all projections of the elbow a line through the center of the shaft of the radius should intersect the center of the capitellum; failure to do so may indicate dislocation[158]; the anterior humeral line describes a line drawn along the anterior border of the humerus in the lateral projection; under normal circumstances the line should intersect the middle third of the capitellum[139]; anterior displacement of the line may indicate supracondylar fracture

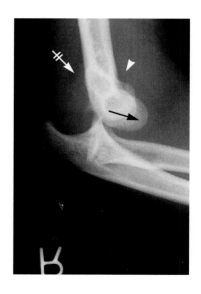

Anterior dislocation of the elbow *(arrow)*. Notice the posterior *(crossed arrow)* and anterior *(arrowhead)* elevated fat pads. (Courtesy Steven P. Brownstein, Springfield, NJ.)

Pulled elbow (nursemaids' elbow)

May be caused by a sudden jerk on a toddler's pronated elbow; this may cause dislocation of the proximal radius with entrapment of the annular ligament within the joint space[144]; radiographs are typically negative

TABLE 12-5
Fractures, Dislocations, and Soft Tissue Injuries of the Upper Extremities—cont'd

Injury	Comments

Forearm
Fractures
Essex-Lopresti fracture[47] — Comminuted fracture of the radial head with dislocation of the distal radioulnar joint[33,45]

Galeazzi (Piedmont,[74] reversed Monteggia) fracture[132] — Fracture of the distal radius with dislocation of the distal radioulnar joint[110,171]

Monteggia fracture[6] — Fracture of the proximal ulna with dislocation of the radial head; although dislocation may occur in any direction, an anterior dislocation was first described and is most common when found with the ulna fracture[19]

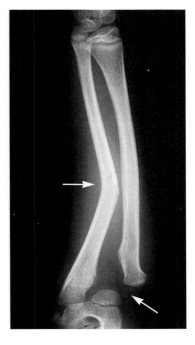

Fracture through the proximal diaphysis of the ulna with dislocation of the radial head (Monteggia fracture-dislocation) *(arrows)*. (Courtesy Jack C. Avalos, Davenport, Iowa.)

Nightstick (parry) fracture — Fracture to the distal,[42] or less often middle, third of the ulnar shaft; this fracture is often secondary to raising one's forearm overhead in an attempt to protect the head or face from a strike from a nightstick or club

Ulna and radius (both bone, or bb) fracture — Concurrent fractures of the radius and ulna most often are found in the middle third of the bones and often result in marked limb angulation and rotation

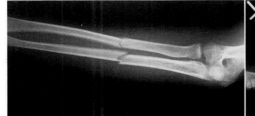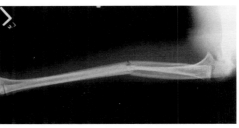

Anteroposterior **(A)** and lateral **(B)** fracture of the ulna and the radius known as a both bone (BB) fracture. (Courtesy Steven P. Brownstein, Springfield, NJ.)

Continued

TABLE 12-5
Fractures, Dislocations, and Soft Tissue Injuries of the Upper Extremities—cont'd

Injury	Comments

Wrist
Fractures
Chauffeur's (backfire, Hutchinson) fracture

Usually undisplaced[24] fracture of the radial styloid, named for the occupational hazard of experiencing a backfire while attempting to start an automobile with a hand crank

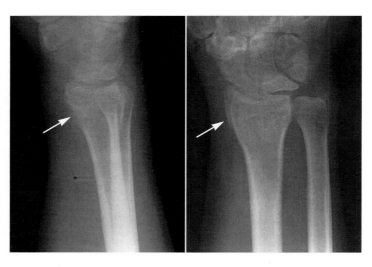

Chauffeur's fracture *(arrows)*. (Courtesy Tim Mick, St. Paul, Minn.)

Colles' fracture

Hyperextension injury following fall on outstretched hand,[173] consisting of a fracture of the distal radius with posterior angulation of the distal fragment producing dinner fork or silver fork deformity; increasing incidence occurs with increasing age; 60% of these fractures are accompanied by fracture of the ulnar styloid process; Colles' fractures are most common among the elderly, particularly women[3]; wrist injury due to a fall on an outstretched hand (FOOSH mechanism) results in a torus or greenstick fracture in children, epiphyseal injuries in adolescents, scaphoid fractures in adults, and Colles' fractures in the elderly

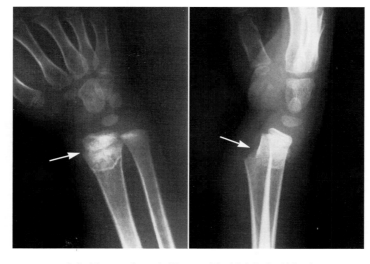

Colles' fracture *(arrows)*. (Courtesy Tim Mick, St. Paul, Minn.)

TABLE 12-5
Fractures, Dislocations, and Soft Tissue Injuries of the Upper Extremities—cont'd

Injury	Comments
Wrist—cont'd	
Fractures—cont'd	
Greenstick fracture	Incomplete fracture of a long bone with marked angulation of the fragments at the site of fracture
Hamate fracture	Common to golf,[165] baseball,[23] and racquet sports,[155] usually involving the hamulus, which if injured appears sclerotic, ill-defined, or absent[119]
Rim (Barton's) fracture	Involves the posterior rim of the distal radius; reversed Barton's fractures involve the anterior rim
Scaphoid (navicular)	Most common carpal bone fracture, usually occurs between 15 and 40 years of age; this type of fracture is rare in children; it is the most common occult fracture[63]; 70% of fractures occur at the waist of the bone[63]; care is warranted with radiographic positioning; it is helpful to distract the wrist to the ulnar side for a better view of the scaphoid; because the principal blood supply for the scaphoid enters at its waist, more proximal fractures risk avascular necrosis (up to 15% of fractures[180]) or nonunion (up to 30% of fractures[139]) of the proximal pole; often fractures are difficult to detect; the presence of carpal injury is suggested by distortion of the fat pad associated with the pronator quadratus along the ventral carpus (MacEwen's sign); 90% of scaphoid fractures will have obliteration of fat stripe overlying[163]; MRI is helpful in the detection of radiographically occult scaphoid fractures and also helps delineate the complication of osteonecrosis; MRI is the most sensitive modality for the detection of osteonecrosis and is more sensitive than radionuclide studies in the early detection of this pathology[170]; MRI findings of osteonecrosis are variable, depending on the stages of ischemia; typical findings include low signal intensity within the bone marrow on T1-weighted images with regions of increased signal intensity on the T2-weighted images with the T2 feature thought to represent hemorrhage or edema

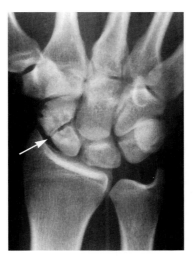

Scaphoid fracture *(arrow)*. (Courtesy Tim Mick, St. Paul, Minn.)

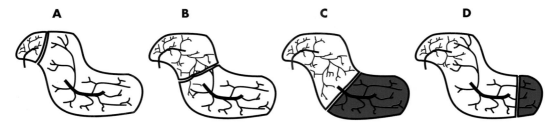

The scaphoid is nourished by two vessels, one entering its distal pole and one entering its waist. Fracture through the distal pole (**A** and **B**) does not interrupt blood flow to any part of the scaphoid, making avascular necrosis unlikely. However a fracture through the waist (**C**) or proximal portion (**D**) of the scaphoid interrupts the main blood supply to the portion of the scaphoid proximal to the fracture. Because of the altered perfusion, the proximal fragment has a tendency to undergo avascular necrosis when the fracture is proximal to the waist. (Modified from Rogers LF: *Radiology of skeletal trauma,* ed 2, vol 2, New York, 1992, Churchill Livingstone.)

Continued

TABLE 12-5
Fractures, Dislocations, and Soft Tissue Injuries of the Upper Extremities—cont'd

Injury	Comments

Wrist—cont'd
Fractures—cont'd

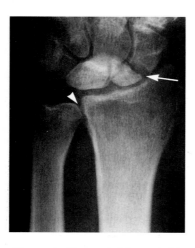

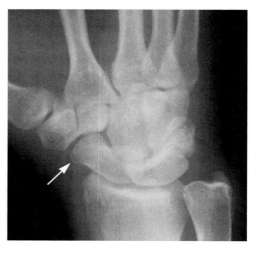

Scaphoid fracture. The proximal fragment of the scaphoid and the lunate appears radiodense, which is consistent with avascular necrosis *(arrow)*. Negative ulnar variance is also noted *(arrowhead)*. (Courtesy Jack C. Avalos, Davenport, Iowa.)

Small avulsion fracture from the distal pole of the scaphoid *(arrow)*. (Courtesy Steven P. Brownstein, Springfield, NJ.)

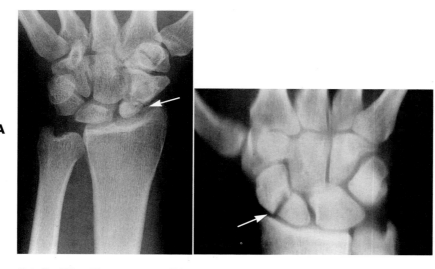

Plain film **(A)** and linear tomogram **(B)** demonstrating fracture through the waist of the scaphoid in different patients *(arrows)*. The proximal fragment of the first patient **(A)** appears condensed and mildly sclerotic, which is suggestive of avascular necrosis.

TABLE 12-5

Fractures, Dislocations, and Soft Tissue Injuries of the Upper Extremities—cont'd

Injury	Comments

Wrist—cont'd

Fractures—cont'd

Smith's (reversed Colles')   Caused by a direct blow to the back of the wrist, resulting in a fracture of the distal radius with an-
    fracture   terior (volar) angulation of the distal fragment

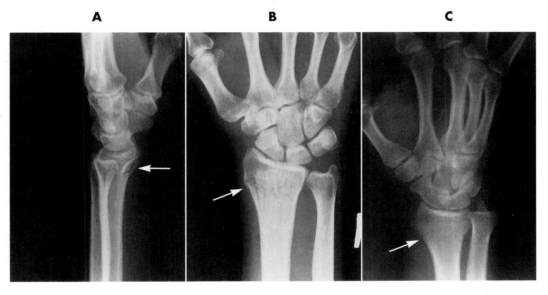

Lateral **(A),** posteroanterior **(B),** and oblique **(C)** wrist projections demonstrating multiple fracture lines in the distal radius with slight ventral angulation of the distal fragment, denoting Smith's fracture *(arrows).* The fractures are less well noted on the oblique projection, emphasizing the need for multiple projections. (Courtesy Joseph W. Howe, Sylmar, Calif.)

Torus fracture   Incomplete fracture of the distal radius appearing as a bulged, buckled, or folded cortex; this is probably the most common wrist fracture that occurs during the ages of 6 to 10 years

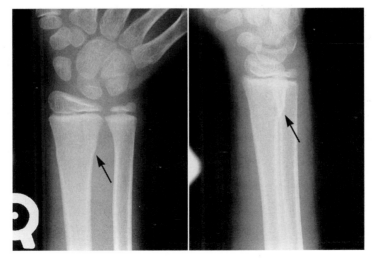

Torus fracture *(arrows).* (Courtesy Tim Mick, St. Paul, Minn.)

Continued

TABLE 12-5
Fractures, Dislocations, and Soft Tissue Injuries of the Upper Extremities—cont'd

Injury	Comments

Wrist—cont'd
Fractures—cont'd
Triquetrum fracture

Second most common carpal bone fracture[43]; usually a dorsal avulsion is mediated by the radiotriquetral and ulnotriquetral ligaments (Fisher's fracture), seen best in the lateral view

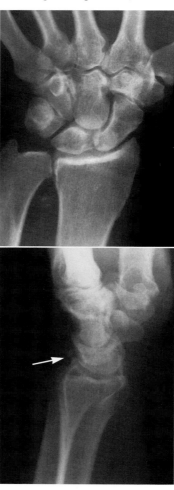

Fragment at the posterior aspect of the wrist representing fracture of the triquetrum (arrow). The lunate is dorsally flexed consistent with dorsal intercalated segment instability (DISI). (Courtesy Tim Mick, St. Paul, Minn.)

Dislocations
Carpal dislocations

Facilitate detecting carpal dislocations by examining three carpal arcs for discontinuity in the PA projection[60]: arc I along the proximal articular surfaces of the proximal row of carpals, arc II along the distal articular surfaces of the proximal row of carpals, and arc III along the proximal articular surfaces of the distal row of carpals (hamate and capitate, mostly); one or several bones may be involved with dislocations; the lunate is the most common single bone dislocation, appearing triangular in shape ("pie" sign) in the PA projection; rotational subluxations of the scaphoid present with a classic ringlike radiodensity (signet ring sign) and wide scapholunate joint space (greater than 2 to 3 mm) in the PA projection; the appearance in the lateral projection of multiple carpal dislocations is described in three patterns: perilunate dislocations involve dorsal dislocation of the capitate on the lunate, midcarpal dislocations involve dorsal dislocation of the capitate on the lunate and partial anterior dislocation of the lunate on the radius, lunate dislocations involve complete dislocation of the lunate with the radius and the capitate while the capitate remains in axial alignment with the radius; the three patterns are interrelated; over time some patients progress from perilunate to midcarpal to lunate patterns of dislocation

TABLE 12-5
Fractures, Dislocations, and Soft Tissue Injuries of the Upper Extremities—cont'd

Injury	Comments

Wrist—cont'd
Dislocations—cont'd

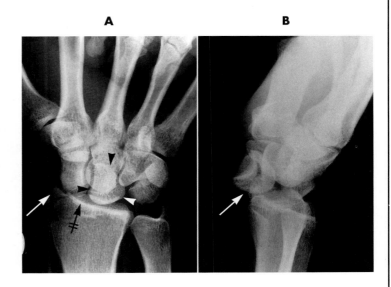

Radial styloid fracture with lunate dislocation. **A,** Posteroanterior projection of the wrist denoting fracture of the radial styloid process *(arrow)* with a triangular "pie sign" appearance to the lunate *(arrowheads)*. The scapholunate joint space is increased, suggesting intercarpal ligament damage *(crossed arrow)*. **B,** The lateral projection reveals anterior displacement of the lunate *(arrow)* from its normal alignment with the distal radius and capitate. (Courtesy Jack C. Avalos, Davenport, Iowa.)

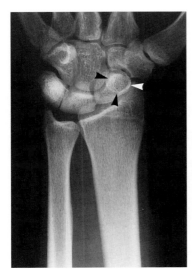

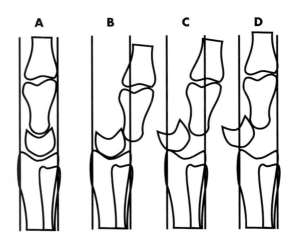

PA wrist projection with apparent foreshortening of the longitudinal axis of the scaphoid and noticeable circular density present ("signet ring" sign) *(arrowheads)*. Both findings are suggestive of rotatory subluxation of the scaphoid. This patient demonstrates no subluxation. The appearance is an artifact caused by radial deviation of the wrist. The wrist should be slightly ulnar-deviated to correctly assess for rotatory subluxation. Also, the scapholunate joint is not diastased, a common finding in scaphoid subluxation. (Courtesy Authur W. Holmes, Foley, Ala.)

A, Normally the longitudinal axes of the radius, lunate, and capitate align. **B,** Perilunate dislocation is marked by posterior dislocation of the capitate-lunate joint and normal alignment of the lunate-radius joint. **C,** Midcarpal dislocation is noted by posterior dislocation of the capitate-lunate joint and anterior dislocation of the lunate-radial joint. **D,** Lunate dislocation is noted by anterior dislocation of the lunate with normal alignment of the capitate and radius.

Carpal instability (see Triquetrum fracture)	Commonly follow ligamentous injury[50,62,96]; the most common is scapholunate disassociation noted by a gap of more than 2 to 3 mm on the PA wrist radiograph (the gapped appearance is known as the Terry Thomas or David Letterman tooth sign); increased dorsal flexion of the lunate on the lateral radiograph suggests a dorsal instability termed *dorsal intercalated segment instability (DISI);* increased palmar flexion of the lunate on the lateral radiograph suggests a ventral instability termed *ventral intercalated segment instability (VISI)*[56]; DISI and the less common VISI[61] may or may not accompany scapholunate disassociation

TABLE 12-5
Fractures, Dislocations, and Soft Tissue Injuries of the Upper Extremities—cont'd

Injury	Comments

Wrist—cont'd
Soft tissue injuries (ligaments and cartilage)

Carpal tunnel syndrome — Structural alterations of the carpal tunnel, inflammatory tenosynovitis, presence of a tumor or other mass, may lead to compression of the median nerve as it travels through the carpal tunnel; an axial MRI image clearly delineates the structures within the carpal tunnel; carpal tunnel syndrome is the most common nerve compression syndrome; MRI features of compression of the median nerve include flattening, swelling, increased signal intensity of this structure, and palmar bowing of the transverse ligament

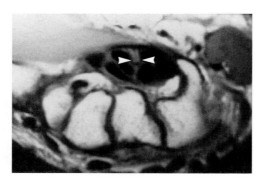

Axial T1-weighted magnetic resonance scan of the wrist, demonstrating alteration of the normally oval median nerve *(arrowheads)*, which suggests compression within the carpal tunnel.

Interosseous ligament injuries — The scapholunate and lunotriquetral interosseous ligaments are probably the most clinically important intrinsic ligaments of the wrist; injury to these structures may lead to carpal dissociation and instability syndromes such as dorsal or volar intercalated segment carpal instability; with rupture of these interosseous ligaments, the scaphoid has a tendency to rotate volarly and the triquetrum dorsally, the lunate typically rotates opposite the bone adjacent the ligament rupture; scapholunate interosseous ligament ruptures often follow fractures of the radial styloid; carpal intervals more than 1 mm deserve investigation, those more than 2 to 3 mm are likely abnormal, and intervals more than 4 mm are nearly always abnormal

Triangular fibrocartilage (TFC) injuries — The TFC absorbs axial loading and lends stability to the ulnar aspect of the wrist; most tears of the triangular fibrocartilage are degenerative in etiology, making it vulnerable to biomechanical forces; high-resolution MRI will show tears of the triangular fibrocartilage with the T2-weighted images differentiating degenerative from traumatic tears

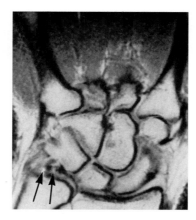

Coronal T1-weighted magnetic resonance scan of the wrist demonstrating hyperintense linear defects signifying tears *(arrows)* through the normal hypointense triangular fibrocartilage.

TABLE 12-5

Fractures, Dislocations, and Soft Tissue Injuries of the Upper Extremities—cont'd

Injury	Comments

Hand
Fractures
Metacarpal fracture

Typically transverse fractures; fractures located in the shafts of the second or third metacarpals are termed *boxer's fractures,* those of the fourth or fifth metacarpal are termed *bar room fractures;* Bennett's fracture is an intraarticular fracture at the base of the first metacarpal with posterolateral dislocation of the first metacarpocarpal joint[10]; Rolando fracture is a comminuted Bennett's fracture[125]

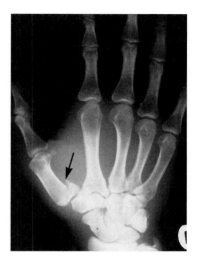

Fracture through the base of the first metacarpal (Bennett's fracture) with posterolateral dislocation of the first digit *(arrow).* (Courtesy Steven P. Brownstein, Springfield, NJ.)

A   **B**

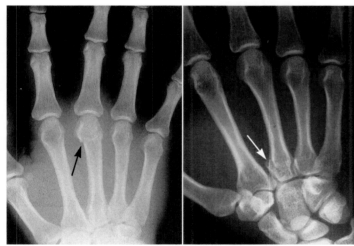

A, Fracture through the neck of the third metacarpal (boxer's fracture) *(arrow).* **B,** Fracture through the base of the third metacarpal *(arrow).* (**B,** Courtesy Steven P. Brownstein, Springfield, NJ.)

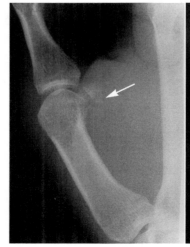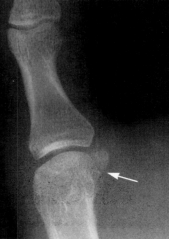

Fracture of a first metacarpophalangeal sesamoid bone *(arrows).*

Continued

TABLE 12-5
Fractures, Dislocations, and Soft Tissue Injuries of the Upper Extremities—cont'd

Injury	Comments

Hand—cont'd

Fractures—cont'd

| Phalanges fracture (see Comminuted Fractures, p. 519) | Probably the most common site of skeletal injury[137]; fractures of the distal phalanges are more common than those of the proximal or middle phalanges; dorsal chip fractures of the inserting extension tendons of the distal phalanges result in flexion deformity of the finger ("mallet" or "baseball" finger)[103]; swan neck deformity may develop, appearing as simultaneous flexion of the distal interphalangeal joint and extension of the proximal interphalangeal joint,[174] fractures of the palmar surface (or volar plate) of the middle phalanges may result in loss of digit flexion; boutonniere deformity results from rupture of the middle slip of the extensor tendons and appears as flexion of the proximal interphalangeal joint with extension of the distal interphalangeal joint |

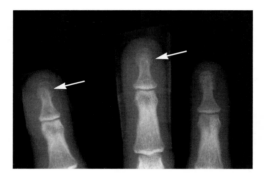

Multiple fractures of the ungual tufts of the distal phalanges *(arrows).*

Dislocations

| Phalanges dislocation | May occur in any location; posterior dislocation following hyperextension injury is most common; interphalangeal dislocations are rarely multiple[172] |

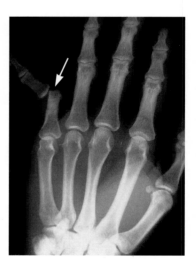

Dislocation of the proximal interphalangeal joint of the fifth digit *(arrow).*

| Gamekeeper's thumb | Disruption of the medial collateral ligament of the first metacarpophalangeal joint with resulting joint instability; anecdotally this dislocation is attributed to breaking the neck of game animals (rabbits and birds) between the thumb and forefinger[21]; contemporarily this dislocation is related to an incorrect grasp of a ski pole |

TABLE 12-6
Fractures, Dislocations, and Soft Tissue Injuries of the Pelvis and Lower Extremities

Injury	Comments
Pelvis	
Fractures	
Acetabular fractures	Can be divided into five types: anterior (iliopubic) and posterior (ilioischial) column, acetabular rim (anterior, posterior, and superior), transverse[95,164] and central or explosion; central fracture-dislocation describes displacement of the femoral head into the pelvis; most fractures of the acetabulum fit into more than one category[70]; fractures typically require great forces, such as those occurring in auto accidents; "dashboard" fractures refer to fractures of the posterior rim secondary to forces applied to the knee when the femur is flexed and adducted during auto accidents
Coccygeal fractures	Most commonly transverse fractures; these fractures are often accompanied by anterior angulation and soft tissue swelling (more than 1 cm presacral space in lateral projection); anterior angulation often occurs as a normal variant and alone does not indicate trauma
Double vertical contralateral (bucket-handle) fracture-dislocations	Fracture of the pelvic ring, consisting of fractures of both the superior and inferior pubic rami with fracture near, or separation of, the contralateral sacroiliac joint[44]
Double vertical ipsilateral (Malgaigne's) fracture-dislocations	Fracture of the pelvic ring consisting of fractures of both the superior and inferior pubic rami with a fracture near, or separation of, the ipsilateral sacroiliac joint; this is the most common fracture of the pelvis[139]
Double vertical pubic (straddle) fracture	Bilateral fractures of all four pubic rami; patients often have concurrent injury to the pelvic viscera[28]
Iliac wing (Duverney's) fracture	Transverse, oblique, or vertical orientation; this fracture does not involve the pelvic ring; it results from a direct lateral blow to the ilium

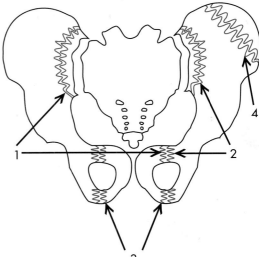

Bucket-handle fracture of the pelvis *(1)*.
Malgaigne's fracture of the pelvis *(2)*.
Straddle fracture of the pelvis *(3)*.
Duverney's fracture of the pelvis. *(4)*.

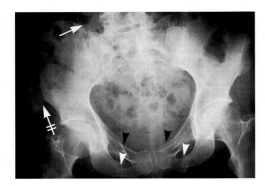

Multiple fractures of the pelvis occurring lateral to the right sacroiliac joint *(arrow)*, iliac crest *(crossed arrow)*, superior and inferior pubic rami bilaterally *(arrowheads)*. Duverney's, bucket-handle, Malgaigne's and straddle fractures are all represented.

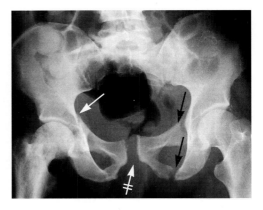

Straddle fracture of the pelvis noted by the bilateral fracture through the superior and inferior pubic rami *(arrows)* with diastasis of the pubic symphysis *(crossed arrow)*. (Courtesy Steven P. Brownstein, Springfield, NJ.)

Continued

TABLE 12-6
Fractures, Dislocations, and Soft Tissue Injuries of the Pelvis and Lower Extremities—cont'd

Injury	Comments

Pelvis—cont'd
Fractures—cont'd

Pelvic avulsion fractures — May be avulsed secondary to muscular traction; the avulsion may occur in various places: avulsion of anterior superior iliac spine (ASIS) at the insertion of the sartorius muscle, avulsion of the anterior inferior iliac spine (AIIS) at the insertion of the rectus femoris, avulsion of the ischial tuberosity at the insertion of the leg flexors (hamstrings), the avulsed segment of bone has been termed *rider's bone;* however, rider's bone is also used to describe localized myositis ossificans of the thigh adductors; injuries are common among hurdlers, cheerleaders, long jumpers, sprinters, and other athletes

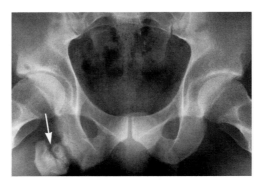

Old avulsion fracture of the right ischial apophysis with residual bulbous deformity *(arrow)*. (Courtesy Jack C. Avalos, Davenport, Iowa.)

Ramus fracture — Common, representing more than 20% to 50% of pelvic fractures, usually seen in older individuals following minor falls[75,105]; single fractures to the pelvic rim are generally stable; however, usually fractures of the superior or inferior ramus are present; bilateral double ramus fractures are straddle fractures

Sacral fractures — Transverse fractures usually occurring in lower sacrum, related to direct trauma or falls on the buttocks; transverse fractures of the upper sacrum are related to high falls ("suicidal jumper" fracture); vertical sacral fractures are often found in combination with other fractures of the pelvic ring[112,175] and are often associated with damage to the pelvic viscera; sacral fractures are difficult to detect on plain film because of overlying gas and fecal matter; tracing the cortices of the sacral foramina is helpful to detect subtle changes of bone structure

Dislocations

Sprung (open book) pelvis — Diastasis of the pubic symphysis with dislocation of one or both of the sacroiliac joints; this injury is secondary to anterior compression injury and is often associated with damage to the pelvic viscera

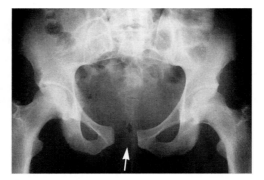

Sprung pelvis noted by the widened pubic symphysis *(arrow)* and probable dislocation of one or both sacroiliac joints. The width of the pubic symphysis joint space should not exceed 6 mm in females and 7 mm in males. (Courtesy Steven P. Brownstein, Springfield, NJ.)

TABLE 12-6

Fractures, Dislocations, and Soft Tissue Injuries of the Pelvis and Lower Extremities—cont'd

Injury	Comments
Hip	
Fractures	
Extracapsular fracture	Fracture of the greater and lesser trochanters, intertrochanteric, and subtrochanteric regions; because the arterial supply remains intact, extracapsular fractures are less often complicated by avascular necrosis and nonunion than are intracapsular fractures
Intracapsular fracture	Fracture proximal to the trochanters; this type includes fractures just below the femoral head (subcapital, which is the most common type),[55] through the femoral neck (midcervical, which is rare), and at the base of the femoral neck (basicervical, uncommon); pathological fractures commonly occur at the femoral neck, usually in a basicervical location; the circumflex arteries may tear with capsular damage resulting in complication of avascular necrosis and nonunion[7,8,77]; fractures of the proximal femur are most common among osteoporotic elderly females

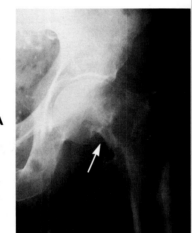 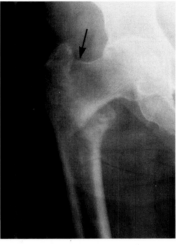

A, Subcapital fracture with loss of apposition and superior displacement of the femur *(arrow).* **B,** Basicervical fracture with a narrowed femoral angle *(arrow).*

Dislocation	
Hip dislocation	Primarily posterior (80% to 85%), most often resulting from a force to the knee while the hip is in flexion as occurs in a motor vehicle accident when the knee strikes the dashboard[46,146]; fracture of the posterior column or posterior rim of the acetabulum, degeneration,[46] or avascular necrosis[94] often accompanies the dislocation; anterior dislocations are caused by hyperextension and abduction injuries
Knee	
Fractures	
Distal femur fracture	Supracondylar fracture resulting from axial loading with varus or valgus stress forces; fractures are oblique or transverse, often comminuted, and may extend into the joint[59,116,117]; fractures involving the condyles often appear as T- or Y-shaped with varying degrees of comminution
Fibula fracture	Commonly occurs in the middle and distal thirds of the fibula; isolated fracture of the proximal fibula is uncommon and is usually accompanied by ligamentous or fractures about the knee and ankle; compartment syndrome may develop secondary to accumulations of hemorrhage and edema within the anterior, posterior, or lateral compartment

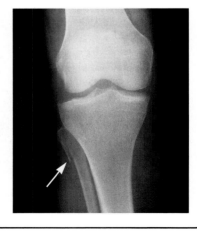

Fracture through the neck of the fibula *(arrow).* (Courtesy Steven P. Brownstein, Springfield, NJ.)

Continued

TABLE 12-6
Fractures, Dislocations, and Soft Tissue Injuries of the Pelvis and Lower Extremities—cont'd

Injury	Comments

Knee—cont'd
Fractures—cont'd

| Flake fracture | Fracture of the posterior patellar surface following patellar dislocation |
| Floating knee fracture | Supracondylar femur fracture in combination with proximal tibia fracture |

Patella fracture

Secondary to direct trauma or indirect forces from contraction of the quadriceps,[98] producing vertical, transverse (most common, 50% to 90%), or stellate (comminuted) fractures; distinguished from the bi- or multipartite normal variants by such characteristics as history of trauma and nonbilateral presentation

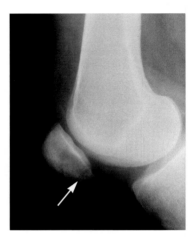

Fracture of the patella *(arrow)*. (Courtesy Tim Mick, St. Paul, Minn.)

Proximal tibia

Fracture of the medial (20%) or lateral (80%) tibial plateau from varus or valgus strain, respectively, with vertical and rotational forces also present; 25% of these result from pedestrians struck by an automobile ("bumper" or "fender" fractures); ligamentous injuries often accompany plateau fractures[150]; occasionally fractures such as those about the knee, shoulder, or elbow extend to the subarticular space, allowing fatty marrow elements to enter the joint space; when this occurs, often a fat-blood interface (FBI sign) is noted in the lateral projection, indicating lipohemarthrosis; lipohemarthrosis is most common in the knee, shoulder, and elbow

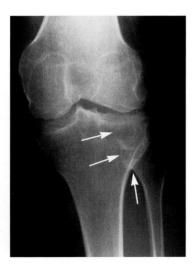

Fracture of the tibial plateau *(arrows)*. (Courtesy Tim Mick, St. Paul, Minn.)

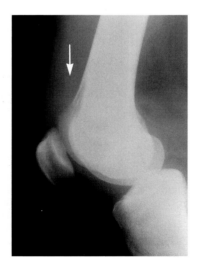

Radiodense suprapatellar effusion *(arrow)*. (Courtesy Tim Mick, St. Paul, Minn.)

TABLE 12-6
Fractures, Dislocations, and Soft Tissue Injuries of the Pelvis and Lower Extremities—cont'd

Injury	Comments

Knee—cont'd
Fractures—cont'd

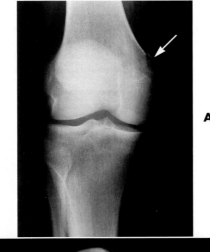

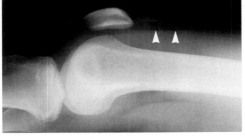

A, Avulsion of the adductor tubercle *(arrow)* with intraarticular fracture of the proximal tibia and medial femoral condyle. Because the fracture extends into the knee joint, bone marrow may extend into the joint. **B,** The intraarticular fatty marrow is less dense and lays above the water-based edema and blood in the joint forming a fat-blood interface (FBI sign) on a recumbent projection *(arrowheads).* (Courtesy Steven P. Brownstein, Springfield, NJ.)

Injury	Comments
Segond's fracture	Avulsion of the lateral capsular ligament secondary to internal tibial rotation while the knee is flexed; this must be distinguished from the more anterior and inferior fragment created by avulsion of the iliotibial band from Gerdy's tubercle; a Segond's fracture is distinguished by the presence of a fracture donor site on the tibial condyle in the frontal projection[139]
Trampoline fracture	Fracture of proximal tibial metaphysis in children
Dislocations	
Knee dislocation	Rare injury resulting from severe trauma, high morbidity secondary to torn ligaments, vessels, and other tissues[85,101,120,131]; classified by position of tibia with respect to femur: anterior (most common, occurring 50% of the time), posterior, medial, lateral, and rotary
Patellar dislocation	Usually lateral[71], often associated with osteochondral flake fracture of the articular surfaces of the patella[140]; lateral dislocation is associated with rapidly changing directions while running[64]; MRI diagnosis of patellar dislocation consists of a typical triad of patellar bone bruise, femoral bone bruise, and associated tearing of the medial retinacular attachments; a large degree of effusion is seen with acute dislocation; the condition is associated with hypoplastic lateral femoral condyle, genu valgum, abnormal lateral insertion of the patellar tendon and patella alta

Continued

TABLE 12-6
Fractures, Dislocations, and Soft Tissue Injuries of the Pelvis and Lower Extremities—cont'd

Injury	Comments

Knee—cont'd

Soft tissue injuries (ligaments and cartilage)

Anterior cruciate ligament (ACL) tear — Normally of intermediate to low signal intensity and is best seen on the sagittal images; the most common site for tears is at the midlength of the ligament; on occasion avulsion occurs, usually at the femoral attachment; coexistent injuries to the meniscus and the medial collateral ligament should be considered; diagnostic accuracy of MRI reaches 95% in the evaluation of anterior cruciate ligament tears[49]; classic features of complete ACL ruptures include increased curvature, or buckling, of the posterior cruciate ligament and anterior tibial subluxation; signs of partial tear include thinning of the fibers of the ACL, hematomas about the intact fibers of the ACL, and increased signal intensity within the ACL, which still has intact fibers

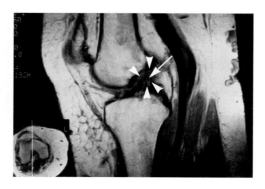

T1-weighted MRI with disruption of the anterior cruciate ligament *(arrow)*. The ACL normally appears as a smooth hypointense (black) oblique band. This case shows disruption of the band and surrounding mixed signal of hemorrhage and edema *(arrowheads)*. (Courtesy Steven P. Brownstein, Springfield, NJ.)

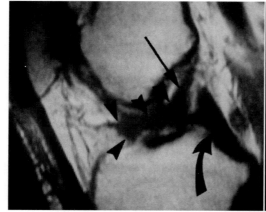

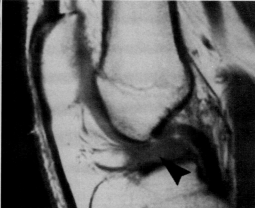

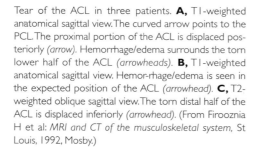

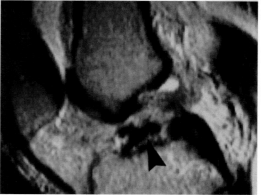

Tear of the ACL in three patients. **A,** T1-weighted anatomical sagittal view. The curved arrow points to the PCL. The proximal portion of the ACL is displaced posteriorly *(arrow)*. Hemorrhage/edema surrounds the torn lower half of the ACL *(arrowheads)*. **B,** T1-weighted anatomical sagittal view. Hemor-rhage/edema is seen in the expected position of the ACL *(arrowhead)*. **C,** T2-weighted oblique sagittal view. The torn distal half of the ACL is displaced inferiorly *(arrowhead)*. (From Firooznia H et al: *MRI and CT of the musculoskeletal system,* St Louis, 1992, Mosby.)

TABLE 12-6

Fractures, Dislocations, and Soft Tissue Injuries of the Pelvis and Lower Extremities—cont'd

Injury	Comments

Knee—cont'd

Soft tissue injuries (ligaments and cartilage)—cont'd

Posterior cruciate ligament (PCL) tear

Moderately thicker and approximately twice as strong as the ACL; consequently, PCL tears are less common than ACL tears; the PCL is of lower signal intensity than the ACL and normally assumes a slightly arcuate course; tears of the PCL are most common at the mid-length of the ligament with avulsion occurring at the tibial insertion; isolated PCL tears are uncommon and associated injuries to the anterior cruciate ligament or the menisci should be sought; bone contusions are often noted about the knee and are associated with complete tears of the ACL and are located on the posterolateral tibial plateau and the lateral femoral condyle because of impaction of the lateral femoral condyle into the posterior tibia

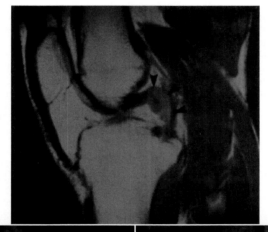

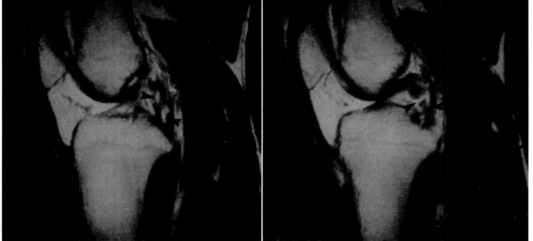

PCL tear. **A,** A sagittal anatomical T1-weighted image. Note the markedly irregular, thickened, and buckled PCL *(arrowheads)*, with its nonhomogeneously increased internal signal intensity (SI). The ACL was also torn in this patient. **B** and **C,** T2-weighted anatomical sagittals. The multiple zones of increased SI in the substance of the PCL indicate tears of the ligament *(arrowheads)*. (From Firooznia H et al: *MRI and CT of the musculoskeletal system,* St Louis, 1992, Mosby.)

Continued

TABLE 12-6

Fractures, Dislocations, and Soft Tissue Injuries of the Pelvis and Lower Extremities—cont'd

Injury	Comments
Knee—cont'd	
Soft tissue injuries (ligaments and cartilage)—cont'd	
Chondromalacia patella	Patellofemoral joint pain accentuated on flexion of the knee, which commonly affects young adults and adolescents; axial MRI studies show early cartilage thinning or erosion of the cartilaginous surface along with focal regions of edema and later marked hypointensity on T1 and T2 (sclerosis) of the subchondral bone
Collateral ligament injuries	Medial collateral ligament (MCL) injuries: secondary to a valgus stress applied to the flexed knee; injuries to the MCL are best evident on coronal images with T2-weighted images demonstrating edema and hemorrhage about the usually low-signal intensity fibers of the ligament; complete tears are seen as a loss of continuity of the ligament fibers; lateral collateral ligament (LCL) injuries often occur with the leg in internal rotation with a varus stress
Meniscal tears	Arise from multiple etiologies: degenerative joint disease, sports injuries, joint tracking disorders, intraarticular fractures, and other joint diseases; the intact meniscus is of low signal intensity on all imaging sequences; the diagnosis of meniscal tear requires evidence of an abnormal linear signal intensity extending to an articular surface of the meniscus; tears are named for their location, shape, and direction of the tear: vertical, horizontal, bucket handle, parrot beak, peripheral, radial, meniscocapsular separation, and tear with truncation; three grades of abnormal signal intensity are associated with abnormal menisci: grade I is a globular foci of abnormal signal correlating with mucinous degeneration; the signal does not extend to the meniscal articular surface; grade II is a linear, horizontal region of increased signal intensity that does not extend to the articular surface; grades I and II menisci are arthroscopically normal; grade III is an abnormal signal intensity (often linear) that extends to an articular surface

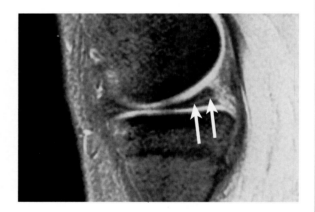

Grade II meniscal signal. Linear signal intensity *(arrows)*, which may communicate with the capsular margin but not with an articular surface, is seen on this radial gradient-echo image (SE 700/14/25 degrees). (From Stark DD, Gradley WG: *Magnetic resonance imaging,* ed 2, St Louis, 1992, Mosby.)

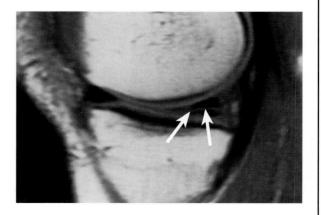

Grade III meniscal signal. Horizontal cleavage tear of the posterior horn of this medial meniscus is visualized as a region of grade III signal *(arrows)*. (SE 2000/20). (From Stark DD, Gradley WG: *Magnetic resonance imaging,* ed 2, St Louis, 1992, Mosby.)

TABLE 12-6

Fractures, Dislocations, and Soft Tissue Injuries of the Pelvis and Lower Extremities—cont'd

Injury	Comments
Knee—cont'd	
Soft tissue injuries (ligaments and cartilage)—cont'd	
Osteochondritis dissecans	Affects younger patients, primarily in the non-weight-bearing lateral surface of the medial femoral condyle; low signal intensity subchondral foci are present on both the T1 and T2; conventional radiographic findings are usually absent early in the disease; features also include in situ bone and cartilage fragment with or without evidence of displacement or migration
Ankle	
Fractures	
Bimalleolar fracture	Medial and lateral malleolar fractures, representing tensile forces on one side and compressive forces on the other side

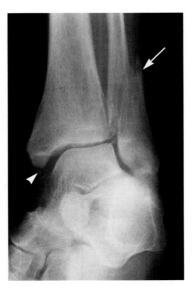

Bimalleolar fracture of the ankle. A small avulsion fracture is noted from the medial malleolus *(arrowhead)* with an oblique fracture through the distal fibula *(arrow),* and lateral displacement of the talus in relation to the tibia evidenced by the increased medial joint space. The fractures are consistent with an eversion injury, causing tension on the medial side (developing an avulsion of the tibia) and compression on the lateral side (developing an oblique or spiral fracture of the distal fibula. At times the fibular fracture may occur higher and may be missed on an ankle series. (Courtesy Steven P. Brownstein, Springfield, NJ.)

Injury	Comments
Dupuytren's fracture	Fracture of the distal fibula proximal to the distal tibiofibular syndesmosis resulting from pronation-external rotation injury; usually a wide separation of the tibial and fibula occurs with lateral displacement of the talus
Lateral malleolus fracture	Usually spiral fracture resulting from outward or external rotation of the foot; fractures proximal to the tibiotalar joint imply damage to the tibiofibular ligaments, representing more unstable injuries than fractures occurring distal to the tibiotalar joint space
Maisonneuve fracture	Fracture of the proximal fibula with rupture of the distal tibiofibular ligaments and interosseous membrane extending proximal to the fibular fracture; this occurs secondary to external rotation of foot; because of its proximal location, it is often missed on the radiographs of the ankle[123]

PART TWO Bone, Joints, and Soft Tissues

Continued

TABLE 12-6
Fractures, Dislocations, and Soft Tissue Injuries of the Pelvis and Lower Extremities—cont'd

Injury	Comments
Ankle—cont'd	
Fractures—cont'd	
Medial malleolus fracture	Transverse or oblique fractures resulting from compressive forces from talus, or tensile forces and avulsion of the deltoid ligament

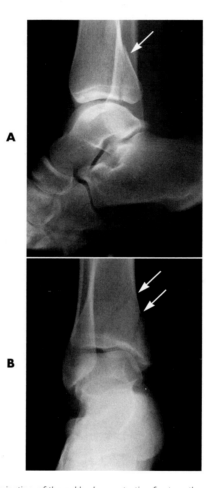

A, Lateral projection of the ankle demonstrating fracture through its lower posterior margin *(arrow)*. B, On the oblique projection the medial malleolus is separated from the tibia *(arrows)*. Two fracture lines *(arrows)* appear because the fracture line is not parallel to the x-ray beam, yielding a double projection. (Courtesy Steven P. Brownstein, Springfield, NJ.)

Injury	Comments
Pilon (pestle) fracture	Compression injury that drives the talus into the tibial plafond similar to a pestle into a mortar,100 most often accompanies other ankle or skeletal trauma
Tillaux's fracture	Fractures of the anterior tibial tubercle, medial and lateral malleoli
Trimalleolar (Cotton's) fracture	Fracture of the medial and lateral malleolus and posterior lip of the distal tibia (sometimes referred to as the *third malleolus*)[102]
Triplane fracture	Describes three planes of fracture: horizontal fracture within the epiphyseal plate, sagittal fracture of the epiphysis, and an oblique vertical fracture in the posterior distal tibial metaphysis[38]
Dislocation	
Ankle dislocation	Fractures accompanying medial and lateral dislocations; anterior and posterior (most common) may occur without fracture

TABLE 12-6

Fractures, Dislocations, and Soft Tissue Injuries of the Pelvis and Lower Extremities—cont'd

Injury	Comments

Ankle—cont'd

Soft tissue injuries (ligaments and cartilage)

Achilles tendon tear — Largest tendon in the body, formed from the gastrocnemius and soleus muscles; ruptures are clearly demonstrated on MRI, whereas clinical examination can miss rupture of the Achilles tendon in up to 25% of cases; radiography is not effective in identifying abnormalities in the Achilles tendon; injuries to the tendon are often secondary to athletic activity and are frequently observed in middle-age males; with rupture of the Achilles tendon the proximal and distal portions of the torn tendon can be delineated; associated hemorrhage within the tendon sheath can also be appreciated; because conservative management of tendon tears is possible, the MRI examination is critical in documenting the degree of apposition in the disrupted tendon and allows early identification of patients who are candidates for surgical intervention

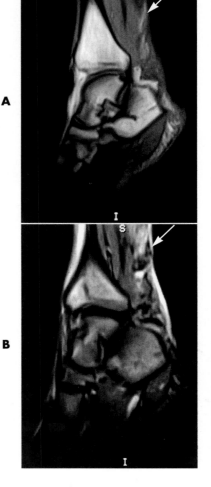

T1-weighted **(A)** and T2-weighted **(B)** MRI scan of a calcaneal (Achilles) tendon rupture. The arrows point to tissue remnants and the area where the hypointense (black) tendon should be found *(arrows)*. (Courtesy Joseph W. Howe, Sylmar, Calif.)

Transchondral injuries — Include osteochondral fractures, osteochondritis dissecans, and talar dome fractures; the latter is usually found to involve either the medial or lateral talar dome with extension into both the articular cartilage and subchondral bone; associated focal cartilaginous signal alteration and joint effusion; MRI is helpful in the evaluation of osteochondral lesions of the ankle, because neither conventional radiography or CT scans can fully assess the integrity of hyaline articular cartilage; further, early x-rays of transchondral fracture may be negative until a necrotic focus is demarcated

Continued

TABLE 12-6

Fractures, Dislocations, and Soft Tissue Injuries of the Pelvis and Lower Extremities—cont'd

Injury	Comments
Foot	
Fractures	
Calcaneal fracture	Most common tarsal fracture; when secondary to compressive injuries, this may reduce the arc of the superior margin of the calcaneus (Boehler's angle, normally 30 to 35 degrees); beak fractures involve the superior calcaneal tuberosity, often secondary to avulsion of the Achilles tendon insertion[99]

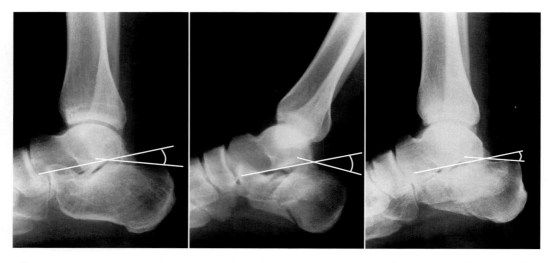

Three cases of calcaneal fracture. In each instance the angle across the superior margin of the calcaneous (Boehler's angle) is reduced to less than 28 degrees. (Courtesy Steven P. Brownstein, Springfield, NJ.)

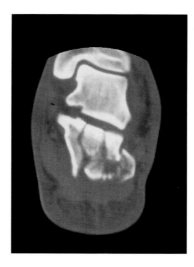

Comminuted fracture of the calcaneus noted on the CT.

TABLE 12-6

Fractures, Dislocations, and Soft Tissue Injuries of the Pelvis and Lower Extremities—cont'd

Injury	Comments

Foot—cont'd
Fractures—cont'd
Metatarsal fracture

Usually the result of a heavy object falling on the foot; stress fractures are common at the second or third metatarsal (march fractures); dancer's or Jones fractures are fractures of the base of the fifth metatarsal that appear transverse, to be distinguished from the normal longitudinal radiolucency often noted at the base of the metatarsal, representing nonunion of the secondary growth center in children

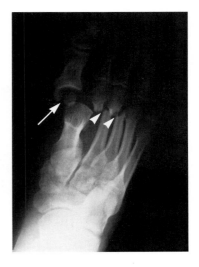

Fracture of the second and third metatarsals *(arrowheads)* with medial dislocation of the first metatarsophalangeal joint *(arrow)*. (Courtesy Steven P. Brownstein, Springfield, NJ.)

A **B**

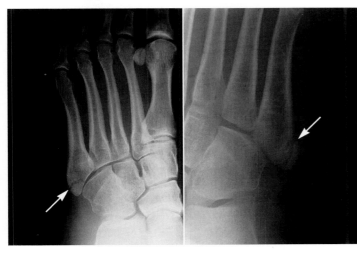

A, Oblique projection of the foot with a fracture of the proximal fifth metatarsal (dancer's or Jones fracture) *(arrow)*. Do not confuse this fracture with the normal growth center found in this proximity. **B,** The radiolucent line of the growth center is found parallel to the long axis of the metatarsal *(arrow)*, the fracture is transverse to the long axis (**A,** arrow). (**B,** Courtesy Joseph W. Howe, Sylmar, Calif.)

Phalangeal fracture

Secondary to kicking or "stubbing" injury (bedroom fracture), or when the foot is struck by heavy falling object; configuration may be oblique, transverse, or comminuted; hallux rigidus refers to a stiff, painful first digit following trauma

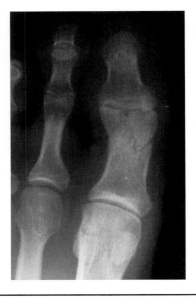

Comminuted fracture of the big toe. (Courtesy Tim Mick, St. Paul, Minn.)

Continued

TABLE 12-6

Fractures, Dislocations, and Soft Tissue Injuries of the Pelvis and Lower Extremities

Injury	Comments

Foot—cont'd
Fractures—cont'd

Talus fracture — Second most common tarsal fracture, usually avulsion; aviator's fracture or aviator's astragalus is a fracture through the neck of the talus, which may occur as the pilot's foot hits the steering pedals during an aircraft crash; a subcortical radiolucent line within the dome of the talus (Hawkins sign) following injury indicates good vascularity, and that avascular necrosis is unlikely to complicate the injury

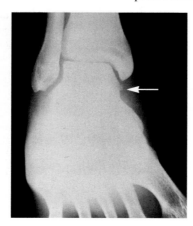

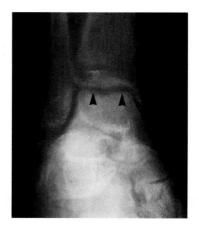

Fracture of the medial malleolus *(arrow)*. (Courtesy Tim Mick, St. Paul, Minn.)

Subtalar lucent zone indicating good vascular supply (Hawkin's sign) *(arrowheads)*. (Courtesy Tim Mick, St. Paul, Minn.)

Dislocations

Midtarsal (Chopart's) dislocation — Rare separation of the hindfoot from the midfoot at the talonavicular and calcaneocuboid joints; the distal foot is typically displaced medially

Phalangeal, metatarsal dislocation (see Metatarsal Fracture, p. 571) — Usually posterior and may be found in combination with fractures of the phalanges and metatarsals

Subtalar dislocation — Simultaneous dislocations of the talonavicular and talocalcaneal joints, produced by compression injuries applied while the foot is inverted,[20] usually displacing the calcaneus, navicular, and forefoot medially respective to the talus

Tarsometatarsal (Lisfranc's) dislocation — Lateral displacement of the metatarsal bases at their articulation with the tarsals; the separation may be associated with fractures, particularly the base of the second metatarsal[51,177]

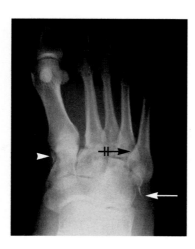

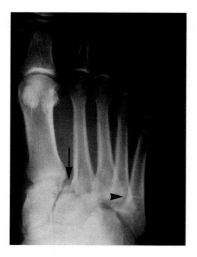

Fracture of the cuboid *(arrow)* and medial cuneiform *(arrowhead)* with lateral dislocation of the second through fifth metatarsals at their articulation with the tarsals (Lisfranc's dislocation) *(crossed arrow)*. (Courtesy Steven P. Brownstein, Springfield, NJ.)

Lateral dislocation of the second through fifth metatarsals *(arrowhead)* at the metatarsotarsal joint with fracture of the proximal medial portion of the second metatarsal *(arrow)*. (Courtesy Steven P. Brownstein, Springfield, NJ).

Joint injuries. Joint injury may result in subluxation, dislocation, diastasis, or fracture. Subluxation is the displacement of a bone in relation to the adjacent bone, resulting in partial loss of articulation of the opposing bone ends. A chiropractic subluxation is a clinical entity that may or may not involve bone misalignment. A dislocation is a displacement of a bone in relation to the adjacent bone, producing a complete loss of articulation between the opposing bone ends. Simple or comminuted intraarticular fractures may involve only the articular cartilage (chondral fractures) or extend into the subjacent bone (osteochondral fractures) (Fig. 12-3). Intraarticular fragments may dislodge or remain in situ. Diastasis describes separation of the adjacent joint surfaces of a fibrous or cartilaginous joint.

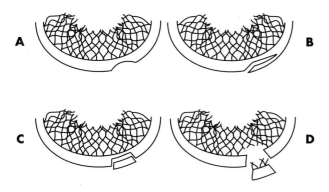

FIG. 12-3 Injuries to the articular surface of a joint appear as indented **(A)**, hinged **(B)**, or detached **(C)** chondral defects. Detached fractures of the articular cartilage and underlying bone **(D)** are known as *osteochondral fractures*. Detached chondral and osteochondral fractures may remain in situ or dislodge to become free bodies within the joint. (Modified from Rogers LF: *Radiology of skeletal trauma*, ed 2, New York, 1992, Churchill Livingstone.)

Fracture healing. Successful fracture healing depends on fragment apposition, fracture fixation, and ample blood supply. For purposes of exposition, bone healing is often divided arbitrarily into five stages (Fig. 12-4):

1. Hematoma. Following trauma, vessels are damaged, and subsequently the damaged bone ends and surrounding soft tissues bleed. A blood clot develops. Osteocytes, imprisoned in their lacunae near the fracture site, lose their blood supply and undergo necrosis (see Fig. 12-4, *A*).

2. Inflammation. Within several hours of the injury an acute inflammatory reaction develops with proliferation of cells from beneath the periosteum and endosteum of the traumatized area. Proliferating granulation tissue surrounds and bridges the fracture fragments. The hematoma is slowly resorbed, and new capillary buds invaginate the injured areas (see Fig. 12-4, *B*).

3. Callus. Around 3 weeks following the initial trauma, the proliferating fibroblasts of the granular tissue show metaplasia to collagenoblasts, chondroblasts, and osteoblasts. This cellular reaction raises the periosteum away from the bone cortex and an osteoblastic collar is formed around the bone fragments, representing primitive woven bone laid in an indiscriminate fashion. Although still mobile, the callus causes the fracture to become more stable. It is visible on a radiograph and may be felt as a firm mass on palpation (see Fig. 12-4, *C*).

4. Consolidation. Osteoclasts are introduced by the penetrating capillary buds. They help the osteoblasts to alter the bone callus from woven to lamellar bone. The healing bone can withstand normal loads and should not move, a state referred to as "clinically united"(see Fig. 12-4, *D*).

5. Remodeling. Over a period of months the bony bridge is remodeled to the pretrauma size and shape, or as near to it as possible. Excessive callus is removed, and the medullary canal is recanalized. Children have greater powers of remodeling and may correct deformities and even discrepancies of length after a fracture (see Fig. 12-4, *E*).

The time required for union varies with the age and health status of the patient in addition to the type of bone that is injured. Typically, cancellous bone requires 6 weeks and cortical bone requires 15 weeks to heal in adults. Children require about half as long as adults to heal.

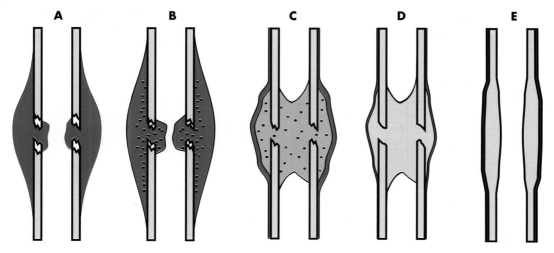

FIG. 12-4 Stages of fracture healing. **A,** Hematoma. **B,** Inflammation. **C,** Callus. **D,** Consolidation. **E,** Remodeling.

Fracture complications. Fracture complications are divided into early or late consequences. For the most part, early complications affect soft tissues and late complications affect bone. Early complications are noted within a few days following the injury, and late complications take months to appear. Some of the more common complications are listed in Table 12-7.

IMAGING FINDINGS

By itself, the patient's clinical presentation is not reliable in determining the presence or absence of skeletal injury. Radiographic examination is necessary to determine the presence or absence of clinically suspected fractures. It should involve at least two opposing projections of the region of interest. Often the clinical circumstances warrant a second radiographic examination to exclude suspected occult fractures. Reexamination is recommended after 7 to 10 days, which gives the osteoclasts time to remove necrotic bone from around the fracture site, producing a more visible radiolucent fracture line than may have been present on the initial radiographs.

To exclude related joint injuries, minimal radiographic studies should include the joint closest to the patient's complaint of pain in the field of view. Tomography (linear and computed) and MRI are

---

TABLE 12-7
Early and Late Fracture Complications

Complication	Description
Early	
Compartmental (Volkmann's) syndrome	Results from hemorrhage or edema, which may increase the osteofascial intracompartmental pressure following trauma, reducing arterial flow producing avascular muscle ischemia; a viscous cycle results as the muscle ischemia causes more edema, leading to a greater reduction in arterial flow, and more ischemic contracture results from damaged, contracted muscle following prolonged ischemia
Hemarthrosis	Bleeding into the joint space results in early arthritis
Infection	Occurs in 12% to 16% of open fractures[36,56]; femur and tibia are the most common sites; the dominant organism is *Staphylococcus aureus*
Loss of function	Loss of limb or digit mobility caused by avulsions of tendons and ligaments; notoriously loss of function follows apparently innocuous chip fractures of the phalanges, which represent avulsions of the extensor or flexion tendon groups
Nerve injury	Open fractures often associated with severed nerves
Spinal cord injury	Requires meticulous neurological examination, with any fracture of the spine, however trivial it may appear to be; this establishes whether the spinal cord or nerve roots have been damaged and documents baseline data for later comparison if neurological signs should develop
Vascular injury	Compressed, cut, or contused vessels by associated trauma; this type of injury most often occurs in the extremities about the knee and elbow
Visceral injury	Caused by trauma to the trunk; abdominal and pelvic viscera are injured, namely puncture of the lung with development of pneumothorax following rib fractures, and rupture of the bladder or urethra with pelvic fractures; it is important to inquire about urinary function; if a urethral or bladder injury is suspected, diagnostic urethrography may be necessary
Late	
Algodystrophy (Sudeck's atrophy)	Condition of altered bone growth typically seen in the hand or foot often after trivial injury
Avascular necrosis	Because they have a precarious blood supply, the scaphoid, femoral head, and other areas of the skeleton are predisposed to ischemia and resulting avascular necrosis following trauma
Delayed union	Delayed healing, resulting from an inadequate blood supply or fixation of fragments; if radiographic evidence of bone callus does not exist within 3 months, internal fixation and bone grafting may be necessary
Growth disturbance	Abnormal growth and deformity caused by trauma to the epiphyseal growth plates in children
Joint stiffness	Reduced joint motion, most often developing in the knee, elbow, and small joints of the hand, resulting from adhesion following hemarthrosis or prolonged immobilization
Malunion	Unsatisfactory healing, usually referring to poor alignment or unacceptable deformity
Myositis ossificans	Heterotropic bone formation developing in soft tissues; although it is most often related to injury, the condition is also seen in nontraumatic conditions such as paraplegia or coma

especially helpful to define areas of complex anatomy (e.g., spine, wrist, and ankle); radionuclide bone scintigraphy is helpful to locate fractures and is especially useful in evaluating the presence of stress fractures.

The radiographic features vary, depending on the interval between the injury and radiographic examination. Initial radiographic findings may lag 2 to 6 days behind the onset of symptoms. Radionuclide bone scintigraphy more accurately denotes the presence of fracture during this interval.

For the most part, fractures appear radiographically as radiolucent lines traversing bone. Frequently, soft tissue swelling accom-

panies fractures. Stress fractures appear as radiodense bands, indicating the bony proliferation occurring in response to the repetitive stress.

CLINICAL COMMENTS

Immediate clinical concern is directed toward first aid of the patient. Measures should be taken to limit pain and prevent further damage by limiting movement of the fragments by supporting or splinting the area. Fractures to long bones may be associated with considerable blood loss, requiring compression.

In general, four levels of treatment exist: reduction, immobi-

TABLE 12-7 Early and Late Fracture Complications—cont'd	
Complication	**Description**
Late—cont'd	
Nonunion	No healing, resulting from an inadequate blood supply, poor fixation, loss of apposition, and the presence of interposed cartilage, muscle, or periosteum between bone fragments; the fracture site is filled in with fibrous tissue that may form a rudimentary joint (pseudoarthrosis) if motion continues at the fracture site; nonunion that appears with large callous formation is termed *hypertrophic nonunion,* whereas nonunion with little callous is termed *atrophic nonunion*

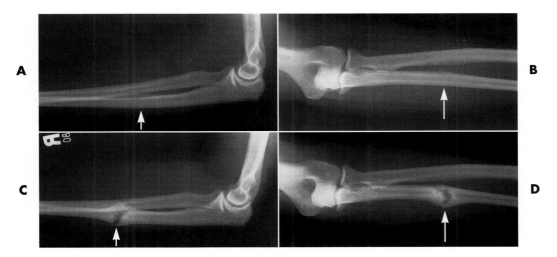

Fracture of the midshaft of the ulna (**A** and **B**), developing nonunion and pseudoarthrosis (**C** and **D**) on subsequent films *(arrows).*

Osteoarthritis	Secondary to hemorrhage or trauma, which may alter the smooth articular joint surfaces leading to degeneration

lization or fixation, bony union, and functional restoration. Closed reduction refers to nonsurgical manipulation or traction of the fracture fragments. Open reduction involves internal manipulation of the fragments. K wires, plates, intramedullary rods, and bone screws may be inserted for internal fixation at the fracture site. Most fractures are treated initially with closed reduction. To ensure a successful outcome, a soft tissue bridge (i.e., periosteum) must be in place. Once bony union occurs, the patient must undergo a vigorous rehabilitation program to achieve rapid and full recovery from the injury.

▋KEY CONCEPTS

- *Plain film radiography is the first modality for most skeletal trauma, CT offers better osseous detail and allows intracranial imaging, and MRI best illustrates bone marrow and soft tissue injuries.*
- *A fracture is a break in the structural continuity of bone, manifesting as minor cracks, crumpling, splintering, or complete disruption of the cortex.*
- *Fractures are often described on the basis of skin puncture (closed or open), etiology (acute, stress, pathologic, or insufficiency), or direction of the fracture plane (oblique, spiral, or transverse).*
- *Description of a fracture should include the following information: identity of injured bone, location of fracture in the bone, fragment apposition (shift), alignment (tilt), rotation (twist), distraction (separation), and any resulting alteration in limb length.*
- *Epiphyseal injuries are described with the Salter-Harris classification (types I through V).*
- *Joint injury may result in subluxation (partial misalignment), dislocation (complete misalignment), diastasis (separation), or fracture (chondral, osteochondral, or osseous).*
- *Healing phases include hematoma, inflammation, callus, consolidation, and remodeling.*
- *Treatment occurs at four levels: reduction, immobilization or fixation, bony union, and functional restoration.*

Myositis Ossificans

BACKGROUND

Myositis ossificans (heterotropic bone formation) presents in two forms: circumscripta and progressiva. The circumscribed form is a benign, solitary, self-limiting disorder representing metaplasia of soft tissue to bone.[92] It is usually related to trauma (myositis ossificans traumatica), but it may also be idiopathic in nature (myositis ossificans idiopathica). The trauma is most often to the muscle, and less commonly fascia, tendon, and joint capsules are involved. Only rarely is fatty tissue implicated. The exact pathogenesis is unknown, and contrary to the name, no primary muscle inflammation is present.[92]

The progressive form, also known as *Muchmeyer's disease* or *fibrodysplasia ossificans progressiva,* is a rare hereditary connective tissue disorder of unknown etiology. The disease is believed to be an autosomal dominant trait with complete penetrance and variable expressivity.[17]

IMAGING FINDINGS

In its early stages, myositis ossificans may appear similar to osteosarcoma or other bone malignancies. Therefore, it is important to recognize the radiographic features of circumscribed myositis ossificans to aid its differentiation. On plain radiographs, myositis ossificans circumscripta may be present as faint tissue calcifications within 2 to 6 weeks after the onset of symptoms.[1] Within 6 to 8 weeks the center of the lesion becomes more radiolucent as the periphery develops a surround radiodense ring (Fig. 12-5). This is re-

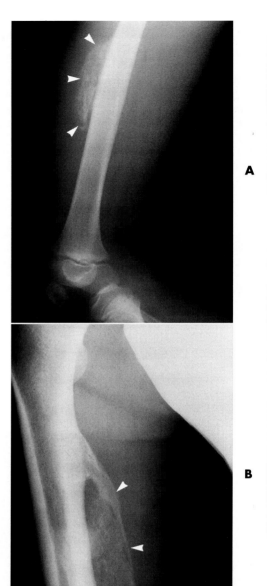

FIG. 12-5   Myositis ossificans appearing as a calcific soft tissue mass in the anterior **(A)** and medial **(B)** regions of the thigh in different patients. The perimeter of each mass *(arrowheads)* appears more radiodense than the center identifying the zonal phenomena characteristic of myositis ossificans. (**A,** Courtesy Steven P. Brownstein, Springfield, NJ.)

ferred to as a *zonal phenomenon* and is more easily noted on CT. A reversal of this zonal pattern is noted in some malignancies. A malignancy may present with a more radiodense center and with a surrounding radiolucent periphery about the lesion. In addition, malignancies are not clearly separated from their parent bone as is myositis ossificans.

Myositis ossificans circumscripta may occur anywhere but is most common in the following: brachialis (fencer's bone), adductor longus (rider's bone), soleus (dancer's bone), and adductor magnus tendon.[167] Myositis ossificans progressiva appears as extensive ossification of the connective tissues of the limbs and spine with mi-

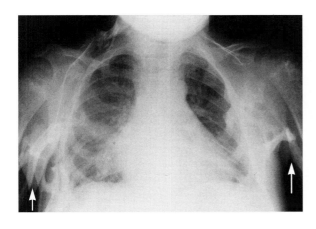

FIG. 12-6 Soft tissue ossifications most prominent in the axillary regions (*arrows*) of a patient with myositis ossificans progressiva. (Courtesy Jack C. Avalos, Davenport, Iowa.)

crodactyly, usually the big toe (90%) and thumbs (50%) are involved (Fig. 12-6). Fusion of the vertebrae and ossification of the voluntary muscle may be complete by age 20 years. The hands, sphincters, diaphragm, and viscera are spared.[31]

CLINICAL COMMENTS

A history of trauma is present in up to 60% of circumscribed presentations. Supportive care (e.g., reduced mobility) is the accepted conservative management.[22,34] However, occasionally surgical removal of ectopic bone may be necessary.[106] The progressive form usually presents in the first year of life as neck stiffness with concurrent edematous subcutaneous nodules. The symptoms progress to the shoulders and upper limbs, and later to the lower extremities. Commonly paraplegics demonstrate circumscribed areas of myositis ossificans in the paralyzed regions, usually hips or thighs.

KEY CONCEPTS

- *Myositis ossificans traumatica is related to history of trauma, presenting with zonal phenomena, separation from bone, and predictive development of radiographic pattern, all of which helps to differentiate it from malignancy.*
- *Zonal phenomena is marked by the appearance of a radiolucent center and radiodense periphery of the involved region.*
- *Reverse zonal phenomena is apparent in some malignancies.*
- *Myositis ossificans idiopathica appears similar to the traumatica variety.*
- *Myositis ossificans progressiva is rare; it begins in the first year of life with neck stiffness and advances to near total body ossification by age 20 years.*

Osteochondritis Dissecans

BACKGROUND

Osteochondritis dissecans is a fragmentation of a portion of the articular surface of a joint, involving articular cartilage and possibly subjacent bone. It follows acute osteochondral fracture, or it may be a consequence of repeated stresses, representing a fatigue fracture.[2] However, because many of the separated fragments appear necrotic, some authorities question a purely traumatic etiology, believing instead that avascular necrosis is a primary reason for the development of osteochondritis dissecans.[114] The fragment of bone and cartilage may remain in place (in situ) or dislodge to become a free fragment within the joint space. Occasionally those remaining in situ renew their blood supply and heal. Osteochondritis dissecans occurs most often between the ages of 5 and 50 years, with peak incidence in young adults immediately following the closure of the growth plates (adolescence).

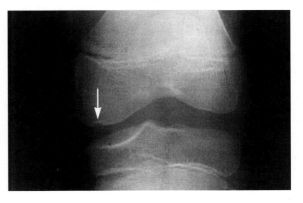

FIG. 12-7 Osteochondritis dissecans of the central medial femoral condyle (*arrow*). (Courtesy Joseph W. Howe, Sylmar, Calif.)

IMAGING FINDINGS

Osteochondritis dissecans is predisposed to target areas of the skeleton. The most common site is the distal femur, involving the medial condyle (usually the lateral portion) 85% of the time and medial condyle 15% of the time (Figs. 12-7 through 12-9). Approximately 20% of presentations are bilateral. Less common sites include: patella, tibial plateau, convex surfaces of metatarsals, talus, capitellum, and femoral head (Figs. 12-10 through 12-12).

CLINICAL COMMENTS

Symptoms are variable, ranging from completely asymptomatic to pain on movement with resulting limitations of motions, joint locking, and stiffness. It is usually not possible to trace the presenting defect to a single traumatic event. MRI is valuable in assessing the stability of the fragment,[180] which has implications for the viability of healing.

KEY CONCEPTS

- *Authorities disagree whether osteochondritis dissecans has a traumatic or avascular etiology.*
- *Osteochondritis dissecans is predisposed to target areas of the skeleton.*
- *Most commonly, this disease occurs at the lateral margin of the medial femoral condyle.*
- *Osteochondritis dissecans typically occurs between the ages of 5 and 50 years with peak incidence during adolescence.*

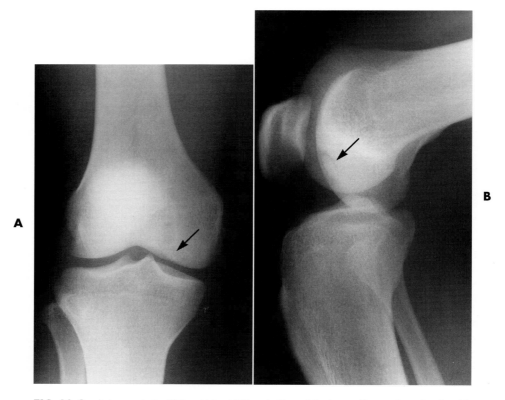

FIG. 12-8   Anteroposterior **(A)** and lateral **(B)** projections of the knee with revealing osteochondritis dissecans on the lateral aspect of the medial femoral condyle *(arrows).* (Courtesy Joseph W. Howe, Sylmar, Calif.)

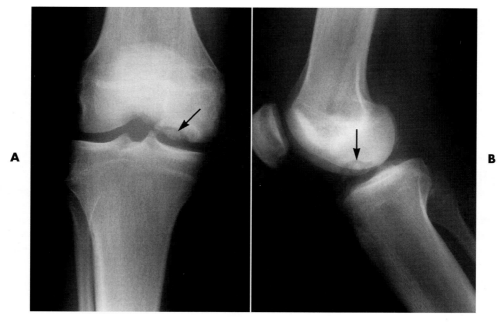

FIG. 12-9   Osteochondritis dissecans of the knee *(arrows).* (Courtesy Steven P. Brownstein, Springfield, NJ.)

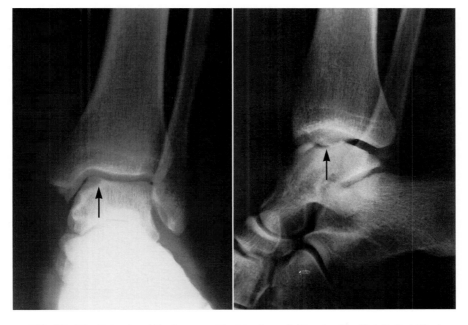

FIG. 12-10 Osteochondritis dissecans of the talus *(arrows)*. (Courtesy Tim Mick, St. Paul, Minn.)

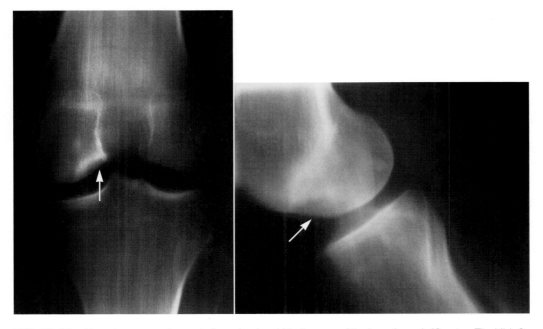

FIG. 12-11 Linear tomograms demonstrating osteochondritis dissecans of the knee *(arrows)*. (Courtesy Tim Mick, St. Paul, Minn.)

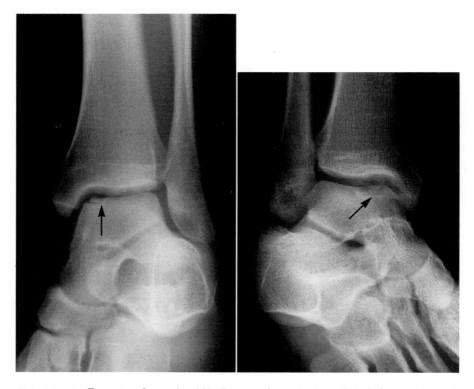

FIG. 12-12   Two cases of osteochondritis dissecans of the talus *(arrows)*. (Left, Courtesy Steven P. Brownstein, Springfield, NJ.)

Slipped Capital Femoral Epiphysis

BACKGROUND

Slipped capital femoral epiphysis (SCFE) is a posteromedioinferior[73] displacement of the proximal femoral epiphysis occurring during childhood. The defect represents a type I Salter-Harris epiphyseal injury. Although the etiology is not clearly defined, the following causes have been implicated: trauma, hormonal influences,[175] adolescent growth spurts,[66] bodyweight,[16,127] vertical orientation of the growth plate,[127] retroversion of the proximal femur,[58,127] renal osteodystrophy,[41] and physical activity.

The condition is more prevalent among blacks,[69,84] males, and those who are overweight[15] and of short stature.[82,83] The peak age is early adolescence. Males typically exhibit this condition between the ages of 10 and 17 years with a peak incidence at 12 years of age; females between the ages of 8 and 15 years with peak incidence at 11 or 12 years of age.[133]

IMAGING FINDINGS

The condition is more common on the left side and is noted bilaterally in 20% to 35% of individuals.[153] The lateral (frog-leg) projection is more sensitive than the frontal projection for demonstrating early changes (Figs. 12-13 and 12-14). To aid recognition, some advocate the use of a line drawn along the lateral cortical margin of the femoral neck (Klein's line). Normally this line should intersect the lateral portion of the femoral capital epiphysis; failure to do so indicates medial slippage of the epiphysis. When compared with the normal side, the slipped epiphysis may appear irregular with decreased vertical height. Buttressing of the lateral femoral neck (Herndon's hump), rounded deformity of the proximal femur (pistol-grip femur), and beaking of the medial epiphysis are other radiographic clues of SCFE.

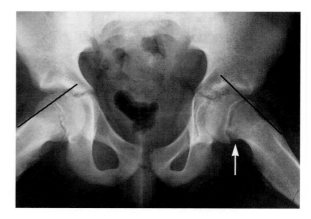

FIG. 12-13   Frog-leg projection demonstrating slipped capital epiphysis on the patient's left *(arrow)*. Kline's line, drawn along the lateral margin of the femoral neck, is a useful aid in the determination of SCFE. (Courtesy Jack C. Avalos, Davenport, Iowa.)

CLINICAL COMMENTS

Clinical symptoms are present in 90% of patients and only 50% have a history of trauma. The usual presentation is that of hip pain and limp. Referred pain to the knee is less common. Limitations of hip motion, particularly in abduction and internal rotation, are usual. SCFE is classified as acute if symptoms are present 3 weeks or less and chronic if longer than 3 weeks. The goal of treatment is stabilization and reduction of further slippage. In situ pinning is the most common treatment.[113,160] A poor outcome may lead to one or more identifiable complications: severe varus deformity, shorten-

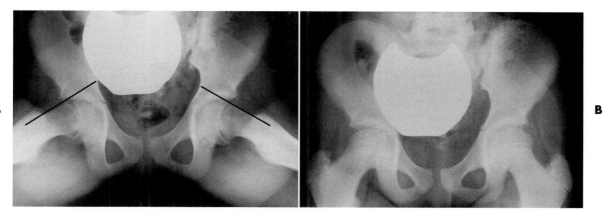

FIG. 12-14 Frog-leg projection **(A)** demonstrating a bilateral presentation of slipped capital femoral epiphysis. The anteroposterior projection **(B)** appears normal. *(Left, Courtesy Steven P. Brownstein, Springfield, NJ.)*

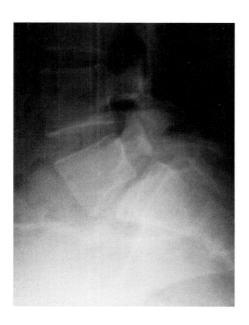

FIG. 12-15 Grade II spondylolisthesis of L5, denoting forward translation of L5 on sacrum.

ing and broadened femoral neck, osteonecrosis,[109] chondrolysis,[76] and precocious degenerative joint disease.[29]

KEY CONCEPTS
- *Posteriomedioinferior displacement of the proximal femoral epiphysis occurs during early adolescence.*
- *Frog-leg (lateral) projection is more sensitive to early slippage.*
- *Hip pain with limp is the typical clinical presentation.*
- *Slipped capital femoral epiphysis has a higher incidence among males, blacks, and those who are overweight.*

Spondylolisthesis

BACKGROUND

Pathogenesis. Spondylolisthesis is an anterior displacement of a vertebrae (and those above it) in relation to the segment immediately below (Fig. 12-15). Spondylolysis denotes disruption of the pars interarticularis, occurring uni- or bilaterally and with (spondylotic spondylolisthesis) or without (prespondylolisthesis)

anterior displacement of the vertebral body. In the lumbar spine the defect usually occurs at the L5 level (67% of the time).[133] In the cervical spine the C6 level is most common.

The incidence of spondylolisthesis is 5% to 7%. Higher incidence occurs among males,[115] whites,[136] Eskimos,[157] Japanese,[91] and those involved in gymnastics, football, weight-lifting, pole-vaulting, and diving.[141] Some authors feel that precocious weight-bearing posture, resulting from infant carriers and walkers, may be a precipitant factor for developing spondylolysis.[179]

Classification. Wiltse, Newman, and MacNab developed a widely used classification system that is based on the etiology and anatomy involved[177]:

Type I: Congenital, developmental abnormalities of the neural arch resulting in deformity and anterior vertebral displacement (Figs. 12-16 and 12-17)

Type II: Isthmic, defect of the pars interarticularis (Fig. 12-18)
  A. Stress fracture through pars interarticularis
  B. Elongated pars interarticularis
  C. Acute fracture of the pars interarticularis

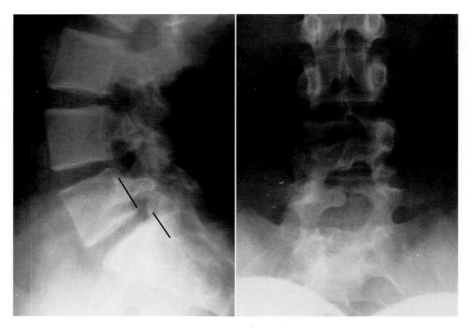

FIG. 12-16   Congenital type I spondylolisthesis of L5 resulting from dysplasia of the posterior arch *(lines)*.

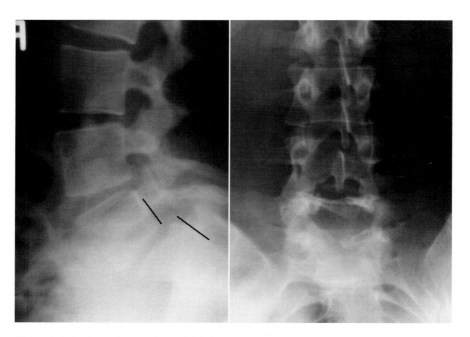

FIG. 12-17   Congenital type I spondylolisthesis of L5 resulting from dysplasia of the posterior arch *(lines)*.

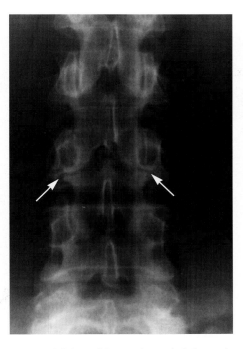

FIG. 12-18   Bilateral defects of the pars interarticularis noted at the L3 level on an anteroposterior projection *(arrows)*. (Courtesy Joseph W. Howe, Sylmar, Calif.)

Type III: Degenerative, segmental instability secondary to advanced degeneration of the intervertebral disc and posterior joints (Figs. 12-19 through 12-21)

Type IV: Traumatic, acute fractures involving the neural arch other than at the pars interarticularis

Type V: Pathologic, osseous deformity secondary to local or systemic pathology (e.g., Paget's disease, metastatic bone disease, osteopetrosis) (Fig. 12-22)

A sixth type, known as *iatrogenic spondylolisthesis* or *spondylolisthesis acquisita* may be used to describe those lesions developing secondary to spinal surgery (e.g., laminectomies, spinal fusions).[179] Of those presenting before the age of 30 years, the mean age of diagnosis is 16 years.[35] Type IIa spondylolisthesis occurring at the L5 level is the most common variety in younger individuals. In older patients, a degenerative etiology (type III) is more common secondary to posterior joint deformity and intervertebral disc laxity. Degenerative spondylolistheses are more common in women and typically occur at the L4 level.[14] In the cervical spine, congenital etiology is most common, and it may be accompanied by spina bifida occulta (Fig. 12-23).

IMAGING FINDINGS

The presence of anterior displacement is best evaluated in a lateral projection. The most noteworthy finding is disruption of the posterior body (George's) line at the level of anterior displacement. An alternative, less sensitive method involves constructing a line along the sacral base and a second line perpendicular to the sacral base line (Ulmann's line). If the second line intersects the vertebral body of L5, a spondylolisthesis is present.

The degree of anterior displacement is qualified by the Meyerding system (Fig. 12-24).[107] This system segments the sacral base into four equal divisions. The degree of spondylolisthesis is described by which of the imaginary sacral base divisions that the posterior body line intersects. For example, if the body of L5 slips forward between 0% and 25% of the total length of the sacral base so that a line drawn along the posterior margin of the L5 body interrupts the most posterior division of the sacral base, it is designated as a grade 1 spondylolisthesis. A grade II spondylolisthesis represents anterior displacement of 26% to 50% of the total sacral base length so that the posterior body line of L5 intersects the second from the most posterior quadrant of the sacral base. Grade III denotes 51% to 75% displacement and grade IV, 76% to 100% displacement. If the L5 vertebra extends beyond the front of the sacrum and into the pelvic cavity, it is designated as a grade V spondylolisthesis, also termed a *spondyloptosis*. The Meyerding system can be used at other levels, and the scale of measurement can be quantified by reporting the percentage of displacement instead of the grades when Meyerding's system is applied to other levels, the segment immediately below the segment displaced is divided into quadrants.

In the frontal projection, spondylolistheses of L5 may demonstrate a characteristic configuration in which the vertebral body resembles an inverted Napoleon hat or inverted bow (bowline of Brailsford). The spinous process at the level of spondylolisthesis is often deviated.[130] Often the transverse processes of an L5 spondylolisthesis overlaps the upper sacrum (Fig. 12-25).

In the oblique lumbar projection the neural arch resembles a Scottish terrier, in which the dog's neck represents the pars interarticularis. Disruption of the pars interarticularis appears as a dog wearing a collar. An additional clue to the presence of spondylolisthesis in the oblique projection is a disruption of the normal progression of each facet joint placed slightly anterior to the segment immediately above (called the *stepladder sign*). A unilateral pars defect often presents with hypertrophy of the intact contralateral pars.

Radionuclide bone scanning is helpful in determining if spondylolysis is active in patients with chronic low back pain.[168] If the region of the pars interarticularis demonstrates increased uptake of the radiopharmaceutical, an active stress fracture or healing fracture is suspected. Single photon emission computed tomography (SPECT) relates better detail than conventional radionuclide bone

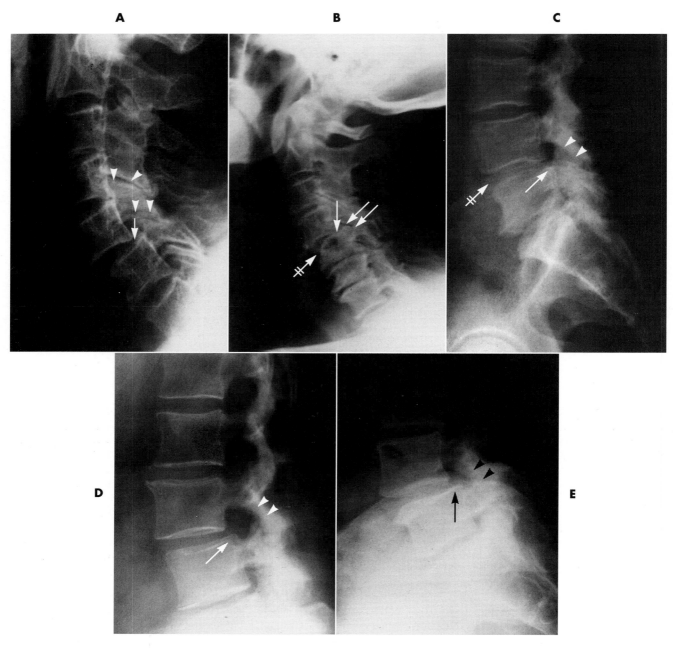

FIG. 12-19 Grade I degenerative spondylolisthesis in the cervical (**A** and **B**), (*arrows*) and lumbar spine (**C** through **E**, *arrows*). Degenerative spondylolisthesis are a consequence of degenerative disc disease (*crossed arrows*) and posterior joint arthrosis (*arrowheads*). Disc degeneration is noted by the reduced disc space and osteophytes. Posterior joint arthrosis is recognized by the increased radiopacity and irregularity of the facet region. (**A,** Courtesy Joseph W. Howe, Sylmar, Calif.)

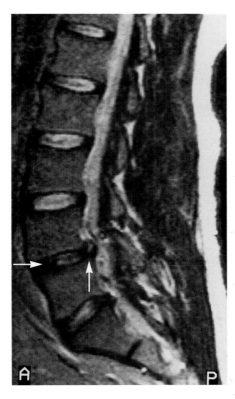

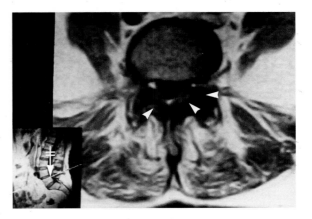

FIG. 12-20 Sagittal T2-weighted magnetic resonance image noting grade I degenerative spondylolisthesis of L3 *(arrows)*. In addition, deceased nuclear signal intensity of the L4, and to a lesser extent the L5, intervertebral discs corresponding to degeneration. (Courtesy Ian D. McLean, Davenport, Iowa.)

FIG. 12-21 Axial T1-weighted magnetic resonance image at the level of the lower L4 disc. The posterior joints appear large and hypointense (dark) secondary to arthrosis with hypertrophic changes *(arrowheads)*. The smaller insert scout image demonstrates anterior translation of the L4 degenerative spondylolisthesis *(crossed arrow)*.

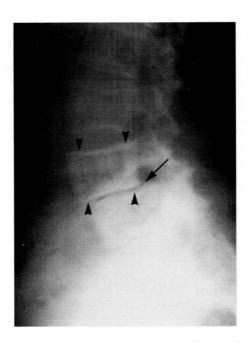

FIG. 12-22 Pathological (type V) spondylolisthesis of L4 on L5 in a patient with Paget's disease *(arrow)*; observe the picture frame vertebra *(arrowheads)* and degenerative disc disease with vacuum phenomena of the L4 disc. (Courtesy Robert C. Tatum, Davenport, Iowa.)

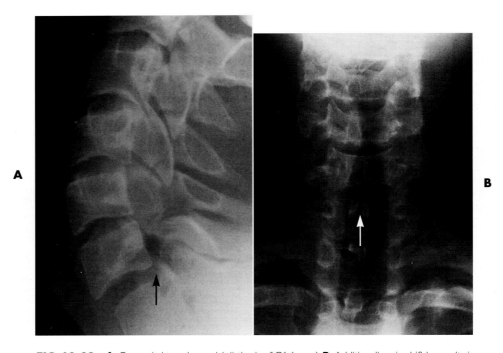

FIG. 12-23　**A,** Congenital type I spondylolisthesis of C6 *(arrow)*. **B,** Additionally, spina bifida occulta is noted at the C6 level *(arrow)*. Spina bifida occulta often accompanies cervical spondylolisthesis. (Courtesy John A.M. Taylor, Portland, Ore.)

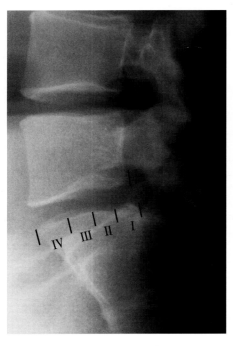

FIG. 12-24　Mild anterolisthesis of L5 on S1. The anterolisthesis is limited to less than 25% of the sacral base corresponding to a grade I using the Meyerding system. Grade II denotes 26% to 50% displacement, grade III is 51% to 75% displacement, and grade IV is 76% to 100% displacement. Some individuals designate a total forward displacement of the vertebra (spondyloptosis) as a grade V spondylolisthesis.

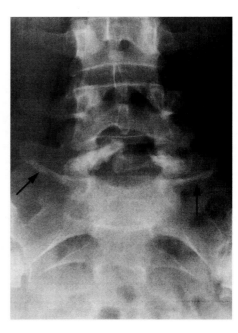

FIG. 12-25　An overlap of the transverse process with the superior margin of the sacrum on the frontal projection provides a clue to the presence of spondylolisthesis *(arrows)*. (Courtesy Arthur W. Holmes, Foley, Ala.)

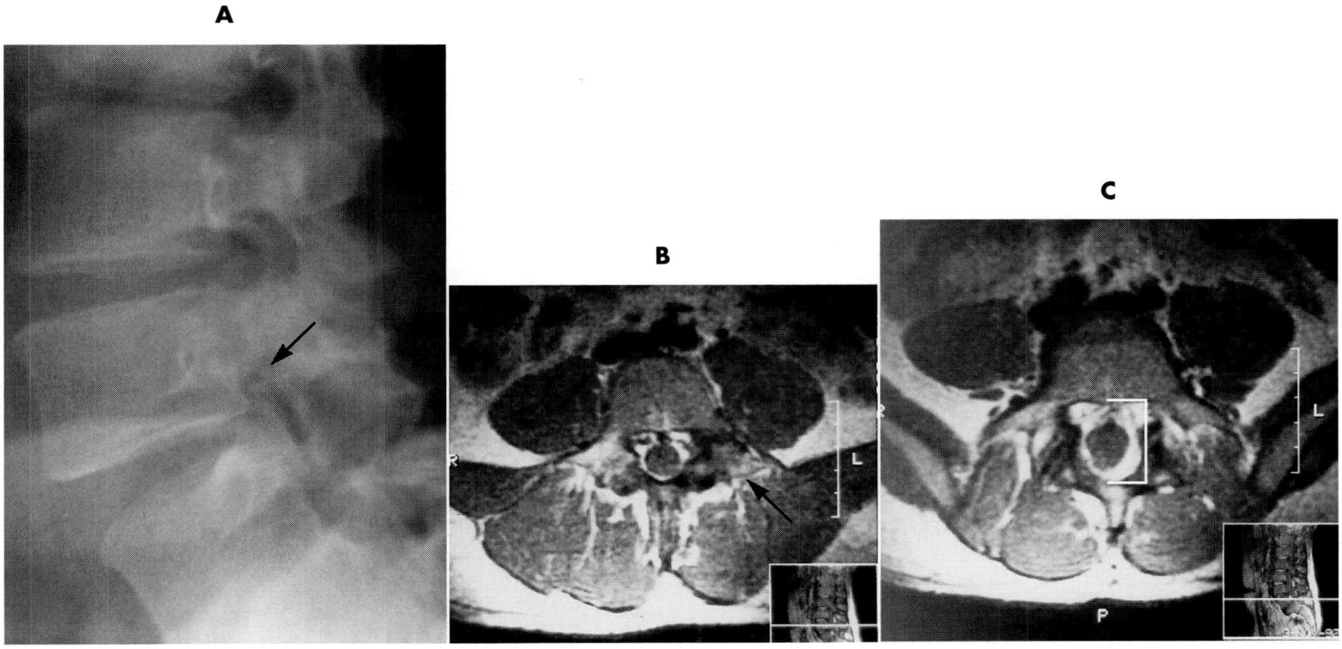

FIG. 12-26 Spondylolytic spondylolisthesis of L4 on L5 with minimal anterolisthesis. **A,** Pars interarticularis is noted on the plain film *(arrow)* and **(B)** MRI axial scan at the L4 level *(arrow).* **C,** The MRI slice at the upper L5 vertebral body best demonstrates the enlarged canal *(bracket).* (Courtesy Jeannie A. Santoro, Pittsburgh, Penn.)

scanning. Specialized imaging demonstrates an enlarged spinal canal in the axial plane in patients with spondylolytic spondylolisthesis (Fig. 12-26).[169]

CLINICAL COMMENTS

Spondylolisthesis is usually discovered during childhood. It may or may not be painful. Most spondylolistheses are due to pars stress fractures and may heal if the patient is immobilized by bracing.[9,108,124] Unfortunately healing rarely occurs, because the fracture may go unnoticed for some time. Spondylolysis has been implicated as a possible source of back pain.[147] However, no correlation seems to exist between the presence or degree of anterior displacement (spondylolisthesis) and back pain.[168] Only 50% of those with spondylolisthesis develop back pain.[118] Physical examination may reveal joint crepitus and palpatory "step defect" at the level of displacement.[179]

The majority of progression is thought to occur during early adolescence. Predisposing factors for progression include rounded sacrum promontory,[161] trapezoidal configuration of the displaced vertebra,[161] narrowed disc space,[145] increased sacral angle, and advanced degree of displacement. Others feel these are the result of slippage and not the cause of it,[133] and that no radiographic findings exist that can accurately predict future displacement.[53] It is rare for spondylolisthesis with degenerative etiology to progress beyond a stage I category.

In general, patients who demonstrate a spondylolisthesis beyond the age of 10 years may continue to participate in athletics without fear of further displacement.[52,149,179] In patients under the age of 10 years activity should be curtailed until serial flexion and extensive lateral lumbar radiographs rule out instability.[179] However, all patients who demonstrate the following conditions may warrant further clinical evaluation: persistent symptoms, an active pars interarticularis defect as noted by a positive SPECT bone scan, and instability as defined by excessive translation (greater than or equal to 4 mm) on flexion/extension or compression/traction lateral radiographs.[81]

KEY CONCEPTS

- *Spondylolisthesis is an anterior displacement of a vertebrae (and those above it) in relation to the segment immediately below, occurring in 5% to 7% of the population.*
- *Spondylolysis denotes unilateral or bilateral disruption of the pars interarticularis.*
- *Spondylolistheses are classified by etiology (type I, congenital; type II, pars interarticularis defect; type III, degenerative; type IV, traumatic; type V, pathologic; type VI, surgical) and degree of anterior displacement (grade I, 0% to 25%; grade II, 26% to 50%; grade III, 51% to 75%; grade IV, 76% to 100%).*
- *Spondylolisthesis is usually due to a stress fracture of the pars interarticularis when presenting in younger individuals and degeneration of the facet and intervertebral disc when presenting in older individuals.*
- *Disruption of the posterior body (George's) line on the lateral projection is the best method of assessment.*
- *No correlation is apparent between the presence or degree of anterior displacement and back pain.*

References

1. Ackerman LV: Extra-osseous localized non-neoplastic bone and cartilage formation (so-called myositis ossificans), *J Bone Joint Surg Am* 40:279, 1958.
2. Aichroth PM: Osteochondritis dissecans of the knee: a clinical survey, *J Bone Joint Surg Br* 53B:440, 1971.
3. Alffram P, Bauer GCH: Epidemiology of fractures of the forearm, *J Bone Joint Surg Am* 44:105, 1962.
4. Asher MA: Dislocations of the upper extremity in children, *Orthop Clin N Am* 7:583, 1976.
5. Atlas SW et al: The radiographic characterization of burst fractures of the spine, *AJR* 147:575, 1986.
6. Bado JL: The Monteggia lesion, *Clin Orthop* 50:71, 1967.
7. Barnes R et al: Subcapital fractures of the femur, *J Bone Joint Surg Br* 58:2, 1976.
8. Bayliss AP, Davidson JK: Traumatic osteonecrosis of the femoral head following intracapsular fracture: incidence and earliest radiological features, *Clin Radiol* 28:407, 1977.
9. Bellah RD et al: Low back pain in adolescent athletes: detection of stress injury to the pars interarticularis with SPECT, *Radiology* 180:509, 1991.
10. Bennett EH: On fracture of the metacarpal hone of the thumb, *Clin Orthop* 220:3, 1987.
11. Bernstein L, McClurg FL: Mandibular fractures: a review of 156 consecutive cases, *Laryngoscope* 87:957, 1976.
12. Berquist TH: *Imaging of orthopedic trauma and surgery,* Philadelphia, 1986, WB Saunders.
13. Bledsoe RC, Izenstark JL: Displacement of fat pads in disease and injury of the elbow: a new radiographic sign, *Radiology* 73:717, 1959.
14. Bolesta MJ, Bohlman HH: Degenerative spondylolisthesis. Instructional Course Lectures, 38:157, 1989.
15. Brenkel IJ et al: Hormone status in patients with slipped capital femoral epiphysis, *J Bone Joint Surg Br* 71:33, 1989.
16. Brenkel IJ et al: Thyroid hormone levels in patients with slipped capital femoral epiphysis, *J Pediatr Orthop* 8:22, 1988.
17. Bridges AJ et al: Fibrodysplasia (myositis) ossificans progressiva [Review], *Semin Arthritis Rheum* 24:155, 1994.
18. Brogdon BG, Crow NE: Little leaguer's elbow, *AJR* 83:671, 1960.
19. Bruce HE, Harvey JP Jr, Wilson JC Jr: Monteggia fractures, *J Bone Joint Surg Am* 56:1563, 1974.
20. Buckingham WW: Subtalar dislocation of the foot, *J Trauma* 13:753, 1973.
21. Campbell CS: Gamekeeper's thumb, *J Bone Joint Surg Br* 37:148, 1955.
22. Carlson WO, Klassen RA: Myositis ossificans of the upper extremity: a long-term follow-up, *J Pediatr Orthop* 4:693, 1984.
23. Carter PR, Eaton RG, Littler JW: Un-united fracture of the hook of the hamate, *J Bone Joint Surg Am* 59:583, 1977.
24. Cautilli RA et al: Classifications of fractures of the distal radius, *Clin Orthop* 103:163, 1974.
25. Chessare JW et al: Injuries of the medial epicondylar ossification center of the humerus, *AJR* 129:49, 1977.
26. Cisternino SJ et al: The trough line: a radiographic sign of posterior shoulder dislocation, *AJR* 130:951, 1978.
27. Cohn I: Observations of the normally developing elbow, *Arch Surg* 2:455, 1921.
28. Conolly WB, Hedberg EA: Observations of fractures of the pelvis, *J Trauma* 9:104, 1969.
29. Cooperman DR et al: Post-mortem description of slipped capital femoral epiphysis, *J Bone Joint Surg Br* 74:595, 1992.
30. Crawley DB, Reckling FW: Supracondylar fracture of the humerus in children, *Am Fam Physician* 5:113, 1972.
31. Cremin B, Connor JM, Beighton P: The radiological spectrum of fibrodysplasia ossificans progressiva, *Clin Radiol* 33:499, 1982.
32. Crotty JM, Monu JU, Pope TL: Magnetic resonance imaging of the musculoskeletal system, *Clin Orthop* 330:288, 1996.
33. Curtis RJ Jr, Corley FG Jr: Fractures and dislocations of the forearm, *Clin Sports Med* 5:663, 1986.
34. Danchik JJ, Yochum TR, Aspegren DD: Myositis ossificans traumatica, *J Manipulative Physiol Ther* 16:605, 1993.
35. Danielson BI, Frennered AK, Irstam LK: Radiologic progression of isthmic lumbar spondylolisthesis in young patients, *Spine* 16:422, 1991.
36. Dellinger EP et al: Risk of infection after open fracture of the arm or leg, *Arch Surg* 123:1320, 1988.
37. Dent JA, Paterson CR: Fractures in early childhood: osteogenesis imperfecta or child abuse? *J Pediatr Orthop* 11:184, 1991.
38. Dias LS, Giegerich CR: Fractures of the distal tibial epiphysis in adolescence, *J Bone Joint Surg Am* 65:438, 1983.
39. Dolan KD, Jacoby CG: Facial fractures, *Sem Roentgenol* 13:37, 1978.
40. Dolan D, Jacoby C, Smoker W: The radiology of facial fractures, *Radiography* 4:577, 1984.
41. Drake DG, Griffiths HJ: Radiologic case study. Slipped epiphysis associated with renal osteodystrophy, *Orthopedics* 12:1489, 1989.
42. Du Toit FP, Grabe RP: Isolated fractures of the shaft of the ulna, *S Afr Med J* 56:21, 1979.
43. Dunn AW: Fractures and dislocations of the carpus, *Surg Clin N Am* 52:1513, 1972.
44. Dunn AW, Morris HD: Fractures and dislocations of the pelvis, *J Bone Joint Surg Am* 50:1639, 1968.
45. Edwards GS Jr, Jupiter JB: Radial head fractures with acute distal radioulnar dislocation, Essex-Lopresti revisited, *Clin Orthop* 234:61, 1988.
46. Epstein HC: Traumatic dislocations of the hip, *Clin Orthop* 92:116, 1973.
47. Essex-Lopresti P: Fractures of the radial head with distal radio-ulnar dislocation, *J Bone Joint Surg Br* 33:244, 1951.
48. Fahey JJ: Fractures of the elbow in children, *Instr Course Lect* 17:13, 1960.
49. Fischer SP et al: Accuracy of diagnoses from magnetic resonance imaging of the knee, *J Bone Joint Surg Am* 73:2, 1991.
50. Fisk GR: The wrist, *J Bone Joint Surg Br* 66:396, 1984.
51. Foster SC, Foster RR: Lisfranc's tarsometatarsal fracture-dislocation, *Radiology* 120:79, 1976.
52. Fredrickson BE et al: The natural history of spondylolysis and spondylolisthesis, *J Bone Joint Surg Am* 66:669, 1984.
53. Frennered AK, Danielson BI, Nachemson AL: Natural history of symptomatic isthmic low-grade spondylolisthesis in children and adolescents: a seven-year follow-up study, *J Pediatr Orthop* 11:209, 1991.
54. Garcia C, Zaninovic A: Battered child syndrome, X-ray findings, *Rev Chilena Pediatr* 62:273, 1991.
55. Garden RS: Reduction and fixation of subcapital fractures of the femur, *Orthop Clin N Am* 5:683, 1974.
56. Garth WP, Hofammann DY, Rooks MD: Volar intercalated segment instability secondary to medial carpal ligamental laxity, *Clin Orthop* 201:94, 1985.
57. Gehweiler JA, Osborne RL, Becker RF: *The radiology of vertebral trauma,* Philadephia, 1980, WB Saunders.
58. Gelberman RH et al: The association of femoral retroversion with slipped capital femoral epiphysis, *J Bone Joint Surg Am* 68:1000, 1968.
59. Giles JB et al: Supracondylar-intercondylar fractures of the femur treated with a supracondylar plate and lag screw, *J Bone Joint Surg Am* 64:864, 1982.
60. Gilula LA: Carpal injuries: analytic approach and case exercises, *AJR* 133:503, 1979.
61. Gilula LA, Weeks PM: Post-traumatic ligamentous instabilities of the wrist, *Radiology* 129:641, 1978.
62. Gilula LA, Weeks PM: Wrist arthrography. The value of fluroscopic spot viewing, *Radiology* 146:555, 1983.
63. Green DP, Terry GC: Complex dislocation of the metacarpophalangeal joint, *J Bone Joint Surg Am* 55:1480, 1972.

64. Gross RM: Acute dislocation of the patella: the Mudville mystery, *J Bone Joint Surg Am* 68:780, 1986.

65. Grossart KWM, Samuel E: Traumatic diastasis of cranial sutures, *Clin Radiol* 12:164, 1961.

66. Hägglund G et al: Growth of children with physiolysis of the hip, *Acta Orthop Scand* 58:117, 1987.

67. Harris JH, Edeiken-Monroe B: *The radiology of acute cervical spine trauma*, ed 2, Baltimore, 1987, Williams & Wilkins.

68. Harris RD, Harris JH: The prevalence and significance of missed scapular fractures in blunt chest trauma, *AJR* 151:747, 1988.

69. Henrikson B: The incidence of slipped capital femoral epiphysis, *Acta Orthop Scand* 40:365, 1969.

70. Hofmann AA, Dahl CP, Wyatt RWB: Experience with acetabular fractures, *J Bone Joint Surg* 24:750, 1984.

71. Hohl M, Luck JV: Fractures of the tibial condyle: a clinical and experimental study, *J Bone Joint Surg Am* 38:1001, 1956.

72. Horne JG, Tanzer TL: Olecranon fractures: a review of 100 cases, *J Trauma* 21:469, 1981.

73. Howorth B: History of slipping of the capital femoral epiphysis, *Clin Orthop* 48:11, 1966.

74. Hughston JC: Fracture of the distal radial shaft, *J Bone Joint Surg Am* 39:249, 1957.

75. Huittinen VM, Slatis P: Fractures of the pelvis. Trauma mechanism, types of injury and principles of treatment, *Acta Chir Scand* 138:563, 1972.

76. Ingram AJ et al: Chondrolysis complicating slipped capital femoral epiphysis, *Clin Orthop* 165:99, 1982.

77. Iversen BJ, Aalberg JR, Naver LS: Complications of fractures of the femoral neck, *Ann Chir Gynaecol* 75:341, 1986.

78. Jaudes PK: Comparison of radiography and radionuclide bone scanning in the detection of child abuse, *Pediatrics* 73:166, 1984.

79. Jones HK, McBride GG, Mumhy RC: Sternal fractures associated with spinal injury, *J Trauma* 29:360, 1989.

80. Juhl JH, Crummy AB: *Paul and Juhl's Essentials of radiologic imaging*, ed 6, Philadephia, 1993, JB Lippincott.

81. Kalebo P et al: Stress views in the comparative assessment of spondylolytic spondylolisthesis, *Skeletal Radiol* 17:570, 1989.

82. Kelsey JL: Epidemiology of slipped capital femoral epiphysis: a review of the literature, *Pediatrics* 51:1042, 1973.

83. Kelsey JL, Acheson RM, Keggi KJ: The body build of patients with slipped capital epiphysis, *Am J Dis Child* 124:276, 1972.

84. Kelsey JL, Keggi KJ, Southwick WO: The incidence and distribution of slipped capital femoral epiphysis in Connecticut and Southwestern United States, *J Bone Joint Surg Am* 52:1203, 1970.

85. Kennedy JC: Complete dislocation of the knee joint, *J Bone Joint Surg Am* 45:889, 1963.

86. Kilcoyne RF et al: Thoracolumbar spine injuries associated with vertical plunges: reappraisal with computed tomography, *Radiology* 146:137, 1982.

87. Kleinman PK: Diagnostic imaging in infant abuse, *AJR* 155:703, 1990.

88. Kleinman PK, Marks SC, Blackbourne B: The metaphyseal lesion in abused infants: a radiologic histopathologic study, *AJR* 146:895, 1986.

89. Knight RA: Fractures of the humeral condyles in adults, *South Med J* 48:1165, 1955.

90. Kohn AM: Soft tissue alterations in elbow trauma, *Am J Roentgenol* 82:867, 1959.

91. Kono S, Hayashi M, Kashahara T: A study on the etiology of spondylolysis with reference to athletic activities (Japanese), *J Jpn Orthop Assoc* 49:125, 1975.

92. Kransdorf MJ, Meis JM, Jelinek JS: Myositis ossificans: MR appearance with radiologic-pathologic correlation, *AJR* 157:1243, 1991.

93. Kristensen S, Tveteras K: Zygomatic fractures: classification and complications, *Clin Otolaryngol* 11:123, 1986.

94. Larsen CB: Fracture dislocations of the hip, *Clin Orthop* 92:147, 1973.

95. Letournel E: Acetabulum fractures: classification and management, *Clin Orthop* 151:81, 1980.

96. Linscheid RL et al: Traumatic instability of the wrist, diagnosis, classification and pathomechanics, *J Bone Joint Surg Am* 54:1612, 1972.

97. Loder RT, Bookout C: Fracture patterns in battered children, *J Orthop Trauma* 5:428, 1991.

98. Lotke PA, Ecker ML: Transverse fractures of the patella, *Clin Orthop* 158:180, 1981.

99. Lowy M: Avulsion fractures of the calcaneus, *J Bone Joint Surg Br* 51:494, 1969.

100. Mast JW, Spiegel PG, Pappas JN: Fractures of the tibial pilon, *Clin Orthop* 230:68, 1988.

101. McCutchan JDS, Gillham NR: Injury to the popliteal artery associated with dislocation of the knee: palpable distal pulses do not negate the requirement for arteriography, *Br J Accident Surg* 20:307, 1989.

102. McDaniel WJ, Wilson FC: Trimalleolar fractures of the ankle: an end result study, *Clin Orthop* 122:37, 1977.

103. McMinn DJW: Mallet finger and fractures, *Injury* 12:477, 1981.

104. Melmed EP, Koonin AJ: Fractures of the mandible: a review of 909 cases, *Plast Reconstr Surg* 56:323, 1975.

105. Melton LJ et al: Epidemiologic features of pelvic fractures, *Clin Orthop* 155:43, 1981.

106. Merchan EC et al: Circumscribed myositis ossificans. Report of nine cases without history of injury, *Acta Orthop Belg* 59:273, 1993.

107. Meyerding HW: Low backache and sciatic pain associated with spondylolisthesis and protruded intervertebral disc, *J Bone Joint Surg Am* 23:461, 1941.

108. Micheli LJ, Hall JE, Miller ME: Use of modified Boston brace for back injuries in athletes, *Am J Sports Med* 8:5, 1980.

109. Mickelson MR et al: Aseptic necrosis following slipped femoral epiphysis, *Skel Radiol* 4:129, 1979.

110. Mikic, ZDJ: Galeazzi fracture-dislocations, *J Bone Joint Surg Am* 57:1071, 1975.

111. Miller WE: Comminuted fractures of the distal end of the humerus in the adult, *J Bone Joint Surg Am* 46:644, 1964.

112. Moed BR, Morawa LG: Displaced midline longitudinal fracture of the sacrum, *J Trauma* 24:435, 1984.

113. Moreau MJ: Remodeling in slipped capital femoral epiphysis, *Can J Surg* 30:440, 1987.

114. Nambu T et al: Deformation of the distal femur: a contribution towards the pathogenesis of osteochondrosis dissecans in the knee joint, *J Biomech* 24:421, 1991.

115. Nathan H: Spondylolysis, *J Bone Joint Surg Am* 41:303, 1959.

116. Neer CS, Shelton ML: Supracondylar fractures of the adult femur: a study of one hundred and ten cases, *J Bone Joint Surg Am* 49:591, 1967.

117. Newman JH: Supracondylar fractures of the femur, *Injury* 21:280, 1990.

118. Newman PH, Stone KH: The etiology of spondylolisthesis, *J Bone Joint Surg Br* 45:39, 1963.

119. Norman A, Nelson, Green S: Fracture of the hook of the hamate: radiographic signs, *Radiology* 154:49, 1985.

120. Ogden JA: Dislocation of the proximal fibula, *Radiology* 105:547, 1972.

121. Ogden JA: Injury to the growth mechanisms of the immature skeleton, *Skel Radiol* 6:237, 1981.

122. Ogilvie-Harris DJ, Hons CB, Fornaiser VL: Pseudomalignant myositis ossificans: heterotropic new-bone formation without a history of trauma, *J Bone Joint Surg Am* 62:1274, 1980.

123. Pankovich AM: Maisonneuve fracture of the fibula, *J Bone Joint Surg Am* 58:337, 1977.

124. Papanicolaou N et al: Bone scintigraphy and radiography in young athletes with low back pain, *AJR* 145:1039, 1985.

125. Pellegrini VD Jr: Fractures at the base of thumb, *Hand Clin* 4:87, 1988.

PART TWO Bone, Joints, and Soft Tissues

126. Pierce GE, Maxwell JA, Boggan MD: Special hazards of first rib fractures, *Trauma* 15:264, 1975.

127. Pritchett JW, Perdue KD: Mechanical factors in slipped capital femoral epiphysis, *J Pediatr Orthop* 8:385, 1988.

128. Protzman RR: Dislocation of the elbow joint, *J Bone Joint Surg Am* 60:539, 1978.

129. Radkowski MA, Merten DF, Leonidas JC: The abused child: criteria for the radiologic diagnosis, *Radiographics* 3:262, 1983.

130. Ravichandran G: A radiological sign in spondylolisthesis, *AJR* 134:113, 1980.

131. Reckling JW, Peltier LF: Acute knee dislocations and their complications, *J Trauma* 9:181, 1969.

132. Reckling FW, Peltier LF: Riccardo Galeazz and Galeazzi's fracture, *Surgery* 58:453, 1965.

133. Resnick D: *Diagnosis of bone and joint disorders,* ed 3, vol 5, Philadelphia, 1995, WB Saunders.

134. Richardson JD, McElvein RB, Trinkle JK: First rib fracture: a hallmark of severe trauma, *Ann Surg* 181:251, 1975.

135. Robinson AE, Meares BM, Goree JA: Traumatic sphenoid sinus effusion: an analysis of 50 cases, *Am J Roentgenol* 101:795, 1967.

136. Roche MB, Rowe GG: The incidence of separate neural arch and coincidental bone variations, *Anat Rec* 109:233, 1951.

137. Rockwood C, Green D: *Fractures,* Philadelphia, 1975, JB Lippincott.

138. Rogers LF: The radiography of epiphyseal injuries, *Radiology* 96:289, 1970.

139. Rogers LF: *Radiology of skeletal trauma,* ed 2, New York, 1992, Churchill Livingstone.

140. Rorabeck CH, Bobechko WP: Acute dislocation of the patella with osteochondral fracture: a Review of 18 cases, *J Bone Joint Surg Br* 58:237, 1976.

141. Rossi F: Spondylolysis, spondylolisthesis and sports, *Sports Med* 18:317, 1978.

142. Ruwe PA et al: Can MR imaging effectively replace diagnostic arthroscopy? *Radiology* 183:335, 1992.

143. Salter RB, Harris WR: Injuries involving the epiphyseal plate, *J Bone Joint Surg Am* 45:587, 1963.

144. Salter RB, Zaltz C: Anatomic investigations of the mechanism of injury and pathologic anatomy of "pulled elbow" in young children, *Clin Orthop* 77:134, 1971.

145. Saraste H: Long-term clinical and radiological follow-up of spondylolysis and spondylolisthesis, *J Pediatr Orthop* 7:631, 1987.

146. Sarmiento A, Laird CA: Posterior fracture-dislocation of the femoral head, *Clin Orthop* 92:143, 1973.

147. Schneiderman GA et al: The pars defect as a pain source: a histologic study, *Spine* 20:1761, 1995.

148. Schultz RC, Oldham RJ: An overview of facial injuries, *Surg Clin N Am* 57:987, 1977.

149. Semon RL, Spengler D: Significance of lumbar spondylolisthesis in college football players, *Spine* 6:1972, 1981.

150. Shelton ML, Neer CS, Grantham SA: Occult knee ligament ruptures associated with fractures, *J Trauma* 11:853, 1971.

151. Sherk HH, Nicholson JT: Fractures of the atlas, *J Bone Joint Surg Am* 52:1017, 1970.

152. Siffert RS: The effect of trauma to the epiphysis and growth plate, *Skel Radiol* 2:21, 1977.

153. Sorensen KH: Slipped upper femoral epiphysis, clinical study on aetiology, *Acta Orthop Scand* 39:499, 1968.

154. Siegel S, White LM, Brahma S: Magnetic resonance imaging of the musculoskeletal system part 5: the wrist, *Clin Orthop* 332:281, 1996.

155. Stark HH et al: Fracture of the hook of the hamate in athletes, *J Bone Joint Surg Am* 59:575, 1977.

156. Stevens DB: Postoperative orthopaedic infections, *J Bone Joint Surg Am* 46:96, 1964.

157. Stewart TD: The age incidence of neural-arch defects in Alaskan natives, considered from the standpoint of etiology, *J Bone Joint Surg Am* 35:937, 1953.

158. Store G: Traumatic dislocation of the radial head as an isolated lesion in children. Report of one case with special regard to roentgen diagnosis, *Acta Chir Scand* 116:144, 1958.

159. Sty JR, Starshak RJ: The role of bone scintigraphy in the evaluation of the suspected abused child, *Radiology* 146:369, 1983.

160. Swiontkowski MF: Slipped capital femoral epiphysis, complications relative to internal fixation, *Orthopaedics* 6:705, 1983.

161. Taillard WF: Etiology of spondylolisthesis, *Clin Orthop* 117:30, 1976.

162. Taveras Jm, Wood EH: *Diagnostic neuroradiology,* ed 2, Baltimore, 1976, Williams & Wilkins.

163. Terry DW, Ramin JE: The navicular fat stripe. A useful roentgen fracture for evaluating wrist trauma, *AJR* 124:25, 1975.

164. Thaggard A, Harle TS, Carlson V: Fractures and dislocations of bony pelvis and hip, *Semin Roentgenol* 13:117, 1978.

165. Torisu T: Fracture of the hook of the hamate by a golf swing, *Clin Orthop* 83:91, 1972.

166. Trapnell DH: The "magnification sign" of the triple mandibular fracture, *Br J Radiol* 50:97, 1977.

167. Tsuno MM, Shu GJ: Myositis ossificans [Review], *J Manipulative Physiol Ther* 13:340, 1990.

168. Turner RH, Bianco AJ: Spondylolysis and spondylolisthesis in children and teenagers, *J Bone Joint Surg Am* 53:1298, 1971.

169. Ulmer JL et al: Distinction between degenerative and isthmic spondylolisthesis on sagittal MR images: importance of increased anteroposterior diameter of the spinal canal ("wide canal sign"), *AJR* 163:411, 1994.

170. Vlarkisz JA et al: Segmental patterns of avascular necrosis of the femoral heads: early detection with MR imaging, *Radiology* 162:717, 1987.

171. Walsh HPJ, McLaren CAN, Owen R: Galeazzi fractures in children, *J Bone Joint Surg Br* 69:730, 1987.

172. Watson FM: Simultaneous interphalangeal dislocation in one finger, *J Trauma* 23:65, 1982.

173. Weber ER: A rational approach for the recognition and treatment of Colles' fracture, *Hand Clin* 3:13, 1987.

174. Wehbe MA, Schneider LH: Mallet fractures, *J Bone Joint Surg Am* 66:658, 1984.

175. Wiesel SW, Zeide MS, Terry RL: Longitudinal fractures of the sacrum: case report, *J Trauma* 19:70, 1979.

176. Wilcox PG, Weiner DS, Leighley B: Maturation factors in slipped capital femoral epiphysis, *J Pediatr Orthop* 8:196, 1988.

177. Wiley JJ: The mechanism of tarso-metarsal joint injuries, *J Bone Joint Surg Br* 53:474, 1971.

178. Wiltse LL, Newman PH, Macnab I: Classification of spondylolysis and spondylolisthesis, *Clin Orthop* 117:23, 1976.

179. Woodring JH, Goldstein SJ: Fractures of the articular processes of the cervical spine, *AJR* 139:341, 1982.

180. Yochum TR, Rowe LJ: *Essentials of skeletal radiology,* ed 2, Baltimore, 1996, Williams & Wilkins.

181. Yulish BS et al: MR imaging of osteochondral lesions of the talus, *J Comput Assist Tomogr* 11:296, 1987.k

chapter 13

Hematologic Bone Disorders

GARY D SCHULTZ

Avascular Necrosis	Hereditary Spherocytosis	Sickle Cell Anemia
Hemochromatosis	Leukemia	Thalassemia
Hemophilia		

Vascular conditions that affect bone may manifest through alterations in the blood supply or changes in the skeletal architecture due to abnormal activation of the hematopoietic potential within bone marrow. Unfortunately, the slow metabolic rate of bone significantly delays visualization of quantitative, qualitative, and morphological changes in the skeleton. The limited number of skeletal responses to hematologic alterations often impairs the physician's ability to render a specific diagnosis based on plain films alone. In general, vascular conditions of the skeleton often have a chronic history of development and nonspecific radiographic findings. Consequently, all radiographic clues must be correlated with historical and laboratory findings. Typically, the clinical findings will suggest the correct diagnosis long before plain film radiographs are useful.

Avascular Necrosis

BACKGROUND

Avascular necrosis is the most common hematologic condition affecting the skeleton. Pathologically, this condition is simply bone death due to an inadequate blood supply. Avascular necrosis is more likely to develop when the blood supply to bone is tenuous or little collateral circulation is present. Many conditions and disorders can be responsible for the interruption of blood supply to a segment of bone.[6] These causes may be divided into three categories: (1) conditions resulting in external blood vessel compression near or within the bone, (2) disorders resulting in blood vessel occlusion because of thickening of the vessel wall, and (3) disorders resulting in blood vessel blockage from a thromboembolic process.[10] (Causes of avascular necrosis are listed in Box 13-1.)

For conditions that result in external blood vessel compression, the mechanism is either marrow edema causing compression of the vessel in an enclosed region or excessive packing of the marrow through the deposition of abnormal tissue or material (e.g., fat in steroid administration or hyperlipidemia). (Box 13-2 lists in descending order of frequency the common causes of ischemic necrosis in children and adults.)

Bone ischemia can have several presentations. Infarction affecting a focal segment of the articular surface is termed *osteochondritis dissecans* in the growing skeleton. This defect may occur in adults and children, and it more frequently affects weight-bearing bones. The lateral aspect of the medial femoral condyle is the most common location of the infarction, followed by the talar dome. Trauma is believed to be the precipitating mechanism, although patients commonly report no history of trauma.

The term *medullary bone infarction* is used to describe ischemic necrosis localized to the medullary portion of a long bone. This infarction is generally not of primary therapeutic interest because it causes no significant symptoms or alterations in osseous shape or integrity. However, the medullary bone infarction is associated with metabolic conditions such as alcoholism, diabetes, and renal disease.

An infarction that affects the entire epiphysis of a skeletally immature long bone is termed *epiphyseal ischemic necrosis*. The proximal femur is by far the most common location for this event. When the proximal femur is affected, the condition is referred to as *Legg-Calvé-Perthes disease* (Box 13-3) in the child and *Chandler's disease* in the adult. Early diagnosis of Legg-Calvé-Perthes is important in prevention of postischemic deformity and functional impairment. Most cases of Legg-Calvé-Perthes disease have an idiopathic origin, although slipped femoral capital epiphysis, trauma, developmental dysplasia of the hip, and other pathologies are also associated with this process.

BOX 13-1
Causes of Skeletal Ischemic Necrosis

External vessel compression
Trauma or surgery
Steroid administration
Idiopathic
Regional infection
Neuropathic joint
Gaucher's disease
Hyperlipidemia

Vessel wall disorders
Systemic lupus erythematosus
Polyarteritis nodosa
Giant cell arteritis
Radiation therapy

Thromboembolic disorders
Alcoholism
Arteriosclerosis
Steroid administration
Thromobembolic syndrome
Diabetes
Trauma
Sickle cell disease

Although ischemia of any segment of a bone is possible, certain locations are more likely to be affected because of their vascular supply (Table 13-1). An avascular etiology has been disproved for some epiphyseal conditions previously attributed to an avascular origin (Table 13-2).

The histological changes in bone necrosis are essentially the same, regardless of location. Pathologically, absence of a blood supply results in bone death within 48 hours; a predictable sequence of events then ensues: inflammatory reaction to the dead bone, neovascular infiltration into the dead segment of bone, resorption of dead bone and deposition of new bone, and remodeling of the resultant bone. This process may take 1 to 8 years to complete.

BOX 13-2
Most Frequent Causes of Ischemic Necrosis

Children
Idiopathic origin
Trauma
Infection

Adults
Drugs and other substances (steroids, alcohol, immunosuppressants)
Trauma
Inflammatory arthritis
Metabolic conditions (diabetes, Cushing's syndrome, pregnancy)

BOX 13-3
Legg-Calvé-Perthes Disease

Background
Idiopathic osteonecrosis of the proximal femoral capital epiphysis in children
Trauma, endocrine abnormality, and infection implicated as possible causes
More common among boys, whites, and those between 3 and 5 years of age

Imaging
Bilateral in approximately 15% of patients
MRI and bone scans more sensitive to early disease than plain film radiographs
Bone scans cold during avascular phase and hot during revascular phase
MRI scans revealing replacement of normal marrow by necrosis
Plain film findings of capsular distention, a small fragmented epiphysis, osteosclerosis (snowcap sign), subchondral collapse (crescent sign), and growth deformity leading to a wide, short femoral neck with an enlarged (coxa magna), flattened (coxa plana) femoral head (mushroom) deformity

Clinical
Slowly evolving painless limp with limited abduction and internal rotation
Clinical outcome worse if weight-bearing area of bone involved
Osteoarthritis secondary to incongruent articular surfaces representing a significant complication
Treatment options of avoidance of full weight-bearing, bracing, and possible surgical realignment

---

IMAGING FINDINGS

Osteochondritis dissecans. Osteochondritis dissecans (local subchondral infarction) generally first manifests radiographically, the plain film showing a subarticular defect accompanied by a free-floating fragment of bone that formerly filled the defect. The defect is characteristically smooth and regular, corresponding to the borders of the fragment (Fig. 13-1). The fragment may be displaced from the parent bone defect. Marginal sclerosis is always present at the defect and blends into the subchondral bone peripherally (Fig.

TABLE 13-1
Common Locations for Ischemic Necrosis

Location	Disorder
Metatarsal head	Freiberg's disease
Tarsal navicular	Köhler's bone disease
Talus	Diaz's disease
Patella (secondary ossification center)	Sinding-Larsen Johansson disease
Medial femoral condyle	Spontaneous osteonecrosis of the knee (SONK)
Femoral head (child)	Legg-Calvé-Perthes disease
Phalanges of hand	Thiemann's disease
Metacarpal head	Mauclaire's disease
Carpal lunate	Kienböck's disease
Carpal scaphoid	Preiser's disease
Capitellum of the humerus	Panner's disease
Humeral head	Hass's disease
Vertebral body	Kümmel's disease

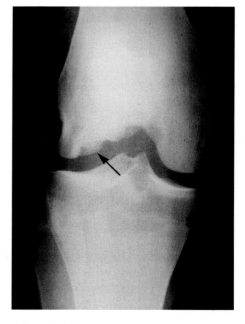

FIG. 13-1 Osteochondritis dissecans. Focal osteochondral infarction of the lateral femoral condyle demonstrating smooth margins and a clear articular defect (*arrow*).

13-2). These findings assist in differentiation of focal subchondral infarction from an acute, traumatic insult. Intraarticular swelling is often noted, but its severity varies considerably.

Medullary bone infarction. The plain film radiograph generally demonstrates no evidence of a medullary bone infarction in the acute phase. After resolution and revascularization, the infarction is seen radiographically as discontinuous, longitudinally oriented, wavy or serpiginous calcific opacities that lie centrally in the medullary cavity (Figs. 13-3, 13-4, and 13-5). The infarction does not result in periosteal reaction, alteration in the cortical thickness, or expansion of the bone. Differentiating a medullary bone infarction from a benign enchondroma of bone can be impossible on plain film images. However, definitive differentiation is generally unnecessary because both conditions are benign.

Epiphyseal necrosis

Avascular phase. From both therapeutic and prognostic standpoints, epiphyseal necrosis is a significantly more important condition than medullary bone infarction. During the avascular phase of epiphyseal necrosis, plain film radiographic skeletal changes are absent[11] (Fig. 13-6). Intraarticular effusion may be visible, but the degree of effusion varies, making it an unreliable sign.

Changes in marrow signal can be identified with magnetic resonance imaging (MRI), which is considered the most sensitive imaging modality for the detection of early bone infarction. The MRI study will demonstrate a loss in the epiphyseal marrow signal, particularly on T1-weighted images, even in the earliest phases of the disease (Fig. 13-7).[9,19]

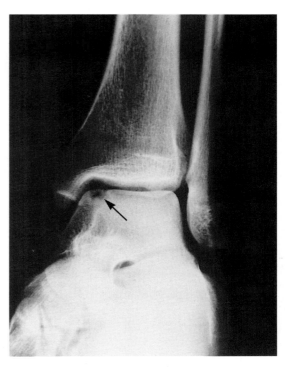

FIG. 13-2   Osteochondritis dissecans of the ankle. Note the in situ osseous fragment at the superomedial aspect of the talar dome *(arrow)*. (From Deltoff MN, Kogon PL, *The portable skeletal x-ray library*, St Louis, 1998, Mosby.)

TABLE 13-2
Epiphyseal Conditions Unrelated to Avascular Necrosis

Condition	Etiology	Description
Blount disease (tibia vara)	Trauma	Local growth alteration of the medial portion of the proximal tibial epiphysis; infantile and adolescent presentation; depressed medial metaphysis of the tibia with an osseous overgrowth noted; shortening of involved leg; usually, a tibia vara deformity
Osgood-Schlatter disease	Trauma	Altered appearance of the tibial tuberosity occurring mostly between the ages of 11 and 15 years; more common among boys and girls who participate in sports such as soccer and weight lifting; fragmentation and soft tissue swelling of the tibial tuberosity evident on radiographs; pain and tenderness over the region; tibial tuberosity possibly fragmented as a normal variant and distinguishable from Osgood-Schlatter disease by lack of pain and soft tissue swelling
Scheuermann's disease*	Trauma	Posttraumatic defect of vertebral endplate maturation first seen during adolescence with three or more levels of wedged vertebrae, narrowed anterior disk space, multiple Schmorl's nodes, and vertebral endplate irregularity; middle and lower thoracic spine are the usual locations; back pain is common; more severe kyphosis possibly necessitates bracing or, in a few cases, surgery to arrest or partially correct the resulting deformity
Sever's phenomenon	Variation in ossification	Irregularity and fragmentation of the secondary ossification center of the calcaneous; generally considered a normal variant and unrelated to any heel pain in the adolescent
Sinding-Larsen-Johansson	Trauma	Fragmented appearance of the lower pole of the patella, most commonly occurring between 10 and 14 years of age; soft tissue swelling and tenderness common and exacerbated by activity

*See Chapter 10.

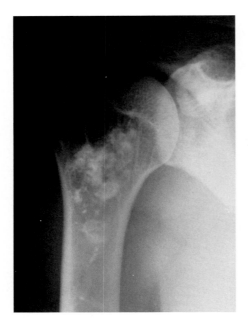

FIG. 13-3   Irregular patchy sclerosis of a medullary bone infarction.

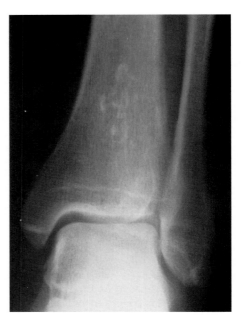

FIG. 13-4   Subtle serpiginous calcifications in a medullary bone infarction.

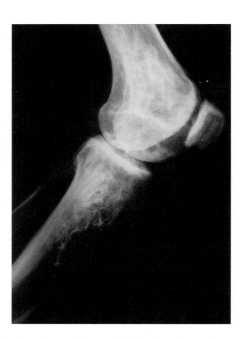

FIG. 13-5   Extensive serpiginous calcificaiton involving the femur and tibia in a patient with longstanding diabetes mellitus. Note the vascular calcification of the posterior tibial artery.

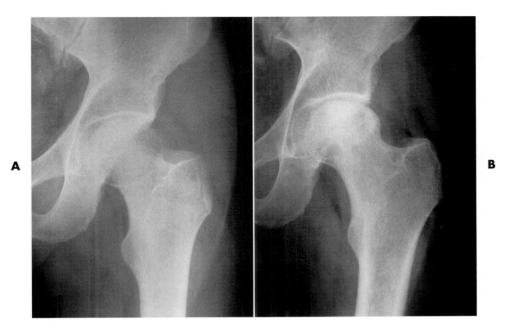

FIG. 13-6 A, Normal plain films in a patient with a painful hip. **B,** Plain films 3 months later demonstrating increased radiodensity and a mottled appearance of the femoral head. These are typical signs of avascular necrosis of the femoral head.

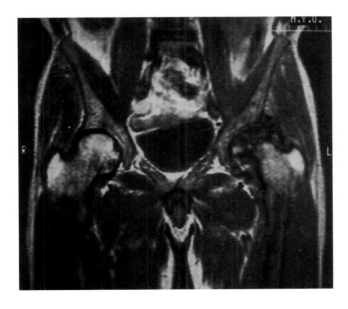

FIG. 13-7 Avascular necrosis of the patient's left *(reading right)* hip with severe secondary osteoarthritis on a coronal T1-weighted MRI scan. (From Firooznia H et al: *MRI and CT of the musculoskeletal system,* St Louis, 1992, Mosby.)

Early epiphyseal infarction can also be detected by radionuclide scintigraphy, which demonstrates focal photopenia affecting the avascular segment. Generally, a zone of increased radionuclide uptake is present in the region surrounding the avascular segment, presumably due to hyperemia[5] (Fig. 13-8).

Inflammatory phase. As the avascular phase gives way to the inflammatory response in epiphyseal necrosis, plain films may demonstrate periarticular osteopenia affecting all but the involved segment of bone. This may create the plain film appearance of sclerosis of the avascular segment, but it is not an infallible radi-

ographic finding (Fig. 13-9). The inflammatory phase may persist for weeks.

During this time the dead bone begins to soften and may collapse under the stresses of use. With this collapse the involved articular surface becomes deformed. Subchondral fractures allowing joint fluid to intrude into the subchondral ischemic bone may produce the "crescent sign" on plain films. This sign appears as a lucent defect in the subchondral bone that parallels the subchondral cortical surface (Fig. 13-10). The crescent sign is considered the most reliable early plain film sign of epiphyseal infarction.[11]

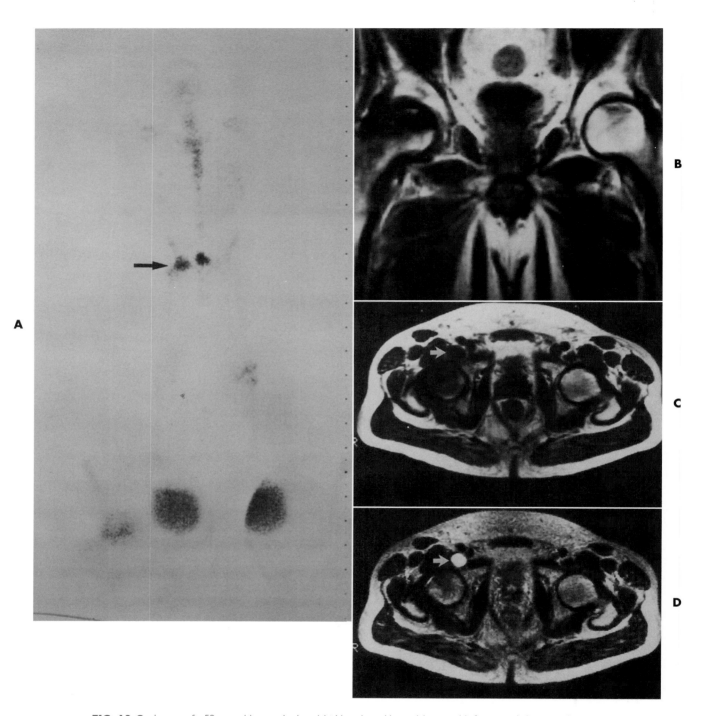

FIG. 13-8 Images of a 52-year-old man who has right hip pain and is receiving steroids for systemic lupus erythematosus. **A,** A technetium Tc 99m pyrophosphate bone scintigram shows increased uptake in the right hip *(arrow)* and a normal left hip. **B,** A coronal T1-weighted MRI shows obvious avasular necrosis on the right and subtle characteristic avascular necrosis changes on the left. Core biopsies confirmed bilateral avascular necrosis. **C,** Axial T1-weighted MRI. **D,** Axial T2-weighted MRI. Fluid is shown *(arrows)* in the right iliopsoas bursa. Iliopsoas bursitis may accompany avascualar necrosis and cause a variety of symptoms. (From Firooznia H et al: *MRI and CT of the musculoskeletal system,* St Louis, 1992, Mosby.)

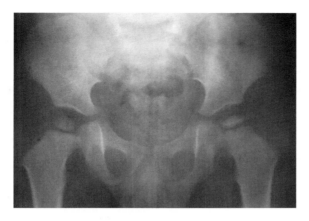

FIG. 13-9   Anteroposterior projection of the pelvis demonstrating a small radiodense epiphysis on the reading right. These changes indicate ischemic necrosis of the epiphysis.

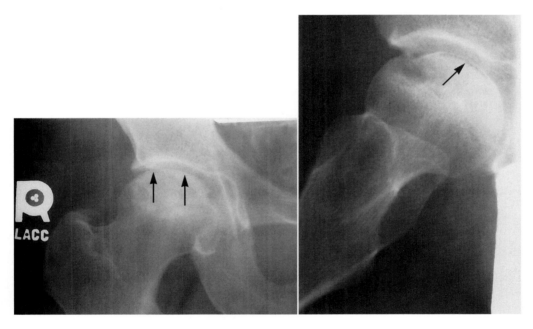

FIGS. 13-10   Ischemic necrosis indicated by a radiolucent crescent sign is faintly visible on the anteroposterior view of the hip but is obvious on the frog-leg lateral view *(arrows)*. Mottled bone sclerosis of the femoral head is also noted.

Revascularization phase. As revascularization continues, the dead bone is resorbed while new bone matrix is being deposited to replace it. On radiographs this process is seen as apparent fragmentation of the epiphysis. In addition, sclerosis begins to appear at the margin of the necrotic segment. Articular collapse is common (Fig. 13-11). The fragmentation gradually recedes as the new epiphyseal bone ossifies.

Any deformity that has occurred during the process of necrosis or early revascularization forms the substrate for the new epiphyseal bone (Fig. 13-12). The result is deformity of the repaired epiphysis in the approximate shape left by the necrotic segment of bone. In most cases the deformity manifests as a flattened and widened epiphysis. Widening of the metaphysis of the involved

bone may accompany the epiphyseal deformity. In the adult skeleton, subchondral infarctions can result in significant deformity of the articular morphology (Figs. 13-13, 13-14, and 13-15).

CLINICAL COMMENTS

The earliest clinical signs of avascular necrosis of the epiphysis are related to the synovitis and inflammatory response or a mechanical deformity. Children complain of hip or knee pain. In either location the pain is generally dull, achy, and boring and is exacerbated with activity. Orthopedic testing of the involved joint often suggests an intraarticular problem. The pain is generally intense enough to cause ambulation with a limp, and it worsens with activity. A child with bilateral, Legg-Calvé-Perthes disease has a "wad-

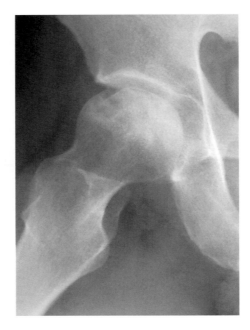

FIG. 13-11   Articular collapse in a patient with adult-onset ischemic necrosis of the femoral head.

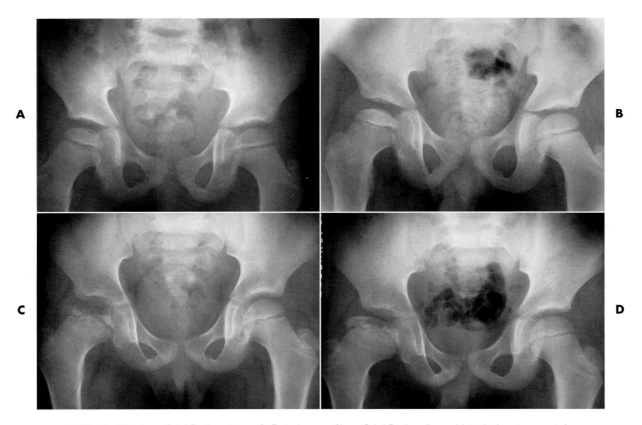

FIGS. 13-12   Legg-Calvé-Perthes disease. **A,** Early changes of Legg-Calvé-Perthes disease. Note the lucent crescent sign at the superior aspect of the femoral epiphyseal surface. **B-D,** Six-month progression of Legg-Calvé-Perthes disease. Note the progression of articular collapse. The fragmentation of the epiphysis is evidence of revascularization.

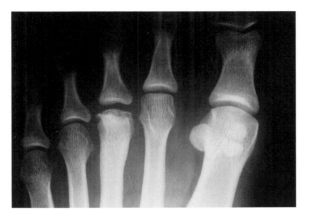

FIG. 13–13   Ischemic necrosis of the third metatarsal head (Freiberg's disease).

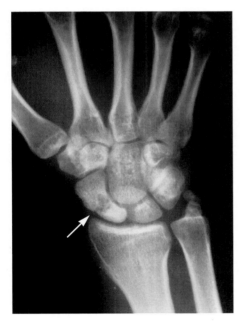

FIG. 13–14   Ischemic necrosis of the proximal pole of the scaphoid secondary to fracture through the waist of the scaphoid *(arrow)*.

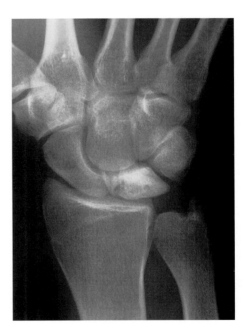

FIG. 13–15   Ischemic necrosis of the lunate (Kienböck's disease) marked by increased radiodensity and fissures.

TABLE 13-3
Staging Osteonecrosis

Stage or class	Findings
Based on radiographs*	
Stage 0	No clinical manifestations, normal radiographs
Stage I	Clinical manifestations, normal to regions of slight osteopenia on the radiographs
Stage II	Clinical manifestations, regions of osteopenia and osteosclerosis on the radiograph
Stage III	Clinical manifestations, early subchondral bone collapse (crescent sign)
Stage IV	Clinical manifestations, late bone collapse and flattened deformity
Based on MRI†	
Class A	Normal marrow, high signal intensity on T1-weighted scans and intermediate signal intensity on T2-weighted scans
Class B	Subacute hemorrhage, high signal intensity on both T1- and T2-weighted scans
Class C	Fluid accumulation, low signal intensity on T1-weighted scans and high signal intensity on T2-weighted scans
Class D	Fibrosis and sclerosis, low signal intensity on both T1- and T2-weighted scans

*Ficat RP, Arlet J: Necrosis of the femoral head. In Hungerford DS, ed: *Ischemia and necrosis of the bone,* Baltimore, 1980, Williams and Wilkins.
†Mitchell DG, Rao VM, Dalinka MK: Femoral head avascular necrosis: correlation of MR imaging, radiographic staging, radionuclide imaging and clinical findings, *Radiology* 162:709-715, 1987.

dling" gait because of the abduction and external rotation of the hips. (Patients with osteonecrosis may be staged using the systems listed in the Table 13-3. These systems are typically applied to avascular necrosis of the femoral head.)

Patients with osteochondritis dissecans generally first report swelling and pain in the involved joints. The symptoms may develop gradually, or they may become apparent after a specific episode or traumatic event. The severity of the symptoms can vary considerably. Objective signs may be difficult to demonstrate if the joint is difficult to palpate or muscular dysfunction accompanies the joint disease. If cartilage integrity is violated or the ischemic segment is displaced, crepitus, clicking, or locking of the joint will occur.

Medullary bone infarctions are asymptomatic conditions that may not be detected on radiographs for months to years. Although these infarctions are generally considered self-limited problems, they can indicate the presence of more ominous overlying conditions. When medullary bone infarctions are bilateral and symmetrical, the clinician should search for an overlying metabolic or vascular disease.

KEY CONCEPTS

- *Avascular necrosis is bone death secondary to an inadequate blood supply.*
- *Pathophysiologic changes are marked by stages of ischemia, revascularization, repair, deformity, and osteoarthritis.*
- *Osteochondritis dissecans is a focal region of bone necrosis secondary to trauma and commonly occurs at the lateral aspect of the medial femoral condyle.*
- *Medullary bone infarcts are seen radiographically as serpiginous calcifications following avascularity within the medullary canal.*
- *Epiphyseal necroses occurring in the skeletally immature (Legg-Calvé-Perthes disease) are potentially serious clinical conditions that may lead to subchondral fracture, bone deformity, and premature joint degeneration.*
- *No reliable radiographic signs exist during the avascular stage of epiphyseal necrosis, but signs during later stages may include increased sclerosis, fragmentation, altered bone contour, and osteoarthritis.*
- *Magnetic resonance imaging demonstrates a loss of marrow signal in the region of bone ischemia early in the disease.*

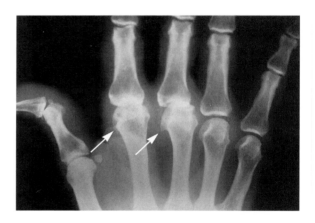

FIG. 13-16   Narrowing and subchondral sclerosis of the second and third metacarpophalangeal joints accompanied by subtle chondrocalcinosis (of the third metacarpophalangeal joint) and subchondral cyst formation (of the second metacarpal head). Small beaklike osteophytes are noted from the second and third metacarpal heads *(arrows)*.

Hemochromatosis

BACKGROUND

Hemochromatosis is a congenital (caused by hepatic xanthine oxidase deficiency) or an acquired disorder of excessive iron deposition within tissues. Patients with this condition generally have liver disease that is of greater long-term significance than the articular disease.

IMAGING FINDINGS

Articular manifestations of hemochromatosis are present in 20% to 50% of cases. The metacarpophalangeal joints of the second and third digits are the most common location, with the wrists, elbows and shoulders less frequently affected. The radiographic manifestations of this disorder are the result of degenerative disease sec-

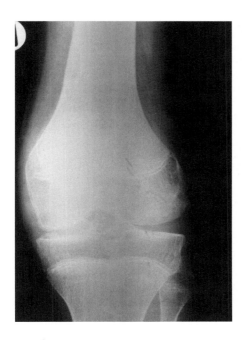

FIG. 13-17 Roughening and squaring of the femoral condyles in a child with hemophilia.

ondary to calcium pyrophosphate dihydrate (CPPD) deposition disease. Hemochromatosis is suspected when unusual distributions of degenerative disease are encountered. Chondrocalcinosis is commonly present and is the result of CPPD within the afflicted joints. The exact association between CPPD and hemochromatosis remains unclear. Morphologically, degenerative disease associated with hemochromatosis demonstrates as flattening of the metacarpal heads along with prominent cyst formation and small beak-like osteophytes, most prominently in the metacarpophalangeal joints[1] (Fig. 13-16).

CLINICAL COMMENTS

Clinically, the articular manifestations of hemochromatosis are typical of secondary degeneration. Symptoms are intermittent, and joint function is generally impaired. Considerable joint destruction may be encountered.

KEY CONCEPTS

- *Hemochromatosis represents excessive iron deposits within tissues.*
- *Articular manifestations are common and include both osteoarthritis and chondrocalcinosis.*

Hemophilia

BACKGROUND

The term *hemophilia* is applied to a class of recessive X-linked disorders that are the result of insufficient clotting factors. Only males manifest clinically evident disease, whereas females are classically carriers of the disease.

Several types of hemophilia have been identified. Hemophilia A (classic hemophilia) is a deficiency of clotting factor VIII and is the most common type. The second most common type is hemophilia B (Christmas disease), which is a deficiency of clotting factor IX. The clinical manifestations of hemophilia generally become apparent in the first year of life and have the most severe impact during childhood. Radiographic manifestations may appear in infancy but generally are not present until the childhood years.[18]

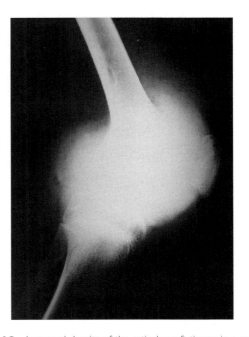

FIG. 13-18 Increased density of the articular soft tissues in a patient with chronic hemophiliac hemarthrosis.

IMAGING FINDINGS

The earliest plain film finding of hemophilia is intraarticular soft tissue swelling, with the large joints usually affected initially and most significantly. The knees, elbows, and ankles are, in decreasing order of frequency, the most commonly affected joints. Joint changes consisting of articular irregularity, epiphyseal overgrowth, and early physeal closure cause the femoral condyles and inferior patella to appear "squared."[18] Generalized osteopenia is present (Fig. 13-17). The synovium increases in thickness and density because of hemosiderin deposition, which accompanies resolution of the intraarticular hemorrhagic episodes (Figs. 13-18 and 13-19).

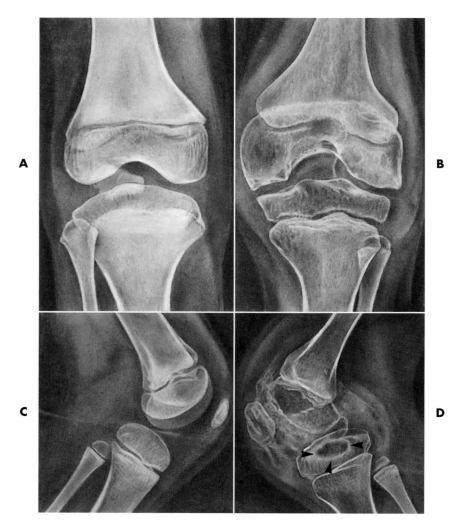

FIG. 13-19   Hemophilia panarthritis in a 7-year-old boy. **A** and **C,** Normal right knee. **B** and **D,** Hemarthrotic left knee—frontal and lateral projections. In the left knee the soft tissues are swollen and more dense. In addition, marked generalized rarefaction of the epiphyses and shafts and atrophy of the shafts is present. However, the epiphyseal centers and patella are enlarged on the left side; the intercondylar notch is deepened and the juxtaarticular surfaces of the bones are ragged. In **D** a large intraosseous hematoma is visible in the tibial epiphysis *(arrowheads)*. (From Caffey J: *Pediatric x-ray diagnosis: an integrated imaging approach,* St Louis, 1993, Mosby.)

Soft tissue changes outside the joints generally relate to hemorrhage and its resolution. Myositis ossificans is relatively unusual at the location of previous hematomas, but it can be present. Intramuscular hemorrhage most commonly occurs in the iliopsoas muscles.

In rare cases the skeleton demonstrates rapidly expanding lytic lesions of bone referred to as *pseudotumors of hemophilia.* The etiology of these lesions is obscure, but their development is probably related to unabated hemorrhage in an intraosseous location.[8] Pseudotumors tend to be painless masses in the pelvis and femur. However, when these lesions are peripheral, they may expand the bone sufficiently to produce bone pain.

CLINICAL COMMENTS

Patients with hemophilia are seen early in life with excessive and spontaneous bleeding. Bone pain and arthralgia with swelling are common complaints. As the disease becomes chronic, degenerative disease may greatly affect articulations. Osteophytic growth is not prominent, but joint thinning and subchondral cyst formation are quite obvious. Chronic inflammatory reactions lead to fibrosis and scarring of the synovium. As a consequence of this, the joints become stiff.

KEY CONCEPTS

- *Hemophilia results from insufficient clotting factors. Females are carriers for disease; clinically significant disease develops only in males.*
- *Knees, elbows, and ankles are the most commonly affected joints in hemophilia.*
- *Joint changes include articular irregularity, epiphyseal overgrowth, epiphyseal squaring, generalized osteopenia, radiodense effusions, and degenerative changes.*

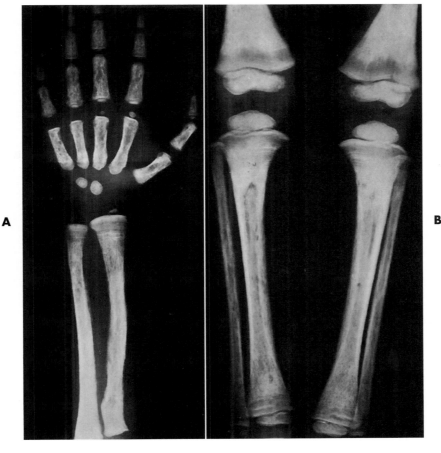

FIG. 13-20   Leukopenic lymphatic leukemia in a 2-year-old boy. **A,** Hand and forearm. **B,** Lower limbs; irregular destruction of all the bones is evident. Deep transverse zones of diminished density occupy the ends of the shafts. In addition to these destructive features, numerous large and small irregular patches of sclerosis are present, indicating a massive osteoblastic reaction. (From Caffey J: *Pediatric x-ray diagnosis: an integrated imaging approach,* St Louis, 1993, Mosby.)

Hereditary Spherocytosis

BACKGROUND

Hereditary spherocytosis is a curious condition in which the red blood cells are spherical rather than biconcave. Because of their shape, the cells are fragile and have a reduced capacity to carry oxygen. Consequently, the half-life of the red blood cells is considerably shortened.

IMAGING FINDINGS

Radiological findings are uncommon in hereditary spherocytosis. However, if the disorder is severe, mild changes of marrow hyperplasia, including osteopenia and expansion of the marrow cavity in the proximal extremities and the axial skeleton, may be seen.

CLINICAL COMMENTS

The spleen may be enlarged, and laboratory values may reflect elevated hemolysis.

▐ KEY CONCEPTS

- *Hereditary spherocytosis is a condition marked by morphological alterations of red blood cells that reduce their ability to carry oxygen.*
- *Radiographic findings are uncommon, but changes may develop secondary to marrow hyperplasia in severe cases.*

Leukemia

BACKGROUND

Leukemia, the most common childhood cancer, has both acute and chronic forms. Although adults may also develop this cancer, the vast majority of leukemia patients are younger than 5 years of age. Lymphoblastic leukemia is the histological variety in approximately 80% of cases.

IMAGING FINDINGS

Plain film findings are abnormal in nearly 50% of children with leukemia. The most common radiological manifestation of this cancer is generalized osteopenia. The earliest radiographic findings are transmetaphyseal lucent bands near the physes of long bones such as the femur and tibia (Fig. 13-20). Rather than leukemic infiltrates, these bands appear to represent a metabolic reaction to the process. Alternatively, they may develop because pressure on the physis from the neoplastic infiltrates alters bony maturation at the zone of provisional calcification.

Discrete bony lesions may be present in the metaphysis or diaphysis where they create a "moth-eaten" or permeative pattern of destruction. Periostitis may also develop with the discrete bone lesions. In some cases, focal, spotty sclerosis is noted after chemotherapy or radiation treatment. Diffuse sclerosis of the bones has been encountered, but it is thought to be secondary myelofibrosis resulting from therapeutic interventions.[3]

Infiltration of the meninges of the brain creates a separation of the skull sutures in a small percentage of patients with leukemia. Based on the radiographic findings alone, differentiation of infiltration of the meninges from neuroblastoma metastasis to the skeleton can be challenging because both conditions cause periostitis and separations of the sutures.

Focal accumulations of leukemic cells have been identified in a small number of patients with acute myelogenous leukemia. Because of their green color, these cells have been termed *chloromas*. Most commonly, chloromas accumulate outside the skeleton. Skeletal accumulations most often develop in the face, sternum, and ribs.[14]

CLINICAL COMMENTS

Patients with leukemia generally have a number of systemic complaints, including fever, malaise, and weakness. The musculoskeletal findings in leukemia include diffuse bone and joint pain, similar to the findings in juvenile rheumatoid arthritis. Joint and soft tissue swelling should alert the physician to the presence of a more serious condition. The laboratory finding of blast cells in the peripheral blood smear is strongly suggestive of leukemia, and bone marrow biopsy is diagnostic.

KEY CONCEPTS
- *Leukemia is the most common childhood cancer.*
- *Radiographic findings include generalized osteopenia, transmetaphyseal lucent bands, and occasionally, osteolytic bone lesions with a moth-eaten or permeative pattern of destruction.*
- *Clinical findings include fever, malaise, weakness, and joint pain.*

Sickle Cell Anemia

BACKGROUND

Sickle cell anemia is the most common disorder in a class of hemoglobinopathies known as *hemolytic anemias*.[16] This autosomal dominant condition is caused by the substitution of valine for glutamic acid at position 6 on the β-globin molecule. The clinically relevant result of this substitution is that red blood cells flatten and become sickle shaped during episodes of low oxygen tension. The sickling is reversible in mild cases but not in more severe cases.

The worldwide prevalence of sickle cell disease is considerable, with as many as 50% of East Africans having some variant of the disease. In North America, the prevalence of sickle cell anemia is estimated to be nearly 9%, and African-Americans are the most commonly affected. The homozygous form of sickle cell disease is present in approximately 1 in 600 African Americans in the United States.[7]

Pathologically, sickle cells aggregate into clumps of deformed red cells that obstruct blood vessels. Not only do these cells tend to deform, they are also quite fragile, and their life span is dramatically shortened. This in turn necessitates accelerated hematopoiesis.

IMAGING FINDINGS

The frequency and severity of the skeletal manifestations in sickle cell anemia depends on the degree of genetic penetrance of the disease. More pronounced radiographic changes are demonstrated at an earlier phase in patients who are homozygous for sickle cell disease than in those who are heterozygous.

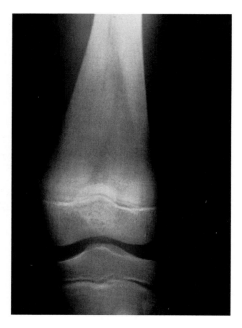

FIG. 13-21 Marrow hyperplasia manifesting as flaring of the metaphysis in a child with sickle cell disease.

The radiographic findings of sickle cell disease relate to marrow hyperplasia and infarction.[4] Marrow hyperplasia appears as an accentuation of the marrow, particularly in the long bones. Long bones demonstrate varying degrees of undertubulation (widening of the diaphysis), and the marrow takes on a somewhat lacelike or reticulated appearance (Fig. 13-21).

In sickle cell anemia, bone density is universally reduced because of cortical thinning and reduced concentration of trabeculae in the medullary bone. In the skull, marrow hyperplasia results in a widening of the diploë with accentuation of the trabeculae. This imparts a "hair-on-end" appearance to the calvarium. In the spine, marrow hyperplasia causes coarsening of the trabeculae and overall osteopenia. The osteopenia may be severe enough to increase the likelihood of spinal compression deformities.[17]

Because of the protective presence of hemoglobin F in the blood, infarctions rarely occur before the age of 6 months in infants with sickle cell anemia. As hemoglobin F recedes from the blood and is replaced by hemoglobin S, infarctions begin to occur. If sickle cell anemia is severe, hemoglobin S may constitute 70% to 99% of circulating hemoglobin. In these instances, infarctions occur early in life. In milder sickle cell anemia, infarctions may be less numerous and they may occur much later in life.

Sickle cell infarctions affect the tubular bones of the hands and feet, most commonly in very young patients. Within these bones, infarctions generally affect the diaphysis or metaphysis. In larger bones such as the humerus and femur, epiphyseal infarction is more common and produces the typical changes of epiphyseal ischemic necrosis (Fig. 13-22). Epiphyseal infarctions can also occur in other long bones and the spine. Interestingly, the skull is an unusual site for sickle cell infarctions.

The earliest plain film evidence of skeletal infarction in the young is an aggressive-appearing lytic destructive process at the site of infarction. At this early stage, differentiation of an infarction from an infection or a neoplasm is difficult based on the radio-

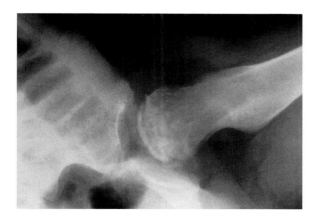

FIG. 13-22 Epiphyseal ischemic necrosis in a patient suffering from sickle cell disease.

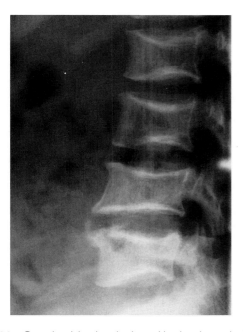

FIG. 13-23 Central endplate invaginations with sclerotic margins in a patient with sickle cell anemia *(H vertebrae sign)*.

graphic appearance. Radionuclide scintigraphy is useful because infarctions demonstrate focal photopenia, whereas other destructive processes generally increase radiopharmaceutical uptake. Once periostitis develops days to weeks later, the differential diagnosis of infection is more difficult, even with scintigraphy.[12] Likewise, distinguishing acute infarction from acute infection with MRI remains difficult.[15] Skeletal deformity and pathological fracture may occur as the infarction progresses.

Old, quiescent infarctions are characterized by mottled sclerosis and irregularity of the medullary bone architecture. Large infarctions may develop marginal sclerosis parallel to the outer surface of the bone, which creates a "bone-within-a-bone" appearance. Quiescent diaphyseal infarctions may extend through a considerable length of bone and generally demonstrate parallel tracks of sclerosis adjacent to but distinct from the diaphyseal cortex. When in-

farctions are epiphyseal or pathological fracture has occurred, the deformity that is present when the bone begins to revascularize persists as a permanent alteration in the bone structure. A classic but not pervasive example of this phenomenon occurs in the spine, where endplate infarctions result in central collapse of the vertebral bodies, which when healed, are accentuated by focal sclerosis at the infarction. These central depressions can alter the overall appearance of the vertebral segments, with the term *H vertebrae* used to describe the biconcavity of the phenomenon (Fig. 13-23). However, this finding is present in only about 50% of sickle cell cases.[17]

CLINICAL COMMENTS

The clinical manifestations of sickle cell disease are usually related to the hemolytic aspect of the disorder. Skeletally, bilateral pain and swelling in the hands and feet are characteristic of the "hand-foot syndrome," which is the result of infarctions in the small tubular bones of the distal extremities. This syndrome generally occurs between the first and second years of life in patients with severe sickle cell disease. In the gastrointestinal tract, infarctions of the mesenteric arteries create symptoms of bowel perforation or obstruction. These bowel infarctions predispose patients to infections at distant sites in the body by allowing gastrointestinal flora, particularly *Salmonella paratyphi,* entrance to the circulatory system. Salmonella osteomyelitis, which tends to affect the diaphysis of the long bones, is considered a classic complication of sickle cell disease. Jaundice and hyperbilirubinemia are constant findings that result from high red cell turnover. Hepatosplenomegaly may be present but is usually minor. Eventually, the infarctions cause involution of the spleen that will progress to autosplenectomy. Renal papillary necrosis and high-output cardiac failure may also result from sickle cell disease.

KEY CONCEPTS

- *Sickle cell anemia is the most common form of hemolytic anemia.*
- *Approximately 1 of every 600 African-Americans has homozygous sickle cell disease.*
- *Radiographic findings are secondary to marrow hyperplasia (coarse trabeculation, osteopenia, long bone undertubulation, and "hair-on-end" appearance of the skull) and vascular occlusion (avascular necrosis, H-shaped vertebrae, and epiphyseal growth disturbances).*
- *Bowel infarctions mimic perforation or obstruction and predispose the individual to Salmonella infections at distant sites.*

Thalassemia

BACKGROUND

Thalassemia represents a spectrum of hematological disorders that are characterized by varying degrees of hypochromic microcytic anemia. The principal abnormality in thalassemia is an excess of hemoglobin F. The disorder is inherited through autosomal dominant transmission. Severe (homozygous) thalassemia is also known as *Cooley's anemia* or *Mediterranean anemia*. Patients with severe manifestations of thalassemia generally die during childhood.

IMAGING FINDINGS

The primary radiographic manifestations of thalassemia are the result of marrow hyperplasia. Signs of the disease are often present on plain films obtained in the first year of life. In the peripheral skeleton, severe osteopenia is the most common and consistent finding. Expansion of the marrow cavity is recognized through undertubulation of the long bones as well as cortical thinning. With severe thalassemia, remodeling of long bones may include Erlenmeyer flask deformities of the metaphyseal regions. The trabecular pattern, particularly in the small tubular bones of the hands and feet, has a lacelike appearance typical of severe osteopenia.[2]

In the axial skeleton, signs of profound osteopenia include trabecular paucity, cortical thinning, and overall loss of bone density (Fig. 13-24). Insufficiency fractures may occur. In severe thalassemia, ballooning of the vertebral bodies may be a manifestation of marrow hyperplasia. Extramedullary hematopoiesis, seen by computed tomography, arises from the vertebral bodies or ribs.

The changes in the skull are characteristic. Because of severe marrow proliferation, the sinuses fail to pneumatize but are filled with a proliferation of marrow. This creates overgrowth of the maxillary region and protrusion of the maxillary incisors, producing the "rodent facies" of thalassemia. Hypertelorism resulting from marrow proliferation in the frontal bones is also noted. Diploic marrow proliferation causes the calvaria to demonstrate varying degrees of the "hair-on-end" appearance,[13] which terminates abruptly at the external occipital protuberance and does not extend into the petrous portion of the occipital bone because the bone segment has no active marrow potential. Infarctions are distinctly unusual. Radiographically, this helps in distinguishing thalassemia from Gaucher's disease and sickle cell anemia.

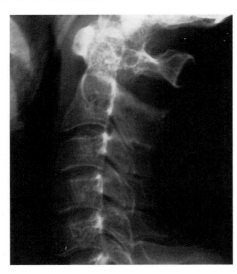

FIG. 13-24　Severe osteopenia in a young adult with thalassemia. The trabecular pattern is coarse, and there is mild expansion (ballooning) of the C2 vertebral body from marrow hyperplasia.

CLINICAL COMMENTS

Patients with severe thalassemia do not have a normal life span. Growth is retarded, and epiphyses may close early as a result of marrow proliferation across the physis and pressure on the physeal margin by the marrow. Skeletal deformities are generally the result of insufficiency fractures; these fractures may be spontaneous or may be a consequence of minor trauma. Hepatosplenomegaly is present, and jaundice is a constant finding. Increased levels of the by-products of red blood cell catabolism are present in the stool, blood, and urine.

KEY CONCEPTS

- *The homozygous form of thalassemia is known as Cooley's anemia or Mediterranean anemia.*
- *Marrow hyperplasia may cause coarse trabeculation, osteopenia, undertubulation of long bones, maxillary overgrowth, and a hair-on-end appearance of the skull.*
- *Rodent facies describes maxillary overgrowth and protrusion of the maxillary incisors.*
- *Hepatosplenomegaly and jaundice are constant findings in patients with thalassemia.*

References

1. Adamson T et al: Hand and wrist arthropathies of hemochromatosis and calcium pyrophosphate deposition disease: distinct radiographic features, *Radiology* 147:377, 1983.
2. Baker D: Roentgen manifestations of Cooley's anemia, *Ann N Y Acad Sci* 119:641, 1964.
3. Benz G, Brandeis W, Wilich E: Radiological aspects of leukemia in childhood: an analysis of 89 children, *Pediatr Radiol* 4:201, 1976.
4. Bohrer S: Bone changes in the extremities in sickle cell anemia, *Semin Roentgenol* 22:176, 1987.
5. Bonnarenz F, Hernandez A, D'Ambrosia R: Bone scintigraphic changes in osteonecrosis of the femoral head, *Orthop Clin North Am* 16:697, 1985.
6. Crues R: Osteonecrosis of bone: current concepts as to etiology and pathogenesis, *Clin Orthop* 208:30, 1986.
7. Gaston M: Sickle cell disease: an overview, *Semin Roentgenol* 22:150, 1987.
8. Gilbert M: Characterizing the hemophilic pseudotumor, *Ann N Y Acad Sci* 240:311, 1975.
9. Gillespy T, Genant H, Helms C: Magnetic resonance imaging of osteonecrosis, *Radiol Clin North Am* 24:193, 1986.
10. Hungerford D, Lennox D: The importance of increased intraosseous pressure in the development of osteonecrosis of the femoral head: implications for treatment, *Orthop Clin North Am* 16:635, 1985.
11. Kenzora J, Glimcher M: Pathogenesis of idiopathic osteonecrosis: the ubiquitous crescent sign, *Orthop Clin North Am* 16:681, 1985.
12. Kim H et al: Differentiation of bone and bone marrow infarcts from osteomyelitis in sickle cell disorders, *Clin Nucl Med* 14:249, 1989.
13. Orzincola C et al: Circumscribed lytic lesions of the thalassemia skull, *Skeletal Radiol* 17:344, 1988.
14. Pomeranz S et al: Granulocytic sarcoma (chloroma): CT manifestations, *Radiology* 155:167, 1985.
15. Rao V et al: Painful sickle cell crisis: bone marrow patterns observed with MR imaging, *Radiology* 161:211, 1986.
16. Reed M: *Pediatric skeletal radiology,* Baltimore, 1992, Williams & Wilkins.
17. Reynolds J: Sickle cell disease: the skull and spine, *Semin Roentgenol* 22:168, 1987.
18. Stein H, Duthie R: The pathogenesis of chronic hemophilic arthropathy, *J Bone Joint Surg Br* 63:601, 1981.
19. Toby E, Kiman L, Bechtold R: Magnetic resonance imaging of pediatric hip disease, *J Pediatr Orthop* 5:665, 1985.

chapter 14

Infections

D ROBERT KUHN

Nonsuppurative Infections

Blastomycosis

BACKGROUND

Blastomycosis, also called *Gilchrist's disease* or *North American blastomycosis,* is produced by the fungus *Blastomyces dermatitidis.*[1,13] *B. dermatitidis, is inhaled by the patient into the lungs and causes pneumonitis.*[13,40] Although blastomycosis affects immunocompromised individuals, it can affect healthy individuals as well. Hematogenous spread may lead to involvement of the skin and osseous structures. The disease can also cause the patient to develop asymptomatic bone lesions.

Blastomycosis is endemic in the central and Great Lakes regions and the Ohio and Mississippi River valleys[46] of the United States and to regions of Canada.[1] Blacks and Native American Indians are more commonly affected than whites.[46] Men are affected more often than women, with the ratio of men to women ranging from 4:1 to 15:1.[46] Infections often develop in people who have contact with soil, work outside, or frequently engage in outdoor activities[13,32,46]; some cases of human-to-human infection transmission have been noted. Blastomycosis develops less frequently than other dimorphic fungi infections in immunocompromised individuals.[13]

IMAGING FINDINGS

Skeletal infections develop in up to 60% of blastomycosis cases, representing 25% of the extrapulmonary infections.[1,13] Bone is the third most commonly infected site after the pulmonary system and skin[32]; in some cases, the disease may spread to the prostate.[13] The vertebral bodies, ribs, and skull are the most commonly affected bones. Features of blastomycosis bone invasion include eccentric, well-circumscribed lesions that cause no significant periosteal reactions and have little cortical penetration.[32] Punched-out lesions are occasionally reported, but sequestration rarely occurs.[32] Whereas the vertebrae may be significantly damaged, the intervertebral discs may be spared. The infection may spread along the anterior longitudinal ligament and skip a vertebral level—a feature that is also associated with tuberculosis.[46]

Blastomycosis joint involvement is usually monoarticular; however, polyarticular presentations may be seen. Systemic or pulmonary disease may concurrently develop.[13] The knee is most commonly infected, followed by the ankle, elbow, wrist, and hand.[1,13] In some cases, blastomycosis presents as a soft tissue mass that is solid, has punctate calcifications, and is very similar to a synovial cell sarcoma.[1] A soft tissue neoplasm cannot be differentiated from this fungal lesion by plain film radiography.[3,46] In addition, neither ultrasound, magnetic resonance imaging (MRI), nor bone scanning can properly diagnosis blastomycosis. Accurate diagnosis is based on a combination of radiographic localization, biopsy, and culture.[32]

CLINICAL COMMENTS

Signs and symptoms of blastomycosis include subclinical infections and signs and symptoms that are similar to those of acute histoplasmosis. Typical features include joint and muscle pain, a productive cough, and chest pain that resolves spontaneously.[13] Other signs and symptoms include fever, weight loss, night sweats, and pleuritic pain.[40] Patients with blastomycosis who have essentially normal laboratory profiles (i.e., normal complete blood count [CBC], erythrocyte sedimentation rate [ESR], and differential count) may have draining ulcers.[46] In certain cases, the hematocrit values may indicate the presence of chronic infection.[46] No skin test exists for blastomycosis—biopsy and culture are the keys to the diagnosis.[40,46] Silver methenamine is used to detect the fungus. The culture may take 1 to 2 weeks to grow.[46] Historically, mortality rates in treated patients in whom the disease had disseminated were as high as 23%.[46] Patients with untreated disease have an 80% mortality rate.[1]

Treatment protocols for blastomycosis include debridement and administration of oral imidazole, ketoconazole, itraconazole, or amphotericin B. A 6-month course of treatment is typical. Patients who are prescribed amphotericin B must be closely monitored[1]; side effects include anorexia, nausea and vomiting, fever with chills, anemia, and nephrotoxicity. In spite of the numerous side affects, the benefits of using amphotericin B outweigh the risks.

KEY CONCEPTS

- *Blastomycosis is produced by the fungus Blastomyces dermatitidis. The fungus is inhaled by the patient and produces pneumonitis.*
- *Hematogenous transport is the likely means by which the infection is disseminated to the skin and osseous structures.*
- *It is endemic to the central and Great Lakes regions of the United States, the Ohio and Mississippi River valleys, and Canada.*
- *Radiographic features include a geographic region of lytic destruction and in some cases punched-out lesions.*
- *The vertebrae may be severely damaged even when the discs are not.*
- *The infection may skip a vertebral level and involve a subjacent segment.*
- *Radiographic localization followed by biopsy and culture are the most accurate methods of diagnosis.*
- *Clinical features include joint and muscle pain, a productive cough, and chest pain that resolves spontaneously.*

Coccidioidomycosis

BACKGROUND

Coccidioidomycosis, which is also called *valley fever* and *desert rheumatism,*[4,51] is a systemic infection caused by the soil fungus *Coccidioides immitis.* It is endemic to the southwestern United States, the San Joaquin Valley, Mexico, and in regions of Central and South America.* The fungus spores are typically inhaled into the lungs, which are the primary site of infection.[39,59] Many patients have mild or no symptoms, so the infection is found incidentally.[26]

Individuals who are older than 65 years of age or have AIDS are the primary populations at risk for becoming infected.[39] Other individuals at risk are those being treated with steroids or chemotherapy. Some evidence suggests that individuals can be genetically predisposed to contracting the infection.[24] Although dissemination is rare, an increased risk for spread of the disease exists among Filipinos, blacks, Mexicans, pregnant females, children younger than 5 years of age, adults older than 50 years of age, and immunosuppressed individuals.[13,59] The skin and subcutaneous tissues are the most common sites of dissemination from pulmonary disease.[59] The next most common site is the mediastinum,[59] followed by the skeletal system.[59] The incidence of coccidioidomycosis has dramatically increased since 1991.[24] Currently, 50,000 patients a year are diagnosed with the infection.[13]

IMAGING FINDINGS

Skeletal lesions are seen in 10% to 50% of the cases in which the disease has spread. Coccidioidomycosis may affect multiple sites, producing osteolytic lesions in cancellous and cortical bone and soft tissue swelling. A periosteal reaction is possible but uncommon.[13,24,59] Previously, bony prominences were considered common sites for coccidioidomycosis infection. More recent studies have failed to document this association and have found that involvement of the axial skeletal is more common.[13,26] In the appendicular skeleton the ankles and knees are more frequently affected; remission occurs in 2 to 4 weeks, and no residual damage remains.[13]

During the initial stages, plain film radiography may not detect infection. Findings of decreased joint space and areas of localized osteopenia may be early signs.[13,26] Ankylosis can be an end result of joint infection.[13] A bone scan is sensitive and can typically detect the infection in the early stages.[26,59] MRI may demonstrate a large, poorly marginated mass with an intermediate signal and lower cen-

tral signal. MRI also typically demonstrates a decreased signal on T1-weighted images and an increased signal on T2-weighted images,[59] together a sign of abscess or necrosis.[33] MRI and computed tomography (CT) are useful for detection and surgical planning.[35] A positive bone scan should be followed by CT or MRI.[59] A decreased disc space and gibbous formation may be seen, but they are much less common than they are in patients with tuberculosis.[59] CT demonstrates low-attenuation lesions that may appear bubbly and expansile.[59]

Septic arthritis secondary to coccidioidomycosis may develop and is usually seen as (1) synovitis with joint effusion, (2) periarticular bone destruction similar to that in patients with tuberculosis or neuropathic joints, and (3) well-defined periarticular erosions resembling pigmented villonodular synovitis. Periosteal reactions are typically associated with a permeative destructive pattern.[59] Soft tissue swelling and osteoporosis may also be seen in conjunction with permeative destructive lesions. A periosteal reaction is not commonly associated with punched-out lesions. Some lesions demonstrate a thin, sclerotic margin surrounding the area of bone involvement, indicating reactive sclerosis.[47]

CLINICAL COMMENTS

Coccidioidomycosis infection of bone and joints is uncommon. Therefore it is frequently overlooked as an initial diagnostic option,[26] resulting in frequent delays in diagnosis.[26] The clinical presentation may closely mimic that of tuberculosis.[5] Two thirds of the patients recover uneventfully and may be asymptomatic throughout the course of their infection. One third will develop symptoms that usually include a self-limiting pneumonitis caused by the inhaled airborne spores. Of those, 40% of patients present with the symptoms within 2 to 3 weeks of exposure. The most common signs and symptoms reported by 80% of the infected patients are fatigue, coughing, night sweats, and fever, a presentation that can significantly resemble the flu.[51] Pneumonia that does not respond to antibiotics may be part of an infected patient's history.[24] Other signs and symptoms are a general achiness, a sore throat, peripheral eosinophilia, erythema nodosum, and erythema multiform.[13] If arthralgia develops. It is usually polyarticular and migratory; tenderness and pain when the affected joint is moved through its range of motion is common, but effusion is not typical.[13] In approximately 1% of the cases the disease will spread to the skin, bones, joints, lymph nodes, and in rare cases the central nervous system.[13,24,26,38] Spread of the disease has been reported to occur months to years after the primary infection.[13]

A brief visit to an area in which coccidioidomycosis is endemic is all that is needed to contract the infection.[26] In one study, 24 out of 25 patients with symptomatic coccidioidomycosis lived in endemic regions and/or were immunocompromised.[26] Exposure and subsequent infection can begin insidiously.

An effective skin test can be used to detect previous coccidioidomycosis infection.[24] A definitive diagnosis of an emerging case of coccidioidomycosis requires biopsy and culture.[26] A tissue biopsy of an infected individual contains necrotic debris composed of polymorphonuclear leukocytes and often Langerhans cells. A culture takes 2 to 5 days to yield results. A microscopic exam is quicker but less sensitive.[26] During the laboratory exam, methenamine silver is used to blacken the capsules of spherical fungi such as *Coccidioides.*[5,24] Lab findings may include elevations in the white blood cell (WBC) count and ESR, but these results are not consistent.[26]

Once the diagnosis of coccidioidomycosis in osseous or joint structures is made, surgical debridement is mandatory.[26] Itracona-

---

*References 4, 6, 24, 28, 53, 59.

zole is slow but effective, and fluconazole was found to be effective in nonmeningeal coccidioidomycosis.[13] Amphotericin B should be reserved for severe infections with skeletal involvement.[13] Open drainage, synovectomy, arthrodesis, and sometimes amputation are reserved for later stages of severe cases.[13] If a timely diagnosis is made and proper treatment is instituted, patients with coccidioidomycosis have excellent outcomes, although in rare instances of treated individuals, fatalities still occur.[26]

KEY CONCEPTS

- *Coccidioidomycosis—also called valley fever or desert rheumatism—is caused by the fungus Coccidioides immitis.*
- *Individuals at risk are individuals older than 65 years of age or who have AIDS.*
- *Many patients demonstrate no symptoms and signs; the infection is found incidentally.*
- *When the disease spreads, it most commonly affects the skin, subcutaneous tissues, mediastinum, and skeleton.*
- *Plain film radiography often does not detect the early stages of infection but does reliably demonstrate the later changes of decreased joint space and osteopenia.*
- *Performing a tissue biopsy and staining biological samples with silver methenamine are diagnostic methods.*
- *Early diagnosis and treatment are associated with excellent outcomes.*

Maduromycosis (Mycetoma or Eumycetoma)

BACKGROUND

Maduromycosis was first discovered in Madura, India, some time between 1842 and 1846.[47] It predominantly affects the feet,[30,43] which are infected by a penetrating trauma.[53] Eumycetoma is a disease that is usually found in the tropics, with only a few cases being reported in temperate climates.[30,44] The organism that causes the disease has been isolated in soil and on thorns—the most likely sources of infection. Mycetoma is produced by a number of organisms that are distributed in two distinct groups:[12] *eumycetes,* or true fungi, and *actinomycetes,* or false fungi, which is a filamentous bacteria. The organism that is usually responsible for maduromycosis in the United States and Canada is *Petriellidium boydii;* in Africa and India, it is *Madurella mycetomi;* in Mexico, it is *Nocardia brasiliensis,* and in Japan, it is *Nocardia asteroides.*[12] Maduromycosis is rare in the United States; it is slightly more common in Mexico, Guatemala, and other parts of South America.[43] Because pharmacologic treatments are frequently unsuccessful, surgical resection or amputation is often required.[4]

IMAGING FINDINGS

Radiographic characteristics of maduromycosis include mottled osseous destructive patterns with a periosteal reaction[12,43] and marked soft tissue swelling, often resulting in permanent deformities.[43] When the periosteum is breached, a laminated, or spiculated, periosteal reaction is typically seen.[30] The cortex is often eroded. Eumycotic lesions tend to be fewer in number and produce larger bone cavities that are greater than 1 cm, and a periosteal reaction occurs in about 50% of the cases.[30] Actinomycetes produce more numerous, smaller lesions, and a periosteal reaction is seen approximately 75% of cases.[30] In all cases, a soft tissue mass is seen.[30] The sequestrum associated with other types of osteomyelitis is not a feature of maduromycosis.[12] Loss of cortical margins followed by erosion and adjacent sclerosis is more typical.[12] If the infection

develops near a joint, the cartilage is typically spared[12]; however, ankylosis may develop as an end result of this process.[12] Osteopenia is very rare, possibly because patients can walk on even a severely infected foot—evidence that this type of infection is typically painless.[30]

CLINICAL COMMENTS

General signs and symptoms of maduromycosis include the presence of multiple, crusted nodules surrounded by hyperpigmented tissue. The common clinical triad consists of a sinus track, granules (colonies), and nodular enlargements of infected body parts.[43] Hematologic laboratory values are usually normal. Patients with maduromycosis often have long histories associated with the development of the disease; one documented case lasted for 18 years.[43]

The disease is almost painless, and few constitutional symptoms are seen unless a secondary infection has developed.[44] The bacteria initially invade soft tissue around superficial and deep fascia. The first sign is typically a small bump, and the foot then becomes swollen (but not painful).[12] The affected limb becomes deformed as a result of microbial colonies forming grains and intercommunicating sinuses that may drain onto the skin's surface.[30] The grains extrude and form colonies that vary in color according to the infecting species.[30] The lesion is usually confined to the soft tissues for years before bone infection occurs.[30] When the disease breaks into the bone in the much later stages, it is usually painless. Hematogenous spread is rare.[12]

An antimicrobial treatment may be sufficient while the infection is limited to the soft tissues.[30] Once the bones are involved, a cure may be impossible and amputation may be necessary, although it is considered to be a last resort.[12,30] Differentiation between eumycetomas and an actinomycetomas is important, because the most effective treatments for each type are different.[44] Some actinomycetomas respond to high doses and long-term usage of antibiotics.[12] In particular, *Nocardia* organisms seem to be sensitive to some of the sulfonamides. Use of solely surgical debridement and resection rarely cures the infection.[12] Some recent progress has been made using itraconazole for 6 months.[43]

KEY CONCEPTS

- *Maduromycosis is the most common fungal infection worldwide.*
- *The organism that causes the infection has been isolated in soil and on thorns—the typical sources of infection.*
- *The feet are usually involved.*
- *Painless soft tissue swelling is one of the early findings.*
- *A painless swollen foot will often reveal sinus tract formation and extrusion of grain colonies, with various colors depicting the primary infecting species.*
- *Treatment consist of antimicrobial agents and amputation.*

Syphilis

BACKGROUND

Syphilis is a chronic systemic infection caused by the spirochete *Treponema pallidum.*[45] Infections are capable of involving any organ or tissue and are classified as either congenital or acquired.[41] Congenital syphilis is contracted by transplacental exposure of the fetus to the infection after about the fourth month of pregnancy. It is categorized into early and late presentations. Early congenital syphilis is diagnosed in children who are younger than 2 years of age, whereas late congenital syphilis is diagnosed in children who are 2 years and older.[41] Acquired syphilis is contracted by close physical (usually sexual) contact with an infected individual's skin lesions or mucous membranes. The disease initially develops as a chancre with local lymphadenopathy. The infection progresses over a period of several months and becomes systemic, or secondary, syphilis. After a latent period of 5 to 15 years, the disease progresses to the tertiary stage, which is characterized by gumma formation. Gummas are rubbery, soft, destructive lesions of various sizes that contain necrotic caseous material and affect bone, skin, viscera, the central nervous system, and other organs and tissues.

Although the incidence of syphilis decreased for many years after World War II, it increased through the 1970s and 1980s and peaked in 1988.[9,20] It has been on the decline through 1997. The increase in the number of congenital syphilis cases has been attributed to an associated rise in the number of women with syphilis who subsequently became pregnant but did not receive adequate prenatal care.[9] Drug addiction has also been associated with the increase, because individuals who abuse drugs have impaired immune systems and are less likely to take protective measures against sexually transmitted diseases while engaging in sexual activity.[20] A clear association has been made between the use of crack cocaine and an increased incidence of syphilis.[20] It was reported in 1988 that congenital syphilis had reached its highest levels since widespread use of penicillin began.[45] The increase is particularly high among homosexual males. Many cases of congenital and especially acquired syphilis are never reported. It is likely that morbidity and mortality figures for both varieties are underestimated.[45]

Yaws is caused by another species of *Treponema—Treponema pertenue—* that is very similar to *T. pallidum*. Yaws primarily develops in children, is an acquired disease through direct contact, but is rarely transmitted sexually. The radiographic findings are similar to those of syphilis, but symptoms tend to be more severe.

IMAGING FINDINGS
Congenital syphilis

Early. Some radiographic evidence of the disease can usually be obtained from most symptomatic newborns with syphilis.[9] Early manifestations of congenital syphilis include osteochondritis or metaphysitis, periostitis, and diaphyseal osteitis. Polyostotic, symmetrical bone involvement is characteristic of congenital syphilis.[18,41,48,56] The long bones, pelvis, vertebrae, and small tubular bones are involved.[18]

The first stage of osteochondritis, or metaphysitis, leads to fragmentation of the metaphysis, with transverse lucencies arising subjacent to the epiphyseal plate (Fig. 14-1). Invading granulation tissue is responsible for the metaphysitis[48] and is particularly common around the large joints, knees, shoulders, and elbows. Horizontal radiolucent metaphyseal bands are seen in the early stages of the disease. The ossification of the epiphyseal cartilage may be impeded and a zone of rarefaction may be present at the epiphyseal line, indicating the presence of syphilitic granulation tissue.[56] This tissue can weaken the bone and cause a pathological fracture.[56] Metaphyseal abnormalities are seen in more than 90% of infants with symptomatic congenital syphilis.[9] The most common radiographic finding in patients with congenital syphilis is lucent metaphyseal bands.[20]

Metaphysitis results in erosive bone destruction, producing a characteristic saw-tooth pattern of bone destruction. Although the saw-tooth appearance of the metaphyseal margin is characteristic, it is generally uncommon.[41] Radiographic examination of the destructive pattern of metaphysitis (which follows longitudinal bone growth) may reveal streaking radiolucent bands extending centrally

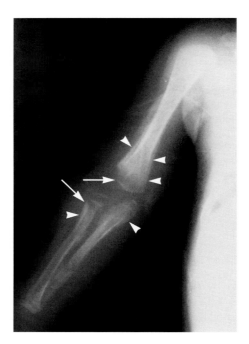

FIG. 14-1   Congenital syphilis. Note the transverse metaphyseal radiolucent band *(arrows)* and solid periostitis along the metadiaphyseal shaft of the humerus, ulna, and radius *(arrowheads)*. (Courtesy Gary M. Guebert, Maryland Heights, Mo.)

from the physis, an appearance that resembles a celery stalk. Destructive metaphysitis is particularly common along the medial margin of the proximal tibia, a finding known as *Wimberger's sign* (Fig. 14-2).[41] Although this sign is a characteristic of syphilis, it is not pathognomonic.

The second stage of early congenital syphilis is marked by bilateral, symmetrical, diffuse periostitis that affects the long tubular bones but usually spares the short tubular bones of the hands and feet.[6,41,56] Although it is less common, a third stage may develop that exhibits radiolucent long bone defects consistent with osteitis. Osteitis is commonly associated with a diffuse region of the diaphysis that has a moth-eaten appearance.[41] These changes can occur in any bone, but the femur and humerus are most commonly affected.[56] Reparative periostitis during this phase may produce prolific changes along the anterior margin of the tibia, creating a saber shin deformity.

Late. Late manifestations of congenital syphilis include destruction of and periostitis in the tibia, skull, jaw, nose, maxilla, and other superficial osseous structures. These changes are noted in patients in their late teens or early 20s. Periostitis is most pronounced along the anterior surface of the tibia bilaterally, creating a saber shin deformity. The destructive changes result from osteomyelitis, which may be associated with gumma formations. *Clutton's joints* refer to the joints that undergo the particular pattern of destruction, and the abnormally peg-shaped teeth secondary to syphilis are known as *Hutchinson's teeth*.

Acquired syphilis. Radiographic findings are mostly confined to the tertiary stages of acquired syphilis. Less than 10% of patients with acquired syphilis ever develop an osseous lesion. The changes that do occur mimic those associated with late congenital

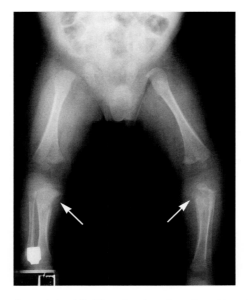

FIG. 14-2 Congenital syphilis. Bilateral periosteal reaction with medial, proximal erosion of the tibia known as *Wimberger's sign (arrows)*. (Courtesy Gary M. Guebert, Maryland Heights, Mo.)

syphilis. The most pronounced radiographic findings consist of proliferative and destructive changes affecting superficial osseous structures, particularly the tibia, clavicle, jaw, maxilla, and skull. It is extremely uncommon to encounter disseminated skeletal lesions in either infants or adults, and it is particularly rare to encounter them in patients who live in developed countries.[55] The proliferative changes manifest as prolific periostitis that is especially prominent along the anterior surface of the tibia, producing bilateral anterior bowing or a saber shin deformity. Destructive changes are secondary to gumma formations that most commonly appear in the skull, nose, and diaphysis of long bones.

CLINICAL COMMENTS

Congenital syphilis should be suspected in a newborn whose mother has positive serologic evidence of syphilis and is receiving inadequate or no treatment.[20] Anemia, hepatosplenomegaly, skin lesions, and rhinitis are the predominant signs and symptoms of affected newborns. Some infants also have gastroenteritis, bronchopneumonia, septicemia, meningitis, pseudoparalysis, and joint swelling. A small number of children may have polydactylias, pathological fractures, and signs and symptoms mimicking brachial plexus lesions.[41] Thermal instability, mucocutaneous lesions, snuffles, hepatosplenomegaly, adenopathy, anemia, hydrops fetalis, pathological jaundice, and pseudoparalysis are consistent with syphilis.[9]

Babies with congenital syphilis are 4 times more likely to have low birth weights. Approximately 62% of patients with congenital syphilis are symptomatic at birth.[48] Microhemagglutination tests are usually used to make a diagnosis,[20] but patients who have none of the typical gummatous lesions or spirochetes are diagnosed by exclusion.[55] The periostitis and osteochondritis seen are often self-limiting and usually heal within a few months even with no treatment.[56]

KEY CONCEPTS

- *The organism associated with syphilis is* Treponema pallidum.
- *The highest rate of increase is in drug-addicted individuals.*
- *There are two forms of syphilis, congenital and acquired.*
- *Congenital syphilis is divided into early and late categories.*
- *Radiographic signs of congenital syphilis include metaphysis fragmentation and transverse lucencies subjacent to the epiphyseal plate; the most common radiographic finding is bilateral symmetrical periostitis.*
- *The osteitis stage may produce the classic saber shin deformity.*
- *Congenital syphilis should be suspected in any newborn whose mother has positive serologic evidence of syphilis.*
- *Chronic signs and symptoms of congenital syphilis include anemia, hepatosplenomegaly, skin lesions, and rhinitis.*
- *Infants born with syphilis are 4 times more likely to have low birth weights.*
- *Microhemagglutination tests are fundamental to the diagnosis.*
- *The neurotrophic disease associated with syphilis is secondary to the damage done to the nervous system.*

Tuberculosis

BACKGROUND

Mycobacterium tuberculosis, Mycobacterium bovis, and *Mycobacterium africanum* are all capable of producing tuberculosis in humans.[20] The infection is spread almost exclusively by human-to-human airborne transmission, and the lungs are its primary target.[19]

Tuberculosis has been a documented human disease for centuries. Hippocrates described features consistent with tuberculosis as early as 450 BC, and typical characteristics were seen in a mummy whose remains dated 3000 BC. Following a long period of decline, the incidence of tuberculosis has been increasing since 1985, with its current rate being 14% in the United States.[48,58] The largest increase has been among Hispanics and blacks.[45]

Several factors are related to the increased incidence, including the HIV epidemic and introduction of tuberculosis cases of a foreign origin.[45] The cities with the highest incidences of AIDS have had a concomitant increase in the incidence of tuberculosis. The incidence of tuberculosis infection in AIDS patients is 500 times the incidence in the general population.[58] In the late 1980s and early 1990s, 60% of tuberculosis cases were of a foreign origin. Some evidence suggests that the number of foreign tuberculosis cases is beginning to decline.[58]

Skeletal tuberculosis develops in 1% to 3% of all patients with tuberculosis and comprises about 10% of all extrapulmonary forms reported.[46] Skeletal tuberculosis is slightly more common in females than males. All races are affected equally, but a higher incidence has been found among adults living in developed countries.[46] In less developed countries, all ages are equally affected.[2]

IMAGING FINDINGS

Despite its nonspecific findings, plain film radiography is the best initial imaging modality for detecting tuberculosis.[58] Tuberculosis can involve any of the bones or joints but is often confined to one location.[58] In long bones, it begins in the epiphysis and results in a secondary infection of the trabeculae.[58] As the infected mass enlarges, the trabecular fibers are resorbed, and tuberculosis granulation tissue is formed.[58] Over time, caseation and liquefaction may develop and produce an abscess cavity containing pus and bone fragments.

Skeletal tuberculosis is secondary to hematogenous dissemination from a lesion that is usually pulmonary in origin. The lung lesion is often located in the upper or apical regions (Fig. 14-3). The spine is affected in 50% of cases (Fig. 14-4), the hip in 15%, and the knee in 15%.[21] Various bones are affected in the remaining 20% of

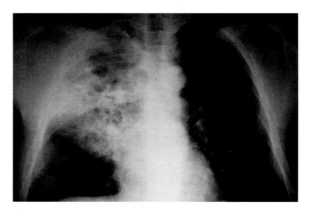

FIG. 14-3   Tuberculosis infection in the right upper lobe.

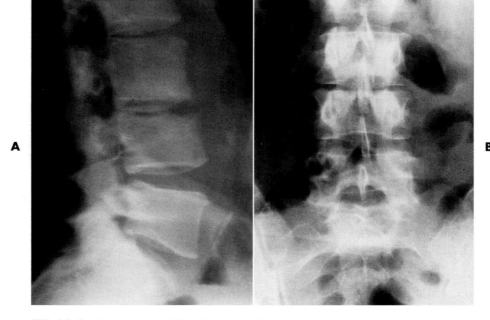

FIG. 14-4   Tuberculosis spondylitis with intervertebral disc involvement. Shown are the typical features of disc space narrowing and endplate destruction on the frontal **(A)** and lateral **(B)** radiographs.

the cases (Fig. 14-5).[58] Joint involvement is similar to the pattern associated with septic arthritis of causes other than tuberculosis. However, the following triad (Phemister's triad) of findings have historically suggested tubercular arthritis[42]:

1. Juxtaarticular osteoporosis
2. Peripherally located osseous erosions
3. Gradually narrowing joint space

In cases involving the spine, the anterior portion of the vertebral body is the most commonly affected region.[31] The most common spinal joint affected is the intervertebral disc.[6] Tuberculosis osteomyelitis in the thoracic or thoracolumbar region can produce an angular kyphosis referred to as a *gibbous formation* (Fig. 14-6).[6] The

average value of the gibbous angle is 113 degrees, as compared with normal kyphotic angles of 20 to 40 degrees (depending on the patient's age).[52] A characteristic paraspinal cold abscess develops as a result of slow development and little inflammation.[6] Healed paraspinal abscesses may calcify, making them readily visible on plain film (Fig. 14-7).[6] If the cervical spine is involved, the soft tissue mass that forms may become large enough to produce dysphagia.[6]

In the majority of cases the lesion will spread and produce an inflammatory reaction that is followed by granulation tissue (pannus) formation (Fig. 14-8). Subligamentous spread of tuberculosis produces scalloping of the vertebral bodies. An effusion can develop and rice bodies, or fibrin precipitates, may be seen. The pan-

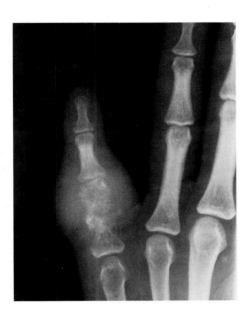

FIG. 14-5 Tuberculosis dactylitis demonstrating an expanded proximal phalanx of the fifth digit with marked surrounding soft tissue enlargement.

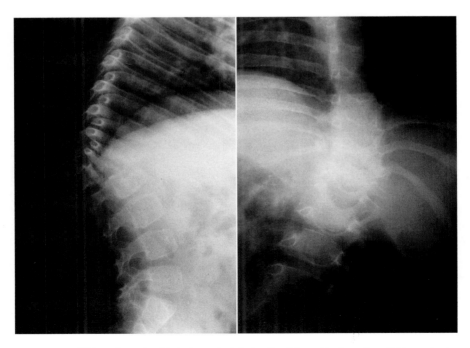

FIG. 14-6 Gibbous formation. Marked vertebral destruction followed by formation of this angular deformity is a hallmark. Compressive myelopathy may result in Pott's paraplegia. (Courtesy Gary M. Guebert, Maryland Heights, Mo.)

nus will then erode and destroy cartilage, eventually affecting the underlying bone and leading to progressive, local demineralization. The cartilage is destroyed peripherally, so relatively normal joint spaces can remain for a period of time.[58]

CLINICAL COMMENTS

The most remarkable clinical feature of tuberculosis can sometimes be its lack of symptoms. When the presenting signs and symptoms of tuberculosis are insidious, diagnosis is often delayed. Associated drug addiction or chronic alcoholism may also delay diagnosis.[45] When symptoms are present, they are nonspecific and include anorexia, weight loss, night sweats, and fever.[2,58] As the disease progresses, pulmonary complaints become more prominent.[2] A small percentage of patients have extrapulmonary symptoms such as back pain. Tenderness may develop in the affected bones and joints,[2] and stiffness and a change in range of motion may be noted.

The tuberculosis skin test is positive in 90% to 100% of nonanergic patients.[2,58] Chest radiographs show some evidence of previous or active pulmonary tuberculosis in approximately 50% of the cases.[58] Definitive diagnosis depends on bone biopsies and synovial fluid cultures. Bone biopsies are 90% sensitive to tuberculosis, whereas synovial fluid cultures are 95% sensitive.[58]

Without proper treatment, tuberculosis can produce a cold abscess in surrounding tissues.[58] As healing takes place, fibrous or osseous ankylosis of the joint may occur.[15] Once an accurate diagnosis has been made, treatment must begin as soon as possible to be effective. Treatment durations are typically between 9 and 12 months; in some cases, surgery may be used to débride or repair the deformity.[58] Acquired drug resistance can be caused by unsuccessful therapy, a situation that usually arises because therapy is inadequate or a patient is not compliant.[28] Forms of tuberculosis that are resistant to multiple drugs are significant concerns because they increase the risk of mortality.[45]

KEY CONCEPTS

- *Skeletal tuberculosis is a relatively uncommon indolent infection that develops secondary to hematogenous spread of pulmonary infections.*
- *Disseminated osteomyelitis involving the skeleton affects the spine in 50% of cases, hip in 15%, and knee in 15%. In the remaining 20% of cases, various other bones are affected.*
- *Tubercular osteomyelitis may be surrounded by prominent abscess formation. Young children and debilitated elderly patients usually account for the bulk of tuberculosis cases.*
- *The most remarkable clinical feature of tuberculosis can be its lack of symptoms.*
- *Symptoms are not specific and include anorexia, weight loss, night sweats, and afternoon fevers.*
- *As the disease progresses, pulmonary complaints increase.*
- *Definitive diagnosis of tuberculosis involving osseous structures depends on synovial samples and/or bone biopsy and culture.*
- *Once tuberculosis is diagnosed, treatment must begin immediately. Treatments last between 9 and 12 months.*
- *Surgery may be used to débride the wound or repair an acquired deformity.*

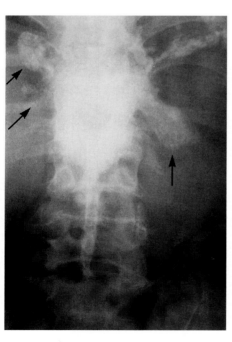

FIG. 14-7   Cold abscess. Healed paraspinal abscess in the thoracolumbar region (arrows).

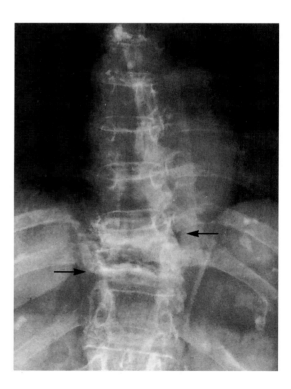

FIG. 14-8   An anteroposterior view of the thoracolumbar junction in a patient with a known paraspinal tuberculosis abscess. Note the loss of height of the T10 and T11 vertebral bodies, as well as the marked bony sclerosis (arrows). These findings suggest a relatively chronic destructive process.

Suppurative Infections

Brodie's Abscess

BACKGROUND

A Brodie's abscess, or "cystic osteomyelitis," is a distinct presentation of subacute or chronic osteomyelitis. It is believed to result from lack or inadequate treatment of osteomyelitis.[47,10] The infection is named after Sir Benjamin Brodie, who in 1832 described localized lesions of tibial metaphyses of children and young adults.[47] *Staphylococcus* organisms are the most common cause of infection.[7] Most affected patients are younger than 25 years of age, and males are slightly more likely than females to become infected.[37]

IMAGING FINDINGS

Imaging studies reveal a Brodie's abscess to be an area of radiolucency surrounded by a varying degrees of bone reaction, or surrounding sclerosis (Fig. 14-9). The surrounding sclerosis is usually well-defined on the inside and less well-defined outside. The lesion is usually slightly eccentric, is metadiaphyseal, varies in size, and is located in intramedullary bone, but it also affects the cortex (Fig. 14-10).[47,49] The femur and tibia are the bones that are most commonly involved.[49]

MRI of a Brodie's abscess reveals well-demarcated lesions with low signal intensity on T1-weighted sequences that brighten on T2-weighted sequences. The sclerotic edge of a Brodie's abscess has a low signal on both T1- and T2-weighted images. Bone marrow edema surrounding the lesion exhibits a poorly defined high signal band on T2-weighted images. The bright/dark/bright appearance on T2-weighted images is known as the *double line sign,* a sign also found in patients with avascular hip necrosis.[15,47] CT reveals a region of trabecular destruction of low attenuation surrounded by bone sclerosis.

CLINICAL COMMENTS

Patients with a Brodie's abscess may have no fever or leukocytosis and often have no signs or symptoms whatsoever.[33] One of the symptoms patients may have is an affected limb that is warm to the touch and tender when palpated.[33] Pain is the most common complaint associated with a Brodie's abscess. The pain is often persistent, but it may increase and decrease in severity and often worsens at night. Aspirin may dramatically relieve the pain, making it more difficult to differentiate an osteoid osteoma from a Brodie's abscess based solely on clinical symptoms. Although it is not a characteristic that can be used to definitively distinguish the two, the radiolucent nidus and surrounding sclerosis of a Brodie's abscess are more pronounced than those of an osteoid osteoma. Angiography can be used to confidently distinguish a Brodie's abscess from an osteoid osteoma. Osteoid osteomas demonstrate an opaque vascular blush that is not associated with a Brodie's abscess.

Progressive, nocturnal pains that may waken patients are classic features of a Brodie's abscess.[34] Biopsy and examination of fluid from an abscess may help in its diagnosis, but if the sample is purulent or mucoid, it may be impossible to detect the infective organism.[33] Classic treatment for a Brodie's lesion involves aseptic drainage, curettage, and administration of systemic antibiotics. Three consecutive negative cultures are a sign of resolution.[33]

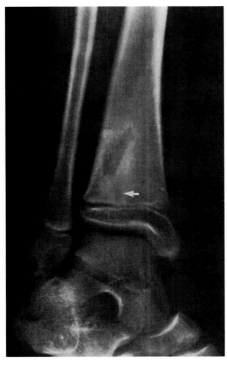

FIG. 14-9 Brodie's abscess. An example of a walled-off or aborted form of suppurative osteomyelitis *(arrow).* (From Blickman JG: *Pediatric radiology: the requisites,* St Louis, 1994, Mosby.)

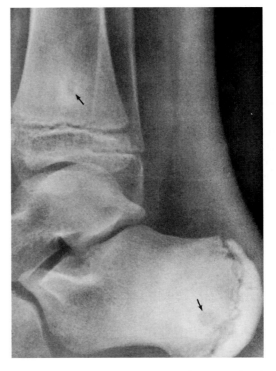

FIG. 14-10 Brodie's abscess in the distal tibia *(upper arrow)* and calcaneus *(lower arrow).* (From Silverman FN, Kuhn JP: *Caffey's pediatric x-ray diagnosis: an integrated imaging approach,* ed 9, 1993, Mosby.)

KEY CONCEPTS

- *A Brodie's abscess is caused by subacute or chronic osteomyelitis that has resulted from lack of or inadequate treatment for preexisting osteomyelitis.*
- *Plain film radiographic evidence of a Brodie's abscess consists of a geographic region of osteopenia surrounded by a rim of sclerosis, with lesions that are typically slightly eccentric, metadiaphyseal, and varied in size.*
- *The femur and tibia are most commonly involved.*
- *The most common chief complaint is persistent pain with periods of exacerbation and remission.*
- *Patients often describe the pain as being worse at night; it may be dramatically alleviated by aspirin (as can the pain caused by osteoid osteomas).*
- *In some cases the patient may have no fever, evidence of leukocytosis, or any other symptoms.*
- *The classic treatment for a Brodie's abscess is aseptic drainage, curettage, and administration of systemic antibiotics.*

Septic Arthritis

BACKGROUND

Septic arthritis is an articular manifestation of an infection. A joint may become infected as a result of hematogenous dissemination or contiguous spread (e.g., from epiphyseal osteomyelitis) or directly through surgery or trauma. Hematogenous dissemination is the most common means by which the infection spreads. Septic arthritis causes joint damage and disability, with the knee, hip, shoulder, and wrist being common sites. Usually only one joint is involved.

Septic arthritis tends to affect young children and elderly individuals. Although *Staphylococcus aureus* is the most common causative agent, certain populations are predisposed to becoming infected by a particular microbe. For instance, individuals who abuse drugs intravenously are predisposed to *Pseudomonas aeruginosa* infections of the axial skeleton joints.[8] Salmonellae commonly cause septic arthritis in patients with sickle cell disease. However, *S. aureus* is still the most common causative agent in this population overall. Although uncommon, infections in prosthetic joints are devastating, leading to loosening, failure, and advanced derangement of the joints.

IMAGING FINDINGS

Early radiographic findings of patients with joint infection include distention of the joint capsule, soft tissue swelling, and osteopenia. Intermediate and late changes are marked by the less distinct cortical bone, permeative or moth-eaten bone destruction, loss of joint space, joint derangement, and bony ankylosis. Hip involvement may distend the lateral (gluteus medius), superomedial (obturator internus), or inferomedial (iliopsoas) muscle-fat interfaces. Waldenström's sign may be seen. Waldenström's sign is defined as lateral displacement of the femoral head from the medial wall of the acetabulum (also known as the *teardrop distance*) by more than 11 mm (or more than 2 mm from the contralateral side) secondary to hip effusion. This finding does not specifically indicate the presence of infection and may be seen in association with other causes of hip effusion (e.g., trauma).[25]

CLINICAL COMMENTS

Joint infections typically cause pain and tenderness, loss of function, and possibly a fever. A high degree of clinical suspicion and proper radiographic evaluation usually lead to the appropriate diagnosis. Administration of antibiotics is the first component of therapy, with surgical debridement, joint replacement, or amputation

indicated for advanced or unresponsive disease. Antibiotic selection is based on the patient's age and history and results of a culture. The duration and modification of the antibiotic therapy is based on the patient's response. The duration of the symptoms, age of the patient, and degree of immunocompetence are all important factors that are used to predict the patient's outcome.

KEY CONCEPTS

- *Septic arthritis is a joint infection that transmitted directly through surgery or trauma, through contiguous spread, or most commonly through hematogenous dissemination.*
- *The knee, hip, shoulder, and wrist are the most commonly affected sites.*
- *Young children and elderly individuals are most commonly affected.*
- *Staphylococcus aureus is the most common infecting organism.*
- *Radiographic findings include joint space alterations, bone destruction, and in later stages, ankylosis.*
- *Conservative management entails antibiotic therapy. In rare cases, amputation may be required.*

Suppurative Osteomyelitis

BACKGROUND

Osteomyelitis is an infection of bone and bone marrow. Although it is usually caused by bacteria, it can also be caused by fungi and other microbes.[15] Osteomyelitis is categorized as either suppurative (pyogenic, or pus producing) or nonsuppurative (nonpyogenic, or non–pus producing). Suppurative osteomyelitis is further classified as either acute, subacute, or chronic based on its clinical progression.

Region of involvement. Normal bone is generally extremely resistant to infection, which usually develops when a large population of microbes is introduced by trauma or surgery.[29] Although any bone can develop an infection (Fig. 14-11),[50] the bones of the knee (Fig. 14-12), hip, and shoulder (Fig. 14-13) are more commonly affected.[50] Osteomyelitis tends to affect long bones, particularly those in the lower extremities.[45] In children, hematogenous osteomyelitis is usually located in the metaphyseal region of long bones (Fig. 14-14), with the most commonly affected bones being the femur and tibia.[6] The epiphysis is more commonly involved in neonates and adults than in children. From the first year of life until skeletal maturity, the physis acts as a barrier to circulatory vessels and therefore limits epiphyseal infections (Fig. 14-15). Infections of the epiphysis increase the likelihood of developing a septic joint.[15]

Suppurative osteomyelitis involves flat bones in about 30% of cases. Infective spondylitis, a combined infection of the vertebrae and intervertebral disc space, is a rare condition that affects older individuals.[16] The average age of a patient with suppurative osteomyelitis of the spine is 61.5 years.[7] Vertebral osteomyelitis may lead to conditions such as cauda equina syndrome that involve neurological compression secondary to a fracture or large infective mass that compresses the neuroanatomical structures.[16,36] Like the symphysis pubis and sacroiliac joints, the apophysis, articular cartilage, and fibrocartilage are all potential targets.[6] Although only one site is typically infected, multiple sites can become infected, especially in neonates.[6,19]

In adults the location of the infection depends on the mechanism by which the infection is established and the presence of an underlying disorder. For instance, diabetes mellitus is more commonly associated with osteomyelitis in lower extremities, whereas patients with spinal cord injuries may develop decubitus ulcers and subsequent pelvic osteomyelitis. Batson's plexus, the valveless venous network in the spine, provides an entryway for spinal infections

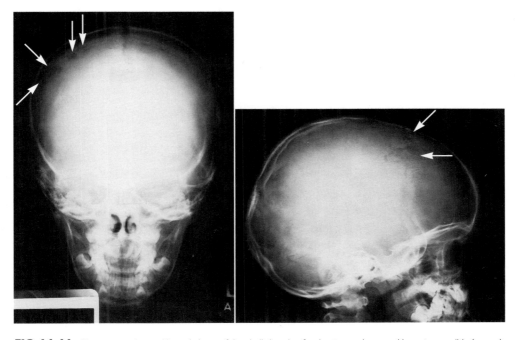

FIG. 14-11 Posteroanterior and lateral views of the skull showing focal osteopenia caused by osteomyelitis *(arrows)*.

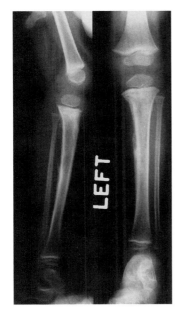

FIG. 14-12 Anteroposterior and lateral views of the lower leg demonstrating cortical and medullary destruction associated with periosteal reaction.

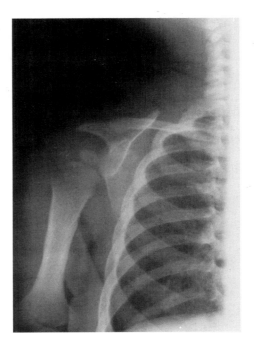

FIG. 14-13 Anteroposterior view of a shoulder with osteomyelitis involving the metaphysis of the proximal humerus.

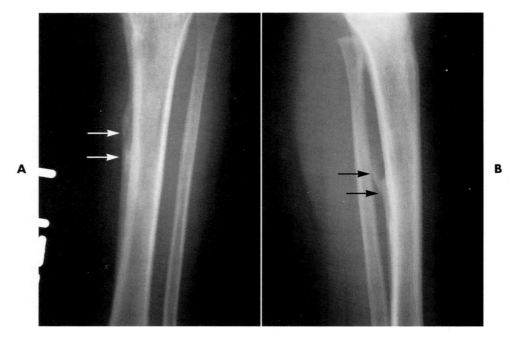

FIG. 14-14   Frontal **(A)** and lateral **(B)** leg projections demonstrating hematogenous osteomyelitis with early osseous destruction and prominent periosteal lifting caused by periostitis *(arrows).*

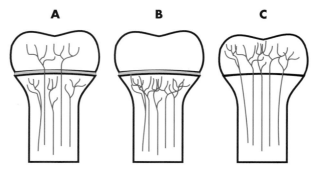

FIG. 14-15   Age-related vascular supply patterns. **A,** Before the age of 1 year a few vessels extend from the metaphysis to the epiphysis. **B,** During childhood and adolescence, the growth plate isolates the epiphysis from metaphyseal blood vessels. **C,** Skeletal maturity leads to closure of the growth plate, allowing revascularization of the epiphysis by metaphyseal vessels. Because of the blood vessel patterns, hematogenous extensions of infections develop less often in the epiphysis while the physis is open. (Modified from Resnick D: *Diagnosis of bone and joint disorders,* ed 3, Philadelphia, 1995, WB Saunders.)

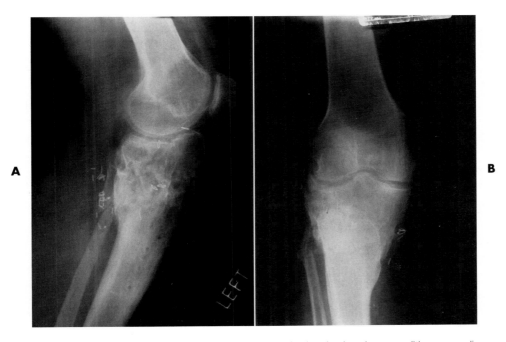

FIG. 14-16 Frontal **(A)** and lateral **(B)** views of a knee that has developed osteomyelitis as a complication of surgery.

secondary to urinary tract infections, intravenous drug abuse, abscesses, and bacterial endocarditis.[15]

Causative agents. The organisms that cause osteomyelitis vary according to age and health status. *S. aureus* is the most common cause of osteomyelitis among all individuals.[6,14,16,35] Some strains of *S. aureus* have an excellent ability to lodge in bone marrow, which may explain why this bacteria is frequently identified as the infectious agent in patients with osteomyelitis.[35] Other causes include *M. tuberculosis,* various fungi, and pneumococcal disease secondary to chronic respiratory infection.[15] Neonates usually develop *S. aureus* and streptococci infections,[6] whereas *S. aureus* is usually the source of infection in the elderly. Fungal osteomyelitis may develop as a complication of a fungal infection caused by catheterization, drug abuse, or prolonged neutropenia.

The presence of underlying conditions or diseases and external factors also influence the type of organism that causes osteomyelitis. Examples include the following:

- *P. aeruginosa* has been isolated from patients who develop osteomyelitis from dwelling catheters.
- *Bartonella henselae* has been associated with infection in patients with HIV.
- Aspergilli, mycobacteria, or *Candida albicans* can infect immunocompromised patients.[21]
- *P. aeruginosa, Klebsiella pneumoniae,* and *C. albicans* commonly infect individuals who are abusing drugs.
- Gram-negative microorganisms are usually the cause of nosocomial osteomyelitis.
- Urogenital surgery is associated with *Escherichia coli* infections.
- Patients with diabetes mellitus or a history of long-term antibiotic therapy may develop *C. albicans* infections; premature infants may also develop *C. albicans* osteomyelitis.

Dissemination. Osteomyelitis is spread by three major routes: (1) hematoge-nous, (2) direct (i.e., implantation by trauma or surgery) (Fig. 14-16), and (3) contiguous.[15,54] Infections of joints or long bones are usually a result of hematogenous spread, with the common primary sources including urinary tract infections, pneumonia, and skin abscesses.[50] Hematogenous osteomyelitis introduces viable organisms into the medullary portion of the bone. If the infected medullary cavity lies within a joint capsule, septic arthritis is more likely to develop, a phenomena that occurs in the hips and shoulders. In adults, it is less common for hematogenous osteomyelitis to develop in the tubular bones; it commonly spreads to the spine and pelvis—as compared with the pattern of dissemination in children, which is usually in the metaphysis of long bones.

The two most common types of trauma that produce osteomyelitis are open fractures and surgical bone reconstruction (Fig. 14-17). In addition, infections associated with prosthetic implantation are common, and staphylococcal organisms cause 75% of these infections.[29]

Risk factors. Individuals who have had urinary tract infections are predisposed to developing osteomyelitis. Approximately 40% of infective spondylitis cases are secondary to urinary tract infections. The lumbar spine is commonly involved and considered to be the result of spread through Batson's venous plexus. Neurological abnormalities and paraplegia are also risk factors for osteomyelitis, as are sickle cell anemia and diabetes mellitus. Patients with a compromised immune system caused by conditions such as lymphoma or a connective tissue disease or who have overused broad-spectrum antibiotics may develop osteomyelitis from atypical organisms.[6,50] Patients who are elderly, are alcoholics, have active rheumatoid arthritis, or have recently received a prosthetic joint all have higher rates of osteomyelitis.[50] Drug addiction is also

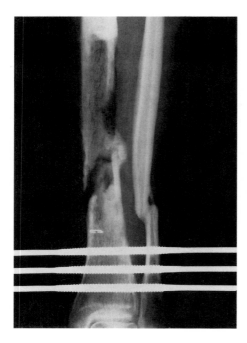

FIG. 14-17   Posttraumatic osteomyelitis. In this case, it is unclear whether the bone infection was caused by the surgery or the compound fracture. (Courtesy Gary M. Guebert, Maryland Heights, Mo.)

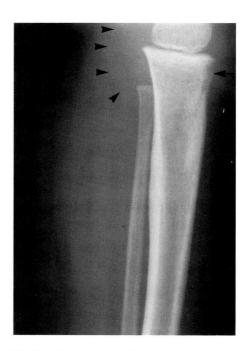

FIG. 14-18   Plain film radiography often does not detect early stages of osteomyelitis. Retrospectively, capsular swelling *(arrowheads)* and localized osteopenia *(arrow)* were noted.

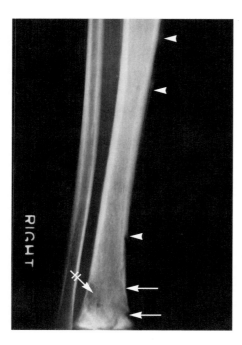

FIG. 14-19   Anteroposterior view of osteomyelitis of the tibia. Note the periosteal reaction *(arrowheads)* and cortical *(arrows)* and medullary *(crossed arrow)* osseous destruction.

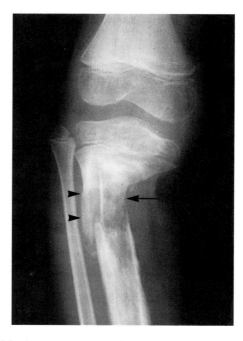

FIG. 14-20   Anteroposterior view of the knee showing residual dead bone, or sequestra *(arrow)*, and the florid periosteal response, or involucrum *(arrowheads)*. A sample was taken, and the culture that was performed revealed the presence of *P. aeruginosa.* (Courtesy Gary M. Guebert, Maryland Heights, Mo.)

highly associated with spondylitis, and individuals who use the drugs intravenously seem to develop *P. aeruginosa* infections more often than individuals of other subpopulations. Pseudomonads tend to affect the S joints, which include the spine, sacroiliac, symphysis pubis, and sternoclavicular joints.[45,50]

Garré's chronic sclerosing osteomyelitis. In 1893 a Swiss surgeon named Garré described the sclerosing type of osteomyelitis found in young adults that is now known as *Garré's osteomyelitis.*[23] This form of osteomyelitis is characterized by an insidious onset of pain and marked sclerotic lesions on radiographic images. The absence of central radiolucent nidus helps distinguish it from osteoid osteoma or a Brodie's abscess. The shafts of the femur and tibia are commonly affected.

IMAGING FINDINGS

Plain film radiography. Plain film radiography (Fig. 14-18) may not detect the early stages of bone infection, the features of which often do not appear for several weeks or even months after implantation[6]; repeat examinations are usually required.[29] One of the earliest signs of osteomyelitis is deep soft tissue swelling. Three to ten days after infection, distortion or obliteration of fat planes and subcutaneous edema may be evident.[6,15] Focal osteopenia within the medullary cavity typically occurs first, followed by cortical destruction in a focal or multifocal presentation.

During the middle stage of osteomyelitis, a cortical breach develops and leads to periostitis approximately 3 to 6 weeks after infection (Fig. 14-19). As suppurative osteomyelitis develops, pus moves into the vascular channels, raising the intramedullary pressure and impairing blood flow.[6,29] Ischemic necrosis hastens the damage and results in pockets of dead bone called *sequestra* (Fig. 14-20).[29]

In the late stages of osteomyelitis the remaining sequestra may be surrounded by a florid periosteal reaction called an *involucrum* (see Fig. 14-20); an opening in the involucrum is called a *cloaca.* The sequestra and involucrum appear no earlier than 3 weeks after infection.[6] Communication with the skin surface occurs through sinus tracts, and pus and bony debris may migrate to the surface. A rare complication of osteomyelitis is a Marjolin's ulcer, which develops as the tissue associated with the cloaca and sinus tract degenerate into a squamous cell carcinoma. The latent period may be as long as 20 to 30 years.[6]

Chronic osteomyelitis can be used to describe osteomyelitis in a patient who has had the disease for many years or chronic osteomyelitis that is revealed for the first time. The disease typically presents as bony sclerosis. Viable organisms capable of producing infection can survive in necrotic abscesses or fragments of necrotic bone for months or years.[47] Continuous bouts with mild infections are typical.

Infections have the ability to cross joint spaces, whereas other aggressive bone diseases such as bone tumors typically do not exhibit this ability.[6] Spinal infections usually involve the intervertebral disc. The vertebral body is more commonly affected and may develop endplate erosion.[11] In cases of spondylitis, the facet joints are rarely involved. Although the discs of some young children heal after the infection, residual deformities are typical in the elderly.

The radiographic differentiation of pyogenic infection from a tuberculosis infection or a tumor may not be possible.[6] Unlike tuberculosis, pyogenic spinal infections demonstrate less paravertebral soft tissue involvement.[7] The paravertebral involvement is seen as a cuff around the involved vertebrae and discs.[7] Plain film radiography has a high incidence of false negative examinations (Fig. 14-21). Bone scanning and CT have improved sensitivity rates, but delays in diagnosis remain a problem.

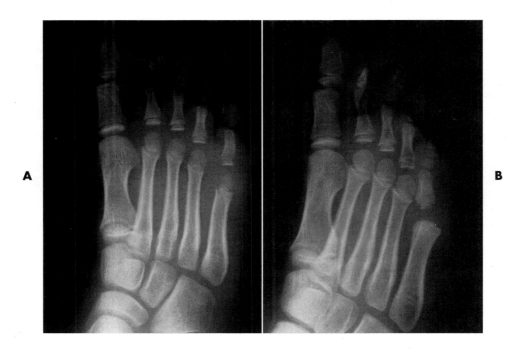

FIG. 14-21 **A,** Anteroposterior projection of a foot with no visible abnormalities. **B,** Two months later, destructive bone changes and periostitis secondary to infection of the fifth metatarsophalangeal joint can be seen.

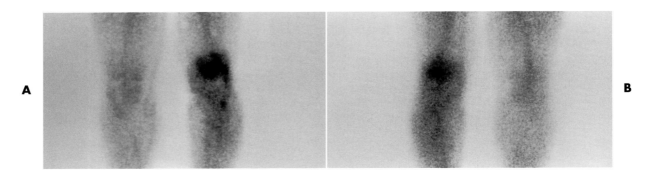

FIG. 14-22 Anterior **(A)** and posterior **(B)** bone scans demonstrating evidence of increased bony uptake in a patient with osteomyelitis.

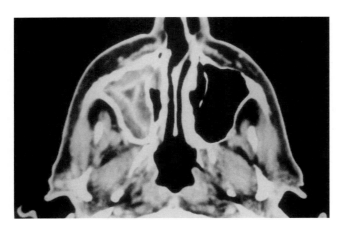

FIG. 14-23 Axial CT scan showing an obstructed right maxillary sinus. In the center of the sinus is a triangular area of dense mucus composed of trapped sinus secretions. The inflamed sinus mucosa surrounds this region and is seen on the scan as a thin, uniform enhancement. Between the mucosa and bony sinus wall is a zone of submucosal edema. (From Som PM, Curtin HD: *Head and neck imaging*, ed 3, St Louis, 1996, Mosby.)

Specialized imaging. Specialized imaging provides a more sensitive evaluation of a clinically suspected infection than is possible with plain film radiography. Whereas plain films of the early stages of infection may be essentially normal, bone scanning and MRI detect abnormalities.[45] Detection with plain film radiographs may lag 10 to 14 days behind the onset of clinical symptoms,[15] whereas bone scans typically detect abnormalities within 24 hours of clinical onset. The classic positive sign of osteomyelitis from a three-phase bone scan is increased blood flow during the angiogram phase, focal hyperemia in the blood pool phase, and increased bony uptake in the bone activity phase. Bone scintigraphy is useful during the early stages of infection, but clinical correlation is essential (Fig. 14-22).[6,12] Some authors have suggested that in cases of suspected osteomyelitis, a bone scan is not cost effective. Seldom are surgeons satisfied with the ability of bone scans to define an image, therefore MRI and/or CT are needed to define the lesions' dimensions and features.[22]

CT is useful in assessing the extent of damage and detecting soft tissue extensions (Fig. 14-23).[6] CT and MRI provide excellent resolution and can provide information regarding medullary and cortical destruction, articular damage, and periosteal and soft tissue in-

volvement.[29] MRI may detect osteomyelitis before a bone scan because of its superior ability to monitor bone marrow changes.[29]

The typical MRI findings associated with osteomyelitis during standard T1- and T2-weighted images are a low signal intensity on T1-weighted images and an abnormally bright signal on T2-weighted images (Fig. 14-24).[29,33] With regard to osteomyelitis, MRI sensitivity is 88% and specificity is 93%, whereas bone scan sensitivity is 61% and specificity is 33%.[22] MRI may also detect articular involvement and the presence of sinus tracts (cloaca) during the early stages.[15] Evidence of epidural infection extension may be best seen using gadolinium-enhanced imaging.[7] MRI shows intervertebral disc involvement as a decreased signal on T1-weighted images and an increased signal on T2-weighted images, characteristics similar to other findings related to osteomyelitis.[15,24] However, a decreased signal from an intervertebral disc on a T2-weighted image does not rule out osteomyelitis.[14]

Other MRI findings include joint effusion, thickened synovium, and ill-defined margins of the lesion.[15] The synovium is typically enhanced with gadolinium infusion.[15] Articular cartilage destruction may be also seen on MRI images.[15] Acutely evolving neuropathic arthropathy has a presentation that is similar to osteomyelitis. Chronic neuropathic arthropathy is easily distinguished from osteomyelitis by a decreased signal intensity that is not affected by pulse sequencing.[33]

Performing a proper work-up of patients with suspected osteomyelitis requires cooperation between the clinician and radiologist.[6] In equivocal cases or cases in which abscess formation is suspected, radionuclide imaging using white blood cells tagged with gallium 67 is useful to investigate the presence of osteomyelitis.[6,15] In patients with diabetes, scans using leukocytes labeled with indium In 111 have shown great sensitivity and specificity.[15,54] Some large studies have suggested that an ^{111}In scan is superior to a three-phase technetium 99m scanning.[54] However, MRI is usually less costly than the combined cost of a bone scan and an ^{111}In or a ^{67}Ga scan.[15]

CLINICAL COMMENTS

Signs and symptoms of osteomyelitis are often vague and may be present for a long time. Subacute presentations are becoming more common, possibly because of the increased use of antibiotics. In particular, patients with pyogenic spinal infections often experience a long delay in receiving their diagnosis.[11] The symptoms are not specific, and the disease is often not considered when the infection is in its early stages.[11] A delay in diagnosis may cause excessive and extensive tissue destruction and abscess formation.[11,50]

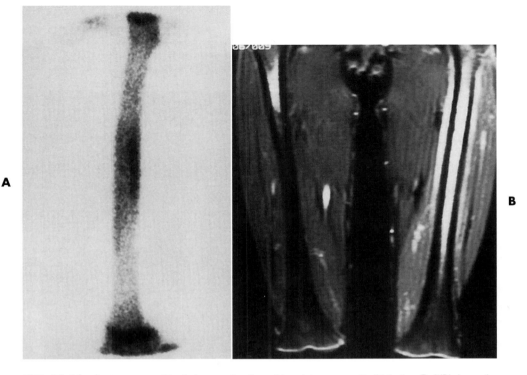

FIG. 14-24 Acute osteomyelitis. **A,** Increased radionuclide uptake as a result of infection. **B,** MRI shows the marrow and soft tissue involvement and more accurately detects the multiple sites of infection. (From Blickman JG: *Pediatric radiology: the requisites,* St Louis 1994, Mosby.)

The most common complaint from patients with vertebral osteomyelitis is back pain that has been increasing in severity for several days. Laboratory data such as WBCs and ESR elevations may indicate the presence of an inflammation, but these findings are variable and nonspecific.[11,49] Most studies report an average delay in diagnosis of 2 to 6 months after the onset of symptoms.[11] The nonspecific nature of laboratory and radiographic findings and the ubiquitous nature of back pain make diagnosis a challenge.[11]

The classic clinical features of hematogenous suppurative osteomyelitis are chills, fever, malaise, local pain, and swelling. Loss of function or decreased range of motion in the affected region often develops.[29] Skin lesions are clear evidence of septicemia and vasculitis.[50] Possible osteomyelitis should be viewed as a medical emergency and be addressed immediately.[50]

The major objective of a work-up for a bone or joint infection is identification of the infectious organism,[50] which is essential for proper treatment.[29] Surgical sampling or a needle biopsy provides indispensable information.[29] Information provided by swabs from ulcers or fistulae may be misleading. Assessment of stained histopathological bone biopsy samples is the most reliable way to accurately identify the infectious agent.[29]

Attempting to diagnose osteomyelitis in a patient with a diabetic foot is very difficult both from a clinical and an imaging point of view (Fig. 14-25). A concomitant neuropathic osteoarthropathy may be present and could produce a delay in diagnosis. Neuropathic joint destruction may simulate infection, and to further complicate the presentation, osteomyelitis can coexist with the neuropathy. The infection often starts as an ulcer in the dermal layer that later burrows into the underlying bone.[29,33,50] Osteomyelitis caused by vas-

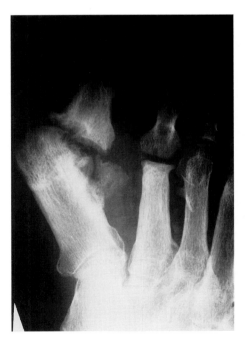

FIG. 14-25 Advanced arthropathy associated with diabetic osteomyelitis of the foot.

cular insufficiency or diabetes is found exclusively in the feet.[29] A physical examination may reveal that patients with neuropathy have little or no pain whereas patients whose pain sense is intact and have rapid osseous destruction may experience excruciating pain. MRI may provide early information, and a bone biopsy is confirmatory of disease.[29] Fifteen percent of diabetic patients develop osteomyelitis as a result of a combination of vascular insufficiency and peripheral neuropathy.[33] Early diagnosis of osteomyelitis in patients with diabetes may help prevent the need for amputation.[33] More limb-saving procedures are currently being used in an effort to improve patients' quality of life.[15]

KEY CONCEPTS

- *Osteomyelitis is an infection of bone and bone marrow that is usually caused by bacteria but can also be caused by fungi and other microbes. Staphylococcus aureus is the most common cause.*
- *Populations at risk for osteomyelitis include infants and young children, the elderly, and those who have diabetes or are immunocompromised.*
- *Radiographic findings include disruption of the surrounding fat planes and intramedullary bone and eventually endosteal scalloping, cortical destruction, and periosteal reactions.*
- *Sequestra are pockets of dead bone; an involucrum is the result of a florid periosteal response and surrounds the infective mass.*
- *The cloaca is a channel through the involucrum that may connect to a sinus and allow migration of pus and bloody bone debris onto the skin surface.*
- *The bone and joint structures of some young children heal after infection, whereas older patients usually have residual deformities.*
- *There is often a delay of 3 to 6 weeks between implantation and expression of signs and symptoms.*
- *A rare complication of osteomyelitis that can develop in later stages is a Marjolin's ulcer—cloaca and sinus tract tissue that has developed into a squamous cell carcinoma; the latent period for carcinoma development may be as long as 20 to 30 years.*
- *Classic clinical features of suppurative osteomyelitis are chills, fever, malaise, local pain and swelling, and loss of function or decreased range of motion in the affected region.*

References

1. Albert MC, Zachary SV, Alter S: Blastomycosis of the forearm synovium in a child, *Clin Orthop* 317:223, 1995.
2. Antunes JL: Infections of the spine, *Acta Neurochir* 116:179, 1992.
3. Banner AS: Tuberculosis. Clinical aspects and diagnosis, *Arch Intern Med* 139:1387, 1979.
4. Batra P, Batra RS: Thoracic coccidioidomycosis, *Semin Roentgenol* 31:28, 1996.
5. Bharucha NE et al: All that caseates is not tuberculosis, *Lancet* 348:1313, 1996.
6. Bonakdar-Pour A, Gaines VD: The radiology of osteomyelitis, *Orthop Clin North Am* 14:21, 1983.
7. Brailsford JF: Brodie's abscess and its differential diagnosis, *Br Med J* 120:119, 1938.
8. Brankos MA et al: Septic arthritis in heroin addicts, *Semin Arthritis Rheum* 21:81, 1991.
9. Brion LP et al: Long-bone radiographic abnormalities as a sign of active congenital syphilis in asymptomatic newborns, *Pediatrics* 88:1037, 1991.
10. Brodie BC: An account of some cases of chronic abscess of the tivia, *Trans Med Chiro Soc* 17:239, 1832.
11. Carragee EJ: The clinical use of magnetic resonance imaging in pyogenic vertebral osteomyelitis, *Spine* 22:780, 1997.
12. Ching BY, Maraczi G, Urbina D: Madura foot. A case presentation, *J Am Podiatr Med Assoc* 81:443, 1991.
13. Cuellar ML et al: Other fungal arthritides, *Rheum Dis Clin North Am* 19:439, 1993.
14. Dagirmanjian A et al: MR imaging of vertebral osteomyelitis revisited, *AJR* 167:1539, 1996.
15. Deely DM, Scheitzer ME: MR imaging of bone marrow disorders, *Radiol Clin North Am* 35:193, 1997.
16. Faraj A, Krishna M, Mehdian SMH: Cauda equina syndrome secondary to lumbar spondylodiscitis caused by *Streptococcus milleri, Eur Spine J* 5:134, 1996.
17. Foster MR, Friedenberg ZB, Passero F: Lumbar *Petriellidium boydii* osteomyelitis with a systemic presentation, *J Spinal Disord* 7:356, 1994.
18. Giacola GP, Wood BP: Radiological case of the month. Congenital syphilis, *Am J Dis Child* 145:1045, 1991.
19. Gold R: Diagnosis of osteomyelitis, *Pediatr Rev* 12:292, 1991.
20. Greenberg SB, Bernal DV: Are long bone radiographs necessary in neonates suspected of having congenital syphilis?, *Radiology* 182:637, 1992.
21. Gropper GR, Acker JD, Robertson JH. Computed tomography in Pott's disease, *Neurosurgery* 10:506, 1982
22. Haygood TM: Magnetic resonance imaging of the musculoskeletal system: part 7, the ankle, *Clin Orthop* 336:318, 1997.
23. Jacobsson S, Heyden G: Chronic sclerosing osteomyelitis of the mandible, Histologic and histochemical findings, *Oral Surg Oral Med Oral Pathol* 43:357, 1977.
24. Johnston JO, Genant HK, Rosenam W: Ankle pain and swelling in a 30-year-old man, *Clin Orthop* 314:281, 1995.
25. Keats TE: Atlas of roentgenographic measurement, ed 6, St Louis, 1990, Mosby.
26. Kushwaha VP et al: Musculoskeletal coccidioidomycosis. A review of 25 cases, *Clin Orthop* 332:190, 1996.
27. Leff A, Geppert EF: Public health and preventive aspects of pulmonary tuberculosis. Infectiousness, epidemiology, risk factors, classification, and preventive therapy, *Arch Intern Med* 139:1405, 1979.
28. Lester TW: Drug-resistant and atypical mycobacterial disease. Bacteriology and treatment, *Arch Intern Med* 139:1399, 1979.
29. Lew DP, Waldvogel FA: Osteomyelitis, *N Engl J Med* 336:999, 1997.
30. Lewall DB, Ofole S, Bendl B: Mycetoma, *Skeletal Radiol* 14:257, 1985.
31. Lin-Greenberg A, Cholankeni J: Vertebral arch destruction in tuberculosis: CT feature, *J Comput Assist Tomogr* 14:300, 1990.
32. MacDonald PB, Black GB, MacKenzie R: Orthopaedic manifestations of blastomycosis, *J Bone Joint Surg Am* 72:860, 1990.
33. Marcus CD et al: MR imaging of osteomyelitis and neuropathic osteoarthropathy in the feet of diabetics, *Radiographics* 16:1337, 1996.
34. Mascola L et al: Congenital syphilis revisited, *Am J Dis Child* 139:575, 1985.
35. Matsushita K et al: Experimental hematogenous osteomyelitis by *Staphylococcus aureus, Clin Orthop* 334:291, 1997.
36. McHenry MC et al: Vertebral osteomyelitis presenting as spinal compression fracture, *Arch Intern Med* 148:417, 1988.
37. Miller WB, Murphy WA, Gilula LA: Brodie abscess. Reappraisal, *Radiology* 132:15, 1979.
38. Mirels LF, Stevens DA: Update on treatment of coccidioidomycosis, *West J Med* 166:58, 1997.
39. Mosley D et al: From the Centers for Disease Control and Prevention. Coccidioidomycosis—Arizona, 1990-1995, *JAMA* 277:104, 1997.
40. Proctor ME, Davis JP: Blastomycosis—Wisconsin, 1986-1995, *MMWR* 45:601, 1996.
41. Rasool MN, Goender S: The skeletal manifestations of congenital syphilis. A review of 197 cases, *J Bone Joint Surg Br* 71:752, 1989.
42. Resnick D: *Diagnosis of bone and joint disorders,* ed 3, Philadelphia, 1995, WB Saunders.

43. Resnik BI, Burdick AE: Improvement of eumycetoma with itraconazole, *J Am Acad Dermatol* 33:917, 1995.
44. Restrepo A: Treatment of tropical mycoses, *J Am Acad Dermatol* 31(suppl):91, 1994.
45. Richter RW: Infections other than AIDS, *Neurol Clin* 11:591, 1993.
46. Riegler HF, Goldstein LA, Bett RF: Blastomycosis osteomyelitis, *Clin Orthop* 100:225, 1974.
47. Rogoff RS Tinkle JD, Bortis DG: Unusual presentation of calcaneal osteomyelitis. Twenty-five years after inoculation, *J Am Podiatr Med Assoc* 87:125, 1997.
48. Rosenfeld SR, Weinert CR, Kahn B: Congenital syphilis. A case report, *J Bone Joint Surg Am* 65:115, 1983.
49. Ruppert D, Barron BJ, Madewell JE: Osteomyelitis, acute and chronic, Radiol Clin North Am 25:1171, 1987.
50. Schmid FR: Infectious arthritis and osteomyelitis, *Prim Care* 11:295, 1984.
51. Schneider E et al: A coccidioidomycosis outbreak following the Northridge, Calif, earthquake, *JAMA* 277:904, 1997.
52. Smith IE et al: Kyphosis secondary to tuberculosis osteomyelitis as a cause of ventilatory failure. Clinical features, mechanisms, and management, *Chest* 110:1105, 1996.
53. Stevens DA: Coccidioidomycosis, *N Engl J Med* 332:1077, 1995.
54. Sutter CW, Shelton DK: Three-phase bone scan in osteomyelitis and other musculoskeletal disorders, *Am Fam Physician* 54:1639, 1996.
55. Ushigome S et al: Case report 308. Diagnosis: disseminated syphilitic osteomyelitis (presumptively proved), *Skeletal Radiol* 13:239, 1985.
56. Waldrogel FA, Vasey H: Osteomyelitis: the past decade, *N Engl J Med* 303:360, 1980.
57. Winer-Muram HT, Vargus S, Slabod K: Cavitary lung lesions in an immunosuppressed child, *Chest* 106:937, 1994.
58. Wright T, Sundaram M, McDonald D: Radiologic case study. Tuberculosis osteomyelitis and arthritis, *Orthopedics* 19:699, 1996.
59. Zeppa MA: Skeletal coccidioidomycosis: imaging findings in 19 patients, *Skeletal Radiol* 25:337, 1996.
60. Zimmerman MR. Pulmonary and osseous tuberculosis in an Egyptian mummy. *Bull N Y Acad Med* 55:604, 1979.

chapter 15

Bone Neoplasms

DENNIS M MARCHIORI
DAVID J SARTORIS

Bone tumors are one of the most serious diagnostic possibilities in patients with musculoskeletal complaints. The evaluation of a bone lesion or soft tissue mass requires careful assessment of the patient's history and clinical studies to develop a concise list of different possibilities. Diagnostic imaging plays a major role in developing and narrowing this list.

Imaging

Plain film remains the chief imaging modality for the initial assessment of bone tumors. Sometimes the radiographic presentation reveals a lesion that is nonaggressive with classic characteristics, necessitating no further examination and leading to an immediate diagnosis. However, further assessment is necessary with poorly defined lesions or any benign-appearing lesion that is not consistent with the patient's clinical complaint.

By providing a view of thin axial slices of anatomy, computed tomography (CT) is particularly helpful in defining the spine and other regions of complex anatomy. Although they lack specificity, radionuclide bone scans are sensitive to the presence of early disease and are widely used to assess the possibility of multiple lesions. Magnetic resonance imaging (MRI) has the ability to demonstrate abnormality of the bone marrow and delineate extraosseous involvement. Replacement of normal marrow by pathological processes (e.g., metastasis, multiple myeloma, osteomyelitis) is readily demonstrated and provides an early sign of disease. However, MRI remains inferior to both plain film and CT for detailing calcification, ossification, cortical destruction, and periosteal reaction. Radiographic evidence provides information regarding the rate of growth and aggressiveness of a lesion but will not establish a histological diagnosis with the same accuracy as a biopsy.

When the radiographic appearance suggests the presence of an aggressive lesion, the practitioner should give immediate consideration to the possibility of a polyostotic disease process. It is important to determine if the process involves one or multiple bones; this helps to narrow the diagnostic list of possibilities. In most instances, the large field of view and sensitivity of radionuclide imaging make it the best means of identifying a pathology as polyostotic. However, radionuclide imaging is insensitive to some disease processes (e.g., multiple myeloma). In these cases, radiographic surveys or multiregional MRI studies are needed to assess the possibility of multiple lesions. Plain film radiographs and CT scans of the chest help to assess the possibility of pulmonary metastasis, the presence of which may alter the treatment plan. If needed, CT and MRI can be used to better define the extent or stage of the lesion. And lastly, biopsy is used typically to establish the histologic diagnosis and complement the imaging studies.

Laboratory Tests

In general, laboratory tests are less helpful in diagnosing tumors than imaging is. Benign bone tumors demonstrate normal values, and malignant tumors often demonstrate normal values. However, some characteristic laboratory findings may be noted with malignancy. Following advanced bone destruction, metastatic bone disease may exhibit increased serum calcium levels. Osteosarcoma, osteoblastic metastasis, and other bone-proliferating malignancies are often accompanied by increased serum alkaline phosphatase levels. Serum electrophoresis exhibits characteristic changes in cases of multiple myeloma.

Bone Biopsy

Bone biopsy is the removal of suspect tissue from the body for examination by a pathologist. In almost every circumstance, a biopsy provides the most accurate diagnosis possible, typically more accurate than can be obtained by imaging. Although a biopsy provides the most accurate method of assessing the histologic tissue of a lesion, a biopsy is less helpful in assessing its rate of growth and aggressiveness. The latter qualities are best assessed by conventional and specialized imaging modalities. Therefore, a biopsy and imaging studies are complementary, leading to an end diagnosis.

Tissue should be collected from the most aggressive and viable portion of the lesions. This often necessitates an open biopsy approach. However, open biopsy is associated with higher complication rates than is a percutaneous approach.[138] The accuracy of the results depends on such critical decisions as which region of the lesion should be collected, who performs the biopsy, and under which clinical circumstances a biopsy takes place.

Signs and Symptoms

Clinically important lesions are usually detected secondary to the patient's complaint of pain or palpable mass. Less frequently, asymptomatic bone lesions are detected on radiographs obtained for unrelated reasons.

TUMOR DISCRIMINATORS

Many tumors and tumorlike conditions produce similar radiographic changes. The following list of radiographic and clinical pa-

rameters assists in narrowing the broad number of pathological possibilities for a given radiographic appearance. In addition, the following parameters assist in evaluating the aggressiveness and clinical importance of a lesion.

Patient age. The age of the patient is an important clue to assist the examiner in differentiating between lesions that may look the same but are unique to certain age groups. Conversely, the patient's age may suggest a diagnostic possibility that would not otherwise be considered from the radiographic appearance because of an atypical presentation. Age is more helpful when the age range associated with the tumor is narrow. Given only the patient's age, an examiner can determine which tumor is present with a high degree of accuracy.[60] (Tables 15-1 and 15-2 present the ages at which common benign and malignant tumors, respectively, develop.)

Location. Individual tumors are often more prevalent in certain types of bones (Table 15-3). Probably even more important is the lesion's position within any single bone. Some tumors are associated with specific areas of the longitudinal areas of bones (diaphysis, metadiaphysis, metaphysis, and epiphysis) (Fig. 15-1) and transverse axes of bones (central or eccentric medullary, cortical, periosteal, and parosteal) (Fig. 15-2 and Table 15-4).

TABLE 15-1	
Typical Ages for the Development of Selected Benign Tumors	
Age (in years)	**Tumor**
5 to 20	Simple bone cyst
10 to 20	Chondroblastoma, nonossifying fibroma, osteoid osteoma
10 to 30	Aneurysmal bone cyst, chondromyxoid fibroma, osteoblastoma, osteochondroma
15 to 35	Enchondroma, osteoma
20 to 40	Giant cell tumor
30 to 50	Lipoma
40 to 50	Hemangioma

TABLE 15-2	
Typical Ages for the Development of Selected Malignant Tumors	
Age (in years)	**Tumor**
Less than 1	Metastatic neuroblastoma
1-30	Ewing's sarcoma, osteosarcoma
20-40	Giant cell tumor, parosteal osteosarcoma
30-50	Chordoma, chondrosarcoma, fibrosarcoma, malignant fibrous histiocytoma, primary lymphoma of bone
Greater than 40	Chondrosarcoma, metastatic disease, multiple myeloma

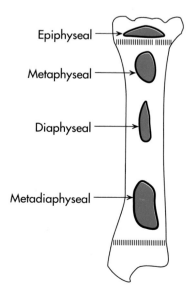

FIG. 15-1   Longitudinal location.

TABLE 15-3
Most Common Sites for the Development of Selected Tumors[43,165]

Tumor	Location
Bone	
Benign	
Bone island	Femur, innominate, rib
Osteoblastoma	Vertebra*, tibia, femur
Osteoma	Skull, facial bone, paranasal sinus
Osteoid osteoma	Femur, tibia, foot
Malignant	
Osteosarcoma	Femur, tibia, humerus
Cartilage	
Benign	
Chondroblastoma	Femur, humerus, tibia
Chondroma	Hand, wrist, humerus
Chondromyxoid fibroma	Tibia, femur, foot
Osteochondroma	Femur, humerus, tibia
Malignant	
Chondrosarcoma	Femur, innominate, humerus
Fibrous	
Benign	
Fibrous cortical defect, nonossifying fibroma	Femur, tibia, fibula
Malignant	
Fibrosarcoma	Femur, jaw, tibia
Malignant fibrous histiocytoma	Femur, tibia, humerus
Other	
Benign	
Aneurysmal bone cyst	Tibia, femur, vertebra*
Giant cell tumor	Femur, tibia, radius
Hemangioma	Skull, spine, ribs
Lipoma	Fibula, foot, femur
Simple bone cyst	Humerus, femur, tibia
Malignant	
Chordoma	Skull (clivus), vertebra* (sacrum and C2 body)
Ewing's sarcoma	Femur, innominate, tibia
Lymphoma of bone	Femur, innominate, vertebrae, humerus
Multiple myeloma/ plasmacytoma	Vertebra, rib, innominate, femur

*Including sacrum and coccyx.

TABLE 15-4
Location of Selected Tumors within a Bone

Location	Comment
Longitudinal	
Diaphysis	Round cell lesions (Ewing's sarcoma, primary lymphoma of bone, multiple myeloma), malignant fibrous histiocytoma, adamantinoma
Diametaphysis	Osteoblastoma, chondromyxoid fibroma, nonossifying fibroma, Ewing's sarcoma
Metaphysis	Aneurysmal bone cyst, chondrosarcoma, enchondroma, fibrosarcoma, giant cell tumor, osteosarcoma
Epiphysis	Chondroblastoma, giant cell tumor
Axial	
Central	Central chondrosarcoma, Ewing's sarcoma, fibrous dysplasia, primary lymphoma of bone, solitary bone cyst
Eccentric	Aneurysmal bone cyst, fibrosarcoma, giant cell tumor nonossifying fibroma
Cortical	Fibrous cortical defect
Parosteal	Parosteal chondrosarcoma, periosteal chondroma

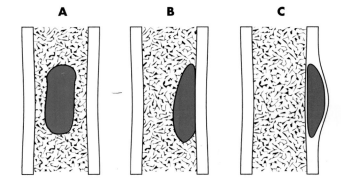

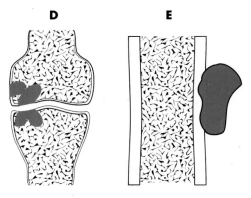

FIG. 15-2   Axial location. **A,** Central. **B,** Eccentric. **C,** Cortical. **D,** Intraarticular. **E,** Parosteal. (Modified from Juhl JH, Crummy AB: *Paul and Juhl's Essentials of radiologic imaging,* ed 6, Philadelphia, 1993, JB Lippincott.)

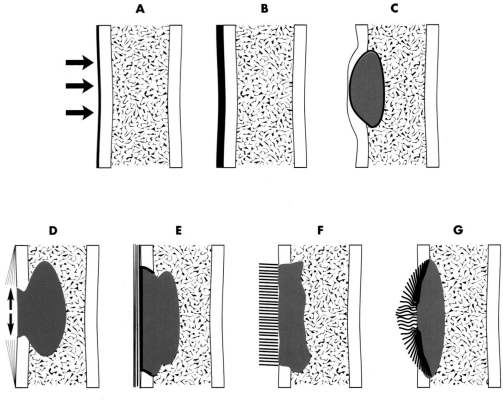

FIG. 15-3   Periosteal reaction. **A,** Thin lamellar. **B,** Thick lamellar. **C,** Cortical buttressing. **D,** Codman's angles (arrows). **E,** Aggressive lamellar. **F,** Hair-on-end spiculated. **G,** Sunburst. Patterns D through G are associated with aggressive lesions of bone. (Modified from Juhl JH, Crummy AB: Paul and Juhl's Essentials of radiologic imaging, ed 6, Philadelphia, 1993, JB Lippincott.)

TABLE 15-5
Radiographic Characteristics of Tumor Grades

Aggressiveness	Characteristics
Low grade— nonaggressive	Geographic destruction surrounded by sclerotic rim of bone
Medium grade— moderately aggressive	Geographic destruction, short transition zone, possible sclerotic rim, possible bone expansion, possible thick periosteal reaction
High grade— highly aggressive	Permeative or moth-eaten destruction, wide transition zone, no surrounding sclerosis, possible bone expansion, aggressive periosteal reaction

Soft tissue involvement. A soft tissue mass, created when the tumor mass breaks through the host bone's cortex, suggests an aggressive tumor. A soft tissue mass related to tumors distorts but does not disrupt intramuscular soft tissue planes as do soft tissue masses secondary to infections.

Host bone reaction. A number of pathological processes are capable of accentuating or reviving normal mechanisms of bone growth resulting in periosteal or endosteal reactions. The appearance of the periosteal and endosteal reactions relates to the aggressiveness, intensity, and duration of the inciting process.

Periosteal and endosteal reactions must mineralize to be visible on radiographs; several patterns are identified (Fig. 15-3). Mineralization takes between 1 and 3 weeks. If the inciting process is indolent (e.g., vascular stasis), a thick, wavy periosteal reaction develops. Layered or lamellar periosteal reactions indicate a mildly aggressive underlying pathology (e.g., acute osteomyelitis). Aggressive pathology (e.g., osteosarcoma) may disrupt the periosteum, producing a radiating (sunburst) or parallel (hair-on-end) spiculated pattern (Fig. 15-4, A). The disrupted periosteum may form an acute angle with the cortex of the bone (Codman's triangle) (Fig. 15-4, B). Endosteal reactions are more limited, appearing thickened or scalloped in response to pathology within the medullary canal. Radiological tumor grades based on the reaction of the host bone are presented in Table 15-5.

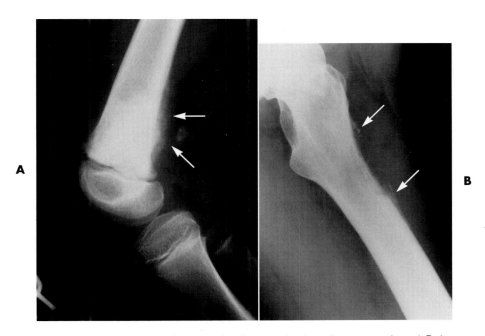

FIG. 15-4 **A,** Aggressive periosteal reaction demonstrating the sunburst pattern *(arrows).* **B,** Aggressive periostitis with Codman's triangles *(arrows)* secondary to lymphoma of the proximal femur. (Courtesy Joseph W. Howe, Sylmar, Calif.).

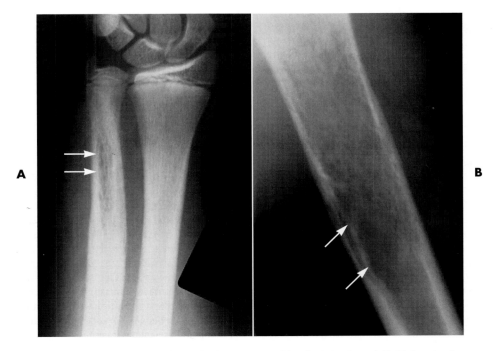

FIG. 15-5 **A,** Moth-eaten destructive bone pattern of the distal ulna *(arrows).* **B,** Moth-eaten *(arrows)* and more permeative pattern of bone destruction. (Courtesy Joseph W. Howe, Sylmar, Calif.).

Pattern of bone destruction. A number of explanations exist as to why tumors produce bone destruction. Tumors may stimulate osteoclastic activity by direct pressure, local hyperemia, or invasion. Bone destruction may be permeative, moth-eaten (Fig. 15-5), or geographical (Fig. 15-6). Geographical lesions are generally less aggressive than the more subtle moth-eaten destructive pattern, which is generally less aggressive than the nearly imperceptible permeative pattern.

An observer's ability to recognize bone destruction depends primarily on the size and location of the lesion. Destructive lesions in cortical bone are more easily recognized than those in cancellous bone because greater contrast exists between osteolytic lesions and

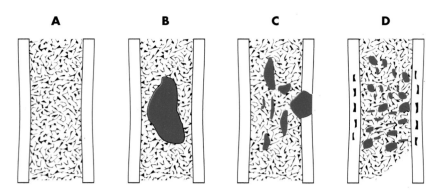

FIG. 15-6 Patterns of bone destruction. **A,** Normal bone. **B,** Geographic. **C,** Moth-eaten. **D,** Permeative. (Modified from Juhl JH, Crummy AB: *Paul and Juhl's Essentials of radiologic imaging,* ed 6, Philadelphia, 1993, JB Lippincott.)

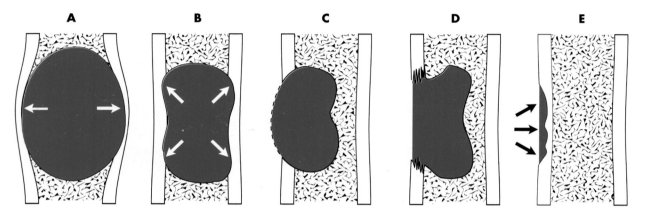

FIG. 15-7 Cortical bone reaction. **A,** Expansile. **B,** Endosteal scalloping. **C,** Thin, nearly imperceptible. **D,** Destructive. **E,** Saucerization. (Modified from Juhl JH, Crummy AB: *Paul and Juhl's Essentials of radiologic imaging,* ed 6, Philadelphia, 1993, JB Lippincott.)

compact bone than osteolytic lesions and cancellous bone (Fig. 15-7). Although technical factors need to be considered, in general, lesions in cancellous bone that are less than 1 cm in diameter are difficult to recognize. Moreover, between 30% and 50% of cancellous bone may be destroyed before an osteolytic lesion is recognized.[31,35,59] Osteolytic lesions in the diaphysis are more easily recognized because of the higher proportion of compact bone.

Size of the lesion. Each tumor has a unique growth rate influenced, in part, by the nature of the lesion and the response of the host bone. Markedly expansile lesions result when endosteal bone reabsorption of the inner cortex occurs in concert with periosteal appositional, intramembranous, new bone growth of the outer cortex. Although it is generally true that larger lesions are more aggressive than smaller ones, one should be careful not to judge a tumor's clinical importance by size alone. (See Fig. 15-7 for patterns of cortical destruction.

Rate of growth. The rate of growth is a very important characteristic for assessing the aggressiveness of a lesion. Benign lesions grow slowly and have thick margins. Malignant lesions grow quickly and have less defined margins. Although highly important, the assessment of a lesion's growth rate is difficult because of the usual lack of available serial studies.

Margination. The appearance of the zone of bone surrounding a lesion and the margins of the lesion are determined by the lesion's aggressiveness and the response of the host bone (Fig.

15-8). Malignant tumors are typically poorly marginated, exhibiting a wide zone of transition (Figs. 15-9 and 15-10). Conversely, a lesion is most likely benign if surrounded by a sclerotic rim of varying thicknesses producing a narrow zone of transition. The presence of a thick margin is always accompanied by a short zone of transition and represents an attempt of the host bone to surround and limit a lesion's growth. However, a short zone of transition is not always accompanied by a thick margin (e.g., giant cell tumor).

Tumor matrix. The radiographic appearance of the tumor's matrix, or substance, assists its categorization as primarily bone, fibrous, or cartilage forming. Most bone tumors have a radiolucent matrix. Only when the matrix is sufficiently mineralized with hydroxyapatite crystals will it become radiographically visible. Bone-producing tumors are radiodense. Highly aggressive bone-producing tumors appear less dense, with poorly formed osteoid material, than do nonaggressive bone-producing tumors. Tumors with a purely fibrous matrix appear radiolucent or slightly hazy. Cartilage tumors are usually accompanied by irregular ringlike, flocculent, stippled, or flecklike radiodensities within the matrix.

Multiplicity. Multiple lesions suggest different diagnostic possibilities than single lesions. Generally, radionuclide bone scanning will determine if multiple lesions exist. Because radionuclide imaging is sensitive but not specific, plain film radiographs are usually taken at regions of increased radionuclide uptake. Radiographs are usually directed at evaluating a lesion rather than finding it. MRI and CT are

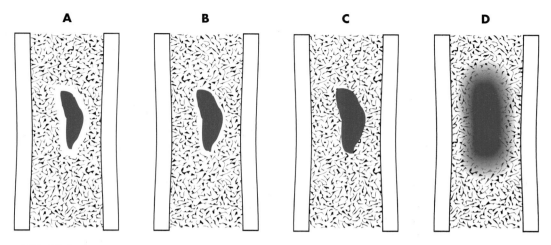

FIG. 15-8 Margination of bone lesion. **A,** Thick. **B,** Thin. **C,** Absent. *A through C* demonstrate a short zone of transition between normal bone and the lesion. **D,** Ill-defined. **D** demonstrates a long zone of transition between normal bone and the lesion. A long zone of transition is most often associated with an aggressive lesion. (Modified from Juhl JH, Crummy AB: *Paul and Juhl's Essentials of radiologic imaging,* ed 6, Philadelphia, 1993, JB Lippincott.)

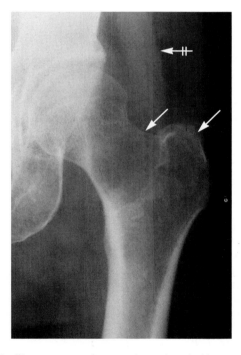

FIG. 15-9 Fibrosarcoma causing a poorly marginated, wide zone of transition of normal bone to the subtle decrease in bone density in the superior aspect of the femoral neck and greater trochanter *(arrows).* Incidentally noted, is a prominent gluteal muscle shadow *(crossed arrow).* (Courtesy Joseph W. Howe, Sylmar, Calif.)

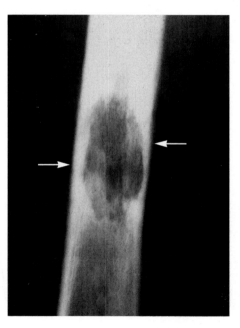

FIG. 15-10 Malignant fibrous histiocytoma in the diametaphysis of the femur, producing a poorly marginated lesion with a wide zone of transition *(arrows).* (Courtesy William E. Litterer, Elizabeth, NJ.)

applied less commonly to resolve uncertain findings of the radionuclide bone scan and plain films. The presence of multiple lesions limits the differential diagnosis. Common aggressive polyostotic diseases include metastatic bone disease and multiple myeloma, and less commonly, multicentric osteosarcoma and multifocal infections. Common nonaggressive polyostotic lesions include fibrous dysplasia, Paget's disease, histocytosis, hereditary multiple exostosis (HME), multiple enchondromas (Ollier's disease), and osteomyelitis.

Treatment Options

Treatment options include surgery, chemotherapy, and radiation; all may be applied alone or in combination. Surgical options extend from curettage for benign lesions to wide resection and possible amputation for highly malignant lesions. Each treatment approach is associated with complications, tumor recurrence, and varying success rates dependent on the patient's clinical status and the type and stage of the lesions.

PART TWO Bone, Joints, and Soft Tissues

Benign Tumors

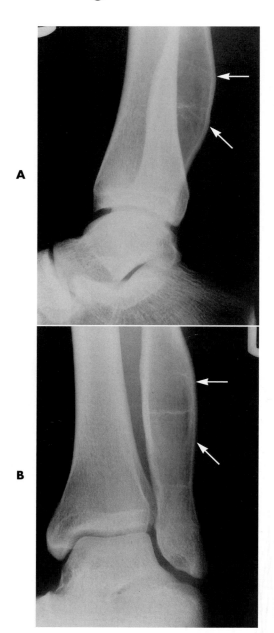

FIG. 15-11 Lateral **(A)** and oblique **(B)** projections of the ankle demonstrating an expansile, central aneurysmal bone cyst *(arrows)* in the distal fibula. (Courtesy Jack C. Avalos, Davenport, Iowa.)

Aneurysmal Bone Cyst

BACKGROUND

An aneurysmal bone cyst (ABC) is a solitary, expansile, benign osteolytic lesion of the metaphysis of long bones. The tumor represents blood-filled spaces that are separated by fibrous tissue containing multinucleated giant cells. ABCs may appear as primary lesions or are found in association with past trauma or other tumors. In about 30% of cases, concurrent lesions are clearly identified. Giant cell tumors (GCTs) are probably the most common concurrent lesions, although fibrous dysplasia, osteoblastoma, angioma, chondroblastoma, chondromyxoid fibroma, solitary bone cyst, and osteosarcoma also occur. Approximately 80% of patients with an ABC are younger than 20 years old.[105,174]

IMAGING FINDINGS

The radiographic appearance is characterized by an eccentric location with cortical thinning producing a blown out or "ballooned" contour of the host bone (Fig. 15-11), geographic bone destruction with well-defined edges, and absence of periosteal reaction, visible matrix, or floating debris (fallen fragment sign)[74,174] Aneurysmal bone cysts range in size from 2 to 25 cm.

At times the cortical expansion may appear very thin (Fig. 15-12) and mimic an aggressive periosteal change suggestive of a primary malignant tumor (Fig. 15-13). Aneurysmal bone cysts are most often found in the metaphysis of long bones.[105] The spine accounts for 10% to 30% of lesions, typically found in the posterior osseous elements (Figs. 15-14, 15-15, and 15-16). The pelvis accounts for half of all flat bone lesions.[105]

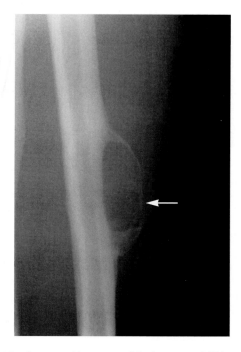

FIG. 15-12 Aneurysmal bone cyst of the humerus exhibiting an expanded and a very thin cortex *(arrow)*. (Courtesy Joseph W. Howe, Sylmar, Calif.)

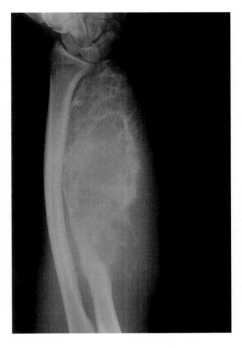

FIG. 15-13 Grossly expansile aneurysmal bone cyst of the distal ulna. (Courtesy Joseph W. Howe, Sylmar, Calif.)

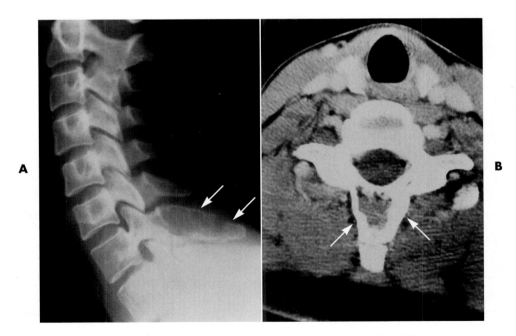

FIG. 15-14 **A,** Plain film cervical projection revealing cystic enlargement of the C7 spinous process *(arrows)* with fracture through its distal portion. **B,** Computed tomogram confirming the expanded cortex consistent with aneurysmal bone cyst *(arrows)*.

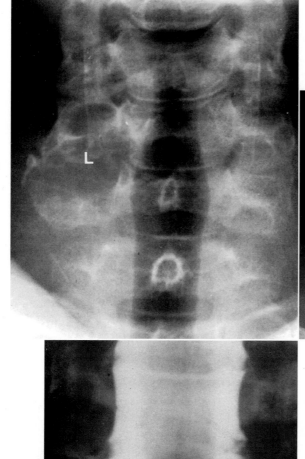

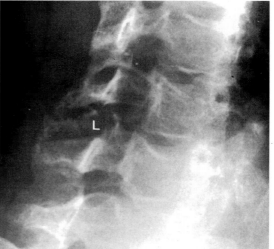

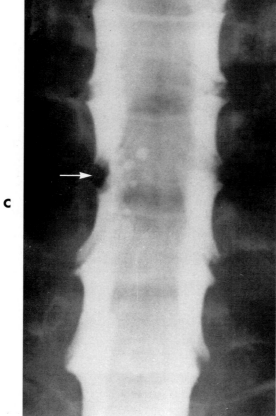

FIG. 15-15   Aneurysmal bone cyst arising from the posterior elements of the cervical spine. **A** and **B,** Frontal and oblique radiographs demonstrate expansile osteolytic areas involving the pillars and facet joints at C5-C6. **C,** Myelography documents encroachment on the adjacent C6 nerve root *(arrow).* Differential diagnosis should include consideration of osteoblastoma, metastatic disease (particularly from renal and thyroid primaries), plasmacytoma, indolent infection, and tophaceous gout. (From Sartoris DJ: *Musculoskeletal imaging: the requisites,* St Louis, 1993, Mosby.)

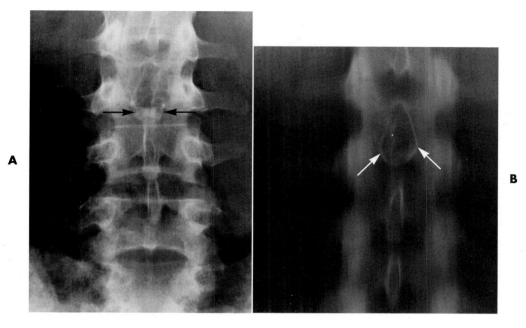

FIG. 15-16 Plain film **(A)** and linear tomogram **(B)** of an aneurysmal bone cyst of the L3 spinous process *(arrows).*

CLINICAL COMMENTS

Most patients complain of pain, swelling, and tenderness of less than 6 months' duration.[105] Their complaint is related to the lesion itself or an associated pathological fracture. The lesion's expansile nature may lead to stenosis of the vertebral canal or intervertebral foramen.[81] Intralesional excision with adjunctive cryosurgery is an effective method for the treatment of aneurysmal bone cysts.[124]

KEY CONCEPTS

- *Aneurysmal bone cysts (ABCs) occur as primary or secondary (e.g., GCT) lesions.*
- *ABCs are solitary, grossly expansile, eccentric lesions of the metaphysis of long bones.*
- *Patients are usually younger than 20 years of age.*

Bone Island (Enostosis), Osteoma, and Osteopoikilosis

BACKGROUND

A bone island (enostosis) is a commonly encountered entity, representing a region of compact bone located in cancellous bone (Fig. 15-17).[103] It may appear as a single defect or as multiple defects with a variety of shapes. Osteomas differ from enostosis in that the former protrude from the surface of the affected bone and are found in the skull. Also, bone islands are encountered in all age groups with no apparent gender predilection, while osteomas are discovered typically in the adult patient.

Osteopoikilosis is a nonpainful condition of multiple enostoses; their distribution is predominantly around joints with a symmetrical distribution (Fig. 15-18). Multiple osteomas may be one component of Gardner's syndrome, comprising colonic polyposis, osteomatosis, dental lesions, and soft tissue tumors.[3,181]

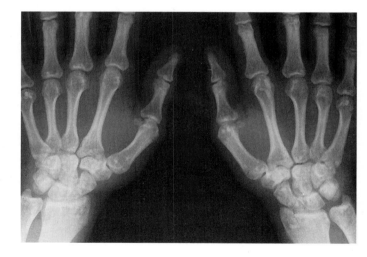

FIG. 15-17 Bilateral hand projection demonstrating multiple bone islands (osteopoikilosis) most notable in the wrist. (Courtesy Steven P. Brownstein, Springfield, NJ.)

IMAGING FINDINGS

Enostoses are radiodense lesions that occur in all bones, although they are more common in the pelvis, proximal femora, and ribs (Figs. 15-19 and 15-20). They usually have a characteristic horny or spickled border, which blends into normal trabeculae, producing a characteristic whiskered or "brush border" appearance. Osteomas are dense radiopacities found almost exclusively in the skull and facial bones (Figs. 15-21, 15-22, and 15-23).

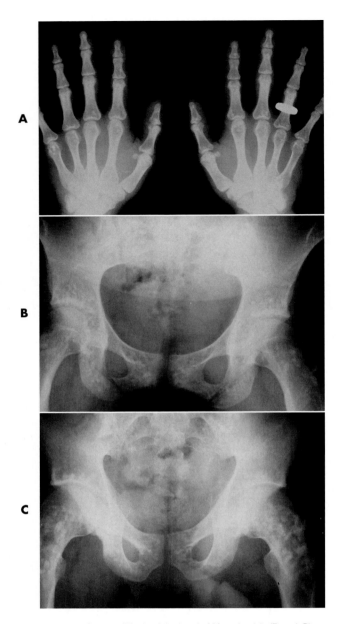

FIG. 15-18   Osteopoikilosis of the hands **(A)** and pelvis (**B** and **C**), presenting as bilateral, symmetrical, periarticular bone islands.

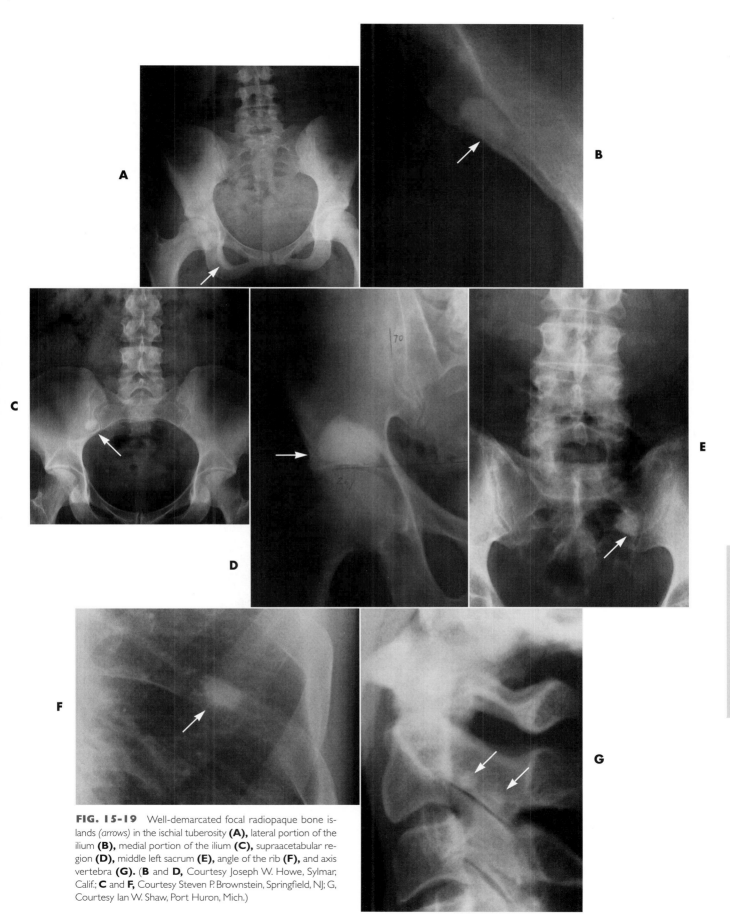

FIG. 15-19 Well-demarcated focal radiopaque bone islands *(arrows)* in the ischial tuberosity **(A),** lateral portion of the ilium **(B),** medial portion of the ilium **(C),** supraacetabular region **(D),** middle left sacrum **(E),** angle of the rib **(F),** and axis vertebra **(G).** (**B** and **D,** Courtesy Joseph W. Howe, Sylmar, Calif.; **C** and **F,** Courtesy Steven P. Brownstein, Springfield, NJ; G, Courtesy Ian W. Shaw, Port Huron, Mich.)

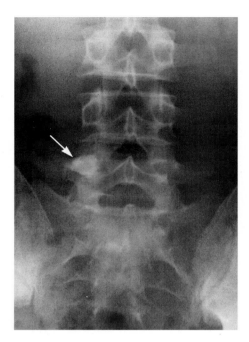

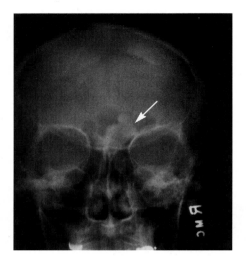

FIG. 15-20   Radiodense L5 pedicle shadow *(arrow)* representing a bone island. Additionally, initial consideration was given to osteoid osteoma and congenital bone hypertrophy.

FIG. 15-21   Osteoma near the frontal sinus *(arrow).*

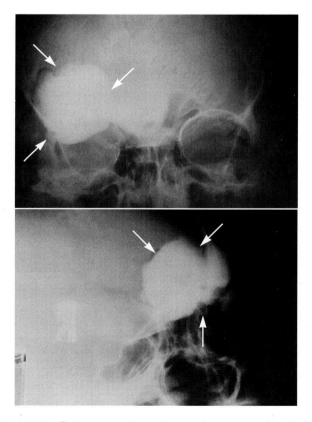

FIG. 15-22   Osteoma appearing as a dense radiopaque mass above the right orbit *(arrows).* (Courtesy Ian D. McLean, Davenport, Iowa.)

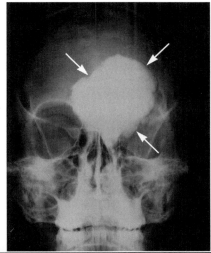

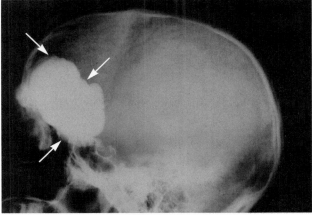

FIG. 15-23 Osteoma near the left frontal sinus *(arrows)*. (Courtesy Steven P. Brownstein, Springfield, NJ.)

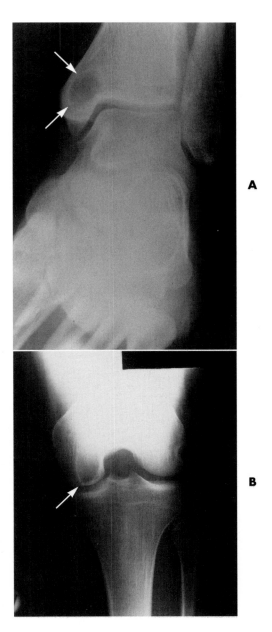

FIG. 15-24 Chondroblastoma *(arrows)* of the medial malleolus **(A)** and medial femoral condyle **(B)**. The lesions both have the characteristic appearance of an oval, geographic, radiolucent defect in the epiphysis. (Courtesy Joseph W. Howe, Sylmar, Calif.)

CLINICAL COMMENTS

Occasionally enostoses grow, necessitating differentiation from an aggressive neoplasm (e.g., osteoblastic metastasis). The absence of pain and usually normal radionuclide bone scan are characteristic of enostosis.[149,179] Osteomas become clinically significant if they enlarge and interfere with sinus drainage.

KEY CONCEPTS

- *Enostoses are very common, clinically silent lesions.*
- *Osteomas are found in skull and facial bones, usually in adult patients.*
- *Enostoses occur at all ages and in all bones; they are particularly common in the pelvis, femur, and ribs.*

Chondroblastoma

BACKGROUND

A chondroblastoma (Codman's tumor) is a rare, benign primary bone tumor usually occurring in secondary centers of enchondral ossification. Lesions appear most frequently in long, tubular bones and less frequently in short tubular and flat bones.[24,58,198] Up to 15% of lesions are found in combination with an aneurysmal bone cyst.[40] Ninety percent of lesions occur in patients who are between the ages of 5 and 25 years. Men are affected more than women, at a 1.5 or 2:1 ratio.[58]

IMAGING FINDINGS

The imaging findings of those lesions within long bones are highly characteristic, consisting of a centric or eccentric, osteolytic region of less than 5 cm, well defined by a thin rim of sclerosis, and located within an epiphysis or apophysis. The proximal femur, distal femur, proximal tibia, and proximal humerus are the most common sites of involvement (Figs. 15-24 and 15-25). Calcific foci within the matrix are common. Its appearance in nontubular bones is less characteristic (Fig. 15-26).

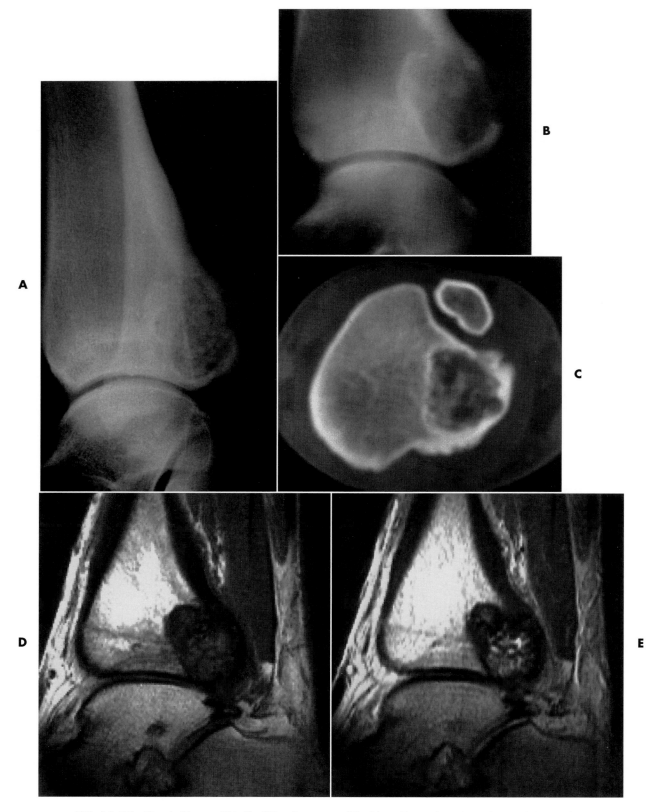

FIG. 15-25   Chondroblastoma. Plain film **(A)** and tomogram **(B)** of the ankle reveal a well-marginated lytic lesion of the distal tibial epiphysis with prominent lesional calcification. **C,** CT scan defines the cortical expansion. **D,** T1-weighted MRIs demonstrate diffuse low signal intensity. **E,** T2-weighting reveals mixed areas of high and low signal intensity. The high intensity probably represents uncalcified cartilage, and the low signal corresponds to areas of calcified matrix. (From Stark DD, Gradley WG: *Magnetic resonance imaging,* ed 2, St Louis, 1992, Mosby.)

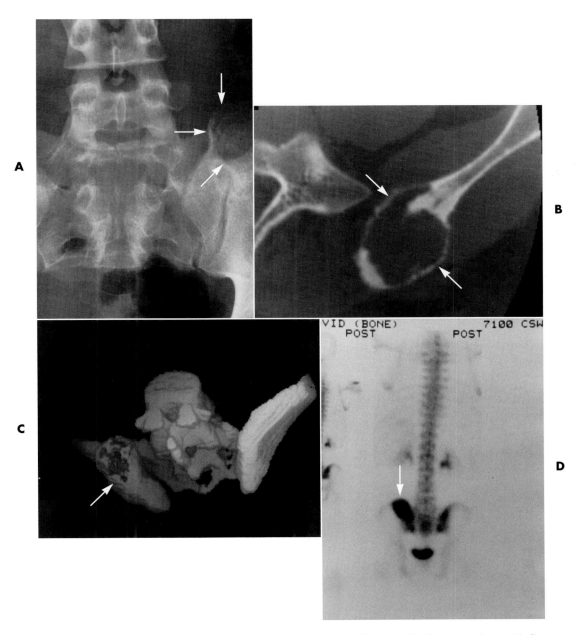

FIG. 15-26 A 24-year-old patient with local pain resulting from a chondroblastoma of the ilium presenting on plain film (**A**) as a well-circumscribed radiolucent defect in the iliac crest *(arrows).* The lesion appears expansile on conventional (**B,** *arrows*) and three-dimensional reformatted CT (**C,** *arrow*). The ilium appears as a hot spot on the posterior view of the radionuclide bone scan (**D,** *arrow*). This is not a typical location of chondroblastoma.

CLINICAL COMMENTS

Local pain, tenderness, and swelling of the involved region is often reported. Complete curettage with bone grafting is the preferred treatment.[194]

KEY CONCEPTS

- *This rare, benign bone tumor is located within an epiphysis or apophysis.*
- *It is most commonly found around the knee.*
- *Chondroblastoma usually presents between 5 and 25 years of age and is more common among men.*

Chondroma, Ollier's Disease, and Maffucci's Syndrome

BACKGROUND

A chondroma is a cartilage tumor found within the medullary canal (enchondroma) (Fig. 15-27) or adjacent to the cortex beneath the periosteal membrane (periosteal or juxtacortical chondroma, or perichondroma) (Fig. 15-28) of enchondrally formed bones. Chondromas represent discrete islands of hyaline cartilage surrounded by lamellar enchondral bone.

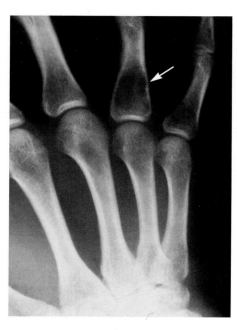

FIG. 15-27   Central enchondroma in the proximal phalanx of the fourth digit *(arrow).*

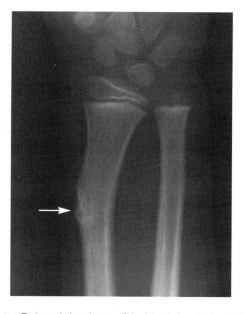

FIG. 15-28   Periosteal chondroma of the lateral diametaphysis of the radius *(arrow).* (Courtesy Joseph W. Howe, Sylmar, Calif.)

Enchondroma is the most common tumor occurring in the phalanges and is, after osteochondroma, the second most common benign cartilage neoplasm of bone.[77] The presence of multiple enchondromas (enchondromatosis, or Ollier's disease) (Fig. 15-29) increases the risk of malignant transformation by 30%.[14,38,175] The combination of multiple enchondromas and subcutaneous hemangiomas is termed *Maffucci's syndrome* (Fig. 15-30) and is associated with a 30% or greater increased risk for malignant transformation than occurs with solitary enchondromas.[4,97,195] The malignant transformation is usually to a chondrosarcoma.

Enchondromas most often present in patients between the ages of 20 and 30 years, with an equal gender distribution. Juxtacortical chondromas are found in patients predominantly before the age of 30 years,[20] appearing more commonly in males than females, at a ratio of 2:1.

IMAGING FINDINGS

Chondromas, whether medullary or juxtacortical, solitary or multiple, are usually found in the small bones of the hands, particularly the proximal phalanges, and less commonly the feet. The humerus,

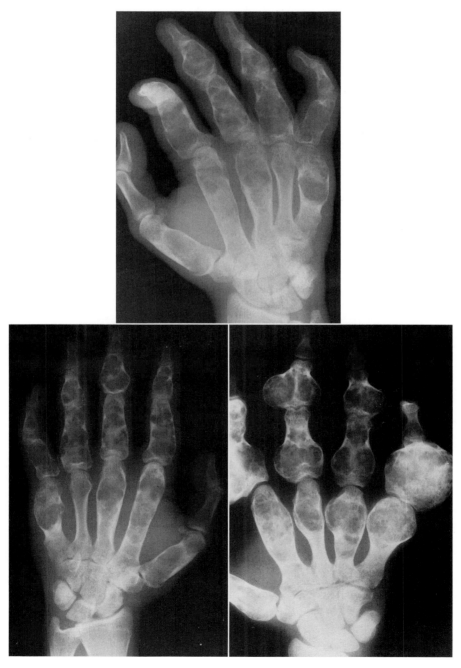

FIG. 15-29 Three cases of multiple enchondromatosis (Ollier's disease). Each case exhibits multiple, expansile enchondromas in the small bones of the hand. Most of the individual lesions exhibit stippled matrix calcification, characteristic of cartilage tumors. (Courtesy Joseph W. Howe, Sylmar, Calif.)

femur (Fig. 15-31), and tibia are also involved. An enchondroma appears as a well-defined medullary lesion, most often with some degree of calcification (Figs. 15-32 and 15-33), endosteal scalloping (Fig. 15-34), and bone expansion. Periosteal chondromas appear as soft tissue masses with erosion or saucerization of the adjacent cortex (Figs. 15-35 and 15-36). Calcification is noted in 50% of periosteal chondromas.[202]

CLINICAL COMMENTS

Chondromas are typically asymptomatic. The presence of associated pain increases the clinical suspicion for the presence of pathological fracture (Fig. 15-37) or malignant transformation, usually to chondrosarcoma. Additionally, any chondroma that exhibits continued growth in a skeletally mature patient should be closely scrutinized to exclude malignant transformation.

KEY CONCEPTS

- *Chondromas are the most common tumor of the phalanges.*
- *Chondromas have a medullary (enchondroma) or juxtacortical (perichondroma) location.*
- *They usually occur in patients younger than age 30 years.*
- *Matrix calcification occurs in 50% of patients with chondromas.*
- *Malignant transformation to a chondrosarcoma is a rare occurrence (1% of patients) unless multiple lesions are present (30% of patients).*

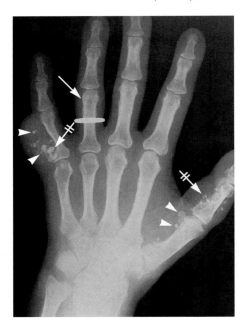

FIG. 15-30   Maffucci's syndrome noted by the enchondroma *(arrow)* with soft tissue hemangioma *(crossed arrows)* involving the first and fifth digits. Phleboliths are noted within the soft tissue hemangioma *(arrowheads).* (Courtesy Steven P. Brownstein, Springfield, NJ.)

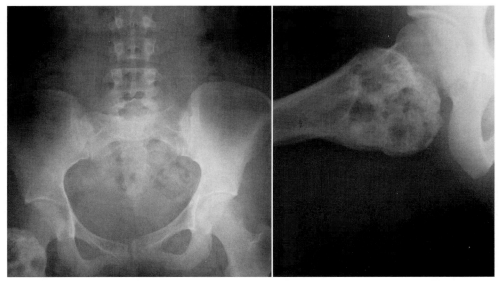

FIG. 15-31   Intertrochanteric enchondroma of the right femur. This case emphasizes the importance of reading the entire film, avoiding the tendency to underinterpret the corners.

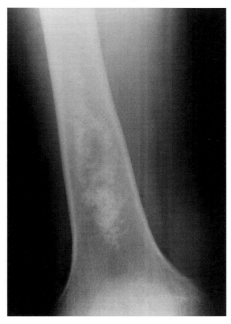

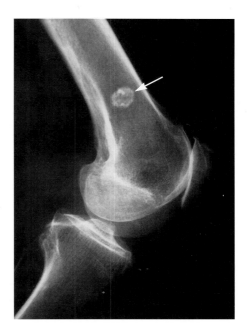

FIG. 15-32 Enchondroma of the distal femur presenting with patchy medullary calcification. This appearance of an enchondroma is very similar to medullary infarct and central chondrosarcoma, often making distinction difficult. (Courtesy Joseph W. Howe, Sylmar, Calif.)

FIG. 15-33 Calcific enchondroma of the distal femur *(arrow)*. (Courtesy Jack Avalos, Davenport, Iowa.)

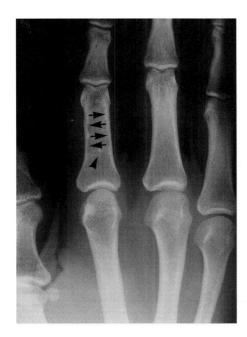

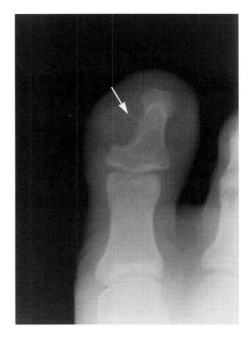

FIG. 15-34 Enchondroma of the proximal phalanx of the second digit presenting with endosteal scalloping *(arrows)* and a single focus of calcification *(arrowhead)*. (Courtesy Robert C. Tatum, Davenport, Iowa.)

FIG. 15-35 Periosteal chondroma of the distal phalanx of the great toe exhibiting soft tissue mass and cortical saucerization *(arrow)*. (Courtesy Ian D. McLean, Davenport, Iowa.)

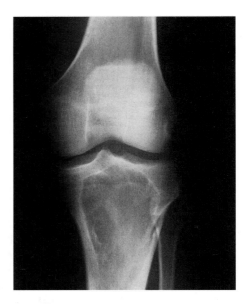

FIG. 15-38 Chondromyxoid fibroma of the proximal tibia.

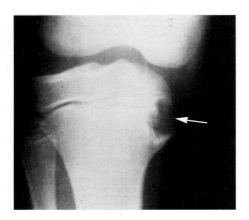

FIG. 15-36 Periosteal chondroma (*arrow*) of the medial portion of the proximal tibia. (Courtesy Steven P. Brownstein, Springfield, NJ.)

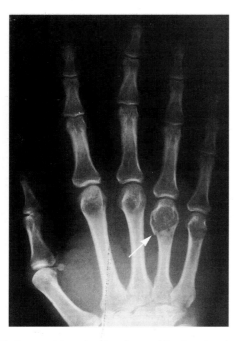

FIG. 15-37 Fractured (*arrow*) enchondroma of the distal fourth metacarpal.

Chondromyxoid Fibroma

BACKGROUND

A chondromyxoid fibroma (CMF) is the least frequent benign cartilage neoplasm.[118,151] Its basic composition is cartilage, but varying degrees of myxoid and fibrous tissues are also present. CMF most often occurs in patients before the age of 30 years.

IMAGING FINDINGS

Long, tubular bones of the lower extremity, namely the proximal tibia and fibula and proximal and distal femur, are most often in-

volved (Fig. 15-38). CMFs characteristically appear as 2- to 10-cm oval, eccentric, metaphyseal, noncalcified, osteolytic lesions. Because of the scalloped inner margins of the host bone, the lesions may appear chambered by thick trabeculation.[68]

CLINICAL COMMENTS

Pain, tenderness, swelling, and restricted motion of the involved region are common clinical complaints. Lesions rarely undergo malignant transformation, and less than 5% demonstrate pathological fracture.[77]

KEY CONCEPTS
- *Chondromyxoid fibroma (CMF) is a rare tumor of mixed histology.*
- *CMF is usually located in the proximal tibia and usually occurs in patients before the age of 30 years.*
- *CMF is a 2- to 10-cm, eccentric, oval, osteolytic lesion.*

Fibrous Cortical Defect and Nonossifying Fibroma

BACKGROUND

Fibrous cortical defect (FCD) and nonossifying fibroma (NOF) are histologically identical development defects of bone. Collectively they are referred to as *fibrous xanthomas* or *metaphyseal fibrous defects*. They differ in age of presentation, size, frequency, and region of bone that is involved.

FCD is found on the cortical surface and NOF is eccentrically placed within the medullary cavity. Both may present as multiple lesions,[142] although multiple FCDs are more common than multiple NOFs.[87] Multiple lesions may be associated with neurofibromatosis[67] and Jaffe-Campanacci syndrome. The latter is a complex marked by café au lait spots, mental retardation, hypogonadism, and ocular abnormalities.[26]

FCDs are much more common than NOFs. FCDs have been estimated to occur in 30% to 40% of children. They are typically found in patients between the ages of 4 and 8 years and are twice as frequent in males. NOFs are found in patients between the ages of 2 and 20 years, with a slight male predominance.

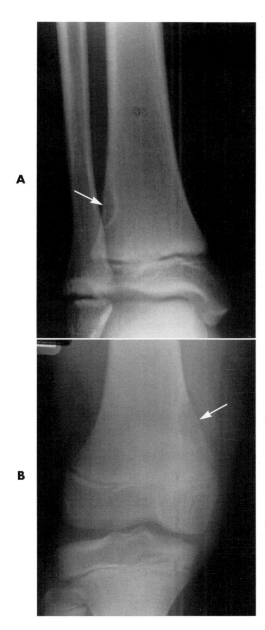

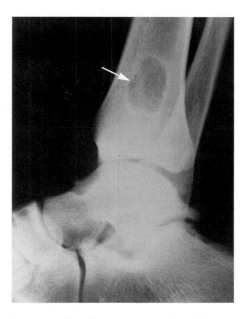

FIG. 15-40 Nonossifying fibroma of the distal tibia, demonstrating a margin characteristic of a benign lesion *(arrow)*. (Courtesy Joseph W. Howe, Sylmar, Calif.)

FIG. 15-39 Well-defined cortical lesion *(arrows)* representing fibrous cortical defects of the lateral margin of the distal tibia **(A)** and the medial aspect of the distal femur **(B)**. (**A,** Courtesy Ian D. McLean, Davenport, Iowa; **B,** Courtesy Ronnie L. Firth, East Moline, Ill.)

IMAGING FINDINGS

FCDs and NOFs are common in the lower extremities, particularly around the knee. An FCD appears as a 1- to 4-cm, round or oval geographic radiolucency eroding the cortical surface of the metaphysis of a long bone (Fig. 15-39).[113] It is sharply marginated by a thin rim of surrounding sclerosis (Fig. 15-40). An NOF appears similarly, except it is found in the medullary cavity, more often appears multiloculated, and is larger than an FCD (Figs. 15-41 and 15-42).[41]

CLINICAL COMMENTS

Both FCD and NOF are usually clinically silent. They generally heal spontaneously as the peripheral rim of reactive sclerosis thick-

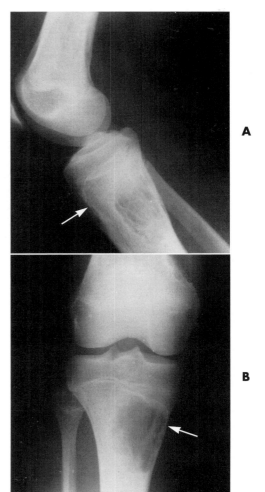

FIG. 15-41 Lateral **(A)** and anteroposterior **(B)** projections of the knee demonstrating a multiloculated, eccentric, well-marginated lesion *(arrows)* consistent with nonossifying fibroma.

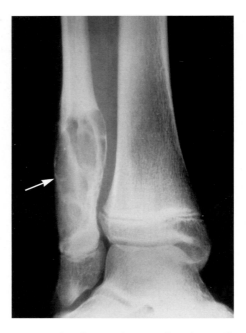

FIG. 15-42   Nonossifying fibroma of the distal fibula *(arrow)*. (Courtesy Steven P. Brownstein, Springfield, NJ.)

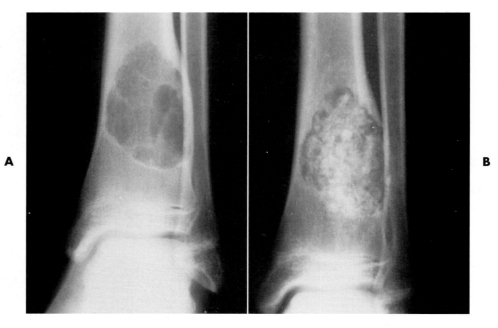

FIG. 15-43   Before **(A)** and after **(B)** prophylactic curettage and bone grafting of a large, nonossifying fibroma of the distal tibia. (Courtesy Steven P. Brownstein, Springfield, NJ.)

ens, reducing the central radiolucent region. If large, NOFs may fracture, occasionally necessitating prophylactic curettage and bone grafting (Fig. 15-43).[6]

KEY CONCEPTS

- *FCDs are very common and are seen in patients between the ages of 4 and 8 years.*
- *NOFs are common, are larger than FCDs, and occur in patients between the ages of 2 and 20 years.*
- *Both FCDs and NOFs are usually clinically silent, osteolytic lesions, most often found around the knee.*
- *Both FCDs and NOFs heal spontaneously.*

Fibrous Dysplasia

BACKGROUND

Fibrous dyplasia (FD) is a nonneoplastic disturbance of bone maintenance. Bone undergoing normal physiological lysis becomes replaced by fibrous tissue containing small, abnormally arranged bone trabeculae. The condition may be confined to a single bone (monostotic fibrous dysplasia) or involve multiple bones (polyostotic fibrous dysplasia). These forms of the disease differ clinically, but the individual osseous lesions are pathologically and radiographically identical. The monostotic form occurs three to four times as frequently as the polyostotic form. Approximately 3% of patients with polyostotic FD exhibit concurrent endocrinopathies, such as Albright's syndrome.

Albright's syndrome comprises a triad that includes the classic FD bony lesions in unilateral and polyostotic form, precocious puberty, and cutaneous pigmentation located on the same side as the polyostotic lesions.[4,71,185] Mazabraud's syndrome is made up of multiple fibrous and fibromyxomatous soft tissue tumors occurring in association with polyostotic FD.[189]

Fibrous dysplasia affects men and women equally. A wide range of age is observed, affecting those from 1 to 75 years, although most cases are identified before the age of 20 years and most cases of polyostotic FD are identified before the age of 8 years.[23] The presence of concurrent endocrinopathies may lead to an earlier discovery of polyostotic FD.

IMAGING FINDINGS

FD most often occurs in the femur (Fig. 15-44), tibia, craniofacial bones, pelvis, or ribs (Fig. 15-45).[84,88] Involvement of the pelvis typically occurs with the polyostotic form, where concurrent lesions are usually present in the femur. Spine involvement is uncommon in polyostotic FD and rare as a monostotic lesion (Fig. 15-46). Polyostotic FD has a peculiar predisposition to affect multiple bones on one side of the body.[117] The individual osseous lesions vary in size from 1 to 30 cm.

The radiographic appearance depends on the bone involved. Tubular bones appear mildly expansile, with an osteolytic or mildly sclerotic inner matrix (Fig. 15-47). Mild sclerosis has been likened to the appearance of ground glass and results from the primitive bone trabeculation within the lesion (Fig. 15-48). Surrounding bony sclerosis is usually, but not always, present. "Shepherd's crook" deformity is a lateral bowing and coxa vara deformity occurring in the proximal femur secondary to remodeling of pathological microfracture. Skull bones appear densely sclerotic and often enlarged with FD. Involvement of the pelvis results in a distinctive bubbly appearance. MRI demonstrates low signal intensity medullary lesions on both T1- and T2-weighted images (Fig. 15-49).

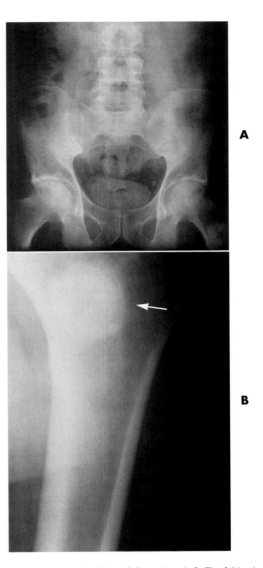

FIG. 15-44 Fibrous dysplasia of the left femoral neck. **A,** The full lumbopelvic projection demonstrates an obscure alteration of bone density in the patient's left intertrochanteric region. **B,** A spot projection reveals a radiodense lesion *(arrow)* of the intertrochanteric region consistent with fibrous dysplasia. The proximal femur is a common location for the lesion; most lesions are not this dense. (Courtesy Ian D. McLean, Davenport, Iowa.)

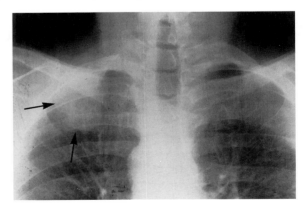

FIG. 15-45 Sclerotic appearance of the right first rib resulting from fibrous dyplasia *(arrows)*. (Courtesy Joseph W. Howe, Sylmar, Calif.)

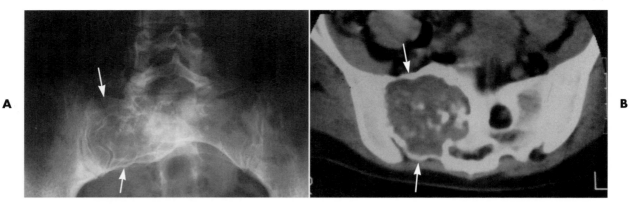

FIG. 15-46 Plain film **(A)** and CT scan **(B)** of a mildly expansile lesion of the right sacral ala *(arrows)* thought to represent fibrous dysplasia. (Courtesy Joseph W. Howe, Sylmar, Calif.)

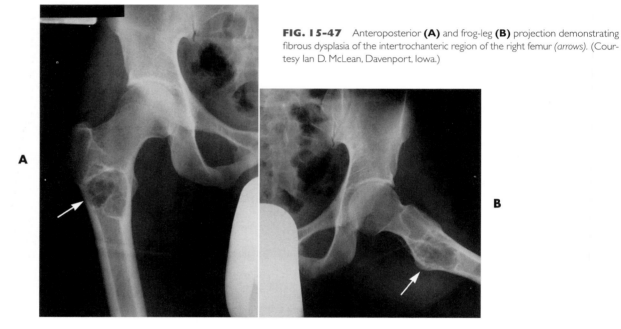

FIG. 15-47 Anteroposterior **(A)** and frog-leg **(B)** projection demonstrating fibrous dysplasia of the intertrochanteric region of the right femur *(arrows)*. (Courtesy Ian D. McLean, Davenport, Iowa.)

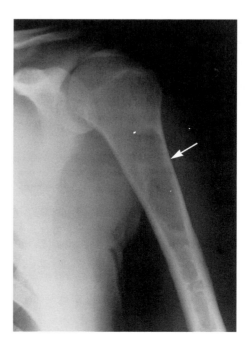

FIG. 15-48 Fibrous dyplasia of the upper humerus *(arrow)*. The matrix of the lesion appears mildly sclerotic, which is consistent with the ground glass density characteristic of fibrous dysplasia. (Courtesy Joseph W. Howe, Sylmar, Calif.)

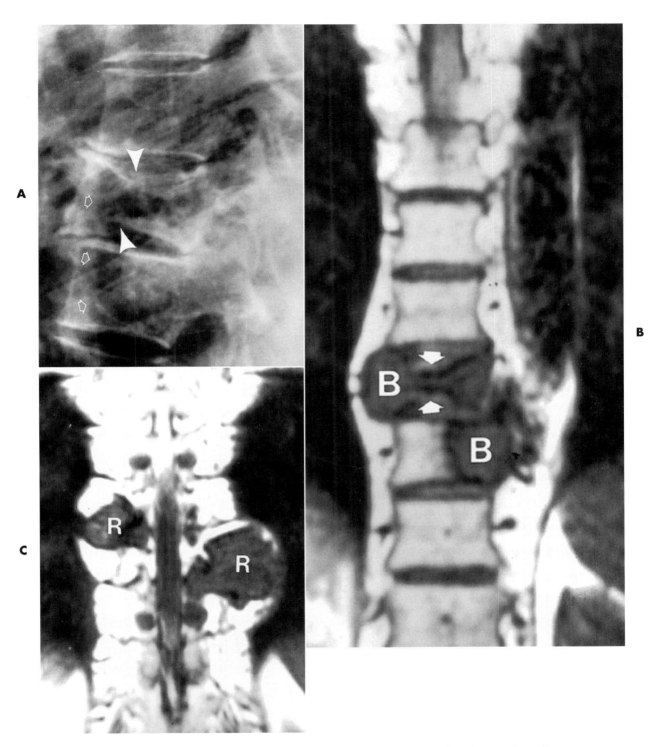

FIG. 15-49 Polyostotic fibrous dysplasia. **A,** Lateral radiograph demonstrates osteolytic involvement of two adjacent vertebral bodies *(open arrows)*, along with irregular endplate deformities *(arrowheads)*. **B** and **C,** Coronal T1-weighted MRIs reveal expansile low signal intensity areas within the vertebral bodies *(B)* and proximal ribs *(R)*. Arrows point to the pathological fracture. Differential diagnosis should include consideration of metastatic disease and indolent infection. (From Sartoris DJ: *Musculoskeletal imaging: the requisites*, St Louis, 1993, Mosby.)

PART TWO
Bone, Joints, and Soft Tissues

CLINICAL COMMENTS

Symptoms are more common when long tubular bones are involved, believed to result from microfracture. Polyostotic FD is associated with café au lait spots, the borders of which appear irregular, rather than smooth as occurs with spots associated with neurofibromatosis. Endocrinopathies including Albright's syndrome (noted above), Cushing's syndrome, diabetes mellitus, acromegaly, and hyperparathyroidism are associated with polyostotic FD. Pathological fracture is noted in up to 85% of patients with the polyostotic form of the disease.[84] Patient treatment is directed to any presenting fractures, deformity, or pain.

▌ KEY CONCEPTS

- *Fibrous dysplasia is a nonneoplastic, tumorlike disturbance of bone.*
- *The polyostotic form is often unilateral, associated with Albright's syndrome and cutaneous abnormalities.*
- *Although a wide age range exists, the monostotic form usually occurs in patients before the age of 20 years and the polyostotic form usually before the age of 8 years.*
- *Lesions of both forms appear osteolytic and expansile, most often involving the femur and tibia.*
- *Skull lesions appear sclerotic.*

Giant Cell Tumor

BACKGROUND

A giant cell tumor (GCT) is a sometimes malignant, osteolytic tumor believed to originate from undifferentiated cells within the supporting tissues of bone marrow. It is composed of mostly large mononuclear cells and fewer giant multinucleated cells.[187] Uncommonly, GCTs are associated with Paget's disease[15,153] and aneurysmal bone cysts.[126] Less than 5% of GCTs are malignant.[5,57] Most malignant lesions represent conventional GCTs, which transform into fibrosarcoma, or less commonly osteosarcoma, following irradiation.

Few GCTs are malignant from their onset. Unlike most osseous neoplasms, GCTs demonstrate a slight female predominance.[79,127,140] GCT is rare among the skeletally immature or the elderly.[79,169] Most lesions occur in patients between the ages of 20 and 40 years.

IMAGING FINDINGS

Although controversial in the past, it is now generally accepted that GCTs arise within the metaphysis.[104,204] As they enlarge, 84% to 98% extend to within 1 cm of the subarticular cortex.[91,128] Almost half of all GCTs are found around the knee in either the distal femur or proximal tibia (Fig. 15-50).[111] In decreasing order of frequency, some other sites include distal radius (Fig. 15-51), proximal femur, distal tibia, sacrum (Fig. 15-52), distal ulna, proximal fibula, and pelvis (Fig. 15-53). Spinal sites above the sacrum are rare.

The classic radiographic description of a GCT includes an eccentric osteolytic lesion with a narrow zone of transition and without surrounding sclerosis that arises in the metaphysis and extends to the epiphyseal subarticular cortex, usually around the knee in young adults. A malignant GCT is suggested by the presence of cortical breakthrough and soft tissue mass (Fig. 15-54).

CLINICAL COMMENTS

Patients complain of pain, limited range of motion, swelling, and tenderness. Treatment for GCT usually involves marginal (Fig. 15-55) or wide resection. Marginal resection is associated with a high rate of recurrence,[55] whereas wide resection typically compromises the function of the affected limb. Wide resection is indicated for recurrent or malignant lesions.[55]

▌ KEY CONCEPTS

- *Giant cell tumor (GCT) appears as an osteolytic, nonmarginated, eccentric lesion, located in the metaphysis with subarticular extension.*
- *GCT occurs in patients between 20 and 40 years of age and is occasionally malignant, suggested by painful soft tissue mass.*

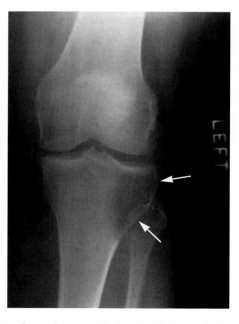

FIG. 15-50   Giant cell tumor with characteristic imaging findings of a subarticular, eccentric, nonmarginated, well-defined, osteolytic lesion around the knee (*arrows*). (Courtesy Steven P. Brownstein, Springfield, NJ.)

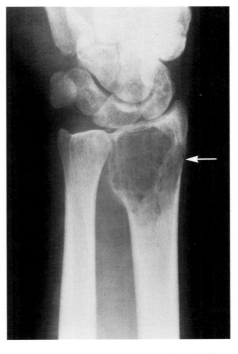

FIG. 15-51 Giant cell tumor of the distal radius *(arrow).* (Courtesy Steven P. Brownstein, Springfield, NJ.)

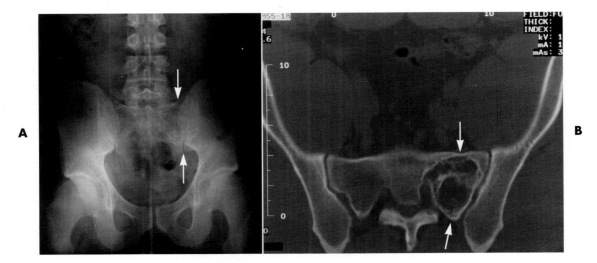

FIG. 15-52 Plain film **(A)** and computed tomogram **(B)** of an osteolytic lesion of the sacrum *(arrows).* The lesion is consistent in appearance with giant cell tumor and fibrous dyplasia.

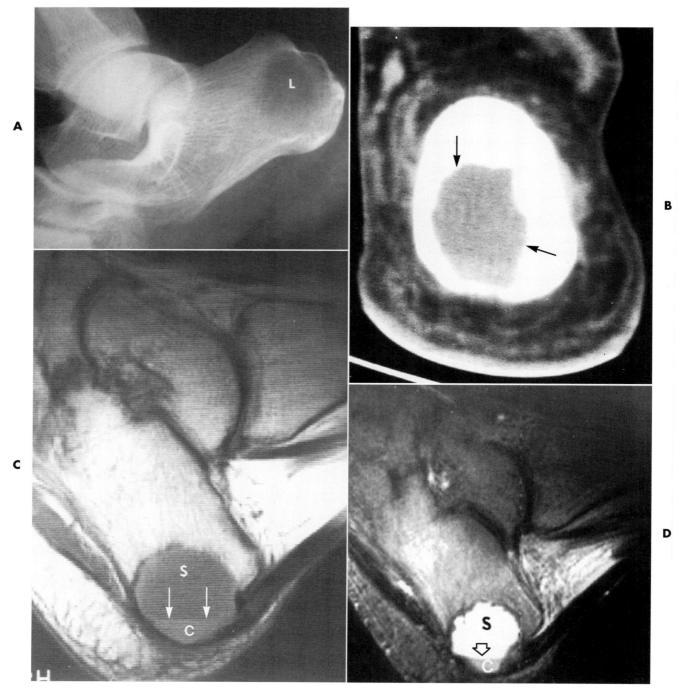

FIG. 15-53   Giant cell tumor. **A,** A poorly defined lytic lesion *(L)* is present in the calcaneal tuberosity. **B,** CT demonstrates a homogenous tissue-density process *(arrows)* without radiodense matrix. **C,** Sagittal T1-weighted MRI reveals a fluid-fluid level *(arrows)* within the lesion, indicating a hematocrit effect *(S, serum; C, cells).* **D,** The finding *(arrow)* is confirmed on a sagittal T2-weighted image, where the serum *(S)* manifests high signal intensity *(C, cells).* Fluid-fluid level indicates a blood-filled lesion, the differential diagnosis of which should include consideration of aneurysmal bone cyst, hemorrhagic metastasis, and other vascular tumors. (From Sartoris DJ: *Musculoskeletal imaging: the requisites,* St Louis, 1993, Mosby.)

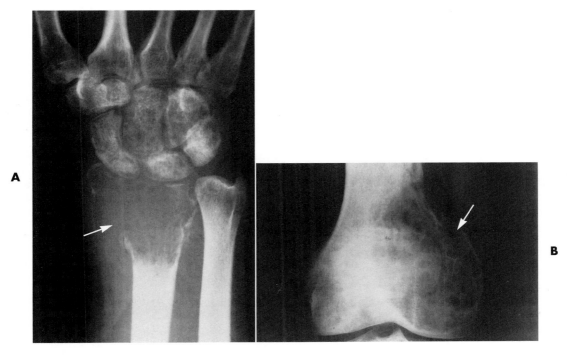

FIG. 15-54 Malignant degeneration of a giant cell tumor in the distal radius **(A)** and distal femur **(B).** Note the cortical breakthrough and soft tissue mass *(arrows).* (*A*, Courtesy Steven P. Brownstein, Springfield, NJ; *B*, Courtesy Joseph W. Howe, Sylmar, Calif.)

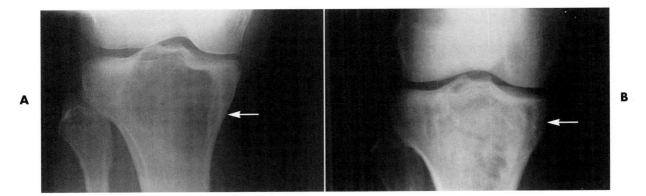

FIG. 15-55 Giant cell tumor *(arrows)* before **(A)** and following **(B)** marginal excision and bone grafting. (Courtesy Joseph W. Howe, Sylmar, Calif.)

Hemangioma of Bone

BACKGROUND

A hemangioma is a congenital anomaly in which a proliferation of vascular endothelium leads to a benign mass that resembles neoplastic tissue. Hemangiomas occur in bone, skin, and viscera. They are considered the most common benign tumors of the spine. In general, osseous hemangiomas are predominantly of two broad categories: capillary hemangiomas, which consist of haphazardly arranged, capillary-sized vessels, and the more common cavernous hemangiomas, which contain dilated vessels, lined with attenuated endothelial cells. Less commonly, osseous hemangiomas demonstrate a histological appearance consistent with venous soft tissue lesions.[150]

Hemangiomas may be encountered in patients of any age, although most are recognized in the fifth decade with a 3:2 female-to-male predominance.[52]

IMAGING FINDINGS

More than 50% of osseous hemangiomas are in the spine (Figs. 15-56 through 15-59),[176] 20% are in the skull, and the remaining lesions are found in the ribs, patella, long bones, and short tubular bones of the hands and feet. Hemangiomas usually occur as solitary lesions.

Capillary hemangiomas appear most commonly in the frontal bone, appearing as radiating radiolucent striations from a central radiolucent focus (sunburst appearance). Cavernous hemangiomas are most commonly seen in the vertebral bodies of the lower tho-

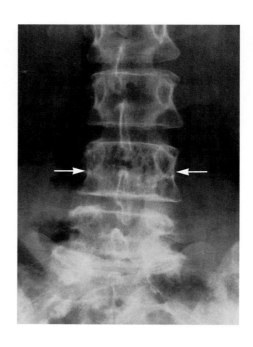

FIG. 15-56   Anteroposterior projection of the lumbar spine demonstrating the coarsened trabecular pattern indicative of hemangioma at the L4 level *(arrows)*. (Courtesy Ian D. McLean, Davenport, Iowa.)

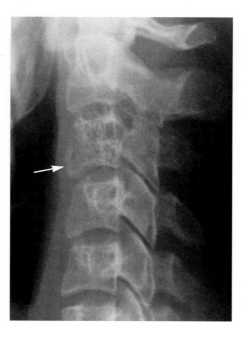

FIG. 15-57   Hemangioma of C3 *(arrow)*. (Courtesy Joseph W. Howe, Sylmar, Calif.)

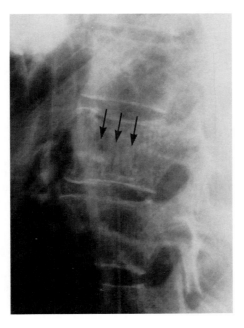

FIG. 15-58 Vertical striations characteristic of hemangioma *(arrows)*. (Courtesy Ian D. McLean, Davenport, Iowa.)

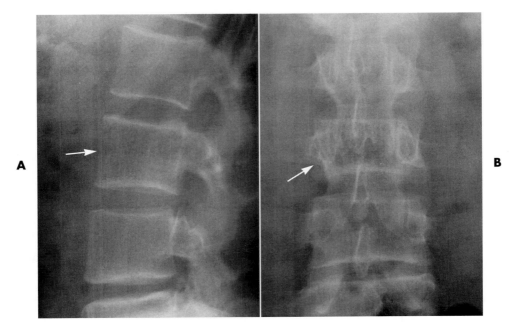

FIG. 15-59 **A,** Hemangioma of the L3 segment appearing with faint vertical prominence of the trabecular pattern in the lateral projection *(arrow)*. **B,** In the frontal projection the trabecular pattern appears coarsened *(arrow)*. (Courtesy Ian D. McLean, Davenport, Iowa.)

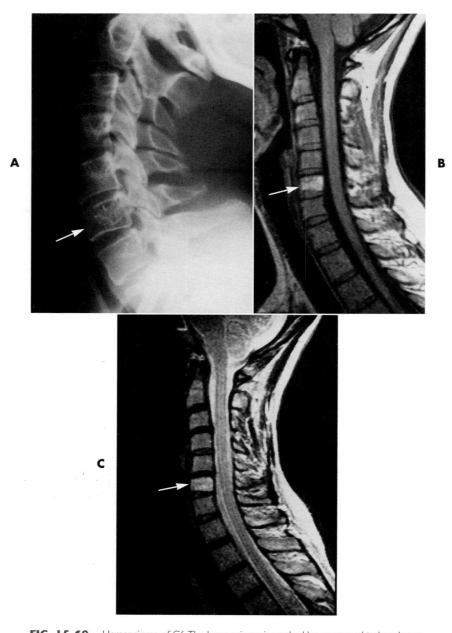

FIG. 15-60   Hemangioma of C6. The hemangioma is marked by coarsened trabeculae on the plain film **(A)** and a hyperintense signal on both the T1-weighted **(B)** and T2-weighted **(C)** MRI scan *(arrows)*. (Courtesy Ian D. McLean, Davenport, Iowa.)

racic and upper lumbar spine[206] and are marked by exaggerated vertical radiopaque striations of the involved vertebral body (accordion, corduroy cloth, or jailbar pattern). Less commonly, the vertebral body will have a honeycomb appearance. Infrequently, lesions extend into the neural arch.

Contrary to most tumors, hemangiomas demonstrate increased signal intensity on both T1- and T2-weighted magnetic resonance images (Fig. 15-60).[169]

CLINICAL COMMENTS

As evidenced by the large number of asymptomatic lesions found at autopsy (10% to 12%), most hemangiomas are unnoticed.[206] Symptoms are usually secondary to pathological fracture, occurring in

long bones. Rarely, an expanding spinal lesion may cause spinal canal stenosis. No treatment is applied to asymptomatic lesions. The treatment for painful lesions depends on their location and degree of osseous involvement. Radiation alleviates painful lesions, although the radiographic appearance remains unchanged.[123]

KEY CONCEPTS

- *Hemangiomas are common bone lesions located in the skull (capillary) and spine (cavernous) and are clinically silent.*
- *The radiographic appearance of a spine lesion is marked by thick vertical striations.*
- *Hemangiomas exhibit increased signal intensity on both the T1- and T2-weighted MRIs.*

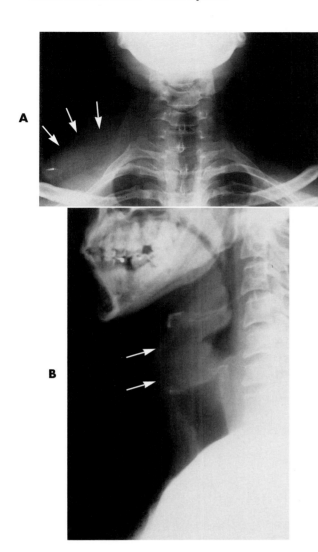

FIG. 15-61 Soft tissue lipoma presenting as a suprascapular mass *(arrows)* on the frontal projection **(A)** and extending as an anterior neck mass on the lateral projection **(B)**. (Courtesy William E. Litterer, Elizabeth, NJ.)

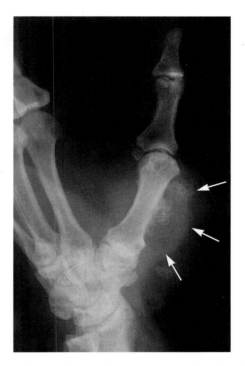

FIG. 15-62 Parosteal lipoma with several scattered foci of calcification *(arrows)*. The appearance is similar to a soft tissue hemangioma with phleboliths. (Courtesy Steven P. Brownstein, Springfield, NJ.)

Lipoma

BACKGROUND

A lipoma is a common, benign collection of mature fat cells within subcutaneous tissue, nerves, synovium, and between or within muscles. Rarely, lipomas occur as intraosseous, cortical, or parosteal lesions.[116,133,144] Soft tissue lesions typically occur as palpable, compressive, moveable, subcutaneous masses, most often found in women. Osseous lesions usually occur during middle age, with no gender predilection.

IMAGING FINDINGS

Soft tissue lipomas appear as radiolucent regions of fat radiodensity surrounded by the less radiolucent water density of the adjacent soft tissues (Fig. 15-61). They usually involve the extremities (Fig. 15-62).

Intraosseous lesions appear radiolucent, surrounded by a thin sclerotic rim of bone. Often a centrally located radiodense nidus of calcification is noted within the radiolucency (Fig. 15-63).[33] Osseous lesions are found predominately in the proximal femur and calcaneus (Figs. 15-64 and 15-65).

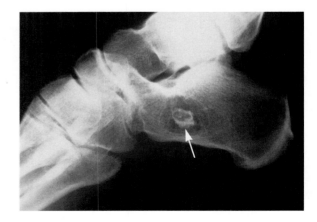

FIG. 15-63 Interosseous lipoma of the calcaneus demonstrating a central nidus of calcification *(arrow)*. (Courtesy Steven P. Brownstein, Springfield, NJ.)

PART TWO Bone, Joints, and Soft Tissues

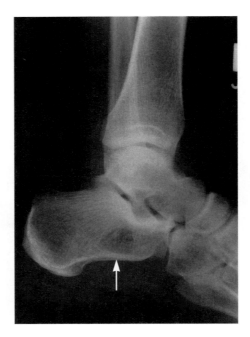

FIG. 15-64 Interosseous lipoma of the calcaneus *(arrow)*.

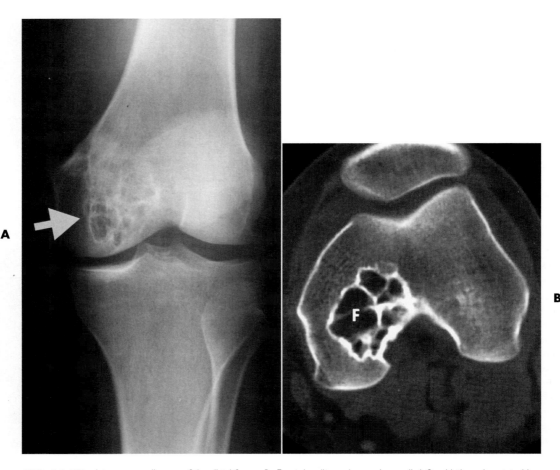

FIG. 15-65 Interosseous lipoma of the distal femur. **A,** Frontal radiograph reveals a well-defined lytic and septated lesion *(arrow)* in the epiphysis. Differential diagnosis for lytic epiphyseal lesions should include consideration of chondroblastoma, giant cell tumor, intraosseous ganglion, clear-cell chondrosarcoma, infection, and (rarely) eosinophilic granuloma. **B,** CT eliminates these possibilities by documenting low-density fat *(F)* within the lesion. (From Sartoris DJ: *Musculoskeletal imaging: the requisites,* St Louis, 1993, Mosby.)

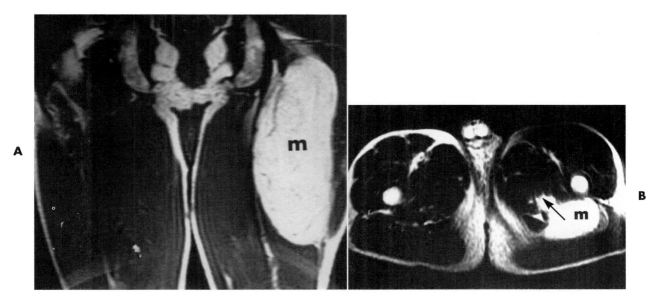

FIG. 15-66   Soft tissue lipoma of the thigh. **A,** Coronal T1-weighted MRI documents a large, relatively homogeneous fat-containing mass (m) in the posterior compartment. **B,** Transaxial T2-weighted image demonstrates predominant displacement of the adductor magnus muscle (arrow) by the mass (m). Differential diagnosis should include consideration of well-differentiated liposarcoma. (From Sartoris DJ: *Musculoskeletal imaging: the requisites,* St Louis, 1993, Mosby.)

Lipomas demonstrate a fat signal intensity on MRIs. The lesions are bright on T1-weighted images and bright to isointense on T2-weighted images (Fig. 15-66).

CLINICAL COMMENTS

Lipomas are usually asymptomatic, but localized pain, tenderness, and a soft tissue mass can occur, often exacerbated by activity of the affected region.[112] Multiple lesions may be associated with systemic hyperlipoproteinemia.[75]

KEY CONCEPTS

- *Soft tissue lipomas are radiolucent lesions usually seen in the extremities.*
- *Interosseous lesions are uncommon but when present, they appear as radiolucent lesions with a thin, sclerotic rim and often have a radiodense, calcific nidus.*
- *They occur most often in the proximal femur and calcaneus.*

Osteochondroma and Hereditary Multiple Exostosis

BACKGROUND

An osteochondroma (exostosis) is a benign outgrowth of bone covered by a cartilaginous cap of varying thickness. Osteochondromas are the most common benign skeletal neoplasm[85] and may arise in any bone that is preformed in cartilage.

Osteochondromas develop from a small dysplastic fragment of the epiphyseal growth plate and therefore stop growing when the patient reaches skeletal maturity. Growth beyond skeletal maturity suggests malignant degeneration. Malignant degeneration has been reported to occur in 1% to 2% of solitary lesions and from 1% to 3% or up to 25% of multiple lesions.[57,157,203] A cartilage cap of greater than 2 cm strongly suggests malignant transformation.[91]

Multiple inherited lesions are referred to as *hereditary multiple exostoses (HME)* or *diaphyseal aclasis* (Figs. 15-67 and 15-68). The term *diaphyseal aclasis* refers to the altered growth patterns of the

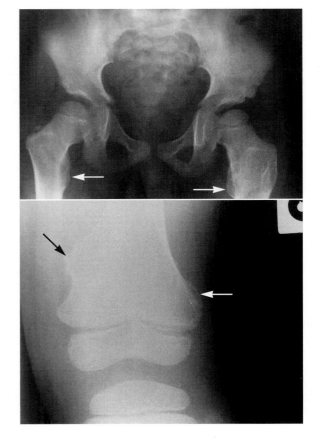

FIG. 15-67   Multiple osteochondromas and growth deformity of the proximal and distal tibia femora secondary to HME (arrows).

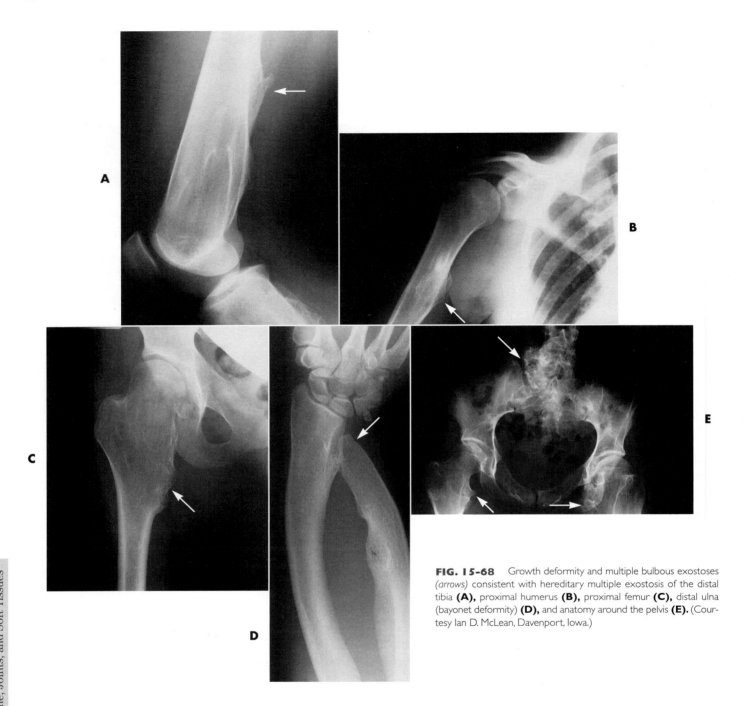

FIG. 15-68   Growth deformity and multiple bulbous exostoses *(arrows)* consistent with hereditary multiple exostosis of the distal tibia **(A)**, proximal humerus **(B)**, proximal femur **(C)**, distal ulna (bayonet deformity) **(D)**, and anatomy around the pelvis **(E)**. (Courtesy Ian D. McLean, Davenport, Iowa.)

involved bones. Wrist and ankle deformities are associated with relative shortening and bowing of the ulna and fibula.[157] Specifically, shortening of the ulna and outward bowing of the radius are referred to as a *bayonet deformity.* Multiple lesions are usually polyostotic and only rarely occur as multiple lesions within a single bone.

Single or multiple osteochondromas are usually discovered in patients before the age of 20 years.[20] A slight male predominance is noted.

IMAGING FINDINGS

Osteochondromas are found in the metaphyses of long bones, affecting the lower extremities more commonly than the upper extremities.[90,110] Most lesions occur around the knee.

Osteochondromas arise from the cortex and grow outward, pointing away from the nearest joint. They most often appear pe-

dunculated, with the pedicle blending in smoothly with the host bone's cortex (Figs. 15-69 through 15-72). Less often the lesion appears broad and flat, which is known as a *sessile osteochondroma.* It has been reported that the sessile configuration is more closely aligned with malignant transformation.[142]

FIG. 15-69   Solitary pedunculated osteochondromas *(arrows)* extending from the lesser trochanter **(A)**, lower scapula **(B)**, middle phalanx **(C)**, upper scapula **(D)**, femur **(E** and **F)**, lumbar vertebra **(G)**, and iliac fossa (seen en face) **(H)**. (*B* and *C,* Courtesy Ian D. McLean, Davenport, Iowa; *D* and *F,* Courtesy Steven P. Brownstein, Springfield, NJ; *E,* Courtesy William E. Litterer, Elizabeth, NJ; *H,* Courtesy Joseph W. Howe, Sylmar, Calif.)

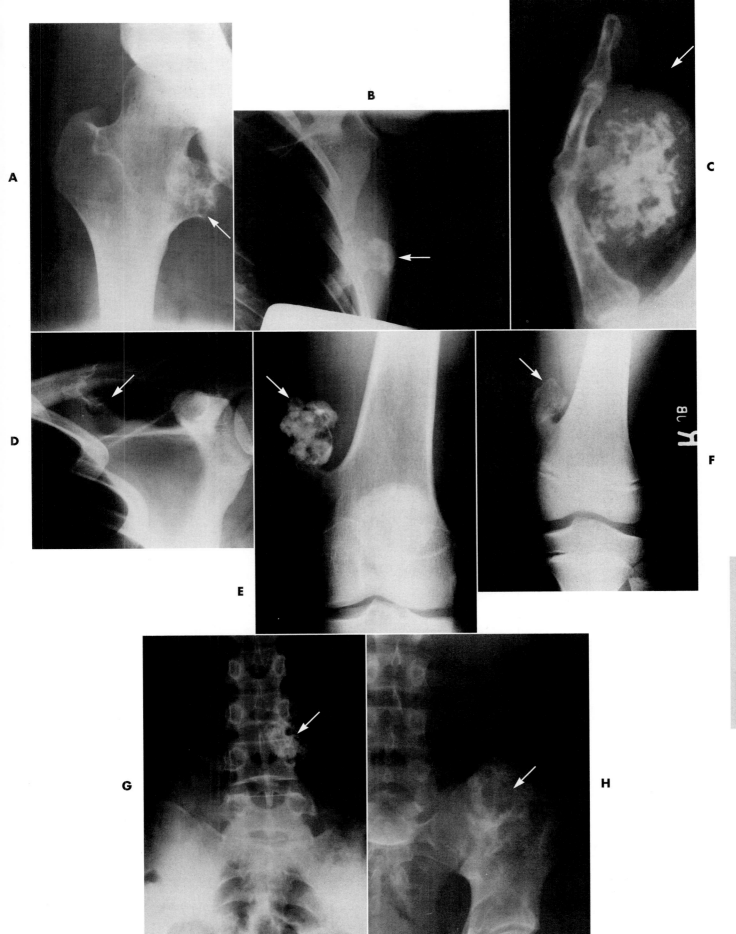

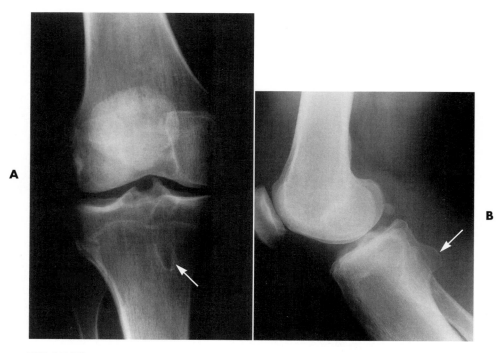

FIG. 15-70   Anteroposterior and lateral projection of the knee demonstrating a central radiolucent region in the proximal tibia (**A,** *arrow*) corresponding to the osteochondroma projection from the posterior surface of the proximal tibia (**B,** *arrow*). (Courtesy Ian D. McLean, Davenport, Iowa.)

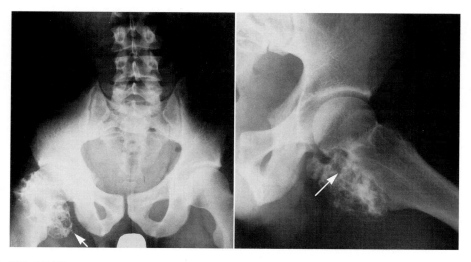

FIG. 15-71   Large "cauliflower" exostosis projecting anteriorly from the intertrochanteric region of the right femur. The appearance is characteristic of a pedunculated osteochondroma *(arrows)*.

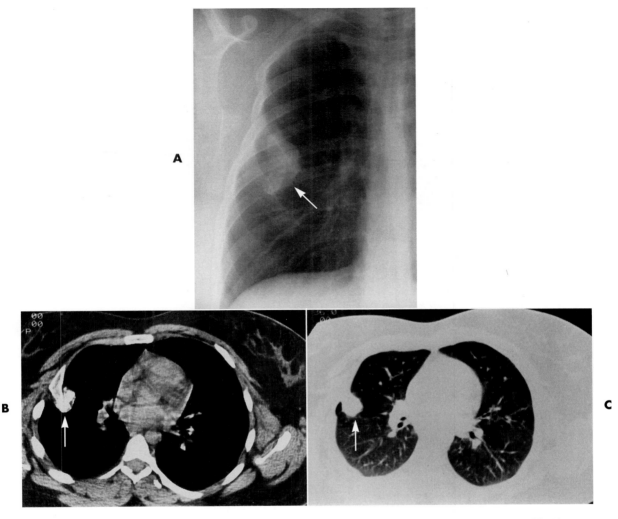

FIG. 15-72 Solitary osteochondroma projection inward *(arrows)* from the right chest wall on plain film **(A)** and CT with bone **(B)** and soft tissue windows **(C).** The axial image provided by CT demonstrates the extent of the lesion much better than plain film radiography. (Courtesy Jack C. Avalos, Davenport, Iowa.)

MRI and CT are useful to define the extent of the lesion, especially if malignant transformation is suspected or if the lesion originates from regions that are difficult to image with plain film (i.e., vertebral arch, ribs) (see Fig. 15-72). Radionuclide bone imaging may not accurately differentiate benign osteochondroma from malignant transformation to chondrosarcoma.[90,110]

CLINICAL COMMENTS

Patients typically present with a palpable mass, with or without pain. Pressure on the adjacent neurovascular bundle may produce neuropathy or vascular disturbance.[19,62] An enlarging painful osteochondroma suggests malignant degeneration. When necessary, treatment consists of surgical excision.

KEY CONCEPTS

- *Osteochondromas are the most common primary skeletal neoplasm.*
- *They are found in metaphyses of long bones, particularly around the knee.*
- *Osteochondromas are discovered usually in patients younger than 20 years of age.*
- *Malignant degeneration occurs in up to 2% of solitary and 25% of multiple lesions.*

Osteoid Osteoma and Osteoblastoma

BACKGROUND

An osteoid osteoma and osteoblastoma are histologically similar, benign bone lesions that differ in size and usually in radiographic appearance. Each consists of a highly vascularized nidus of connective tissue with interlacing trabeculae of osteoid and calcified bone surrounded by osteoblasts. Reactive bone response is variable and most often more pronounced on the cortical side of the lesions (less pronounced in osteoblastoma). Toward the center of the lesion, trabeculae merge into a mass of calcified bone. Osteoid osteomas and osteoblastomas usually occur in patients between the ages of 10 and 25 years, with a 2:1 male predominance.

IMAGING FINDINGS

Osteoid osteoma appears as a small (less than 1.5 cm in diameter) osteolytic lesion with surrounding reactive sclerosis (Fig. 15-73). The central radiolucent nidus may be only a few millimeters in diameter and often contains a small focus of calcification. The surrounding reactive sclerosis may become so prominent that it completely obscures the radiolucent nidus completely. Osteoid

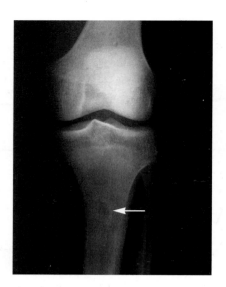

FIG. 15-73   Osteoid osteoma presenting as a central radiolucent region with thick surrounding sclerosis *(arrow)*. Brodie's abscess has a similar radiographic appearance. (Courtesy Steven P. Brownstein, Springfield, NJ.)

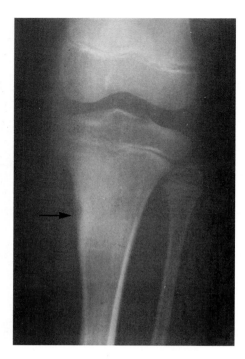

FIG. 15-75   Osteoid osteoma appearing with a central radiolucent nidus and surrounding sclerosis in the medial cortex of the proximal tibia *(arrow)*. (Courtesy Joseph W. Howe, Sylmar, Calif.)

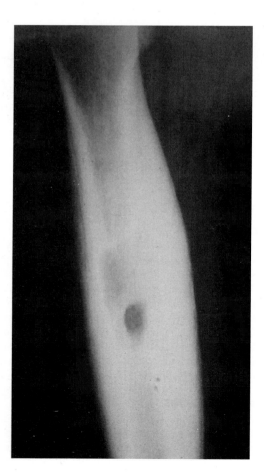

FIG. 15-74   The femur represents another frequent site for the development of an osteoid osteoma. (From Deltoff MN: *The portable skeletal x-ray*, St Louis, 1997, Mosby.)

osteomas are most commonly located in the cortex of long bones, usually the proximal femur (Fig. 15-74) or tibia (Fig. 15-75). Other locations include the posterior elements of the spine (e.g., concave side of painful scoliosis) (Fig. 15-76), humerus, hand, and talus. Osteoid osteomas are usually based in the cortex, but medullary, subperiosteal, and intracapsular locations do occur.[98]

Osteoblastoma appears as a larger (greater than or equal to 1.5 cm in diameter), geographical, expansile, generally nonaggressive, eccentric medullary lesion. It may exhibit a sclerotic component. Osteoblastomas are most commonly located in the posterior elements of the spine[125] (Fig. 15-77) and less frequently in the proximal femur, tibia, talus, ribs, and hands (Fig. 15-78).[129]

Because osteoid osteomas and osteoblastomas are richly vascularized, an intense uptake is noted on radionuclide bone scans. CT is valuable to further delineate the lesions and demonstrate a radiolucent nidus. This is particularly true when imaging areas of complex anatomy, such as the spine.

CLINICAL COMMENTS

Patients with osteoid osteomas and osteoblastomas often describe pain in the affected region. The pain begins as intermittent and vague, progressing to a dull and boring quality, which is typically not related to activity. Patients with osteoid osteomas often report a worsening of pain at night, which is characteristically alleviated by aspirin.[173]

Osteoid osteomas of the spine are typically located on the concave side of a painful scoliosis.[100] Osteoblastomas are also associated with scoliosis but do not exhibit a predilection for the concave side.[107] Markedly expansile osteoblastomas may cause canal stenosis. Clinically, an osteoid osteoma in a cortical location of the medial femoral neck may mimic an impeding stress fracture or infection. Excision is the preferred treatment for both lesions. Often the excision of the radiolucent nidus of an osteoid osteoma is followed by dramatic relief of the patient's complaint.[137]

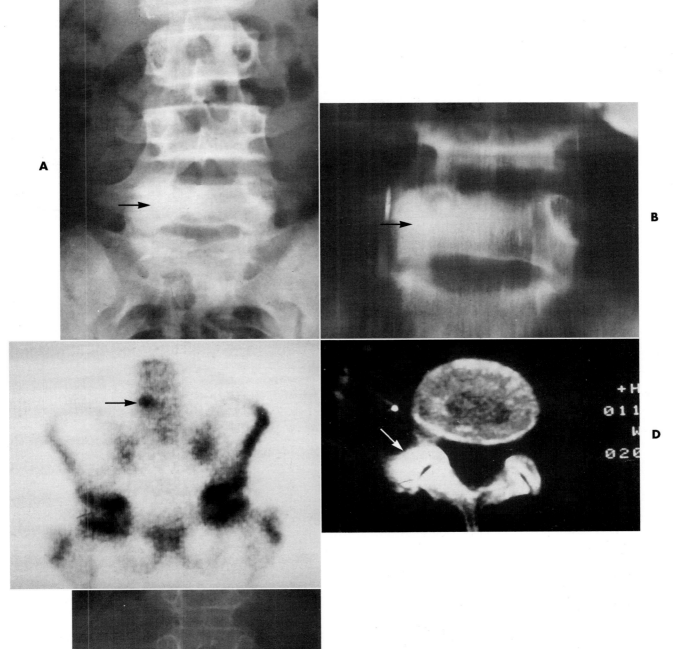

FIG. 15-76 **A,** The pedicle is a predilectory site for the development of an osteoid osteoma of the spine *(arrow)*. **B,** A tomogram manifests the homogenous sclerosis associated with an osteoid osteoma, suggesting a "bright" pedicle *(arrow)*. **C,** Increased radioisotopic uptake is noted in the presence of a pedicular osteoid osteoma *(arrow)*. **D,** A computed axial tomographic scan exhibits the presence of an osteoid osteoma in the vertebral arch *(arrow)*. **E,** Note the dense, homogeneous sclerosis, representing the "bright" pedicle associated with an osteoid osteoma of the neural arch. (From Deltoff MN: *The portable skeletal x-ray*, St Louis, 1997, Mosby.)

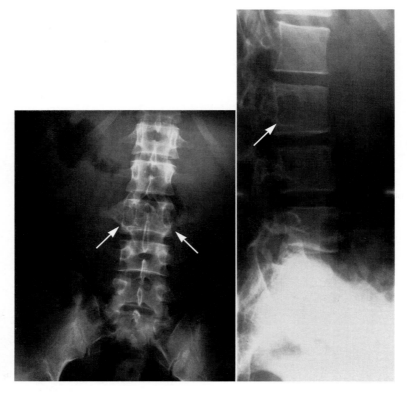

FIG. 15-77   Osteoblastoma presenting as an expansile osteolytic lesion of the vertebral body and arch of L3 *(arrows)*. (Courtesy Steven P. Brownstein, Springfield, NJ.)

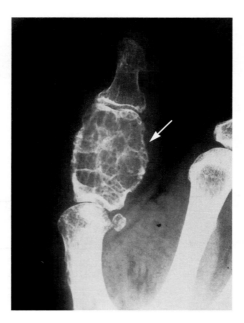

FIG. 15-78   Expansile, multilocular appearance of the proximal phalanx of the first digit resulting from an osteoblastoma *(arrow)*. (Courtesy Steven P. Brownstein, Springfield, NJ.)

Simple Bone Cyst

BACKGROUND

A simple (solitary or unicameral) bone cyst is a common, nonneoplastic, osteolytic, fluid-filled bone lesion of uncertain etiology. Its development may be related to a local disturbance of venous drainage, leading to increased intraosseous pressure, bone resorption, and replacement with intracellular fluid.[32,200] Cysts have been classified as active, demonstrating continued growth, when they abut the epiphyseal plate (Fig. 15-79), or inactive (latent) when they are separated from the plate by normal cancellous bone (Fig. 15-80). However, even cysts separated from the plate can continue to grow.[152] Growth is likely more related to the patient's age than location within the bone.

The majority of cases are discovered in patients before the age of 20 years, with an average age of 9 years.[21] Males are more commonly affected than females at a ratio of 3:1. Lesions in the ilium and calcaneus (Fig. 15-81) occur in a slightly older patient population than lesions in long bones.

IMAGING FINDINGS

Ninety percent of simple bone cysts are found in the proximal humerus and femur, with nearly a 2:1 ratio of the former to the latter. The ilium and calcaneus[182] are involved, usually in a slightly older patient population.

Simple cysts appear as mildly expansile, well-marginated, geographic osteolytic lesions in the metaphysis, less frequently the diaphysis, or rarely the epiphysis. The cortex is thinned but remains intact (Fig. 15-82).[119] The cyst's long axis parallels that of the host bone. A "fallen fragment" sign describes the appearance of bony fragments in the gravity-dependent portion of a fractured cyst and is present in up to 20% of all simple cysts.[188] A similar phenomenon occurring with an incomplete fracture is termed a *trap door sign*. The interior of the cyst often has ridges that may anchor true fibrous septations, and therefore use of the term *unicameral* (meaning monolocular, or one chamber) to describe simple bone cysts should be discouraged.

CLINICAL COMMENTS

Two thirds of patients seek clinical attention because of a pathological fracture of the cyst (Figs. 15-83 and 15-84).[2] Clinical signs

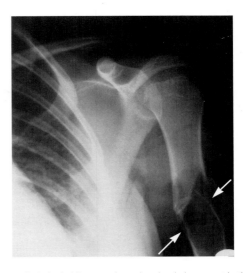

FIG. 15-80 Pathological fracture through a simple bone cyst in the diaphysis of the humerus *(arrows)*. (Courtesy Ian D. McLean, Davenport, Iowa.)

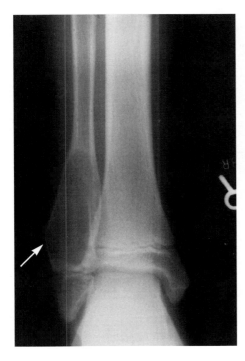

FIG. 15-79 Expansile, centrally located osteolytic lesion abutting the epiphyseal growth plate in the distal fibula *(arrow)*. (Courtesy Joseph W. Howe, Sylmar, Calif.)

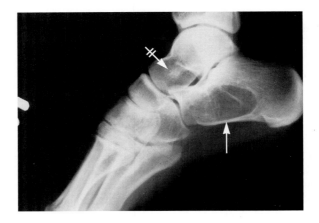

FIG. 15-81 Simple bone cyst in the calcaneus *(arrow)*. Incidentally, a bone island is noted in the talus *(crossed arrow)*. (Courtesy Steven P. Brownstein, Springfield, NJ.)

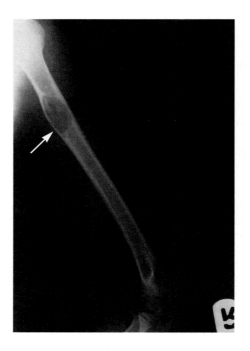

FIG. 15-82　Simple bone cyst in the diametaphyseal region of the humerus *(arrow)*. (Courtesy Ian D. McLean, Davenport, Iowa.)

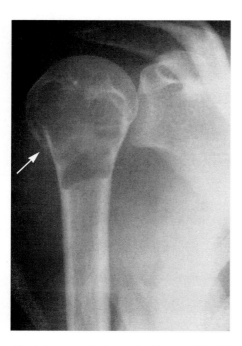

FIG. 15-83　Simple bone cyst in the proximal humerus. The thinned outer cortex of the lesion has fractured *(arrow)*. (Courtesy Steven P. Brownstein, Springfield, NJ.)

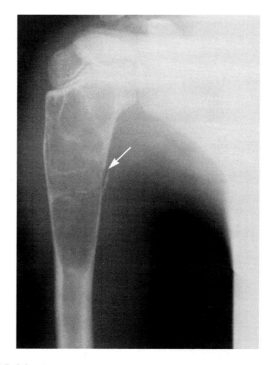

FIG. 15-84　Simple bone cyst in the proximal humerus with pathological fracture of the thinned medial cortex *(arrow)*. (Courtesy Ian D. McLean, Davenport, Iowa.)

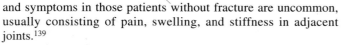

and symptoms in those patients without fracture are uncommon, usually consisting of pain, swelling, and stiffness in adjacent joints.[139]

Simple cysts in tubular bones often require treatment to prevent recurring pathological fractures and possible deformity. Treatment includes curettage and grafting, excision, saucerization, and more recently, percutaneous steroid injection.[78,139,145] Recurrence rates after curettage are around 18% to 20%.[8,21]

KEY CONCEPTS

- *Simple bone cysts are common benign tumors, 90% of which are found in the proximal humerus and femur.*
- *Patients are usually younger than 20 years of age.*
- *Lesions appear as central geographic lesions in the metaphysis, migrating to the diaphysis over time.*

Malignant Tumors

Adamantinoma

BACKGROUND

An adamantinoma (angioblastoma) is a rare, locally aggressive or malignant lesion composed of epithelium-like cells in dense fibrous stroma.[93] Similar appearing lesions of the mandible or maxilla are known as *ameloblastomas*. Adamantinomas typically occur between the ages of 25 and 40 years and are slightly more common in females.[165]

IMAGING FINDINGS

Ninety percent of lesions are found in the middle third of the tibia; less common sites include the fibula, ulna (Fig. 15-85), carpals, and metacarpals. They appear as central or eccentric, slightly expansile, well-circumscribed, osteolytic lesions. Rarely, multifocal lesions are found.[11]

CLINICAL COMMENTS

Patients often relate a history of trauma with clinical findings of swelling and pain in the involved extremity. Lesions tend to recur following excision.

KEY CONCEPTS

- *Adamantinomas are rare, locally aggressive lesions usually located in the tibial diaphysis.*
- *Adamantinomas occur between 25 and 40 years of age and demonstrate a high rate of reoccurrence following excision.*

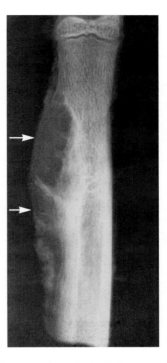

FIG. 15-85   Cadaveric specimen demonstrating expansile lesion of the ulna representing an adamantinoma *(arrows)*. (Courtesy Steven P. Brownstein, Springfield, NJ.)

Ameloblastoma

BACKGROUND

An ameloblastoma is an extremely rare, locally aggressive, odontogenic epithelial neoplasm that histologically mimics embryonal enamel but does not form hard dental tissue. Men and women are affected equally. The average patient age is 36 years,[162] and most patients are between the ages of 30 and 50 years.

IMAGING FINDINGS

An ameloblastoma appears as a slowly growing, expansile, well-defined, radiolucent lesion occurring most commonly in the molar regions of the mandible and less commonly in the maxilla (5:1 ratio).[99,146,162] Less often, ameloblastoma has a peripheral, nonosseous, mucosal location within the jaw.[7,10,147] Adamantinoma or angioblastoma has a similar radiographic appearance but occurs in the long bones of the skeleton, primarily the tibia.

CLINICAL COMMENTS

Lesions are often accompanied by painless swelling and a slow-growing mass in the jaw. A marked tendency exists for lesions to reoccur if inadequately excised. Radiographic unilocular lesions are treated less aggressively than multiloculated lesions.

KEY CONCEPTS

- *Ameloblastoma is a rare, radiolucent, slightly expansile lesion of the mandible.*
- *It is usually found in patients who are between 30 and 50 years of age.*

Chondrosarcoma

BACKGROUND

Chondrosarcomas are a heterogeneous group of bone neoplasms of which the basic neoplastic tissue is cartilaginous.[49] Chondrosarcomas are classified by histological subtype (clear-cell, mesenchymal, skull base, soft tissue, or soft parts), by histological grade or aggressiveness (low, medium, or high grade), by location (central or peripheral), or by the presence of a precursor lesion (primary or secondary).[186] They represent the third most common primary malignant tumor of bone, following multiple myeloma and osteosarcoma. The higher the histological grade, the more likely metastasis is to occur.

Primary chondrosarcomas arise de novo. Secondary chondrosarcomas develop from solitary or multiple enchondromas (Ollier's disease), solitary or multiple osteochondromas (hereditary multiple exostosis), synovial osteochondrometaplasia, chondromyxoid fibromas, and chondroblastomas. Because of this association, growing or painful preexisting benign cartilaginous tumors warrant particular clinical attention. The secondary chondrosarcoma is the most malignant of the chondrosarcomas, associated with an extremely high risk of distant metastasis.

Central chondrosarcomas arise within the medullary canal, and peripheral lesions arise from the surface of the bone. Primary chondrosarcomas are virtually always central.

Chondrosarcomas are more common in males, at a ratio of 3:2.[160] Although presentation ranges widely, most patients are between the ages of 50 and 70 years. Peripheral chondrosarcomas tend to occur in slightly younger patients.[76]

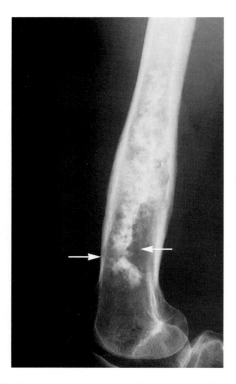

FIG. 15-86 Central chondrosarcoma of the distal femur. The lesion demonstrates stippled calcification and endosteal cortical bone destruction *(arrows)*. (Courtesy Steven P. Brownstein, Springfield, NJ.)

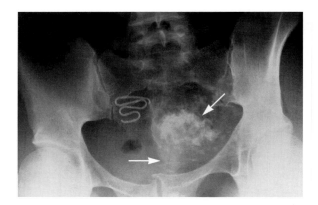

FIG. 15-88 Chondrosarcoma of the sacrum demonstrating soft tissue mass, stippled matrix calcification, and bone destruction *(arrows)*. (Courtesy Joseph W. Howe, Sylmar, Calif.)

IMAGING FINDINGS

Although chondrosarcomas may involve any bone, most are found in the pelvis, proximal femur, proximal humerus, distal femur, proximal tibia, and ribs.[43,65,76,170] The radiographic appearance is varied, depending on the type of chondrosarcoma. Primary, central chondrosarcomas appear most often as metaphyseal regions of bone destruction with scattered stippled calcification (Fig. 15-86)[164] and periosteal reaction. Endosteal cortical thinning is noted, but rarely is the cortex destroyed. The more aggressive types exhibit extraosseous soft tissue masses (Figs. 15-87 and 15-88). Matrix calcification is characteristic but may be absent in up to 30% of cases. Often, chondrosarcomas appear relatively nonaggressive (Fig. 15-89).

On MRI examination, the low-grade lesions often appear as lobulated hyaline cartilage masses with increased signal intensity on the T2-weighted scans (Fig. 15-90). High-grade lesions may demonstrate inhomogeneous increased signal intensity on the T2-weighted scans. MRI demonstrates the degree of soft tissue involvement. CT is better to detect the presence of calcification or ossification within the matrix of the lesion.

CLINICAL COMMENTS

The most common presenting clinical complaint is progressive, but not debilitating, pain in the hip and buttocks of more than 3 months' duration. The pain often occurs at night and is not alleviated by rest. Aside from a slight limp and limited range of motion, the patient appears in excellent health. Laboratory findings are typically normal.

Resection is the preferred treatment for all chondrosarcomas. The prognosis depends on the histological grade of the tumor and on the adequacy of the resection. Irradiation and chemotherapy play minimal roles.[64,86] MRI provides the most accurate assessment of the extent of involvement and most often precedes resection.

KEY CONCEPTS

- *Chondrosarcomas are the third most common malignant primary bone tumor, arising as primary lesions or secondary to benign cartilaginous tumors (such as enchondromas and osteochondromas).*
- *Chondrosarcomas are common in the pelvis, proximal femur, and proximal humerus.*
- *They most often occur in patients between the ages of 50 and 70 years.*
- *Matrix calcification is usually present and may appear nonaggressive.*

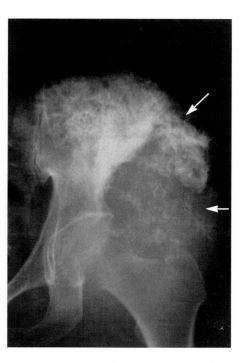

FIG. 15-87 Chondrosarcoma of the ilium with a large soft tissue mass, stippled matrix calcification, and bone destruction *(arrows)*. (Courtesy Joseph W. Howe, Sylmar, Calif.)

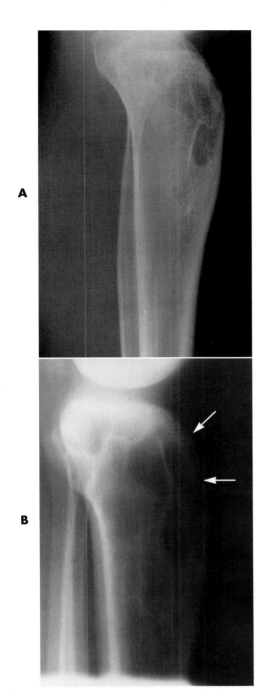

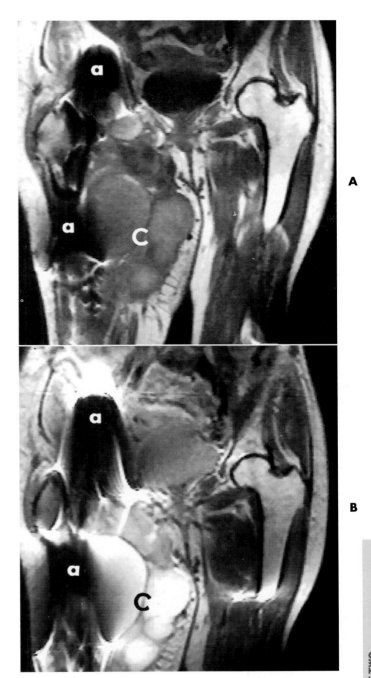

FIG. 15-89   Plain film **(A)** and linear tomogram **(B)** of a chondrosarcoma in the proximal tibia exhibiting a relatively nonaggressive appearance *(arrows)*. (Courtesy Joseph W. Howe, Sylmar, Calif.)

FIG. 15-90   Recurrent chondrosarcoma following surgical resection. **A,** Coronal T1-weighted MRI demonstrates a lobulated mass *(C)* of low signal intensity arising from the femoral diaphysis *(a,* artifact from orthopedic hardware). **B,** The lesion *(C)* exhibits high signal intensity on a corresponding T2-weighted image *(a,* artifact from orthopedic hardware). Differential diagnosis should include consideration of other osseous and soft tissue malignancies. (From Sartoris DJ: *Musculoskeletal imaging: the requisites,* St Louis, 1993, Mosby.)

Chordoma

BACKGROUND

A chordoma is a rare, solitary, malignant neoplasm that develops from remnant portions of the notochord.[191] The cells of the tumor are arranged in lobules with abundant quantities of extracellular mucus. Some of the cells contain vacuoles of mucus that resemble soap bubbles, known as *physalipherous cells*. Chordomas are slow-growing, recurring neoplasms that incapacitate by locally aggressive growth; less than 10% of cases demonstrate distal metastasis. Parachordoma describes an extraaxial, soft tissue tumor that is histologically similar to a chordoma.[95,171,178]

Chordomas may develop in men and women of all ages.[101] Sacrococcygeal chordomas occur most often in patients between the ages of 40 and 70 years, with greater male predominance in a ratio of 2:1. Sphenoocciput lesions occur most often in patients between the ages of 30 and 60 years, with equal gender distribution.

IMAGING FINDINGS

In the sacrococcygeal region, 48% of chordomas arise, in the sphenoocciput 39%, and in the mobile spine less than 13%.[16] Rarely, chordomas have been noted in the mandible, maxilla, and scapula. Chordomas are twice as common in the cervical spine as the other mobile spinal regions; C2 vertebral body is the most common site.

Chordomas are midline lesions, characterized by the presence of bone destruction and a large soft tissue mass (Fig. 15-91). Calcification is noted in up to 40% of lesions on plain films. Although most of the calcification is probably dystrophic tissue calcification, undoubtedly some also represent bony debris. Contrary to other neoplasms, chordomas may cross the intervertebral disc to involve adjacent segments.

CLINICAL COMMENTS

Regardless of the location, lesions may produce local pain and soft tissue mass. Sphenoocciput chordomas may have accompanying headaches, sinus pain, and symptoms related to the eyes (diplopia is characteristic), ears, or throat.[72,136] Bowel and bladder dysfunction may accompany sacrococcygeal lesions.[1] Radiation is applied to those lesions that cannot be resected.[18,201]

KEY CONCEPTS

- *Chordomas are tumors histologically derived from notochord.*
- *Approximately 48% of chordomas appear in the sacrococcygeal region, 39% in the sphenoocciput region, and 13% in the mobile spine (usually C2 body).*
- *Most lesions occur in patients between 30 and 70 years of age.*

Ewing's Sarcoma

BACKGROUND

Ewing's sarcoma is a small, malignant round cell neoplasm of uncertain origin. Traditionally, Ewing's sarcoma was thought to originate from noncommitted mesenchymal cells; however, more recent studies suggest an association between Ewing's sarcoma and a neuroectodermal origin.[47,120,208] Ewing's sarcoma is the fourth most common primary malignant tumor of bone after multiple myeloma, osteosarcoma, and chondrosarcoma.

Although Ewing's sarcoma has been reported in patients from ages 5 months to 79 years, 90% of cases involve patients younger than 30 years of age.[61,148] It exhibits a strong predilection for whites[114,134] and a slight predilection for males.

IMAGING FINDINGS

Ewing's sarcoma may occur in any bone of the body, although the majority of cases occurs in the pelvis (Fig. 15-92) and long bones of the lower extremities. A diaphyseal location is classic, but a metadiaphysis is more common (Fig. 15-93).[44,61]

The radiographic appearance is marked by permeative osteolytic bone destruction, cortical erosion or saucerization, laminated or "hair-on-end" periosteal reaction, and a large soft tissue mass (Fig.

FIG. 15-91 Sacrococcygeal chordoma appearing as a midline osteolytic lesion with dystrophic calcification with the matrix *(arrows)*. Surgical vascular clips and contrast from intravenous pyelogram are incidentally noted. (Courtesy Joseph W. Howe, Sylmar, Calif.)

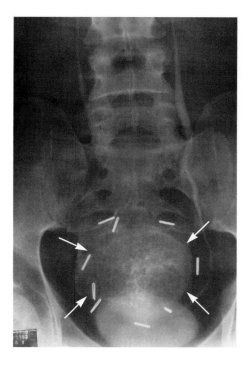

15-94).[163] Ewing's sarcoma is less commonly a mixed osteolytic and sclerotic lesion (Fig. 15-95). Only rarely does Ewing's sarcoma appear as a predominantly sclerotic lesion. Ewing's tumor may appear similar to other round cell tumors, including lymphoma and metastatic neuroblastoma.

CLINICAL COMMENTS

Usually patients experience a lengthy history of diffuse pain and swelling involving the affected region. Other symptoms frequently include an elevated sedimentation rate, erythema, leukocytosis, and fever, mimicking osteomyelitis. The prognosis is poor. Treatment includes chemotherapy, radiation, and resection.

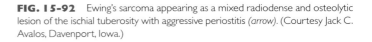

KEY CONCEPTS

- *Ewing's sarcoma is the fourth most common primary malignant tumor.*
- *Patients are usually younger than 30 years of age.*
- *The clinical presentation may mimic an infection.*
- *Ewing's sarcoma typically presents as a metadiaphyseal permeative osteolytic lesion with cortical saucerization and aggressive periosteal changes, and less commonly appears as an osteosclerotic lesion.*

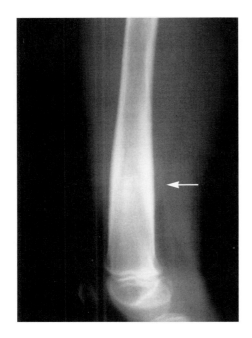

FIG. 15-92   Ewing's sarcoma appearing as a mixed radiodense and osteolytic lesion of the ischial tuberosity with aggressive periostitis *(arrow)*. (Courtesy Jack C. Avalos, Davenport, Iowa.)

FIG. 15-93   Ewing's sarcoma presenting as increased radiodensity and periosteal irregularity of the diametaphyseal region of the distal femur *(arrow)*. (Courtesy Steven P. Brownstein, Springfield, NJ.)

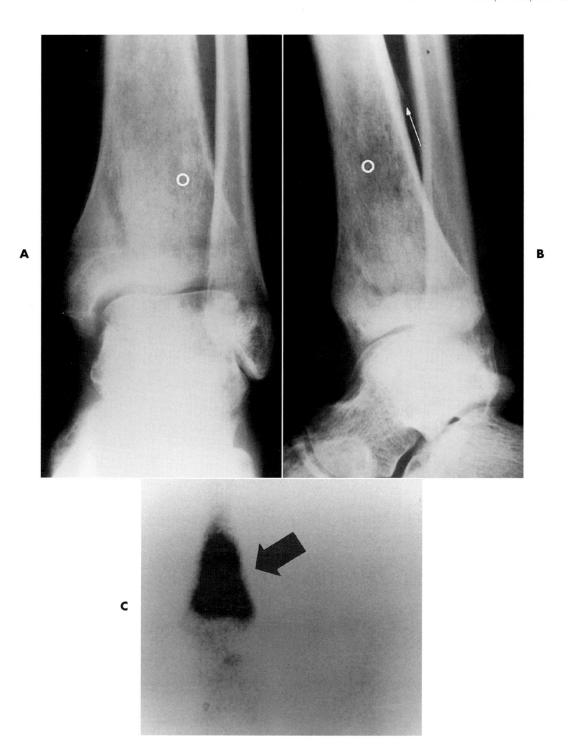

FIG. 15-94   Ewing's sarcoma. **A** and **B,** Frontal and lateral radiographs reveal permeative osteolysis *(o)* in the distal tibia with an associated Codman's triangle *(arrow).* **C,** The process exhibits increased activity *(arrow)* on a radionuclide bone scan. (From Sartoris DJ: *Musculoskeletal imaging: the requisites,* St Louis, 1993, Mosby.)

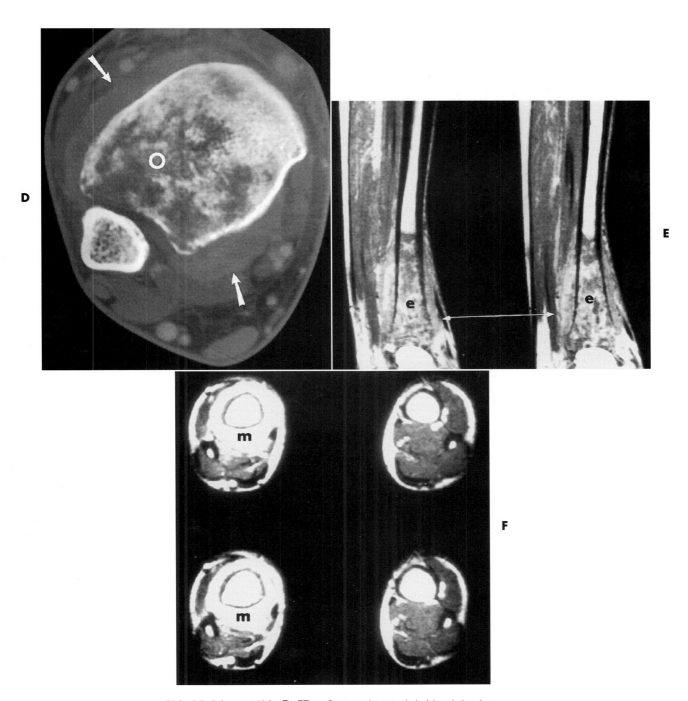

FIG. 15-94—cont'd **D,** CT confirms patchy osteolysis *(o)* and also documents a soft tissue mass *(arrows)*. **E,** Coronal T1-weighted MRIs demonstrate inhomogeneous marrow replacement *(e)* with soft tissue extension *(double-headed arrow)*. **F,** Transaxial T2-weighted images reveal homogeneous high signal intensity within both the marrow and soft tissue mass *(m)*. Differential diagnosis should include consideration of metastatic disease, fibrosarcoma, lymphoma, and other round cell neoplasms.

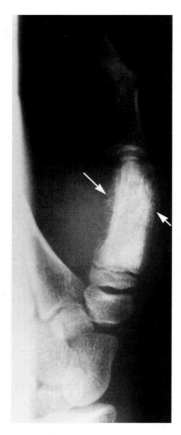

FIG. 15-95   Mixed radiodense and osteolytic lesion of the first metacarpal. Aggressive periostitis is noted *(arrows)* and consistent with Ewing's tumor. (Courtesy Ian D. McLean, Davenport, Iowa.)

Fibrosarcoma and Malignant Fibrous Histiocytoma

BACKGROUND

A fibrosarcoma is an uncommon malignant tumor derived from deep fibrous tissue. It is characterized by the presence of immature fibroblasts with variable amounts of collagen formation. Fibrosarcomas produce no osteoid in either the primary bone lesion nor in their metastatic deposits.

A malignant fibrous tumor that contains both fibroblasts and histiocytes is termed *malignant fibrous histiocytoma (MFH).*[27,69,183,184] MFH is more commonly a lesion within soft tissue than bone (Fig. 15-96). Malignant fibrous tumors arise de novo, or in association with other lesions, including marrow infarct[135] previous radiation therapy, Paget's disease[37] enchondroma, chronic osteomyelitis,[42] and prosthetic replacement.[82]

Fibrosarcoma affects the sexes equally; the typical patient age is between 10 and 50 years. MFH demonstrates a 1.5:1 male predominance; the typical patient age is between 10 and 70 years.

IMAGING FINDINGS

Fifty percent of fibrosarcomas and MFH of bone are found in the distal femur, and less commonly the proximal tibia, humerus (Fig. 15-97), fibula, radius, and pelvis.[13,161] Up to 80% of lesions are found around the knee. Both malignant fibrous lesions appear similarly. They demonstrate geographic (Fig. 15-98), moth-eaten (Figs. 15-99 and 15-100), or permeative (Fig. 15-101) osteolytic destruc-

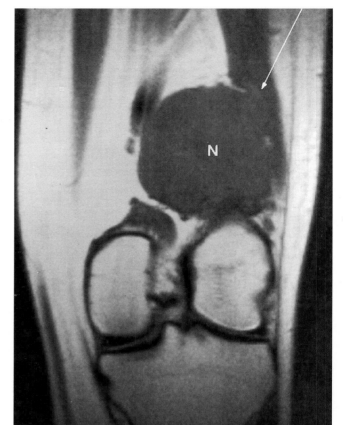

A

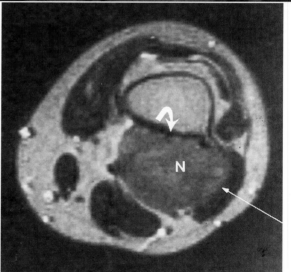

B

FIG. 15-96   Low-grade malignant fibrous histiocytoma. **A,** Coronal T1-weighted MRI demonstrates a well-defined soft tissue neoplasm *(N)* of low signal intensity superior to the femoral condyles and with displacement of the adjacent biceps femoris muscle *(arrow).* **B,** Transaxial T2-weighted image reveals intermediate signal intensity within the lesion *(N),* which has invaded the biceps femoris muscle *(arrow)* and posterior femoral cortex *(curved arrow).* Differential diagnosis should include consideration of fibrosarcoma, desmoid tumor, and other soft tissue neoplasms of predominantly fibrous composition. (From Sartoris DJ: *Musculoskeletal imaging: the requisites,* St Louis, 1993, Mosby.)

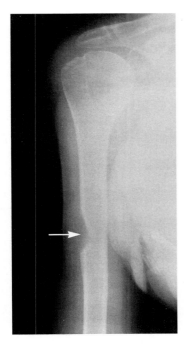

FIG. 15-97 70-year-old woman with outer cortical saucerization of the humeral diaphysis secondary to fibrosarcoma *(arrow)*. (Courtesy Steven P. Brownstein, Springfield, NJ.)

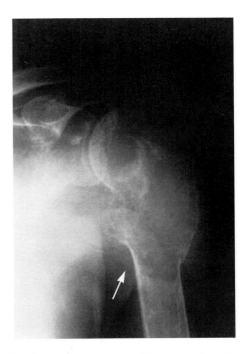

FIG. 15-98 Geographic bone lesion with poor margins and cortical breakthrough with soft tissue mass *(arrow)* secondary to fibrosarcoma. (Courtesy Joseph W. Howe, Sylmar, Calif.).

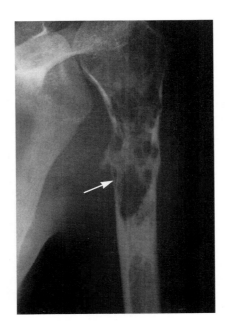

FIG. 15-99 Malignant degeneration of fibrous dysplasia to fibrosarcoma. The lesion demonstrates moth-eaten bone destruction of the proximal humerus without visible matrix calcification *(arrow)*. (Courtesy Steven P. Brownstein, Springfield, NJ.)

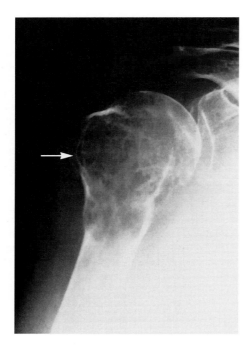

FIG. 15-100   Malignant fibrous histiocytoma with moth-eaten destruction of the proximal humerus *(arrow).* (Courtesy Steven P. Brownstein, Springfield, NJ).

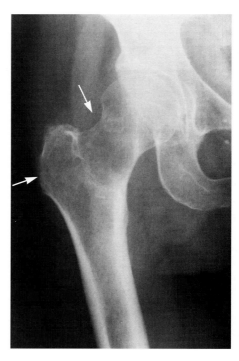

FIG. 15-101   Fibrosarcoma with permeative destruction of the femoral neck and greater trochanter *(arrows).* (Courtesy Joseph W. Howe, Sylmar, Calif.).

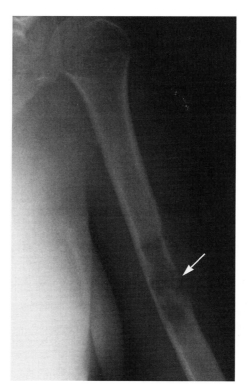

FIG. 15-102   Cortical destruction of the humeral diaphysis secondary to malignant fibrous histiocytoma *(arrow).* (Courtesy Joseph W. Howe, Sylmar, Calif.)

tion. They are typically located in the metaphysis, often extending into the diaphysis. Cortical destruction (Fig. 15-102), extraosseous mass, and periosteal reaction are often present. The tumor matrix does not exhibit calcification, although occasional bony fragments may be present. Central fibrosarcomas are more common than peripheral lesions.

CLINICAL COMMENTS

Typically patients complain of pain, tenderness, and soft tissue swelling in the involved region. One third of patients demonstrate pathological fracture. Fibrosarcomas and MFH are aggressive lesions and carry poorer prognoses with soft tissue involvement.

KEY CONCEPTS

- *Fibrosarcomas and malignant fibrous histiocytomas are aggressive osteolytic tumors developing as primary or secondary lesions.*
- *Fibrosarcoma occurs in patients between 10 and 50 years of age.*
- *MFH occurs in patients between 10 and 70 years of age.*
- *MFH is more commonly a lesion of soft tissue.*
- *Fibrosarcomas and MFH usually occur around the knee.*

Liposarcoma

BACKGROUND

A liposarcoma is a malignant tumor of adults, usually occurring in the deep intermuscular or periarticular planes of the buttocks, thigh, calf, and retroperitoneal tissues. Liposarcomas are the second most common soft tissue sarcoma, following malignant fibrous histiocytoma (MFH). Liposarcoma of bone is extremely rare. Liposarcoma usually occurs in patients between 30 and 50 years of age.

IMAGING FINDINGS

The appearance is variable, from a highly aggressive lesion with soft tissue density to a well-defined mass often of fat radiodensity. They appear most commonly in the buttocks, thigh (Fig. 15-103), calf, and retroperitoneal space. Often, dystrophic calcification or ossification can be observed within the soft tissue mass.

The MRI appearance is marked by increased signal intensity on the T2-weighted image and mixed to increased signal intensity on the T1-weighted images. Most aggressive soft tissue lesions demonstrate a high signal on the T2-weighted images (Figs. 15-104 and 15-105), but the increased signal intensity on the T1-weighted scans is characteristic of the fatty tissues of the liposarcoma, although this appearance is not seen necessarily in all liposarcomas.

CLINICAL COMMENTS

Liposarcomas are often asymptomatic during early stages of development and therefore may be extremely large at clinical presentation. Once the lesion has been identified, surgery is indicated and accomplished through wide excision, which is often combined with chemotherapy. Recurrence and metastasis, usually to the lungs, is common.

KEY CONCEPTS

- *Liposarcoma is the second most common soft tissue sarcoma.*
- *Common locations for liposarcoma include the buttocks, thigh, calf, and retroperitoneal tissues.*
- *Patients are usually between 30 and 50 years of age.*
- *Liposarcomas are often asymptomatic initially and therefore may be large when clinically recognized.*

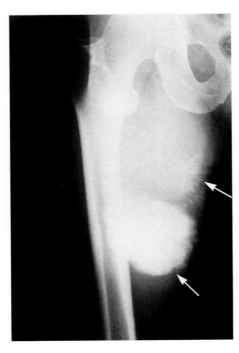

FIG. 15-103 Liposarcoma presenting as a large soft tissue mass of the inner thigh (*arrows*). (Courtesy Steven P. Brownstein, Springfield, NJ.)

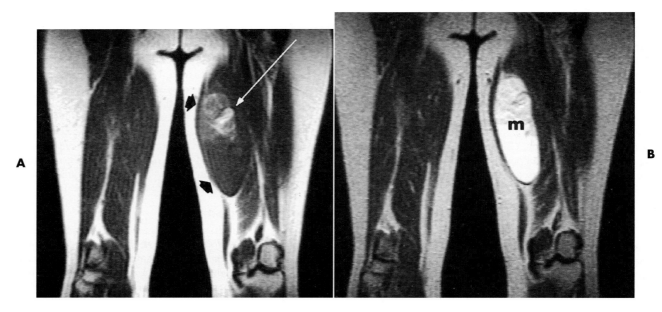

FIG. 15-104   Liposarcoma of the thigh. **A,** Coronal T1-weighted MRI reveals a heterogeneous fat-containing *(white arrow)* mass *(black arrows),* suggesting the correct diagnosis. **B,** The mass *(m)* exhibits uniformly high signal intensity on a corresponding T2-weighted image. Other fat-containing soft tissue lesions include lipoma, macrodystrophia lipomatosa, hemangioma, and neurofibromatosis. (From Sartoris DJ: *Musculoskeletal imaging: the requisites,* St Louis, 1993, Mosby.)

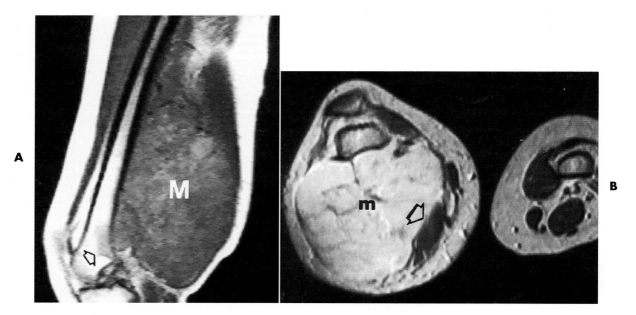

FIG. 15-105   Poorly differentiated liposarcoma of the thigh. **A,** Sagittal T1-weighted MRI demonstrates a large inhomogeneous mass *(M)* containing only sparse fat with early invasion of the distal femur *(arrow).* **B,** Transaxial T2-weighted image reveals predominantly high signal intensity within the mass *(m),* which has invaded and displaced the semimembranous muscle *(arrow).* Differential diagnosis should include consideration of other soft tissue sarcomas. (From Sartoris DJ: *Musculoskeletal imaging: the requisite,* St Louis, 1993, Mosby.)

Lymphoma

BACKGROUND

A lymphoma is a malignant tumor composed of lymphocytes, and less commonly histiocytes, that arises from lymph nodes, the spleen, or other sites of lymphoid tissue anywhere in the body. Lymphomas are classified by cell type, degree of differentiation, and nodular or diffuse pattern of distribution. Hodgkin's disease (HD) is a distinctive form of lymphoma, separated from the larger, more common spectrum of non-Hodgkin's lymphoma (NHL) on the basis of the characteristic appearance of cellular morphology exhibited (Reed-Sternberg cells).

Lymphoma involves bone as either a primary focus or secondary to systemic lymphoma. Primary lymphoma of bone is incorporated within the NHL classification and is often referred to as *reticulum cell sarcoma of bone*. By definition, primary lymphoma of bone is nonsystemic. Lymphoma is classified as a primary bone lesion if the single osseous lesion, with occasional minimal regional metastasis, is the only lymphoma lesion found in the body. Burkitt's lymphoma is a type of primary bone lymphoma (Fig. 15-106). Secondary lymphoma of bone may develop from systemic NHL and HD.

Primary NHL lymphoma of bone occurs at any age and affects men more often than women.[156] The average age is 34 years and 50% of patients are between 10 and 30 years of age.[22,39,70,177] Secondary bone involvement from systemic NHL or HD is more common among children with the former and adults with the latter.

IMAGING FINDINGS

Eighty-eight percent of patients with primary lymphoma of bone present with a single osseous lesion that fulfills the definition of primary NHL of bone.[39] Four percent of all patients with systemic NHL present with a concurrent skeletal lesion. Twenty percent of patients with HD demonstrate concurrent osseous lesions.[12,199]

Osseous lesions caused by primary NHL of bone are radiographically indistinguishable from metastatic osseous lesions caused by systemic NHL and HD.[121] All types of lymphoma usually exhibit a permeative pattern of osteolytic bone destruction (Fig. 15-107). Osteoblastic lesions are more common secondary to HD, often presenting as "ivory vertebra" (Fig. 15-108). Soft tissue masses are common and periosteal reactions are infrequent.[166]

Primary lymphoma of bone predominates in the lower extremities (Fig. 15-109). Secondary (metastatic) bone involvement from systemic NHL and HD most commonly involves the spine, pelvis, and ribs. Burkitt's lymphoma is most common in the mandible and maxilla (see Fig. 15-106).[25]

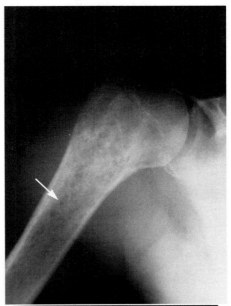

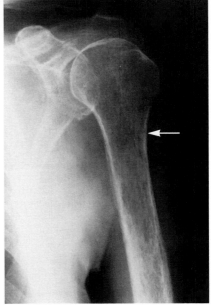

FIG. 15-107   Two cases of lymphoma presenting as a permeative osteolytic process involving the proximal humerus *(arrows)*. (*Top,* Courtesy Joseph W. Howe, Sylmar, Calif.; *Bottom,* Courtesy Steven P. Brownstein, Springfield, NJ.)

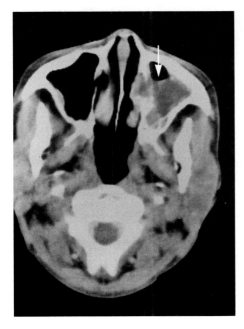

FIG. 15-106   CT scan of a patient with Burkitt's lymphoma. The scan demonstrates partial filling of the left maxillary sinus with thickening and irregularity of the medial sinus wall *(arrow)*. (Courtesy Steven P. Brownstein, MD, Springfield, NJ.)

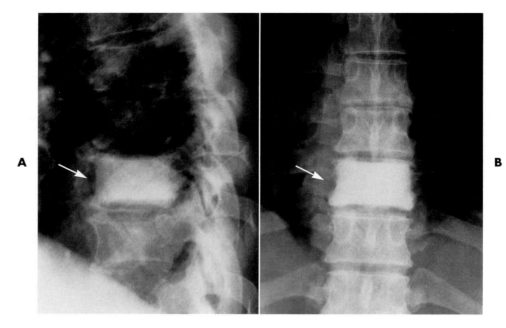

FIG. 15-108   Lymphoma presenting as a radiodense "ivory vertebra" lesion of the lower thoracic spine in the lateral **(A)** and anteroposterior **(B)** projection *(arrows).*

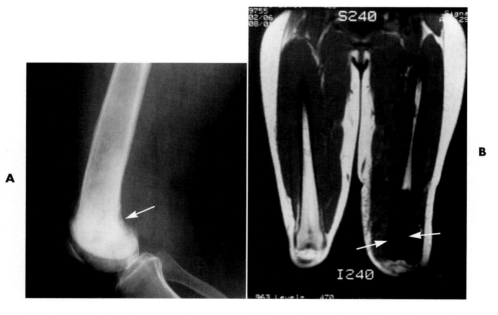

FIG. 15-109   Lymphoma presenting as a sclerotic lesion in the lower femur **(A)** and demonstrating decreased marrow signal intensity on the T1-weighted MRI **(B)** consistent with marrow replacement in the distal region of the left femur secondary to lymphoma *(arrows).* (Courtesy Ian D. McLean, Davenport, Iowa.)

CLINICAL COMMENTS

Patients with osseous lymphoma typically complain of pain in the region of involvement but otherwise appear healthy. Radiation therapy, with or without adjuvant chemotherapy, may control the local bone lesions for years.

■ KEY CONCEPTS

- *Primary lymphoma of bone and secondary lymphoma of bone (systemic NHL and HD) appear as permeative radiolucent lesions of the lower extremities, pelvis, and spine.*
- *Although generally osteolytic, bone lesions secondary to HD are the most common to appear osteosclerotic ("ivory vertebra").*
- *Lymphoma of bone occurs in patients over a wide age range.*

Metastatic Bone Disease

BACKGROUND

Dissemination. Metastatic bone disease represents the osseous dissemination of cells originating from a primary malignant neoplasm. Cells are most often transported to bone by antegrade hematogenous means secondary to venous or lymphatic access, and are less commonly transported by direct extension or retrograde venous flow. The lungs, liver, and red marrow are common initial sites of metastasis via hematogenous seeding. The high frequency of metastasis to the axial skeleton is explained by its rich supply of red marrow.[106,130]

Skeletal distribution. Metastasis is more common in the lumbar and thoracic spine than the cervical spine. Skeletal involvement distal to the elbows or knees, referred to as *acral metastasis,* is unusual and when present is usually from a primary lung neoplasm.

Cellular origin. Skeletal metastases are much more common than primary malignant neoplasms of bone. Although deriving an accurate prevalence ratio is complicated by patient age[73], cell type, bones involved and other sampling factors, the overall ratio of metastatic lesions to primary bone malignancies has been reported at 25:1.[122] Not all primary malignant neoplasms have an equal propensity to metastasis to bone. Metastatic bone disease most often originates from primary lesions in the prostate, breast, kidney, thyroid, and lung. Sixty percent of metastatic bone disease in males arises from prostate neoplasms and 70% in women arises from primary neoplasms of the breast.

In children, metastasis is most often associated with neuroblastomas, retinoblastoma, Ewing's tumor, osteosarcoma, and lymphoma. In patients with known metastases, the primary lesion is not always easy to find. In one survey, less than 50% of primary lesions could be established in those with known metastatic disease.[180]

Age. Although metastasis may occur at any age, the disease predominantly affects those over the age of 40 years.

Sensitivity of imaging. Plain film radiology is relatively insensitive to alterations of osseous density. Lesions are radiographically apparent when 30% to 50% of bone destruction is present.[31,35,59] In contrast, radionuclide studies can demonstrate as little as 5% to 10% osseous change.[154] Although the sensitivity of radionuclide imaging is much greater during early stages of metastases, the difference in practical circumstances is probably less pronounced. Because most patients present with advanced disease, both the radionuclide imaging and the plain films are likely to be positive.[193] However, with early metastatic disease, up to 40% of patients with positive bone scans have normal radiographs.[30,114]

In diffuse metastatic disease, the radioisotope accumulation of a bone scan may be so uniform that the pattern mimics a normal scan.

This phenomenon, known as a *superscan,* is distinguished from a normal scan by a superscan's near lack of radioisotope collection in the kidneys and bladder. Radionuclide imaging is sensitive but not specific for metastatic disease. In fact, up to 30% of solitary abnormalities detected on bone scans of patients with primary malignancy have been shown to be benign processes.[36] Often, positive scans require follow-up biopsies,[34] radiographs, or other specialized imaging studies to identify the pathological process.

Although bone scans and plain film imaging are most dominant in assessing patients for metastatic disease, CT and MRI are helpful in further delimiting the extent of involvement. However, because of their smaller region of study and higher cost, CT and MRI are rarely the first imaging choice.

IMAGING FINDINGS

The imaging findings reflect the aggressiveness of the primary lesion. An enlarging metastatic mass of primary tumor cells elicits varying amounts of osteoclastic bone resorptive and osteoblastic bone deposition response. Depending on which of these processes predominates, an osteolytic (Figs. 15-110 and 15-111), osteoblastic (Figs. 15-112 and 15-113), or mixed (Figs. 15-114 and 15-115) radiographic appearance evolves. Overall, osteolytic lesions are much more common than either osteoblastic or mixed appearances.

Metastatic bone disease typically appears as a polyostotic moth-eaten pattern of destruction with poorly defined zones of transition surrounding the lesions (Fig. 15-116). Periosteal reaction and soft tissue masses are usually small or absent. Spinal metastases may present radiographically as only an indistinct compression fracture. Metastasis has a propensity to involve the vertebral body (Figs. 15-117 through 15-124) and pelvis (Figs. 15-125, through 15-130). The pedicle region is also predisposed. Bilateral pedicle destruction causes a "blind" vertebra (Fig. 15-131), and unilateral destruction causes a "one-eyed" vertebra (Fig. 15-132 and 15-133). An

Text continued on p. 696

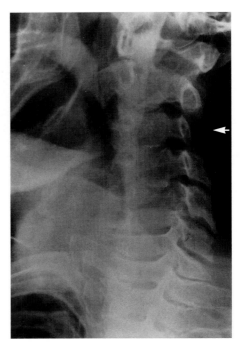

FIG. 15-110   Osteolytic metastasis to the articular pillar of C3 *(arrow).* (Courtesy Joseph W. Howe, Sylmar, Calif.).

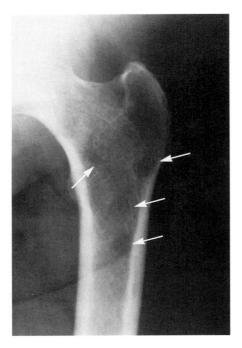

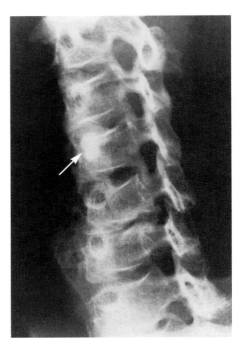

FIG. 15-111   Several foci of osteolytic metastasis involving the proximal femur in a patient with primary breast malignancy *(arrows).* (Courtesy Joseph W. Howe, Sylmar, Calif.)

FIG. 15-112   Osteoblastic metastasis of the C4 pedicle *(arrow).* (Courtesy Joseph W. Howe, Sylmar, Calif.)

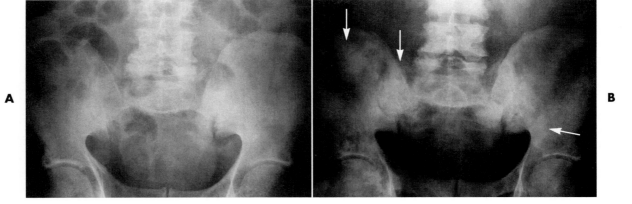

FIG. 15-113   Osteoblast metastasis of the pelvis *(arrows).* The condition has progressed from the initial film **(A)** to the film taken 16 months later **(B).** (Courtesy Steven P. Brownstein, Springfield, NJ.)

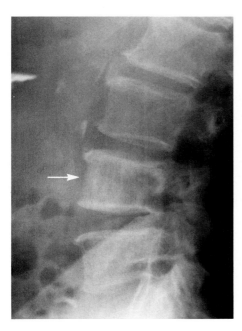

FIG. 15-114 Mixed osteolytic and osteoblastic metastasis of the L4 vertebral body *(arrow)*. (Courtesy Ian D. McLean, Davenport, Iowa.)

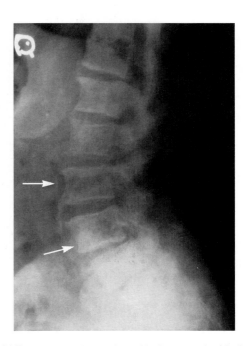

FIG. 15-115 Mixed osteolytic and osteoblastic metastasis of the lumbar spine *(arrows)*. (Courtesy Ian D. McLean, Davenport, Iowa.)

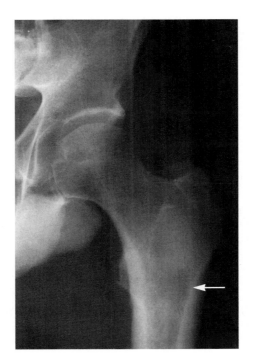

FIG. 15-116 Patient with primary lung carcinoma and focal osteolytic bone metastasis to the proximal femoral bone *(arrow)*. (Courtesy Joseph W. Howe, Sylmar, Calif.)

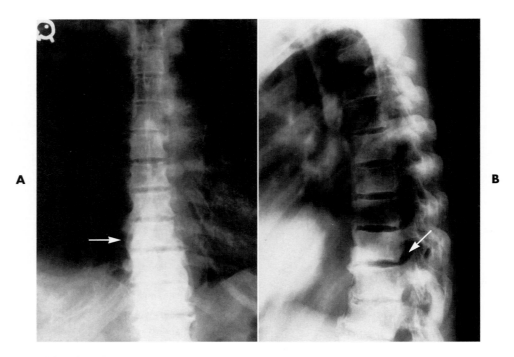

FIG. 15-117 Anteroposterior **(A)** and lateral **(B)** lumbar projections demonstrating generalized osteoblastic of the thoracolumbar spine *(arrows)*. (Courtesy Ian D. McLean, Davenport, Iowa.)

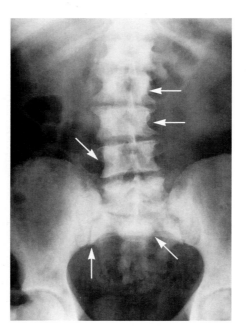

FIG. 15-118 Generalized osteoblastic metastasis in a 72-year-old male with a primary malignancy of the prostate *(arrows)*. (Courtesy Steven P. Brownstein, Springfield, NJ.)

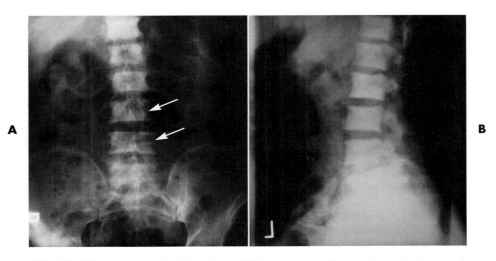

FIG. 15-119 Anteroposterior **(A)** and lateral **(B)** lumbar spine radiographs demonstrating generalized increased bone density consistent with predominantly osteoblastic metastasis. The left pedicle shadows of L3 and L4 are indistinct *(arrows)*.

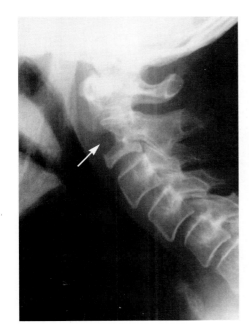

FIG. 15-120 Osteolytic bone metastasis of the anterior portion of the C2 vertebral body *(arrow)*. (Courtesy Steven P. Brownstein, Springfield, NJ.)

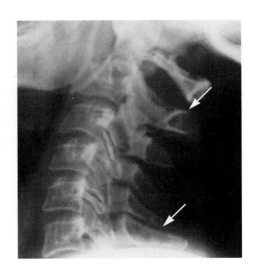

FIG. 15-121 "Punched-out" osteolytic metastasis involving the spinous processes of C2 and C7 *(arrows)*. (Courtesy Ian D. McLean, Davenport, Iowa.)

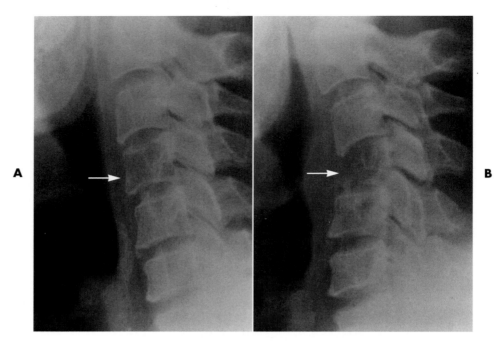

FIG. 15-122   Initial **(A)** and 3 months following **(B)** lateral cervical projections of a patient with osteolytic metastasis arising from a primary thyroid malignancy. In a short period of time the radiographic changes have significantly advanced *(arrows)*. (Courtesy Joseph W. Howe, Sylmar, Calif.).

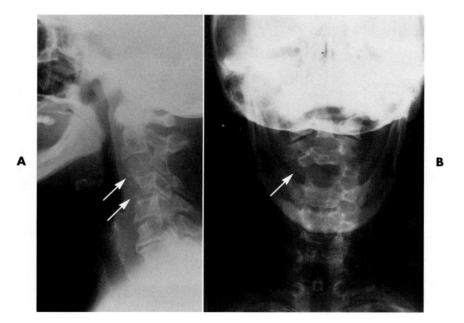

FIG. 15-123   A, Osteolytic metastasis involving the C3 and C4 vertebral bodies *(arrows)*. **B,** In the anteroposterior projection the right side of the C3 segment is nearly completely destroyed *(arrow)*. (Courtesy Ian D. McLean, Davenport, Iowa.)

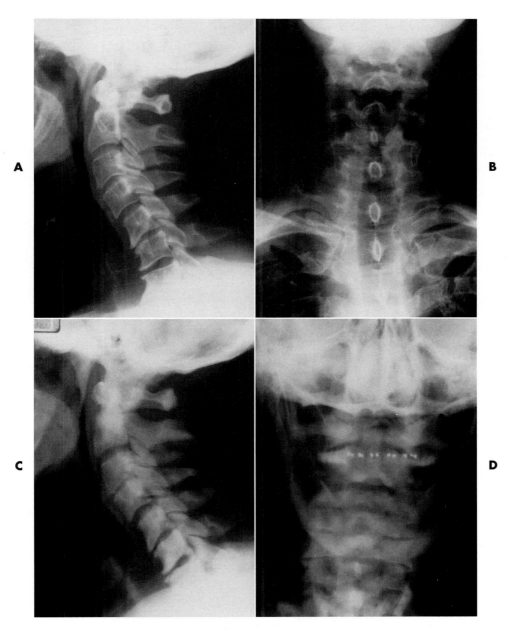

FIG. 15-124 Blastic metastasis. **A** and **B**, Initial lateral and frontal cervical projections demonstrate only kyphosis and spondylosis; the bone density is normal. Approximately 17 months later, the same projection (**C** and **D**) presents a generalized increase in the bone density. (Courtesy Steven P. Brownstein, Springfield, NJ.)

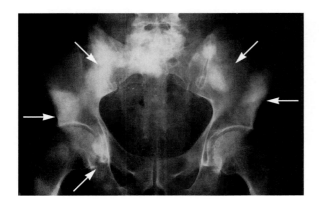

FIG. 15-125 Well-defined osteoblastic metastasis occurring throughout the pelvis (arrows). (Courtesy Joseph W. Howe, Sylmar, Calif.)

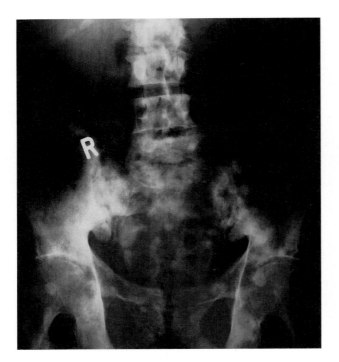

FIG. 15-126   Widely disseminated osteoblastic metastasis of the pelvis. (Courtesy Ian D. McLean, Davenport, Iowa.)

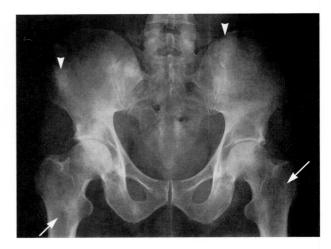

FIG. 15-127   Mixed osteolytic *(arrows)* and osteoblastic *(arrowheads)* metastatic bone disease.

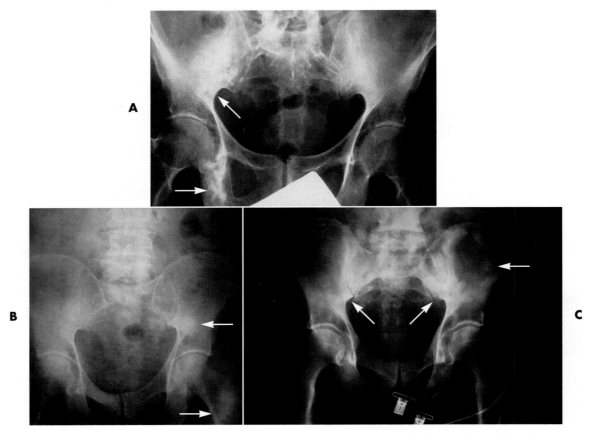

FIG. 15-128   Osteoblastic metastasis in three patients. **A,** Osteoblastic metastasis of the right ischium and lower ilium *(arrows).* **B,** Osteoblastic metastasis occurring in the left ilium and the intertrochanteric region of the left femur *(arrows).* **C,** Radiodense metastatic nodules scattered throughout the pelvis *(arrows).*

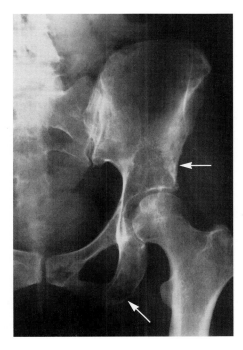

FIG. 15-129   Radiolucent osteolytic bone lesions secondary to metastasis *(arrows)*. (Courtesy Joseph W. Howe, Sylmar, Calif.)

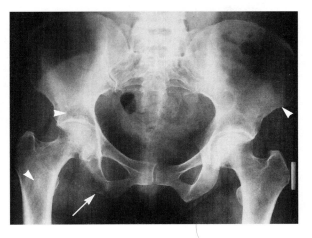

FIG. 15-130   Mixed osteolytic *(arrow)* and osteoblastic *(arrowheads)* metastasis to the pelvis. (Courtesy Steven P. Brownstein, Springfield, NJ.)

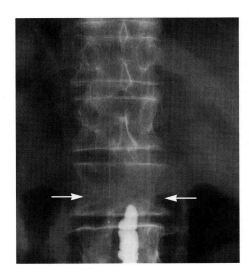

FIG. 15-131   Osteolytic metastasis destroying both pedicles at the L2 level (blind vertebra) *(arrows)*. (Courtesy Steven P. Brownstein, Springfield, NJ.)

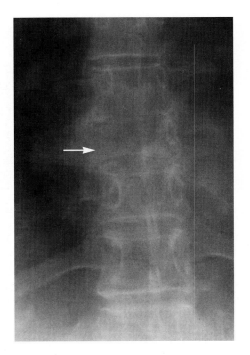

FIG. 15-132   Osteolytic metastasis causing destruction of one pedicle, relating a one-eyed vertebra or winking owl sign *(arrow)*. (Courtesy Joseph W. Howe, Sylmar, Calif.)

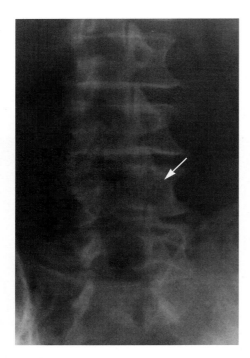

FIG. 15-133 Osteolytic metastasis causing expansion and destruction of the left L4 pedicle *(arrow)*. (Courtesy Joseph W. Howe, Sylmar, Calif.)

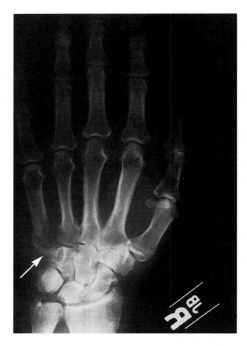

FIG. 15-135 Osteolytic bone metastasis of the proximal fifth metacarpal *(arrow)*. Metastasis is rare distal to the elbows and knees. When it occurs it is known as *acral metastasis* and often arises from primary lung malignancies. (Courtesy Steven P. Brownstein, Springfield, NJ.)

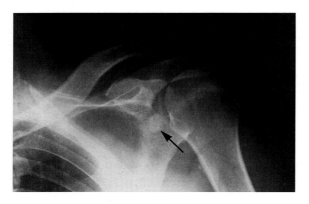

FIG. 15-134 Solitary focus of osteoblastic metastasis occurring in the left body of the scapula *(arrow)*. Metastasis uncommonly occurs as a solitary focus. (Courtesy Joseph W. Howe, Sylmar, Calif.)

atypical presentation of expansile, bubbly, solitary geographic lesions is associated with primary lesions of the thyroid and kidney.[53] Purely osteoblastic lesions occur most often from breast, prostate, GI, bladder, and lung neoplasms. Extremities are uncommonly involved (Fig. 15-134), especially distal to the knees and elbows (acral metastasis) (Fig. 15-135).

On MRI, metastatic lesions are noted as regions with hypointense signal on the T1-weighted scans, which become hyperintense on the T2-weighted sequence (Figs. 15-136 and 15-137). This appearance is consistent with marrow replacement by tumor tissue. CT is very helpful to further delineate cortical bone involvement (Fig. 15-138). On bone scintigraphy, the metastatic lesions appear as hot spots often widely disseminated throughout the skeleton (Fig. 15-139). Chest radiography may reveal pulmonary

abnormality in a patient in whom skeletal metastasis is suspected. The pulmonary pattern is characteristically marked by multiple nodules or masses. In addition, rib metastasis may lead to an extrapleural sign (Figs. 15-140 and 15-141).

CLINICAL COMMENTS

A high index of clinical suspicion for the presence of metastasis accompanies patients with spinal pain who are over the age of 40 or who have a known primary malignancy. Characteristically the pain they experience is not related to trauma or appreciably affected by activity. It is commonly more severe at night, often reported to awaken the patient. Expanding osseous lesions may encroach on the spinal canal, producing neurological signs and symptoms.

At first, with metastases, laboratory parameters remain normal. As the disease progresses, an increased erythrocyte sedimentation rate (ESR), serum alkaline phosphatase, and serum calcium concentration are often found, although their absence does not exclude disease. Once metastasis has occurred, the prognosis is typically poor. Treatment is directed at alleviating the patient's pain and includes radiotherapy,[102] corticosteroids, and decompressive laminectomy.[48]

KEY CONCEPTS

- *Skeletal metastasis is 25 times as common as primary malignant tumors of bone.*
- *The most common mechanism is hematogenous seeding from primary tumors; the breast gives rise to 70% of female lesions, and prostate 60% of male lesions.*
- *Skeletal metastasis has a predilection for the axial skeleton and is rarely found distal to elbows or knees.*
- *Patients are typically older than 40 years of age.*
- *Lesions appear as areas of osteolytic destruction with no or small soft tissue mass and periosteal reaction.*

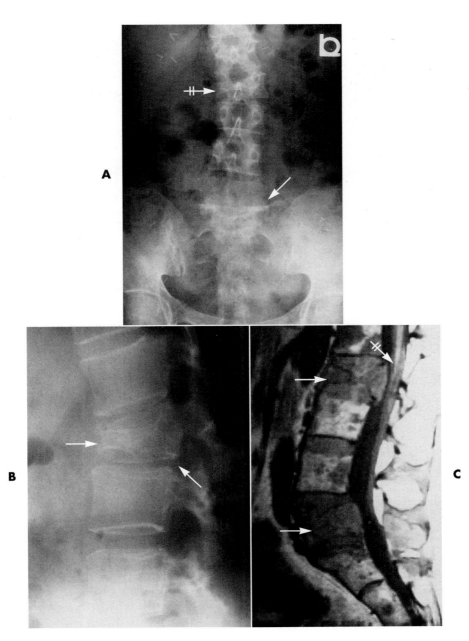

FIG. 15-136 Osteolytic metastatic bone disease. The frontal projection **(A)** shows multiple regions of osteolytic bone destruction in the sacrum, missing pedicle shadows at L5 *(arrow)*, and compression fracture of L2 *(crossed arrow)*. In the lateral projection **(B),** the compressed vertebrae is posteriorly displaced *(arrows)*. The T1-weighted MRI scan **(C)** reveals mild effacement of the thecal sac *(crossed arrow)*, and multiple hypointense regions where normal hyperintense marrow has been replaced by tumor tissue *(arrows)*. This is particularly the case at L5, which appears homogeneously hypointense. (Courtesy Robert C. Tatum, Davenport, Iowa.)

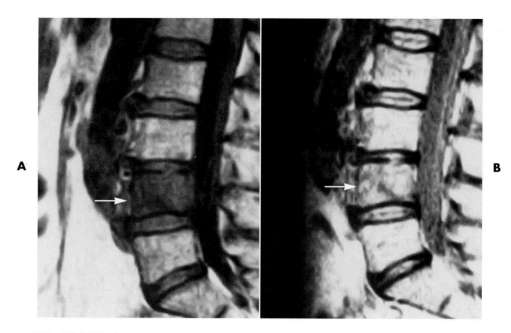

FIG. 15-137 Metastatic bone disease. **A,** T1-weighted sagittal MRI demonstrating hypointense signal from the L4 vertebra body secondary to tumor replacement of the normally bright bone marrow *(arrow)*. **B,** On the T2-weighted sagittal MRI the L4 vertebrae demonstrates a bright signal intensity, indicating the presence of a water-based pathology representing the tumor *(arrow)*.

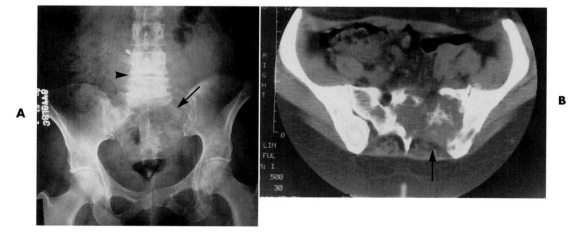

FIG. 15-138 Plain film **(A)** and CT scan **(B)** of mixed osteolytic *(arrows)* and osteoblastic *(arrowhead)* metastasis to the pelvis and lumbar spine.

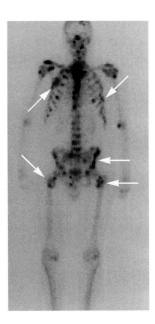

FIG. 15-139 Multiple, asymmetrical areas of increased radionuclide uptake ("hot spots") widely distributed throughout the spine, ribs, skull, and pelvis *(arrows)*. (Courtesy Ian D. McLean, Davenport, Iowa.)

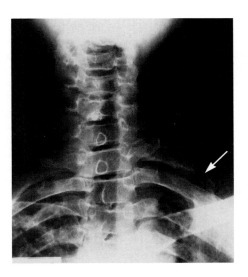

FIG. 15-140 Osteolytic metastasis to the lateral angle of the left first rib *(arrow)*. (Courtesy Steven P. Brownstein, Springfield, NJ.)

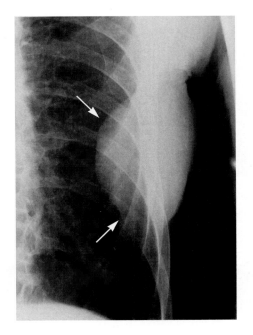

FIG. 15-141 Inward soft tissue mass of the chest wall *(arrows)* secondary to rib metastasis. (Courtesy Steven P. Brownstein, Springfield, NJ.)

Multiple Myeloma and Plasmacytoma

BACKGROUND

A multiple myeloma (MM) is a malignant proliferation of plasma cells occurring predominately in the red marrow of various bones. Numerous diffuse foci or larger nodular accumulations of malignant plasma cells are surrounded by areas of increased osteoclastic activity. It is believed that the abnormal plasma cells produce osteoclastic-activating factors[167] and osteoblastic inhibitory factor, which leads to increased bone resorption and decreased bone formation.[9,56] Initially MM invades the axial skeleton, progressing to the appendicular skeleton over time. It represents the most common primary malignant tumor of bone. Most patients with MM are between the ages of 50 and 70 years; rarely are those under the age of 30 years affected.[94] A slight male predominance is often reported.

IMAGING FINDINGS

Rarely, MM presents as one or more sclerotic lesions (Fig. 15-142), typically part of a larger syndrome known as *POEMS. POEMS* is an acronym for *p*olyneuropathy, *o*rganomegaly, *e*ndocrinopathy, *m*yeloma, and *s*kin changes.

Up to 30% of MM patients exhibit a solitary lesion of bone, known as a *plasmacytoma* (Figs. 15-143 through 15-146). Plasmacytomas appear as large (typically larger than 4 cm in diameter), expansile, cystic lesions, which may progress to MM (Figs. 15-147 and 15-148).

Most commonly, MM occurs as multicentric (polyostotic) lesions of punch-out or moth-eaten patterns of bone destruction (Figs. 15-149 and 15-150). Less commonly, MM presents as diffuse osteopenia without focal bone destruction—probably the most difficult presentation to recognize, because it mimics osteoporosis.[29]

MM lesions exhibit a short zone of transition and no surrounding sclerosis, have no visible matrix (except in POEMS), and are usually less than 4 cm in diameter. MM originates in bones that are high in red marrow content. The skull, vertebral bodies, ribs, and proximal humerus and femurs are most commonly involved. Extraosseous manifestations are rare, found in fewer than 5% of patients.[80,143]

Plain film radiography appears more sensitive than radionuclide bone scanning; however, both miss a significant portion of cases. MRI is highly sensitive and is used in cases of negative radiographic and radionuclide imaging.[192]

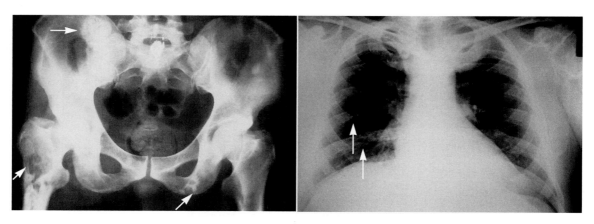

FIG. 15-142   Mixed osteolytic and osteosclerotic lesions of the ribs and pelvis of a patient with multiple myeloma *(arrows)*. (Courtesy Steven P. Brownstein, Springfield, NJ.)

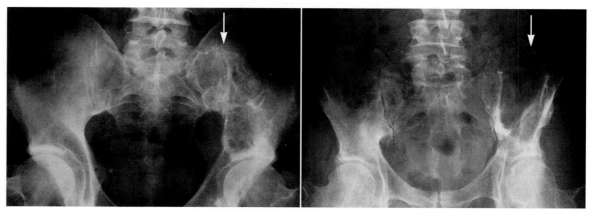

FIG. 15-143   Plasmacytoma presenting as expansile cystic lesions of the left ilium in different patients *(arrows)*. (*Left,* Courtesy Ian D. McLean, Davenport, Iowa; *Right,* Courtesy Steven P. Brownstein, Springfield, NJ.)

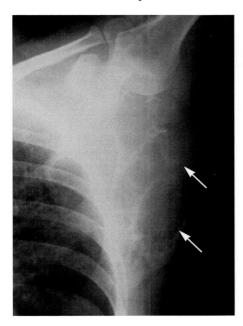

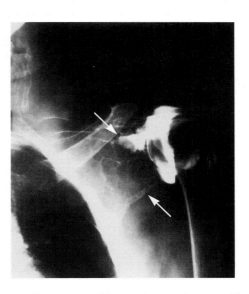

FIG. 15-144 Expansile cystic lesion of the scapula representing plasmacy-toma *(arrows)*. (Courtesy Steven P. Brownstein, Springfield, NJ.)

FIG. 15-145 Plasmacytoma of the scapula presenting as a multiloculated ex-pansile lesion *(arrows)*. This lesion was discovered accidentally during arthrography examination. (Courtesy Steven P. Brownstein, Springfield, NJ.)

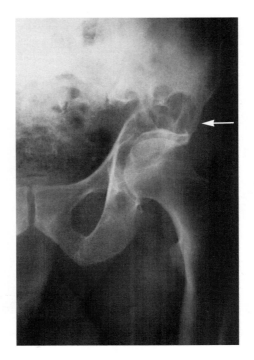

FIG. 15-146 Plasmacytoma of the left ilium, producing the characteristic ap-pearance of a multiloculated expansile lesion with a sclerotic margin *(arrow)*. Plas-macytomas are most common to the spine and pelvis. (Courtesy Joseph W. Howe, Sylmar, Calif.)

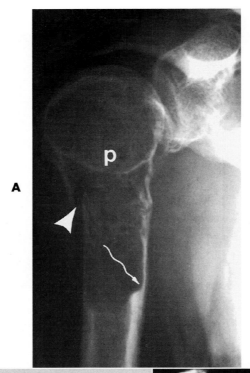

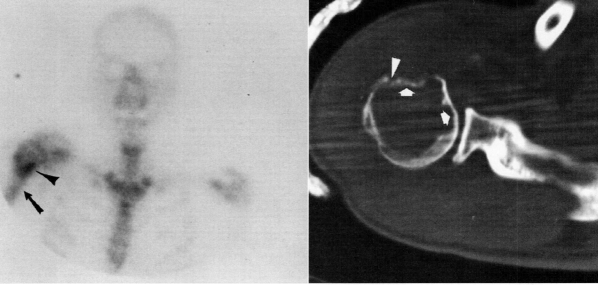

FIG. 15-147 Plasmacytoma of the proximal humerus. **A,** Radiography reveals a septate lytic lesion *(p)* with endosteal scalloping *(curved arrow)* and pathological fracture *(arrowhead)*. **B,** Increased activity is present within the lesion *(arrow)* and particularly at the site of fracture *(arrowhead)* as seen on a radionuclide bone scan. **C,** CT optimally demonstrates the degree of cortical thinning *(arrows)*, as well as the fracture *(arrowhead)*. (From Sartoris DJ: *Musculoskeletal imaging: the requisites,* St Louis, 1993, Mosby.)

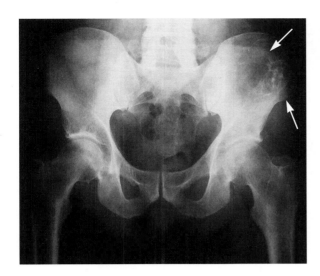

FIG. 15-148 Cystic lesion of the left ilium, representing plasmacytoma *(arrows)*.

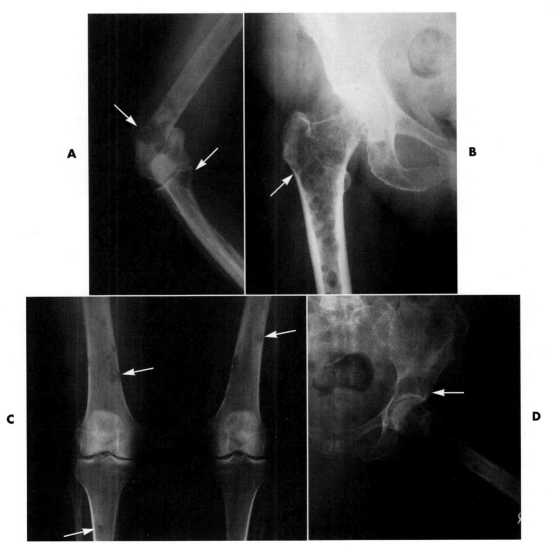

FIG. 15-149 Multiple myeloma causing punch-out osteolytic defects *(arrows)* of the humerus **(A)**, ulna **(A)**, proximal femora **(B)**, distal femur **(C)**, and ilium **(D)**.

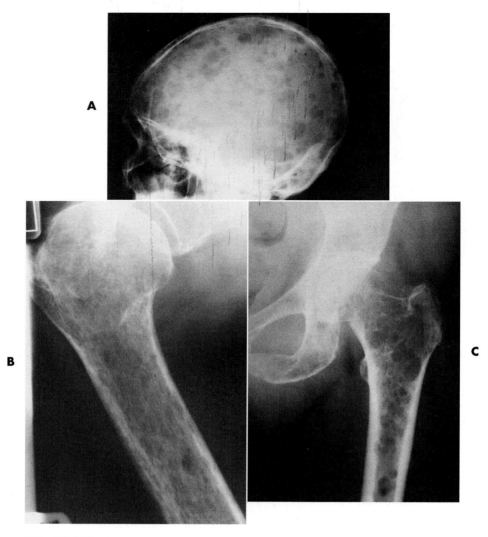

FIG. 15-150 Different patients exhibiting multiple osteolytic lesions of the skull **(A),** proximal humerus **(B),** and proximal femur **(C),** which are characteristic of multiple myeloma. (Courtesy Joseph W. Howe, Sylmar, Calif.)

CLINICAL COMMENTS

Clinical findings are secondary to excessive plasma cell production. Pain is the most common patient complaint, reported in up to 70% of cases. Pathological fractures are common. MM is associated with amyloidosis, hemorrhages, recurrent infections, and general weakness.[108] In rare instances, patients may remain asymptomatic.[50,51]

Laboratory examination may reveal hypercalcemia, hyperuricemia, elevated creatine, anemia, and thrombocytopenia. The abnormal plasma cells produce altered proteins in the serum and urine (Bence Jones proteins). The serum abnormality consists of hyperglobulinemia with a reversal of the albumin-globulin (A/G) ratio. Most patients produce an overabundance of the immunoglobulin G (IgG) type. Serum abnormalities are recognized by electrophoresis and are considered central to the diagnosis of the disease.

MM is diagnosed by a high index of clinical suspicion, with radiographic and laboratory correlation. Once a lesion is identified, a biopsy for histological examination is necessary. Although variable, the usual course of the disease is that of gradual progression with a median survival of 3 years.[109] Treatment includes radiation and chemotherapy.

KEY CONCEPTS

- *Multiple myeloma (MM) is the most common primary malignant tumor of bone.*
- *Most patients are between 50 and 70 years of age.*
- *Bone scans are notoriously insensitive because of suppressed osteoblastic activity.*
- *MM exhibits a predilection for the axial skeleton.*
- *Most commonly, MM presents as multicentric (polyostotic) lesions of punch-out or moth-eaten patterns of bone destruction.*
- *Solitary lesions are termed* plasmacytomas *and appear less aggressive and are expansile.*

Osteosarcoma

BACKGROUND

An osteosarcoma is a highly aggressive, malignant tumor of bone. Osteosarcomas are the second most common primary malignant tumor of bone, after multiple myeloma. Although all osteosarcomas produce osteoid matrix, the proportion of chondroid and fibroid histological constituents is variable. Only about 50% of osteosarco-

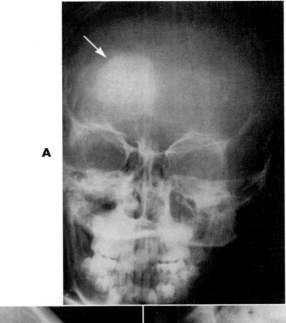

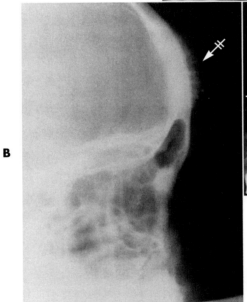

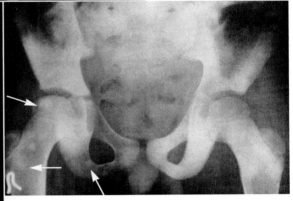

FIG. 15-151 **A** and **B,** Osteosarcoma of the frontal bone with increased radiodensity *(arrow)* and aggressive periostitis *(crossed arrow).* **C,** Additional regions of increased radiodensity are noted in the pelvis *(arrows).* (Courtesy Steven P. Brownstein, Springfield, NJ.)

mas contain predominantly osteoid matrix, appearing osteoblastic on the radiographs. Osteosarcoma can be classified into intraosseous, surface, extraosseous, secondary, and multicentric types.[17]

Intraosseous osteosarcoma. Conventional and telangiectatic osteosarcomas are subtypes of the intraosseous classification. Conventional osteosarcomas account for 75% to 85% of all osteosarcomas. Conventional osteosarcomas arise within cancellous bone and then grow aggressively, extending into the medullary canal and penetrating the cortex to invade the soft tissues. Telangiectatic osteosarcoma is an aggressive, rare variant of osteosarcoma. It is characterized by large, blood-filled cavities and thin septations.[93]

Surface osteosarcoma. Periosteal and parosteal (juxtacortical) osteosarcomas are subtypes of surface osteosarcoma clas-

sification that arise from the cortex, subperiosteal tissue, or periosteum. They are marked by outward growth toward the soft tissues of the involved limb. Parosteal osteosarcoma is more common and exhibits large amounts of osteoid production. Periosteal osteosarcoma is rare and difficult to distinguish from periosteal chondrosarcoma because of the large amounts of chondroid and scant osteoid tissue that may be present in the lesion.

Other osteosarcomas. Extraosseous osteosarcomas are soft tissue tumors with the same histological composition as conventional osteosarcomas. Secondary osteosarcoma most commonly occurs in elderly patients with Paget's disease, infarcts, fibrous dysplasia, or past regions of radiation therapy.[168,207] Multicentric osteosarcoma defines symmetrically distributed, multiple synchronous osteosarcomas of similar size and development (Fig. 15-151).[155]

Patient age.   Conventional and telangiectatic osteosarcomas have a slight male predominance and occur most commonly between the ages of 10 and 25 years, with a second peak in incidence over the age of 60 years with conventional osteosarcoma. Periosteal osteosarcomas are seen most often between the ages of 10 and 20 years, more commonly in females. Parosteal osteosarcomas occur in a slightly older age group than conventional or parosteal osteosarcomas. The average age of patients with extraosseous os-

teosarcomas is 45 years. Multicentric osteosarcoma occurs during the first decade.

IMAGING FINDINGS

Conventional osteosarcomas most commonly arise in the metaphysis of long bones, usually the distal femur (40%) (Fig. 15-152), proximal tibia (20%), humerus (9%), pelvis (5%) (Fig. 15-153), facial bones (5%), fibula (4%) (Fig. 15-154), and patella (less than

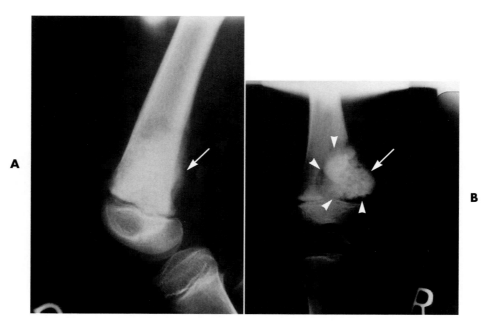

FIG. 15-152   **A,** Osteosarcoma in the distal femur with aggressive spiculated periostitis *(arrow)*. **B,** A band of osteolytic destruction *(arrowheads)* surrounding the radiodense matrix of the lesion *(arrow)* in the frontal projection.

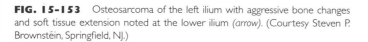

FIG. 15-153   Osteosarcoma of the left ilium with aggressive bone changes and soft tissue extension noted at the lower ilium *(arrow)*. (Courtesy Steven P. Brownstein, Springfield, NJ.)

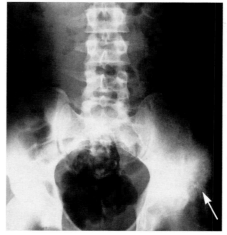

1%). Older patients exhibit a higher incidence of osteosarcoma in flat bones. The radiographic appearance of conventional osteosarcomas begins with a medullary osteolytic (25%), osteoblastic (25%), or mixed (50%) lesion in the metaphysis, often extending into the epiphysis or diaphysis. Ninety percent have a large, cloud-like density representing tumor bone (Fig. 15-155) and an aggressive (laminated, sunburst, hair-on-end, or Codman's triangles) periosteal reaction. A large soft tissue mass is typical.

Telangiectatic osteosarcoma usually appears as an osteolytic, expansile lesion in the diaphysis of the femur, tibia, or humerus. It is characterized by periosteal reaction with a large soft tissue mass and lack of visible bone production.

Parosteal osteosarcoma usually appears as a lobular, radiodense mass arising from a sessile base to surround the metaphysis of the host bone. A thin radiolucent line is present, but rarely seen, separating the tumor from the host bone. Nearly 70% of parosteal os-

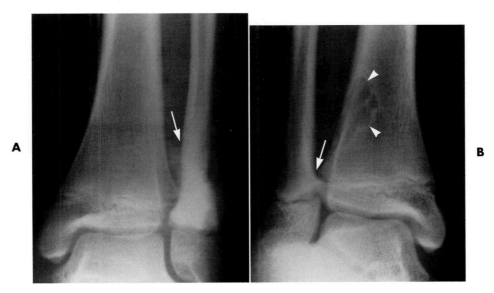

FIG. 15-154 The anteroposterior **(A)** and oblique **(B)** ankle projections reveal an aggressive osteosclerotic lesion of the distal fibula. Aggressive periosteal and soft tissue extension is noted on the medial side of the fibula *(arrow)*. **B,** Incidentally noted is a nonossifying fibroma in the distal tibia, best seen on the oblique projection *(arrowheads)*.

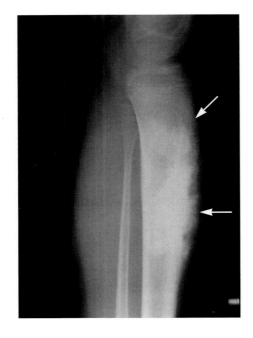

FIG. 15-155 Osteosarcoma of the proximal tibia appearing osteosclerotic with aggressive periostitis *(arrows)*. (Courtesy Steven P. Brownstein, Springfield, NJ.)

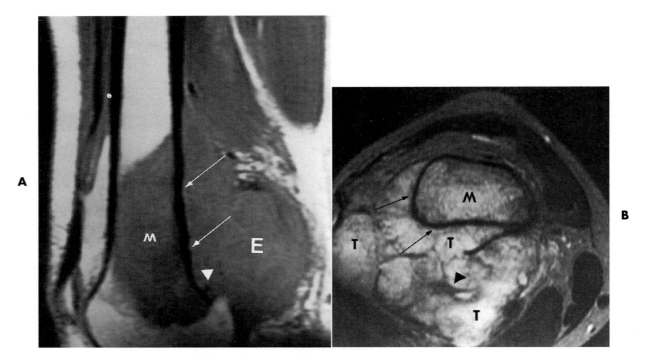

FIG. 15-156   Distal femoral osteosarcoma. **A,** Sagittal T1-weighted MRI demonstrates low signal intensity marrow involvement *(M)* with prominent posterior extension *(E)*. **B,** Transaxial T2-weighted image reveals predominantly high signal intensity within both the marrow *(M)* and soft tissue *(T)* components of the lesion. Areas of intact cortex *(arrows)* are evident on both images, along with tumor bone formation *(arrowheads)*, suggesting the correct diagnosis. (From Sartoris DJ: *Musculoskeletal imaging: the requisites,* St Louis, 1993, Mosby.)

teosarcomas are metaphyseal, arising from the posterior surface of the distal femur; other sites include the proximal tibia and humerus. Periosteal reaction is rare. Periosteal osteosarcomas present as soft tissue masses extending from the diaphysis of long bones, usually femur or tibia, which may have small bones, perpendicular bone spicules, or amorphous calcification within the tumor mass. The endosteal margin is not involved.

Secondary osteosarcomas appear as destructive lesions usually indistinguishable from conventional osteosarcomas, occurring in the region of primary disease. Extraosseous osteosarcomas appear as large soft tissue masses most often in the buttocks and thigh.[66] More than half of the lesions demonstrate radiographic evidence of calcification. These lesions are best demonstrated by MRI.[197] Multicentric osteosarcoma is accompanied by multiple, symmetrically distributed radiodensities in the metaphyses.

For the most part, primary osseous lesions are well defined on conventional radiographs. CT and MRI are used to assess the extent of the lesion and evaluate its relationship to adjacent anatomy (Figs. 15-156 and 15-157).

CLINICAL COMMENTS

Patients with osteosarcoma present with pain, swelling, and sometimes limited joint motion of the involved limb. Symptoms are usu-

ally present a few months prior to presentation. Serum alkaline phosphatase levels may be elevated. An initial complaint of pathological fracture is more common with telangiectatic osteosarcoma. Multicentric, telangiectatic, and conventional osteosarcomas have poorer prognoses than surface osteosarcomas.

Conventional treatment includes the application of one or some combination of the following: excision, amputation, chemotherapy, and radiation.[46,132,159,190,205] Patient survival rates range from promising, with parosteal osteosarcoma, to poor, with multicentric osteosarcoma, and depend on the type of osteosarcoma, applied treatment, and general patient health status.

KEY CONCEPTS

- *Osteosarcoma is the second most common primary malignant tumor of bone.*
- *Osteosarcoma occurs most often between the ages of 10 and 25, with a later age group for the parosteal subtype.*
- *Osteosarcomas are very aggressive, including bone, periosteal, and soft tissue manifestations; 50% have radiodense matrices.*
- *These tumors most commonly arise from the metaphysis of long bones around the knee.*
- *Symptoms include pain, swelling, and limited motion of the limb that is involved.*

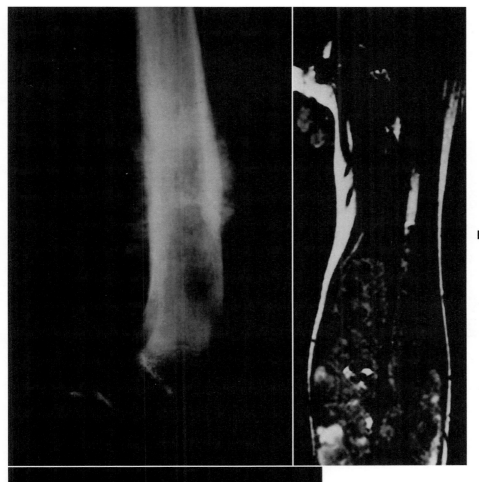

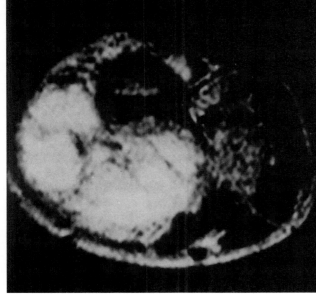

FIG. 15-157 Characteristic appearance of osteosarcoma in the distal femur of a 15-year-old boy. **A,** The involved portion of bone has a mixed sclerotic and lytic appearance with periostosis and a soft tissue mass. Note the sunburst appearance caused by radially oriented linear ossification. **B,** A coronal T1-weighted image demonstrates the relatively low signal tumor extending to the middiaphysis. The signal intensity of the tumor contrasts well with the normal bright signal of the yellow marrow. The rather low signal from the proximal diaphysis is caused by partial volume averaging of the cortical and medullary signal. The low signal in the proximal metaphysis is secondary to the presence of the normal red marrow. Note the loss of the signal void of the distal femoral cortex resulting from destruction (and replacement) by a tumor. The signal intensity of the tumor is only marginally different than the normal skeletal muscle. The bright signal areas represent areas of hemorrhage. **C,** This T2-weighted image better defines the high signal intensity of the tumor from the surrounding low signal muscle vessels. (From Firooznia H et al: *MRI and CT of the musculoskeletal system,* St Louis, 1992, Mosby.)

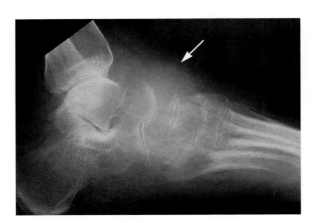

FIG. 15-158   Synovial sarcoma (synovioma) of the dorsum of the foot, causing aggressive osteolytic bone destruction with associated soft tissue mass *(arrow)*. (Courtesy Steven P. Brownstein, Springfield, NJ.)

Synovial Sarcoma

BACKGROUND
Synovial sarcoma (synovioma) is an uncommon malignant soft tissue tumor arising from the mesenchyme rather than mature synovial tissues.[28] They express epithelial and supporting tissue features.[28,172] Synovial sarcoma occurs most often in patients between the ages of 15 and 40 years[5,63] and more predominantly in males.[96]

IMAGING FINDINGS
Synovial sarcomas occur more often as extraarticular lesions in the lower extremities, appearing as a soft tissue mass with associated calcifications and bony erosions.[89,96] Common sites include the knee, hip, thigh, ankle, elbow, wrist, hands, and feet (Figs. 15-158 and 15-159).

CLINICAL COMMENTS
Pain is a very common clinical complaint, often preceeding the clinical recognition of the tumor by several years.[63] Treatment includes surgical excision with or without radiation and/or chemotherapy.[131]

KEY CONCEPTS
- *Synovial sarcoma is an uncommon, soft tissue mass in the lower extremities, usually around the knees.*
- *Synovial sarcoma is often calcified.*
- *Synovial sarcoma usually occurs between the ages of 15 and 40 years.*

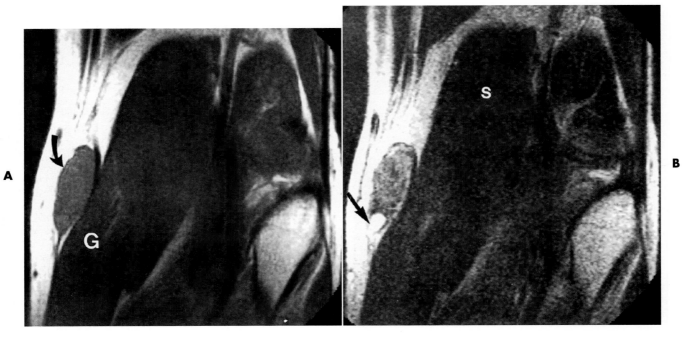

FIG. 15-159   Synovial sarcoma. **A,** Coronal T1-weighted MRI reveals a well-defined mass of low signal intensity *(arrow)* adjacent to the medial head of the gastrocnemius muscle *(G)*. **B,** Corresponding T2-weighted image demonstrates an inhomogeneous appearance, with high signal intensity in the inferior portion of the lesion *(arrow)* (s, semimembranosus muscle). Differential diagnosis should include consideration of other benign and malignant soft tissue neoplasms. (From Sartoris DJ: *Musculoskeletal imaging: the requisites,* St Louis, 1993, Mosby.)

References

1. Aguilar JL et al: Difficult management of pain following sacro-coccygeal chordoma: 13 months of subarachnoid infusion, *Pain* 59:317, 1994.
2. Ahn JI, Park JS: Pathological fractures secondary to unicameral bone cysts, *Int Orthop* 18:20, 1994.
3. Albregts AE, Rapini RP: Malignancy in Maffucci's syndrome, *Dermatol Clin* 13:73, 1995.
4. Albright F et al: Syndrome characterized by osteitis fibrosa disseminata, areas of pigmentation and endocrine dysfunction, with precocious puberty in females, *N Engl J Med* 216:727, 1937.
5. Amble FR et al: Head and neck synovial cell sarcoma, *Otolaryngol Head Neck Surg* 107:631, 1992.
6. Arata MA, Peterson HA, Dahlin DC: Pathological fractures through nonossifying fibromas, *J Bone Joint Surg Am* 63:980, 1981.
7. Baden E, Doyle JL, Petriella V: Malignant transformation of peripheral ameloblastoma, *Oral Surg Oral Med Oral Pathol Oral Radiol Endod* 75:214, 1993.
8. Baker DM: Benign unicameral bone cyst, *Clin Orthop* 71:140, 1970.
9. Bataille R, Chappard D, Klein B: Mechanisms of bone lesions in multiple myeloma, *Hematol Oncol Clin North Am* 6:285, 1992.
10. Batsakis JG, Hicks MJ, Flaitz CM: Peripheral epithelial odontogenic tumors, *Ann Otol Rhinol Laryngol* 102:322, 1993.
11. Benevenia J et al: Imaging rounds. Multifocal adamantinoma of the tibia and fibula, *Orthop Rev* 21:996, 1992.
12. Bennett MH et al: Classification of non-Hodgkin's lymphomas, *Lancet* 2:405, 1974.
13. Bertoni F et al: Primary central (medullary) fibrosarcoma of bone, *Semin Diagn Pathol* 1:185, 1984.
14. Bessler W, Grauer W, Allemann J: Case report 726. Enchondromatosis of the left femur and hemipelvis (Ollier's disease), *Skeletal Radiol* 21:201, 1992.
15. Bhambhani M et al: Giant cell tumors in mandible and spine: a rare complication of Paget's disease of bone, *Ann Rheum Dis* 51:1335, 1992.
16. Bjornsson J et al: Chordoma of the mobile spine, a clinicopathologic analysis of 40 patients, *Cancer* 71:735, 1993.
17. Bloem JL, Kroon HM: Osseous lesions, *Radiol Clin North Am* 31:261, 1993.
18. Bohm B et al: Our approach to the management of congenital presacral tumors in adults, *Int J Colorectal Dis* 8:134, 1993.
19. Borges AM, Huvos AG, Smith J: Bursa formation and synovial chondrometaplasia associated with osteochondromas, *Am J Clin Pathol* 75:648, 1981.
20. Boriani S et al: Periosteal chondroma. A review of twenty cases, *J Bone Joint Surg Am* 65:205, 1983.
21. Boseker EH, Bickel WH, Dahlin DC: A clinicopathological study of simple unicameral bone cysts, *Surg Gynecol Obstet* 127:550, 1968.
22. Braunstein EM, White SJ: Non-Hodgkin lymphoma of bone, *Radiology* 135:59, 1980.
23. Brenner RJ, Hattner RS, Lilien DL: Scintigraphic features of nonosteogenic fibroma, *Radiology* 131:727, 1979.
24. Brien EW, Mirra JM, Ippolito V: Chondroblastoma arising from a nonepiphyseal site, *Skeletal Radiol* 24:220, 1995.
25. Burkitt DP: A sarcoma involving the jaws in African children, *Br J Surg* 46:218, 1968.
26. Campanacci M, Laus M, Boriani S: Multiple nonossifying fibromata with extraskeletal anomalies: a new syndrome? *J Bone Joint Surg Br* 65:627, 1983.
27. Capanna R et al: Malignant fibrous histiocytoma of bone, *Cancer* 54:177, 1984.
28. Carrillo R, Rodriquez-Peralto JL, Batsakis JG: Synovial sarcomas of the head and neck, *Ann Otol Rhinol Laryngol* 101:367, 1992.
29. Carson CP, Ackerman LV, Maltby JD: Plasma cell myeloma: clinical, pathologic and roentgenologic review of 90 cases, *Am J Clin Pathol* 25:849, 1955.
30. Charkes ND, Malmud LS, Caswell T: Preoperative bone scans: use in women with early breast cancer, *JAMA* 233:516, 1975.
31. Charkes ND, Young J, Sklaroff DM: The pathologic basis of the strontium bone scan, *JAMA* 206:2482, 1968.
32. Chigira M et al: The aetiology and treatment of simple bone cysts, *J Bone Joint Surg Br* 65:633, 1983.
33. Chow LT, Lee KC: Intraosseous lipoma. A clinicopathologic study of nine cases, *Am J Surg Pathol* 16:401, 1992.
34. Collins JC et al: Percutaneous biopsy following positive bone scans, *Radiology* 132:439, 1979.
35. Copeland MM: Metastases to bone from primary tumors in other sites, *Proc Natl Cancer Conf* 6:743, 1970.
36. Corcoran RJ et al: Solitary abnormalities in bone scans of patients with extraosseous malignancies, *Radiology* 121:663, 1976.
37. Cossetto D, Nade S, Blackwell J: Malignant fibrous histiocytoma in Paget's disease of bone: a report of seven cases, *Aust N Z J Surg* 62:52, 1992.
38. Cowan WK: Malignant change and multiple metastases in Ollier's disease, *J Clin Pathol* 18:650, 1965.
39. Craver LF: Lymphosarcoma: a review of 1269 cases, *Medicine (Baltimore)* 40:31, 1961.
40. Crim JR et al: Case report 748: chondroblastoma of the femur with an aneurysmal bone cyst, *Skeletal Radiol* 21:403, 1992.
41. Cunningham JB, Ackerman LV: Metaphyseal fibrous defects, *J Bone Joint Surg Am* 38:797, 1956.
42. Czerwinski E, Skolarczyk A, Fransik W: Malignant fibrous histiocytoma in the course of chronic osteomyelitis, *Arch Orthop Trauma Surg* 111:58, 1991.
43. Dahlin DC: *Bone tumors: general aspects and data on 6,221 cases,* ed 3, Springfield, Ill, 1978, Charles C Thomas.
44. Dahlin DC, Coventry MB, Scanlon PW: Ewing's sarcoma: a critical analysis of 165 cases, *J Bone Joint Surg Am* 43:185, 1961.
45. Dahlin DC: Giant cell tumor of bone: highlights of 407 cases, *AJR* 144:955, 1985.
46. Damron TA, Pritchard DJ: Current combined treatment of high-grade osteosarcomas, *Oncology* 9:327, 1995.
47. Dehner LP: Primitive neuroectodermal tumor and Ewing's sarcoma, *Am J Surg Pathol* 17:1, 1993.
48. Dewald RL et al: Reconstructive spinal surgery as palliation for metastatic malignancies of the spine, *Spine* 10:21, 1985.
49. Dijkhuizen T et al: Cytogenetics as a tool in the histologic subclassification of chondrosarcomas, *Cancer Genet Cytogenet* 76:100, 1994.
50. Dimopoulos MA et al: Risk of disease progression in asymptomatic multiple myeloma, *Am J Med* 94:57, 1993.
51. Dimopoulos MA et al: Solitary plasmacytoma of bone and asymptomatic multiple myeloma, *Hematol Oncol Clin North Am* 6:359, 1992.
52. Dorfman HD, Steiner GC, Jaffe HL: Vascular tumors of bone, *Hum Pathol* 2:349, 1971.
53. Dorn W, Gladden P, Ranken EA: Regression of a renal-cell metastatic osseous lesion following treatment, *J Bone Joint Surg Am* 57:869, 1975.
54. Du YK et al: Dedifferentiated chondrosarcoma arising from osteochondromatosis. A case report, *Chang Keng I Hsueh* 14:130, 1991.
55. Duncan CP, Morton KS, Arthur JS: Giant cell tumor of bone: its aggressiveness and potential for malignant change, *Can J Surg* 26:475, 1983.
56. Durie BGM, Salmon SE, Mundy GR: Relation of osteoclast activating factor production to extent of bone disease in multiple myeloma, *Br J Haematol* 47:21, 1981.

57. Eckardt J, Grogan T: Giant cell tumor of bone, *Clin Orthop* 204:45, 1986.

58. Edel G et al: Chondroblastoma of bone. A clinical, radiological, light and immunohistochemical study, *Pathol Anat Histopathol* 421:355, 1992.

59. Edelstyn GA, Gillespie PJ, Grebbell FS: The radiological demonstration of osseous metastases: experimental observations, *Clin Radiol* 18:158, 1967.

60. Edeiken J: *Roentgen diagnosis of diseases of bone,* ed 3, Baltimore, 1981, Williams & Wilkins.

61. Eggli KD, Quiogue T, Moser RP: Ewing's sarcoma, *Radiol Clin North Am* 31:325, 1993.

62. EI-Khoury GY, Bassett GS: Symptomatic bursa transformation with osteochondromas, *AJR* 133:895, 1979.

63. Enterline HT: Histopathology of sarcomas, *Semin Oncol* 18:133, 1981.

64. Eriksson AL, Schiller A, Mankin HJ: The management of chondrosarcoma of bone, *Clin Orthop* 153:44, 1980.

65. Evans HL, Ayala AG, Romsdahl MM: Prognostic factors in chondrosarcoma of bone. A clinicopathologic analysis with emphasis on histologic grading, *Cancer* 40:818, 1977.

66. Fang Z et al: Extraskeletal osteosarcoma: a clinicopathologic study of four cases, *Jap J Clin Oncol* 25:55, 1995.

67. Fauré C et al: Multiple and large nonossifying fibromas in children with neurofibromatosis, *Ann Radiol* 29:396, 1986.

68. Feldman F, Hecht HL, Johnson AD: Chondromyxoid fibroma of bone, *Radiology* 94:249, 1970.

69. Feldman F, Lattes R: Primary malignant fibrous histiocytoma (fibrous xanthoma) of bone, *Skeletal Radiol* 1:145, 1977.

70. Ferrant A et al: Detection of skeletal involvement in Hodgkin's disease: a comparison of radiography, bone scanning, and bone marrow biopsy in 38 patients, *Cancer* 35:1346, 1975.

71. Feuillan PP: McCune-Albright's syndrome, *Curr Ther Endocrinol Metab* 5:205, 1994.

72. Forsyth PA et al: Intracranial chordomas: a clinicopathological and prognostic study of 51 cases, *J Neurosurg* 78:741, 1993.

73. Francis KC, Hutter RVP: Neoplasms of the spine in the aged, *Clin Orthop* 26:54, 1963.

74. Freeby JA, Reinus WR, Wilson AJ: Quantitative analysis of the plain radiographic appearance of aneurysmal bone cysts, *Invest Radiol* 30:433, 1995.

75. Freiberg RA et al: Multiple intraosseous lipomas with type IV hyperlipoproteinemia, *J Bone Joint Surg Am* 56:1729, 1974.

76. Gitelis S et al: Chondrosarcoma of bone. The experience at the Istituto Ortopedico Rizzoli, *J Bone Joint Surg Am* 45:1450, 1981.

77. Giudici MA, Moser RP, Kransdorf MJ: Cartilaginous bone tumors, *Radiol Clin North Am* 31:237, 1993.

78. Goel AR et al: Unicameral bone cysts: treatment with methylprednisolone acetate injections, *J Foot Ankle Surg* 33:6, 1994.

79. Goldenberg RR, Campbell CJ, Bonfiglio M: Giant cell tumor of bone. An analysis of 218 cases, *J Bone Joint Surg Am* 52:619, 1970.

80. Green T et al: Multiple primary cutaneous plasmacytomas, *Arch Dermatol* 128:962, 1992.

81. Gupta VK et al: Aneurysmal bone cysts of the spine, *Surg Neurol* 42:428, 1994.

82. Haag M, Adler CP: Malignant fibrous histiocytoma in association with hip replacement, *J Bone Joint Surg Br* 71:701, 1989.

83. Harned RK et al: Extracolonic manifestations of the familial adenomatous polyposis syndromes, *AJR* 156:481, 1991.

84. Harris WH, Dudley HR, Barry RV: The natural history of fibrous dysplasia, *J Bone Joint Surg Am* 44:207, 1962.

85. Harsha WN: The natural history of osteocartilaginous exostoses (osteochondroma), *Am Surg* 20:65, 1954.

86. Harwood AR, Krajbich JL, Fornasier VL: Radiotherapy of chondrosarcoma of bone, *Cancer* 45:2769, 1980.

87. Hatcher CH: The pathogenesis of localized fibrous lesions in the metaphysis of long bones, *Ann Surg* 122:1016, 1945.

88. Henry A: Monostotic fibrous dysplasia, *J Bone Joint Surg Br* 51:300, 1969.

89. Horowitz AL, Resnick D, Watson RC: The roentgen features of synovial sarcomas, *Clin Radiol* 24:481, 1973.

90. Hudson TM, Chew FS, Manaster BJ: Scintigraphy of benign exostoses and exostotic chondrosarcoma, *AJR* 140:581, 1983.

91. Hudson TM et al: Benign exostoses and exostotic chondrosarcomas: evaluation of cartilage thickness by CT, *Radiology* 152:595, 1984.

92. Hudson TM et al: Radiology of giant-cell tumors of bone: computed tomography, arthro-tomography, and scintigraphy, *Skeletal Radiol* 11:85, 1984.

93. Huvos AG et al: Telangiectatic osteogenic sarcoma: a clinicopathologic study of 124 patients, *Cancer* 49:1979, 1982.

94. Ishida T, Dorfman HD: Plasma cell myeloma in unusually young patients: a report of two cases and review of the literature, *Skeletal Radiol* 24:47, 1995.

95. Ishida T et al: Parachordoma: an ultrastructural and immunohistochemical study, *Pathol Anat Histopathol* 422:239, 1993.

96. Jong B et al: Imaging and differential diagnosis of synovial sarcoma, *J Belge Radiol* 75:335, 1992.

97. Kaplan RP et al: Maffucci's syndrome: two case reports with a literature review, *J Am Acad Dermatol* 29:894, 1993.

98. Kattapuram SV et al: Osteoid osteoma: an unusual cause of articular pain, *Radiology* 147:383, 1983.

99. Katz JO, Underhill TE: Multilocular radiolucencies, *Dent Clin North Am* 38:63, 1994.

100. Keim HA, Reina EG: Osteoid osteoma as a cause of scoliosis, *J Bone Joint Surg* 57A:159, 1975.

101. Keneko Y et al: Chordoma in early childhood: a clinicopathological study, *Neurosurg* 29:442, 1991.

102. Khan FR et al: Treatment by radiotherapy of spinal cord compression due to extradural metastases, *Radiology* 89:495, 1967.

103. Kim Sk, Barry WF: Bone islands, *Radiology* 90:77, 1968.

104. Kransdorf MJ et al: Giant cell tumor in skeletally immature patients, *Radiology* 184:233, 1992.

105. Kransdorf MJ, Sweet DE: Aneurysmal bone cyst: concept, controversy, clinical presentation, and imaging, *AJR* 164:573, 1995.

106. Krishnamurthy GT et al: Distribution pattern of metastatic bone disease: a need for total body skeletal image, *JAMA* 237:2504, 1977.

107. Kroon HM, Schuurmans J: Osteoblastoma: clinical and radiologic findings in 98 new cases, *Radiology* 175:783, 1990.

108. Kyle RA: Diagnostic criteria of multiple myeloma, *Hematol Oncol Clin North Am* 6:347, 1992.

109. Kyle RA: Prognostic factors in multiple myeloma, *Stem Cells (Dayt)* 13(suppl):56, 1995.

110. Lange RH, Lange TA, Rao BK: Correlative radiographic, scintigraphic, and histologic evaluation of exostoses, *J Bone Joint Surg Am* 66:1454, 1984.

111. Larsson SE, Lorentzon R, Boquist L: Giant-cell tumor of bone, *J Bone Joint Surg Am* 57:167, 1975.

112. Lauf E et al: Intraosseous lipoma of distal fibula. Biomechanical considerations for successful treatment, *J Am Podiatry Assoc* 74:434, 1984.

113. Laus M, Vicenzi G: Hiostiocytic fibroma of bone (a study of 170 cases), *Ital J Orthop Traumatol* 5:343, 1979.

114. Lee YTN: Bone scanning in patients with early breast carcinoma: should it be a routine staging procedure? *Cancer* 47:486, 1981.

115. Li FB et al: Rarity of Ewing's sarcoma in China, *Lancet* 1:1255, 1980.

116. Liapi-Avgeri G et al: Intraosseous lipoma. A report of three cases, *Arch Anat Cytol Pathol* 42:334, 1994.

117. Lichtenstein L: Polyostotic fibrous dysplasia, *Arch Surg* 36:874, 1938.

118. Lichenstein L, Bernstein D: Unusual benign and malignant chondroid tumors of hone, *Cancer* 12:1422, 1959.

119. Lodwick GS: Juvenile unicameral bone cyst, *AJR* 80:495, 1958.

120. Loizaga JM: What's new in Ewing's tumor? *Pathol Res Pract* 189:616, 1993.

121. Malloy PC, Fishman EK, Magid D: Lymphoma of bone, muscle, and skin: CT findings, *AJR* 159:805, 1992.

122. Manaster BJ. Handbook of Skeletal Radiology, Second Edition, Mosby Year Book, St. Louis, 1997.

123. Manning JH: Symptomatic hemangioma of the spine, *Radiology* 56:58, 1951.

124. Marcove RC et al: The treatment of aneurysmal bone cyst, *Clin Orthop* 311:157, 1995.

125. Marsh BW et al: Benign osteoblastoma: range of manifestations, *J Bone Joint Surg Am* 57:1, 1975.

126. Martinez V, Sissons HA: Aneurysmal bone cyst: a review of 123 cases including primary lesions and those secondary to other bone pathology, *Cancer* 61:2291, 1988.

127. McDonald DJ et al: Giant cell tumor of bone, *J Bone Joint Surg Am* 68:235, 1986.

128. McInemey DP, Middlemiss JH: Giant-cell tumor of bone, *Skeletal Radiol* 2:195, 1978.

129. McLeod RA, Dahlin DC, Beabout JW: Spectrum of osteoblastoma, *Am J Roentgenol* 126:321, 1976.

130. McNeil BJ: Value of bone scanning in neoplastic disease, *Semin Nucl Med* 14:277, 1984.

131. Menendez LR, Brien E, Brien WW: Synovial sarcoma. A clinicopathologic study, *Orthop Rev* 21:465, 1992.

132. Mertens WC, Bramwell V: Osteosarcoma and other tumors of bone, *Curr Opin Oncology* 7:349, 1995.

133. Miller MD, Ragsdale BD, Sweet DE: Parosteal lipomas: a new perspective, *Pathology* 24:132, 1992.

134. Miller RW: Contrasting epidemiology of childhood osteosarcoma, Ewing's tumor and rhabdomyosarcoma, *Monogr Natl Cancer Inst* 56:9, 1981.

135. Mirra JM et al: Malignant fibrous histiocytoma and osteosarcoma in association with bone infarcts. Report of four cases, two in caisson workers, *J Bone Joint Surg Am* 56:932, 1974.

136. Mizerny BR, Kost KM: Chordoma of the cranial base: the McGill experience, *J Otolaryngol* 24:14, 1995.

137. Moberg E: The natural course of osteoid osteoma, *J Bone Joint Surg Am* 33:166, 1951.

138. Moore TM et al: Closed biopsy of musculoskeletal lesions, *J Bone Joint Surg Am* 61:375, 1979.

139. Moreau G, Letts M: Unicameral bone cyst of the calcaneus in children, *J Pediatr Orthop* 14:101, 1994.

140. Moser RP: *Cartilaginous tumors of the skeleton,* Philadephia, 1990, Hanley and Belfus.

141. Moser RP et al: Giant cell tumor of the upper extremity, *Radiographics* 10:83, 1990.

142. Moser RP et al: Multiple skeletal fibroxanthomas: radiologic-pathologic correlation of 72 cases, *Skeletal Radiol* 16:353, 1987.

143. Moulopoulos LA et al: Extraosseous multiple myeloma: imaging features, *AJR* 161:1083, 1993.

144. Murphey MD et al: Parosteal lipoma: MR imaging characteristics, *AJR* 162:105, 1994.

145. Mylle J, Burssens A, Fabry G: Simple bone cysts. A review of 59 cases with special reference to their treatment, *Arch Orthop Trauma Surg* 111:297, 1992.

146. Nastri AL et al: Maxillary ameloblastoma: a retrospective study of 13 cases, *Br J Oral Maxillofac Surg* 33:28, 1995.

147. Naula JM et al: Peripheral ameloblastoma. A case report and review of the literature, *Int J Oral Maxillofac Surg* 21:40, 1992.

148. Neff JR: Nonmetastatic Ewing's sarcoma of bone: the role of surgical therapy, *Clin Orthop* 204:111, 1986.

149. Ngan H: Growing bone islands, *Clin Radiol* 23:199, 1972.

150. Niechajev IA, Stemby NH: Diagnostic accuracy and pathology of vascular tumors and tumor-like lesions, *Chir Maxillofac Plast* 7:153, 1983.

151. Nimityongskul P, Anderson LD, Dowling EA: Chondromyxoid fibroma, *Orthop Rev* 21:863, 1992.

152. Norman A, Schiffman M: Simple bone cysts: factors of age dependency, *Radiology* 124:779, 1977.

153. Nusbacher N, Sclafani SJ, Birla SR: Case report 155: polyostotic Paget disease complicated by benign giant cell tumor of left clavicle, *Skeletal Radiol* 6:233, 1981.

154. O'Mara RE: Bone scanning in osseous metastatic disease, *JAMA* 229:1915, 1974.

155. Parham DM et al: Childhood multifocal osteosarcoma, clinicopathologic and radiologic correlates, *Cancer* 55:2653, 1985.

156. Parker BR, Marglin S, Castellino RA: Skeletal manifestations of leukemia, Hodgkin disease and non-Hodgkin lymphoma, *Semin Roentgenol* 15:302, 1980.

157. Peterson HA: Multiple hereditary osteochondromata, *Clin Orthop* 239:222, 1989.

158. Picci P et al: Giant-cell tumor of bone in skeletally immature patients, *J Bone Joint Surg Am* 65:486, 1983.

159. Picci P et al: Treatment recommendations for osteosarcoma and adult soft tissue sarcomas, *Drugs* 47:82, 1994.

160. Pritchard DJ et al: Chondrosarcoma: a clinicopathologic and statistical analysis, *Cancer* 45:149, 1980.

161. Pritchard DJ et al: Fibrosarcoma of bone and soft tissues of the trunk and extremities, *Orthop Clin North Am* 8:869, 1977.

162. Reichart PA, Philipsen H P, Sonner S: Ameloblastoma: biological profile of 3677 cases, *Eur J Cancer B Oral Oncol* 31B:86, 1995.

163. Reinus WR, Gilula LA: Radiology of Ewing's sarcoma: intergroup Ewing's sarcoma study (IESS), *Radiographics* 4:929, 1984.

164. Reiter FB, Ackerman LV, Staple TW: Central chondrosarcoma of the appendicular skeleton, *Radiology* 105:525, 1972.

165. Resnick D: *Diagnosis of bone and joint disorders,* ed 3, Philadelphia, 1995, WB Saunders.

166. Rodman D, Raymond AK, Phillips WC: Case report 201: primary lymphoma of bone (PLB) - left fibula, *Skeletal Radiol* 8:235, 1982.

167. Roodman GD: Osteoclast function in Paget's disease and multiple myeloma, *Bone* 17(suppl 2):575, 1995.

168. Rosenberg ZS et al: Osteosarcoma: subtle, rare, and misleading plain film features, *AJR* 165:1209, 1995.

169. Ross JS et al: Vertebral hemangiomas: MR imaging, *Radiology* 165:165, 1987.

170. Sanerkin NF, Gallagher P: A review of the behavior of chondrosarcoma of bone, *J Bone Joint Surg Br* 61:395, 1979.

171. Sangueza OP, White CR: Parachordoma, *Am J Dermatopathol* 16:185, 1994.

172. Santavirta S: Synovial sarcoma. A clinicopathological study of 31 cases, *Arch Orthop Trauma Surg* 111:155, 1992.

173. Saville DP: A medical option for the treatment of osteoid osteoma, *Arthritis Rheum* 23:1409, 1981.

174. Schmidt RG, Kabbani YM, Mayer DP: Aneurysmal bone cyst, *J Am Podiatric Med Assoc* 83:595, 1993.

175. Schwartz HS et al: The malignant potential of enchondromatosis, *J Bone Joint Surg Am* 69:269, 1987.

176. Sherman RS, Wilner D: The roentgen diagnosis of hemangioma of bone, *AJR* 86:1146, 1961.

177. Sherman RS, Wolfson Sl: Roentgen diagnosis of lymphosarcoma and reticulum cell sarcoma in infancy and childhood, *AJR* 86:693, 1961.

178. Shin HJ et al: Parachordoma, *Ultrastruct Pathol* 18:249, 1994.

179. Sickles EA, Genant HK, Hoffer PB: Increased localization of 99mTc-pyrophosphate in a bone island: case report, *J Nucl Med* 17:113, 1976.

180. Simon MA, Bartucci EJ: The search for the primary tumor in patients with skeletal metastases of unknown origin, *Cancer* 58:1088, 1986.

181. Small IA et al: Gardner's syndrome with an unusual fibro-osseous of the mandible, *Oral Surg* 49:477, 1980.

PART TWO Bone, Joints, and Soft Tissues

182. Smith SB, Shane HS: Simple bone cyst of the calcaneus. A case report and literature review, *J Am Podiatr Med Assoc* 84:127, 1994.

183. Spanier SS, Enneking WF, Enrique P: Primary malignant histiocytoma of bone, *Cancer* 36:2084, 1975.

184. Spanier SS: Malignant fibrous histiocytoma of bone, *Orthop Clin North Am* 8:947, 1977.

185. Sposto MR et al: Albright's syndrome: review of the literature and case report, *J Nihon Univ School Dent* 36:283, 1994.

186. Springfield DS, Gebhardt MC, McGuire MH: Chondrosarcoma: a review, *J Bone Joint Surg Am* 78A:141, 1996.

187. Steiner HJ, Shosh L, Dorfman HD: Ultrastructure of giant cell tumors of bone, *Hum Pathol* 3:569, 1972.

188. Struhl A et al: Solitary (unicameral) bone cyst: the fallen fragment sign revisited, *Skeletal Radiol* 18:261, 1989.

189. Sundaram M, McDonald DJ, Merenda G: Intramuscular myxoma: a rare but important association with fibrous dysplasia of bone, *AJR* 153:107, 1989.

190. Szendroi M: New aspects in the treatment of bone sarcomas, *Acta Med Hungarica* 50:237, 1994.

191. Tashiro T et al: Intradural chordoma: case report and review of the literature, *Neuroradiology* 36:313, 1994.

192. Tertti R, Alanen A, Remes K: The value of magnetic resonance imaging in screening myeloma lesions of the lumbar spine, *Br J Haematol* 91:658, 1995.

193. Thrall JH, Ellis BI: Skeletal metastases, *Radiol Clin North Am* 25:1155, 1987.

194. Turcotte RE et al: Chondroblastoma, *Hum Pathol* 24:944, 1993.

195. Unroe BJ, Kissel CG, Rosenberg JC: Maffucci's syndrome. Review of the literature and case report, *J Am Podiatr Med Assoc* 82:532, 1992.

196. van Loon CJ et al: Aneurysmal bone cyst: long-term results and functional evaluation, *Acta Orthop Belg* 61:199, 1995.

197. Varma DG et al: MRI of extraskeletal osteosarcoma, *J Comput Assist Tomogr* 17:414, 1993.

198. Varvares MA et al: Chondroblastoma of the temporal bone. Case report and literature review, *Ann Otol Rhinol Laryngol* 101:763, 1992.

199. Vieta JO, Friedell HL, Craver LF: A survey of Hodgkin's disease and lymphosarcoma of the bone, *Radiology* 39:1, 1942.

200. Watanabe H, Arita S, Chigira M: Aetiology of a simple bone cyst. A case report, *Int Orthop* 18:16, 1994.

201. Weber AL et al: Chordomas of the skull base. Radiologic and clinical evaluation, *Neuroimaging Clin North Am* 4:515, 1994.

202. Wheelhouse WW, Griffin PP: Periosteal chondroma, *South Med J* 75:1003, 1982.

203. Wicklund CL et al: Natural history study of hereditary multiple exostoses, *Am J Med Genet* 55:43, 1995.

204. Willis RA: Pathology of osteoblastoma of bone, *J Bone Joint Surg Br* 31:236, 1949.

205. Winkler K et al: Treatment of osteosarcoma: experience of the Cooperative Osteosarcoma Study Group (COSS), *Cancer Treat Res* 62:269, 1993.

206. Wold LE, Swee RG, Sim FH: Vascular lesions of bone, *Pathol Ann* 20:101, 1985.

207. Young JW, Liebscher LA: Postirradiation osteogenic sarcoma with unilateral metastatic spread within the field of irradiation, *Skeletal Radiol* 8:279, 1982.

208. Yunis EJ: Ewing's sarcoma and related small round cell neoplasms in children, *Am J Surg Pathol* 10(suppl 1):54, 1986.

chapter 16

Endocrine, Metabolic, and Nutritional Disorders

D ROBERT KUHN

ENDOCRINE DISORDERS
Acromegaly
Cushing's Syndrome
Giantism (Gigantism)
Hyperparathyroidism
Hypoparathyroidism

Pseudohypoparathyroidism
Pseudopseudohypoparathyroidism
Hypothyroidism

METABOLIC DISORDERS
Osteoporosis

NUTRITIONAL DISORDERS
Hypervitaminosis A
Hypervitaminosis D
Osteomalacia
Rickets
Scurvy (Hypovitaminosis C)

Endocrine Disorders

Acromegaly

BACKGROUND

Acromegaly is marked by the oversecretion of growth hormone (somatotropin) in a skeletally mature patient. Oversecretion is caused by an adenoma in the anterior lobe of the pituitary. Anterior pituitary tumors account for about 18% of all intracranial tumors. The incidence of acromegaly is reportedly 50 to 60 cases per million and the prevalence 3 to 4 cases per million per year.[2] Acromegaly has no gender bias. If the level of growth hormone increases, it produces overgrowth of bone, particularly those bones that are formed intramembranously, principally the skull and mandible. Enlarged joint spaces and soft tissue swelling is typical, producing enlarged hands and feet with thickening of the tongue.

Because the growth centers have not closed, increased levels of growth hormone in skeletally immature patients result in giantism.[2,68,76] Giantism patients with persistent increases in growth hormone also demonstrate acromegalic features. Complications include degenerative joint disease (DJD), increased risk for colonic polyps and colon cancers, and death caused by cardiovascular and cerebral vascular disease. Patients who exhibit diabetes mellitus or hypertension have the highest mortality rate.[2,76]

IMAGING FINDINGS

Increased disc spaces and other joint spaces are demonstrated early. This is followed by generalized osteoporosis and DJD in advanced cases. Increased AP diameter of the thorax and enlargement of the ribs at the costochondral junction is typical.[2,68,76] Sella turcica expansion (Fig. 16-1) and/or destruction, enlarged sinus cavities, malocclusion, and widened mandibular angle (prognathism) are common (Fig. 16-2). The hands and feet exhibit thickening of the tubular bones and prominent ungual tufts. Soft tissue thickening may be seen at the heel pad, (Fig. 16-3) measuring 20 mm or more.[2,76] Although this measure varies, the heel pad thickness should not exceed 23 mm among female and 25 mm among male patients.

CLINICAL COMMENTS

Acromegaly is a gradually progressive disorder in which the symptoms often precede diagnosis by 5 to 10 years. The classic features are a prominent forehead, malocclusion associated with a wide mandibular angle, thickening of the tongue, and large hands and feet. Soft tissue swelling may produce neural compression in the carpal tunnel. Barrel chest, seborrhea, sweating, hypertrichosis, hyperglycemia, hypertension, and cardiomyopathy are frequently occurring features.[2,68,76] Diagnosis is accomplished by documenting excess growth hormone secretion. In cases of episodic excess of growth hormone, documentation of oral glucose administration that fails to suppress growth hormone secretion is helpful. Magnetic resonance imaging or computed tomography documentation of pituitary hyperplasia is suggested.[2,76] Treatment revolves around removal or destruction of the pituitary tumor, reversal of hypersecretion, and maintenance of normal anterior and posterior pituitary function.[2,76]

KEY CONCEPTS

- *Acromegaly is excessive secretion of growth hormone from the anterior lobe of the pituitary gland in a skeletally mature patient.*
- *Excessive secretion of growth hormone from the anterior lobe in a skeletally immature patient results in giantism.*
- *Acromegaly leads to an elaboration of intramembranously formed bone (skull, hands, feet, chondral tissues).*
- *Thickening of the skin overlying the calcaneus can be assessed through the heel pad sign.*
- *Acromegaly is associated with diabetes mellitus, premature degenerative joint disease, increased mortality, colon cancer, hypertension, and artherosclerosis.*

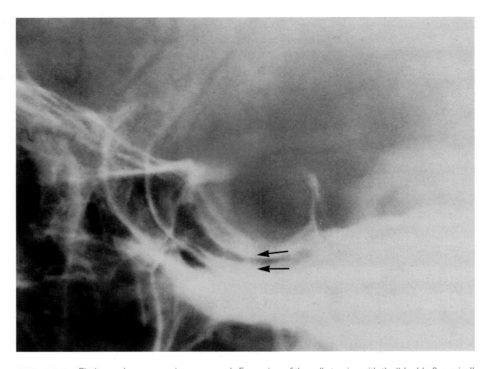

FIG. 16-1 Pituitary adenoma causing acromegaly. Expansion of the sella turcica with the "double floor sign" *(arrows)*. (Modified from Eisenberg RL, Dennis CA: *Comprehensive radiographic pathology,* ed 2, St Louis, 1995, Mosby.)

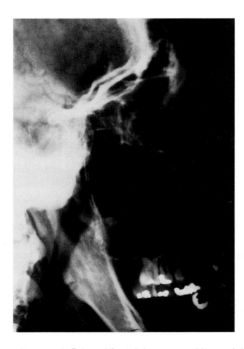

FIG. 16-2 Acromegaly. Enlarged frontal sinus, prognathism, and dental caries.

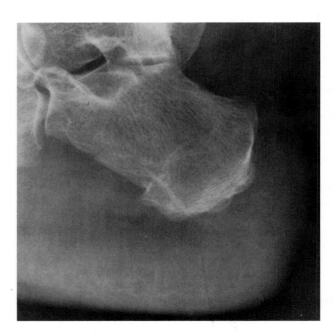

FIG. 16-3 Acromegaly. Positive heel pad sign measuring 32 mm. (From Eisenberg RL, Dennis CA: *Comprehensive radiographic pathology,* ed 2, St Louis, 1995, Mosby.)

Cushing's Syndrome

BACKGROUND

Cushing's syndrome (CS) is hyperadrenocorticism secondary to anterior lobe pituitary tumors, tumors that secrete ectopic adrenocorticotropic hormone (ACTH), adrenal cortex tumors, or as a complication of glucocorticoid therapy (Fig. 16-4). Cushing's disease adds an additional component, hypothalamic-pituitary dysfunction. The incidence of adrenal tumors in the United States is 0.5 per million people per year.[39] Pituitary tumors producing CS are more frequent.[72] Women are more commonly affected, and a wide age distribution is seen.[22,34,39] Growth retardation and suppressed sexual maturation are most notable in children. Additional characteristics include rapid weight gain associated with abnormal fat distribution. A thick layer of facial fat rounds out the cheeks, producing the typical circular "moon face" appearance. In addition, a prominent fat pad is deposited over the upper thoracic spine, producing a mass called a "buffalo hump". The abdomen is typically pendulous. Patients may also demonstrate hypertension, rapid hair growth,[19,48] muscular atrophy,[33] and striae.[39,48]

IMAGING FINDINGS

The hallmark radiographic sign is generalized osteoporosis typified by marked loss of trabecular bone and less evident loss of cortical bone. Also evident is an increased number of insufficiency fractures of the vertebrae, scapula, ribs, and pubic bones.[19,22,34,48,76] Corticosteroid therapy producing CS may also lead to osteonecrosis[48,76] and insufficiency fractures.[48]

CLINICAL COMMENTS

Excessive production of cortisol is due to ACTH hypersecretion by pituitary adenomas and occasionally ectopic ACTH-secreting tumors or autonomous adrenal corticoid tumors.

Characteristic features. These features include facial-trunk obesity (buffalo hump, moon face), abdominal striae, growth retardation, rapid hair loss, and muscular atrophy.* Generalized osteopenia, insufficiency fractures, and occasional osteonecrosis are the primary imaging findings.[19,22] Enlarged sella turcica or evidence of pituitary hypertrophy[29] may be present but is not a routine finding.[9] Plain films of the skull, chest, and abdomen are often normal. Computed tomography (CT), magnetic resonance imaging (MRI), and ultrasound (US) are often required.[9,40] Angiography and venous sampling are useful to document the hypovascularity that is typical of endocrine tumors.[40,72] Occult secretory tumors may be found with scintigraphy.[33] In cases of recurrent Cushing's disease, the treatment of choice is transphenoidal pituitary adenectomy. Surgery is followed by irradiation (4,000 to 5,000 RAD). Surgical success rate is 90% for skilled neurosurgeons.[38] Hypercortisolemia, external pituitary irradiation, and posttreatment hypopituitarism may increase the risk of brain infarction.[42]

KEY CONCEPTS

- *Cortisol levels are elevated secondary to glucocorticoid therapy or a pituitary or adrenal cortex tumor.*
- *The physical appearance is marked by a rounded moon face and buffalo hump fat accumulation along the upper back.*
- *Other findings include hypertension, abdominal striae, retarded growth maturation in children, inappropriate osteopenia, possibly osteonecrosis, and insufficiency fractures.*
- *Surgery and occasional use of irradiation are highly successful.*

*References 19, 22, 33, 34, 39, 72.

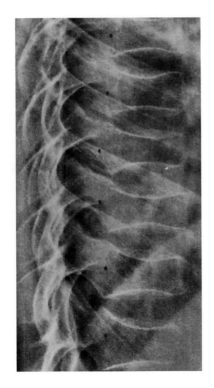

FIG. 16-4   Cushing's syndrome produced by prolonged administration of adrenocorticoids. Generalized osteopenia and bone softening produce deep end-plate concavities (codfish vertebra) and loss of vertical height by repeated microfractures. (From Silverman F, Kuhn J: *Caffey's pediatric x-ray diagnosis: an integrated imaging approach,* ed 9, St Louis, 1993, Mosby.)

Giantism (Gigantism)

BACKGROUND

Hypersecretion of growth hormone (GH) occurring in a skeletally immature patient produces excessive proportional bone growth, known as *giantism*. This unusual condition is produced typically by adenomas of the anterior lobe of the pituitary gland or, less commonly, by diffuse hyperplasia of acidophilic cells elsewhere. Organomegaly and commensurate hypertrophy of muscles and connective tissue are associated findings.

IMAGING FINDINGS

The hallmark imaging findings of true giantism are of proportional, yet exaggerated, skeletal growth. The bones are increased in both length and diameter.[5,17] Enlargement of the sella turcica or evidence of pressure erosion may be seen occasionally on plain film or, more reliably, with CT. MRI better demonstrates the abnormal pituitary gland. Combinations of imaging may be required to identify ectopic sources of GH.[77]

CLINICAL COMMENTS

Remarkable, proportional growth is typical. The skeletal maturation of patients with giantism may exceed that of their age-related peers by 11 standard deviations. A case study reported a 3½-year-old boy who demonstrated a level of skeletal maturity consistent with a 10½-year-old. At 7 years of age he was a well-proportioned boy 182 cm (6 feet, ¾ inches) tall, weighing 99.4 kg (219 lb) and wearing size 13EEE shoes.[77] Lab profiles include elevations of 24-hour growth hormone secretion, paradoxical growth response to administered thyrotropin-releasing hormone (TRH), and failure to suppress serum growth hormone levels with oral glucose loading.[5,17,77] Hypercalcemia, hyperphosphaturia, and elevated levels of alkaline phosphatase are consistent findings.

> ## KEY CONCEPTS
> - *Giantism involves hypersecretion of growth hormone occurring in skeletally immature patients.*
> - *This condition is marked by proportional enlargement of the skeleton.*
> - *The abnormal pituitary gland may alter the appearance of the sella turcica.*

Hyperparathyroidism

BACKGROUND

Hyperparathyroidism (HPT) is the condition of elevated levels of parathormone (PT), resulting from a variety of direct and indirect stimuli.[16,66,76] Excess levels of PT produce disorders of calcium, phosphate, and bone metabolism; this is the most common cause of hypercalcemia.[64,66] HPT occurs in approximately 1 in 700 persons. HPT is divided into three categories: primary, secondary, and tertiary.

Primary hyperparathyroidism is most commonly produced by a single adenoma (80% to 85% of cases), less commonly, parathyroid hyperplasia (10% to 15% of cases), multiple adenomas (4% to 5% of cases), and rarely secretory carcinomas (1% to 3% of cases).[23,66] Secondary hyperparathyroidism is due to chronic renal failure in most cases (Fig. 16-5).[27,32,76] PT secretion is stimulated by elevated serum levels of phosphate and reduced ionized serum calcium.[27,76] Diffuse enlargement of all parathyroid glands is typical.[23] Tertiary HPT may be described as a complication of dialysis. Parathyroid glands may act independently of the serum calcium levels.[27,76] In this setting, as serum phosphate levels increase, stimulus for PT secretion also increases.

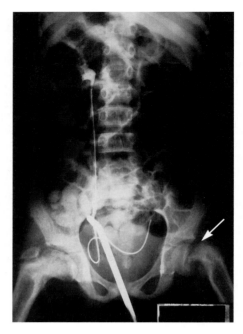

FIG. 16-5   Secondary hyperparathyroidism produced in this child by renal hypoplasia. Also note the slipped capital femoral epiphysis on the reading right *(arrow)*.

"PT acts predominantly on the skeleton, the kidneys and gastrointestinal tract to mobilize skeletal calcium into circulation, reducing the renal excretion of calcium and increasing gastrointestinal absorption of calcium by a diversity of metabolic actions."[23,66] Although primary HPT remains the most common form of hyperparathyroidism, secondary and tertiary HPT are increasing in frequency. This is most likely a result of an increasingly larger geriatric population, more frequent encounters with the causes of secondary and tertiary HPT, and increased longevity. Primary HPT is a disease that affects predominantly middle-age women, one half of whom are postmenopausal. The balance of the cases are equally divided between men and premenopausal women.[16,23,64] It is exceedingly rare to find patients younger than 16 years of age.[66]

IMAGING FINDINGS

It is now recognized that HPT is more common than previously thought[16,23,55,64,66] and is most likely to demonstrate little or no specific signs or symptoms.[16,55,64] The insensitivity of plain film and earlier recognition of HPT by laboratory exam often produce essentially normal radiographs.[55] Bone mineral density assessments using single- or dual-energy x-ray absorbptiometry or quantitative CT are more useful and should be used to investigate asymptomatic hyperparathyroidism.[16,55,76] Bone biopsy is definitive, but it is not used on a routine basis and is primarily a research tool.[27,64]

The radiographic analysis must answer two basic questions. First, what is the cause of the elevations of parathormone? Determining this will establish presurgical localization, treatment of renal disease if possible, and change in dialysis technique if required. Second, what is the clinical status and what skeletal and extraskeletal manifestations are present?

Follow-up examinations monitor successful treatments or identify progressive disease. Experts do not agree on which imaging strategy is best. Successful imaging often includes several complementary modalities. Because the majority of cases of primary hyperparathyroidism is caused by a single adenoma (80% to 85%),

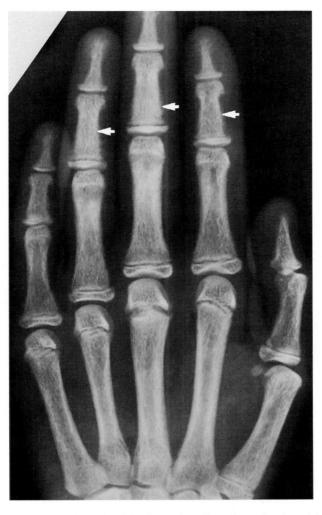

FIG. 16-6 Hyperparathyroidism. Resorption of bone from subperiosteal sites typically located along the radial side of the middle phalanges of second, third, and fourth rays (arrows). This patient also demonstrates acroosteolysis of the terminal tufts. (From Eisenberg RL, Dennis CA: *Comprehensive radiographic pathology*, ed 2, St Louis, 1995, Mosby.)

high-resolution ultrasound by an experienced sonographer is advocated as a first step. This study is considered safe, cost effective, and relatively sensitive. Its value is diminished by small or ectopic lesions.[23,58,64] Scintigraphy in the form of [99M]Tc-Sestamibi localizes parathyroid tumors normally situated and in ectopic locations. It also can determine parathyroid gland functionality.[23,58,64] Magnetic resonance imaging is advocated in cases of hyperparathyroidism with essentially normal parathyroid glands or persistent postsurgical elevations of parathormone. This clinical picture is often associated with ectopic secretory tissue.[23,58] Contrast-enhanced CT, arthrography, and selected venous sampling may be used in difficult cases or if reoperation is contemplated.[40,58,66]

The effects of hyperparathyroidism on the skull and extraskeletal structures are numerous. Some are classically, if not exclusively, associated with HPT. HPT effects on bone probably include a higher remodeling rate of the haversian canals. Ultimately longitudinal defects will appear in cortical bone.[27,37,55,66] Hyperthyroidism, Sudeck's atrophy, and Paget's disease may appear similarly. Cortical endosteal and trabecular resorption also occur.[27] Subperiosteal reabsorption is seen early and most often found along the radial side

of the middle phalanx of the hand. Fine grain screens producing images with great detail[18] are required for early recognition of this virtually pathognomonic sign.* If progression of the disease occurs, ungual tufts (acroosteolysis), proximal phalanges, and metacarpals will be involved[27] (Fig. 16-6).

Reports exist of generalized osteopenia[16] with accentuated trabeculae pattern caused by resorption of nonessential trabeculae and loss of cortical definition. The latter involves both periosteal and endosteal cortices. This produces blurring and irregular, thinned cortices with widened, yet rarified medullary cavities.[27,76] Pseudowidening of the joint space may be seen as resorption of the sacroiliac (Fig. 16-7), acromioclavicular (Fig. 16-8), and pubic joint surfaces.[27,76] The upper medial surface of the humerus, tibia, calcaneus, ischial tuberosities, and the upper border of the ribs may demonstrate resorption.[27] The fine permeative destructive pattern of the skull, known as "salt-and-pepper" skull, is also typical of HPT (Fig. 16-9).[66,76] Resorption of the lamina dura surrounding the tooth

---

*References 16, 27, 32, 49, 55, 66, 76.

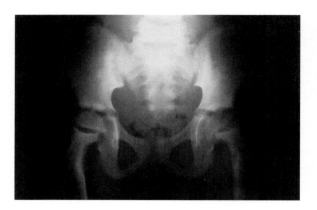

FIG. 16-7   Hyperparathyroidism. Subchondral resorption producing pseudowidening and sclerotic margins. The ilium is affected to a greater extent. (Courtesy Gary M. Guebert, Maryland Heights, Mo.)

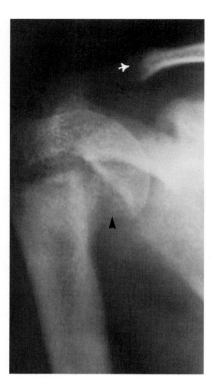

FIG. 16-8   Hyperparathyroidism. Acroosteolysis of the clavicle is common. Subperiosteal resorption of the humerus has led to slipped capital epiphysis *(arrowhead).* (From Eisenberg RL, Dennis CA: *Comprehensive radiographic pathology,* ed 2, St Louis, Mosby, 1995.)

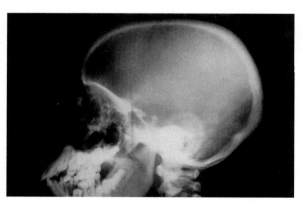

FIG. 16-9   Hyperparathyroidism. "Salt-and-pepper skull" produced by alternating zones of lucency and sclerosis. Loss of trabecular detail in the diploic space blurs the separation between inner and outer tubules. (Courtesy Gary M. Guebert, Maryland Heights, Mo.)

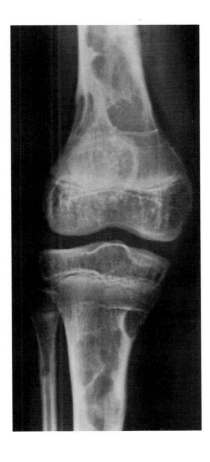

FIG. 16-10 Hyperparathyroidism. Brown tumors, collections of fibrous tissue and giant cells, producing lytic regions within the osseous structures of the knee. (From Eisenberg RL, Dennis CA: *Comprehensive radiographic pathology*, ed 2, St Louis, 1995, Mosby.)

socket is also seen. Administration of vitamin D and calcium leads to accelerated loss of bone mineral density in some patients, and cases of hyperphosphotemia exhibit increased incidence of soft tissue calcification.

Osteitis fibrosa cystica, also referred to as a *brown tumor* (Fig. 16-10), is a collection of fibrous tissue and giant cells in bone that is found in primary and secondary hyperparathyroidism.[9,23,66] These present as geographic lucencies. Slightly expansile, they are most commonly found in the mandible, pelvis, ribs, and femora.[22] Overall, brown tumors are seen infrequently.[64] Soft tissue calcifications are seen in later stages of HPT (Figs. 16-11 and 16-12).[27,76] Nephrocalcinosis is still considered to be a common presenting complaint.[64] Chondrocalcinosis of menisci in the knee as well as other sites is seen. Secondary hyperparathyroidism is thought to produce more frequent soft tissue calcifications of vascular and periarticular structures.[27,40,76] Osteosclerosis of the spine (rugger jersey spine) (Fig. 16-13) is a characteristic, yet unusual, sign.[14,76] In the presence of open growth plates, periarticular condensation of bone may be seen.[14]

CLINICAL COMMENTS

As our understanding of HPT has increased, it has become recognized that the most common presenting sign is hypercalcemia.* Hypercalcemia in the presence of elevated PT by immunoradiometric assay (IRMA) or immunochemoluminescent assay (ICMA) is a definitive diagnosis.[64] Some patients have persistent high normal levels of serum calcium. If this resulted from anything other than pri-

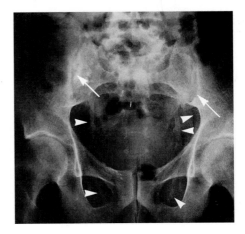

FIG. 16-11 Hyperparathyroidism. Metastatic vascular calcification is seen *(arrowheads)*. Note the pseudowidening of the sacroiliac joints *(arrows)*.

PART TWO Bone, Joints, and Soft Tissues

---

*References 16, 23, 27, 58, 64, 66.

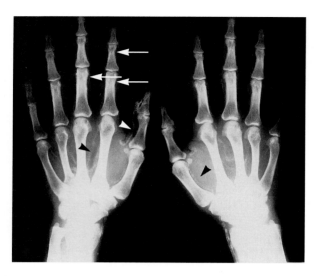

FIG. 16-12   Hyperparathyroidism. Metastatic vascular calcifications in the hand (*arrowheads*). Note the subperiosteal resorption of bone on the radial margins of the middle phalanges (*arrows*).

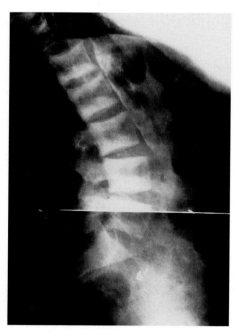

FIG. 16-13   Hyperparathyroidism. Unusual yet characteristic osteosclerosis in the spine (rugger jersey spine).

mary or secondary parathyroid disease, the PT levels would be low or nonexistent.[64] Otherwise a paucity of presenting features exists.[9] Silverberg and Bilezikian found one half of their patients were asymptomatic or demonstrated nonspecific complaints.[64] These may include depression, subjective weakness, memory and sleep abnormalities, constipation, "bone pain," loss of appetite, nausea, vomiting, or polydipsia.[58,64,66] Some report an association between childhood irradiation of the neck and primary hyperparathyroidism.[64] The classic features of HPT are decreased bone density, brown tumors, leontiasis ossea, renal calculi, chondrocalcenosis, and metastatic calcification. These features, although classic, are uncommon presenting features. Of these, renal calculi is the most frequent finding, occurring in 20% of all cases.[32,64]

KEY CONCEPTS

- *Hyperparathyroidism involves hyperactivity of the parathyroid gland, presenting in primary, secondary, and tertiary forms.*
- *It most often affects middle-age females.*
- *The patient may remain asymptomatic.*
- *Classic laboratory findings include hypercalcemia and elevated parathormone levels.*
- *Imaging findings are recognized as periosteal and endosteal resorption of the cortices of the middle phalanges of the second and third digits bilaterally.*
- *Additional radiographic changes include salt-and-pepper skull, acroosteolysis, accentuated trabecular pattern, nephrocalcinosis, vascular calcification, chondrocalcinosis, and resorption of lamina dura.*
- *Bone density may be decreased and can be quantified by photon absorptiometry.*
- *Brown tumors and rugger jersey spine are characteristic but uncommon.*
- *Mild cases are managed by hormone replacement therapy; surgery is indicated in cases of low vertebral bone mass and primary hyperparathyroidism with vitamin D deficiency.*
- *Surgical removal by experienced surgeons produces success rates approaching 95%.*
- *Administration of vitamin D and calcium leads to accelerated loss of bone mineral density in some patients and in cases of hyperphosphotemia exhibits an increased incidence of soft tissue calcification.*

Hypoparathyroidism

BACKGROUND

Hypocalcemia secondary to low or absent parathormone is the hallmark of hypoparathyroidism. Hypoparathyroidism most commonly follows thyroidectomy or radical laryngeal surgery.[17] Cases of hypoparathyroidism have followed radioactive iodine treatments for hyperthyroidism.[10] Reports exist of metastases (typically breast cancer) and transient forms relating to surgical cure for hyperparathyroidism.[14] Sporadic idiopathic and familial idiopathic conditions have a more variable presentation. Familial forms may be associated with pernicious anemia and hypoadrenalism. This is characterized further by circulating antibodies to the parathyroid, thyroid, and adrenal glands, supporting the concept of an autoimmune etiology in some cases.[53] The earliest age of onset is seen in the familial form, often within the first year of life. Sporadic forms are typically found in patients ages 5 through 10 years. The acquired form of hypoparathyroidism occurs later in life.

IMAGING FINDINGS

Generalized or localized sclerosis is the most common skeletal abnormality. Thickened calvarium and hypoplastic dentition, radiodense metaphyseal bands seen in the long bones, iliac crest and vertebral margins are also potential findings. Occasionally reported are osteopenia, typically in pseudohypoparathyroidism. Asymptomatic periarticular calcifications, particularly involving the hips and shoulders, are not rare.[53]

CLINICAL COMMENTS

The predominant features of hypoparathyroidism evolve as a result of chronic hypoglycemia. These include tetany, epilepsy, cataracts, and papilledema with elevated intracranial pressure. Common, yet not absolute, features include short stature and mental impairment. Alopecia occurs in varying degrees. Underdevelopment of the dental roots is a common presenting complaint. Excessive renal reabsorption of phosphorous as a consequence of hypocalcemia is inevitable. Hypocalcemia and hyperphosphatemia combine to suppress 1, 25 dihydroxy vitamin D synthesis to very low levels.

Effective treatment includes calcium and vitamin D analogs. Once the hyperphosphatemia reduces, serum calcium levels rise. Candidiasis of the nail beds or orogenital regions occurs in some sporadic or familial cases.[5,17]

KEY COMMENTS

- *Low or undetectable levels of parathormone leading to chronic hypocalcemia and hyperphosphatemia cause hypoparathyroidism.*
- *Acquired forms occur later in life and may result from neck surgery (often for hyperthyroidism), following iodine treatment of breast metastasis.*
- *Radiology features are marked by osteosclerosis, thickened calvarium, hypoplastic dentition, periarticular calcification around the hips and shoulders.*

Pseudohypoparathyroidism

BACKGROUND

Pseudohypoparathyroidism (PHP) is an X-linked genetic disorder associated with normal or enlarged parathyroid glands and parathyroid target organ (bone, kidney) insensitivity. Often, but not always, a typical skeletal phenotype occurs in addition to parathormone resistance and is referred to as *Albright's hereditary osteodystrophy (AHO) type I*.[5,17,51,61] These skeletal changes include shortened fourth and fifth metacarpals, short stature, round face, premature hair loss, and some degree of mental impairment.[5,61,78]

IMAGING FINDINGS

It is rare to see PHP in the absence of metacarpal shortening; it most frequently affects the first, fourth, and fifth digits. Metatarsals may also be affected. A positive metacarpal sign is frequently observed.[17,51,53,78] A line tangential to the heads of the fourth and fifth metacarpals should be distal to or just contact the head of the third metacarpal. Failure to do so indicates a positive metacarpal index.[51,53] However, variability in the pattern and degree of metacarpal shortening may render the metacarpal index unreliable (Fig. 16-14).[5] In addition, the metacarpals and phalanges, particularly those of the first digit, may appear wide with cone-shaped epiphyses and perpendicularly oriented exostoses.[51,78] Thickening of the skull (Fig. 16-15) and calcification of the basal ganglion (Fig. 16-16)[47] may also be present. Reports of spinal stenosis also exist.

CLINICAL COMMENTS

PHP presents with the classic phenotypic changes, and laboratory studies indicate hypocalcemia, hyperphosphatemia, and elevated

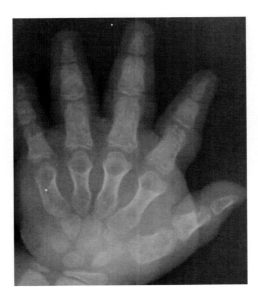

FIG. 16-14   Pseudohypoparathyroidism. Short metacarpals and short, wide phalanges are demonstrated here. The uniform shortening of all the metacarpals prevents demonstration of a positive metacarpal index. (From Taybi H: Pseudohypoparathyroidism [PH], *Semin Roentenol* 8:214, 1973.)

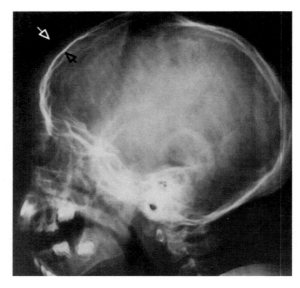

FIG. 16-15   Pseudohypoparathyroidism. A thickened skull *(arrows)* demonstrated in a short, obese 4-year-old. (From Taybi H: Pseudohypoparathyroidism [PH], *Semin Roentenol* 8:214, 1973.)

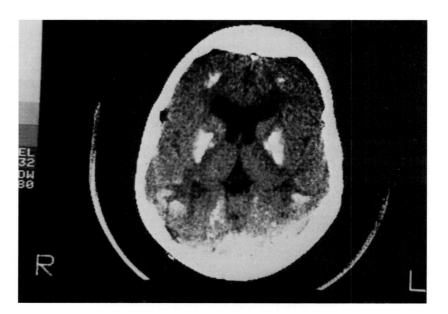

FIG. 16-16   Pseudohypoparathyroidism. Axial CT demonstrates thickening of the cranial vault and several sites of intracerebral calcification. (From Taybi H, Lachman RS: *Radiology of syndromes, metabolic and skeletal dysplasias,* ed 4, St Louis, 1996, Mosby.)

PT levels.[47,78] The renal and osseous PT receptors do not respond.[47,78] Treatment of PHP involves administration of vitamin D derivatives.[17] Short stature, obesity, round face, and early hair loss are typical.[1,47,51]

KEY CONCEPTS

- *Pseudohypoparathyroidism represents an end organ insensitivity to parathormone, also known as Albright's hereditary osteodystrophy type I, when patients exhibit a characteristic phenotype.*
- *Hypocalcemia and hyperphosphatemia occur, despite elevated serum levels of parathormone.*
- *Positive metacarpal index is frequent and suggestive of the condition.*
- *The small bones of the hands and feet appear short, wide, with cup-shaped epiphyses, and exostoses perpendicular to the long axis of the bones.*
- *Those afflicted often exhibit mild mental retardation, round face, obesity, and a short stature.*

Pseudopseudohypoparathyroidism

BACKGROUND

Pseudopseudohypoparathyroidism (PPHP) is the normal calcemic form of pseudohypoparathyroidism (PHP). PPHP and PHP may appear in the same family, suggesting a close genetic similarity.[1,51] These entities share common skeletal and developmental defects without the laboratory findings suggestive of hypothyroidism.[1] Pseudopseudohypoparathyroidism patients, unlike those with PHP, have a normal cyclic adenosine monophosphate (cAMP) response to parathormone in the kidney, suggesting an adequate number of membrane receptors.

IMAGING FINDINGS

The findings of PPHP are indistinguishable from PHP.[51] They share the features of short stature, metacarpal shortening (Fig. 16-17), and shortened, wide phalanges with cupped epiphysis. Exostosis may be seen.[17,51,78]

CLINICAL COMMENTS

The classic radiographic features are also seen in conjunction with obesity, round face, absent knuckles, and a prematurely receding hair line.[17,51,78] Mild mental retardation, abnormal dentition, strabismus, impaired taste, and olfaction complete the clinical picture.[53]

KEY CONCEPTS

- *Pseudopseudohypoparathyroidism is the normocalcemic form of pseudohypoparathyroidism.*
- *Skeletal and phenotypical changes are indistinguishable from PHP, including short metacarpals, positive metacarpal index, and exostoses.*

Hypothyroidism

BACKGROUND

Hypothyroidism involves decreased levels of thyroid hormones, such as triiodothyronine, T3, and thyroxin, T4, in peripheral tissues. The condition results from disorders of the thyroid gland (primary) or decreased stimulating hormone secondary to disorders of the pituitary (secondary) or hypothalmus (tertiary). However, rare, peripheral resistance to the circulating hormone may also occur. A long list of primary, secondary, and tertiary causes have been identified, including dietary deficiencies, gland atrophy and inflammation, or destruction of gland tissue secondary to radioactive iodine treatments, surgery, and infiltrative disorders such as amyloidoses, metastases, and lymphoma.

In endemic regions, dietary deficiencies of iodine pose a significant health problem. Deficiency of dietary iodine represents the most common preventable cause of mental impairment. In 1991 the World Health Organization stated that 20% of the world's population were at risk.[11,35] Although endemic iodine deficiency is the most common cause of goiter and hypothyroidism worldwide, autoimmunity is the most common cause in nonendemic regions. Surgery and radioiodine treatments for thyroid toxicosis account for approximately one third of all cases of hypothyroidism.[5,11,20]

Hypothyroidism in utero produces cretins. Two types are re-

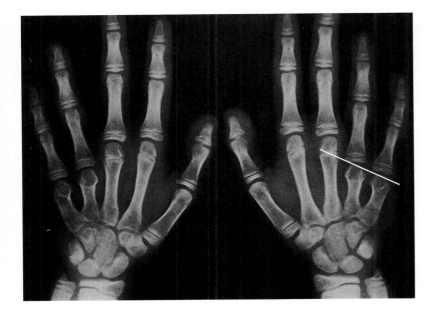

FIG. 16-17   Pseudopseudohypoparathyroidism. A positive metacarpal index *(line)* was demonstrated by this short, but normally proportioned patient with PPHP. (From Silverman F, Kuhn J: *Caffey's pediatric x-ray diagnosis: an integrated imaging approach,* ed 9, St Louis, 1993, Mosby.)

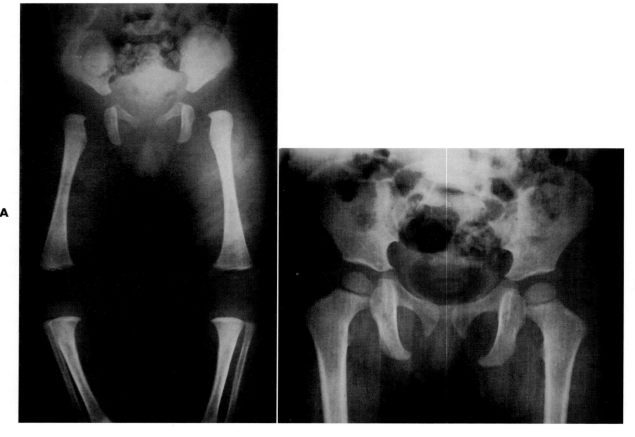

FIG. 16-18   Hypothyroidism. **A,** Delayed ossification of the acetabulum-simulated acetabular dysplasia. **B,** After 30 months of thyroid medication ossification has progressed and no longer appears dysplastic. (From Silverman FN, Currano G. *Metabolism* 9:248, 1960.)

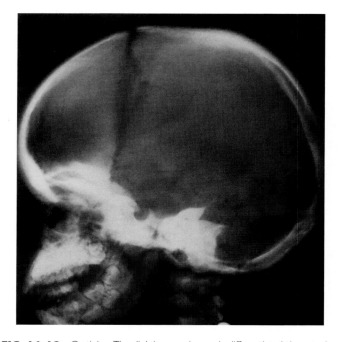

FIG. 16-19   Cretinism. The diploic space is poorly differentiated, the anterior fontanelle shows delayed closure, and the cranial sutures are wide. The pneumatization of the skull is delayed. (From Eisenberg RL, Dennis CA: *Comprehensive radiographic pathology,* ed 2, St Louis, 1995, Mosby.)

ported: myxedematous and neurological.[20] Juvenile myxedema occurs in children with fewer musculoskeletal abnormalities. The pattern of involvement in the adult varies further.

IMAGING FINDINGS

The majority of radiographic abnormalities occurs in the younger patients who demonstrate cretinism or juvenile myxedema. Delayed osseous maturation (Fig. 16-18), persistent sutures with wormian bones, brachycephaly, and enlarged sella turcica are features commonly seen. Prognathism and hypoplasia of the sinuses may be present. Multiple epiphyseal growth centers arise, producing irregular articular surfaces. Coxa vara, coxa valga, and slipped femoral capital epiphysis have all been described.[35,53] The spine may demonstrate a bullet shape, osteoporosis, and delayed development.[20,53] The adult may occasionally demonstrate osteosclerosis (Fig. 16-19) secondary to a decreased rate of turnover.

CLINICAL COMMENTS

Although regions of endemic cretinism exist, it is not a significant problem in North America. The hallmark features of juvenile myxedema include mental retardation, lethargy, constipation, large tongue, abdominal distention, hypotonia, dry hair and skin, and delayed dentition. Adults who acquired hypothyroidism are typically female with dry, coarse skin and hair, easy fatigability, lethargy, edema, hoarseness, constipation, and bradycardia. The most common neurological complaint is carpal tunnel syndrome.

KEY CONCEPTS

- *Deficiency of thyroid hormones (triiodothyronine, T3 and thyroxin, T4) produces a variable clinical picture based on the stage of development.*
- *Hypothyroidism in infants results in cretinism, and in children results in juvenile myxedema.*
- *Osseous changes are predominant in children and may include delayed ossification, persistent sutures, wormian bones, brachycephaly, prognathic jaw, enlarged or altered shape of the sella turcica secondary to pituitary hypertrophy, multiple epiphyseal growth centers, hip abnormalities, bullet-shaped vertebrae, and osteopenia.*
- *Signs and symptoms include lethargy, dry hair and skin, mental retardation, constipation, large tongue, abdominal distention, hypotonia, and delayed dentition.*

 # Metabolic Disorders

Osteoporosis

BACKGROUND

Generalized. *Osteoporosis* is defined as qualitatively normal bone present in deficient quantities. Osteoporosis is the most common cause of generalized metabolic osteopenia. Females are affected to a greater degree than males. It is mostly a disease of older patients; young patients are rarely affected. It is estimated that up to 20 to 25 million individuals are affected in the United States.[74] Osteoporosis is associated with 1.5 million fractures per year in the female population over 40 years of age. The United States spends in excess of 8 billion dollars per year on direct and indirect costs related to osteoporosis.

The three major categories of osteoporosis are the following:
1. Generalized; affecting the majority of the skeleton
2. Regional; affecting one limb or section of the body
3. Localized; producing focal osteopenia in one or multiple discrete portions of bone.

The more common and classic causes of generalized osteoporosis such as immobilization, disuse, and transient regional osteoporosis are discussed in this section (Table 16-1). The balance of the etiologies associated with generalized osteoporosis are discussed in this chapter and elsewhere in the text. Localized osteoporosis, typically produced by neoplastic and infectious bone destruction, as well as periarticular osteopenia, seen in some cases of inflammatory arthritis, are discussed in their respective chapters.

Generalized osteoporosis is typically asymptomatic until a complication, usually fracture, occurs. Decreased bone mineral density (BMD) often leads to fracture.[29,43,53,59] Vertebral fractures are commonly found in the transitional spine regions. The thoracolumbar junction, lumbosacral junction, apex of the thoracic spine, proximal femur, and distal radius are the most common locations.

Regional. Osteoporosis may be limited to a skeletal region following disuse or immobilization, reflex symphathetic dystrophy (Sudeck's atrophy), and as idiopathic transient presentations (transient regional osteoporosis and regional migratory osteoporosis). The most common of these are immobilization and disuse osteoporosis. Casted fractures, central nervous system injury producing motion loss, and bone and joint inflammations[50] are the most frequent causes. These patients demonstrate a negative calcium balance. That is, skeletal loss of calcium in the urine and reduced uptake of dietary calcium occur. Variable patterns of presentation include osteopenia, spotty lucencies, bandlike zones of rarification, and cortical scalloping. These patterns may mimic aggressive osteolytic lesions at times.[53,76] The degree of bone mineral density loss associated with disuse and immobilization may lead to further insufficiency fractures.

Transient regional osteoporosis defines a rapid onset of osteopenia in a periarticular location, which is self-limiting and spontaneously reverses without evident cause.[53,76] This disorder may take the form of transient osteoporosis of the hip or regional migratory osteoporosis.[53,76] They demonstrate similar clinical and radiological features, prompting discussion that these disorders are related to each other, and probably related to reflex sympathetic dystrophy.[53]

Transient osteoporosis of the hip occurs in young adults. Men are more commonly affected than women (Fig. 16-20). Patients present with a painful limp and antalgic gait that predates the radiographic changes. It is well documented yet unexplained that the left hip is almost always involved in females. Full recovery is expected in 3 months to 1 year.[53,76]

Regional migratory osteoporosis, the other form of transient regional osteoporosis,[53,76] involves the hip less frequently. The knee, ankle, and foot are the typical locations.[53] Men are affected more

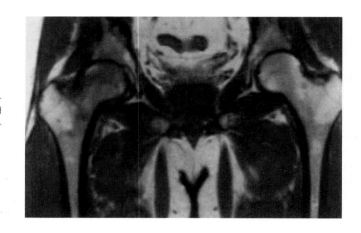

FIG. 16-20   Transient osteoporosis of the hip. Demonstration of diffuse decrease in signal intensity in the right *(reading left)* femur head on this T1-weighted (TR 500, TE 15) image. (From Taybi H, Lachman RS: *Radiology of syndromes, metabolic and skeletal dysplasias,* ed 4, St Louis, 1996, Mosby.)

TABLE 16-1
Pattern of Osteopenia

Pattern	Definition	Classic examples
Generalized	Osteopenia affecting the majority of the skeleton	Senile osteoporosis Postmenopausal Hyperparathyroidism Cushing's disease Widespread malignant disease (e.g., metastasis, multiple myeloma)
Regionalized	Osteopenia affecting one limb or section of the body	Disuse atrophy (immobilization) Reflex sympathetic dystrophy Transient regional osteoporosis Regional migratory osteoporosis
Localized	Focal osteopenia in one or multiple discrete portions of bone	Lytic metastasis Osteomyelitis Inflammatory arthritides

than women.[76] Regional migratory osteoporosis presents in the fourth and fifth decade of life. The progression starts with pain and swelling, typically involving the lower extremity. Radiographic changes appear in weeks to months, then regression occurs within 9 months,[53,76] and involvement of another region may follow. Plain film demonstrates a regional pattern of profound osteopenia and rarified subchondral bone. A bone scan may be positive and MRI demonstrates signal intensity consistent with intraosseous edema.[53,69]

IMAGING FINDINGS

Generalized osteoporosis is demonstrated on the plain film as widespread osteopenia produced by thin cortices and expanded intratrabecular spaces.[4,53,59] The relative insensitivity of plain film requires a decrease in bone mineral density of approximately 30% to 50% before it is demonstrated on the plain films. Bone scans are invariably normal unless fracture repair is present.[29,53,76] Evaluation of bone mineral density is most effective by single photon absorbtiometry, dual photon absorbtiometry, and quantitative computerized tomography. These bone mineral density studies must be age-, gender-, and race-matched to normal values.[15]

By the time osteoporosis is readily apparent on plain film, it is usually beyond the mild or moderate stage and increasingly likely that the classically associated findings are present. The spine, prox-

imal femur, and tubular bones of the extremities display the most characteristic features of osteoporosis. First and foremost is osteopenia.[59] The remaining bone is histologically normal; it is simply rarified. The cortex is thin and porous (Fig. 16-21). Resorption occurs in the horizontal trabeculae, which uncover the fibers that sit predominantly along the lines of stress, thus accentuating their appearance (Fig. 16-22). Piezoelectric activity is thought to account for the disparate resorption rates between horizontal and vertical trabeculae.[50] Use of fine grain screens produces the best detail and demonstrates osseous structures with distinct, sharp cortical margins.[18] This is not a feature of osteomalacia, another common cause of osteopenia.

Change in the shape of a spinal segment may also indicate osteoporosis. Chronic microfractures producing bone remodeling are typically represented by the "fish" or "codfish" vertebrae.[54] This deformity is marked by deepened concavities of the vertebral endplates, without significant alteration of the anterior and posterior vertebral margins.[53,54] The expansile pressures of the intervertebral disc produces the deformity in the weakened vertebrae. On occasion, focal intrusion of nuclear material into the vertebral bodies may be seen (Schmorl's nodes). The wedge-shape fracture[4] and the vertebrae plana, or pancake vertebrae, are signs of abrupt osseous failure resulting from single traumatic events. In cases of severe osteoporosis, trivial trauma such as coughing and sneezing may be

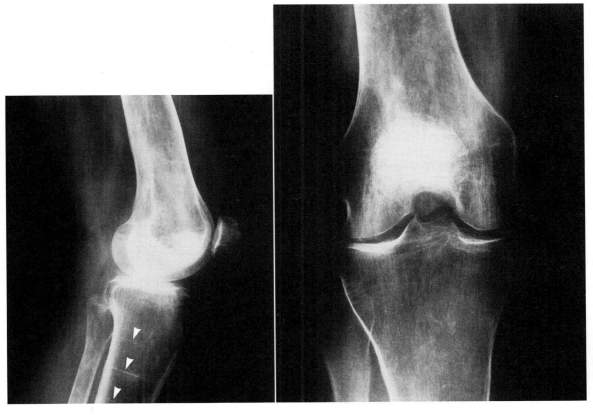

FIG. 16-21 Osteoporosis. Marked cortical thinning and widened medullary cavity are classic features. Note the horizontal bone bars or reinforcement lines (*arrowheads*).

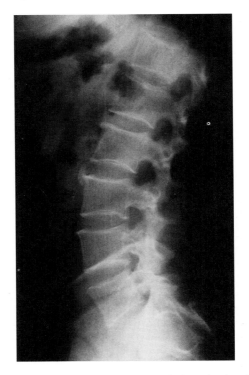

FIG. 16-22 Osteoporosis. Resorption of the horizontal trabeculae has "uncovered" the vertical fibers, accentuating their appearance.

the proximate cause of the spinal fracture and a common cause of localized pain.

The expression of osteoporosis in the proximal femur is in the alteration of Ward's triangle.[28,53,76] Ward's triangle is bordered by three groups of trabecular fibers. The principal compressive group, secondary compressive group, and tensile group make up the boundaries of Ward's triangle (Fig. 16-23). Normally, it is difficult to resolve the individual groups of fibers. As trabecular absorption progresses, these groups are readily visible and Ward's triangle continues to enlarge until the secondary compression group disappears. The last fibers to resorb belong to the principle compressive group.[25,53,76] Femoral neck fracture is a common, serious, potentially life-threatening complication of osteoporosis. The aging population in the United States guarantees that this incidence of femoral neck fracture will increase. This will continue to cost billions of dollars until proper preventive and management protocols are perfected.

CLINICAL COMMENTS

The pathogenesis of osteoporosis is unclear. Studies of the processes associated with senile and postmenopausal osteoporosis have explored theories of primary failure of bone formation as well as excessive bone resorption with conflicting results. Hormone imbalance with loss of estrogenic activity features prominently in today's preventive and therapeutic models.[29,43,53]

Other factors considered are calcium deficiency, fluctuations in gonadal and adrenal cortical hormones, thyroid hormone, and growth hormone. These are known to be influential, but why and to what extent remains unclear.[53] Dietary deficiency of calcium has been strongly supported.[25,43] The type and degree of physical activity demonstrated by the patients during their adolescent and young adult years certainly play a role in developing bone mineral density.[43] Men and women have a positive bone mineral density increase until approximately 30 years of age. After 40 years of age,

men and women lose bone mineral density at a rate of 0.3% per year. This rate continues for men, unless aggravated by some other factor, through the end of their lives. As females reach menopause, the rate of decline in bone mineral density jumps to 3% per year for approximately 8 to 10 years. Over this interval, women lose approximately 30% of their bone mineral density.[25,43,53]

LABORATORY VALUES

Laboratory values are routinely normal with the exception of hydroxyproline found in urine. Osteoporosis most frequently comes to light as a result of some complication of the process. Typically fracture is the elucidating event. In patients with proximal femoral neck fractures, 75% to 80% have demonstrable osteoporosis at the time of the injury. Femoral fractures are associated with a high mortality rate, 10% to 20% in excess of their age-matched peers. Although most patients survive the hip fracture, 20% to 30% still acquire enough disability and dependency that institutionalization occurs.[43]

Although hip fractures are the most devastating, several other sites of fracture are common. Fractures of the distal radius, foot/toe, and vertebrae, although typically cared for in nonhospital settings, still represent significant, yet poorly elucited, morbidity.[43] A less common, but serious, form of vertebral body fracture is the one associated with a retropulsion of an osseous fragment, producing cord injury.

TREATMENT

The burgeoning elderly population in the Unites States guarantees a dramatic rise in the number of fractures, with ever-increasing health care costs. This creates an urgent need for the adoption of adequate preventive programs. Treatment options are numerous and represent the various etiological viewpoints. Estrogen therapy, biphosphonate,[29,30,74] calcium, and vitamin D supplementation are potential therapeutic models. Some combination of the above treatments is often proposed with the additional instruction

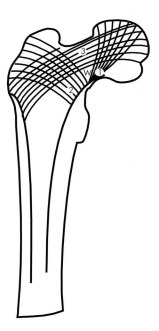

FIG. 16-23 Ward's triangle (*W*) is an area in the lower femoral neck nearly devoid of trabeculae. It is surrounded by three patterns of trabeculae: *1*, principal compressive group; *2*, secondary compressive group; *3*, principal tensile group.

to exercise. Exercise must produce skeletal loading to be effective. Activities such as hill walking, weightlifting, and jogging appear beneficial. Swimming has been demonstrated not to be effective for maintenance or even slowing the loss of bone mineral density. These exercises should be considered by any individual under the age of 30 years who wishes to increase his or her peak bone mineral density.

Calcitonin has demonstrated some ability to slow, if not reverse, bone mineral density loss. Therapeutic agents may be divided into two categories. One group is aimed at slowing or minimally reversing osteoporosis. Because these agents do not significantly reduce the patient's incidence of fracture, this course of action represents an interim course.[29] Sodium fluoride does add new bone, but it is of poor quality. Fracture rates are decreased, yet frequent side effects and a 25% nonresponder rate continues to drive interest in other directions. Currently biphasic treatment models are being explored and may provide significant relief. This treatment model involves both the administration of bone-forming agents followed by treatment protocols in which bone conservation is promoted.[29]

> ### KEY CONCEPTS
> - *Osteoporosis is characterized by decreased quantity, not quality, of bone.*
> - *Females are affected more often than males, and the incidence increases with age.*
> - *Typically those afflicted remain asymptomatic until fractures occur.*
> - *Hip fractures are associated with a 10% to 20% mortality rate; 20% to 30% become institutionalized as a result of their fracture.*
> - *Radiographic appearance is noted by thin cortex with accentuated trabecular pattern.*
> - *Osteoporotic vertebrae may appear biconcave (codfish or fish vertebrae), flat (vertebrae plana), or narrowed anteriorly (wedge fracture).*
> - *Hydroxyproline in urine is a nonspecific sign.*
> - *Diagnosis is achieved by bone mineral density assessments using single photon absorbtiometry, dual photon absorptiometry, or quantitative computerized tomography.*
> - *Regional osteoporosis results most commonly from disuse or immobilization, injury to the central nervous system, and bone and joint inflammation.*
> - *Transient regional osteoporosis and regional migratory osteoporosis are idiopathic, self-limiting types of regional osteoporosis; they are typically evident on plain films and MRI is particularly helpful in the diagnosis.*

 # Nutritional Disorders

Hypervitaminosis A

BACKGROUND
Elevations of vitamin A resulting from dietary excess, common cold prophylaxis, anti-acne therapies, and treatment of keratosis follicularis have been reported.[21,62,76] Hypervitaminosis A affects the central nervous system, skeleton, and integument.[8,62,76]

IMAGING FINDINGS
Painful regions that show subperiosteal cortical thickening (Fig. 16-24)[21,62,76] commonly affect the ulna (Fig. 16-25, *A* and *B*) and metacarpals. Generalized osteoporosis may be seen.

CLINICAL COMMENTS
Vitamin A administration in unknowing conjunction with medical therapy for acne and keratosis follicularis is an important and preventable cause of this entity. Self-administered, high doses of vitamin A also cause this condition.[62] Headache, blurred vision, palsies of cranial nerve VI, and increased intracranial pressure are presenting central nervous system complaints. Chronic toxicity may produce perioral fissures, hair loss, hair coarsening, and desquamation of the skin of the palms and soles. Pruritis may be present.[21,62,76] Hepatosplenomegaly is sometimes observed. The liver must become saturated before toxicity is noted. Elimination of vitamin A and management of the complications of hypervitaminosis A are fundamental to the cure (Fig. 16-25, *C* and *D*).[8,62,76]

> ### KEY CONCEPTS
> - *Hypervitaminosis A results from iatrogenic and dietary excess intake of vitamin A leading to liver saturation.*
> - *Signs and symptoms include hepatosplenomegaly, blurred vision, headache, increased intracranial pressure, cranial nerve IV neuropathy, perioral fissures, hair loss, coarse hair, pruritis, and desquamation of palms and soles.*
> - *Radiographic changes include solid, painful subperiosteal cortical thickening and osteoporosis.*

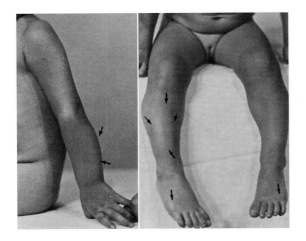

FIG. 16-24   Hypervitaminosis A. Painful swelling *(arrows)* of the forearm and lower leg. (From Silverman F, Kuhn J: *Caffey's pediatric x-ray diagnosis: an integrated imaging approach,* ed 9, St Louis, 1993, Mosby.)

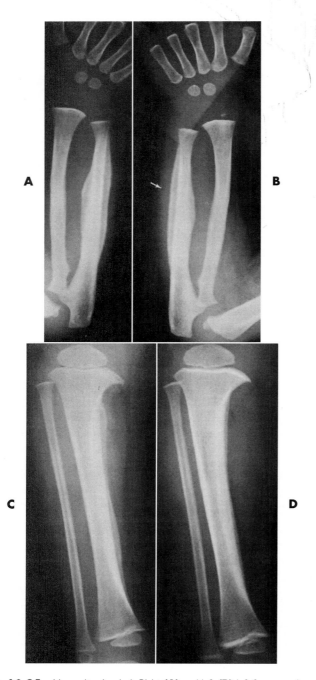

FIG. 16-25 Hypervitaminosis A. Right **(A)** and left **(B)** left forearms showing symmetrical cortical hyperostosis *(arrow)*. **C,** Tibial hyperostosis at the time of diagnosis of hypervitaminosis A. **D,** 5 weeks after removal of dietary vitamin A. (From Silverman F, Kuhn J: *Caffey's pediatric x-ray diagnosis: an integrated imaging approach,* ed 9, St Louis, 1993, Mosby.)

Hypervitaminosis D

BACKGROUND

Hypervitaminosis D is a product of excessive vitamin D intake in children and adults.[7,26,31,60] Nearly 98% of the milk sold today is fortified with vitamin D. This practice began in the 1930s[7] to combat the epidemic presentation of rickets seen in many industrial cities of the United States.[52,56] The current practice is also aimed at preventing the onset of rickets[7,26,31,56,63] but, in addition, is also present to limit senile, postmenopausal, and glucocorticoid-induced osteoporosis. Vitamin D therapies have also been suggested in cases of Paget's disease and rheumatoid arthritis.[53]

Toxic levels of vitamin D have been produced by accidental overfortification,[7,26] prolonged administration of therapeutic levels of vitamin D,[24] and coincidental self-administration of vitamin D. Renal failure and thiazide diuretics lower the threshold for the expression of vitamin D toxicity.[60]

IMAGING FINDINGS

Generalized osteopenia produced by the enhanced resorption of calcium by osteoclasts is evident.[7] In skeletally immature patients, alternating bands of sclerosis and lucencies are seen in the metaphyseal regions of the tubular bones (Fig. 16-26).[53] Appositional bone thickening is produced. Metastatic calcium deposits are found in periarticular locations (Fig. 16-27), vasculature, and a variety of other organs, including the falx cerebri (Fig. 16-28) and tentorium cerebelli.[53]

CLINICAL COMMENTS

Vitamin D toxicity can occur abruptly with high doses or in the presence of renal disease.[60] Toxic levels of vitamin D may accumulate over long periods of time.[31] The effects of hypervitaminosis D include the following: anorexia, weight loss, weakness, fatigue, disorientation, vomiting, dehydration, polyuria, constipation, and bone pain.[7,53] Laboratory findings include hypercalcemia, hyper-

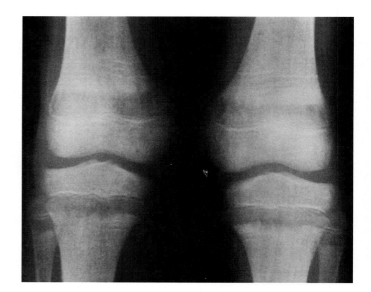

FIG. 16-26 Hypervitaminosis D. Alternating bands of sclerosis and lucency in this 9-year-old who subsequently died of vitamin D toxicity. (From Silverman F, Kuhn J: *Caffey's pediatric x-ray diagnosis: an integrated imaging approach,* ed 9, St Louis, 1993, Mosby.)

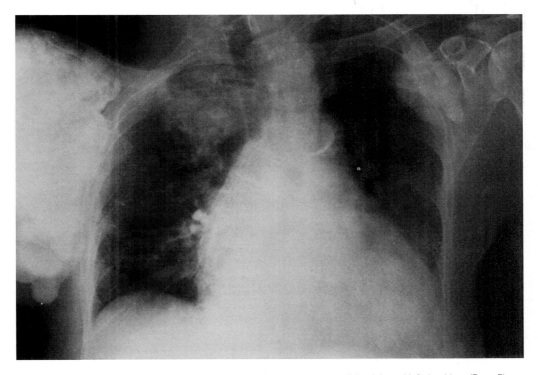

FIG. 16-27 Hypervitaminosis D. Metastatic depositis of calcium in region of the right and left shoulders. (From Eisenberg RL, Dennis CA: *Comprehensive radiographic pathology,* ed 2, St Louis, 1995, Mosby.)

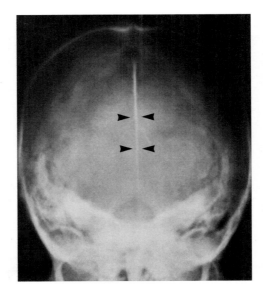

FIG. 16-28 Hypervitaminosis D. Calcification of the falx cerebri *(arrowheads)* and tentorium cerebelli are demonstrated on this Towne view. (From Silverman F, Kuhn J: *Caffey's pediatric x-ray diagnosis: an integrated imaging approach,* ed 9, St Louis, 1993, Mosby.)

BOX 16-1
Etiologies of Osteomalacia

Dietary deficiencies
- Vitamin D
- Calcium
- Phosphate
- Dietary chelator

Malabsorption
- Gastrointestinal
- Hepatobiliary
- Pancreatic

Renal disease
- Chronic renal failure
- Renal tubular disease

Miscellaneous
- Solar irradiation deficiency
- Neoplastic invasion
- Fibrous dysplasia
- Neurofibromatosis
- Hypophosphatasia
- Medications (e.g., anticonvulsants)

calcuria, hematuria, albuminuria, and documentation of elevated levels of vitamin D_2 and/or D_3.[53]

KEY CONCEPTS
- *Hypervitaminosis D occurs secondary to dietary or therapeutic excess.*
- *Renal disease and thiazide diuretics increase the risk of toxicity.*
- *Metastatic calcification is commonly found in viscera, vasculature, muscles, periarticular soft tissues, and the falx cerebri and tentorium cerebelli.*
- *Local or widespread osteoporosis may result; tubular bones demonstrate alternating bands of dense and lucent bone.*

Osteomalacia

BACKGROUND
Osteomalacia, also referred to as *adult rickets*,[45,69] is typified by the presence of poor quality bone. Osteomalacia is more accurately described as a group of entities that can produce similar yet nonspecific radiographic changes. The clinical and biochemical profile of osteomalacia varies. Osteomalacia is often camouflaged by the associated complaints of the various etiological entities. Delayed or inadequate mineralization of the osteoid matrix, demonstrated by bone biopsy, the gold standard diagnostic tool, producing bone rarefaction and osseous deformities classically describes this lesion.[6,45] These findings and alteration of the growth plate and metaphysis represent rickets, which was discussed previously. Although several varied and distinct etiologies are able to produce osteomalacia, the majority of the cases involve abnormal calcium, vitamin D, or phosphorous metabolism (Box 16-1).[6,13,76] These are produced by dietary deficiencies, malabsorption, renal disease, and a small group of miscellaneous diseases.

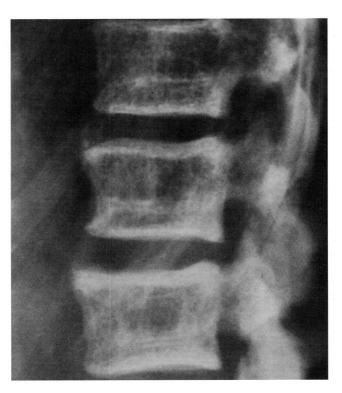

FIG. 16-29   Osteomalacia. Thickened cortical margins and coarsening trabecular patterns without overall enlargement is typical. (From Eisenberg RL, Dennis CA: *Comprehensive radiographic pathology*, ed 2, St Louis, 1995, Mosby.)

IMAGING FINDINGS

Osteomalacia in adults is less severe than rickets, which appears in children.[13] Generalized osteopenia with coarse, hazy-appearing trabeculae is typical. The skeletal detail appears out of focus (Fig. 16-29). Looser's lines, or pseudofractures, a form of insufficiency fracture, occurring perpendicular to and through the cortex, may be present.[13,53,76] Common sites of involvement are the femoral necks, scapulae, pelvis (Fig. 16-30), ribs, occiput, and long bones of the extremities.*

Other bone softening processes also produce this feature. Bowed proximal femoral necks, shepherd's crook deformity, and basilar invagination are findings in Paget's disease, fibrous dysplasia, and rickets, as well as osteomalacia. The periosteal and endosteal cortical margins are blurred. Increased osteoid volumes and expanded, irregular Haversian canals produce intracortical lucencies.[6,45,53]

CLINICAL COMMENTS

Common presenting complaints are bone pain with subjective or objective lower extremity weakness, waddling gait, bony tenderness, and osseous deformity. These features may suggest the diagnosis but are not exclusive to osteomalacia.[6,45,71] Biochemical analysis most often demonstrates elevated alkaline phosphatase and less often hypocalcemia and hypophosphatemia. Other features are deficiencies in the hormone vitamin D, secondary hyperparathyroidism, and elevated hydroxyproline in the urine. "Osteomalacia encompasses many clinical signs and symptoms, biomechanical abnormalities, and radiographic features that are suggestive of the diagnosis; nonetheless, histologic analysis of an iliac crest bone

---

*References 5, 13, 45, 53, 75, 76.

biopsy is often relied on to definitively establish the diagnosis."[6] Attempts are being made to formulate suitable screening examinations for the diagnosis of osteomalacia, yet to date, no procedure has garnered unequivocal support.[6,75]

■ KEY CONCEPTS

- *Osteomalacia is the lack of appropriate mineralization of normal osteoid resulting in poor bone in adults.*
- *Several contributing factors have been identified, including abnormal calcium, vitamin D, or phosphorus metabolism.*
- *Osteopenia is typical; shepherd's crook and basiliar invagination, and pseudofracture deformities are also noted.*

Rickets

BACKGROUND

More than 30 causes of rickets and osteomalacia exist.[13] Rickets is closely related to osteomalacia. Rickets demonstrates additional features of disorganized growth plates and widened epiphysis with rarefication of the zone of provisional calcification (ZPC).[13,45,76] The most frequently encountered cases involve defects in vitamin D, calcium, or phosphate absorption or metabolism.[46]

IMAGING FINDINGS

Typically generalized osteopenia occurs.[13,45,46,76] The remaining trabeculae are coarse.[45,76] The flared metaphysis may be cupped and the epiphysis is enlarged in all planes (Fig. 16-31). The costochondral junction is enlarged and demonstrates the "rosary bead" appearance (Fig. 16-32).[13,45,46,76] Pectus carinatum, with notching found at the diaphragmatic attachment sites and hyperkyphosis, is

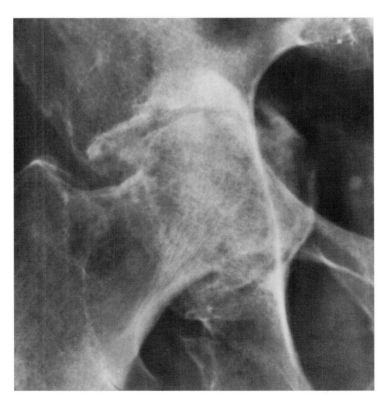

FIG. 16-30   Osteomalacia. Weak and poor quality bone producing acetabular protrusion in this patient. (From Eisenberg RL, Dennis CA: *Comprehensive radiographic pathology,* ed 2, St Louis, 1995, Mosby.)

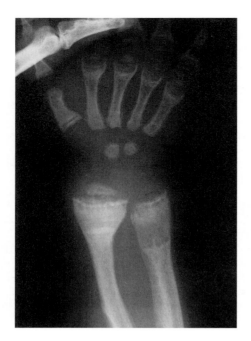

FIG. 16-31   Rickets (vitamin D resistant). The typical flaring and cupping of the metaphysis is seen. (Courtesy Gary M. Guebert, Maryland Heights, Mo.)

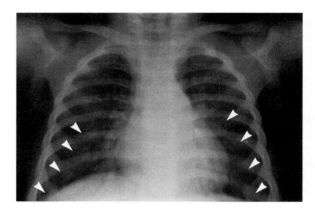

FIG. 16-32   Rickets (vitamin D resistant). Enlargement of the costochondral junction *(arrowheads)* produces the rosary bead chest. (Courtesy Gary M. Guebert, Maryland Heights, Mo.)

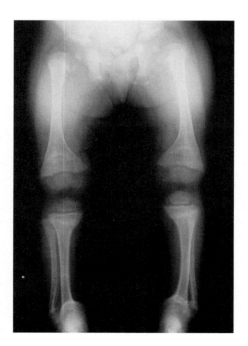

FIG. 16-33   Rickets (vitamin D resistant). Underdevelopment of the long bones and wide, irregular metaphysis is typical. The ZPC is rarified and disorganized. The long bones are bowed. (Courtesy Gary M. Guebert, Maryland Heights, Mo.)

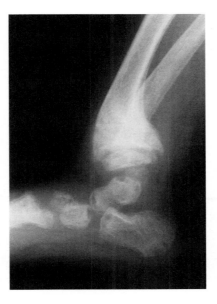

FIG. 16-34   Rickets (vitamin D resistant). The lateral view redemonstrates the flared, cupped tibial metaphysis with bowing of the long bones. (Courtesy Gary M. Guebert, Maryland Heights, Mo.)

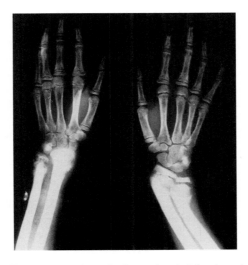

FIG. 16-35   Renal osteodystrophy. Osteosclerosis deformity and disorganization of the growth centers are demonstrated by this young patient.

seen.[13] As the child becomes ambulatory, bowing of the long bones is typical (Fig. 16-33 and 16-34).[46,63,70]

CLINICAL COMMENTS

Vitamin D deficiency existed in epidemic proportions in the United States until the early 1920s.[63,56] Rickets, in several forms, continues to plague our society, although in greatly reduced numbers.[63] High-risk populations are listed in Box 16-2.

Vitamin D deficiency rickets is a thoroughly preventable disease.[63] Mild cases are effectively treated with standard vitamin D supplements of 400 IU per day. Other causes of rickets include renal osteodystrophy, vitamin D resistant rickets, and renal hypophosphatemia rickets. Renal osteodystrophy produces features of hyperparathyroidism in addition to rickets (Fig. 16-35).[3] Vita-

---

BOX 16-2
Risk Factors for Developing Rickets

1. Deeply pigmented skin
2. Dietary deficiencies
   - Prolonged breastfeeding in infants
   - Vegetarian diets with inadequate intake of vitamin D or calcium
   - Vitamin D deficiency in mothers who are breastfeeding
   - Diet composed of soy-based products without vitamin D
   - Supplementation
   - Fad diets
3. Inadequate exposure to sunlight
4. Vitamin D3 resistance
5. Renal hypophosphatemia

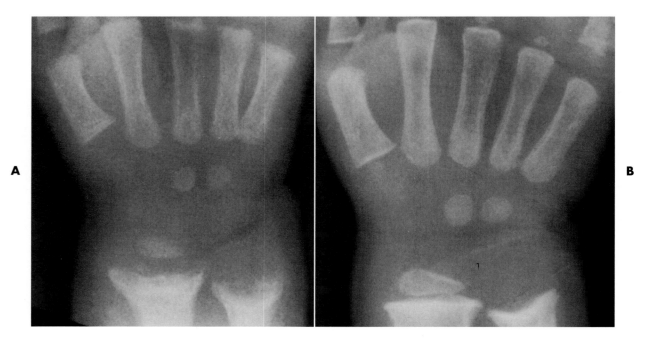

FIG. 16-36   Rickets. Pretreatment **(A)** posttreatment **(B)** radiographs demonstrate the increasing density of the ZPC, a sign of successful treatment. (From Eisenberg RL, Dennis CA: *Comprehensive radiographic pathology,* ed 2, St Louis, 1995, Mosby.)

min D resistance is typified by end organ insensitivity to the hormone vitamin D_3 and the inability to respond to vitamin D supplementation.[24] Failure of renal resorption of phosphate-producing hypophosphatemia leads to deficient mineralization.[57] Successful treatment produces remineralization of metaphyseal bone and the ZPC returns (Fig. 16-36).

KEY CONCEPTS
- *Rickets is a lack of appropriate mineralization of normal osteoid resulting in poor bone quality in children.*
- *Radiographic changes are most marked at areas of rapid growth: wide, irregular, cupped metaphyses; wide, lucent zones of provisional calcification; and osseous deformities.*
- *Deficiencies of vitamin D, calcium, or phosphate intake or metabolism are the most frequent causes.*
- *Rickets is a largely preventable disease.*

Scurvy (Hypovitaminosis C)

BACKGROUND
Dietary deficiency of vitamin C for a duration of 4 months or more leads to the typical changes of scurvy. Infantile and adult forms have been identified. Infantile scurvy is infrequent and adult scurvy is rare.

IMAGING FINDINGS
Infantile scurvy leads to reduced osteoblast function, producing intraosseous collagen and a disorganized growth plate, which causes a widened metaphysis and a sclerotic zone of provisional calcification (ZPC) (Fig. 16-37). Beaklike metaphyseal outgrowths (Pelken's spurs) and a radiodense band surrounding ossification centers (Wimberger's sign of scurvy) are typical findings (Fig. 16-38). Subperiosteal hemorrhage, localized or generalized, may lift the periosteal layer (Fig. 16-39). Hemarthrosis may be found in the larger, lower joints. Permanent reduction in growth is infrequent.[12,53,76]

CLINICAL COMMENTS
Persons affected fall into one of several groups: infants who are fed exclusively pasteurized or boiled milk, the elderly with chronic dietary insufficiencies, patients with malabsorption of water-soluble vitamins, and widespread dietary deficiencies in developing nations. Signs and symptoms include irritability, petechiae, swollen and bleeding gums, scorbutic rosary, periarticular swelling, and tenderness of the lower limbs. Interarticular hemorrhage may lead to infants assuming a frog-leg position to decrease the pain.[12,44]

KEY CONCEPTS
- *Scurvy results from deficient vitamin C intake, occurring primarily in infants fed pasteurized or boiled milk.*
- *Radiographic abnormalities include growth plate abnormalities, wide metaphyses, sclerotic zones of provisional calcification, Wimberger's sign, Pelken's spurs, and periosteal lifting resulting from hemorrhage.*
- *Clinically, patients exhibit bleeding gums, irritability, rosary bead chest, and periarticular soft tissue swelling.*

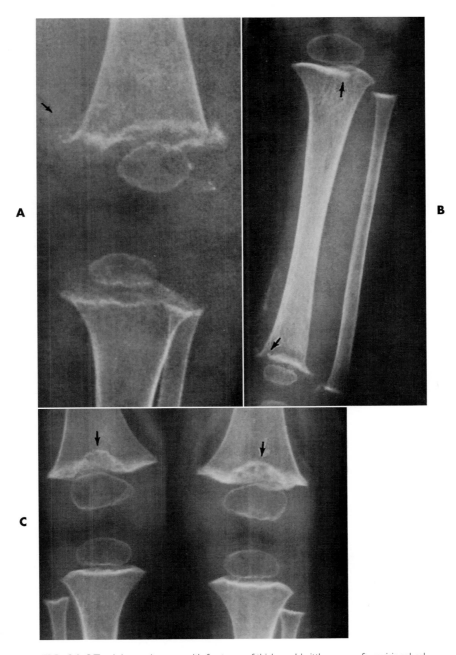

FIG. 16-37   Advanced scurvy with fractures of thickened, brittle zones of provisional calcification. **A,** Multiple infarctions in the provisional zone, with peripheral spurring and beginning subperiosteal ossification *(arrow)* of the terminal segment of the shaft by the externally displaced periosteum. The osteogenetic layer is lifted by hemorrhage and continues to form normal cortical bone. The bones generally are rarefied, but the provisional zones of the femur, tibia, and ulna and of the femoral and tibial ossification centers are thickened. **B,** Longitudinal fractures of provisional zones and distal ends of the tibia *(arrows)*. **C,** Crumpling fractures of proximal and distal provisional zones of the ends of the femora, with incomplete cupping of ends of the shafts *(arrows)*. (From Silverman F, Kuhn J: *Caffey's pediatric x-ray diagnosis: an integrated imaging approach,* ed 9, St Louis, 1993, Mosby.)

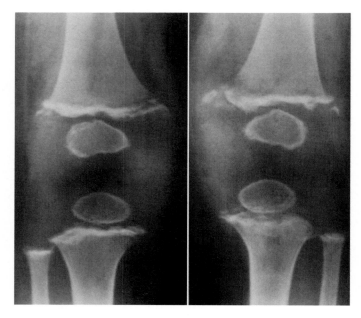

FIG. 16-38   Scurvy. Dense, thick ZPC is characteristic of scurvy. Marginal spurs (Pelken's spur) and dense ring of sclerosis surrounding the impoverished growth center (Wimberger's sign) is present here. (From Eisenberg RL: *Atlas of signs in radiology,* Philadelphia, 1984, Lippincott.)

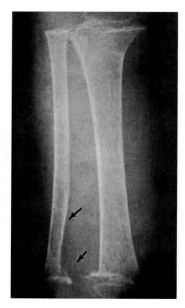

FIG. 16-39   Scurvy. The insecurely attached periosteum is easily lifted in cases of subperiosteal bleeding *(arrows).* (From Silverman F, Kuhn J: *Caffey's pediatric x-ray diagnosis: an integrated imaging approach,* ed 9, St Louis, 1993, Mosby.)

References

1. Ablow RC, Hsia YE, Brandt IK: Acrodysostosis coinciding with pseudohypoparathyroidism and pseudo-pseudohypoparathyroidism, *Am J Roentgenol* 128:95, 1977.

2. Aron DC, Tyrrell J B, Wilson CB: Pituitary tumors: current concepts in diagnosis and management, *West J Med* 162:340, 1995.

3. Ballantyne ES, Findlay GFG: Thoracic spinal stenosis in two brothers due to vitamin D-resistant rickets, *Eur Spine J* 5:125, 1996.

4. Bauer RL: Assessing osteoporosis, *Hosp Pract* 26s:23, 1991.

5. Besser GM, Thorner MO, editors: *Clinical endocrinology,* ed 2, London, 1994, Wolfe.

6. Bingham CT, Fitzpatrick LA: Noninvasive testing in the diagnosis of osteomalacia, *Am J Med* 95:519, 1993.

7. Blank S et al: An outbreak of hypervitaminosis D associated with the overfortification of milk from a home-delivery dairy, *Am J Public Health* 85:656, 1995.

8. Braun L: Vitamin A excess common deficiency, requirements, metabolism, and misuse, *Pediatr Clin North Am* 9:935, 1962.

9. Buchfelder, Nistor R, Fahlbusch, R, Huk WJ: The accuracy of CT and MR evaluation of the sella turcica for detection of adrenocortrophic hormone-secreting adenomas in Cushing disease, *AJNR* 14:1183, 1993.

10. Burch WM, Posillico JT: Hypoparathyroidism after I-313 therapy with subsequent return of parathyroid function, *J Clin Endocrinol Metab* 57:398, 1983.

11. Cao XY et al: Timing of a vulnerability of the brain to iodine deficiency in endemic cretinism, *N Engl J Med* 331:1739, 1994.

12. Capistol PJ et al: Scurvy, presentation of six cases, *Ann Espana Pediatr* 12:745, 1979.

13. Doppelt SH: Vitamin D, rickets and osteomalacia, *Orthop Clin North Am* 15:671, 1984.

14. Genant HK et al: Osteosclerosis in primary hyperparathyroidism, *Am J Med* 59:104, 1975.

15. Grampp S et al: Radiographic diagnosis of osteoporosis, *Radiol Clin North Am* 31:1133, 1993.

16. Grey AB et al: Effect of hormone replacement therapy on bone mineral density in postmenopausal women with mild primary hyperparathyroidism: a randomized, controlled trial, *Ann Intern Med* 125:360, 1996.

17. Grossman A, editor: *Clinical endocrinology,* Boston, 1992, Blackwell Scientific Publications.

18. Guebert GM, Pirtle OL, Yochum TR: *Essentials of diagnostic imaging,* St Louis, 1995, Mosby.

19. Haddad G, Haddad JG, Kaplan FS: Severe symptomatic osteopenia in a man with pigmented micronodular adrenal hyperplasia, *Clin Orthop* 313:220, 1995.

20. Halpern JP et al: The neurology of endemic cretinism: a study of two endemias, *Brain* 114:825, 1991.

21. Hathcock JM et al: Evaluation of vitamin A toxicity *Am J Clin Nutr* 52:183, 1990.

22. Hermus AR et al: Bone mineral density and bone turnover before and after surgical cure of Cushing's syndrome, *J Clin Endocrinol Metab* 80:2859, 1995.

23. Higgins CB: Roll of magnetic resonance imaging in hyperparathyroidism, *Radiol Clin North Am* 31:1017, 1993.

24. Hochberg Z et al: 1,25-dehyroxyvitamin D resistance, rickets, and alopecia, *Am J Med* 77:805, 1984.

25. Jackson DW, editor: *Instructional course lectures,* 1995, American Academy of Orthopedic Surgeons.

26. Jacobus CH et al: Hypervitaminosis D associated with drinking milk, *N Engl J Med* 326:1173, 1992.

27. Jensen PS, Kliger AS: Early radiographic manifestations of secondary hyperparathyroidism associated with chronic renal disease, *Radiology* 125:645, 1977.

28. Kerr R et al: Computerized tomography of proximal femoral trabecular patterns, *J Orthop Res* 4:45, 1986.

29. Kimmel DB, Slovik DM, Lane NE: Current and investigational approaches for reversing established osteoporosis, *Rheum Dis Clin North Am* 20:735, 1994.

30. Kirk JK, Spangler JG: Alendronate: a bisphosphonate for treatment of osteoporosis, *Am Fam Physician* 54:2053, 1996.

31. Kuroume T: Hypervitaminosis D after prolonged defeat with premature formula, *Pediatrics* 92:862, 1993.

32. Lee VS et al: Uremic leontiasis ossea: "big head" disease in humans? Radiologic, clinical, and pathologic features, *Radiology* 199:233, 1996.

33. Lefebvre H et al: Characterization of the somatostatin receptor subtype in a bronchial carcinoid tumor responsible for Cushing's syndrome, *J Clin Endocrinol Metab* 80:1423, 1995.

34. Leong GM et al: The effect of Cushing's disease on bone mineral density, body composition, growth, and puberty: a report of an identical adolescent twin pair, *J Clin Endocrinol Metab* 81:1905, 1996.

35. Maberly GF: Symposium: clinical nutrition in developing countries: toward the application of contemporary concepts and technology iodine deficiency disorders, *Contemp Scientific Iss* 1473(suppl), 1994.

36. Meema S, Banker MC, Meema HE: Preventive effect of estrogen on postmenopausal bone loss, *Arch Intern Med* 135:1436, 1975.

37. Meema HE, Meema S: Microradioscopic bone structure of the hand in thyrotoxicosis, renal osteodystrophy and acromegaly; clinical aspects of metabolic bone disease, *Excerpta Medica* 10:10, 1973.

38. Melby JC: Therapy of Cushing disease: a consensus for pituitary microsurgery, *Ann Intern Med* 109:445, 1988.

39. Mendonca BB et al: Clinical, hormonal and pathological findings in a comparative study of adrenocortical neoplasms in childhood and adulthood, *J Urol* 154:2004, 1995.

40. Miller DL: Endocrine angiography and venous sampling, *Radiol Clin North Am* 31:1051, 1993.

41. Mimouni F: Etiology of nutritional rickets: geographic variations, *J Pediatr* 128:600, 1996.

42. Mizokami T et al: Risk factors for brain infarction in patients with Cushing's disease: case reports, *Angiology* 47:1011, 1996.

43. Nevitt MC: Epidemiology of osteoporosis, *Rheum Dis Clin North Am* 20:535, 1994.

44. Nicol M: Vitamins and immunity, *Allerg Immunol (Paris)* 25:70, 1993.

45. Nugent CA, Gall EP, Pitt MJ: Osteoporosis, osteomalacia, rickets and Paget's disease, *Prim Care* 11:353, 1984.

46. Oginni LM et al: Etiology in rickets in Nigerian children, *J Pediatr* 128:692, 1996.

47. Okada K et al: Pseudohypoparathyroidism-associated spinal stenosis, *Spine* 19:1186, 1994.

48. Ontell FK, Shelton DK: Multiple stress fractures: an unusual presentation of Cushing's disease, *West J Med* 162:364, 1995.

49. Parfitt AM: Hormonal influences on bone remodeling and bone loss: application to the management of primary hyperparathyroidism, *Ann Intern Med* 125:413, 1996.

50. Parfitt AM, Duncan H. In Rothman RH, Simeone FE, editors: *Metabolic bone disease affecting the spine,* Philadelphia, 1975, WB Saunders.

51. Poznanski AK et al: The pattern of shortening of the bones of the hand in PHP and PPHP—a comparison with brachydactylia E, Turner's syndrome, and acrodysostosis, *Radiology* 123:707, 1977.

52. Recker RR: Bone biopsy and histomorphonemtry in clinical practice, *Rheum Dis Clin North Am* 20:609, 1994.

53. Resnick D: Diagnosis of bone and joint disorders, ed 3, Philadelphia, 1995, WB Saunders.

54. Resnick DL: Fish vertebrae, *Arthritis Rheum* 25:1073, 1982.

55. Richardson ML et al: Bone mineral changes in primary hyperparathyroidism, *Skeletal Radiol* 15:85, 1986.

56. Saffran M: Rickets: return of an old disease, *J Am Podiatr Med Assoc* 85:222, 1995.

57. Saggese G, Giampiero IB, Bertelloni S, Perri G: Long term growth hormone treatment in children with renal hypophosphatemic rickets: effects on growth, mineral metabolism, and bone density, *J Pediatr* 127:395, 1995.

58. Santos E, Higgins CB, Clark O: Clinical image: recurrent hyperparathyroidism caused by a parathyroid cystic adenoma: localization by MRI, *J Comput Assist Tomogr* 20:996, 1996.

59. Schneider R: Radiologic methods of evaluating generalized osteopenia, *Orthop Clin North Am* 15:631, 1984.

60. Schwartzman MS, Franck WA: Vitamin D toxicity complicating the treatment of senile, postmenopausal, and glucocorticoid-induced osteoporosis: four case reports and a critical commentary on the use of vitamin D in these disorders, *Am J Med* 82:224, 1987.

61. Shapira H et al: Familial Albright's hereditary osteodystrophy with hypoparathyroidism: normal structural $G_s\alpha$ Gere, *J Clin Endocrinol Metab* 81:1660, 1996.

62. Sharieff GQ, Hanten K: Pseudotumor cerebri and hypercalcemia resulting from vitamin A toxicity, *Ann Emerg Med* 27:518, 1996.

63. Sills IN et al: Vitamin D deficiency rickets: reports of its demise are exaggerated, *Clin Pediatr* 33:491, 1994.

64. Silverberg SJ, Bilezikian JP: Extensive personal experience: evaluation and management of primary hyperparathyroidism, *J Clin Endocrinol Metab* 81:2036, 1996.

65. Star VL, Hochberg MC: Osteoporosis in patient's with rheumatic disease, *Rheum Dis Clin North Am* 20:561, 1994.

66. Stulberg BN, Licata AA, Bauer TW, Belhobek GH: Hyperparathyroidism, hyperthyroidism, and Cushing's disease, *Orthop Clin North Am* 15:697, 1984.

67. Suarez F et al: Expression and modulation of the parathyroid hormone (PTH)/PTH-related peptide receptor messenger ribonucleic acid in skin fibroblasts from patients with type IB pseudohypoparathyroidism, *J Clin Endocrinol Metab* 80:965, 1995.

68. Subbarao K, Jacobson HG: Systemic disorders affecting the thoracic cage, *Radiol Clin North Am* 22:497, 1984.

69. Tannebaum H, Esdacle J, Rosenthall L: Joint imaging in regional migratory osteoporosis, *J Rheumatol* 7:237, 1980.

70. Taylor A, Mandel G, Norman ME: Calcium deficiency rickets in a North American child, *Clin Pediatr* 33:494, 1994.

71. Verbruggen LA, Bruyland M, Shahabpour M: Osteomalacia in a patient with anorexia nervosa, *J Rheumatol* 20:512, 1993.

72. Vincent JM et al: The radiological investigation of an occcult ectopic ACTH-dependent Cushing's syndrome, *Clin Radiol* 48:11, 1993.

73. Wang LD: Preliminary study on nutrition and precancerous lesions of the esophagus in the adolescent, *Chung HUA Chung Liu Tsa Chih* 14:94, 1992.

74. Watts NB: Treatment of osteoporosis with bisphosphonates, *Rheum Dis Clin North Am* 20:717, 1994.

75. Wilton TJ et al: Screening for osteomalacia in elderly patients with femoral neck fractures, *J Bone Joint Surg Br* 69:765, 1987.

76. Yochum TR, Rowe L J: *Essentials of skeletal radiology,* ed 2, Baltimore, 1996, Williams and Wilkins.

77. Zimmerman D et al: Congenital giantism due to growth hormone-releasing hormone excess and pituitary hyperplasia with adenomas transformation, *J Clin Endocrinol Metab* 76:216, 1993.

78. Zung A, Herzenberg JE, Chalew SA: Radiological case of the month: ectopic ossification and calcification in pseudohypoparathyroidism and pseudopseudohypoparathyroidism, *Arch Pediatr Adolesc Med* 150:643, 1996.

chapter **17**

Miscellaneous Bone Diseases

DENNIS M MARCHIORI

Amyloidosis

BACKGROUND

Amyloidosis is a rare systemic disease caused by the extracellular accumulation of insoluble amyloid proteins in various organs and tissues of the body. Although several classifications exist, the simplest divides amyloidosis into primary and secondary forms. Amyloidosis without associated antecedent or coexisting disease is primary (idiopathic). Secondary amyloidosis is associated with chronic systemic disease (i.e., rheumatoid arthritis, Crohn's disease, cystic fibrosis, chronic drug abuse), infections (i.e., familial Mediterranean fever, tuberculosis), and tumors (i.e., multiple myeloma). Usually amyloidosis is systemic; only 10% to 20% of cases demonstrate localized disease.[121] Primary amyloidosis affects men more than women and typically occurs between the ages of 40 and 80 years. The presentation of secondary amyloidosis depends on the associated underlying disorder.

IMAGING FINDINGS

Because a variety of systems, including the musculoskeletal, genitourinary, gastrointestinal, and cardiovascular systems, may be involved, amyloidosis demonstrates a wide spectrum of imaging findings.[50,117]

Osteonecrosis may develop from vessel occlusion following amyloid accumulation around capillaries and endothelial cells of larger blood vessels. Other findings include osteolytic bone destruction, periarticular joint swelling, osteoporosis, pathological vertebral fractures, joint subluxations (i.e., proximal femur and humerus), and coarse trabeculae. Calcification may be seen in the amyloid deposits.

CLINICAL COMMENTS

The clinical presentation depends upon which systems are involved. Amyloid deposits in the heart produce pleural effusion and dyspnea. Gastrointestinal involvement is associated with bowel obstruction and malabsorption. Localized amyloid deposits in the upper respiratory system may cause hoarseness and dysphagia. Definitive diagnosis requires biopsy confirmation; imaging studies are nonspecific.

KEY CONCEPTS

- *Amyloidosis results from localized or systemic protein deposits, known to involve a variety of systems.*
- *It occurs as a primary disease or secondary to multiple myeloma, rheumatoid arthritis, Crohn's disease, and other systemic disorders.*
- *Associated bone changes include osteonecrosis, osteolytic destruction, periarticular joint swelling, and pathological vertebral collapse.*

Dermatomyositis

BACKGROUND

Inflammatory myopathies represent a group of disorders involving chronic inflammation, weakness, and wasting of skeletal muscle tissue. Inflammatory cells surround and destroy muscle fibers by a probable autoimmune-mediated mechanism.[85] Dermatomyositis, polymyositis, juvenile myositis, and inclusion body myositis all represent inflammatory myopathies.[84]

Dermatomyositis represents chronic inflammation of the skeletal muscle and skin, affecting 5 out of every 10,000 people. It is the most easily recognized inflammatory myopathy resulting from the presence of a distinctive reddish rash occurring over the eyelids, cheeks, and nose. It occurs in all ages but is most common in adult females. Dermatomyositis is more common in children than are other myopathies. In adults, it is associated with an elevated incidence of visceral carcinomas; this incidence increases with age.[6,103,104]

IMAGING FINDINGS

The most striking radiographic feature of dermatomyositis is the presence of subcutaneous calcifications. Subcutaneous calcifications appear as linear or curvilinear radiodensities most commonly around the knees, elbows, and fingers (Fig. 17-1). In a few cases, widespread calcifications (calcinosis universalis) develop, severely limiting mobility. Calcification of intramuscular septa occurs in the deep muscles of the proximal limbs.

Dermatomyositis is associated with arthritis primarily in the small joints of the hands, appearing with misalignment and juxtaarticular osteoporosis and soft tissue swelling. Particularly char-

743

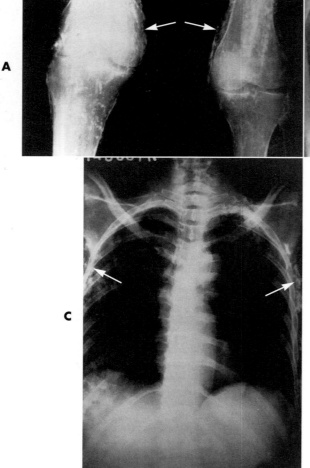
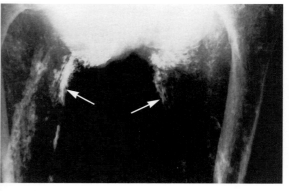

FIG. 17-1   Dermatomyositis presenting as linear cutaneous calcifications *(arrows)* of the knees **(A),** thighs **(B),** and thorax **(C).** (Courtesy Joseph W. Howe, Sylmar, Calif.)

acteristic is the "floppy thumb" sign, indicating subluxation of the interphalangeal joint of the first digit. A diffuse interstitial pattern is often present on the chest radiograph.

Magnetic resonance imaging (MRI) is helpful in localizing focal inflammatory myopathy, muscle atrophy, and fatty replacement of muscle.[86] MRI signal intensity correlates to the activity and distribution of the disease processes.

CLINICAL COMMENTS

Dermatomyositis is often not immediately painful; it may become noticeable only after muscle weakness and atrophy occur. The weakness may interfere with basic movements such as walking and raising arms. The diagnosis is made following an analysis of blood enzyme levels, electromyography, and muscle biopsy.

Steroids (i.e., prednisone) and immunosuppressive drugs (i.e., azathioprine) are given in an attempt to limit inflammation.[42] Passive range of motion and ice are indicated during acute exacerbations. Moderate exercise is advocated beyond the initial inflammatory stages. Muscle stretching appears to limit limb contracture.

The course of the disease is extremely variable, with some rapidly progressing to muscle wasting and weakness in merely days, whereas others take years to progress to this stage. Disease complications include acute renal failure and malignancy.

KEY CONCEPTS

- *Dermatomyositis is a chronic inflammation of the skeletal muscle and skin, probably an autoimmune mechanism.*
- *Malignancy occurs with a higher incidence in adults. Dermatomyositis occurs in people of all ages but is most common in adult females.*
- *Dermatomyositis occurs as a reddish rash occurring over the eyelids, cheeks, and nose.*
- *Linear or curvilinear subcutaneous calcifications may be found, primarily around the knees, elbows, and fingers.*
- *Misalignment, effusion, and osteoporosis of small joints of the hand accompany this disease.*
- *Standard treatment entails steroids, immunosuppressive drugs, passive range of motion, moderate exercise, and muscle stretching.*

Gaucher's Disease

BACKGROUND

Gaucher's disease is a lipid storage disorder resulting from a genetic deficiency of the enzyme glucocerebrosidase (glucosylceramidase), resulting in glucocerebroside accumulations within the cells of the reticuloendothelial system.[76] Gaucher's disease is the most common hereditary metabolic storage disorder.[15]

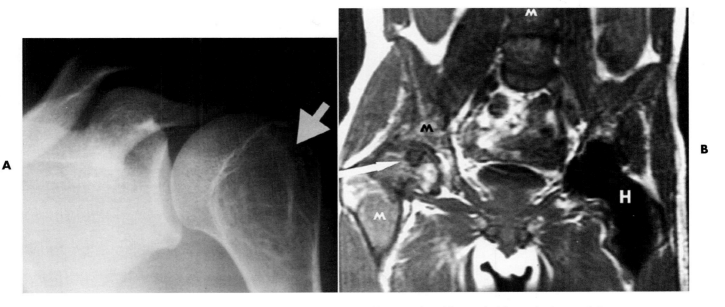

FIG. 17-2   Gaucher's disease. **A,** A lytic lesion in the proximal humerus *(arrow)* has resulted from a focal accumulation of lipid-laden cells. **B,** Coronal T1-weighted MRI demonstrates diffuse low signal intensity within the bone marrow *(M),* along with osteonecrosis of the right femoral head *(arrow)* and contralateral hip replacement *(H)* for the same process. The combination of findings is virtually diagnostic of the disease. (From Sartoris DJ: *Musculoskeletal imaging: the requisites,* St Louis, 1996, Mosby.)

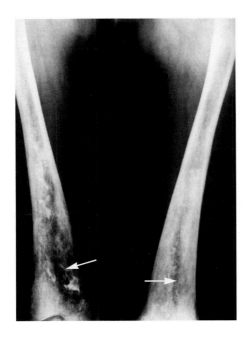

FIG. 17-3   Gaucher's disease. Marrow infarct of the distal femora appearing as serpiginous calcifications in the distal femora *(arrows).* (Courtesy Steven P. Brownstein, Springfield, NJ.)

The disease may develop in individuals in any age, but it is more severe in children and especially infants. A higher incidence of the disease is seen in individuals who have an Ashkenazic ancestry.[15]

IMAGING FINDINGS

Accumulations of glucocerebroside may suppress bone marrow activity and cause destructive bone lesions and enlargements of the liver, spleen, and lymph nodes. The distal femur may exhibit thinned cortex and bone expansion (Erlenmeyer flask deformity). Single or multiple osteolytic lesions may occur and mimic the presentation of an infection or neoplasm (Fig. 17-2). Osteonecrosis may result from vascular occlusion, which follows the increase in the reticulum component of bone marrow (Fig. 17-3). The femoral head, humeral head, and wrist are particularly susceptible. Similar changes may produce H-shaped vertebrae at multiple levels (Fig. 17-4). MRI is useful to assess the extent and activity of bone marrow involvement (Fig. 17-5).[10,57]

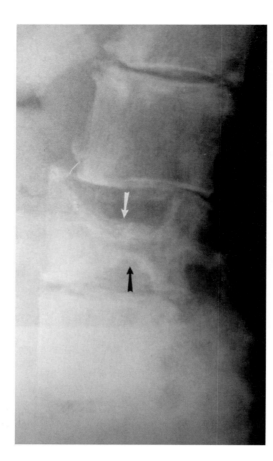

FIG. 17-4   H-shaped vertebra in Gaucher's disease. Central depression of the endplates *(arrows)* with sparing of the periphery is characteristic and occurs secondary to bone infarction. Differential diagnosis should include consideration of sickle cell anemia and sickle-thalassemia. (From Sartoris DJ: *Musculoskeletal imaging: the requisites,* St Louis, 1993, Mosby.)

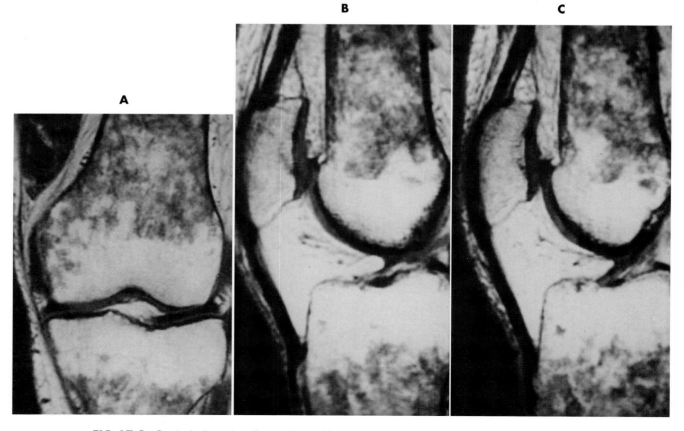

FIG. 17-5   Gaucher's disease in a 63-year old man. Note the patchy decreased signal from the marrow of the distal femur and proximal tibia on the coronal **(A)** and sagittal **(B** and **C)** T1-weighted images. (From Firooznia H et al: *MRI and CT of the musculoskeletal system,* St Louis, 1992, Mosby.)

CLINICAL COMMENTS

The clinical presentation of Gaucher's disease is divided into three forms based on phenotype.[15] All three types are marked by hepatosplenomegaly and the presence of Gaucher's cells in the bone marrow. Bone changes are more apparent in the chronic forms of the disease. In infants, the disease is more severe because of cerebroside accumulations in neurons. All patients are predisposed to osteomyelitis. Intravenous infusion of glucocerebrosidase is an effective therapy but its application is limited because of costs.[80]

KEY CONCEPTS

- *Gaucher's disease is a lipid storage disorder resulting from a genetic deficiency of the enzyme glucocerebrosidase; it is rare.*
- *Findings include anemia, hepatosplenomegaly, Erlenmeyer flask deformity, solitary or multiple osteolytic defects, osteonecrosis (usually femoral head), and H-shaped vertebrae.*

Heavy Metal Poisoning

BACKGROUND

Poisoning may develop from the injection, implantation, ingestion, or inhalation of aluminum, bismuth, copper, lead, arsenic, phosphorus, mercury, or zinc. Lead is the most prevalent, sometimes referred to as the "silent epidemic." Lead accumulates in the body over time, affecting multiple systems but principally the brain. Exposure is highest among occupations associated with extracting and processing lead, and among children who live in dilapidated housing, whose exposure is related to peeling paint (Fig. 17-6). Lead-contaminated dust and soil are other potential threats of exposure for children.[73]

IMAGING FINDINGS

The most striking radiographic feature of lead, phosphorus, copper, or bismuth heavy metal poisoning is the presence of transverse radiodense lines in the metaphyses of long bones, especially around the knee.[11,129] The density of the bands is similar to that of cortical bone. Similar lines are noted with treated rickets, scurvy, and congenital syphilis, but they may also represent a normal variant. Copper, zinc, and aluminum toxicity are associated with altered bone mineralization and osteopenia.

CLINICAL COMMENTS

Heavy metal poisoning is associated with a wide variety of nonspecific clinical findings, including anorexia, irritability, apathy, abdominal colic, vomiting, diarrhea, headaches, convulsions, and others. Toxic exposures damage the central nervous system, blood-forming organs, gastrointestinal tract, and other systems.[95,100]

KEY CONCEPTS

- *Lead, phosphorus, copper, and bismuth poisoning are associated with transverse, radiodense metaphyseal bands.*
- *Copper, zinc, and aluminum toxicity are associated with altered bone mineralization and osteopenia.*

Histiocytosis

BACKGROUND

Langerhans cell histiocytosis, formerly known as *histiocytosis X,* is the abnormal proliferation of histiocytes, resulting in focal or systemic manifestations. Although the true etiology is not known, the prevailing opinion is that Langerhans histiocytosis represents a reactive rather than neoplastic process.[127] Recently, a better understanding of the disease has resulted from advances in specialized imaging and the development of immunohistochemical, morphological, and clinical standards of diagnosis.[40]

Langerhans cell histiocytosis describes three clinical syndromes: eosinophilic granuloma (60% to 80% of cases), Hand-Schüller-Christian disease (15% to 40% of cases), and Letterer-Siwe disease (10% of cases). Eosinophilic granuloma is the least aggressive form, usually seen in patients between the ages of 5 and 15 years.

Hand-Schüller-Christian disease is the chronic disseminated variety, characterized by multifocal bone lesions and extraskeletal involvement of the reticuloendothelial system. It is typically seen in children between the ages of 1 and 5 years. Uncommonly (in 10% of cases), a clinical triad of exophthalmus, diabetes insipidus, and lytic skull lesions is present.

Letterer-Siwe disease represents an acute, disseminated, fulminant variety of the disease, seen in children younger than 2 years of age. Its aggressive clinical presentation may mimic leukemia. Most cases are fatal.

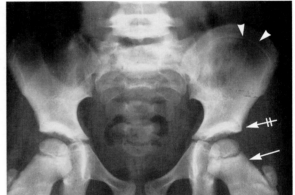

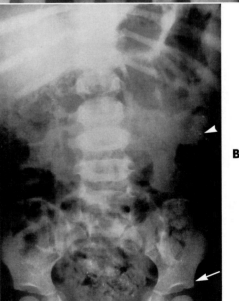

FIG. 17-6 Lead intoxication. **A,** Radiodense bands in the ilium (*arrowheads*), proximal metaphyses of the femora (*arrow*), acetabuli (*crossed arrow*) and L5 vertebra secondary to lead intoxication. **B,** Another case of lead intoxication demonstrating mild radiodense lines in the acetabuli (*arrow*). Observe the radiodense ingested lead fragments in the gastrointestinal tract of the left upper abdominal quadrant (*arrowhead*).

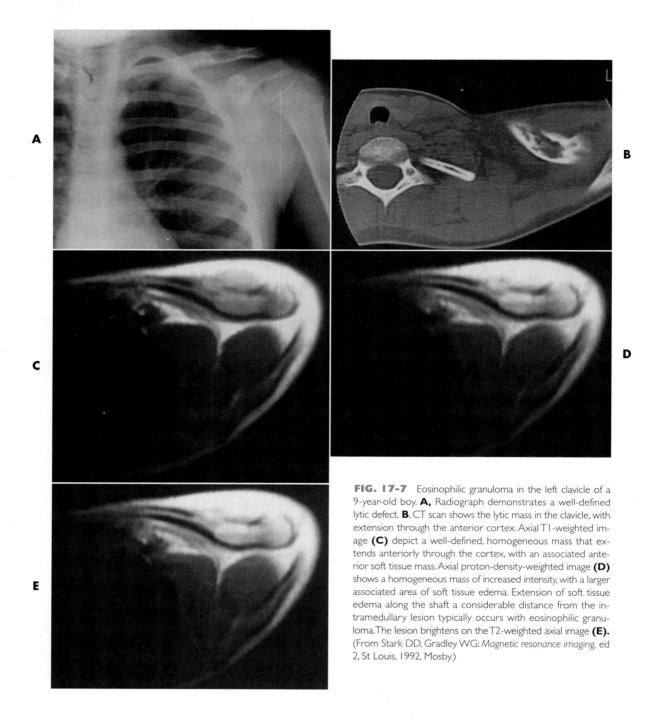

FIG. 17-7   Eosinophilic granuloma in the left clavicle of a 9-year-old boy. **A,** Radiograph demonstrates a well-defined lytic defect. **B**, CT scan shows the lytic mass in the clavicle, with extension through the anterior cortex. Axial T1-weighted image **(C)** depict a well-defined, homogeneous mass that extends anteriorly through the cortex, with an associated anterior soft tissue mass. Axial proton-density-weighted image **(D)** shows a homogeneous mass of increased intensity, with a larger associated area of soft tissue edema. Extension of soft tissue edema along the shaft a considerable distance from the intramedullary lesion typically occurs with eosinophilic granuloma. The lesion brightens on the T2-weighted axial image **(E).** (From Stark DD, Gradley WG: *Magnetic resonance imaging,* ed 2, St Louis, 1992, Mosby.)

IMAGING FINDINGS

The osseous lesions of eosinophilic granuloma, Hand-Schüller-Christian, and Letterer-Siwe diseases are very similar. They appear as one or more medullary-based, lytic lesions with geographic destruction (Figs. 17-7 and 17-8), lobular contour, endosteal scalloping (Fig. 17-9), periosteal reaction (long bone lesions only) (Fig. 17-10), and well-defined, uneven, or beveled margins.[43] Matrix calcification and subarticular extension are not characteristic.[43] Alternatively, sclerotic lesions with or without periosteal reactions may occur.

Overall, more than 50% of osseous lesions occur in the flat bones of the skull, pelvis, and ribs (Figs. 17-11); about 30% of lesions occur in long bones (Fig. 17-11).[115] Spinal involvement usually spares the vertebral arch and may lead to advanced vertebral collapse (vertebral plana). As the lesions heal, the diminished vertebral height may reconstitute (Fig. 17-13). Soft tissue masses may occur, representing extension from adjacent bone marrow involvement.[60] Advanced bony destruction of the mandible produces an isolated, "floating" appearance of the teeth. Pulmonary manifestation of eosinophilic granuloma includes a reticulonodular pattern of the middle and upper lung zones, often progressing to honeycomb lung.

Osseous lesions occurring with Letterer-Siwe disease are typically limited to the skull, often appearing as widespread, multiple osteolytic lesions. Eosinophilic granuloma typically presents as a solitary lesion and involves the appendicular skeleton more often than Letterer-Siwe or Hand-Schüller-Christian disease. Each of the three types, and especially Letterer-Siwe, may appear permeative with widespread bone destruction, mimicking findings of leukemia, Ewing's sarcoma, or infection. In general, Langerhans histiocytosis has such a variable appearance that it should be considered in every destructive bone lesion that appears in patients younger than age 30 years.

Although radionuclide scintigraphy is more sensitive than radiographic skeletal surveys in detecting histiocytic lesions in the spine, pelvis, and ribs, and it is less sensitive in identifying lesions in the skull.[37]

CLINICAL COMMENTS

Pain, fever, elevated erythrocyte sedimentation rate, progressive anemia, hepatosplenomegaly, lymphadenopathy, and diabetes insipidus may be present.[36] The clinical presentation may mimic an infection. Overall, the prognosis of Langerhans cell histiocytosis is excellent in children with either localized or multifocal disease occurring in the absence of organ dysfunction, chronic disease, new-onset pituitary involvement, or long-term pulmonary fibrosis.[1,75] Current therapeutic approaches involve chemotherapies, immunosuppressives, bone marrow transplant, and gene therapy.[1]

Text continued on p. 752

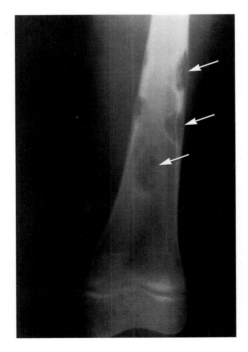

FIG. 17-8 Several well-defined osteolytic regions secondary to eosinophilic granuloma (*arrows*). (Courtesy Joseph W. Howe, Sylmar, Calif.)

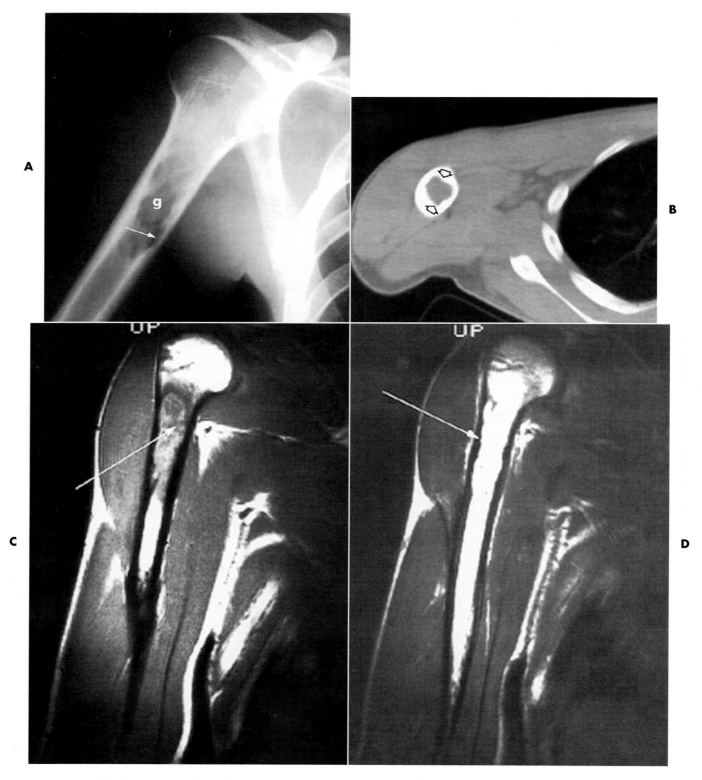

FIG. 17-9   Eosinophilic granuloma. **A,** Radiography demonstrates a well- defined lytic lesion *(g)* in the proximal humeral diaphysis with endosteal scalloping *(arrow)*. **B,** CT documents endosteal erosion *(arrows)* to better advantage. **C,** Coronal T1-weighted MRI reveals predominantly low signal intensity *(arrow)* within the lesion. **D,** The lesion exhibits high signal intensity *(arrow)* on a corresponding T2-weighted image. Differential diagnosis should include consideration of fibrous dysplasia, plasmacytoma, metastatic disease, and indolent infection. (From Sartoris DJ: *Musculoskeletal imaging: the requisites,* St Louis, 1996, Mosby.)

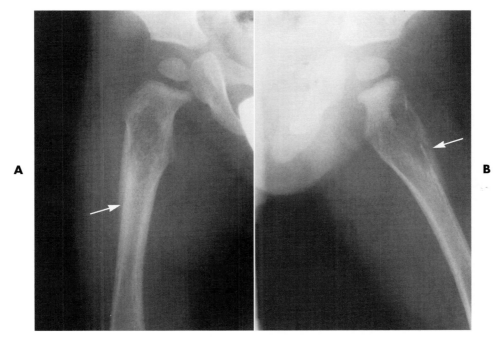

FIG. 17-10 Anteroposterior **(A)** and frogleg **(B)** projections of an aggressive osteolytic lesion in the proximal femur resulting from eosinophilic granuloma. Also noted is parallel periostitis of the lateral femur (*arrows*). (Courtesy Joseph W. Howe, Sylmar, Calif.)

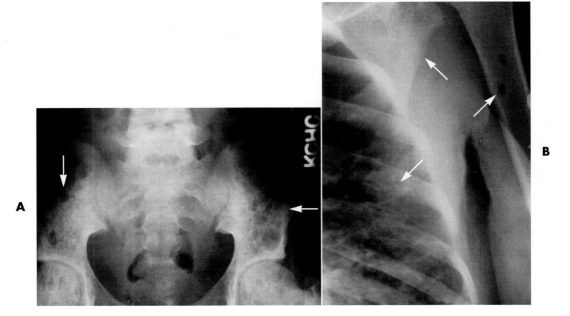

FIG. 17-11 Eosinophilic granuloma marked by multiple osteolytic defects causing a cystic appearance to the pelvis (**A,** *arrows*). The same patient exhibits two well-defined osteolytic changes in the proximal humerus, ribs, and scapula (**B,** *arrows*). (Courtesy Steven P. Brownstein, Springfield, NJ.)

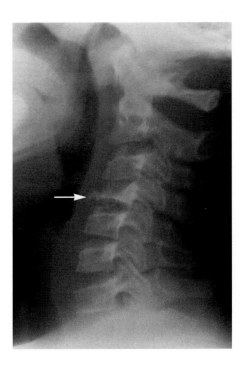

FIG. 17-12 Eosinophilic granuloma presenting as a solitary collapse of the vertebra (vertebra plana) *(arrow)*. (Courtesy Joseph W. Howe, Sylmar, Calif.)

A   **B**

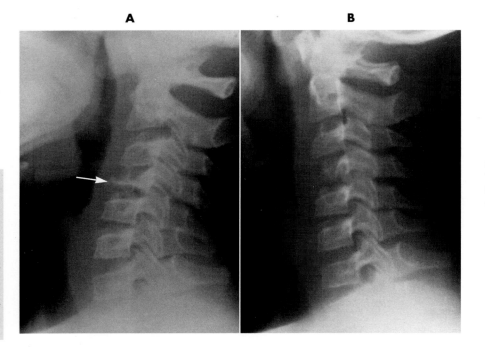

FIG. 17-13 Eosinophilic granuloma leading to flattened C4 vertebral body (**A,** *arrow*). On a later film (**B),** the C4 vertebral body has partially reconstituted. (Courtesy Steven P. Brownstein, Springfield, NJ.)

KEY CONCEPTS

- *Langerhans histiocytosis is marked by an abnormal proliferation of histiocytes.*
- *Langerhans histiocytosis lesions demonstrate a wide variety of osseous presentations and should be considered as a diagnostic differential in every destructive bone lesion occurring in patients younger than age 30 years.*
- *Letterer-Siwe disease, which occurs in 10% of these cases, is the acute disseminated variety occurring in children younger than 2 years of age. Osseous lesions usually consist of multiple lytic skull lesions.*

- *Hand-Schüller-Christian disease, which occurs in 15% to 40% of these cases, is the chronic disseminated variety occurring in children between 1 and 5 years of age. Osseous lesions are typically multiple geographic osteolytic lesions, occurring in the skull, pelvis, and long bones.*
- *Eosinophilic granuloma (which occurs in 60% to 80% of cases) is the least aggressive form, usually seen in patients between the ages of 5 and 15 years. Osseous lesions are usually solitary geographic osteolytic lesions, occurring in the skull, pelvis, long bones, mandible, and spine.*

Hypertrophic Osteoarthropathy

BACKGROUND

Hypertrophic osteoarthropathy describes a primary (pachydermoperiostosis or Touraine-Solente-Golé syndrome) or secondary (Pierre-Marie-Bamberger syndrome) disorder accompanied by digital clubbing, painful swollen joints, and a symmetrical, undulated, periosteal reaction.[9,72] All features of the disorder may not be present. Although the etiology remains elusive, vascular flow, vascular endothelium, and platelet-derived growth factors have all been implicated.[35,64,71] The primary form is less common (occurring in 3% to 5% of cases), has an adolescent onset and a predominance for males and blacks, and is associated with a thickened appearance of the skin of the face and scalp.

Secondary hypertrophic osteoarthropathy is associated with bronchogenic carcinoma (which occurs in up to 12% of cases),[126] pulmonary abscess, pulmonary metastasis, Hodgkin's disease,[88] emphysema, cystic fibrosis, heart disease, and occasionally in other acute and chronic disorders.[23,112] Lesions of the abdominal cavity (i.e., dysentery, Crohn's disease, biliary atresia) may produce secondary hypertrophic osteoarthropathy; however, intrathoracic causes, especially bronchogenic carcinoma, predominate. The age of onset is related to the underlying pathology.

IMAGING FINDINGS

The radiographic features of primary and secondary hypertropic osteoarthropathy are similar. Both are marked by periosteal reaction occurring most commonly in the tubular bones of the extremities, especially the tibia, fibula, radius, and ulna. Less commonly, the wrist, ankle, and small bones of the hands and feet are involved. The periosteal reaction is nonaggressive, thick, and widespread, occurring in the diaphysis and metaphysis (Fig. 17-14). The thickness of the periosteal reaction may increase proportionally to the duration of the disease.

The differences between the primary and secondary forms are that the periosteal reaction occurring in patients with primary hypertrophic osteoarthropathy involves the epiphyses (secondary does not) and appears more "fluffy," "shaggy," or less well-defined than does the reaction that associated with secondary osteoarthropathy. Ligamentous calcifications and bony excrescences are features of primary hypertrophic osteoarthropathy, often involving the calcaneus, patella, and interosseous membrane between the radius and ulna.

Traditionally, the diagnosis of hypertrophic osteoarthropathy has been made on plain film radiographs. However, radionuclide bone scintigraphy provides a sensitive method of detection that correlates well to the clinical presentation.[12,29]

CLINICAL COMMENTS

The clinical onset of primary hypertrophic osteoarthropathy is insidious, marked by clubbing of the distal hands and feet. The skin of the face and scalp appears thickened (pachydermia). The clinical presentation of secondary osteoarthropathy is similar but is also very dependent on the underlying condition. A clinical presentation of vague bone pain and joint swelling occurs more commonly in the secondary form of the disease. The primary form is usually self-limiting after many years of involvement.

KEY CONCEPTS

- *Primary hypertrophic osteoarthropathy is marked by a solid, thick, shaggy periosteal reaction involving the epiphysis, metaphysis, and diaphysis of the tibia, fibula, radius, and ulna. Clubbing of the fingers, ligamentous calcification, and skin changes of the scalp and face are noted.*
- *Secondary hypertrophic osteoarthropathy occurs secondary to underlying disease (usually bronchogenic tumor) and demonstrates a solid, thick, well-defined periosteal reaction involving the metaphysis and diaphysis of the tibia, fibula, radius, and ulna. Clubbing of the fingers and joint swelling are common clinical features.*

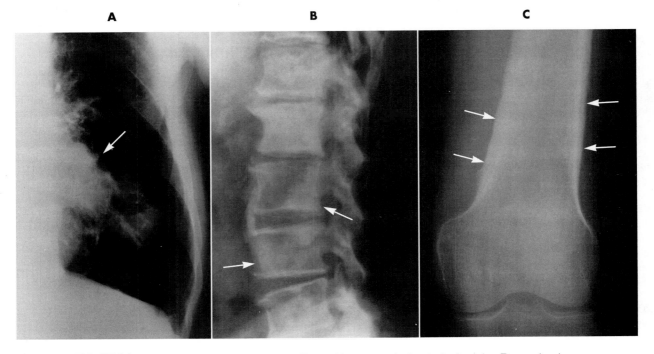

A **B** **C**

FIG. 17-14 Bronchogenic carcinoma of the lung (**A,** *arrow*) has metastasized to the lumbar spine (**B,** *arrows*) and manifested with hypertrophic osteoarthropathy by producing thick periostitis along the distal femora (**C,** *arrows*). (Courtesy Joseph W. Howe, Sylmar, Calif.)

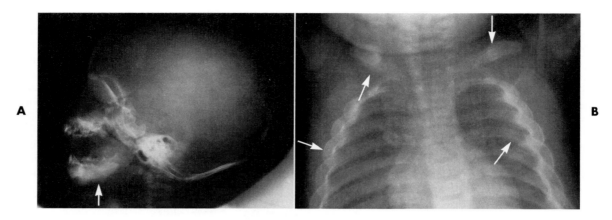

FIG. 17-15   Infantile cortical hyperostosis (Caffey's disease) presenting with bilaterally symmetrical, thick, periostitis (*arrows*) of the mandible **(A)**, clavicles, and ribs **(B)**. (Courtesy Ian D. McLean, Davenport, Iowa.)

Infantile Cortical Hyperostosis

BACKGROUND

Infantile cortical hyperostosis (Caffey's disease, Caffey-Silverman syndrome) is an uncommon familial or sporadic syndrome marked by subperiosteal bone formation. The etiology is unknown, and it usually manifests before 6 months of age, with equal incidence in males and females.[7,46,63]

IMAGING FINDINGS

The radiographic features include symmetrical, thick periosteal reaction most commonly involving the mandible (80% of cases), clavicle, ulna, and less commonly the ribs, scapulae, calvarium, or diaphysis of tubular bones (Fig. 17-15).[46] Although the mandible is the most commonly affected bone in the sporadic form, the tibia is the predominant bone affected in patients with the familial form.[14]

Physiological periostitis is a much more common cause of periosteal reaction in an infant younger than 6 months of age. A similar appearance may occur in rickets and scurvy but rarely before 6 months of age, and each demonstrates additional metaphyseal findings. Pleural effusion may accompany rib involvement. Radionuclide scintigraphy may be useful to further delineate the extent of skeletal involvement. MRI is useful to assess the presence and extent of subperiosteal hemorrhage.[102]

CLINICAL COMMENTS

The clinical manifestation is marked by fever, hyperirritability, soft tissue swelling over the involved bone, and often an elevated erythrocyte sedimentation rate. On palpation, the masses of involved bone and soft tissue swelling are hard and painful. The clinical course is typically self-limiting within a few months.[14]

KEY CONCEPTS

- *Infantile cortical hyperostosis occurs before 6 months of age.*
- *Fever, hyperirritability, and painful soft tissue swelling over affected bones are clinical symptoms.*
- *This disease most commonly involves the mandible and clavicle.*

Mastocytosis

BACKGROUND

Mastocytosis is a term used collectively to describe a heterogeneous group of disorders all characterized by an abnormal proliferation and accumulation of mast cells in various tissues and organs.[113,122] The etiology is largely unknown, but limited evidence points to an abnormality of stem cell factor receptors.[45] Mastocytosis is usually limited to the skin (90% of cases), but rarely it may become systemic, involving primarily the bone marrow and gastrointestinal tract.[33,45,51] Systemic disease usually manifests in adults, although a pediatric form of systemic disease exists.[66] Men and women are equally affected.

IMAGING FINDINGS

The radiographic appearance of systemic mastocytosis is variable. Histamine and heparin released from the mast cells may produce generalized osteopenia similar to osteoporosis.[31,61] Less commonly, localized osteopenic or osteolytic defects are observed. The osteolytic lesions occur most often in the ribs, skull, and long tubular bones. Mast cell proliferation and infiltration may cause reactive sclerosis of the host bone, producing multiple osteosclerotic foci. The osteosclerotic lesions are more common in the axial skeleton and may be accompanied by thickened trabeculae. The osteolytic and osteosclerotic regions often coexist (Fig. 17-16). Radionuclide bone scintigraphy may be helpful to determine the full extent of skeletal involvement.

CLINICAL COMMENTS

Systemic mastocytosis comprises a wide spectrum of clinical features, depending on the organs involved, age of onset, and associated hematological diseases.[45] Clinical features are related to the release of mast-cell–derived mediators (i.e., heparin, histamine, platelet-activating factor, prostaglandin, and peptide leukotrienes) and include vomiting, flushing, diarrhea, hepatosplenomegaly, weight loss, and skin lesions.[90] Treatment is directed toward symptom relief and the prognosis is dependent on the extent of involvement.

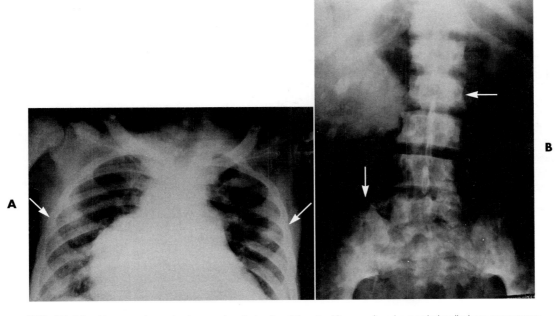

FIG. 17-16   Mastocytosis causing increased radiodensity of the ribs (**A,** *arrows*) and a mottled radiodense appearance (**B,** *arrows*) in the lumbar spine and pelvis. (Courtesy Steven P. Brownstein, Springfield, NJ.)

KEY CONCEPTS

- *Mastocytosis involves the rare proliferation of mast cells, typically affecting adults.*
- *This disease involves general or local osteopenia, local osteosclerosis, or a mixed pattern of presentation.*
- *The clinical symptoms of mastocytosis are vomiting, flushing, weight loss, and diarrhea.*

Neurofibromatosis

BACKGROUND

Neurofibromatosis is the most common of a heterogeneous group of diseases, known as *phakomatoses*. Phakomatoses are disorders of embryological neuroectoderm tissue derivatives and are characterized by hamartomas of various tissues. Other phakomatoses include Lindau's disease, Sturge-Weber syndrome, and tuberous sclerosis.

Neurofibromatosis is a genetic disorder affecting primarily the cell growth of neural tissue.[79] At least eight presentations of the disease exist; however, only two are widely recognized: neurofibromatosis type I (von Recklinghausen's disease, peripheral neurofibromatosis, or NF-1) and neurofibromatosis type II (central neurofibromatosis, or NF-2).[109] Both types have an autosomal dominant pattern of inheritance, no sexual or racial predilection, and are marked by nerve sheath tumors. Each appears to be influenced by hormones, and females may notice exacerbations during pregnancy. Other than these common points the two types appear very different clinically and reflect defects of two different genes (chromosome 17 in NF-1 and chromosome 22 in NF-2).

Neurofibromatosis type I (NF-1).   NF-1 is the most common form of the disorder, affecting approximately 1 in 4000 individuals.[79] It is diagnosed when at least two of the following criteria are present:

1. Six or more cutaneous macules (café-au-lait spots), larger than 5 mm before puberty, larger than 15 mm after puberty

2. Two or more neurofibromas
3. One or more plexiform neurofibromas
4. Axillary or inguinal flecking
5. Optic gliomas
6. Two or more iris hamartomas (Lisch nodules)
7. One or more characteristic bone lesions
8. First-degree relative (parent, child, or sibling) with the disease[80]

NF-1 is associated with a variety of intracranial hamartomatous and neoplastic lesions of the white matter and globus pallidus, including optic nerve and parenchymal gliomas.[87] Those afflicted exhibit characteristic nonelevated, brownish cutaneous hyperpigmentations, known as *café-au-lait spots*. The hyperpigmentations exhibit smooth margins, as opposed to the jagged margins of similar hyperpigmentations that occur with polyostotic fibrous dysplasia. Other cutaneous lesions include the presence of multiple, widely dispersed, soft nodules, known as *fibroma molluscum*. In addition to the intracranial and cutaneous lesions, patients with neurofibromatosis type I exhibit osseous defects of the skull, spine, and extremities, which are detailed under Imaging Findings.[53]

Neurofibromatosis type II (NF-2).   NF-2 is a much less common form of neurofibromatosis than NF-1; 1 in 50,000 individuals are affected.[79] It is diagnosed by the presence of bilateral acoustic schwannomas, or a unilateral acoustic schwannoma occurring in a patient who has a first-degree relative (parent, child, or sibling) with the disease.[79] It is common for patients to develop unilateral acoustic schwannomas unrelated to neurofibromatosis. In addition to acoustic schwannomas, patients often develop schwannomas of other cranial nerves, and solitary or multiple meningiomas.[116] In contrast to NF-1, cutaneous and osseous changes are not characteristic of NF-2.

IMAGING FINDINGS

Although many of the skeletal changes occurring with NF-1 are clearly seen on plain film radiography, plain film radiography offers

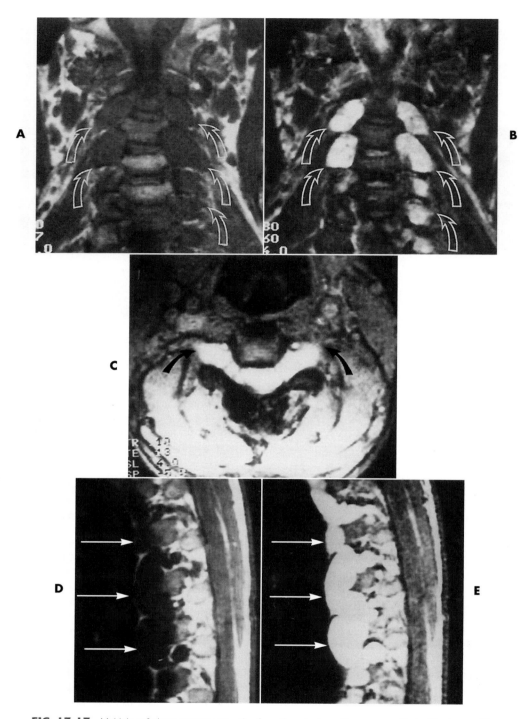

FIG. 17-17   Multiple soft tissue masses emanating from the spinal canal in a young patient with a known history of neurofibromatosis. **A,** A T1-weighted coronal image through the cervical spine shows that the masses are both intradural and extradural *(arrows)*. **B,** A T2-weighted image through the same region demonstrates increased signal within the lesions. Some have ill-defined areas of decreased signal, characteristic of neurofibromas *(arrows)*. **C,** A 10-degree FISP gradient-echo (fast imaging with steady-state precession) image shows widening of the cervical neural foramina by the high-signal lesions *(arrows)*. **D,** A T1-weighted parasagittal image through the thoracic spine reveals multiple septated cavities just lateral to the canal *(arrows)*. **E,** Homogeneously increased signal consistent with a thoracic meningocele *(arrows)*. (From Modic et al: *Magnetic resonance imaging of the spine,* St Louis, 1994, Mosby.)

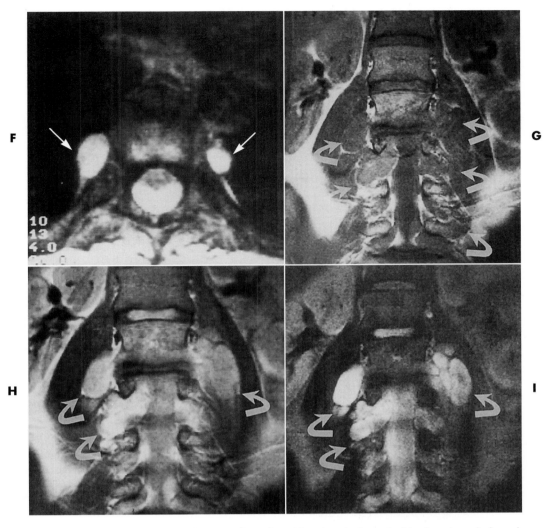

FIG. 17-17—cont'd **F,** The 10-degree gradient-echo axial study again shows the lateral meningocele *(arrows)*. **G,** A T1-weighted coronal image through the lumbar spine demonstrates multiple intradural and extradural "dumbbell" neurofibromas that have the signal intensity of soft tissue *(arrows)*. **H,** A proton-density weighted coronal scan through the lumbar spine shows the dumbbell shape of the neurofibromas, which now are of increased signal intensity *(arrows)*. **I,** A T2-weighted coronal scan through the lumbar spine reveals the high-signal neurofibromas, some of the which have a lower signal intensity within *(arrows)*.

little in the evaluation of the intracranial manifestations of NF-1 or NF-2. Rarely an enlarged internal acoustic or optic canal may be seen, but these osseous changes are always better delineated with computed tomography. MRI offers superb imaging of intracranial and spinal lesions (Fig. 17-17). Patients with NF-1 often show hyperintense foci in the areas of brain involvement on T2-weighted images. The intensity of these areas varies over serial studies. Neurofibromas often demonstrate a characteristic pattern of peripheral hyperintensity and central hypointensity on T2-weighted images (target sign). The intracranial lesions of NF-2 (acoustic schwannomas and less frequent associated meningiomas) are also best imaged by MRI. On MRI, schwannomas are hypointense or isointense relative to brain parenchyma on T1-weighted scans, are hyperintense on T2-weighted scans, and enhance following gadolinium.[94]

Skull. Congenital deficiency of the greater and lesser wing of the sphenoid and posterosuperior orbital wall creates a "bare orbit"

appearance (Fig. 17-18). This abnormality allows the temporal lobe of the brain to directly contact the soft tissues around the eye, producing pulsatile exophthalmus.[20] Other changes include a radiolucent cranial defect at the lambdoidal suture (asterion defect) just posterior to the junction of the parietomastoid and occipitomastoid sutures (Fig. 17-19). This defect is more common on the left side and may be associated with ipsilateral hypoplasia of the mastoid. Enlargement of cranial foramen may be present, especially of the optic and internal auditory canals. Enlargement of the entire skull (macrocranium) is a common and prominent feature in up to 75% of individuals. An additional finding may be the presence of scattered calcifications over the temporal lobe similar to those that occur in the choroid plexus.[131]

Spine. The spine is commonly affected.[69,130] Kyphoscoliosis is seen in 50% of patients and is marked by a short segment; angular, progressive curvature most often occurs in the thoracic spine

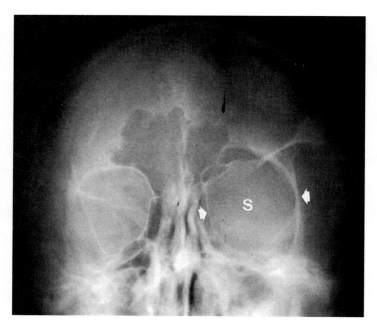

FIG. 17-18   Unilateral absence of the sphenoid wing *(s)* with orbital enlargement *(arrows)* in neurofibromatosis. The findings are virtually specific for this condition and occur secondary to mesodermal dysplasia. (From Sartoris DJ: *Musculoskeletal imaging: the requisites,* St Louis, 1996, Mosby.)

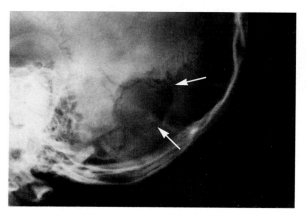

FIG. 17-19   Neurofibromatosis with lambdoidal suture (asterion) defect *(arrows).*

(Fig. 17-20). The kyphoscoliosis may lead to paraplegia. Scalloping of the posterocentral portion of the vertebral body is related to dural ectasia. Neurofibromas of the exiting nerve roots may cause scalloping defects of the posterior vertebral body and other borders of the corresponding intervertebral foramen (Figs. 17-21, 17-22, and 17-23). Large, scalloped osseous defects and paraspinal masses occur with intrathoracic meningoceles, which represent lateral protrusions of the spinal canal's meninges into the extrapleural space.

Ribs.   Ribs may appear irregular, twisted, ribbonlike, or eroded. These changes are related to either adjacent intercostal neurofibromas or mesodermal dysplasia.

Extremities.   Osseous dyplasia of the long bones (Fig. 17-24) manifests as bowing deformity and thin cortices, with or without pseudofractures of the convex cortex. Pseudoarthrosis of long bones results from loose periosteum and poor callus response following pathological fracture. Bowing deformity and pseudoarthrosis most often involve the tibia. A peculiar feature of the disease is focal giantism involving a single bone or the entire extremity. Occasionally multiple cystic bone defects, thought to represent nonossifying fibromas, are encountered.

CLINICAL COMMENTS

A suspected diagnosis of NF-1 should be accompanied by a review of the patient's history for the following: psychomotor deficits, pain, vision problems, progressive neurologic deficits, and constipation.[79] A review of family history for others afflicted is important.

Further manifestations of NF-1 (eye, CNS, PNS, bone) should be evaluated with plain film radiography, MRI, appropriate laboratory tests, and consultation with a specialist. Therapeutic options include surgical intervention, chemotherapy, and radiation therapy. All are used sparingly. The prognosis of the disease is poorly defined and may include serious complications (i.e., disfigurement, language disorders, hypertension, malignancies) in some individuals. The associated hypertension type is usually "essential," but renal artery stenosis and pheochromocytoma should be excluded. Leukemia and lymphoma are more common in children with NF-1.[114] Most patients with NF-1 have normal intelligence, although about half experience some degree of learning disability.[110]

A suspected diagnosis of NF-2 warrants a review of the patient's history for dizziness, headaches, tinnitus, loss of balance, seizures, and hearing loss.[79] Again the family history is important and physical examination should include a detailed neurological assessment of the eighth cranial nerve. Audiograms and tests of vestibular func-

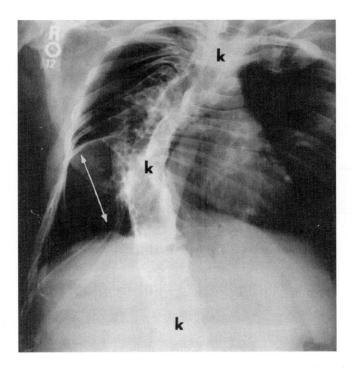

FIG. 17-20 Severe kyphoscoliosis *(k)* with associated rib deformities *(arrows)* in neurofibromatosis. Although this is the most common musculoskeletal manifestation of the disease, the differential diagnosis should include consideration of idiopathic scoliosis, Marfan's syndrome, Ehlers-Danlos syndrome, spondyloepiphyseal and spondylometaphyseal dysplasias, and a large number of other congenital malformation syndromes. (From Sartoris DJ: *Musculoskeletal imaging: the requisites,* St Louis, 1993, Mosby.)

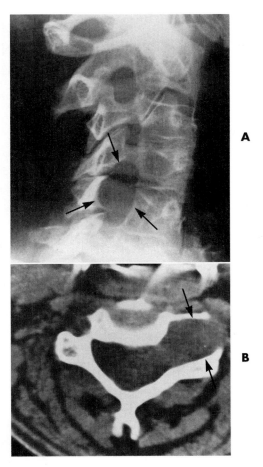

FIG. 17-21 Oblique radiograph demonstrating an enlarged C4-C5 and C5-C6 left intervertebral foramen with complete destruction of the C5 pedicle and posterior scalloping of the vertebral body of C4 and C5 (**A,** *arrows*) caused by an solitary neurofibroma noted on CT (**B,** *arrows*). (Courtesy Ian D. McLean, Davenport, Iowa.)

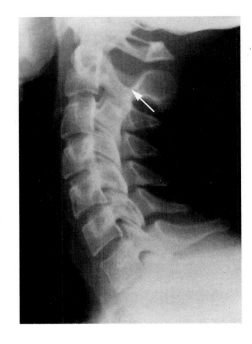

FIG. 17-22 Neurofibroma causing erosive defect of the vertebral arch of C2 *(arrow).* (Courtesy Steven P. Brownstein, Springfield, NJ.)

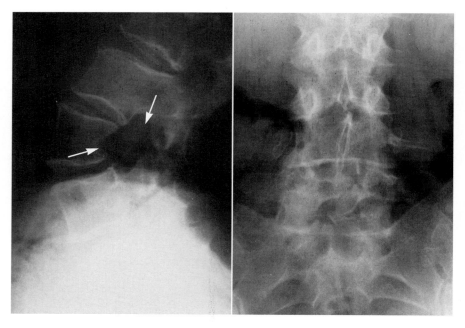

FIG. 17-23   Posterior vertebral scalloping, enlarged intervertebral foramen secondary to neurofibroma *(arrows).* (Courtesy Robert C. Tatum, Davenport, Iowa.)

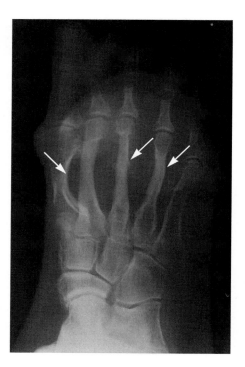

FIG. 17-24   Osseous irregularity and soft tissue masses noted in a patient with neurofibromatosis *(arrows).* (Courtesy Joseph W. Howe, Sylmar, Calif.)

tion are commonly applied. Patients often experience total loss of hearing and marked balance disturbance as the disease progresses. Therapeutics include surgery, stereotactic radiation therapy, and hearing augmentation with mechanical aids.

KEY CONCEPTS

- *Neurofibromatosis is the most common of four diseases collectively known as phakomatoses.*
- *One of the most common genetic diseases, neurofibromatosis has no sexual or racial predilection.*
- *Two widely recognized types include neurofibromatosis type I (von Recklinghausen's disease) and neurofibromatosis type II (central neurofibromatosis).*
- *Neurofibromatosis type I manifests as changes in the nervous system (optic nerve gliomas, neurofibromas of the spinal and peripheral nerves), skin (café-au-lait spots, fibroma molluscum), and bones (erosions of vertebrae and ribs; kyphoscoliosis; dysplasia of the sphenoid, ribs, and long bones; lambdoid suture defects).*
- *Neurofibromatosis type II is marked by bilateral acoustic schwannomas, often with one or more concurrent meningiomas.*
- *Magnetic resonance imaging offers the best imaging of the intracranial- and spine-related manifestations.*

Paget's Disease

BACKGROUND

Paget's disease (osteitis deformans) is a relatively common familial disorder, characterized by abnormal remodeling, hypertrophy, and structure of bone, leading to pain and deformity.[67,74] Determining the true incidence of Paget's disease is problematic, because most cases go unnoticed due to of a lack of symptoms.[83] Autopsy studies have estimated the incidence at 3% of those over the age of 40 years, and slightly more common in men.[26,39] The incidence decreases with decreasing age. Less than 4% of patients with Paget's disease are under the age of 40 years.[5] It is more common in England, Australia, New Zealand, and the northern United States and rare in Asia, Africa, and Scandinavia.[4,34,107]

In Paget's disease, osteoclasts are morphologically abnormal and contain viral-like nuclear inclusions.[98] Although a viral etiology is widely suspected, it has not been confirmed. A rare disease of similar radiographic appearance occurs in childhood and has been termed *juvenile Paget's disease.* However, this disease results from hyperphosphatasia and does not share a similar pathogenesis with Paget's disease.

Traditionally, the pathophysiology of Paget's disease is divided into three phases of bone involvement: lytic, mixed, and blastic. At any one time, multiple phases may exist in the same patient and the rate of progression from one phase to the next is highly variable. The initial or osteolytic phase is marked by bone resorption secondary to increased osteoclastic activity. Osteoblastic activity increases in response, and the two opposing actions lead to concurrent bone formation and resorption, which characterizes the mixed phase of Paget's disease. The third or blastic phase occurs when the osteoclastic activity ceases and osteoblastic activity predominates. Following these actions, a quiescent period usually ensues. The resulting pagetic bone is immature, weak, and hypervascular.

Uncommonly, a locus of pagetic bone may transform into an osteosarcoma (in 50% of malignant cases), fibrosarcoma (in 25% of malignant cases), or chondrosarcoma (in 5% of malignant cases).[94] Malignant transformation (often termed the *fourth phase*) is noted in 1% to 3% of localized Paget's disease and 5% to 10% of generalized Paget's disease (Fig. 17-25).[55,94] Rarely, giant cell tumors of the skull and facial bones are associated with Paget's disease.[8,13]

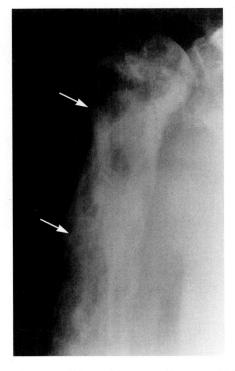

FIG. 17-25   The pagetoid bone of the proximal humerus exhibits a destructive pattern on the lateral aspect resulting from malignant degeneration *(arrows).* (Courtesy Joseph W. Howe, Sylmar, Calif.)

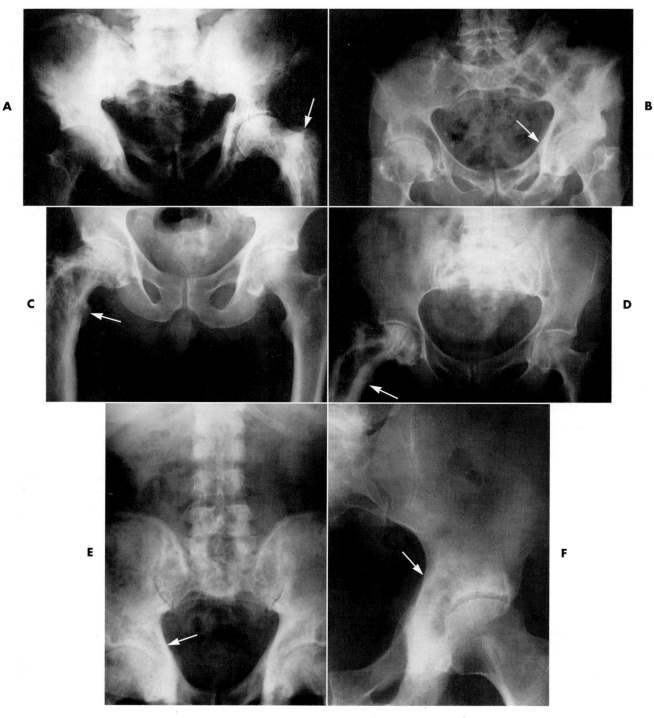

FIG. 17-26   Paget's disease is very common in the pelvis and proximal femora. The appearance is characterized by alteration in bone density, bone enlargement, and thickening of the cortex and trabeculae *(arrows)*. The changes may be predominately bilateral (**A** and **E**) or unilateral (**B, C, D,** and **F**). (*A,* Courtesy Steven P. Brownstein, Springfield, NJ; *B* and *F,* Courtesy Joseph W. Howe, Sylmar, Calif; *D,* Courtesy Jack C. Avalos, Davenport, Iowa.)

IMAGING FINDINGS

Paget's disease may involve any bone. It is typically localized to a bone or skeletal region and is of limited clinical consequence. Less commonly, the disease is widespread, leading to extensive osseous deformity and clinical complications. Transformation from monostotic to polyostotic involvement is not inevitable.

Paget's disease has a predilection to involve the pelvis, sacrum, spine (especially lumbar), skull, and proximal femora. The characteristic radiographic features include osseous enlargement, osteosclerosis, cortical thickening, and thickened, prominent trabeculae (Fig. 17-26). Characteristic features occur at various skeletal regions.

Skull. The lytic phase of Paget's disease of the skull appears with a geographic destructive lesion termed *osteoporosis circumscripta*. This lesion usually begins in the frontal or occipital regions. Mixed and blastic phases produce a "cotton wool" appearance resulting from focal osteosclerosis (Figs. 17-27 and 17-28). Bone softening at the base of the skull often leads to basilar invagination.

Spine. Vertebral involvement is common (occurring in 75% of cases) and is marked by enlargement, endplate thickening ("picture frame"), and increased radiodensity ("ivory vertebrae") of the segments. Bone softening develops biconcave vertebral body endplates. The weakened bone structure predisposes to compression fractures, although loss of vertebral height is more commonly the result of bone deformity than acute fracture.

Pelvis. Cortical thickening of the inner margin (arcuate line) of the ilium is the earliest finding of Paget's disease of the pelvis (Fig. 17-29). The pelvis may appear asymmetrical because of unilateral involvement with Paget's disease. Protrusio acetabuli may follow bone softening.

Extremities. Long bones are involved in about 30% of cases, most often the femur, tibia, and humerus (Fig. 17-30). The hands and feet are rarely involved.[32] The earliest radiographic manifestation of long bone involvement begins as an oval, slanted, V-shaped, osteolytic defect in the subarticular region, which progresses through the length of bone ("flame" or "blade of grass" sign) (Figs. 17-31 and 17-32). Cortical thickening is often present

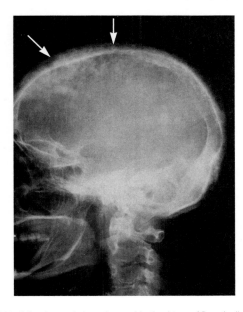

FIG. 17-27 Mixed osteolytic and osteoblastic phase of Paget's disease relating a "cotton wool" appearance to the skull *(arrows)*. (Courtesy Steven P. Brownstein, Springfield, NJ.)

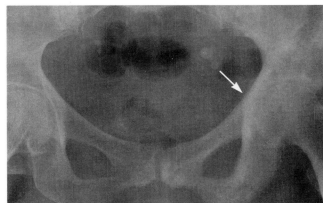

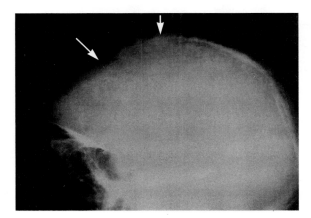

FIG. 17-28 Paget's disease producing a mixed osteoblastic and osteolytic appearance of the skull. The osteolytic destruction is excessive in the region of the frontal bone marking malignant degeneration *(arrows)*. (Courtesy Steven P. Brownstein, Springfield, NJ.)

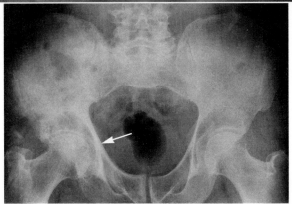

FIG. 17-29 Two cases each with cortical thickening of the inner margin or arcuate line of the pelvis consistent with the "brim" or "rim" sign of the pelvis *(arrows)*. (*Top,* Courtesy Joseph W. Howe, Sylmar, Calif; *bottom,* Courtesy Steven P. Brownstein, Springfield, NJ.)

PART TWO Bone, Joints, and Soft Tissues

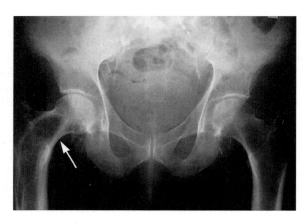

FIG. 17-30   Paget's disease of the right proximal femur marked by thick cortex *(arrow)* and prominent bone trabeculae. (Courtesy Steven P. Brownstein, Springfield, NJ.)

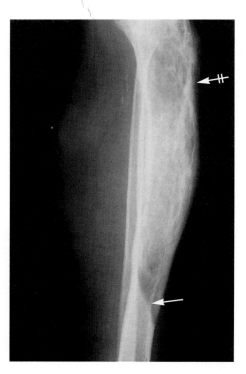

FIG. 17-31   Characteristic appearance of Paget's disease in the tibia. Paget's disease typically begins in one of the bone and progresses as a front of osteolysis *(arrow)* ("blade of grass" sign); the cortex is thick *(crossed arrow)*, and the trabecular pattern is prominent. (Courtesy Steven P. Brownstein, Springfield, NJ.)

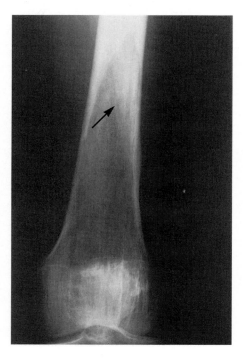

FIG. 17-32   Paget's disease of the distal femur appearing as a well-demarcated osteolytic process ("blade of grass" sign) beginning at the distal end of the femur and proceeding proximally in this case *(arrow)*. (Courtesy Joseph W. Howe, Sylmar, Calif.)

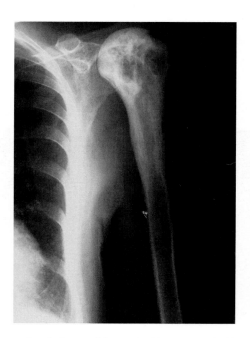

FIG. 17-33   Paget's disease of the proximal humerus marked by cortical enlargement and prominent trabeculae. (Courtesy Steven P. Brownstein, Springfield, NJ.)

(Figs. 17-33, 17-34, and 17-35). Long bones exhibit bowing deformity, which occurs secondary to bone softening, often with pseudofractures fractures on the convex cortex (Figs. 17-36 and 17-37). These lines are distinguished from similarly appearing transverse lucent lines (pseudofractures) occurring on the concave cortex of patient with osteomalacia, fibrous dysplasia, and other disease. Uncommonly, Paget's may begin in the diaphysis, usually the tibia or radius.

The extent of skeletal involvement is assessed by radionuclide bone scans with follow-up radiographs of suspicious areas. Repeated bone scans may be useful to assess the patient's response to therapeutics. MRI and computed tomography (CT) are employed to further delineate osseous or neurological complications. The sole use of MRI to diagnose Paget's without the benefit of plain films may be problematic, owing to the variable appearance of pagetic bone on MRI scans (Fig. 17-38).[94]

CLINICAL COMMENTS

Complications. The clinical features of Paget's disease vary. The localized form of the disease is typically asymptomatic and discovered incidentally.[58] Local pain (worse at night and often unrelated to activity) and tenderness over the involved bone is the most common clinical complaint. Alternatively, patients with advanced disease may complain of severe pain and develop complications of the cardiovascular, skeletal, and neuromuscular systems.

High-output congestive heart failure and temperature differences are cardiovascular complications resulting from the hyperemic pagetic bone.[54] Skeletal complications include progressive osseous enlargement, bowing of long bones, degenerative joint disease, extramedullary hematopoieses, and pathological fractures.[101] Neuromuscular complications are mainly the result of bone enlargement. Deafness may result from eighth cranial nerve compression by an enlarging temporal bone, deformity resulting from basilar impression, or enlarged dysfunctional ossicles. Pathological fracture or enlarged vertebrae may compress the spinal cord leading to muscle weakness, paralysis, and incontinence.

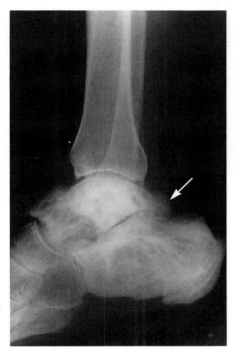

FIG. 17-34   Prominent trabeculae and bone enlargement consistent with Paget's disease of the calcaneous and navicula *(arrow)*. (Courtesy Joseph W. Howe, Sylmar, Calif.)

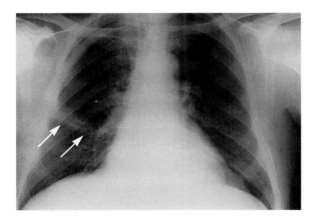

FIG. 17-35   Paget's disease of the right fourth rib *(arrows)*. The rib appears more radiodense and larger than the adjacent ribs. (Courtesy Steven P. Brownstein, Springfield, NJ.)

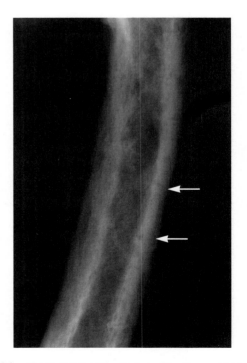

FIG. 17-36   Paget's disease of the diaphysis of the femur, exhibiting thick cortex, prominent trabecular pattern, and bowing deformity. Additionally, radiolucent defects are noted in the cortex, perpendicular to the long axis of the bone *(arrows)*, representing pseudofractures. Pseudofractures represent fibrous tissue replacement of bone and are also seen osteomalacia, fibrous dyplasia, and several other conditions. (Courtesy Joseph W. Howe, Sylmar, Calif.)

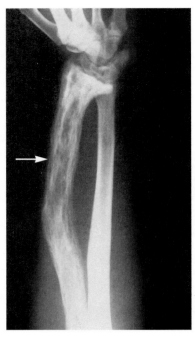

FIG. 17-37   Bone enlargement, cortical thickening, and prominent trabecular pattern *(arrow)* are noted in this radiograph of Paget's disease of the radius.

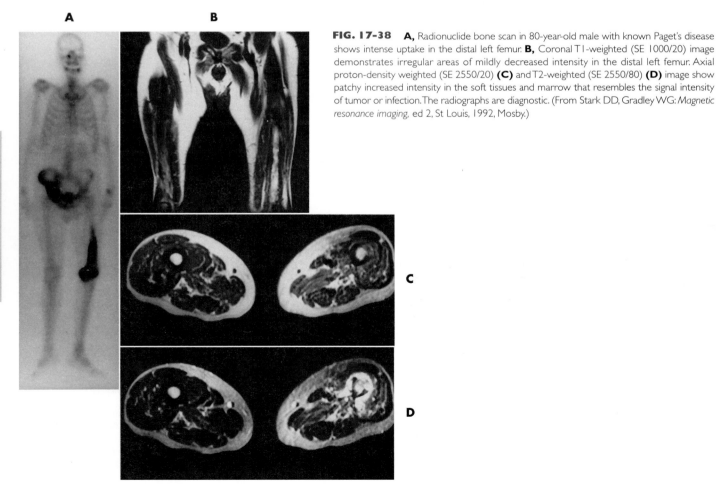

FIG. 17-38   **A,** Radionuclide bone scan in 80-year-old male with known Paget's disease shows intense uptake in the distal left femur. **B,** Coronal T1-weighted (SE 1000/20) image demonstrates irregular areas of mildly decreased intensity in the distal left femur. Axial proton-density weighted (SE 2550/20) **(C)** and T2-weighted (SE 2550/80) **(D)** image show patchy increased intensity in the soft tissues and marrow that resembles the signal intensity of tumor or infection. The radiographs are diagnostic. (From Stark DD, Gradley WG: *Magnetic resonance imaging,* ed 2, St Louis, 1992, Mosby.)

Laboratory values. Laboratory analysis reveals elevated serum alkaline phosphatase resulting from increased bone formation and elevated urinary hydroxyproline levels secondary to bone resorption.[68] Monitoring these laboratory values may provide insight to the activity and progression of Paget's disease.[62] Serum calcium levels are usually not affected, unless pathological fracture occurs.[62]

Treatment. Therapeutics are directed at alleviating pain and slowing the progression of the disease. The risk of progression and complications depends on the age of the patient, skeletal location, and aggressiveness of the Paget's disease.[74] Bisphosphates (e.g., tiludranate, pamidronate, alendronate) and calcitonin are widely used therapeutic agents that may arrest the disease process, partially restore normal bone architecture, and alleviate pain.[91,99,106] Bisphosphates appear to offer longer lasting benefits than can be obtained with calcitonin.[89,91]

KEY CONCEPTS

- *Paget's disease is a relatively common familial disorder, characterized by abnormal remodeling, hypertrophy, and structure of bone, leading to pain and deformity occurring in middle-age and older individuals.*
- *Pathophysiology is divided into lytic, mixed, and blastic phases, replacing normal bone with immature, weak, and hypervascular bone.*
- *Sarcomatous malignant transformation is a severe but uncommon complication may involve any bone; most common in the pelvis, sacrum, spine, skull, and proximal femora characteristic findings include osseous enlargement, osteosclerosis, cortical thickening, and thickened, prominent trabeculae.*
- *Paget's disease may affect the skull (osteoporosis circumscripta, "cotton wool," basilar impression), spine ("picture frame," ivory, and biconcave vertebrae, compression fractures), pelvis ("brim" sign, protrusio acetabuli), and extremities ("flame" or "blade of grass" sign, bowing, transverse fractures).*
- *Diagnosis is made by radionuclide bone scanning and plain film radiographs for initial assessment; MRI and CT are used to image complications (especially neurological).*
- *The localized form is typically asymptomatic; most common clinical complaints are local pain and tenderness over involved bone.*
- *Related complications occur in the osseous (i.e., enlargement, deformity, spinal stenosis), cardiovascular (i.e., congestive heart failure), and neurological (i.e., deafness, paralysis, incontinence) systems.*
- *Laboratory values exhibit elevated serum alkaline phosphatase, elevated urinary hydroxyproline, and normal serum calcium.*
- *Therapeutic agents include bisphosphonates (e.g., tiludranate, pamidronate, alendronate) and calcitonin.*

Pigmented Villonodular Synovitis

BACKGROUND

Pigmented villonodular synovitis (PVNS) is a rare, benign, inflammatory, proliferative disorder of synovium.[49] It is characterized by diffuse or localized hyperplastic outgrowth of the synovial membranes of joints, bursae, or tendon sheaths.[16] Morphologically, the hyperplastic outgrowths may be villous, nodular, or villonodular and consist of undifferentiated connective tissue infiltrated by hemosiderin and lipid-containing macrophages. PVNS is typically monoarticular and occurs in patients between 30 and 50 years of age, without a significant sex predilection.[49] Some authorities report a slight male predominance.[77]

When PVNS involves a synovial tendon sheath, it is often termed *giant cell tumor of the tendon sheath* (Fig. 17-39). How-

ever, some authorities feel it is problematic to include synovial tendons sheath lesions as PVNS.[65]

IMAGING FINDINGS

Radiographic features include soft tissue swelling, preservation of joint space (may decrease over time), presence of well-marginated bone erosions and subchondral cysts, and absence of periarticular osteoporosis.

The spine is rarely involved.[19,47] As a tendon sheath abnormality, PVNS favors the digits. The knee is the joint most commonly involved (Fig. 17-40). Other common joints include the hip, ankle

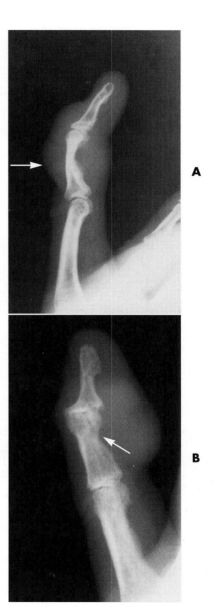

FIG. 17-39 Pigmented villonodular synovitis presenting in the tendon sheaths of the fifth digit **(A)** and first digit **(B)** *(arrows)* of different patients. Some authorities refer to this presentation as *giant cell tumor of the tendon sheath.* (*A*, Courtesy Joseph W. Howe, Sylmar, Calif; *B*, Courtesy Steven P. Brownstein, Springfield, NJ.)

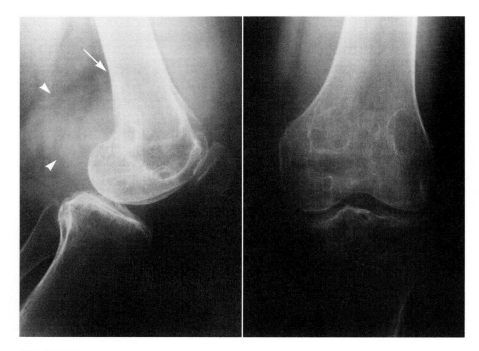

FIG. 17-40   Osseous erosions *(arrow)* and surrounding soft tissue enlargement *(arrowheads)* associated with pigmented villonodular synovitis of the knee. (Courtesy Joseph W. Howe, Sylmar, Calif.)

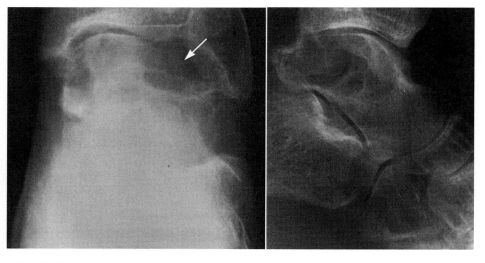

FIG. 17-41   Large cystic defect of the talus *(arrow)* secondary to pigmented villonodular synovitis. (Courtesy Joseph W. Howe, Sylmar, Calif.)

(Fig. 17-41), elbow, and wrist. Erosions and degenerative changes are more likely to occur in the hip and shoulder (Fig. 17-42) than in joints with large synovial recesses such as the knee. The radiographic appearance is very similar to that of noncalcified synovial chondromatosis. Calcification is not a feature of PVNS; its presence suggests synovial osteochondromatosis. Other major radiographic differentials include tuberculosis, hemophilia, and synovial sarcoma.

PVNS has a characteristic appearance on magnetic resonance imaging (MRI) scans. PVNS is hypointense or isointense on T1-weighted images, and mixed hypo- and hyperintense on T2-weighted images (Fig. 17-43).[111] The hyperintense areas represent edema and inflamed synovium. Hemosiderin deposits account for the hypointense regions on both the T1- and T2-weighted images. Correspondingly, large effusions may appear radiodense on plain film radiographs resulting from the hemosiderin deposits.

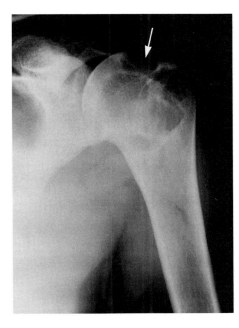

FIG. 17-42 Pigmented villonodular synovitis causing osseous erosions of the proximal humerus (arrow). (Courtesy Steven P. Brownstein, Springfield, NJ.)

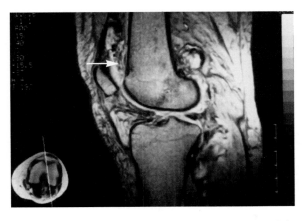

FIG. 17-43 T2-weighted MRI of the knee revealing the characteristic mixed signal intensity of pigmented villonodular synovitis (arrow). (Courtesy Ian D. McLean, Davenport, Iowa.)

In addition to plain film and MRI, ultrasonography, arthrography, and computed tomography may assist in providing critical information toward the correct diagnosis when confronted with an intraarticular abnormality.[24]

CLINICAL COMMENTS

Patients with PVNS most often are accompanied by mechanical pain and limitations of motion.[27] A history of trauma is slightly more often present than not. Joint swelling and joint locking are often present. Optimal treatment is early marginal excision for the local form and total synovectomy for the diffuse form.[44,124] Although recurrence is common,[25] the lesions are not malignant and radical surgical procedures are not indicated.[96]

KEY CONCEPTS

- *Pigmented Villonodular Synovitis (PVNS) is a rare, benign, inflammatory disorder of the synovial membranes of joints, bursae, and tendon sheaths.*
- *PVNS is typically monoarticular (usually involving the knee) and occurs between the ages of 30 and 50 years.*
- *Radiographic features include soft tissue swelling, preservation of joint space (may decrease over time), presence of bone erosions and subchondral cysts, and absence of periarticular osteoporosis.*
- *Common clinical findings include mechanical pain, limitations of motion, and joint swelling.*

Scoliosis

BACKGROUND

Definition. Scoliosis is a lateral curvature of the spine occurring in a coronal plane. The vertebrae involved in the curvature are usually rotated. Because of potential employment and medicolegal ramifications, the term *scoliosis* is typically reserved for lateral curvatures of more than 10 degrees Cobb's angle (see Table 3-2 for Cobb's angle measurement). Kyphosis is a convex posterior curvature and lordosis a convex anterior curvature of the spine, both occurring in a sagittal plane. Kyphoscoliosis refers to spinal curvature, which is both convex lateral and posterior. A sharply angled kyphosis is called a *gibbus*.

Prevalence. The frequency of scoliosis is dependent on the degree of curvature. A study in Montreal indicated a prevalence of 4.5% of curvatures greater than 5 degrees Cobb's angle.[97] Curvatures exceeding 10 degrees Cobb's angle are found in about 2% to 4% of adults in the United States.[18] Curvatures greater than 25 degrees Cobb's angle occur in 1.5 per 1000 individuals in the United States. Overall, the incidence is higher in females. Moreover, the greater the curvature is, the higher the female predilection.[93] Adolescents from 9 to 15 years of age are most at risk.[93]

Classification. Scolioses are broadly divided into structural and nonstructural types. Structural scolioses (Fig. 17-44) are fixed,

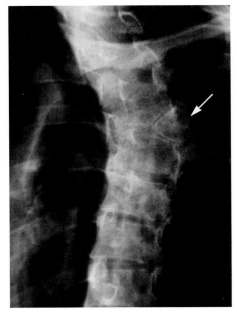

FIG. 17-44 Structural scoliosis created by a left hemivertebra wedged between the T6 and T7 vertebrae (arrow).

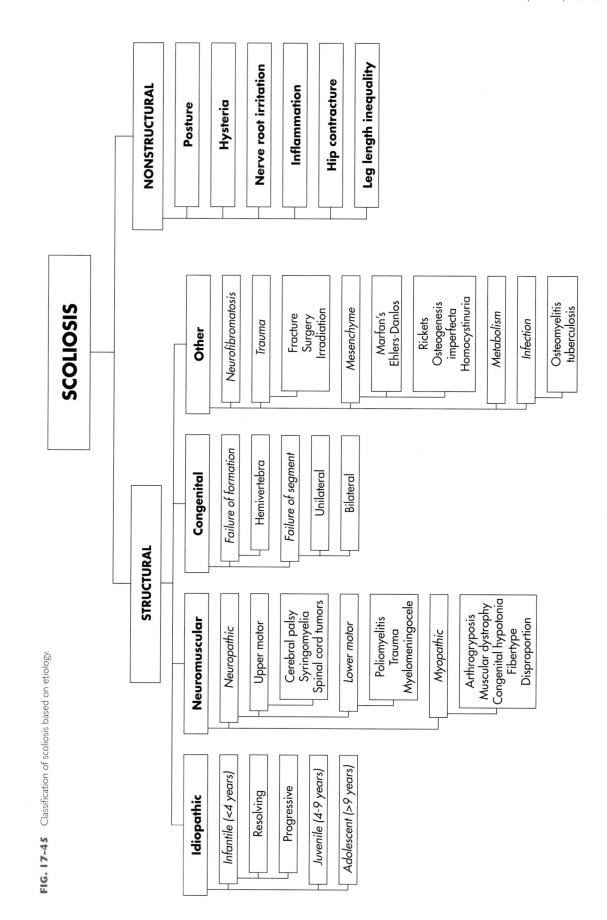

FIG. 17-45 Classification of scoliosis based on etiology.

do not correct on side-bending radiographs, and demonstrate a rib humping on the convex side of the curvature. Nonstructural or functional scolioses lessen or disappear on lateral bending, and any rib humping disappears on forward flexion.

More than 50 conditions are associated with scoliosis. Etiologies and further classifications are listed in Fig. 17-45. In nearly 80% of cases of scoliosis, an etiology cannot be determined. Overall, these idiopathic curvatures are more common to occur in females (a 7:1 ratio of females to males). They are subdivided into infantile (0 to 3 years of age), juvenile (4 to 10 years of age), and adolescent (most common; older than 10 years of age) types based on age of onset. Research efforts are focused on growth and dysfunction of the central nervous system as a possible cause of the currently idiopathic subtype.[21,22,92,105]

Scoliosis may also result from a variety of neurogenic and myogenic causes (see Fig. 17-45). Poliomyelitis and muscular dystrophy are the most common causes respectively. These types typically appear as long-segment, C-type configurations.

Congenital causes of scoliosis are related to abnormal vertebral formation or segmentation. The result is asymmetrical anatomy leading to a lateral curvature (see Fig. 17-44). Because of the proximity of embryonic tissue, developmental defects of the skeletal system are often associated with defects of the genitourinary system. Discovery of skeletal abnormalities necessitates a review of these systems.

IMAGING FINDINGS

Radiographic assessment begins with standing anteroposterior and lateral projections of the spine, preferably each as a single full-spine projection using 14-inch by 36-inch film and cassette.[119] The radiograph should include the entire spine from occiput to sacrum. The degree of spinal curvature is quantified using the Cobb method on the anterolateral projection (Fig. 17-46). An alternative, the Risser-Ferguson method, is less commonly used because of its inaccuracy (Fig. 17-47). Gonadal shielding, rare earth screens, collimation, and a 72-inch to 84-inch focal-film distance are effective in limiting the amount of radiation exposure. If temporal examinations are anticipated as part of long-term treatment, employing a posteroanterior patient position will limit thyroid and gonadal exposure.[59,78]

Lateral bending radiographs are useful to determine the rigidity of the spinal curvature and to differentiate structural from nonstructural curvatures. Compensatory curvatures lessen or disappear on lateral bending films; structural curvatures persist.

The description of the spinal curvature should detail the follow-

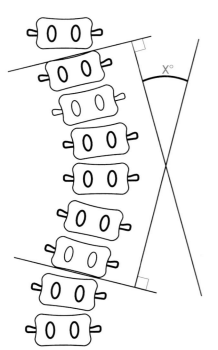

FIG. 17-46   Cobb's method of measuring scoliosis. Line segments are drawn across the superior endplate of the upper and inferior endplate of the lower vertebrae involved with the curvature. These end vertebrae are chosen using the criteria that they tilt most severely toward the scoliosis convexity. Perpendicular lines are drawn from the endplate lines, and the superior or inferior angle at their intersection (X°) is measured.

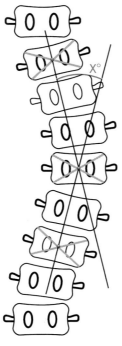

FIG. 17-47   Risser-Ferguson method of measuring scoliosis. Line segments are drawn from the center of the upper vertebra to the center of the vertebra at the apex of the lateral curvature (apical vertebra) and from the center of the lower vertebra to the center of the apical vertebra. The next step is to measure the superior or inferior angle at the intersection of these lines (X°). This method is used less often than Cobb's method.

A   B   C

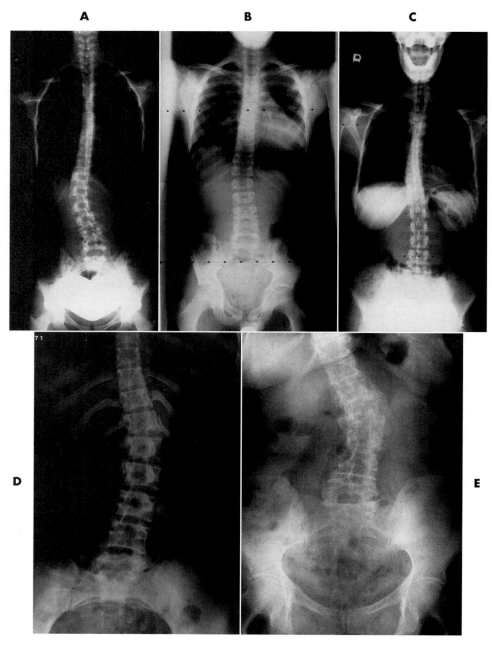

D   E

FIG. 17-48   Scoliosis in five different patients. The curvatures are identified by the direction of the convexity. In each figure the patient's right is on the reader's left. **A** and **B,** Right thoracolumbar. **C,** Right thoracic left lumbar. **D,** Left thoracolumbar. **E,** Left lumbar.

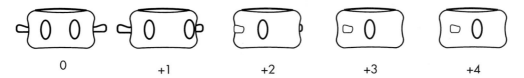

FIG. 17-49 Vertebral rotation is expressed by the pedicle appearance. The normal vertebral alignment is a grade 0. Grade +4 indicates maximum vertebral rotation, leaving only one pedicle visible, and found at the midline on the frontal projection.

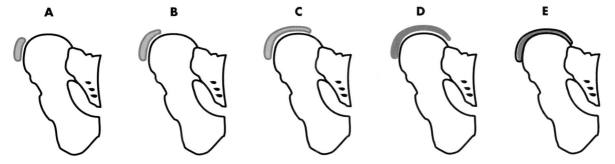

FIG. 17-50 Risser sign. On the anteroposterior projection, the appearance of the iliac apophysis provides a stable indicator of skeletal maturity. If the apophysis is not seen, a grade 0 is designated. The apophysis forms from the lateral aspect and progresses medially along the superior margin of the ilium (**A** through **D,** grades 1 through 4) and eventually fuses (**E,** grade 5).

ing: the spinal region or levels involved (Fig. 17-48), direction of the lateral convexity, degree of curvature, vertebral end used for the measurement, and whether the curvature appears abrupt (short segment, acute) or gradual (long segment, smooth). The most prominent curve is known as *major* or *primary,* concurrent lesser curvatures are referred to as *minor, secondary,* or *compensatory.*

Vertebral bodies. The vertebral bodies involved in the curvature are rotated. The rotation of each vertebra is marked by spinous process rotation opposite the curve's convexity, or alternatively vertebra body rotation toward the curve's convexity (Fig. 17-49). Prolonged vertebral compression on the concave side of the scoliosis leads to a wedged appearance of the vertebrae (Heuter-Volkmann principle) and intervertebral disc. Both are narrowed on the concave side of the scoliosis.

Ribs. The ribs are approximated on the concave side of the curvature. The posterior ribs on the convex side are pushed posteriorly, narrowing the width of the ipsilateral hemithorax and producing rib humping. The rib humping is more obvious upon physical examination of a patient who is in the forward-bending position. On the concave side, the anterior portions of the ribs are pushed anteriorly.

Skeletal maturity. Curvatures progress more rapidly in skeletally immature patients. Radiographs offer several methods to assess the bone maturity of an individual. Radiographs of the hand can be compared with development standards, such as those listed in *Greulich and Pyle's Radiographic Atlas of Skeletal Development of the Hand and Wrist.*[49a,108] A more convenient method consists of qualifying the degree of bone maturity by observing the stage of ossification of the iliac crest apophysis on the anteroposterior projection (Risser sign; Fig. 17-50).

If the iliac crest apophysis is completely ossified to the ilium, the patient is skeletally mature. Although easily obtained, the Risser sign is not as accurate as hand and wrist radiographs and is no more accurate than the use of chronological age alone.[70] The appearance of the vertebral body endplates provides evidence of skeletal maturity (Fig. 17-51). The endplates are completely fused and blend imperceptibly with the vertebral bodies at skeletal maturity.

CLINICAL COMMENTS

Pain and deformity are the most common complaints that bring a patient to a health care provider.[123] The role of the practitioner confronted with scoliosis is to recognize and monitor the condition. Most curvatures can be treated nonoperatively if recognized early. Currently, scoliosis is treated by bracing, electrical stimulation, surgery, or a combination of all three. It is important to not overdiagnose and unnecessarily apply premature bracing or surgery.[128]

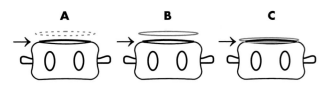

FIG. 17-51   The appearance of the vertebral endplates indicate skeletal maturation. **A,** The endplates are incompletely ossified. **B,** The endplates are ossified but now not fused to vertebra. **C,** The endplates are ossified and fused to the adjacent vertebra, indicating skeletal maturity.

Adolescents and juveniles with curvatures less than 20 degrees should be monitored every 3 to 6 months for progression.[82] Failure to recognize progression of the curve and failure of conservative treatment may delay more aggressive treatment options, possibly leading to increased deformity and complications. Prognostic factors for scoliosis progression include age at time of diagnosis, vertebral rotation, stage of skeletal maturity, early or late menarche, and magnitude and pattern of curvature.[18,51,125] In general, curvatures under 30 degrees will not progress following skeletal maturity.

Braces are widely advocated to limit further progression in skeletally immature patients with flexible curvatures between 20 and 40 degrees.[38,41] The Milwaukee brace is the most widely utilized; others include the Thoracic-Lumbar-Sacral Orthosis (TLSO, Wilmington, Miami, New York, or Boston) and Charleston brace. A brace is not an easy treatment for teenagers who may be more concerned about appearing different from their peers than about their curve progression.

Surgery is considered if the curvature exceeds 50 degrees.[82] However, surgery is based on more than an arbitrary Cobb's measurement. Skeletal maturity, balance, age of onset, location, and size of the curve should be considered.[17,120]

Although chiropractic care lacks explanatory research of its effectiveness in limiting curve progression, various descriptive reports suggest palliative relief of associated symptoms.[2,3,30,82,118] More research is needed to determine chiropractic's full potential in managing patients with scoliosis.

Recent reports have indicated left thoracic curvatures are associated with a higher incidence of neuropathology (i.e., syrinx); however, evidence of sampling bias may exist, indicating that caution should be taken so that preliminary reports are not overinterpreted.[48] Left thoracic curvatures are usually mild and benign and should be viewed as suspicious for neuropathy only if they are severe or rapidly progressive.[48]

KEY CONCEPTS

- Scoliosis is lateral curvature of the spine (greater than 10 degrees); it is often a progressive condition that can lead to significant disability.
- Prevalence is dependent on degree of curvature; overall scoliosis is more common in females. Adolescents from 9 to 15 years of age are most at risk.
- Curvatures greater than 25 degrees Cobb's angle occur in 1.5 per 1000 individuals in the United States.
- Scolioses are broadly divided into nonstructural types and the more common structural type.
- Most structural scolioses are idiopathic and subdivided into infantile (0 to 3 years of age), juvenile (4 to 10 years of age), and adolescent (most common; older than 10 years of age) types, based on age of onset.
- Radiographic assessment begins with standing frontal and lateral projections of the spine, preferably each as a single full-spine projection using 14-inch by 36-inch film and cassette.
- The degree of spine curvature is quantified using the Cobb method, or less accurate Risser-Ferguson method on the anterolateral projection.
- The description of the spinal curvature should include the spinal region or levels involved, the direction of the lateral convexity, degree of curvature, which end vertebrae were used for the measurement, and whether the curvature appears abrupt (short segment, acute) or gradual (long segment, smooth).
- The most prominent curve is known as major or primary, concurrent lesser curvatures are referred to as minor, secondary, or compensatory.
- Curvatures progress more rapidly in skeletally immature patients.
- Pain and deformity are the most common complaints that bring a patient to a health care provider.
- Scoliosis is treated by bracing, electrical stimulation, surgery, chiropractic care or a combination of all four; it is important to not overdiagnose and unnecessarily apply premature bracing or surgery.
- In adolescent and juvenile patients, a curvature less than 20 degrees should be monitored every 3 to 6 months for progression; bracing should be considered with curvatures of 20 degrees to 40 degrees; surgery is considered when curvature is beyond 50 degrees.
- Prognostic factors for scoliosis progression include age at time of diagnosis, vertebral rotation, stage of skeletal maturity, early or late menarche, and magnitude and pattern of curvature.
- Chiropractic care is palliative; further research is needed to assess its role in limiting curve progression.

Synovial Chondromatosis

BACKGROUND

Synovial chondromatosis (synovial osteochondromatosis, joint chondroma) is a benign disorder marked by metaplasia of hyperplastic synovium to hyaline cartilage. The hyaline cartilage calcifies or ossifies and detaches from the synovium to form loose bodies (less than 2 to 3 cm in diameter) within the joint, tendon sheath, or bursae in which it forms. Receiving nutrition from the surrounding synovial fluid, the loose bodies often grow.

The knee is the most common location, but the hip, elbow, shoulder, ankle, and other locations are common. Tendon sheath and bursae involvement is less common.

Men are affected more commonly than women, and usually the disease affects young and middle-age adults.

IMAGING FINDINGS

The radiographic appearance is usually defined by the presence of multiple radiodense loose bodies noted in the confines of the joint capsule (Fig. 17-52). Pressure erosions, widened joint space, and secondary degeneration may be present. Milder forms of the disease may appear similar to the radiodense debris of osteoarthritis or calcium pyrophosphate dihydrate (CPPD) deposition disease. Both CT and MRI are useful to define the intraarticular location (Figs. 17-53 and 17-54).

Less commonly, the loose bodies do not calcify and are not seen on the radiograph. Although the loose bodies are not seen, secondary mechanical bone erosions may be visible, mimicking the appearance of pigmented villonodular synovitis and synovioma.

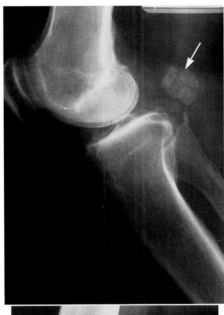

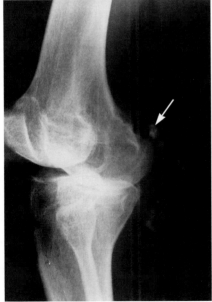

FIG. 17-52 Two cases of synovial osteochondromatosis presenting as multiple loose bodies in the posterior aspect of the knee *(arrows)*. *(Right, Courtesy Joseph W. Howe, Sylmar, Calif.)*

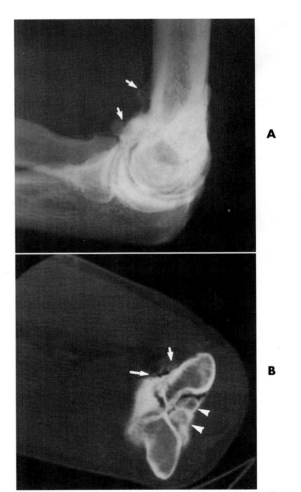

FIG. 17-53 Synovial chondromatosis. **A,** Double-contrast arthrogram showing the granular surface of synovium anteriorly *(arrows)*. Cartilaginous bodies are poorly defined in the posterior part of the joint. **B,** CT-arthrogram. Two large cartilaginous bodies outlined by contrast are seen in the olecranon fossa *(arrowheads)*. Multiple small cartilaginous bodies *(arrows)* are seen anteriorly. (From Firooznia H et al: *MRI and CT of the musculoskeletal system,* St Louis, 1992, Mosby.)

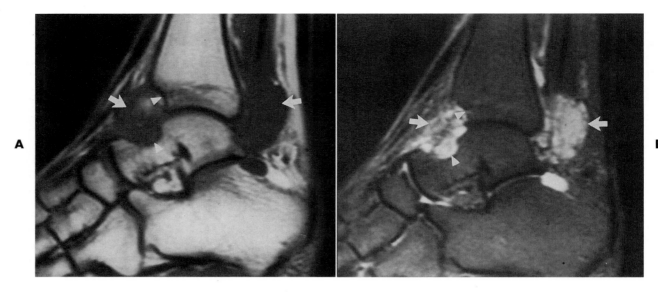

FIG. 17-54　Synovial chondromatosis. **A,** Sagittal T1-weighted image (SE, 500/20) demonstrates abnormal tissue that is isointense to muscle within the joint *(arrows)* and accompanying bony erosions *(arrowheads)*. **B,** Sagittal T2-weighted image (SE, 2500/80) demonstrates the hyperintense mass *(arrows)* and the accompanying bony changes *(arrowheads)*. (From Stark DD, Gradley WG: *Magnetic resonance imaging,* ed 2, St Louis, 1992, Mosby.)

CLINICAL COMMENTS

Symptoms include intermittent pain, joint swelling, stiffness, and episodes of joint "locking." Limitations of movement, synovial thickening, crepitus, and palpable loose bodies are sometimes present. Although the condition is largely self-limiting and may undergo spontaneous regression, the presence of intraarticular loose bodies often produces mechanical derangement and leads to secondary degeneration of the joint. For this reason, surgical excision of the loose bodies and abnormal synovium is often recommended.

KEY CONCEPTS

- *Synovial chondromatosis is a benign disorder of synovial metaplasia to hyaline cartilage.*
- *The knee is the most common location.*
- *It usually affects young and middle-age adults and is more common among men.*
- *The radiographic appearance is usually defined by the presence of multiple radiodense loose bodies noted in the confines of the joint capsule, less commonly a tendon sheath or bursae.*
- *Pressure erosions, widened joint space, and secondary degeneration may be present.*
- *Symptoms include intermittent pain, joint swelling, stiffness, and episodes of joint "locking."*

References

1. Arceci RJ: Treatment options—commentary, *Br J Cancer* 23(suppl):58, 1994.
2. Arthur BE, Nykoliation JW, Cassidy JD: The chiropractic management of adult scoliosis: a case study, *Eur J Chiro* 34:46, 1986.
3. Barge FH: *Idiopathic scoliosis,* vol 3, Davenport, Iowa, 1986, Bawden Bros.
4. Barker DJP: The epidemiology of Paget's disease of bone, *Br Med Bull* 40:396, 1984.
5. Barry HC: *Paget's disease of bone,* Edinburgh, 1969, E & S Livingstone.
6. Bernard P, Bonnetblanc JM: Dermatomyositis and malignancy, *J Invest Dermatol* 100(suppl):128, 1993.
7. Bernstein RM, Zaleske DJ: Familial aspects of Caffey's disease, *Am J Orthop* 24:777, 1995.
8. Bhambhani M et al: Giant cell tumours in mandible and spine: a rare complication of Paget's disease of bone, *Ann Rheum Dis* 51:1335, 1992.
9. Bianchi L et al: Pachydermoperiostosis: study of epidermal growth factor and steroid receptors, *Br J Dermatol* 132:128, 1995.
10. Bisagni-Faure A et al: Magnetic resonance imaging assessment of sacroiliac joint involvement in Gaucher's disease, *J Rheumatol* 19:1984, 1992.
11. Blickman JG, Wilkinson RH, Graef JW: The radiologic "lead band" revisited, *AJR* 146:245, 1986.
12. Boas SR et al: Hypertrophic osteoarthropathy in a child with follicular bronchiolitis, *Clin Nucl Med* 20:49, 1995.
13. Bonakdarpour A, Harwick R, Pickering J: Case report 34, *Skeletal Radiol* 2:52, 1977.
14. Borochowitz Z et al: Familial Caffey's disease and late recurrence in a child, *Clin Genet* 40:329, 1991.
15. Brady RO, Barton NW, Grabowski GA: The role of neurogenetics in Gaucher's disease, *Arch Neurol* 50:1212, 1993.
16. Bravo SM, Winalski CS, Weissman BN: Pigmented villonodular synovitis, *Radiol Clin North Am* 34:311, 1996.
17. Bridwell KH: Surgical treatment of adolescent idiopathic scoliosis: the basics and controversies, *Spine* 19:1095, 1994.

18. Brunnell WP: The natural history of idiopathic scoliosis, *Clin Orthop* 229:20, 1988.

19. Bui-Mansfield LT, Youngberg RA, Coughlin W, Chooljian D: MRI of giant cell tumor of the tendon sheath in the cervical spine, *J Comput Assist Tomogr* 20:113, 1996.

20. Burrows EH: Orbitocranial assymmetry, *Br J Radiol* 51:610, 1978.

21. Burwell RG et al: Pathogenesis of idiopathic scoliosis, the Nottingham concept, *Acta Orthop Belg* 58(suppl 1):33, 1992.

22. Byrd JA: Current theories on the etiology of idiopathic scoliosis, *Clin Orthop* 229:114, 1988.

23. Carcassi U: History of hypertrophic osteoarthropathy (HOA), *Clin Exp Rheumatol* 10 (suppl 7):3, 1992.

24. Cardinal E, Dussault RG, Kaplan PA: Imaging and differential diagnosis of masses within a joint, *Can Assoc Radiol J* 45:363, 1994.

25. Chang YS, Ku MC, Hsu KC, Lee TS: Pigmented villonodular synovitis, *Chin Med J* 52:92, 1993.

26. Collins DH: Paget's disease of bone-incidence and subclinical forms, *Lancet* 2:51, 1956.

27. Cotten A et al: Pigmented villonodular synovitis of the hip: review of radiographic feature in 58 patients, *Skeletal Radiol* 24:1, 1995.

28. Dahlin DC: Classification and general aspects of amyloidosis, *Med Clin North Am* 34:1107, 1950.

29. Daly BD: Thoracic metastases from nasopharyngeal carcinoma presenting as hypertrophic pulmonary osteoarthropathy: scintigraphic and CT findings, *Clin Radiol* 50:545, 1995.

30. Danbert RJ. Scoliosis: biomechanics and rationale for manipulative treatment, *J Manipulative Physiol Ther* 12:38, 1989.

31. de Gennes C, Kuntz D, de Vernejoul MC: Bone mastocytosis. A report of nine cases with a bone histomorphometric study, *Clin Orthop* 279:281, 1992.

32. De Smet L, Roosen P, Zachee B, Fabry G: Monostotic localization of Paget disease in the hand, *Acta Orthop Belg* 60:184, 1994.

33. Debeuckelaele S, Schoors DF, Devis G: Systemic mast cell disease: a review of the literature with special focus on the gastrointestinal manifestations, *Acta Clin Belg* 46:226, 1991.

34. Detheridge FM, Guyer PB, Barker DJP: European distribution of Paget's disease of bone, *Br Med J* 285:1005, 1982.

35. Dickinson CJ: The aetiology of clubbing and hypertrophic osteoarthropathy, *Eur J Clin Invest* 23:330, 1993.

36. DiMaggio LA, Lippes HA, Lee RV: Histiocytosis X and pregnancy, *Obstetr Gynecol* 85:806, 1982.

37. Dogan AS et al: Detection of bone lesions in Langerhans cell histiocytosis: complementary roles of scintigraphy and conventional radiography, *J Pediatr Hematol Oncol* 18:51, 1996.

38. Dutro CL, Keene KJ: Electrical muscle stimulation in the treatment of progressive adolescent idiopathic scoliosis: a literature review, *J Manipulative Physiol Ther* 8:257, 1985.

39. Edeiken J, DePalma AF, Hodes PJ: Paget's disease: osteitis deformans, *Clin Orthop* 146:141, 1966.

40. Egeler RM, D'Angio GJ: Langerhans cell histiocytosis, *J Pediatr* 127:1, 1995.

41. Emans JB: Scoliosis: detecting the curves that mandate treatment, *J Musculoskeletal Med* 2:11, 1985.

42. Euwer RL, Sontheimer RD: Dermatologic aspects of myositis, *Curr Opin Rheumatol* 6:583, 1994.

43. Fisher AJ, Reinus WR, Friedland JA, Wilson AJ: Quantitative analysis of the plain radiographic appearance of eosinophilic granuloma, *Invest Radiol* 30:466, 1995.

44. Flandry F, Norwood LA: Pigmented villonodular synovitis of the shoulder, *Orthopedics* 12:715, 1989.

45. Genovese A, Spadaro G, Triggiani M, Marone G: Clinical advances in mastocytosis, *Int J Clin Lab Res* 25:178, 1995.

46. Gentry RR, Rust RS, Lohr JA, Alford BA: Infantile cortical hyperostosis of the ribs (Caffey's disease) without mandibular involvement, *Pediatr Radiol* 13:236, 1983.

47. Giannini C, Scheithauer BW, Wenger DE, Unni KK: Pigmented villonodular synovitis of the spine: a clinical, radiological, and morphological study of 12 cases, *J Neurosurg* 84:592, 1996.

48. Goldberg CJ, Dowling FE, Fogarty EE: Left thoracic scoliosis configurations: why so different? *Spine* 19:1385, 1994.

49. Goldman AB, DiCarlo EF: Pigmented villonodular synovitis. Diagnosis and differential diagnosis, *Radiol Clin North Am* 26:1327, 1988.

49a. Greulich WW, Pyle SI: *Radiographic atlas of skeletal development of the hand and wrist,* ed 2, Stanford, 1959, Stanford University Press.

50. Grossman RE, Hensley GT: Bone lesions in primary amyloidosis, *AJR* 101:872, 1967.

51. Gruchalla RS: Mastocytosis: developments during the past decade, *Am J Med Sci* 309:328, 1995.

52. Gunnoe BA: Adolescent idiopathic scoliosis, *Orthop Rev* 19:35, 1990.

53. Gupta SK et al: Skeletal overgrowth with modelling error in neurofibromatosis, *Clin Radiol* 36:643, 1985.

54. Guyer PB: Research into Paget's disease: clues to the etiology and clinical significance, *Radiography* 48:185, 1982.

55. Hadjipavlou A, Lander P, Srolovitz H, Enker IP: Malignant transformation in Paget's disease of bone, *Cancer* 70:2802, 1992.

56. Haher TR et al: Meta-analysis of surgical outcome in adolescent idiopathic scoliosis, *Spine* 20:1575, 1995.

57. Hainaux B et al: Gaucher's disease. Plain radiography, US, CT and MR diagnosis of lungs, bone and liver lesions, *Pediatr Radiol* 22:78, 1992.

58. Hamdy RC: Clinical features and pharmacologic treatment of Paget's disease, *Endocrinol Metab Clin North Am* 24:421, 1995.

59. Hellstrom G, Irstam L, Nachemson A: Reduction of radiation dose in radiologic examination of patients with scoliosis, *Spine* 8:28, 1983.

60. Henck ME, Simpson EL, Ochs RH, Eremus JL: Extraskeletal soft tissue masses of Langerhans' cell histiocytosis, *Skeletal Radiol* 25:409, 1996.

61. Huang TY, Yam LT, Li CY: Radiological features of systemic mast-cell disease, *Br J Radiol* 60:765, 1987.

62. Hughes S, Peel-White AL, Peterson CK: Paget's disease of bone: current thinking and management, *J Manipulative Physiol Ther* 15:242, 1992.

63. Jones ET, Hensinger RN, Holt JF: Idiopathic cortical hyperostosis, *Clin Orthop Rel Res* 163:210, 1982.

64. Kahaleh MB: The role of vascular endothelium in fibroblast activation and tissue fibrosis, particularly in scleroderma (systemic sclerosis) and pachydermoperiostosis (primary hypertrophic osteoarthropathy), *Clin Exper Rheumatol* 10(suppl 7):51, 1992.

65. Karasick D, Karasick S: Giant cell tumor of tendon sheath: spectrum of radiologic findings, *Skeletal Radiol* 1992; 21:219.

66. Kettelhut BV, Metcalfe DD: Pediatric mastocytosis, *Ann Allergy Asthma Immunol* 73:197, 1994.

67. Klein RM, Norman A: Diagnostic procedures for Paget's disease. Radiologic, pathologic, and laboratory testing, *Endocrinol Metab Clin North Am* 24:437, 1995.

68. Krane SM, Simon LS: Metabolic consequences of bone turnover in Paget's disease of bone, *Clin Orthop* 217:26, 1987.

69. Leeds NE, Jacobson HG: Spinal neurofibromatosis, *AJR* 126:617, 1976.

70. Little DG, Sussman MD: The Risser sign: a critical analysis, *J Pediatr Orthop* 14:569, 1994.

71. Martinez-Lavin M: Pathogenesis of hypertrophic osteoarthropathy, *Clin Exper Rheumatol* 10 (suppl 7):49, 1992.

72. Matucci-Cerinic M et al: The spectrum of dermatological symptoms of pachydermoperiostosis (primary hypertrophic osteoarthropathy): a genetic, cytogenetic and ultrastructural study, *Clin Exper Rheumatol* 10(suppl 7):45, 1992.

73. McElvaine MD et al: Prevalence of radiographic evidence of paint chip ingestion among children with moderate to severe lead poisoning, St Louis, Missouri, 1989 through 1990, *Pediatrics* 89:740, 1992.

74. Meunier PJ, Vignot E: Therapeutic strategy in Paget's disease of bone, *Bone Suppl* 17:4895, 1995.

75. Meyer JS et al: Langerhans cell histiocytosis: presentation and evolution of radiologic findings with clinical correlation, *Radiographics* 15:1135, 1995.

76. Morales LE: Gaucher's disease: a review, *Ann Pharmacother* 30:381, 1996.

77. Myers BW, Masi AT, Feigenbaum SL: Pigmented villonodular synovitis and tenosynovitis. A clinical epidemiologic study of 166 cases and literature review, *Medicine* 59:223, 1980.

78. Nash CL, Gregg EC, Brown RH, Pillai K: Risks of exposure to x-rays in patients undergoing long term treatment for scoliosis, *J Bone Joint Surg Am* 61:371, 1979.

79. National Institutes of Health Consensus Development Conference: Neurofibromatosis: conference statement, *Arch Neurol* 45, 575, 1988.

80. National Institute of Health Technology Assessment Panel on Gaucher Disease: Gaucher disease: current issues in diagnosis and treatment, *JAMA* 275:548, 1996.

81. *Neurofibromatosis: a handbook for patients, families, and healthcare professionals,* New York, 1990, Thieme Medical Publishers.

82. Nykoliation JW, Cassidy JD, Arthur BE, Wedge JH: An algorithm for the management of scoliosis, *J Manipulative Physiol Ther* 9:1, 1986.

83. O'Doherty DP, Bickerstaff DR, Kanis JA, Russell RGG: Paget's disease of bone, *Curr Orthop* 3:262, 1989.

84. Oddis CV, Medsger TA: Inflammatory myopathies, *Baillieres Clin Rheumatol* 9:497, 1995.

85. Ostezan LB, Callen JP: Cutaneous manifestations of selected rheumatologic diseases, *Am Fam Physician* 53:1625, 1996.

86. Pachman LM: Juvenile dermatomyositis (JDMS): new clues to diagnosis and pathogenesis, *Clin Exper Rheumatol* 12(suppl 10):569, 1994.

87. Parkinson D, Hay R: Neurofibromatosis, *Surg Neurol* 25:109, 1986.

88. Peck B: Hypertrophic osteoarthropathy with Hodgkin's disease in the mediastinum, *JAMA* 238:1400, 1986.

89. Plosker GL, Goa KL: Clodronate. A review of its pharmacological properties and therapeutic efficacy in resorptive bone disease, *Drugs* 47:945, 1994.

90. Ray D, Williams G: Pathophysiological causes and clinical significance of flushing, *Br J Hosp Med* 50:594, 1993.

91. Reginster JY, Lecart MP: Efficacy and safety of drugs for Paget's disease of bone, *Bone Suppl* 17:4855, 1995.

92. Renshaw TS: Idiopathic scoliosis in children, *Curr Opin Pediatr* 5:407, 1993.

93. Renshaw TS: Screening schoolchildren for scoliosis, *Clin Orthop* 229:26, 1988.

94. Resnick D: *Diagnosis of bone and joint disorders,* ed 3, Philadelphia, 1995, WB Saunders.

95. Ringenberg QS et al: Hematologic effects of heavy metal poisoning, *S Med J* 81:1132, 1988.

96. Robinson DL, Blair DW, Lee SS, Ho PK: Pigmented villonodular synovitis presenting as a large lateral knee mass. Case report and review of the literature, *Orthop Rev* 17:59, 1988.

97. Rogala EJ, Drummond OS, Gurr J: Scoliosis: incidence and natural history, *J Bone Joint Surg Am* 60:173, 1978.

98. Roodman GD: Osteoclast function in Paget's disease and multiple myeloma, *Bone Suppl* 17:575, 1995.

99. Rosen CJ, Kessenich CR: Comparative clinical pharmacology and therapeutic use of bisphosphonates in metabolic bone diseases, *Drugs* 51:537, 1996.

100. Rovira M et al: Radiological diagnosis of inorganic lead poisoning, *J Clin Gastroenterol* 11:469, 1989.

101. Ryan MD, Taylor TK. Spinal manifestations of Paget's disease, *Aust N Z J Surg* 62:33, 1992.

102. Sanders DG, Weijers RE: MRI findings in Caffey's disease, *Pediatr Radiol* 24:325, 1994.

103. Scerri L, Zaki I, Allen BR, Golding P: Dermatomyositis associated with malignant melanoma—case report and review of the literature, *Clin Exper Dermatol* 19:523, 1994.

104. Seda H, Alarcon GS: Musculoskeletal syndromes associated with malignancies, *Curr Opin Rheumatol* 7:48, 1995.

105. Shaughnessy WJ: Management of adolescent idiopathic scoliosis, *Curr Opin Rheumatol* 5:301, 1993.

106. Singer FR, Minoofar PN: Bisphosphonates in the treatment of disorders of mineral metabolism, *Adv Endocrinol Metab* 6:259, 1995.

107. Sirikulchayanonta V, Naovaratanophas P, Jesdapatarakul S: Paget's disease of bone—clinico-pathology study of the first case report in Thailand, *J Med Assoc Thai* 75(suppl 1):136, 1992.

108. Skaggs DL, Bassett GS: Adolescent idiopathic scoliosis: an update, *Am Fam Phys* 53:2327, 1996.

109. Smirniotopoulos JG, Murphy FM: The phakomatoses, *AJNR* 13:725, 1992.

110. Solot CB et al: *Communication disorders in children with neurofibromatosis type I.* In Rubenstein AE, Korf BR: *Neurofibromatosis,* New York, 1990, Thieme Medical Publishers.

111. Spritzer CE, Dalinka MK, Kressel HY: Magnetic resonance imaging of pigmented villonodular synovitis: a report of two cases, *Skeletal Radiol* 16:316, 1987.

112. Staalman CR, Umans U: Hypertrophic osteoarthropathy in childhood malignancy, *Med Pediatr Oncol* 21:676, 1993.

113. Stein DH: Mastocytosis: a review, *Pediatr Dermatol* 3:365, 1989.

114. Stiller CA, Chessells JM, Fitchett M: Neurofibromatosis and childhood leukaemia/lymphoma: a population-based study, *Br J Cancer* 70:969, 1994.

115. Stull MA, Kransdorf MJ, Devaney KO: Langerhans cell histiocytosis of bone, *Radiographics* 12:801, 1992.

116. Stull MA et al: Magnetic resonance appearance of peripheral nerve sheath tumors, *Skeletal Radiol* 20:9, 1991.

117. Subbarano K, Jacobson HG. Amyloidosis and plasma cell dyscrasias of the musculoskeletal system, *Semin Roentgenol* 21:139, 1986.

118. Tarola GA: Manipulation for the control of back pain and curve progression in patients with skeletally mature idiopathic scoliosis: two cases, *J Manipulative Physiol Ther* 17:253, 1994.

119. Taylor JAM: Full-spine radiography: a review, *J Manipulative Physiol Ther* 16:460, 1993.

120. Tolo VT: Surgical treatment of adolescent idiopathic scoliosis, *Instr Course Lectures* 38:143, 1989.

121. Urban BA et al: CT evaluation of amyloidosis: spectrum of disease, *Radiographics* 13:1295, 1993.

122. Valent P: Biology, classification and treatment of human mastocytosis, *Wien Klin Wochenschr* 108:385, 1996.

123. van Dam BE: Nonoperative treatment of adult scoliosis, *Orthop Clin North Am* 19:347, 1988.

124. van Meter CD, Rowdon GA: Localized pigmented villonodular synovitis presenting as a locked lateral meniscal bucket handle tear: a case report and review of the literature, *Arthroscopy* 10:309, 1994.

125. Weinstein SL: Adolescent idiopathic scoliosis: prevalence and natural history, *Instr Course Lect* 38:115, 1989.

126. Wierman WH, Clagett OT, McDonald JR: Articular manifestations in pulmonary disease. An analysis of their occurrence in 1024 cases in which pulmonary resection was performed, *JAMA* 155:1459, 1954.

127. Willman CL: Detection of clonal histiocytes in Langerhans cell histiocytosis: biology and clinical significance, *Br J Cancer Suppl* 23:29, 1994.

128. Winter RB: The pendulum has swung too far. Bracing for adolescent idiopathic scoliosis in the 1990s, *Orthop Clin North Am* 25:195, 1994.

129. Woolf DA, Riach IC, Derweesh A, Vyas H:. Lead lines in young infants with acute lead encephalopathy: a reliable diagnostic test, *J Trop Pediatr* 36:90, 1990.

130. Yaghmai I: Spine changes in neurofibromatosis, *Radiographics* 6:261, 1986.

131. Zatz LM. Atypical choroid plexus calcifications associated with neurofibromatosis, *Radiology* 91:1135 1968.

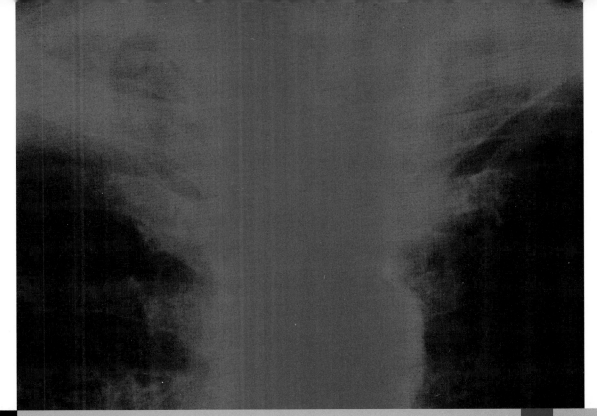

Chest

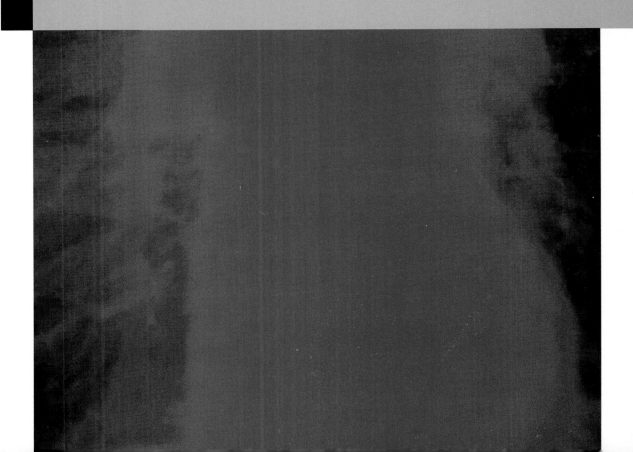

chapter 18

Introduction to Chest Radiography

DENNIS M MARCHIORI*

Chest Radiography
Anatomy

Radiographic Signs
Pattern Recognition

Chest Radiography

Radiographic examination of the chest plays an important role in the diagnosis and management of pulmonary disease. Chest radiographs account for the majority of radiographs taken each year by the medical profession. Chest radiography plays a less dominant but no less important clinical role in chiropractic practice. Although limitations exist, when combined with a thorough history and physical examination, chest radiography offers a sensitive method for detecting serious pathology of the thorax.

The standard radiographic examination of the chest consists of a posteroanterior (PA) and a right or left lateral projection. Oblique, lateral decubitus, and apical lordotic views are some of the more helpful accessory projections that may augment the standard views. The lateral projection adds little as a screening procedure in the younger patient.[14] Consequently, the posteroanterior projection alone is generally accepted as adequate screening of the thorax in young individuals who are without symptoms directly referable to the chest. All patients older than 40 years of age or patients of any age who exhibit clinical findings directly referable to the chest should have both a posteroanterior and lateral projection radiograph taken during routine evaluation.

Because the side of the body closest to the film is demonstrated with better detail and much of the left lung is obscured by the heart in the frontal projection, the left side of the body is customarily positioned next to the film in the lateral projection.[5] However, if pathology is known or suspected on the right, then the right side of the patient is placed next to the film to exhibit the area of concern with better detail.

Chest radiography employs high peak kilovoltage (110 to 150 kVp) exposures during full patient inspiratory effort, with a film-focal distance of 72 inches. In the frontal projection, rotation is present if the clavicles are not equidistant from the patient's midline. Although individual preferences exist, generally a properly exposed chest radiograph should barely outline the thoracic spine through the heart shadow. The radiograph should display the entire thorax and particularly the costophrenic angles on the film. Good

patient inspiratory result is noted by observing the posterior portions of the first 10 ribs (or anterior portions of the first 7 ribs) above the right hemidiaphragm. The position of the left hemidiaphragm is more variable because of the subjacent gastric air bubble. Diagnostic purposes sometimes warrant taking films during patient expiration. For instance, if a "check-valve" bronchial obstruction is present, the involved lung demonstrates a pathological state in which it remains well-inflated on an expiration film.

The criteria for ordering chest films vary and are often individualized at the personal, departmental, or institutional level. Some of the more common indications include chronic cough, hemoptysis, expectoration, shortness of breath, cyanosis, clubbing of the fingers, and pain in the chest, thoracic spine, or upper extremities. Routine chest radiographs in an otherwise healthy patient population are discouraged. However, when these baseline films are available, they offer valuable comparative studies for equivocal radiographic findings on subsequent studies. Often patients exhibit residue of an old or inactive disease, such as healed granulomas, chronic obstructive pulmonary disease (COPD), and pulmonary scarring. Frequently the availability of old films for comparison may eliminate the need for continued evaluation, limiting further cost and patient exposure. Likewise, practitioners should cautiously apply serial radiographs to follow a disease process, and then only at large enough intervals that overirradiation does not become an issue.

Many times it is necessary to augment the information gathered from the chest radiographs with other imaging modalities to more completely evaluate the patient. Fluoroscopy is an often overlooked, but valuable, procedure for localizing pulmonary nodules and evaluating diaphragmatic movement. Computed tomography (CT) is probably the most useful additional procedure and has all but replaced conventional tomography. CT is particularly advantageous when shadows of the chest wall, pleura, lung, hilum, or mediastinum need to be better visualized when partially obstructed by overlying densities. CT is most widely used to delineate and assess neoplastic disease.

Magnetic resonance imaging (MRI) is most often used to distinguish pathology of the hilar and mediastinal lymph node from adjacent vascular anatomy. It has particular advantage over CT for distinguishing mediastinal lymph node involvement from vascular masses, because flowing blood has no signal on MRI and therefore

---

*Special thanks to James C. Reed for his contribution as a reviewer of this material.

appears black, readily distinguishing vessels from the high signal intensity of the lymph nodes. The ventilation and perfusion scans of lung scintigraphy are valuable to the diagnosis of pulmonary embolism, although the more invasive pulmonary angiography remains the imaging standard for questionable scan results.

Anatomy

The bony thorax consists of 12 thoracic vertebrae, 12 pairs of ribs with costal cartilages, and the sternum. The scapulae and clavicles are superimposed over the thorax on the PA chest radiograph. Individual muscles of the thorax are generally not discernible on radiographs. However, absence of large muscles, such as the pectorals, appears as regions of decreased density. The intercostal arteries, veins, and nerves pass along the inferior border of the ribs; enlargements of these structures may cause a characteristic erosion deformity of the inferior rib margin.

The thoracic cavity is divided into two pleural cavities surrounding a centrally located mediastinum. The mediastinum is divided into four anatomical (superior, anterior, middle, and posterior) or three radiographic (anterior, middle, and posterior) areas as depicted in Fig. 18-1. The heart, great vessels, esophagus, thymus, and lymph tissues are all important structures contained within the mediastinum.

Visceral pleura covers the lungs and lines the pulmonary fissures; parietal pleura lines the inside of the pleural cavities. The largely potential pleural space created by these membranes may become enlarged by fluid accumulating in response to disease, known as *pleural effusion*. Visceral pleura also lines the pulmonary fissures. The right oblique and transverse fissures separate the right lung into three lobes (upper, middle, and inferior) and a left oblique fissure separates the left lung into two lobes (upper and lower).

Occasionally, accessory lung fissures are noted. Inferior accessory lung fissures are the most common in autopsy studies but are difficult to recognize on radiographs. The rarer azygous fissure is

actually more commonly seen on radiographs. About 1% of patients demonstrate an azygous fissure. The azygous fissure is created by the downward migration of the azygous vein, taking with it a portion of the apical parietal and visceral pleura of the right upper lobe. It appears as a right-sided, thin, curvilinear structure of several centimeters, which ends inferiorly as a teardrop-shaped radiopacity, representing the invaginated azygous vein (Fig. 18-2). Azygous fissures are normal variants of no clinical significance. The portion of the right upper lobe that is medial to the fissure is termed an *azygous lobe.*

The lower trachea divides into two primary (main) bronchi, one directed to each lung. In addition, each lung is supplied by two pulmonary veins, a single pulmonary artery, a bronchial artery, and multiple nerves and lymph vessels. These structures enter the lung through the hilum (root of the lung). Within the lung the arteries and bronchi follow a similar branching pattern, whereas the veins have an individual path. Reflecting gravitational forces, perfusion is greatest in the lower regions of the lung in the upright patient. This, coupled with the fact that the lung's base is thicker in an anteroposterior dimension than at its apex, accounts for the more prominent appearance of normal vascular markings in the lower regions of the lung. Increased perfusion also results in more blood-borne infections, metastasis, and pulmonary emboli occurring in the lower lung regions. Contrary to perfusion, ventilation is fairly uniform throughout the lung. Stable ventilation and relatively lower perfusion results in a higher PO_2 in the upper lung segments, possibly contributing to the predilection of tuberculosis reinfections in the upper regions of the lung.

AIRWAY

Each primary bronchus divides into secondary or lobar bronchi (two in the left lung and three in the right lung). The secondary bronchi further divide into tertiary or segmental bronchi, each supplying specific sectors of lung, termed *bronchopulmonary segments.* The bronchial branching varies, but typically 8 to 25 gener-

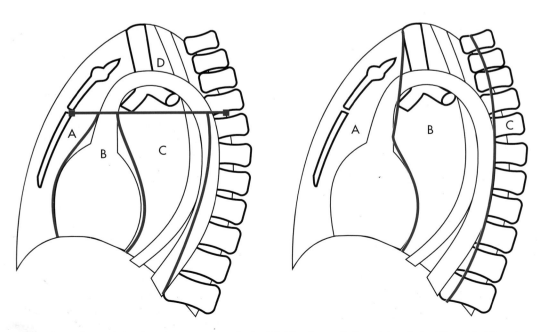

FIG. 18-1   Anatomical and roentgenometric methods of dividing the mediastinum into anterior *(A)*, middle *(B)*, posterior *(C)*, and superior *(D)* portions. The latter is part of the anatomical system only.

ations of divisions exist.[8] Bronchial branching ends with the terminal or lobular bronchioles.

AIR-SPACE

The pulmonary region distal to the terminal bronchial is termed *acinus* or *primary lobule,* representing the basic functional unit of respiration. The aggregation of 4 to 5 primary lobules constitutes a secondary lobule. Secondary lobules are 1 to 2 cm in diameter and are separated from one another by connective tissue layers, known as *interlobular septa.* Accessory pathways of communication exist between adjacent alveoli (pores of Kohn) and between alveoli and distal bronchioles (canals of Lambert). Accessory communications influence the spread of disease through lung parenchyma.

Pulmonary lobules contain respiratory bronchioles, alveolar ducts, and alveolar sacs. The alveolar ducts and sacs are lined with cup-shaped alveoli, functionally representing the area of gas exchange. Two types of epithelial cells, or pneumonocytes, line the alveoli. The type I pneumonocytes comprise 95% of the cell population. They are squamous cells, which lack the ability of mitosis. The second cell type, type II pneumonocytes, are cuboidal cells responsible for maintaining type I pneumonocytes and producing surfactant (a substance that reduces alveoli surface tension, maintaining an open alveolar sac). The normally radiolucent lung tissue becomes radiopaque if the air within the acini is replaced by pathology of water density (such as blood, edema, exudate, tumor cells, and proteins). The resulting radiopaque regions may be completely opaque if the alveolar filling is extensive (homogeneous or complete consolidation) or appears patchy and poorly defined if the alveolar filling is incomplete (heterogeneous or incomplete consolidation).

INTERSTITIUM

The interstitium, also termed *interstitial space,* provides a supporting framework for the delicate alveolar sacs. The interstitium comprises three freely communicating compartments: axial, parenchymal, and peripheral.[1] The axial (or peribronchovascular) space surrounds the primary bronchi and pulmonary artery as they enter the lung. The axial interstitium follows the bronchial and arterial branching, eventually becoming continuous with the interlobular septa, which separate adjacent secondary lobules. The parenchymal or alveolar interstitium provides delicate fibers to support the intralobular air-exchanging portion of the lung. The space between visceral pleura and the lung parenchyma is termed the *peripheral* (or *subplural*) *interstitium* and sends strong supporting fibers to the parenchyma.

An explanation of the arrangement between the capillary and alveolus within the parenchymal interstitium is needed to fully understand the radiographic appearance of interstitial and air-space patterns of lung disease. The cell junctions of the portion of the capillary walls that are in contact with alveoli are tight, maintaining the relative "dryness" of the alveoli by limiting fluid movement from the capillaries to the alveoli. In contrast, the capillary cell junctions are relatively loose where the capillary is not in contact with the alveoli. This allows a slow "drip" of fluid into the surrounding parenchymal interstitium (the space that separates the capillary from neighboring alveoli). Under normal circumstances, fluid entering the interstitium is balanced by the fluid reabsorbed into lymphatics. Because parenchymal interstitium does not contain lymphatics, the excessive fluid flows to the lymphatics of the adjacent axial and subpleural interstitium.

Normally, the interstitium is not seen on radiographs. However, alterations in the amount of fluid entering the interstitium, impairment in the lymphatic clearing mechanism, or alterations in permeability of the capillary walls result in excessive fluid accumulation and distention of the interstitium, producing radiographic linear shadows. Additionally, if the interstitium is distended by space-taking lesions (e.g., blood, edema, pus, tumor) or thickened in response to such disorders as connective tissue disorders, it may become visible on the radiographs. Distention of the axial interstitium appears as peribronchial cuffing and parahilar haze; parenchymal interstitium relates a ground glass appearance, and the peripheral interstitium appears as thick pleura.

Radiographic Signs

SILHOUETTE SIGN

The silhouette sign was popularized by Felson,[4] who summarized the concept as follows: "An intrathoracic lesion touching a border of the heart, aorta, or diaphragm will obliterate that border on the roentgenogram. An intrathoracic lesion not anatomically contiguous with a border of one of these structures will not obliterate that border." Loss of the anatomical border is described as a *positive* silhouette sign.[3] Obscuring lesions may be large or small, positioned within or outside of the lung.

Structures are visualized on the radiograph because they are contiguous with another structure of different density. For instance, the right heart border is seen because it is contiguous with the air-filled right middle lobe. If pathology of similar density to that of the heart filled the right middle lobe, the right heart border would be lost, creating a positive silhouette sign. Absence of anatomical borders aids in localizing lesions within the chest. In general, the left heart border is adjacent to the lingula of the left upper lobe, the right heart border is adjacent to the right middle lobe, the diaphragm is adjacent to the inferior lobes, the ascending aorta is next to the anterior segment of the right upper lobe, and the aortic arch is next to the apical segment of the left upper lobe. Loss of these borders suggests adjacent pathology.

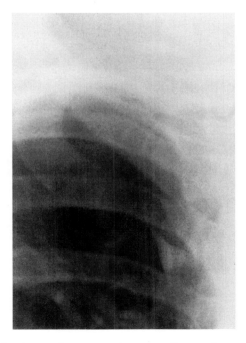

FIG. 18-2   Azygous fissure presenting as a curvilinear radiopaque line in the apex of the right upper lobe ending in a teardrop-shaped radiodensity.

CERVICOTHORACIC SIGN

Because only the apical segments of the upper lobes extend superior to the clavicles, radiographic shadows extending above the clavicle shadows are posteriorly located. Anterior structures entering the neck (e.g., brachiocephalic artery) are not seen above the clavicle shadows and appear cut off at the level of the clavicles.

AIR-BRONCHOGRAM SIGN

Unless they appear on end, intrapulmonary airways are not seen on radiographs. The thin air tubes are surrounded by the air-filled lung parenchyma and therefore are not seen because of the lack of contrast. However, if the lung parenchyma is filled with pathology of water density, and the airways are not involved, they will appear as lucent tubes traversing the region of lung consolidation. The presence of this sign is indicative of air-space pathology, usually pneumonia or pulmonary edema. Air-alveologram describes an air-filled lobule surrounded by consolidated parenchyma.

Pattern Recognition

It is generally more efficient to group abnormal radiographic findings into "patterns of disease" than to describe or conclude on each finding individually. The concept of grouping radiographic findings into patterns of chest disease has been advocated by other authors[4,5,7,10-13,15] and certainly predates this publication.

The radiographic appearance of parenchymal disease of the lung is commonly dichotomized into air-space and interstitial patterns. *Air-space, alveolar,* and *consolidation* are all terms used to describe the poorly marginated parenchymal opacities that follow space-taking lesions within the alveolar sacs. The opacities have a tendency to coalesce and are most commonly segmental or lobar in distribution. Air-alveologram and air-bronchograms are characteristic, appearing respectively as lucent spheres or tubes within the consolidated lung. Diffuse interstitial disease appears as linear, reticular, nodular, or reticulonodular patterns of pulmonary disease. A reticular pattern appears as a "net" overlying the lung. The net may be very fine, or coarse as in "honeycomb" lung, which represents end-stage lung fibrosis. Small, well-circumscribed, homogenous nodules occur alone or may accompany the linear shadows, the latter presentation denoting a reticulonodular pattern.

Although patterns of lung disease are largely descriptive in nature, some degree of radiologic-pathologic correlation exists. In other words, it is possible to anatomically localize pathology to either an interstitial or air-space location based on the radiographic appearance.[8] For instance, a poorly defined region of incomplete consolidation in the peripheral lung field is consistent with an air-space pattern of disease. This is not solely a descriptive "tag"; the appearance most often correlates to pathology within the "air space" of the lung. Unfortunately, this is not always the case. The alveolar stages of sarcoidosis appear as fluffy, ill-defined, air-space filling of the lung, but they actually represent granulomatous deposits within the interstitium, not the air space of the lung.

A more accurate assessment of the underlying pulmonary disease is obtained when the radiographic patterns are combined with clinical information. The pattern's chronicity, complexity, severity, and its correlation to clinical findings will aid in determining the significance and lead to a narrowed list of possibilities. Or at the very least, they will suggest which follow-up examination should be applied to provide the missing information.

The chest section continues the general theme of this book. Radiographic abnormalities are grouped into common radiographic patterns. Each pattern lists diseases that are commonly associated with the radiographic appearance and provides short descriptions of each listing to aid in differential diagnosis between listings. The second portion of the chest section comprises chapters presenting detailed descriptions of the some of the more commonly encountered disease entities that are listed with each pattern.

References

1. Bachofen H, Bachofen M, Weibel ER: Ultrastructural aspects of pulmonary edema, *J Thorac Imaging* 3:1,1988.
2. Burgener FA, Kormano M: *Differential diagnosis in conventional radiology,* New York, 1991, Thomas Medical Publishers.
3. Felson B, Felson H: Localization of intrathoracic lesions by means of the posteroanterior roentgenogram, the silhouette sign, *Radiology* 55:363, 1955.
4. Felson B: A new look at pattern recognition of diffuse pulmonary diseases, *AJR* 133:183, 1979.
5. Felson B: *Chest roentgenology,* Philadelphia, 1973, WB Saunders.
6. Felson B: The roentgen diagnosis of disseminated pulmonary alveolar diseases, *Semin Roentgenol* 2:3, 1967.
7. Fraser RG, Pare JAP: *Tables of differential diagnosis and decision trees.* In Fraser RG, Pare JAP: *Diagnosis of diseases of the chest,* ed 2, Philadelphia, 1979, WB Saunders.

8. Genereux GP: Pattern recognition in diffuse lung disease: a review of theory and practice, *Med Radiog Photog* 61:2, 1985.
9. Horsfield K, Cumming G: Morphology of the bronchial tree in man, *J Appl Physiol* 24:373, 1968.
10. Lillington GA: *A diagnostic approach to chest diseases,* Baltimore, 1987, Williams & Wilkins.
11. Meschan I: *Roentgen signs in clinical diagnosis,* Philadelphia, 1956, WB Saunders.
12. Reed JC: *Chest radiology: patterns and differential diagnosis,* Chicago, 1981, Year Book.
13. Reeder MM: *Reeder and Felson's Gamuts in radiology,* New York, 1993, Springer-Verlag.
14. Sagel SS et al: Efficacy of routine screening and lateral chest radiographs in a hospital-based population, *N Engl J Med* 291:1001, 1974.
15. Simon G: *Principles of chest x-ray diagnosis,* London, 1956, Butterworths.

Chest Disease Patterns

DENNIS M MARCHIORI*

PART THREE
Chest

*Special thanks to James C. Reed for his contribution as a reviewer of this material.

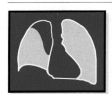

CS 1 | Atelectasis

Atelectasis is defined as incomplete air filling and underexpansion of the lung. It may involve the entire lung or appear localized to a lobe, segment, or subsegment. The collapsed lung may displace the diaphragm, fissures, hila, mediastinum, or other anatomical borders. Occasionally, regions of increased radiopacity and approximation of vascular markings, ribs, or other structures are apparent. Atelectasis is always secondary to underlying pathology; therefore its presence should prompt a vigorous search for a cause. Although several mechanisms of collapse have been identified, obstruction of the airway is the most common.

DISEASE	COMMENTS
Adhesive (adhesion of the alveolar interior walls)	
Hyaline membrane disease	Decreased surfactant production in the neonate
Postoperative	Tissue adhesions related to cardiac or thoracic surgery
Cicatrizing (scarring, fibrosus, and contraction of lung interstitium)	
Connective tissue disease	Widely disseminated radiopacities resulting from tissue fibrosus related to rheumatoid arthritis, scleroderma, idiopathic pulmonary fibrosis, etc.

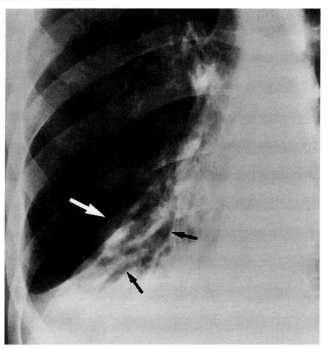

FIG. 19-1   Right lower lobe collapse caused by destruction and fibrosis from past infection. Air in dilated bronchi (black arrows) is an important clue to fibrosis and resulting bronchiectasis as the cause of the collapsed lobe. White arrow points to displaced major fissure. (From Armstrong P et al: *Imaging of diseases of the chest,* ed 2, St Louis, 1995, Mosby.)

Infections [p. 853] **(FIG. 19-1)**	Scattered linear and circular radiopacities in the upper lung fields correlating to history of granulomatous infections (tuberculosis, histoplasmosis, coccidioidomycosis); lesions have a tendency to form irregular thick-walled cavities
Radiation	Nonanatomical regions of involvement that correlate to history and site of past therapeutic radiation exposure
Compressive (intrapulmonary lesions compressing normal lung tissue)	
Bullous emphysema [p. 838]	Large, thin-walled air sacs associated with emphysema and typically found in the upper lung; these sacs may compress adjacent normal lung tissue
Pulmonary mass	Space-occupying mass lesion within the lung (neoplasms, sarcoidosis, etc.)
Obstructive (intrinsic or extrinsic airway obstruction)	
Broncholithiasis	Occurs occasionally when a radiodense, calcified lymph node from prior granulomatous infection erodes through the bronchial wall and obstructs the lumen of the airway
Foreign bodies	Seen in infants, children (marble, peanut, etc.) and adults (dentures, tooth fragments following trauma, nails or screws held in mouth, meat, etc.); usually a characteristic history exists; occasionally patients exhibit an asymptomatic period of hours to days following incident
Mucus plugs	Most often associated with asthma, chronic bronchitis, surgery, and neurological suppression of cough reflex
Tumors [p. 863] **(FIG. 19-2)**	Bronchogenic carcinoma is a common cause of obstruction in patients over the age of 50 years; these patients may exhibit concurrent enlargement of the involved hilum or mediastinum; bronchial carcinoid tumors are more common in younger patients

Continued

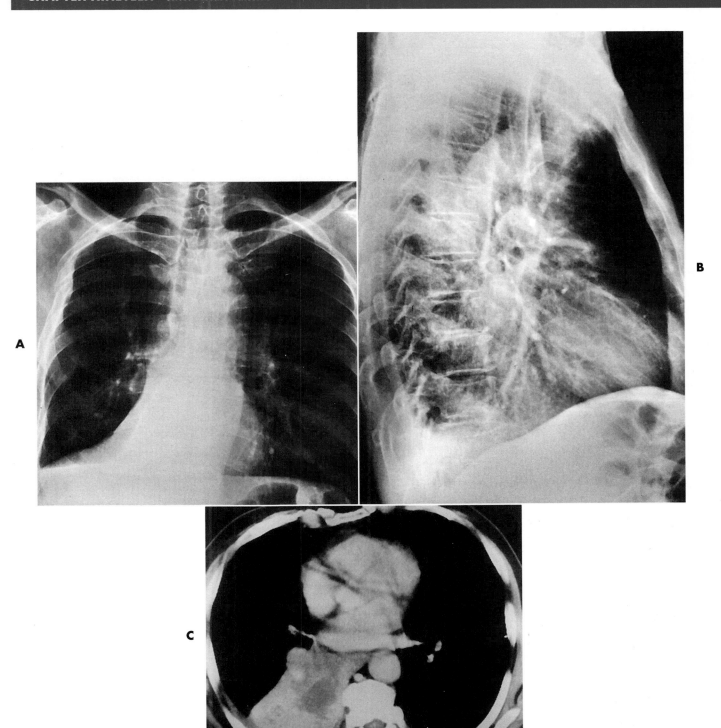

FIG. 19-2   Right lower lobe collapse resulting from bronchial carcinoma. Although the obstructing bronchial lesion is not seen, metastatic bone disease is present in right eighth rib, and there are multiple old fractures of right ribs. **A,** Postero-anterior radiograph. **B,** Lateral radiograph. **C,** Computed tomographic scan in a different patient. (From Armstrong P et al: *Imaging of diseases of the chest,* ed 2, St Louis, 1995, Mosby.)

DISEASE	COMMENTS
Passive (extrapul-monary lesions compressing normal lung tissue)	
Body wall lesions	Expansile rib lesions, pleural-based disease, and intercostal soft tissue lesions
Pleural space filling	Space-taking lesions in the pleural space (edema, chyle, hemorrhage, air, etc.)
Subsegmental, platelike, discoid (linear radio-pacity in periphery of lung) (FIG. 19-3)	
Hospitalization	Resulting from hypoventilation because of painful breathing, anesthesia, pleural effusion, pneumonia, etc
Pulmonary embolism [p. 850]	Commonly involves collapse as a nonspecific finding of acute pulmonary embolism, often associated with pleural effusion; when the collapse occurs in the late manifestions of the disease, it represents pulmonary scar formations

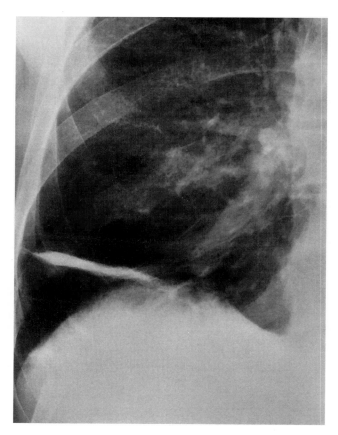

FIG. 19-3   Discoid atelectasis showing a typical bandlike shadow. (From Armstrong P et al: *Imaging of diseases of the chest,* ed 2, St Louis, 1995, Mosby.)

CS2 | Chest Wall Pleural-Based Lesions

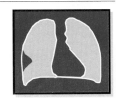

Chest wall and pleural-based lesions are often marked by a characteristic radiographic appearance of a radiopaque convexity extending inward, toward the lung, with sloping superior and inferior tails. The outer border of the lesion is incompletely defined, confirming an extrapulmonary location. A variety of etiologies are responsible, including infections, primary neoplasms, metastasis, and trauma.

DISEASE	COMMENTS
Abscess [p. 853]	Most commonly results from *Staphylococcus* infection, tuberculosis, and actinomycosis; associated characteristics include rib involvement, pulmonary infiltrate, pleural effusion, and a painful, red, subcutaneous mass
Hematoma	Suggested by the presence of pleural effusion, history of trauma, evidence of trauma (i.e., rib fracture), or hemoptysis; retrosternal hematomas are occasionally seen in the lateral projection on those patients experiencing automobile accidents, where the steering wheel inflicts blunt trauma to the chest
Pleural fluid [p. 849]	Free or loculated transudate, exudate, blood, chyle, etc., presenting as a well-defined density in the pleural space

DISEASE	COMMENTS
Rib fracture	Secondary to blunt or penetrating trauma to normal ribs or less forceful trauma to ribs affected by pathology (e.g., tumor or infection); fracture occurs as a thin, vertical radiolucent line with offset of rib cortices, often best seen on an oblique projection; acute fracture warrants a careful search for associated hemothorax or pneumothorax
Rib tumors **(FIG. 19-4)**	Most common benign tumors: osteochondromas, followed by enchondromas and osteoblastomas; metastatic bone disease, chondrosarcoma, and multiple myeloma produce multiple lytic regions; nonneoplastic lesions such as fibrous dysplasia commonly involve the ribs

Continued

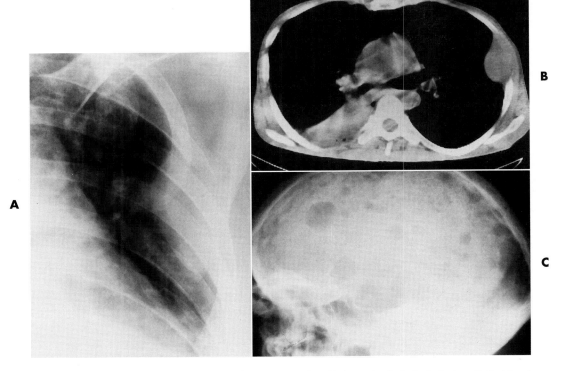

FIG. 19-4 Multiple myeloma of the rib appearing as an extrapleural lesion and pathologic rib fracture. **A,** Peripheral pulmonary radiopacity extending inward from a broad-based chest wall origin (extrapleural sign). **B,** The appearance is better demarcated on computed tomography scans. **C,** Involvement of the skull is also noted in this patient. (Courtesy Steven P. Brownstein, Springfield, NJ.)

PART THREE Chest

DISEASE	COMMENTS
Skin lesions	Soft tissue densities (nipples, moles, neurofibromas, etc.) typically appear with incomplete borders because of region of contact with the skin; examination of the skin surface or repeat radiographs using a radiopaque marker will confirm questionable lesions
Soft tissue benign tumor	Variety of tissue types, appearing as a smooth protruding mass from body wall into lung field; lipomas are most common and may present as intrathoracic or extrathoracic lesions
Soft tissue malignant tumor	Often visible, painful mass with associated bone destruction; the most common malignant soft tissue neoplasms of the chest wall in adults are fibrosarcoma and liposarcoma; metastasis, mesotheliomas, and bronchogenic (Pancoast) tumors may involve the pleura; a past history of radiation therapy is a risk factor

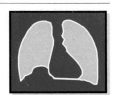

CS3 Diaphragmatic Abnormalities

The right hemidiaphragm is typically one intercostal space higher than the left. With proper inspiratory effort, the right leaf of the diaphragm should be below the level of the posterior portion of the tenth rib or the anterior portion of the seventh rib. The position of the left leaf of the diaphragm is more variable than that of the right because of the subjacent gastric air bubble. Unilateral or bilateral changes of the diaphragm's position may suggest underlying pathology of the thorax or abdomen.

CS3a Depressed Diaphragm

DISEASE	COMMENTS
Increased pulmonary volume (FIG. 19-5)	Unilateral lung overinflation resulting from a large bulla, pulmonary cyst, or in response to a contralateral small lung; chronic bilateral overinflation results from diffuse obstructive emphysema or transient with asthma and expiratory air trapping because of bronchial obstruction
Large pleural effusion [p. 849]	Difficult to detect because the fluid obliterates the diaphragm contour; the position of the gastric air bubble will indicate the position of the left hemidiaphragm
Pneumothorax [p. 884]	Other radiographic findings of pneumothorax: absence of interstitial and bronchovascular lung markings and the characteristic, thin, radiodense line represents visceral pleura; if large, the pneumothorax may invert the dome of the diaphragm

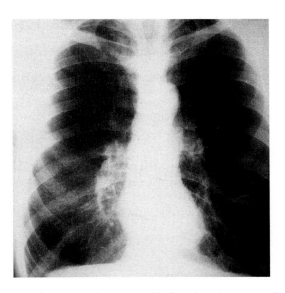

FIG. 19-5 Emphysema demonstrated by hyperlucent, overexpanded lung fields, prominent truncated pulmonary arteries, and flattened hemidiaphragms.

PART THREE Chest

CS3b | Elevated Diaphragm

DISEASE	COMMENTS
Congenital eventration	Represents an elevated segment of the diaphragm, resulting from congenital absence or weakness of a portion of the diaphragmatic musculature; this results in poor contractility and inability to resist infradiaphragmatic visceral pressure; total hemidiaphragm eventration is more common on the left, partial hemidiaphragm eventration is more common on the right and usually involves the anteromedial segment
Diaphragm splinting	Lack of diaphragm excursion in response to pain, fracture, infection, etc.
Diaphragmatic hernia	Most commonly the esophageal hiatal hernia presenting as a centrally located air-fluid level behind the heart shadow in the frontal projection; an esophagram is confirmatory; Bochdalek's hernias typically appear as posterolateral masses above the left hemidiaphragm and represent herniations of retroperitoneal contents; Morgangni's hernias typically appear as anteromedial right-sided masses in the cardiophrenic angles
Intraabdominal mass (FIG. 19-6)	Unilateral elevation resulting from renal, hepatic, or splenic abscess, tumor, cyst, or gas distention of the bowel, stomach, or peritoneal cavity; bilateral elevation results from pregnancy, obesity, and ascites
Phrenic nerve paralysis	Reduces the contractility of hemidiaphragm by damage to the phrenic nerve (surgical transection, pressure from hilar mass, poliomyelitis, and Erb's palsy); the affected diaphragm will exhibit paradoxical motion under fluoroscopic observation by ascending rather than descending movement during inspiration (positive sniff test)
Poor inspiratory result	*Inspiratory effort*: the patient's compliance with inspiratory instructions during the radiographic exposure; *inspiratory result:* a general term encompassing both inspiratory effort and mechanical obstacles to full inspiration, such as obesity, pregnancy, and ascites

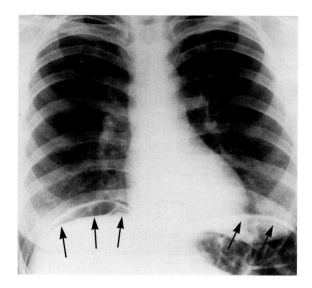

FIG. 19-6   Radiolucent, sickle-shaped air shadows subjacent to the right and left hemidiaphragm secondary to perforated ulcer *(arrows)*. (Courtesy Steven P. Brownstein, Springfield, NJ.)

Reduced pulmonary volume	Loss of lung volume resulting from congenital hypoplasia, pneumonectomy, atelectasis, and other diseases
Ruptured diaphragm (FIG. 19-7)	Significant blunt, crushing, or penetrating thoracoabdominal trauma possibly causing abdominal contents to herniate into the thoracic cavity; the rupture is nearly always left-sided, because the liver dissipates traumatic forces on the right; a ruptured diaphragm appears as a gas-filled bowel or stomach seen in the left lower lung field
Subpulmonary effusion [p. 849]	Pleural fluid under the lung possibly simulating elevation of the diaphragm; commonly the pseudodiaphragm, or dome of the fluid, appears more lateral than its normal position; lateral decubitus projections may aid in differentiating subpulmonary effusion from an elevated diaphragm

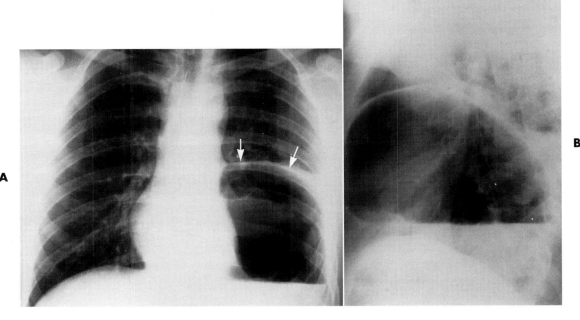

FIG. 19-7 Posteroanterior **(A)** and lateral **(B)** projections demonstrating traumatic rupture of the left hemidiaphragm with herniation of an air-filled portion of the stomach into the thoracic cavity *(arrows)*. As a result, there is a gastric air-fluid level. (Courtesy Steven P. Brownstein, Springfield, NJ.)

PART THREE Chest

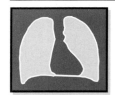

CS4 | Diffuse Alveolar (Air Space) Disease

Diffuse alveolar disease comprises bilateral, widely disseminated opacifications that may appear very dense (homogenous consolidation) and correlate to complete filling of the alveolar space. Alternatively, a patchy and fluffy appearance (heterogeneous consolidation) denotes incomplete filling of the alveolar space.

The opacifications of lung vary in size and exhibit a tendency toward coalescence. Within the regions of opacification, characteristic tubular radiolucent shadows are occasionally seen representing air-filled bronchi transversing water-filled parenchyma (air-bronchogram sign).

Based on history and serial radiography, the diseases are divided into acute and chronic forms. Although an exact timeline is difficult to develop, patterns that remain largely unchanged for several weeks or months are chronic.

DISEASE	COMMENTS
Acute diffuse alveolar disease	
Adult respiratory distress syndrome (ARDS) [p. 881]	Increased capillary permeability resulting from a wide variety of systemic and pulmonary insults (e.g., drug abuse, fractures, smoke inhalation, shock) resulting in excessive fluid accumulation in the alveolar spaces
Near-drowning **(FIG. 19-8)**	May be prevented by laryngeal spasm; otherwise fluid may enter the lung from drowning or submersion events
Pneumonia [p. 853]	Related to aggressive infections of the lung; patients are typically very ill, exhibiting fever, productive cough, difficulty breathing, and malaise; although many organisms may be associated with this presentation, the gram-negative infections are notorious for producing this appearance
Pulmonary edema [p. 850] **(FIG. 19-9)**	Accumulates within the interstitium during the early stages; the resulting linear densities are termed *Kerley's lines* and are subdivided by position within the lung; as fluid accumulates, lymphatic drainage is overwhelmed, and edema spills over to the alveolar lumen relating an alveolar pattern; the appearance may be "cloudlike," diffusely involving the lung fields bilaterally; as pulmonary edema progresses, the alveolar pattern is seen centrally with interstitial extensions to the periphery

Pulmonary hemorrhage	Associated with anticoagulant therapy, pulmonary contusion, or less commonly Goodpasture's syndrome; hemoptysis and patient history are indicative
Chronic diffuse alveolar disease	
Alveolar proteinosis **(FIG. 19-10)**	Bilateral confluent radiopacities, less commonly diffuse nodular pattern; appearance may be transient and there are surprisingly few associated clinical symptoms apart from dyspnea
Radiation pneumonitis	Diffuse pulmonary damage with accompanying history of therapeutic radiation

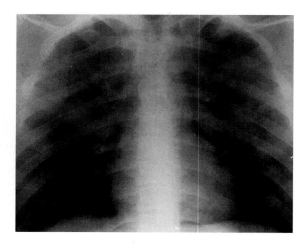

FIG. 19-8   Bilateral, symmetrical, air-space radiodense shadows in a near-drowning victim. (Courtesy Steven P. Brownstein, Springfield, NJ.)

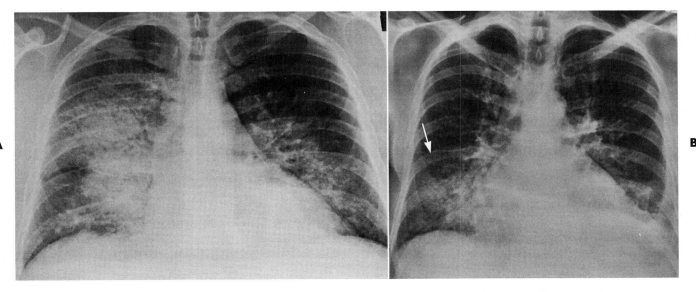

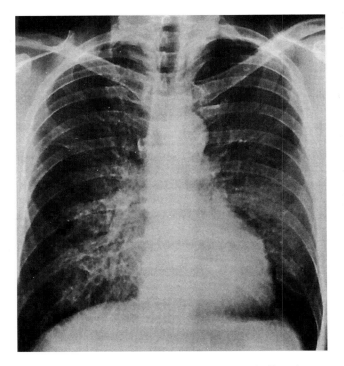

FIG. 19-9   Cardiogenic alveolar edema. **A,** Butterfly pattern. **B,** Bibasilar edema in a different patient showing septal lines and a left pleural effusion. Note also the bronchial wall thickening and thickening of the minor fissure *(arrow)*. (From Armstrong P et al: *Imaging of diseases of the chest*, ed 2, St Louis, 1995, Mosby.)

FIG. 19-10   "Bat's wing" shadowing in alveolar proteinosis. (From Armstrong P et al: *Imaging of diseases of the chest*, ed 2, St Louis, 1995, Mosby.)

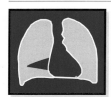

CS5 | Localized Alveolar (Air Space) Disease

Solitary or multiple localized alveolar disease is marked by extensive filling of the alveolar spaces with space-occupying lesions (blood, edema, pus, protein, cells, etc.), relating a complete (homogenous) or partial (heterogeneous) consolidation or opacification of a segment, lobe, or entire lung.

This pattern differs from the previous pattern of diffuse alveolar pattern, because the involved pulmonary region is localized, unilateral, and peripherally well defined. However, similar to the previous pattern of lung disease, it may be separated into acute and chronic presentation based on the patient's history and available serial radiographs. Although an exact timeline is difficult to develop, patterns that remain largely unchanged for several weeks or months are chronic.

DISEASES

COMMENTS

Acute localized alveolar disease

Bronchioloalveolar (alveolar cell) carcinoma [p. 863] **(FIG. 19-11)**

May appear as well-defined consolidation similar to pneumonia; however, it will not respond to appropriate management of pneumonia

Obstructive pneumonitis

Appearance corresponding to alveolar collections of edema and atelectasis of the lung in response to bronchial obstruction; the obstruction may develop slowly (bronchogenic carcinoma, bronchial carcinoid tumors, etc.) or rapidly (foreign body, mucus plug, etc.)

Pneumonia [p. 853] **(FIG. 19-12)**

Consolidation of lung parenchyma (lung, lobe, or segment) resulting from filling of the normally air-filled alveolar sacs with exudate and inflammatory cells of similar radiopacity to water; causative agents include bacteria, fungi, and viruses; clinical feature of malaise, fever, and purulent expectorant typically accompany the radiographic findings; following successful treatment the consolidated area becomes patchy and fades to normal

Pulmonary contusion

Transient dense radiopaque or incompletely consolidated patchy regions that extend from the body wall and represent blood and edema in the alveolar sacs; history of blunt trauma to the chest and presence of rib fractures are strongly indicative

Chronic localized alveolar disease

Atelectasis [p. 833]

Incomplete inflation of a lung (or segment) possibly appearing as a region of increased radiopacity resulting from increased lung density; concurrent finding of incomplete inflation (hilar, diaphragm, or mediastinum displacement) and clinical absence of fever and purulent cough will distinguish atelectasis from pneumonia

Lymphoma [p. 872]

Appearance of radiopacities that represent pulmonary infiltrate of neoplasm or superimposed infection secondary to immunosuppression following treatment; often lymphoma presents with mediastinal widening; pulmonary involvement occurs as a result of direct lymphatic extension from the mediastinum

Pulmonary infarct [p. 850] **(FIG. 19-13)**

Radiopaque parenchymal density (classically pleural-based triangular appearance with apex toward hilum) located most commonly in the peripheral lower lung field; over time the lesions tend to resolve from the periphery, inward to the center, preserving the radiopacity's triangular configuration ("melting" sign)

Radiation pneumonitis

Patchy, irregular areas of incomplete consolidation resulting from tissue "weeping" and edema produced from tissue irradiation; a history of radiation is suggestive; the location corresponds to the radiation port

Sarcoidosis [p. 885]

Patchy, irregular, radiopaque areas representing noncaseating, granulomatous deposits in the interstitium; it appears as an alveolar pattern; parenchymal involvement only is an uncommon presentation of the disease; more commonly, findings include concurrent findings of enlarged hilar lymph nodes, or adenopathy, which precedes the pulmonary disease; sarcoidosis is more common in blacks and women

Tuberculosis [p. 860]

Transmitted by repeated contacts with infected individuals through inhalation; tuberculosis is not easily contracted in immunocompetent individuals; consequently the immunocompromised and those of low socioeconomic scale (AIDS patients, alcoholics, elderly, homeless, etc.) are vulnerable; the radiographic features of the primary infection include consolidation with pleural effusion; any lung segment may be involved and the findings typically resolve without complication; reactivation infections typically involve the upper lobes, often with scarring and a tendency toward cavitation

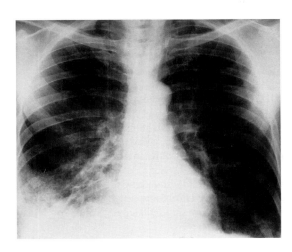

FIG. 19-11 Localized pattern of bronchioloalveolar carcinoma appearing as air-space consolidation in the right lower lung. (Courtesy Steven P. Brownstein, Springfield, NJ.)

A   **B**

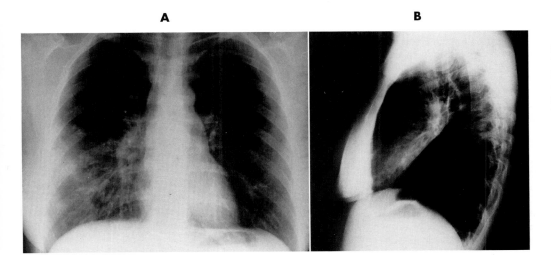

FIG. 19-12 A, PA chest radiograph demonstrating partial consolidation of the lateral portion of the right middle lobe. **B,** The partially consolidated segment is noted as a radiodense zone anterior to the oblique fissure on the overexposed lateral projection.

A   **B**

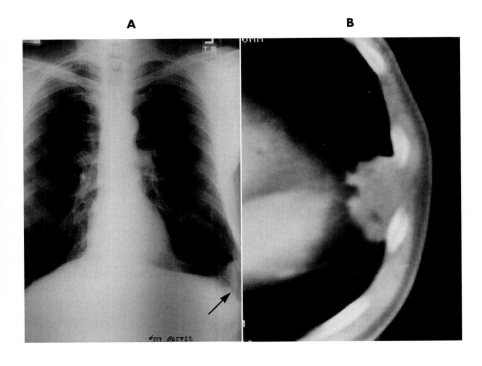

FIG. 19-13 Pulmonary infarct. Posteroanterior radiograph **(A)** and computed tomography scan **(B)** of a pleural-based mass in the left lateral costophrenic angle of the peripheral lung field *(arrow).* (Courtesy Steven P. Brownstein, Springfield, NJ.)

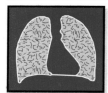

CS6 | Diffuse Interstitial Disease

Diffuse interstitial disease describes a variety of radiographic patterns, more specifically separated into miliary, nodular, reticular, reticulonodular, and honeycomb patterns. These patterns represent disease in the interstitium, although often air-space (alveolar) disease is concurrently present, making the radiographic appearance confusing to the practitioner.

In its uncomplicated presentation, interstitial disease is marked by well-defined linear or nodular radiopacities widely disseminated throughout the lung fields, usually in a bilateral, symmetrical distribution.

Similar to those of an alveolar pattern, the causes of an interstitial radiographic pattern can be divided into acute and chronic, based on history and, in the case of chronicity, serial studies. Although an exact timeline is difficult to develop, patterns that remain largely unchanged for several weeks or months are chronic.

DISEASE	COMMENTS
Acute diffuse interstitial disease	
Infection [p. 853]	Appearance resulting from inflammation and thickening of interstitial spaces often appearing as reticulonodular opacities; an interstitial pattern is an uncommon presentation of pneumonia, seen most commonly with viral or mycoplasmic agents; the appearance is typically more prominent in the lower lung regions with accompanying clinical findings suggestive of infection
Pulmonary edema [p. 850]	During the initial stages, pulmonary edema accumulates within the interstitium; the resulting linear densities are termed *Kerley's lines* and are subdivided by position within the lung; as fluid accumulates, lymphatic drainage is overwhelmed, and edema spills over to the alveolar lumen, relating an alveolar pattern; as pulmonary edema progresses, the alveolar pattern is seen centrally with interstitial extensions at the periphery

DISEASE	COMMENTS
Chronic diffuse interstitial disease	
Connective tissue disorders	Group of systemic disorders causing chronic interstitial patterns that are more pronounced in the lower lung fields; examples include rheumatoid arthritis, dermatomyositis, systemic lupus erythematosus, or scleroderma
Cystic fibrosis **(FIG. 19-14)**	Coarse interstitial pattern with mixed areas of consolidation, atelectasis, and peribronchial thickening; cystic fibrosis is seen in patients younger than 30 years of age
Histiocytosis X (Langerhans cell histiocytosis)	Coarse interstitial appearance more common in the upper lung fields; radiographic changes are often seen in the absence of clinical findings
Idiopathic interstitial fibrosis **(FIG. 19-15)**	Describes a group of conditions of unknown origin associated with a chronic interstitial pattern predominately in the lower peripheral lung regions; the initial presentation is that of diffuse, thin linear densities that progress to thickened cystic "end-stage" or "honeycomb" lung disease; symptoms include dyspnea and cough
Lymphangitic metastasis	Lymph dissemination of primary malignancy (most commonly breast, stomach, thyroid, lung, etc.) through pulmonary tissue; it is more prominent in the lower lung field, commonly associated with hilar enlargement, unilateral presentation, and history of primary malignancy
Pneumoconioses [p. 883]	Chronic inhalation of inorganic dust particles (asbestos, silicon, iron, tin, barium, etc.) is associated with interstitial patterns and varying degrees of clinical complaints; involvement by silicosis is more commonly noted in the upper lung fields, whereas asbestosis has a lower lobe distribution; a history of exposure is usual
Sarcoidosis [p. 885] **(FIG. 19-16)**	Marked by a progression of radiographic appearances from hilar and mediastinal lymphadenopathy to an interstitial pattern; it is characterized by a disparity between the advanced radiographic presentation and the mild patient symptoms; it is more commonly seen in blacks and women

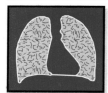

FIG. 19-14 Generalized multiple linear and cystic radiodensities scattered bilaterally through the lung fields indicative of cystic fibrosis. (Courtesy Steven P. Brownstein, Springfield, NJ.)

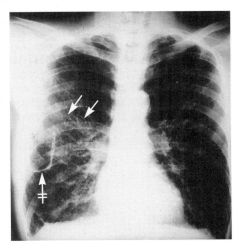

FIG. 19-15   Chronic obstructive pulmonary disease relating linear and cystic radiodense shadows characteristic of an interstitial pattern of parenchymal disease *(arrows)*. Cyst formation is also noted *(crossed arrow)*.

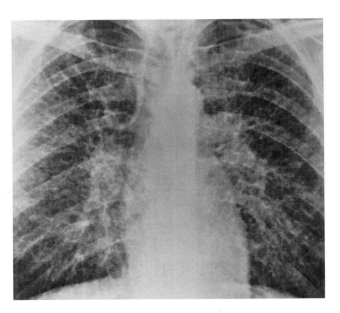

FIG. 19-16   Parenchymal sarcoidosis. Note mild adenopathy and mild hilar elevation. Parenchymal shadowing is reticulonodular with pronounced linear elements that suggest development of scarring. Uniformity of changes in all zones is unusual. (From Armstrong P et al: *Imaging of diseases of the chest,* ed 2, St Louis, 1995, Mosby.)

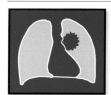

CS7 | Enlarged Hilum

The hilum is the root of the lung, representing the connection between the lung and mediastinum. Anatomically it is a conduit for the primary bronchi, pulmonary artery, bronchial artery, two pulmonary veins, and lymphatics. On the radiograph, the hilum appears as the radiopacity at the central, medial portion of the lung. Alterations in the size, configuration, or density of the hilum may indicate disease process of one of these elements entering the lung.

Minor changes in size are difficult to differentiate from variants of normal. Abnormalities are best detected by comparing questionable appearances to the contralateral hilum or old radiographs. An enlarged or altered hilum may occur alone or in combination with other imaging findings (parenchymal disease, pleural effusion, mediastinal involvement, etc.). In the frontal projection, the normal pulmonary artery alone measures around 16 mm in diameter.

DISEASE	COMMENTS
Airway	
Bronchogenic carcinoma [p. 863] **(FIG. 19-17)**	Represents the most common cause of unilateral hilar enlargement in the adult patient; the tumor arises in the large bronchi and extends to the surrounding lymph nodes, which account for much of the mass seen; obstructive pneumonitis and atelectasis may be the first signs of disease
Bronchial carcinoid tumors [p. 863]	Arise in the central bronchi and are recognized by the appearance of hilar mass or secondary findings of bronchial obstruction, including obstructive pneumonitis and atelectasis
Lymph nodes	
Infectious adenopathy	Tuberculosis, coccidioidomycosis, and histoplasmosis may present as a bilateral or unilateral hilar mass; the involved nodes generally calcify over time and may be associated with unilateral parenchymal disease; more aggressive infections also cause hilar enlargement but are typically dominated by their parenchymal patterns

Leukemia	Bilateral, symmetrical enlargement of hila and mediastinum commonly seen in adults with chronic lymphocytic leukemia, but rarely seen in childhood leukemias; pleural effusion and parenchymal involvement are common and must be differentiated from opportunistic infections and drug reactions
Lymphoma [p. 872] **(FIG. 19-18)**	Characteristic bilateral enlargement for Hodgkin's and non-Hodgkin's types; mediastinal involvement (especially anterior) and pleural effusion are common; patient may also exhibit peripheral lymphadenopathy and splenomegaly and symptoms of weakness and fever
Metastatic adenopathy [p. 873]	Unilateral or bilateral involvement, commonly with accompanying wide mediastinum and sometimes with interstitial pattern resulting from lymphangitic spread

Continued

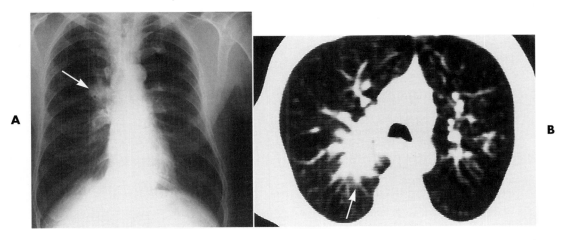

FIG. 19-17 Posteroanterior **(A)** and computed tomography **(B)** studies demonstrating enlargement of the patient's right hilum secondary to bronchogenic carcinoma *(arrows)*. (Courtesy Steven P. Brownstein, Springfield, NJ.)

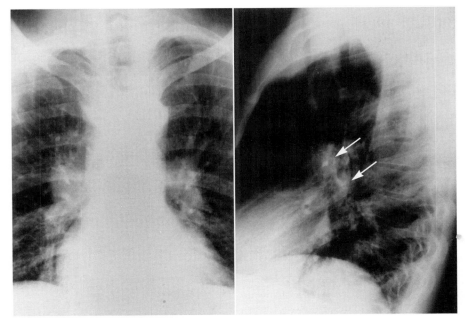

FIG. 19-18 Bilateral hilar enlargement secondary to lymphoma *(arrows)*. (Courtesy Steven P. Brownstein, Springfield, NJ.)

DISEASE	COMMENTS
Sarcoidosis [p. 885] **(FIGS. 19-19 THROUGH 19-21)**	Common early manifestation is bilateral hilar enlargement from large, well-defined "potato nodes"; these nodes may spontaneously regress or the disease may progress to further stages of parenchymal involvement; mediastinal involvement is common and enlarged right paratracheal nodes are characteristic
Vessels	
Pulmonary artery aneurysm **(FIG. 19-22)**	Rare, usually secondary to pulmonary hypertension or infection (i.e., mycotic and bacterial endocarditis)
Pulmonary artery hypertension	Bilateral enlargement of the central pulmonary vessels, which taper peripherally, relating a truncated appearance; additionally, the patient may exhibit cardiomegaly, suggesting a cardiogenic origin of hypertension
Pulmonary embolism [p. 850]	Bilateral or unilateral pulmonary artery enlargement resulting from massive central or multiple peripheral emboli

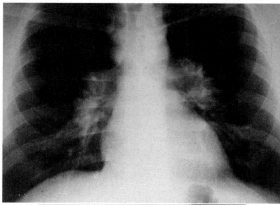

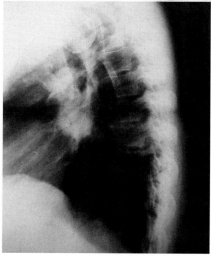

FIG. 19-21   Stage I sarcoidosis presenting with bilateral, symmetrical hilar adenopathy. (Courtesy Robert C. Tatum, Davenport, Iowa.)

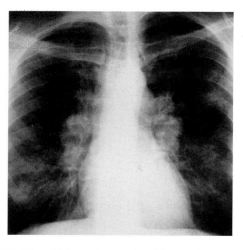

FIG. 19-19   Bilateral hilum enlargement and linear pulmonary radiopacities consistent with stage II sarcoidosis. (Courtesy Steven P. Brownstein, Springfield, NJ.)

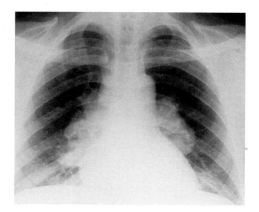

FIG. 19-20   Bilateral hilar adenopathy without parenchymal abnormality consistent with stage I sarcoidosis. (Courtesy Steven P. Brownstein, Springfield, NJ.)

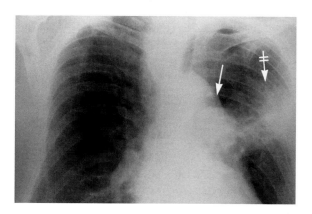

FIG. 19-22   Enlarged left hilum (*arrow*) due to pulmonary artery aneurysm with pneumonitis producing the parenchymal airspace pattern in the periphery of the middle left lung field (*crossed arrow*). (Courtesy Steven P. Brownstein, Springfield, NJ.)

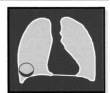

CS8 | Focal Radiolucent Lesions

Holes in the lung are broadly divided into cysts and cavities on the basis of appearance and etiology. Cysts are thin-walled (1 to 3 mm), circular defects of lung appearing alone or in groups. Cavities are defined as areas of radiolucency that represent areas of tissue necrosis and clearing within areas of parenchymal opacification. The radiolucency is surrounded by the remaining opacification, creating a surrounding rim of more than 3 mm. Cavities also appear alone or in groups. The presence of a cavity suggests a more aggressive pathology than can be inferred from the presence of a cyst.

CS8a | Cavities

DISEASE	COMMENTS
Infections (FIGS. 19-23 THROUGH 19-25)	Common for cavitation to become a chronic development among the granulomatous diseases; tuberculosis is the most widely recognized of these diseases and usually involves the lung apices with associated pulmonary findings; cavitation in the presence of clinical
Infections—cont'd	symptoms (e.g., fever, elevated WBC counts, and positive sputum and cultures) strongly suggests an infection from pyogenic agents; these cavitations are referred to as *abscesses*

Continued

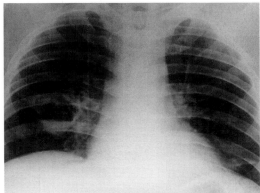

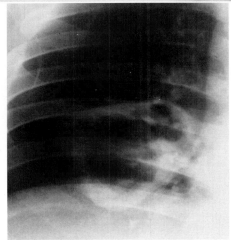

FIG. 19-23 Staphylococcal infection with cavity in right middle lung field. (Courtesy Steven P. Brownstein, Springfield, NJ.)

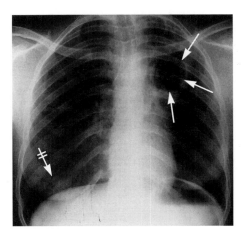

FIG. 19-24 Postinfection cavity in left upper lung field *(arrows)*, adjacent to the aortic knob. Also, a right nipple shadow mimics a pulmonary nodule just above the right hemidiaphragm *(crossed arrow)*. (Courtesy Steven P. Brownstein, Springfield, NJ.)

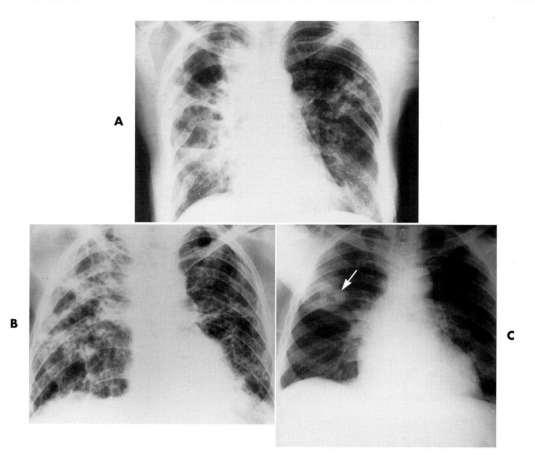

FIG. 19-25 Different patients with multiple (**A** and **B**) and solitary (**C,** *arrow*) infectious pulmonary cavities. Associated volume loss of right lung is marked by the elevated right hemidiaphragm.

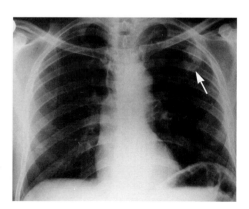

FIG. 19-26 Cavitating squamous cell bronchogenic carcinoma located in the periphery of the left upper lobe *(arrow)*. (Courtesy Steven P. Brownstein, Springfield, NJ.)

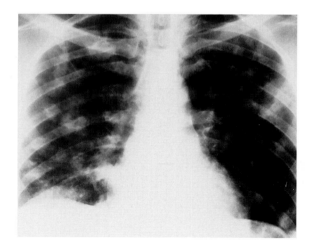

FIG. 19-27 Septic emboli presenting as multiple bilateral pulmonary nodules. (Courtesy Steven P. Brownstein, Springfield, NJ.)

DISEASE	COMMENTS
Neoplasms (FIG. 19-26)	Thick-walled cavities with irregular, lobulated inner margins; they most often occur with bronchogenic carcinomas (especially squamous cell type), lymphoma, and metastasis from various origins
Septic embolism (FIG. 19-27)	Typically multiple in the lower lung regions resulting from shower of emboli; related to right-sided bacterial endocarditis or history of intravenous drug abuse
Wegener's granulomatosis (FIG. 19-28)	Common for cavitation to develop within the multiple granulomatous lesions of Wegener's granulomatosis; often concurrently the kidney and the nasal cavity are involved; cavities may regress with treatment

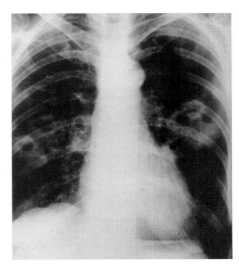

FIG. 19-28   Wegener's granulomatosis, appearing with bilateral cavitating nodules in the central regions of the lungs. (Courtesy Steven P. Brownstein, Springfield, NJ.)

PART THREE Chest

CS8b | Cysts

DISEASE	COMMENTS
Bronchogenic cyst [p. 837]	Appear as solitary, moderately large lesions within the lung or mediastinum; most begin as radiopaque, fluid-filled lesions and become air-filled cysts only after connection to an airway is established
Bulla/bleb	Very thin-walled cysts in the upper lung fields of various sizes; they are associated with emphysema and recurrent pneumothorax; although some authorities use the terms *bulla* and *bleb* interchangeably, others use *bleb* to represent a smaller lesion of subpleural location
Cystic fibrosis	Multiple, ringlike shadows associated with an interstitial pattern; they may be filled with fluid
Hydatid cyst (Echinococcus granulosus)	Typically in the lower lobe; if ruptured, debris may appear floating on the internal fluid ("water-lily sign")
Pneumatocele	Small cyst resulting from a check-valve obstruction of an airway, usually secondary to *Staphylococcus* infection in children
Rheumatoid arthritis (FIG. 19-29)	Single or multiple, thin- or thick-walled peripheral subpleural defects that may be associated with pleural effusion; lesions typically demonstrate smooth inner walls that may regress with remission of the disease
Traumatic lung cyst	Development of single or multiple peripheral subpleural cysts following pulmonary trauma

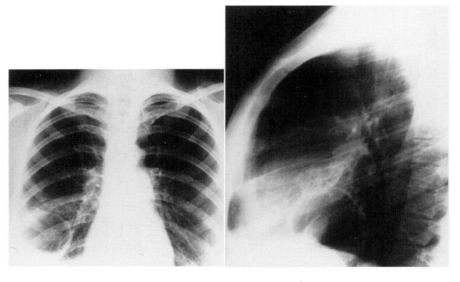

FIG. 19-29   Rheumatoid cyst within the lower right lobe. (Courtesy Steven P. Brownstein, Springfield, NJ.)

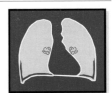

CS9 | Intrathoracic Calcifications

Chest radiographs commonly demonstrate calcification within the thorax. Most often, calcifications are dystrophic, occurring in degenerated or necrotic tissue. Physiological age-related calcification is often present in the costal cartilages and may be present in other tissues. Calcification within masses of the parenchyma and mediastinum is clinically important, often helping to establish the etiology of the lesion.

CS9a | Cardiovascular Calcifications

DISEASE	COMMENTS
Aortic calcification	Linear calcification of the aortic wall, consistent in location with the path of the vessel, most often resulting from atherosclerosis; dilation of the vessel may indicate aneurysm
Aortic annulus or valve calcification	Annular calcification is typically more pronounced than that of the valve, often secondary to rheumatic valve disease
Coronary artery calcification (FIG. 19-30)	Best demonstrated in the lateral projection, typically involves the left circumflex artery
Mitral annulus or valve calcification (FIG. 19-31)	Dense, curved, calcified band secondary to rheumatic valve disease

Continued

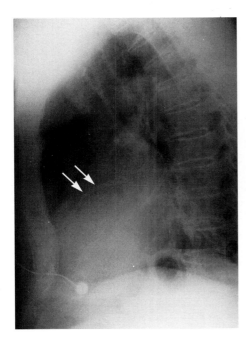

FIG. 19-30 Arterial calcification of the anterior interventricular branch of the left coronary artery *(arrows)*. (Courtesy Steven P. Brownstein, Springfield, NJ.)

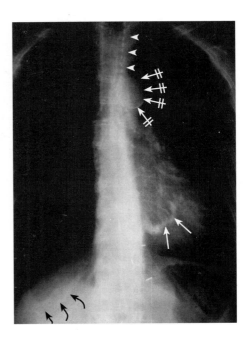

FIG. 19-31 Calcification of the mitral annulus *(arrows)*, tracheal ring cartilage *(arrowheads)*, aortic knob *(crossed arrows)*, and costal cartilages *(curved arrows)* is noted in this posteroanterior chest projection.

DISEASE	COMMENTS
Myocardial calcification (FIG. 19-32)	Secondary to infarct, tumor, aneurysm, trauma, etc.
Pericardial calcification (FIGS. 19-33 AND 19-34)	Calcification most often associated with pericardial infection

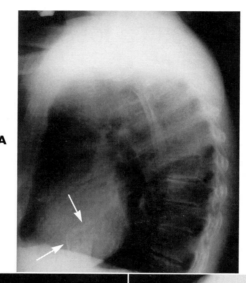

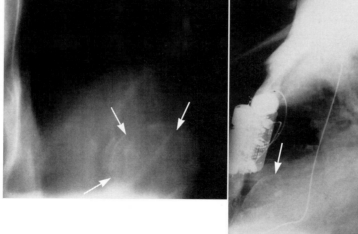

FIG. 19-32   Plain film **(A)** and linear tomogram **(B)** of calcified myxoma in the left ventricle *(arrows)*. In a second patient **(C),** calcification of the left ventricle is noted most prominently at the anterior border, inferior to the pacemaker *(arrow)*. (Courtesy Steven P. Brownstein, Springfield, NJ.)

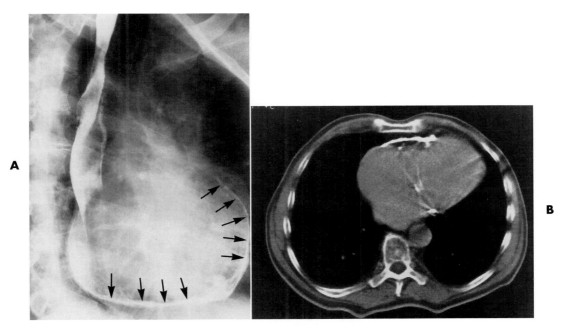

FIG. 19-33 **A,** Plain film demonstrating calcification of the pericardium *(arrows)* and barium in the esophagus. **B,** Computed tomography scan demonstrating calcification of the anterior pericardium. (Courtesy Steven P. Brownstein, Springfield, NJ.)

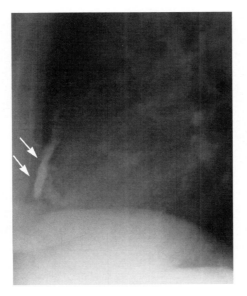

FIG. 19-34 Calcification of the anterior pericardium *(arrows).* (Courtesy William E. Litterer, Elizabeth, NJ.)

CS9b | Hilar/Mediastinal Calcifications

DISEASE	COMMENTS
Granuloma (FIG. 19-35)	Central focal or widespread calcification of involved lymph nodes, occasionally associated with a calcified parenchymal nodule (Ghon's lesion); this is associated with histoplasmosis, tuberculosis, and coccidioidomycosis infections
Calcification secondary to radiation therapy	May result in the presence of multiple calcifications of irradiated lymph nodes
Silicosis	Ring or "eggshell" calcification of the periphery of involved lymph nodes; a similar appearance is noted in sarcoidosis and irradiated nodes with Hodgkin's disease

DISEASE	COMMENTS
Teratoma	Indicated by peripheral calcification, anterior mediastinal location, and the presence of rudimentary dental elements
Thyroid calcification	Peripheral calcification, most often present in the upper anterior mediastinum
Tracheobronchial cartilage calcification	Physiological calcification of the tracheal rings occasionally noted in elderly patients

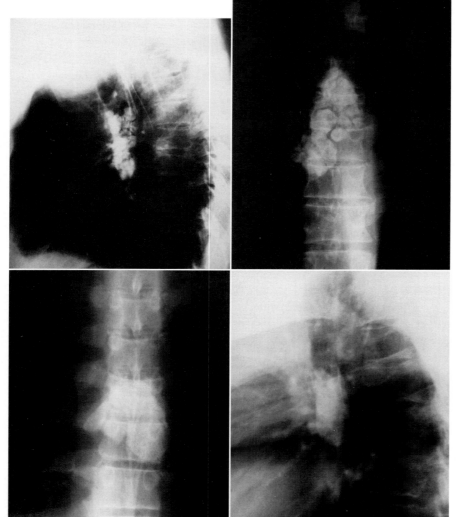

FIG. 19-35 Frontal (**B** and **C**) and lateral (**A** and **D**) chest radiographs demonstrating calcification of the subcarinal lymph nodes secondary to past granulomatous infection in two patients.

CS9c Lung Parenchymal Calcifications

DISEASE	COMMENTS
Fungal ball	Scattered calcification within the mass
Granuloma	Probably the most common intrathoracic calcification; the presence of calcification in a benign pattern and stability of size over time help differentiate from other, more aggressive lesions; often granuloma is associated with other sites of calcification in the lymph nodes or spleen, secondary to histoplasmosis, tuberculosis, and coccidioidomycosis infections
Hamartoma [p. 871]	Benign, focal lung malformation with a "popcorn" or "coma-shaped" pattern of calcification
Metastasis [p. 873]	Calcification of multiple widespread nodules resulting from osteosarcoma or chondrosarcoma
Pneumoconioses [p. 883] **(FIG. 19-36)**	Silicosis demonstrating multiple small densities of calcification scattered throughout the parenchyma with associated "eggshell" calcification of the hilar lymph nodes; asbestosis is associated with pleural plaquelike calcification near the diaphragm
Varicella (chickenpox)	Small, discrete calcifications scattered throughout lower lung fields following varicella infection; typically no lymph node involvement

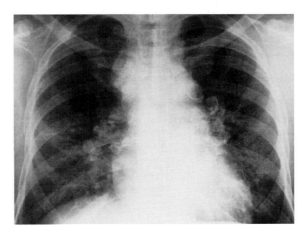

FIG. 19-36 Silicosis presenting with bilateral hilar adenopathy with characteristic "eggshell" calcifications. Similar calcifications are also noted with sarcoidosis and irradiated Hodgkin's nodes. (Courtesy Steven P. Brownstein, Springfield, NJ.)

CS9d Pleural Calcifications

DISEASE	COMMENTS
Empyema [p. 853] **(FIG. 19-37)**	Unilateral board sheet or multiple smaller regions of calcification commonly in a posterolateral location similar to traumatic hemothorax; a history positive for infection and negative for trauma may differentiate between the two entities
Hemothorax	Unilateral broad sheet or multiple smaller regions of calcification accompanying history of trauma; most commonly occurs in a posterolateral location
Pneumoconioses [p. 883]	Asbestos-related pleural disease resulting in bilateral calcified pleural plaques, most commonly appearing parallel to the diaphragm; a similar presentation is seen in talcosis

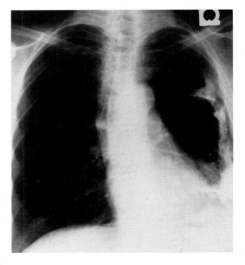

FIG. 19-37 Hemothorax with thick pleural calcifications and left lung atelectasis, causing a shift of the heart shadow to the left.

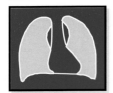

CS10 | Mediastinal Lesions

The mediastinum is the central portion of the thorax. It can be subdivided into anterior and middle parts by an imaginary line drawn posterior to the heart shadow on the lateral projection (see Fig. 18-1). A second line constructed 1 cm posterior to the anterior thoracic vertebral body margins, drawn parallel to the thoracic spine, separates the middle and posterior parts. This method of subdivision, known as the *roentgen divisions,* is commonly employed by radiologists and surgeons.

This system differs from the traditional anatomical divisions, which subdivide the mediastinum into anterior, middle, and posterior parts by constructing lines along the anterior and posterior margins of the cardiac shadow. Using the anatomical approach, a third line extends horizontally from the sternal angle to the T4 intervertebral disc space, creating a superior part of the mediastinum above the line. The roentgen divisions extend to the thoracic inlet, eliminating the superior mediastinal subdivision.

Mediastinal lesions may appear as radiodensities of various sizes and shapes. If possible, there should be an attempt to localize lesions to a division by the radiographic appearance on multiple projection.

CS10a | Anterior Mediastinum

DISEASE	COMMENTS
Ascending aortic aneurysm [p. 841]	Fusiform or saccular in form; it appears as radiopacity continuous with the aortic shadow, seen anteriorly on the lateral projection and to the patient's right on the frontal projection; ascending aortic aneurysm may be atherosclerotic, leutic, mycotic, or traumatic in origin
Lipoma (FIG. 19-38)	Localized fat accumulation often occurring around the heart
Lymphoma [p. 872] (FIG. 19-39)	Follows cardiomegaly as the second most common cause of mediastinal enlargement; accompanying hilar masses are common; although both Hodgkin's disease and non-Hodgkin's lymphoma may occur, the former is more commonly presenting as an anterior mediastinal mass
Morgagni's hernia	Most often in a right posterolateral location, often occurs with a gas-filled loop, representing a herniated bowel; opaque mass correlates with herniation of abdominal omentum or liver; it appears in middle-aged patients and is usually small
Pericardial cyst	Asymptomatic mass in right anterior costophrenic angle, less often left-sided; pericardial cyst appears as a dense, radiopaque, rounded, well-circumscribed mass

Continued

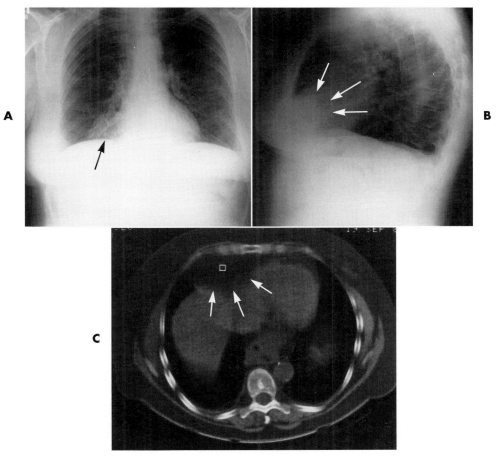

FIG. 19-38   Plain film (**A** and **B**) and computed tomogram (**C**) of a lipoma presenting as a mass in the right cardiophrenic angle *(arrows)*.

PART THREE
Chest

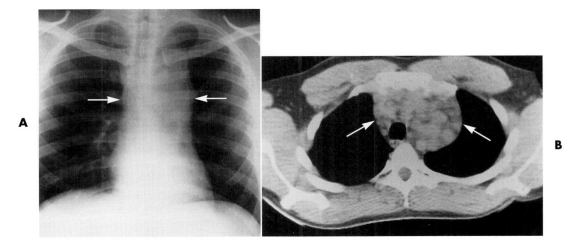

FIG. 19-39   Lymphoma appearing on the posteroanterior radiograph (**A**) and computed tomography scan (**B**) as wide anterior and middle mediastinal compartments *(arrows)*.

DISEASE	COMMENTS
Substernal thyroid (FIG. 19-40)	Smooth, often lobulated mass, which has a propensity to calcify, located at the superior region of the neck; it is more commonly projecting to the patient's right and may deviate the tracheal air shadow on frontal projection
Teratoma [p. 876] (FIG. 19-41)	Appears as mass, often with calcification, teeth, or fat contained within lesion; dense lobulated lesions may be malignant
Thymic masses [p. 876]	Thymic masses including hyperplasia, cysts, and tumors of the gland; the most common is thymoma, which represents a large, smooth mass often associated with myasthenia gravis

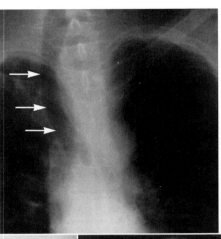

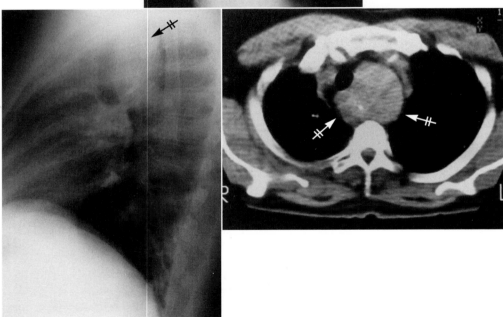

FIG. 19-40 Substernal thyroid *(crossed arrows)* presenting as a mass in the upper middle mediastinal, deviating the tracheal air shadow to the right *(arrows)* on the posteroanterior radiograph and computed tomography scan. (Courtesy Steven P. Brownstein, Springfield, NJ.)

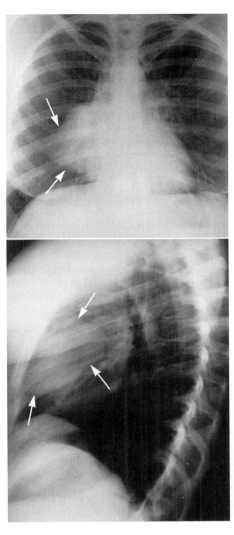

FIG. 19-41   Large teratoma in the anterior portion of the mediastinum (*arrows*).

CS10b | Middle Mediastinum

DISEASE	COMMENTS
Aortic aneurysm [p. 841]	Artheriosclerotic, mycotic, luetic, and traumatic etiologies; it may obliterate the aortic window in the lateral projection and project to either the left or right side in the frontal projection; position and contour are consistent with the vessel's path; hemorrhage will cause symmetrical massive enlargement of the superior mediastinum
Bronchogenic cyst [p. 837]	Round, well-defined fluid-filled cyst usually located just inferior and to the right of the carina; the cyst may be air-filled following communication with the tracheobronchial tree
Esophageal neoplasm **(FIG. 19-42)**	Occasionally large enough to be seen on the radiograph, appearing as a smooth, rounded mass demonstrated best on an esophagram

DISEASE	COMMENTS
Hiatal hernia	Retrocardiac mass of variable size appearing solid or containing an air-fluid level positioned immediately above the diaphragm; in the frontal projection the density can be seen through the cardiac shadow; an esophagram is diagnostic
Lymph node enlargement	Enlargement secondary to neoplasm (metastasis and lymphoma), granulomatous infection (tuberculosis, histoplasmosis, and coccidioidomycosis), pneumoconiosis (silicosis and asbestosis), and sarcoidosis
Mediastinal lipomatosis **(FIG. 19-43)**	Fat deposits resulting in diffuse enlargement of the mediastinum; the condition is associated with hyperadrenocorticism, diabetes, obesity, etc.
Pneumomediastinum (mediastinal emphysema)	Air within the mediastinum, typically secondary to blunt or penetrating trauma

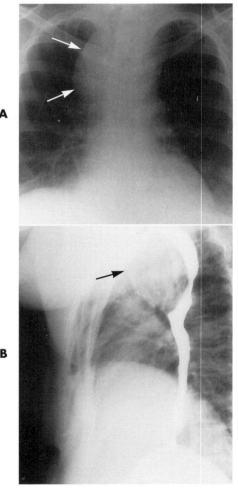

FIG. 19-42 Posteroanterior radiograph **(A)** and lateral projection of esophagram **(B)** revealing a solid middle mediastinal mass of undetermined etiology *(arrows)*. On the esophagram, the column of barium is posteriorly distended around the mass. (Courtesy Steven P. Brownstein, Springfield, NJ.)

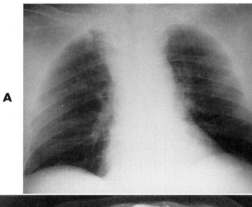

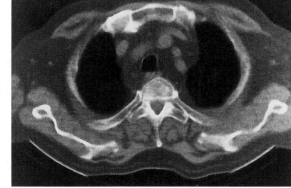

FIG. 19-43 Lipomediastinum. Posteroanterior radiograph **(A)** and computed tomography scan **(B)** show a widened mediastinum and thoracic inlet secondary to fatty infiltrate. (Courtesy Steven P. Brownstein, Springfield, NJ.)

CS10c | Posterior Mediastinum

DISEASE	COMMENTS
Aneurysm of descending aorta [p. 841]	Mass on the left side of the patient's mediastinum that appears continuous with the vascular shadow of the aorta; it may calcify and erode vertebral bodies
Bochdalek's hernia	Radiodense retrocardiac mass nearly always on the left
Extramedullary hematopoiesis	Vertebral bone marrow extrusion seen with the congenital anemias (i.e., thalassemia), producing smooth-appearing paravertebral masses in the posterior mediastinum; it is often accompanied by splenomegaly
Neurogenic neoplasm **(FIG. 19-44)**	Unilateral and paravertebral well-circumscribed mass, often representing neurofibroma and neurolemmoma in adult, or neuroblastoma and ganglioneuromas in children; rib or vertebral erosions may accompany this disease
Spinal neoplasm **(FIG. 19-45)**	Bony destruction resulting from osteochondroma, aneuysmal bone cyst, osteogenic sarcoma, metastasis, etc.; soft tissue paravertebral mass is uncommon

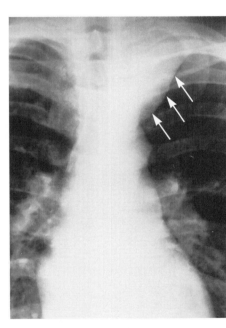
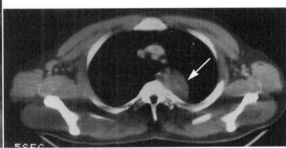

FIG. 19-44 Ganglioneuroma presenting as a posterior mediastinal mass *(arrows)*. (Courtesy Steven P. Brownstein, Springfield, NJ.)

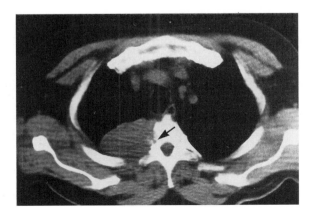

FIG. 19-45 Computed tomography scan demonstrating bronchogenic tumor mass with associated destruction of the adjacent rib and vertebral body *(arrow)*. (Courtesy Steven P. Brownstein, Springfield, NJ.)

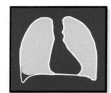

CS11 | Pleural Effusion

Pleural effusion describes larger collections of transudate, exudate, blood, or chyle in the pleural space. Radiographic findings vary from blunting of the costophrenic angles with mild effusion to opacification of the hemithorax with shifting the mediastinum with massive fluid accumulations. Pleural effusion is a nonspecific sign of underlying neoplasm, trauma, embolism, pulmonary edema, or other disease. The presence of pleural effusion should prompt a thorough search for concurrent disease.

DISEASE	COMMENTS
Abdominal diseases	Effusion often accompanies subphrenic abscesses, acute pancreatitis, and hepatitis
Chylothorax	Accumulations of chyle from ruptured thoracic duct secondary to trauma or neoplasm
Collagen diseases	Small, bilateral pleural effusions may accompany rheumatoid arthritis, systemic lupus erythematosus, Sjögren's syndrome, mixed connective tissue diseases, and dermatomyositis
Congestive heart failure (CHF) [p. 845]	Represents the most common cause of transudate effusion; resulting effusion is most often bilateral, but if unilateral, it occurs most commonly on the right side; CHF is accompanied by findings of an enlarged heart shadow, cephalization of pulmonary vascular and pulmonary edema
Empyema [p. 853]	Purulent effusions often result from the spread of infection from contiguous lung structures
Malignancies (FIG. 19-46)	Pleural effusion frequently accompanying primary and metastatic lesions of the pleura or adjacent tissues; malignant effusions typically are massive and rapidly reoccur following aspiration; examples include bronchogenic carcinoma, lymphoma, mesothelioma, and multiple myeloma

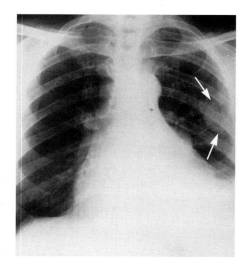

FIG. 19-46   Left-sided pleural effusion secondary to bronchogenic carcinoma appearing at the level of the posterior margin of the sixth left rib *(arrows)*. (Courtesy Steven P. Brownstein, Springfield, NJ.)

Pneumonia [p. 853]	Small unilateral effusion often accompanying radiographic findings of pneumonia; effusion occurs more commonly with bacterial agents	**Renal diseases**	Effusions of varying degrees produced by neoplasms, infections, and failure of the renal system
Pulmonary infarct [p. 850]	Typically small or moderate effusions; they are nonprogressive and may represent the only radiographic findings of a pulmonary infarct; pulmonary infarct is commonly accompanied by localized pleuritic pain or chest wall discomfort	**Trauma**	Chest wall trauma or surgical procedures; these may cause blood or edema accumulations in the pleural space
		Tuberculosis [p. 860] **(FIG. 19-47)**	Effusion is a common early manifestation of primary intrathoracic tuberculosis and is often the only radiographic finding; effusions are typically unilateral and small

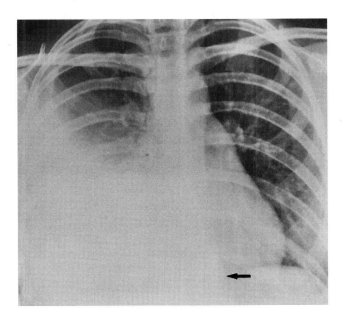

FIG. 19-47 Pleural effusion. Right-sided opacity has the classic feature of free pleural effusion in an erect patient. Opacity is homogeneous, occupies inferior part of chest, and has concave upper margins that extend higher laterally than medially. The medial to lateral limb of meniscus exhibits characteristic haziness without clear upper border. At first glance, shadow low and to the left (arrow) resembles displaced azygoesophageal recesss, as sometimes occurs with pleural effusion. Its configuration is, however, not quite as expected, and it was found to result from tuberculosis paravertebral abscess-cause of the effusion. (From Armstrong P et al: *Imaging of diseases of the chest,* ed 2, St Louis, 1995, Mosby.)

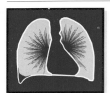

CS12 | Pulmonary Edema

Pulmonary edema represents fluid accumulation in the lungs from increased capillary permeability, increased hydrostatic capillary pressure, or blockage of lymphatic canals. Excessive fluid accumulates in the interstitium, overwhelms the lymphatics, and spills over to the air-space of the lung. The resultant appearance is one of confluent radiopaque perihilar densities with peripheral irregular linear shadows. A symmetrical, bilateral pattern has been referred to as "bat-wing consolidation" or "perihilar haze." Changes in patient position or blood flow (such as are seen in patients with emphysema) may alter the fluid distribution and radiographic appearance. The appearance reflects a combination of interstitial and alveolar patterns.

DISEASE	COMMENTS
Adult respiratory distress syndrome (ARDS) [p. 881] **(FIG. 19-48)**	Hemorrhagic pulmonary edema resulting from a variety of toxic substances ingested, inhaled, or aspirated; findings are related to alterations in capillary permeability and develop 2 to 36 hours after the exposure; this clinical feature helps to differentiate ARDS from other causes of pulmonary edema
Aspiration pneumonia [p. 853]	Bilateral, often asymmetrical pattern resulting from aspiration of vomitus related to anesthesia, alcohol abuse, seizures, coma, or neurological disturbance of the swallowing reflex

Cardiogenic **(FIG. 19-49)**	Represents the most common cause of pulmonary edema, resulting from hydrostatic factors typically secondary to mitral valve disease or left heart failure; although cardiomegaly is common, it does not always indicate cardiogenic disease (i.e., chronic renal failure) nor does its absence rule out cardiogenic disease (i.e., heart arrhythmia); patients may demonstrate dyspnea, orthopnea, and pink frothy sputum; pleural effusions are common

Continued

FIG. 19-48 Lung abscess complicating adult respiratory distress syndrome (ARDS). **A,** Plain chest radiograph shows features of ARDS, but a complicating pneumonia with abscess formation is difficult to recognize. **B,** Computed tomographic (CT) scan shows widespread but patchy distribution of the airspace shadows. **C,** CT section at a lower level shows a large abscess in the middle lobe. Sputum cultures revealed mixed gram-positive and gram-negative bacteria. (From Armstrong P et al: *Imaging of diseases of the chest*, ed 2, St Louis, 1995, Mosby.)

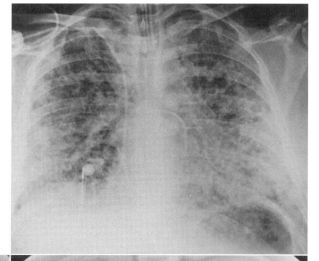

A

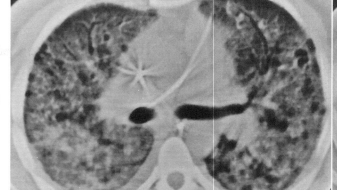

B

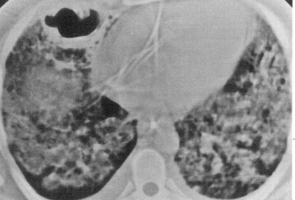

C

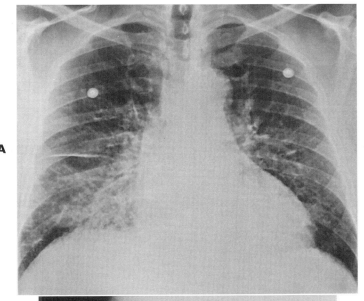

A

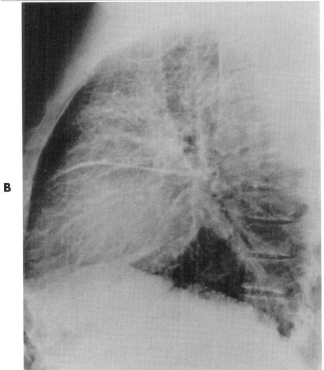

B

FIG. 19-49 Cardiogenic pulmonary edema following myocardial infarction in a 52-year-old man, illustrating widespread fissural thickening and lack of clarity of the intrapulmonary vessels and septal lines. Frank alveolar edema is evident in the right lower zone. The fissural thickening caused by subpleural edema is particularly striking. **A,** Frontal view. **B,** Lateral view. (From Armstrong P et al: *Imaging of diseases of the chest,* ed 2, St Louis, 1995, Mosby.)

DISEASE	COMMENTS
Extrinsic allergic alveolitis (EAA) [p. 882]	Hypersensitivity pneumonitis resulting from inhalation of antigenic organic dusts; a wide variety of agents have been identified, such as moldy hay (farmer's lung) and avian excreta (bird fancier's lung)
Fat embolism	Occurs 12 to 36 hours following trauma, usually a fracture in lower limbs, which releases fatty marrow embolism into the circulation
Near-drowning	Indicated by a history of fresh or saltwater near-drowning; edema results from asphyxia secondary to laryngeal spasm and aspiration of water
Nephrogenic	Occurs secondary to glomerulonephritis and chronic renal failure; heart shadow may be enlarged
Neurogenic (FIG. 19-50)	Observed in individuals with seizures, head trauma, and increased intracranial pressure; atypical distributions of pulmonary edema have been reported; the heart shadow is normal unless concurrent heart disease is present

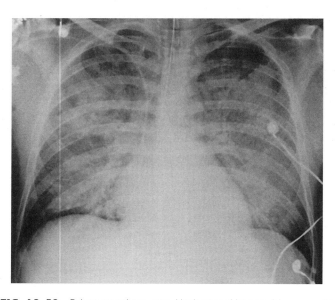

FIG. 19-50   Pulmonary edema caused by increased intracranial pressure following a subarachnoid hemorrhage caused by a ruptured aneurysm. (From Armstrong P et al: *Imaging of diseases of the chest,* ed 2, St Louis, 1995, Mosby.)

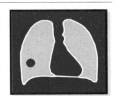

CS13 | Solitary Pulmonary Nodule and Mass

Well-circumscribed pulmonary radiopacities of 3 cm or less in diameter are nodules, and those greater than 3 cm are masses. The presentation of a mass is more serious than a nodule; the larger the lesion, the more likely that it is malignant. Although multiple etiologies have been identified, the differential diagnosis often is between granuloma and malignancy. The growth rate of the lesion, age of patient, presence of calcification, and associated clinical presentation are valuable clues to determine its etiology. Although any calcification is strong evidence against malignancy, periphery calcification may exist in malignant lesions. Central, stippled, laminated, and complete patterns of calcification indicate benign etiology. Early detection of pulmonary nodules and masses is directly related to a successful patient outcome.

DISEASE	COMMENTS
Abscess [p. 853]	Pulmonary abscesses: begin as solid radiopacities that cavitate and then appear as poorly circumscribed masses; most often they are associated with clinical findings consistent with infection
Arteriovenous malformation (AVM) **(FIG. 19-51)**	Congenital defect of capillaries that results in an abnormal vascular communication between a pulmonary artery and vein; AVMs are typically located in the medial portion of the lower lobes; they appear as dense bands extending from the lesion to the hilum, representing a feeding artery and draining vein (rabbit ear sign)
Bronchial carcinoid tumors [p. 863]	Low-grade malignancies most commonly arising from the lobar bronchi, often presenting with radiographic findings of airway obstruction

Continued

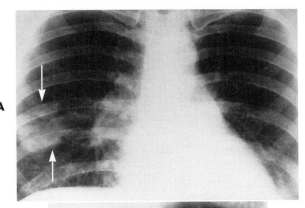

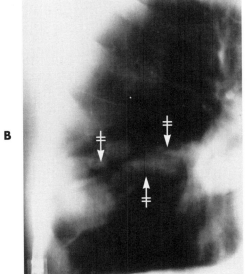

FIG. 19-51 Pulmonary arteriovenous malformation. The peripheral mass (**A,** *arrows*) is formed from a communication between the large artery and vein (**B,** *crossed arrows*), which extend from the hilum. Linear tomogram demonstrating the large artery and vein as cords connecting the hilum to the peripheral mass. (Courtesy Steven P. Brownstein, Springfield, NJ.)

DISEASE	**COMMENTS**
Bronchogenic carcinoma [p. 863] **(FIGS. 19-52 AND 19-53)**	May exhibit fuzzy or lobulated borders, classically never with a laminated, central, or completely calcified pattern, although it may demonstrate focus of peripheral calcification; serial chest films demonstrate increased growth rate over time; bronchogenic carcinoma is seen more commonly in those over 35 years of age; it may relate a history of chronic cough and hemoptysis
Bronchogenic cyst [p. 837]	Sharply defined mass in the lower lung fields representing a fluid-filled cyst; it may appear air-filled if a communication with an adjacent airway is established
Chest wall lesion **(FIGS. 19-54 AND 19-55)**	Not to be confused with moles, nipples, cutaneous neurofibromas, and other skin lesions that may mimic pulmonary lesions; reevaluation with the use of metallic markers is helpful in determining if the location is extrathoracic *Continued*

Continued

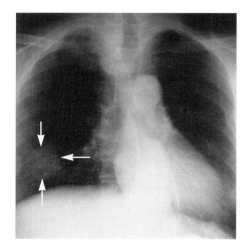

FIG. 19-52 Bronchogenic carcinoma presenting as a solitary mass in the right lower lung field *(arrows)*. (Courtesy Steven P. Brownstein, Springfield, NJ.)

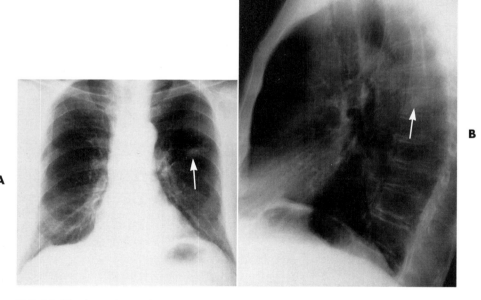

FIG. 19-53 Lung adenocarcinoma presenting as a noncalcified solitary pulmonary nodule *(arrow)* overlying the posterior margin of the left sixth rib on the left **(A)** and the body of the seventh vertebrae **(B).** (Courtesy Steven P. Brownstein, Springfield, NJ.)

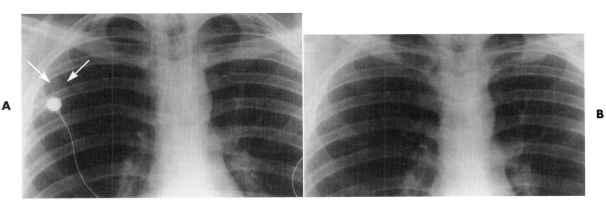

FIG. 19-54   A, Skin artifact resulting from adhesive paste for chest lead mimicking a solitary pulmonary nodule in the second anterior intercostal spaces on the right, immediately above the chest lead *(arrows).* **B,** Artifact disappeared when chest lead was removed. (Courtesy Steven P. Brownstein, Springfield, NJ.)

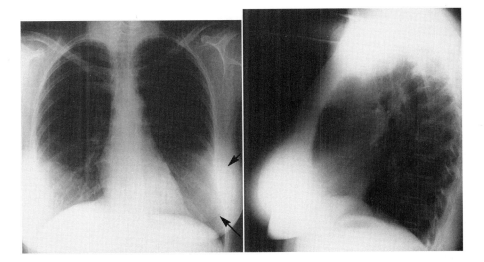

FIG. 19-55   Bilateral radiodense zones of the lower lung fields resulting from breast implants. A double density created by the implant can be seen on the patient's left *(arrows).* (Courtesy Robert C. Tatum, Davenport, Iowa.)

DISEASE	COMMENTS
Granulomas **(FIGS. 19-56** **AND 19-57**	Most common cause of solitary pulmonary nodules, represents nearly 90% of lesions in patients younger than 35 years of age; granulomas are associated with tuberculosis, histoplasmosis, and coccidioidomycosis infections; typically no or little change in size is noted on serial films
Hamartoma [p. 871]	Most common benign lung tumor, commonly calcified (characteristic popcornlike pattern); usually no clinical symptoms emerge, and the growth rate is slow
Intralobar **sequestration** [p. 837]	Sharply defined mass of variable shape in the lower lung field, representing poorly developed pulmonary tissue; lesions are most commonly left-sided, appearing in contact with the diaphragm
Metastasis [p. 873] **(FIG. 19-58)**	May uncharacteristically present as a solitary nodule or mass; calcification is rare, but when present it usually indicates a primary bone tumor
Progressive **massive fibrosus** **(PMF)**	Large, bilateral, slightly asymmetrical masses in the upper portion of the lungs; the lesions begin peripherally and can be seen to migrate toward the hila on serial chest films; the presence of PMF is related to silicosis or coalworker's pneumoconiosis

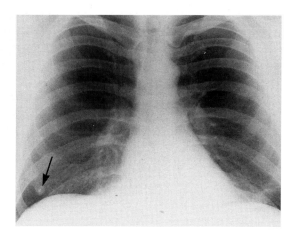

FIG. 19-56   Small nodule in the right lower peripheral lung field. The nodule demonstrates a central focus of calcification (target pattern) typical of histoplasmosis *(arrow)*.

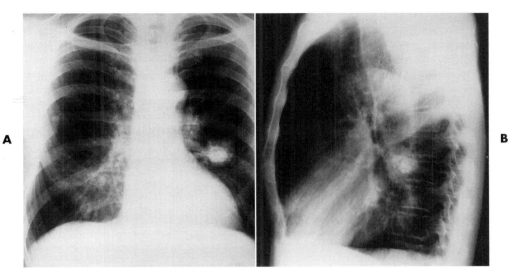

FIG. 19-57 Posteroanterior **(A)** and lateral **(B)** projection demonstrating a calcified giant granuloma and nonspecific thickened interstitium of the medial portion of the right middle lung field. (Courtesy Steven P. Brownstein, Springfield, NJ.)

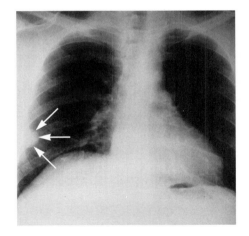

FIG. 19-58 Solitary metastatic pulmonary lesion from seminoma *(arrows)*. (Courtesy Steven P. Brownstein, Springfield, NJ.)

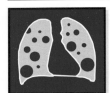

CS14 | Multiple Nodules and Masses

A multiple nodule or mass presentation is strongly suggestive of metastatic lung disease, particularly if a primary tumor has already been established. The primary tumor may originate from any organ system, with the notable exception of the CNS, from which tumors rarely metastasize to the lungs. Although most primary tumors appear as solitary lesions, lymphoma and alveolar cell carcinoma are exceptions, often presenting as multiple lesions.

Pneumonia is the most common cause of noncircumscribed lesions, appearing as fluffy, poorly defined, inhomogeneous consolidation, strongly indicative of alveolar filling (see pattern CS4). The presence of multiple, discrete, calcified nodules suggests granulomatous disease, in particular, coccidioidomycosis, histoplasmosis, and tuberculosis. Thromboemboli may cause ill-defined regions of pulmonary infarct (usually in the lower lung fields adjoining the pleural surface).

DISEASE	COMMENTS
Alveolar cell carcinoma **(FIG. 19-59)**	Subtype of pulmonary adenocarcinoma; it appears as single or multiple poorly defined regions, often resembling pneumonia or other alveolar disease pattern
Granuloma **(FIG. 19-60)**	Well-defined, small lesions related to tuberculosis, histoplasmosis, and coccidioidomycosis infections; calcification is common
Lymphoma [p. 872]	More often in the lower lung regions, appearing as radiopacities with irregular borders; it may be associated with hilar or mediastinal enlargement
Metastasis [p. 873] **(FIG. 19-61)**	Multiple lesions of small (miliary) or large (cannonball) size, more often in the lower lobes; calcification is rare, but when seen is highly suggestive of primary bone tumor (osteosarcoma); cavitation is associated with metastasis from squamous cell neoplasms

Rheumatoid arthritis	Small, well-defined lesions occurring in peripheral subpleural locations; cavitation is common; the lesions regress with remission of the arthritis
Sarcoidosis [p. 885]	Less common presentation of the disease; sarcoidosis is usually associated with hilar or mediastinal lymphadenopathy; sarcoidosis is more common in blacks and females
Wegener's granulomatosis **(FIG. 19-62)**	Widely scattered irregular nodules mostly in the lower lung regions; nodules have a tendency to cavitate, producing shaggy inner margins

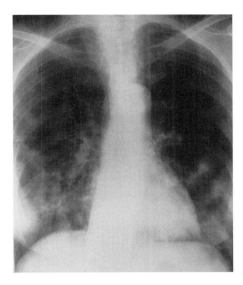

FIG. 19-59 Multiple nodule pattern of bronchoalveolar carcinoma appearing as bilateral nodules in the lower lung fields. (Courtesy Steven P. Brownstein, Springfield, NJ.)

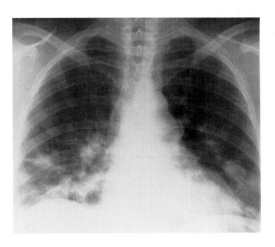

FIG. 19-60 Lymphoid granulomatosis occurring as multiple nodules in the lower lung fields. (Courtesy Steven P. Brownstein, Springfield, NJ.)

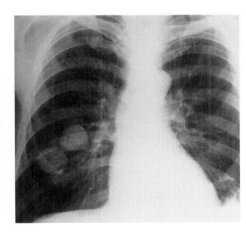

FIG. 19-61 Multiple small masses in the lower lung field, representing pulmonary metastasis from a primary carcinoma of the colon. (Courtesy Steven P. Brownstein, Springfield, NJ.)

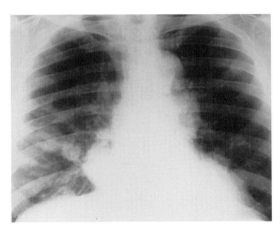

FIG. 19-62 Wegener's granulomatosis occurring with scattered bilateral pulmonary nodules, most notably in the right lower lung field. (Courtesy Steven P. Brownstein, Springfield, NJ.)

Suggested Readings

Burgener FA, Kormano M: *Differential diagnosis in conventional radiology,* New York, 1991, Thieme Medical Publishers.

Dahnert W: *Radiology review manual,* Baltimore, 1991, Williams and Wilkins.

Eisenberg RL: *An atlas of differential diagnosis,* ed 2, Gaithersburg, 1992, Aspen.

Felson B: *Chest roentgenology,* Philadelphia, 1973, WB Saunders.

Felson B: A new look at pattern recognition of diffuse pulmonary diseases, *AJR* 133:183, 1979.

Fraser RG, Pare JAP: *Tables of differential diagnosis and decision trees.* In Fraser RG, Pare JAP: *Diagnosis of diseases of the chest,* ed 2, Philadelphia, 1979, WB Saunders.

Genereux GP: Pattern recognition in diffuse lung disease: a review of theory and practice, *Med Radiog and Photog* 61:2, 1985.

Lillington GA: *A diagnostic approach to chest diseases,* Baltimore, 1987, Williams & Wilkins.

Meschan I: *Roentgen signs in clinical diagnosis,* Philadelphia, 1956, WB Saunders.

Ravin CE, Cooper C, Leder RA: *Review of radiology,* Philadelphia, 1994, WB Saunders.

Reed JC: *Chest radiology: patterns and differential diagnoses,* Chicago, 1981, Year Book.

Reeder MM, Bradley WG: *Reeder and Felson's Gamuts in radiology,* ed 3, New York, 1993, Springer-Verlag.

Simon G: *Principles of chest x-ray diagnosis,* London, 1956, Butterworths.

Weissleder R, Wittenberg J: *Primer of diagnostic imaging,* St Louis, 1994, Mosby.

chapter 20

Diseases of the Airways

DENNIS M MARCHIORI*

Atelectasis	Bronchiectasis	Congenital Bronchogenic Cysts
Bronchial Asthma	Bronchopulmonary Sequestration	Emphysema

Atelectasis

BACKGROUND

General. Atelectasis is defined as incomplete air filling and underexpansion of pulmonary tissue. It should be distinguished from consolidation, which also represents incomplete air filling of the lung. However, in consolidation, the missing air is replaced by blood, edema, pus, or other space-occupying substance, whereas missing air of an atelectatic region is not replaced, resulting in segmental collapse. Atelectasis may involve the entire lung or appear localized to a lobe, segment, or subsegment of the lung. It is not a disease itself, but rather a radiographic sign suggesting the presence of another pathology. Based on the underlying mechanism, atelectasis is divided into five categories: obstructive, passive, compressive, adhesive, and cicatrization.

Obstructive atelectasis. The first and most common type of atelectasis is termed *obstructive* or *resorptive atelectasis*. It is caused by intrinsic or extrinsic obstruction of an airway by such phenomena as the presence of neoplasm, infection, foreign body, and heavy secretions.[2,6] Over time, air distal to the airway obstruction is resorbed and not replaced, leading to an airless, radiolucent, collapsed portion of lung tissue (Fig. 20-1). Often the lung distal to bronchial obstruction exhibits increased radiopacity correlating to replacement of the alveolar air with inflammatory transudate, exudate, or other substance. Less commonly, a check-valve or obstruction develops, creating a hyperlucent, overinflated portion of lung tissue.

A check-valve mechanism involves accumulation of air distal to an airway obstruction. During inhalation, airways dilate, permitting air to pass by a partial bronchial obstruction. During exhalation the airways constrict tightly around an obstruction, effectively limiting the expiration of air distal to the obstruction. With each breathing cycle more air is "pumped" into the overinflated lung tissue distal to the obstruction. Check-valve obstructions in small airways are of limited clinical significance; however, when present in a large airway, they may result in respiratory distress.

Passive atelectasis. Passive (relaxation) atelectasis is the second type of atelectasis and results from the presence of a space-taking lesion external to the lung. Pleural fluid (blood, exudate, transudate, and chyle) or air may accumulate to such an extent that the adjacent lung is "pushed" aside, resulting in partial or complete pulmonary collapse. Diaphragmatic elevation or herniation of abdom-

inal viscera may also compress the lung. The amount of collapse is proportional to the size of the space-taking lesion.

Compressive atelectasis. Compressive atelectasis is a form of passive atelectasis in which the space-taking lesion is located within the involved lung. Large bullae, neoplasms, abscesses, and other large lesions may result in compressive atelectasis of adjacent lung tissue.

Adhesive atelectasis. Adhesive atelectasis refers to the nonobstructive, noncompressive pulmonary collapse secondary to decreased surfactant production by the type II pneumonocytes.[31] Pneumonocyte damage results from genetic defects, general anesthesia, ischemia, or radiation damage. Adhesive atelectasis is seen in neonates afflicted with hyaline membrane disease.

Cicatrization atelectasis. Lastly, cicatrization atelectasis represents scarring and contracture of pulmonary tissue following infection, pneumoconioses, scleroderma, radiation, idiopathic pulmonary fibrosis, and so on. This condition may appear localized (tuberculosis in the lung apices) or generalized (interstitial pulmonary fibrosis).

IMAGING FINDINGS

The presence of atelectasis is suggested by direct and indirect radiographic signs (Box 20-1). Displacements of intralobar fissures are the most reliable findings. The radiographic appearance differs based on the degree of lung involvement, location, and type of atelectasis (Table 20-1). Combined lobar collapse may complicate the radiographic appearance.[16] Rounded atelectasis is a form of peripheral pulmonary collapse that must be differentiated from similarly appearing neoplastic masses.[20,32]

CLINICAL COMMENTS

Whenever atelectasis is noted, it should prompt a vigorous search for a cause. Although several mechanisms of collapse have been identified, obstruction of the airway resulting from neoplasm is a common cause of lobar or segmental atelectasis that should direct patient management.

KEY CONCEPTS

- *Atelectasis is a sign of underlying disease process, defined as incomplete inflation of the lung.*
- *The five categories of atelectasis are obstructive, compressive, passive, adhesive, and cicatrization.*
- *The radiographic appearance depends on the location and extent of collapse; findings include loss of pulmonary volume, increased radiopacity, and distorted anatomical structures.*

---

*Special thanks to James C. Reed for his contribution as a reviewer of this material.

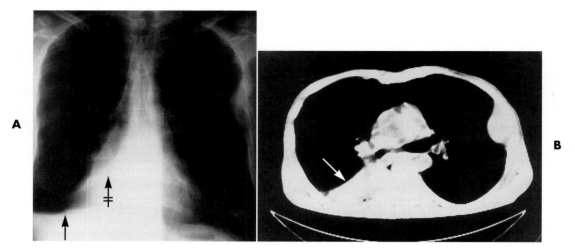

FIG. 20-1 Obstructive atelectasis of the right middle and lower lobe. **A,** The plain film radiograph demonstrates an elevated right hemidiaphragm *(arrow)* and loss of the silhouette of the right heart border *(crossed arrow)*. **B,** Computed tomography reveals an airless lung mass in the right costal angle and left rib mass, representing costal metastasis *(arrow)*.

BOX 20-1
Direct and Indirect Signs of Lobar Atelectasis

Direct signs	**Indirect signs**
Displacement of interlobular fissures	Elevation of the diaphragm (Fig. 20-2)
Increased radiopacity*	Mediastinal displacement
	Hilar displacement
	Overinflation of remaining normal lung
	Approximation of pulmonary vessels
	Approximation of ribs

*Some sources consider increased radiopacity an indirect sign of atelectasis.

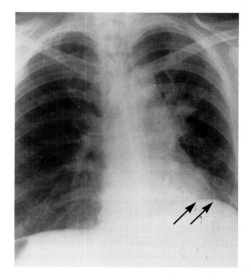

FIG. 20-2 Tracheal carcinoma with left hilar mass and partial obstructive atelectasis of the left lung and elevation of the left hemidiaphragm *(arrows)*. (Courtesy Steven P. Brownstein, Springfield, NJ.)

TABLE 20-1
Radiographic Appearance of Atelectasis

Atelectasis	Imaging findings
Lung	Opacification of the entire hemithorax, compensatory shift of the mediastinum with over-inflation and herniation of opposite lung toward collapsed lung side
Lobe*	
Right upper lobe	Radiodense lobe displaced superomedially, superiorly displaced diaphragm, oblique and horizontal fissures; can see the characteristic reversed "S-shape of Golden sign"[10] when a central mass is found in combination with the displaced horizontal fissure
Right middle lobe	Best demonstrated on the lateral projection, where the minor and major fissure approximate one another, bordering a thin, oblique-to-horizontal density; loss of silhouette of the left heart border on the frontal projection; on frontal projection, lordotic projection best for visualizing a wedge-shaped density with base adjacent to heart border
Right lower lobe	Radiodense lobe displaced posteromedially with posterior displacement of oblique fissure noted on lateral projection
Left upper lobe	Radiodense lobe displaced anterolaterally with overinflation of lower lobe occasionally located between collapsed upper lobe and mediastinum, "Luftsichel" sign[35]
Left lower lobe	Radiodense lobe displaced posteromedially, often obstructed by heart shadow; posterior displacement of the oblique fissure on the lateral projection
Segment	Increased radiodensity and volume loss that correspond to region collapsed and appear less marked than lobe involvement
Subsegment	Also known as platelike, discoid, or linear atelectasis; represents peripheral atelectasis of small areas of pulmonary tissue appearing as 2 to 10 cm horizontal linear density in the lower lung field
Round (folded lung)	Rare form of atelectasis associated with asbestosis-related pleural disease, in which the involved lung appears as a round mass (2 to 7 cm) in the lower lung

*Multiple lobes may be collapsed, yielding a combination of findings.

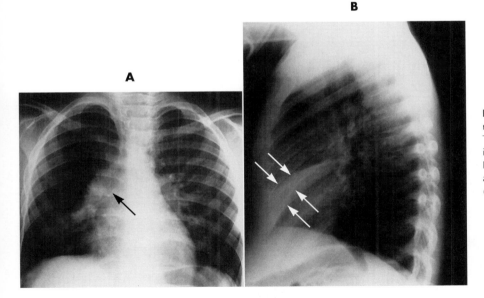

FIG. 20-3   Right middle lobe obstructive atelectasis resulting from a mucous plug in an asthmatic patient. **A,** The right heart border is poorly demarcated because it is in contact with the collapsed lobe (*arrow*). **B,** The collapsed lobe appears as a triangular density with the apex anchored at the hilum in the lateral projection (*arrows*). (Courtesy Steven P. Brownstein, Springfield, NJ.)

Bronchial Asthma

BACKGROUND

Bronchial asthma is characterized by widespread, episodic, reversible narrowing of the airways resulting from smooth muscle spasm, mucosal edema, or excess mucus in the lumen of the bronchi and bronchioles. A wide variety of inciting factors have been identified, including the following: exercise, infection, pharmaceuticals, or hypersensitivity to known allergens, such as pollen, animal fur, and fungi.

IMAGING FINDINGS

Early in the disease process no imaging findings are evident between acute episodes of the disease. However, radiographs taken at the time of an acute attack will demonstrate increased radiolucency secondary to general lung overinflation and depression of the diaphragm.[21,23] Patients who suffer from chronic asthma attacks may demonstrate increased prominence of the central interstitial markings and, when projected on end, bronchial wall thickening greater than 1 mm.[13,18] The radiographic findings may be complicated by the presence of infection or mucous plugs resulting in atelectasis[5] (Fig. 20-3) or consolidation.[3]

CLINICAL COMMENTS

Asthma attacks are characterized by wheezing, prolonged expiration phases of respiration, dyspnea, and cough.[1] Asthma may be complicated by pneumonia, pneumomediastinum, pneumothorax, emphysema, and mucous plugs in the airway.

▌ KEY CONCEPTS

- • *Asthma is a common condition marked by well-defined clinical symptoms.*
- • *The radiographic appearance varies from normal to increased radiolucency of lung fields secondary to overinflation.*
- • *The chronicity, nature of the attacks, and presence of complicating infection influence the radiographic appearance.*

Bronchiectasis

BACKGROUND

Bronchiectasis is chronic, irreversible dilation of bronchi or bronchioles that occurs as a sequel of inflammatory disease,[11,12] obstruction, or congenital alteration in either the smooth muscle or cartilage of an airway. The disease may be localized (i.e., tuberculosis) or generalized (i.e., cystic fibrosis) and predominates in the lower lobes. Based on the macroscopic appearance, cylindrical, varicose, and saccular forms of the disease have been described (Table 20-2).[25]

IMAGING FINDINGS

Imaging findings include alterations in lung volume and thickened bronchial walls, which appear as linear or cystic radiopacities as depicted in Fig. 20-4.[11] The computed tomography and bronchography appearance is more specific and may be characteristic to a morphological type (Table 20-2).

CLINICAL COMMENTS

Patients with localized bronchiectasis may have little or no pulmonary impairment. In the more generalized form, the patient may exhibit shortness of breath and wheezing. The most common associated clinical finding is a chronic cough with purulent expectorant. Often hemoptysis and clubbing of the fingers are present.[7]

TABLE 20-2
Types of Bronchiectasis

Type	Macroscopic and HRCT appearance*
Cylindrical (tubular)	Mild form, mild bronchial dilatation ("tramlines," "signet ring"), normal branching of tracheobronchial tree
Varicose	Moderate bronchial dilatation with intervening constrictions producing a "beaded" appearance, reduced branching of tracheobronchial tree
Saccular (cystic)	Severe form, grossly dilatated bronchi ("string of cysts"), greatly reduced branching of tracheobronchial tree, reduced functional lung parenchyma

*HRCT, high-resolution computed tomography.

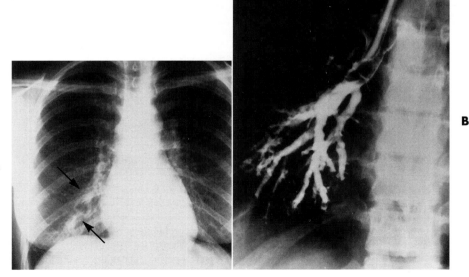

FIG. 20-4   A, Bronchiectasis appearing as prominent, thick bronchial markings in the right paracardiac region of the lung *(arrows).* **B,** Bronchogram demonstrating ectasia and irregularity of the bronchi.

Bronchopulmonary Sequestration

BACKGROUND

Bronchopulmonary sequestration represents congenital malformation of the foregut, resulting in a portion of lung that is not connected to the tracheobronchial tree (Fig. 20-5).[8] The sequestered segment of lung retains its embryonic systemic blood supply and may be found within (intralobar) or, less commonly, outside (extralobar) of the lung's pleural envelope.[27]

IMAGING FINDINGS

An extralobar sequestration appears as a dense mass located immediately above or within the left hemidiaphragm in 90% of cases. Less frequent locations include mediastinum, pericardial, and retroperitoneal spaces. By contrast, 60% of intralobar sequestrations are found on the right and may appear dense or cystic if infection has formed communication with the bronchial tree.[19] Rarely, intralobar lesions are found in the upper regions of the lung.[14]

CLINICAL COMMENTS

Extralobar sequestered regions of lung are asymptomatic, incidental findings. Intralobar types often represent areas of recurrent infection.

Congenital Bronchogenic Cysts

BACKGROUND

Bronchogenic cysts represent anomalous outpouching of the primitive foregut. The outpouchings become separated from the tracheobronchial tree, but unlike bronchopulmonary sequestrations do not undergo further tissue development. Bronchogenic cysts do not communicate with the tracheobronchial tree. The mediastinum contains 80%, and 20% are in a pulmonary, hilar,[30,24] or ectopic location.[22]

IMAGING FINDINGS

The radiographic appearance is that of a well-defined mass in the mediastinum, hilum, or lung (Fig. 20-6). Bronchogenic cysts are typically in close proximity to the large airways. An air-filled cystic appearance may follow infection and resulting communication

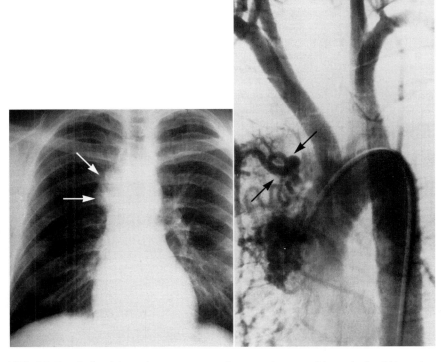

FIG. 20-5 **A,** Extralobar pulmonary sequestration appearing as a solid mass in the right paratracheal region (*arrows*). **B,** The angiogram demonstrates an anomalous systemic blood supply to the sequestration (*arrows*). (Courtesy Steven P. Brownstein, Springfield, NJ.)

PART THREE Chest

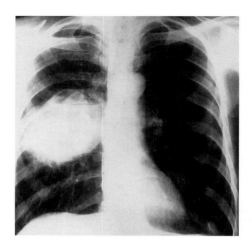

FIG. 20-6 Fluid-filled bronchogenic cyst. (Courtesy Steven P. Brownstein, Springfield, NJ.)

TABLE 20-3
Structural Types of Emphysema

Type	Comments
Centrilobular	Upper lobes, patchy distribution, associated with chronic bronchitis and smoking, involves center of pulmonary acinus
Panacinar	Lower lobes, homogenous distribution, associated with alpha 1-antitrypsin deficiency and smoking, involves all of pulmonary acinus
Distal acinar (paraseptal)	Along septal lines, peripheral distribution, associated with smoking, involves distal portion of acinus
Irregular (para-cicatricial)	No consistent distribution, associated with lung fibrosis, irregular involvement of the acinus

between the cyst and the tracheobronchial tree. The cyst's thin wall will aid its differentiation from an abscess. Calcification is unusual.

CLINICAL COMMENTS

Infants may exhibit respiratory distress secondary to extrinsic airway obstruction.[9] They are typically asymptomatic in the adult.[15]

KEY CONCEPTS

- *A bronchogenic cyst is a developmental mediastinal, hilar, or pulmonary mass.*
- *It is usually solid and may appear as a thin-walled, air-filled cyst following infection.*
- *Bronchogenic cysts are of limited clinical significance in the adult.*

Emphysema

BACKGROUND

Emphysema is defined as chronic dilatation of the air space distal to a terminal bronchiole, an area known as a *primary lobule* or *acinus*. The acinar walls are destroyed, leading to large aggregate air spaces, effectively decreasing the number of acini. Little or no evidence of fibrosis is present.[29] In Table 20-3, emphysema is classified into structural types based on the portion of the acinus most affected. Several types may coexist in the same patient.

Bullae are a prominent feature of emphysema. Bullae represent parenchymal collections of air resulting from advanced tissue destruction and are associated with emphysema, Marfan's syndrome, Ehlers-Danlos syndrome, HIV infection, intravenous drug use, and others. They are typically in a subpleural location and vary from a few centimeters to a lobe or larger in size. Many use the term *bleb* interchangeably with *bulla*. However, *bleb* should be reserved for much smaller interstitial collections of air, typically in a peripheral, subpleural location. Bullous emphysema describes the condition of patients with emphysema in whom bullae are a prominent feature of the radiographic presentation. Spontaneous pneumothorax may result from ruptured blebs and bullae.

IMAGING FINDINGS

The most prominent radiographic findings are due to lung overinflation, which manifests as increased pulmonary radiolucency and a bilaterally flat, depressed hemidiaphragm (below the anterior portion of the seventh rib or the posterior portion of the tenth rib),[17,34] increased retrosternal space (greater than 4.5 cm on the lateral film measured from a point 3 cm below the sternal angle),[28] accentuated kyphosis, and increased intercostal spaces (Figs. 20-7 and 20-8). The number of vessels is decreased in emphysemic tissue. The central pulmonary arteries are more prominent and appear truncated peripherally. Increased prominence of the interstitial markings is often present.[4,33] Bullae may appear as radiolucent air sacs in the periphery of the apex or base of the lungs. Only moderate to severe forms of emphysema are detectable on plain film radiography.[26,33] Computed tomography may identify early manifestations of the disease.

CLINICAL COMMENTS

Emphysema is characterized by breathlessness on exertion, secondary to reduced surface area for gas exchange. The presence of a productive cough is related to chronic bronchitis, which often accompanies emphysema. Physically, patients may exhibit a "barrel chest" appearance, caused by the collapse of small airways with trapping of alveolar gas during expiration, which in turn causes the chest to be held in the position of inspiration with prolonged expiration effort and increased residual volume. Most patients relate a history of cigarette smoking.

KEY CONCEPTS

- *Emphysema results in overinflation of the distal air spaces of the lung.*
- *Emphysema may be divided into the following categories: centrilobular, panacinar, distal acinar, and irregular types.*
- *Radiographic findings include hyperinflation, interstitial changes, vascular changes, and possibly bullae.*

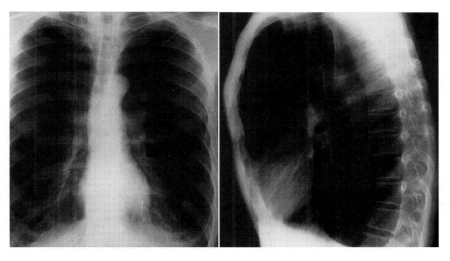

FIG. 20-7 Emphysema marked by hyperinflation, oligemic upper lung fields, prominent truncated pulmonary arteries, enlarged retrosternal clear space, obtuse sternodiaphragmatic angle, and depressed and flattened hemidiaphragms.

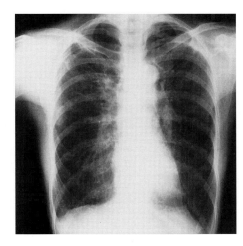

FIG. 20-8 Emphysema demonstrated by hyperlucent, overexpanded lung fields and flattened hemidiaphragms.

References

1. American Thoracic Society: Definitions and classifications of chronic bronchitis, asthma and pulmonary emphysema, *Am Rev Resp Dis* 85:762, 1962.
2. Barbato A et al: Use of fiberoptic bronchoscopy in asthmatic children with lung collapse, *Pediatr Med Chir* 17:253, 1995.
3. Blair DN, Coppage L, Shaw C: Medical imaging in asthma, *J Thorac Imag* 1:23, 1986.
4. Boushy SF et al: Lung recoil pressure, airway resistance, and forced flows related to morphologic emphysema, *Am Rev Respir Dis* 104:551, 1971.
5. Brashear RE, Meyer SC, Manion MW: Unilateral atelectasis in asthma, *Chest* 63:847, 1973.
6. Brooks-Brunn JA: Postoperative atelectasis and pneumonia: risk factors, *Am J Crit Care* 4:340, 1995.
7. Clark NS: Bronchiectasis in childhood, *Br Med J* 1:80, 1963.
8. De Parades CG et al: Pulmonary sequestrations in infants and children: a 20 year experience and review of the literature, *J Pediatr Surg* 5:136, 1970.
9. Eraklis AJ, Griscom NT, McGovern JB: Bronchogenic cysts of the mediastinum in infancy, *N Engl J Med* 281:1150, 1969.
10. Golden R: The effect of bronchostenosis upon the roentgen-ray shadows in carcinoma of the bronchus, *AJR* 13:21, 1925.
11. Gudbjerg CE: Roentgenologic diagnosis of bronchiectasis, *Acta Radiol* 143:209, 1955.
12. Heard BE et al: The morphology of emphysema, chronic bronchitis, and bronchiectasis: definition, nomenclature, and classification, *J Clin Pathol* 32:882, 1979.
13. Hodson CJ, Trickey SE: Bronchial wall thickening in asthma, *Clin Radiol* 11:183, 1960.
14. Hoeffel JC, Bernard C: Pulmonary sequestration of the upper lobe in children, *Radiology* 160:513, 1986.
15. Kirwan WO, Walbaum PR, McCormack RJM: Cystic intrathoracic derivatives of the foregut and their complications, *Thorax* 8:424, 1973.
16. Lee KS et al: Combined lobar atelectasis of the right lung: imaging findings, *AJR* 163:43, 1994.
17. Lennon EA, Simon G: The height of the diaphragm in the chest radiograph of normal adults, *Br J Radiol* 38:937, 1965.
18. Lynch DA et al: Uncomplicated asthma in adults: comparison of CT appearance of the lungs in asthmatic and healthy subjects, *Radiology* 188:829, 1993.

19. Niaidich DP et al: Intra-lobar pulmonary sequestration, MR evaluation, *J Comput Assist Tomogr* 11:531, 1987.
20. Ohri SK, Townsend ER: Folded lung: a masquerader of malignancy, *Scand J Thorac Cardiovasc Surg* 26:213, 1992.
21. Petheram IS, Kerr IH, Collins JV: Value of chest radiographs in severe acute asthma, *Clin Radiol* 32:281, 1981.
22. Ramenofsky ML, Leape Ll, McCauley RGK: Bronchogenic cyst, *J Pediatr Surg* 14:219, 1979.
23. Rebuck AS: Radiological aspects of severe asthma, *Aust Radiol* 4:264, 1970.
24. Reed JC, Sobonya RE: Morphologic analysis of foregut cysts in the thorax, *Am J Roentgenol* 120:851, 1974.
25. Reid LM: Correlation of certain bronchographic abnormalities seen in chronic bronchitis with the pathological changes, *Thorax* 10:199, 1955.
26. Sanders C: The radiographic diagnosis of emphysema, *Radiol Clin North Am* 29:1019, 1991.
27. Savic B et al: Lung sequestration: report of seven cases and review of 540 published cases, *Thorax* 34:96, 1979.
28. Simon G et al: Relation between abnormalities in the chest radiograph and changes in pulmonary function in chronic bronchitis and emphysema, *Thorax* 28:15, 1973.
29. Snider GL et al: The definition of emphysema: report of a National Heart, Lung, and Blood Institute, Division of Lung Diseases workshop, *Am Rev Respir Dis* 132:182, 1985.
30. St-Georges R et al: Clinical spectrum of bronchogenic cysts of the mediastinum and lung in the adult, *Ann Thorac Surg* 52:6, 1991.
31. Sutnick AI, Soloff LA: Atelectasis with pneumonia. A pathophysiologic study, *Ann Intern Med* 60:39, 1964.
32. Szydlowski GW et al: Rounded atelectasis: a pulmonary pseudotumor, *Ann Thoracic Surg* 53:817, 1992.
33. Thurlbeck WM et al: Chronic obstructive lung disease: a comparison between clinical, roentgenologic, functional and morphologic criteria in chronic bronchitis, emphysema, asthma and bronchiectasis, *Medicine* 49:82, 1970.
34. Thurlbeck WM, Simon G: Radiographic appearance of the chest in emphysema, *AJR* 130:429, 1978.
35. Webber M, Davies P: The Luftsichel: an old sign in upper lobe collapse, *Clin Radiol* 32:271, 1981.

chapter 21

Circulation and the Heart

DENNIS M MARCHIORI*

Acquired Valvular Heart Disease   Congenital Heart Disease   Pulmonary Edema
Aortic Aneurysms   Congestive Heart Failure   Pulmonary Thromboembolism
Coarctation of the Aorta   Pleural Effusion

Acquired Valvular Heart Disease

BACKGROUND

Acquired valvular heart disease is caused by rheumatic heart disease,[31] arteriosclerosis,[9] hypertension, or congenital heart defects. The mitral and aortic valves are usually involved.

IMAGING FINDINGS

Chest radiographs of patients with valvular heart disease typically demonstrate changes in the size of the cardiac shadow, alterations in the size and configuration of specific heart chambers, and alterations in pulmonary vascularity (Fig. 21-1). Valvular calcification may also be present, suggesting mitral and aortic stenosis. Specific radiographic findings are listed in Table 21-1. Magnetic resonance imaging (MRI) may be helpful in providing anatomical and functional information about patients with valvular heart disease.[8,17]

CLINICAL COMMENTS

The diagnosis of valvular heart disease is made based on the patient's clinical history, a physical examination, electrocardiography, chest radiography, and echocardiography.[45] In the past, acquired valvular disease was most often caused by rheumatic fever. This is still the case in underdeveloped countries, but in developed countries, other causes predominate today.

KEY CONCEPTS

- *Acquired valvular heart disease presents with a variety of symptoms and findings that vary according to the specific valve involved.*
- *Radiographic changes in the size of the heart and specific chamber, along with the degree of pulmonary blood flow and presence of calcification, will aid in locating the valve involved.*

Aortic Aneurysms

BACKGROUND

Aneurysms are circumscribed dilations of an arterial wall. Saccular aneurysms involve part of the circumference of the vessel, whereas fusiform aneurysms involve the entire circumference. If all three arterial layers (the tunicas intima, media, and adventitia) are affected, the aneurysm is referred to as a *true aneurysm*. False aneurysms disrupt arterial walls but are contained by the surrounding connective tissue. A number of conditions, including athero-

sclerosis, syphilis, mycoses, posttraumatic conditions, congenital conditions, cystic media necrosis, and arteritis, have been named as possible causes of aneurysms (Table 21-2; Figs. 21-2 and 21-3). Atherosclerosis is the most common cause and usually involves the descending aorta.

Aortic dissection occurs when a hematoma in the middle to outer third of the aortic wall longitudinally separates the aortic wall proximally and distally. The hematomas often develop as a result of a vasa vasorum hemorrhage, which is seen in patients with hypertension. The tunica intima may rupture and reconnect the hematoma with its aortic lumen, creating a "double barrel" aorta. A number of classification schemes have been developed to describe the nature and region of aortic involvement (e.g., DeBakey, Stanford).

IMAGING FINDINGS

The radiographic features of an aneurysm are limited to contour changes in the frontal and lateral projections (Figs. 21-4 and 21-5). Although it does not indicate the presence of an aneurysm, vessel calcification provides a means of visualizing distortions of the vessel's wall. Aortic dissection is suggested by mediastinal widening, cardiomegaly, pleural effusion, and (in rare cases) medial displacement of the calcified plaque more than 1 cm inward from the outer vessel wall of the descending aorta (which is referred to as the *calcification sign*).[10,11] MRI and computed tomography (CT) provide the best initial and follow-up evaluations of the aorta.[27,56] Angiography may be used preoperatively to better define the vessel.

CLINICAL COMMENTS

The clinical presentation of an aneurysm depends on its size and location; the majority are asymptomatic.[41] Compression of the vena cava (vena cava syndrome), stridor, hoarseness (caused by laryngeal nerve compression), dysphagia, and sternal chest pain may develop in patients who have a large aneurysm mass.

The risk of rupture is related to the size of the aneurysm. Aneurysms of the aortic arch or descending aorta that have a diameter less than 5 cm rarely rupture. Those exceeding 6 cm have a significant risk of rupturing, with 40% of those greater than 10 cm rupturing. A patient with a rapidly expanding aneurysm of any size has a poor prognosis.[41]

KEY CONCEPTS

- *Aneurysms are localized dilations of all (true aneurysms) or some (false aneurysms) of the arterial wall layers and involve part (saccular aneurysms) or all (fusiform aneurysms) of the vessel's circumference.*
- *Although many have no clinical symptoms, large aneurysms are significant and life-threatening.*

*Special thanks to James C. Reed for his contribution as a reviewer of this material.

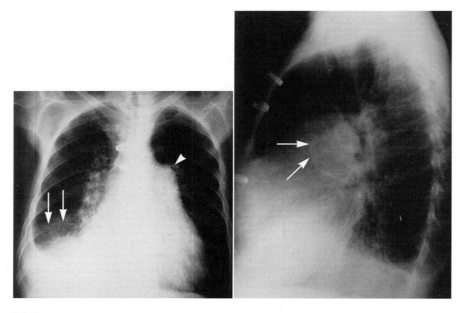

FIG. 21-1　Right-sided pleural effusion, pulmonary artery hypertension *(arrowhead)*, and calcification *(arrows)*. (Courtesy Steven P. Brownstein, Springfield, NJ.)

TABLE 21-1
Radiographic Appearance of Acquired Valvular Heart Disease

Condition	Radiographic appearance
Mitral stenosis	Large left atrium, right ventricle, and pulmonary trunk; long, straight left heart border; cephalization of pulmonary blood flow; narrowed retrosternal clear space and occasional calcification
Mitral insufficiency	Large left atrium and left ventricle, pulmonary edema in severe cases
Mitral prolapse (floppy mitral valve syndrome)	Normal (unless regurgitation develops)
Aortic stenosis	Large left ventricle, prominent ascending arch, small aortic knob, valve calcification
Aortic insufficiency	Large left ventricle, prominent aortic knob
Tricuspid stenosis	Large right atrium
Tricuspid insufficiency	Large right atrium and right ventricle, dilated superior vena cava and dilated azygous vein
Pulmonary stenosis	Large left pulmonary artery, increased left lung vascularity and large right ventricle
Pulmonary insufficiency	Large right ventricle

TABLE 21-2
Types of Aneurysms

Type	Comments
Cystic media necrosis-related	An aneurysm seen in patients with Marfan syndrome, Ehlers-Danlos syndrome, and other diseases in which collagen production is altered; commonly involves the ascending aorta or sinus of Valsalva
Atherosclerotic	An aneurysm in which the vasa vasorum is impaired; often demonstrates calcification; commonly affects the aortic arch or descending aorta (see Fig. 21-2)
Congenital	An aneurysm involving a congenital discontinuity of arterial wall; commonly involves the sinus of Valsalva
Arterites-related	An aneurysm seen in patients with Takayasu's disease and other diseases involving intimal proliferation and fibrosis; most often affects the ascending aorta
Mycotic	A saccular aneurysm caused by infection; does not result in calcification
Posttraumatic	An aneurysm involving a vessel tear; common near the ligamentum arteriosum; has a poor prognosis (see Fig. 21-3)
Syphilitic	An aneurysm in which the vasa vasorum has been impaired by *Treponema* organisms; most commonly affects the ascending aorta and aortic arch

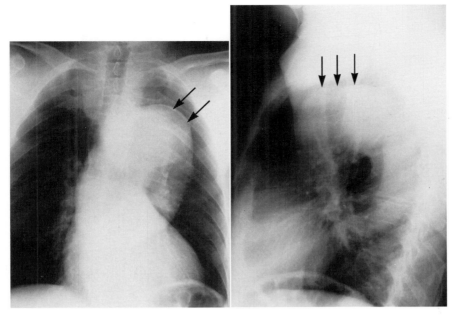

FIG. 21-2   Arteriosclerotic aneurysm in the aortic arch *(arrows)*.

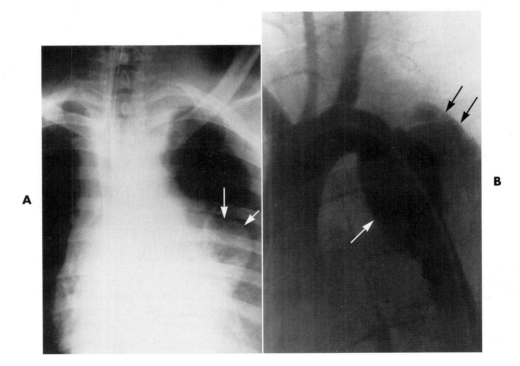

FIG. 21-3   Plain film **(A)** and angiogram **(B)** of 21-year-old car accident victim with a traumatic tear of the proximal descending aorta *(arrows)*. (Courtesy Steven P. Brownstein, Springfield, NJ.)

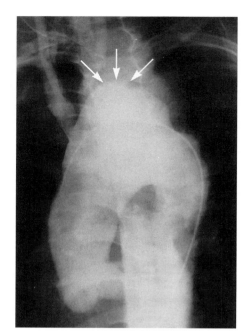

FIG. 21-4 Angiogram showing an aneurysm in the aortic arch *(arrows)*. (Courtesy Steven P. Brownstein, Springfield, NJ.)

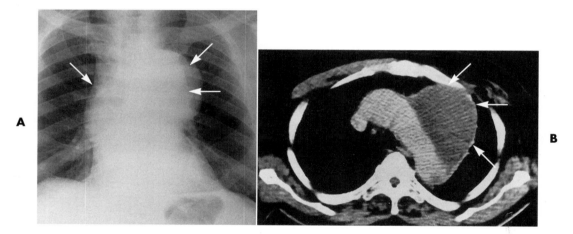

FIG. 21-5 Plain film **(A)** and CT scan **(B)** demonstrating an aneurysm in the aortic arch *(arrows)*.

Coarctation of the Aorta

BACKGROUND

Juxtaductal, or adult type, coarctation of the aorta is a discrete narrowing of the aortic isthmus (the region between the arch and descending aorta) distal to the origin of the left subclavian artery and near the ductus or ligamentum arteriosus.[46] Tubular hypoplasia, or infantile type coarctation of the aorta, is less common and involves narrowing of a segment of the transverse aortic arch. Coarctation is more common in males and often develops in conjunction with other cardiovascular defects, particularly when it is found in infants.

Although the aorta is narrowed, the collateral circulation typically prevents hypoperfusion of the trunk and lower extremities. In one such collateral path, blood from the subclavian arteries (before the coarctation has developed) enters the internal mammary arteries. It flows to the anterior intercostals and across the intercostal anastomoses, reversing the normal blood flow of the posterior intercostals and causing it to enter the aorta distal to the coarctation

that developed. The hypertrophy of the intercostal arteries causes characteristic inferior rib notching.

Pseudocoarctation is kinking of the aorta that is commonly seen secondary to arteriosclerosis in elderly patients.

IMAGING FINDINGS

Imaging features of infants with coarctation of the aorta may include cardiomegaly and possibly increased pulmonary vascular markings. In children and adults a characteristic inward deformity of the proximal descending aorta may be present with bulging of the vessel immediately above and below (the "figure 3" sign) (Fig. 21-6). This sign is uncommonly seen on images of infants because the aortic arch is so difficult to observe. Although not pathognomonic for coarctation, bilateral inferior rib notching is common at the posterior angles of the third through ninth ribs (Fig. 21-7). Rib notching is not seen in the infant. MRI is the modality of choice for further assessment.

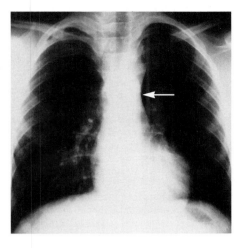

FIG. 21-6 Coarctation of the aorta. The narrowed aorta and immediately distal poststenotic dilation of the descending aorta *(arrow)* combine to form a "figure 3" shape. (Courtesy Steven P. Brownstein, Springfield, NJ.)

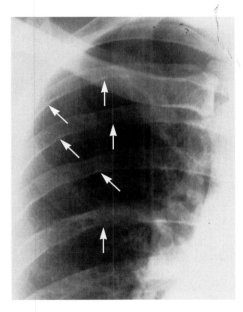

FIG. 21-7 Notching defect at the lower margin of several ribs in a patient with coarctation of the aorta *(arrows)*. (Courtesy Steven P. Brownstein, Springfield, NJ.)

CLINICAL COMMENTS

Most symptomatic infants with coarctation of the aorta have concurrent cardiovascular abnormalities (e.g., aortic stenosis, a patent ductus arteriosus, a ventricular septal defect).[42] Associated cardiac anomalies are uncommon in adults. A blood pressure difference of 20 mm Hg between the arms and legs is strongly indicative of coarctation.[33,42] Treatment involves surgical correction of the deformity.[25]

KEY CONCEPTS

- *Coarctation of the aorta is localized postductal (adult type) or generalized preductal (infantile type) stenosis of the aortic isthmus.*
- *Adult type coarctation of the aorta is characterized by an inward deformity of the proximal descending aorta on frontal projections and typically demonstrates inferior rib notching.*
- *Infantile type coarctation of the aorta is more serious than the adult type, is usually associated with other anomalies, and has few common radiographic features.*

Congenital Heart Disease

BACKGROUND

Congenital heart disease (Table 21-3) encompasses a wide variety of defects that appear at birth as either isolated anomalies or part of larger complexes. Patients with congenital heart disease are categorized based on the presence or absence of cyanosis. Further subdivisions can be made based on the heart size and pulmonary vascularity.

IMAGING FINDINGS

Plain film radiography is used to evaluate pulmonary vascularity, heart size, and configuration of the great vessels.[15,50] Echocardiography, angiocardiography, and MRI are all useful imaging modalities for evaluating congenital heart defects.[13,55]

CLINICAL COMMENTS

Although congenital heart disease can be so severe that an affected unborn fetus cannot survive, it can also be largely asymptomatic. Many infants with the condition seem to be healthy immediately after birth, but their condition changes as the ductus arteriosus closes and adult circulation begins. Some congenital heart diseases may not appear until adulthood (e.g., floppy mitral valve syndrome).

Clinical findings are often nonspecific.[35] Cyanosis, indicated by clubbing of the fingers and toes, hypertrophic osteoarthropathy, and polycythemia, is a prominent feature of many forms of the disease. Congestive heart failure, impaired growth and development, and pulmonary vascular disease may also be found.[21]

KEY CONCEPTS

- *The diagnosis of congenital heart disease is made in part by clinical findings of cyanosis, radiographic appearance of pulmonary vascularity, and specific anatomical defects demonstrated by echocardiography.*
- *The success and application of many surgical and palliative measures depend largely on early recognition.*

Congestive Heart Failure

BACKGROUND

Four factors are involved in heart functioning: preload (the end-diastolic volume), afterload (the ejection resistance), myocardium contractility, and heart rate. Disturbance of one or several of these factors results in heart failure, the mechanical inability of the heart to circulate an adequate supply of blood. In rare cases the four cardiac factors may appear normal, but the heart still cannot meet the tissues' increased metabolic and flow needs; this is referred to as *high-output heart failure* and is seen in patients with conditions such as Paget's disease and severe anemia.

Forward heart failure refers to the inability of the heart to pump an adequate volume of blood. Symptoms of this condition are related to underperfusion of vital organs (e.g., the brain, leading to fatigue; skeletal muscle, leading to weakness). Backward heart failure refers to the inability of the heart to pump blood that enters it through the venous system. Backward failure results in increased venous pressure and produces transudate in the tissues. During left-sided heart failure, blood is not expelled from the left side of the heart at the same rate as it is on the right, and as a consequence the blood backs up and "congests" the pulmonary tissues.[6,36] During right-sided heart failure, blood accumulates on the venous side of the major circulation pathways but typically spares the lungs. Right-sided heart failure is usually caused by left-sided heart failure.

These types of heart failure are not mutually exclusive, but rather are useful categories for conceptualizing the cause and expected dynamics of heart failure.

TABLE 21-3
Summary of Common Congenital Heart Diseases

Defect	Physical appearance*	Pulmonary vascularity**	Frequency†	Comments
Ventricular septal defect (VSD)	A	↑	25%	A defect that is usually in the fibrous portion of the septum; second most common congenital heart defect (with bicuspid aortic valve defect being the most common); asymptomatic if small[30]
Atrial septal defect (ASD)	A	↑	—	Defect of the ostium secundum; most common congenital defect recognized in adults; often asymptomatic
Patent ductus arteriosus	A	↑	15%	Defect in which the ductus arteriosus fails soon after birth, resulting in aortic/pulmonary artery shunt
Coarctation of the aorta	A	=	12%	Localized or generalized stenosis of aortic isthmus; results in a large heart in infants and rib notching in adults[25,43]
Aortic stenosis	A	=	10%	Valvular or vessel stenosis; usually asymptomatic; in severe cases in infants, results in congestive heart failure
Pulmonary stenosis	A	=	10%	Valvular or vessel stenosis; usually asymptomatic; results in loud systolic murmur and poststenotic dilation of pulmonary trunk
Tetralogy of Fallot	C	↓	10%	(1) Obstructed pulmonary outflow tract, (2) ventricular septal defect, (3) right ventricular hypertrophy, (4) aorta overriding interventricular septum[18] (in addition, normal heart size); most common congenital heart defect with cyanosis after 1 year of age
Pentalogy of Fallot	C	↓	—	Defect comprising the tetralogy of Fallot and an ASD; increased heart size
Ebstein anomaly	C	↓	—	Defect in which a caudally displaced tricuspid valve creates an enlarged right atrium and small right ventricle; increased heart size
Tricuspid atresia	C	↓	2%	Absence of tricuspid valve and presence of ASD; increased heart size
Total anomalous pulmonary venous return (TAPVR)	C	↑	—	Aberrant communication between pulmonary and systemic veins; an ASD is needed for the defect to be compatible with life; "figure 8" or "snowman" configuration of heart shadow (Fig. 21-8)
Truncus arteriosus	C	↑	—	Defect in which a failure of septation forces the pulmonary, systemic, and cardiac arteries to share a single cardiac outlet
Transposition of great vessels	C	↑	10%	Defect in which the aorta arises from the right ventricle and the pulmonary trunk arises from the left ventricle; most common cause of neonatal cyanosis; results in a wide heart shadow[55]
Double outlet right ventricle	C	↑	—	Defect in which the aorta and pulmonary trunk arise from the right ventricle; VSD present
Single ventricle	C	↑	—	Defect in which the ventricular septum is absent and associated defects of the atrioventricular valves are present

*A, Acyanotic; C, cyanotic.
**↑, Increased; ↓, decreased: =, normal.
†Frequency of congenital heart disease cases in children.

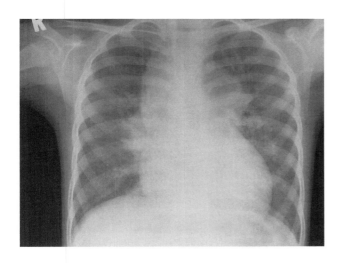

FIG. 21-8 "Figure 8," or "snowman," configuration of total anomalous pulmonary venous return. (Courtesy Steven P. Brownstein, Springfield, NJ.)

TABLE 21-4
Radiographic Appearance of Congestive Heart Failure

Finding	Appearance
Enlarged heart shadow	Suggested if the widest transverse dimension of the cardiac shadow in the frontal projection is more than one half the internal dimension of the hemithorax (spinous process to body wall) (Fig. 21-9)
Left ventricular enlargement	In the frontal projection, an enlarged left lower heart border. In the lateral projection, an enlarged posterior inferior heart border (more than 2 cm posterior to the inferior vena cava shadow)
Left atrial enlargement	In frontal projection, appears more than 7 cm inferolaterally from center of left bronchus (may form right heart border if massive enlargement present)
Cephalization of blood flow	Increased vascular markings in the superior lung fields
Enlarged superior vena cava and azygous vein	Enlarged right mediastinal border
Perivascular cuffing	Hazy, blurred pulmonary vessels
Peribronchial cuffing	Thick, "donut," or on-end appearance of bronchial walls
Kerley lines (A, B, C, etc.)	Interstitial accumulation of fluid (Fig. 21-10)
Thickening of interlobar fissures	Fluid accumulation in fissures
Pleural effusion	Transudate accumulation in the pleural space, common
Pulmonary edema	Perihilar edema accumulations appearing as "bat-wing," "butterfly," or "perihilar haze"

IMAGING FINDINGS

The radiographic features of patients with congestive heart failure are summarized in Table 21-4. One or more chambers of the heart are usually enlarged, and signs of pulmonary congestion and edema are often present. Pleural effusion is often found[29] and may be bilateral or predominantly right-sided. As shown in Fig. 21-11, the radiographic findings change as time passes. Patients with isolated right-sided heart failure may exhibit few pulmonary findings.

CLINICAL COMMENTS

Although symptoms and physical findings are helpful in diagnosing congestive heart failure, they have limited sensitivity and specificity.[26] Common clinical findings include shortness of breath (which often worsens with activity), a chronic and nonproductive cough, nocturia, pulmonary rales, pitting edema, an enlarged and tender liver, and engorged neck veins. The prevalence of congestive heart failure increases with age.[2,23,53] The majority of the patients have irreversible heart damage and a poor prognosis. Drugs combined with modifications in diet and activity are part of most treatment programs.

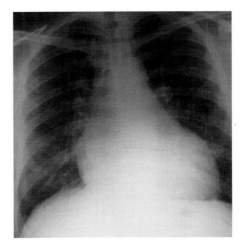

FIG. 21-9 Enlarged heart shadow secondary to congestive heart failure. Also noted are sternal wires that are residua of a previous intrathoracic surgery. (Courtesy Steven P. Brownstein, Springfield, NJ.)

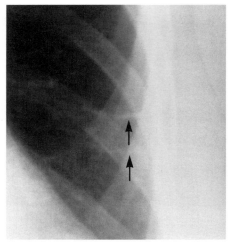

FIG. 21-10 Distention of the subpleural interstitial space appearing as two horizontal, 1-cm long radiodense lines perpendicular to the visceral pleura in the lower periphery of the lung field; these lines are known as *Kerley's B-lines (arrows)*.

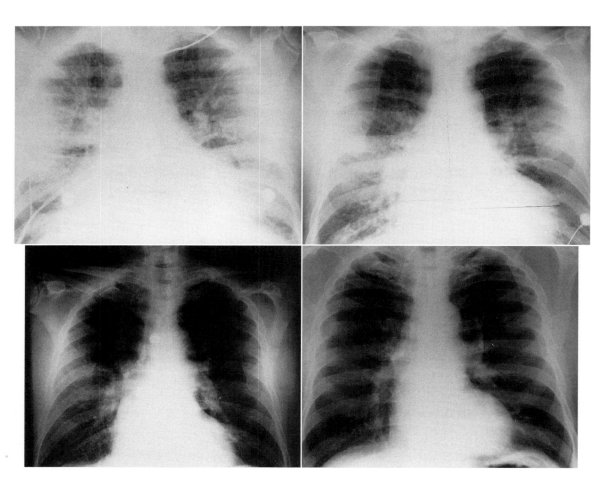

FIG. 21-11 Plain films taken during a 2-week period in a patient with congestive heart failure. The initial film reveals cardiomegaly with a bilateral air-space pattern of radiodensities and haziness of the bronchovascular shadows. These findings become less distinct on subsequent films and are not apparent on the last films of the series, taken 2 weeks after the initial radiograph. (Courtesy William E. Litterer, Elizabeth, NJ.)

PART THREE
Chest

Pleural Effusion

BACKGROUND

Normally, little more than a potential space exists between the visceral and parietal pleurae, containing less than 2 ml of fluid. Pleural effusion is the presence of a larger collection of transudate, exudate, blood, or chyle in this pleural space. More specific terms, such as hydrothorax, hemothorax, or chylothorax, are used if the fluid content is known. The composition of the fluid cannot be determined by its radiographic appearance.

Pleural effusion is typically secondary to diseases of the mediastinum, lungs, or chest wall. Radiographs often provide additional characteristics of a chest disease that may be associated with effusion. In some radiographs, large effusions may obscure part of the lung, so CT is needed to visualize much of the parenchyma.

IMAGING FINDINGS

Pleural fluid can be free or loculated by surrounding fibrosus. Free pleural fluid occupies the most gravity-dependent portion of the lung, making first the posterior costophrenic angle and then the lateral costophrenic angle appear blunted.[14] Capillary pressure may draw the effusion upward along the body wall, creating a meniscus sign. Loculated fluid in an interlobar fissure may appear as a mass ("pseudotumor") that characteristically shrinks and disappears ("vanishing" or "phantom" tumor) as its fluid is absorbed.[22] Loculated effusion is more common in the right lung[12] and typically affects the minor fissures.[22] A pseudotumor can be correctly identified by the way its characteristic tapered margins enter into the fissure.

Occasionally, fluid occupies a subpulmonary location, a condition that mimics an elevated hemidiaphragm. Subpulmonic effusion is more common on the right.[39] Left-sided subpulmonic effusion is more easily recognized because the increased distance (greater than 1 cm) between the gastric air bubble and the top of the subpulmonary fluid presents as an easily recognizable finding. Regardless of the side of the body affected, the pseudodiaphragm created by the top of the subpulmonic fluid appears more lateral than the true dome of the hemidiaphragm.[3]

A lateral decubitus projection (with the affected side placed down) can help the clinician distinguish between pleural effusion and an elevated diaphragm (Fig. 21-12). Free effusion moves to the most gravity-dependent position and spreads out laterally on the dependent side. Lateral decubitus projections provide a more sensitive evaluation of early effusions.[52] Massive effusion may opacify the hemithorax and shift the mediastinum toward the contralateral side.

CLINICAL COMMENTS

Pleural effusion is a nonspecific indication of some other underlying problem, such as a neoplasm, trauma, an embolism, or pulmonary edema. The observation of pleural effusion should prompt a thorough review of the patient's history and concurrent radiographic findings for a cause. Often a pleural tap is necessary to rule out certain significant pathological factors.

The symptoms of patients with pleural effusion often include well-localized, pleuritic pain that is typically described as "stabbing" and may be aggravated by actions such as coughing, inhaling deeply, or sneezing. Severe dyspnea may also develop, necessitating thoracocentesis. Although physical examinations cannot reliably detect small effusions, large effusions may cause certain areas to produce dull or flat sounds during percussion.

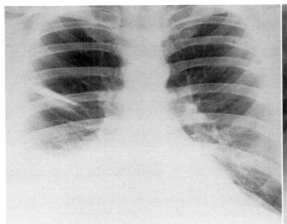
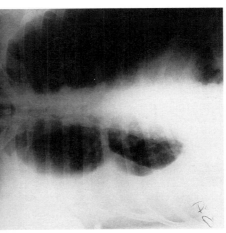

FIG. 21-12 A, Posteroanterior projection demonstrating right-sided pleural effusion in the lower pleural space and loculated pleural effusion in the lateral portion of the horizontal fissure presenting as a linear radiodense shadow in the middle right lung field. **B,** Lateral decubitus projection in which fluid from the effusion spills laterally, creating a fluid level along the right side of the chest wall. (Courtesy William E. Litterer, Elizabeth, NJ.)

Pulmonary Edema

BACKGROUND

Pulmonary edema is excess fluid accumulation in the extravascular lung space. The most common cause of increased fluid accumulation is elevated venous and capillary pressures caused by left-sided heart disease. The increased capillary pressure forces excessive amounts of fluid from vessels to the interstitial spaces. Normally the lymphatics drain excess fluid from the interstitial spaces and transport it back to the systemic circulation. However, interstitial fluid accumulations can become excessive and overwhelm the draining ability of the lymphatics, leading to a breakdown of the tight junctions between adjacent alveolar cells. Consequently, fluid may force its way into the air space of the lungs and accumulate.

Other factors leading to excessive extravascular fluid accumulations include those that increase capillary wall permeability (e.g., noxious substances, high altitude, pancreatitis), cause fluid overload syndromes (e.g., excessive intravenous fluid administration, renal failure), or cause obstruction of the lymphatic vessels (e.g., neoplasms, neurogenic factors).[1,48] (See Chapter 19, pattern CS-12, for a more complete list of causes.)

IMAGING FINDINGS

The radiographic appearance of pulmonary edema is largely based on whether the fluid accumulation is in the interstitial or alveolar spaces (Box 21-1). Interstitial edema precedes alveolar edema, al-

though they can be present concurrently. Identifying the cause of pulmonary edema from the radiographic appearance alone is difficult, but classic appearances of several causes have been identified.

- Cardiac failure presents with a cephalic redistribution of pulmonary blood flow that results in prominent vascular markings in the upper lung zone. An enlarged heart shadow and pleural effusion are also present and are often more prominent on the right side of the patient.[37,57]
- Features of pulmonary edema caused by renal failure may include heart enlargement, normal pulmonary vascular distribution, and symmetrical, bilateral perihilar opacities.
- Typically, pulmonary edema caused by increased vascular permeability is associated with a widespread pattern of alveolar filling and a normal-sized heart shadow and vascular distribution.

CLINICAL COMMENTS

Acute pulmonary edema presents with characteristic symptoms that include severe dyspnea; tachypnea; pink, frothy sputum; diaphoresis; and cyanosis. Examination of the lungs reveals rales and wheezing.

KEY CONCEPTS

- *Pulmonary edema represents increased extravascular fluid accumulations due to hydrostatic, permeability, or lymphatic factors*
- *The radiographic appearance changes rapidly; it is generally seen as an interstitial or air-space pattern depending on the location of the excess fluid.*

BOX 21-1
Radiographic Appearance of Pulmonary Edema

Interstitial pattern

Septal lines

Kerley's A lines: thin, 5-10 cm thin lines seen in the upper lung fields representing distension of the interlobular septa suggesting acute disease.

Kerley's B lines: dense, 1-2 cm horizontal lines perpendicular to the pleura of the lower lung representing distension of the subpleural interlobular septa (see Fig. 21-10).

Kerley's C lines: thin lines which radiate peripherally from the hilum relating a diffuse reticular pattern.

Hilar haze

A loss of definition of the large pulmonary vessels.

Subpleural edema[20,41]

Fluid accumulations immediately beneath the visceral pleura. Appears as linear thickening, thick fissures if interlobular visceral pleura is involved.

Peribronchovascular blurring and cuffing[7]

Loss of definition of the bronchi and vessels due to surrounding fluid accumulations.

Alveolar pattern

Bilateral hilar densities[24]

"Butterfly," "sunburst," "bat's wings" or "fan-shaped" radiopacities extending from the hila bilaterally. The opacification may be partial (appearing patchy and mottled) or complete (appearing homogeneously radiodense).

Air-bronchogram

A radiolucent transverse shadow representing an air-filled bronchi contrasted by surrounding fluid-filled air spaces.

Transient

Typically, air-space patterns of pulmonary edema change rapidly over time.

Pulmonary Thromboembolism

BACKGROUND

Pulmonary emboli arise from thrombi in the venous circulation, tumors in the venous system, or nonvenous sources such as amniotic fluid, bone marrow, or air. Most pulmonary emboli originate from clots in the deep veins of the lower extremities. Predisposing clinical factors for the formation of deep venous thrombi include prolonged standing, obesity, prolonged bed rest, surgery, stroke, congestive heart disease, and fractures of large bones.

Pulmonary emboli become lodged in the pulmonary trunk, pulmonary arteries, or arterial tree. Emboli may have both hemodynamic (i.e., obstructive) and physiological (i.e., vasoconstrictive) effects on blood flow. (The effects of vasoconstriction are probably less clinically significant.[45])

Most pulmonary emboli resolve, restoring pulmonary arterial flow.[5,16,32] Embolism results in pulmonary infarction in up to 15% of patients,[34] typically involving the lower lobes. It appears as pleural-based triangular radiopacities resulting from alveolar filling with edema and hemorrhage.

IMAGING FINDINGS

Although many radiographic findings have been associated with pulmonary embolism, none are specific for or highly sensitive to the disease.[4,19] The pulmonary arteries may appear enlarged (i.e., greater than 16 mm). Oligemia distal to the site of arterial obstruction may appear radiolucent (Westermark's sign) in patients who have a pulmonary embolism but no infarct. A triangular, pleural-based radiopacity is seen in patients with a pulmonary embolism and an infarct. This radiographic feature, referred to as *Hampton's hump,* is an accumulation of blood and edema in the alveolar space of a lung infarct. Over a period of months, the periphery of the hump "melts away," resolving completely or remaining as a small, horizontal, linear tissue scar.

The combination of ventilation and perfusion (V/Q) radionuclide imaging demonstrates the air distribution and blood flow to the lung. Radionuclide imaging is an important imaging modality for use in patients who already show clinical or radiographic evidence indicative of a pulmonary embolism.

CLINICAL COMMENTS

The clinical presentation of a pulmonary embolism depends largely on the size of the embolus and the patient's health status. Up to 80% of patients with a known embolism do not exhibit significant clinical symptoms.[47] However, pulmonary emboli are a major cause of death for up to 15% of adults in acute care hospital settings. Clinical manifestations, when present, are diffuse, poorly defined, and nonspecific,[49] causing many cases to go unnoticed.[43] Common clinical findings include chest pain, dyspnea, cough, hemoptysis, rales, tachypnea, and fever.

KEY CONCEPTS

- *Pulmonary emboli arise from deep venous thrombi, bone marrow, amniotic fluid, air, and other sources. They are more common in the lower portions of the lungs.*
- *Of the patients who develop a pulmonary embolism, 15% also develop a pulmonary infarct, which is often indicated radiographically by a triangular, pleural-based, radiodense region.*
- *Although many patients remain asymptomatic, complaints of dyspnea, cough, hemoptysis, and chest pain are suggestive of a pulmonary embolism.*
- *Ventilation and perfusion (V/Q) radionuclide scanning is helpful in diagnosing patients in whom clinical suspicion of pulmonary embolism is high.*

References

1. Aryre SM: Mechanisms and consequences of pulmonary edema, *Am Heart J* 103:97, 1982.
2. Besse S et al: Is the senescent heart overloaded and already failing? *Cardiovasc Drugs Ther* 8:581, 1994.
3. Bryk D: Infrapulmonary effusion: effect of expiration on the pseudodiaphragmatic contour, *Radiology* 120:33, 1976.
4. Buckner CB, Walker CW, Purnell GL: Pulmonary embolism: chest radiographic abnormalities, *J Thoracic Imaging* 4:23, 1989.
5. Dalen JE et al: Pulmonary angiography in acute pulmonary embolism: indications, techniques, and results in 367 patients, *Am Heart J* 81:175, 1971.
6. Dhalla NS et al: Pathophysiology of cardiac dysfunction in congestive heart failure, *Can J Cardiol* 9:873, 1993.
7. Don C, Johnson R: The nature and significance of peribronchial cuffing in pulmonary edema, *Radiology* 125:577, 1977.
8. Duerinckx AJ, Higgins CB: Valvular heart disease, *Radiol Clin North Am* 32:613, 1994.
9. Duncan AK et al: Cardiovascular disease in elderly patients, *Mayo Clin Proc* 71:184, 1996.
10. Earnest F, Muhm JR, Sheedy PF: Roentgenographic findings in thoracic aortic dissection, *Mayo Clin Proc* 54:43, 1979.
11. Eyler WR, Clark MD: Dissecting aneurysms of the aorta. Roentgen manifestations including a comparison with other types of aneurysms, *Radiology* 85:1047, 1965.
12. Feder BH, Wilk SP: Localized interlobar effusion in heart failure: phantom lung tumor, *Dis Chest* 30:289, 1956.
13. Fellows KE et al: Evaluation of congenital heart disease with MR imaging: current and coming attractions, *AJR* 159:925, 1992.
14. Fleischner FG: Atypical arrangement of free pleural effusion, *Radiol Clin North Am* 1:347, 1963.
15. Foster E: Congenital heart disease in adults, *West J Med* 163:492, 1995.
16. Fred HL et al: Rapid resolution of pulmonary thromboemboli in man, *JAMA* 196:1137, 1966.
17. Globits S, Higgins CB: Assessment of valvular heart disease by magnetic resonance imaging, *Am Heart J* 129:369, 1995.
18. Greenberg SB, Faerber EN, Balsara RK: Tetralogy of Fallot: diagnostic imaging after palliative and corrective surgery, *J Thorac Imaging* 10:26, 1995.
19. Greenspan RH et al: Accuracy of the chest radiograph in diagnosis of pulmonary embolism, *Invest Radiol* 17:539, 1982.
20. Harrison MO, Conte Pl, Heitzman ER: Radiological detection of clinically occult cardiac failure following myocardial infarction, *Br J Radiol* 44:265, 1971.
21. Higgins IT: The epidemiology of congenital heart disease, *J Chronic Dis* 18:699, 1965.
22. Higgins JA et al: Loculated interlobar pleural effusion due to congestive heart failure, *Arch Intern Med* 96:180, 1955.
23. Hixon ME: Aging and heart failure, *Prog Cardiovasc Nurs* 9:4, 1994.
24. Hodsun CJ: Pulmonary edema and bats-wing shadows, *J Fac Radiol* 1:176, 1950.
25. Hougen TJ, Sell JE: Recent advances in the diagnosis and treatment of coarctation of the aorta, *Curr Opin Cardiol* 10:524, 1995.
26. Jimenez MQ: Ten common congenital cardiac defects, *Pediatrician* 10:3, 1981.
27. Karon BL: Diagnosis and outpatient management of congestive heart failure, *Mayo Clin Proc* 70:1080, 1995.
28. Kersting-Sommerhoff BA et al: Aortic dissection: sensitivity and specificity of MRI imaging, *Radiology* 166:651, 1988.
29. Maher GG, Berger HW: Massive pleural effusion: malignant and nonmalignant causes in 46 patients, *Am Rev Respir Dis* 105:458, 1972.
30. Mahoney LT: Acyanotic congenital heart disease. Atrial and ventricular septal defects, atrioventricular canal, patent ductus arteriosus, pulmonic stenosis, *Cardiol Clin* 11:603, 1993.

PART THREE Chest

31. Majeed HA et al: Acute rheumatic fever and the evolution of rheumatic heart disease: a prospective 12 year follow-up report, *J Clin Epidemiol* 45:871, 1992.

33. Mathur VS et al: Pulmonary angiography one to seven days after experimental pulmonary embolism, *Invest Radiol* 2:304, 1967.

34. McNamara DG: Coarctation of the aorta: difficulties in clinical recognition, *Heart Dis Stroke* 1:202, 1992.

35. Moser KM: Pulmonary embolism: state of the art, *Am Rev Respir Dis* 115:829, 1977.

36. Moss AJ: Clues in diagnosing congenital heart disease, *West J Med* 156:392, 1992.

37. Navas JP, Martinez-Maldonado M: Pathophysiology of edema in congestive heart failure, *Heart Dis Stroke* 2:325, 1993.

38. Nessa CB, Rigler LG: The roentgenological manifestations of pulmonary edema, *Radiology* 37:35, 1941.

39. Ober WB, Moore TE: Congenital cardiac malformations in the neonatal period. An autopsy study, *N Engl J Med* 253:271, 1955.

40. Petersen JA: Recognition of infrapulmonary pleural effusion, *Radiology* 74:34, 1960.

41. Pistolesi M, Giuntini C: Assessment of extravascular lung water, *Radiol Clin North Am* 16:551, 1978.

42. Posniak HV, Demus TC, Marsan RE: Computed tomography of the normal aorta and thoracic aneurysms, *Semin Roentgenol* 24:7, 1989.

43. Rao PS: Coarctation of the aorta, *Semin Nephrol* 15:87, 1995.

44. Rosenow EC, Osmundson PJ, Brown ML: Pulmonary embolism: subject review. *Mayo Clin Proc* 56:161, 1981.

45. Ruttley MS: The chest radiograph in adult heart valve disease, *J Heart Valve Dis* 2:205, 1993.

46. Sabiston DC: Pathophysiology, diagnosis, and management of pulmonary embolism, *Am J Surg* 138:384, 1979.

47. Shinebourne EA, Elseed AM: Relations between fetal blood flow patterns, coarctation of the aorta and pulmonary blood flow, *Br Heart J* 36:492, 1974.

48. Spittell JA: Pulmonary thromboembolism—some editorial comments, *Dis Chest* 54:401, 1968.

49. Staub NC: Pulmonary edema due to increased microvascular permeability to fluid protein, *Annu Rev Med* 32:291, 1981.

50. Stein PD, Saltzman HA, Weg JG: Clinical characteristics of patients with acute pulmonary embolism, *Am J Cardiol* 68:1723, 1991.

51. Steiner RM et al: Congenital heart disease in the adult patient: the value of plain film chest radiology, *J Thorac Imaging* 10:1, 1995.

52. Storstein O: Congenital cardiac disease. An analysis of 1,000 consecutive cases, *Acta Med Scand* 176:195, 1964.

53. Vix VA: Roentgenographic recognition of pleural effusion, *JAMA* 229:695, 1974.

54. Walker JE: Congestive heart failure in the elderly, *Conn Med* 7:293, 1993.

55. Webb GD et al: Transposition complexes, *Cardiol Clin* 11:651, 1993.

56. Wexler L, Higgins CB: The use of magnetic resonance imaging in adult congenital heart disease, *Am J Card Imaging* 9:15, 1995.

57. Wolff DA et al: Aortic dissection: Atypical patterns seen at MR imaging, *Radiology* 181:489, 1991.

58. Youngberg AS: Unilateral diffuse lung opacity, *Radiology* 123:277, 1977.

chapter 22

Pulmonary Infections

DENNIS M MARCHIORI*

Empyema
Lung Abscess

Pneumonia
Tuberculosis

*Special thanks to James C. Reed for his contribution as a reviewer of this material.

Empyema

BACKGROUND

Empyema is an intrapleural infection that is distinguished from simple parapneumonic effusions on the basis of positive cultures. The most likely infectious agents are tuberculosis or Staphylococcus, although many others have been identified. Often other radiographic evidence accompanies empyema, including pneumonia, surgery, trauma, and abdominal infections.[2,20]

IMAGING FINDINGS

The radiographic appearance varies from a slight chest wall mass producing an inward deformity and pleural effusion to the presence of a massive radiopacity obscuring most of the hemithorax. The infective process may become extensive, encasing the lung. Computed tomography is instrumental in determining if the infection is largely pleural or pulmonary (Fig. 22-1).

CLINICAL COMMENTS

Fever, chills, chest pain, and other clinical findings consistent with infection are typically present. Thoracentesis may be necessary to establish the causative agent.[4] Most lung abscesses respond to appropriate antimicrobial therapy, with only about 10% requiring external drainage or surgical therapy.[39]

KEY CONCEPTS

- *Empyema most often develops from pulmonary infection.*
- *It is distinguished from pleural effusion by the presence of a positive culture.*

Lung Abscess

BACKGROUND

A lung abscess is a localized suppurative process marked by tissue necrosis. It most commonly results from aspiration and bronchogenic spread of foreign material or infectious debris secondary to oropharyngeal surgery, sinobronchial infections, dental sepsis, and so on. Aspiration is common among patients who have a suppression of the cough reflex from any of a variety of reasons, including alcoholism, coma, general anesthesia, and narcotic use. Antecedent bacterial pneumonias (commonly *Staphylococcus aureus* and *Klebsiella pneumoniae*) may result in abscess formation.

IMAGING FINDINGS

When secondary to aspiration the most gravity-dependent portions of the lung are typically involved—namely, the posterior segment of the upper lobes during an upright posture and the superior segments of the lower lobes during a supine posture. Lesions typically begin as areas of spherical consolidation. If the cavity forms a communication with the adjacent airways, the cavity's fluid is replaced by air (Fig. 22-2), creating an air-fluid level within the once radiopaque cavity.

CLINICAL COMMENTS

The clinical presentation is characterized by cough, fever, and abundant amounts of foul-smelling, purulent, or sanguineous sputum. Chest pain and weight loss are common. Complications result if the infection extends into the pleural space. The radiographic appearance of a lung abscess should alert the interpreter of the radiograph to the possibility of bronchogenic carcinoma, which may arise in long-standing abscesses and empyemas.

KEY CONCEPTS

- *Lung abscesses are aggressive infections of the lung often secondary to aspiration of infectious debris.*
- *Cavitation follows a communication with adjacent airway.*

Pneumonia

BACKGROUND

Pneumonia represents inflammation of the alveolar parenchyma of the lung from a variety of causes (such as infections, inhalation of chemicals, and trauma to the chest wall). Unless otherwise stated, the common usage of the term *pneumonia* implies an infectious etiology. Pneumonias are classified by their causative organism (such as virus, bacteria, mycoplasma, yeasts, or fungi), radiographic appearance (lobar, lobular or bronchostitial, interstitial, and spherical or round), or etiology (community-acquired, nosocomial, immunosuppressed, or aspiration).

Infections are transmitted to the lung parenchyma by one or more of the following pathways: direct extension, hematogenous spread, inhalation of airborne agents, and aspiration of gastric or nasopharyngeal organisms. The characteristics of selected pneumonias are presented in Table 22-1.

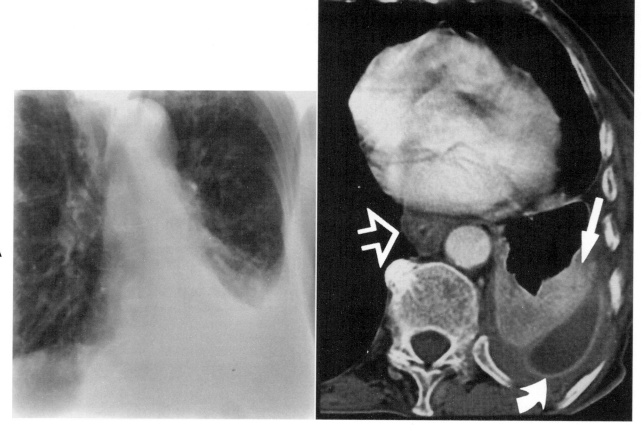

FIG. 22-1 Chest radiograph **(A)** shows consolidation and volume loss of the left lower lobe. An associated left pleural effusion is evident. Contrast-enhanced CT **(B)** shows consolidation of a portion of the left lower lobe *(straight arrow)*. This was an aspiration pneumonia. This patient had an esophageal hiatal hernia that resulted in a Barrett's esophagus. Note the thickened esophageal wall *(open arrow)*. Gastroesophageal reflux resulted in the aspiration pneumonia. The aspiration pneumonia was complicated by a parapneumonic effusion that became infected, and therefore, an empyema *(curved arrow)*. (From Swenson SJ: *Radiology of thoracic diseases: a teaching file*, St Louis, 1993, Mosby.)

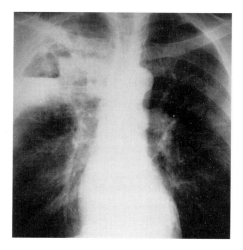

FIG. 22-2 Pneumonia and pulmonary abscess within the right upper lobe. (Courtesy Steven P. Brownstein, Springfield, NJ.)

TABLE 22-1
Characteristics of Selected Pneumonias

Causative agent	Comments
Bacterial (gram-positive)	
Streptococcus pneumoniae (*S. pneumoniae*, pneumococci)	Most common bacterial community-acquired agent[35] and common hospital-acquired pneumonia; it occurs at any age; prototype lobar pneumonia appears as homogenous consolidation[16]; children often demonstrate spherical pattern
Streptococcus pyogenes (*S. pyogenes*)	Seen rarely today, although common in early part of this century, appears as homogenous consolidation, typically of lower lobes; it is often accompanied by large pleural effusion and empyema[5]
Staphylococcus aureus (*S. aureus*)	Commonly results from aspiration of gastric contents; patchy segmental consolidation; cavitation, pneumatoceles, pleural effusion, and empyema are common
Anthrax (*Bacillus anthracis*)	Uncommon in the United States, typically acquired in the Middle East from contact with infected goats; it produces patchy consolidation of the lower lungs with occasional mediastinal widening because of lymphadenopathy[38]
Bacterial (gram-negative)	
Klebsiella pneumoniae (*K. pneumoniae*, Friedländer's disease)	Typically affects individuals with chronic debilitating disease or alcoholism; it appears as homogenous nonsegmental consolidation, often rapidly progressing to involve the entire lobe[17]; regions of lung involvement may appear expanded[14,21]
Legionella pneumophila (*L. pneumophila*)	Found in aquatic environments (humidifiers, water towers, reservoirs, etc.); radiographic appearance begins as patchy peripheral densities, rapidly progressing to involve the entire lobe[12]; pleural effusion is often noted
Pertussis (*Bordetella* [*Haemophilus*] *pertussis*)	Marked by streaking peribronchial consolidation in one or more lobes[3,4]; a tendency exists to involve the right lung to a greater extent
Haemophilus influenzae (*H. influenzae*)	Common in patients with chronic obstructive pulmonary disease,[6] alcoholism, and diabetes mellitus and in children[37]; it exhibits a lower lobe bronchopneumonia pattern; *H. influenzae* is often concomitant with empyema, meningitis, or epiglottitis
Pseudomonas aeruginosa (*P. aeruginosa*)	Common in hospitalized ventilated patients with lowered immunity; it appears as extensive, bilateral, ill-defined opacities in the lower lobes, often with small pleural effusion[22] and abscess formation
Mycobacterial	
Mycobacterium tuberculosis (*M. tuberculosis*)	Distribution largely impacted by social and economic factors; few patients demonstrate signs or symptoms with primary infection; secondary infections are marked by clinical symptoms and radiographic changes in the lung parenchyma, tracheobronchial tree, and hilar and mediastinal lymph nodes (Fig. 22-3)
Mycoplasmal	
Mycoplasma pneumoniae (*M. pneumoniae*)	Exhibits bacterial and viral characteristics; this type is generally recognized as the most common nonbacterial cause of pneumonia[15]; it appears similar to viral pneumonias, with primarily an interstitial pattern in the early stages of the disease,[9] possibly progressing to an air-space pattern (Fig. 22-4)
Viral	
Influenza (Groups A, B, and C)	Usually confined to the upper respiratory tract, rarely produces pneumonia; when present, appears as patchy, bilateral lower lobe consolidation; less commonly, localized consolidation occurs
Varicella zoster	Affects immunosuppressed patients or may complicate lymphoma; the radiographic appearance of acute disease appears as patchy diffuse airspace consolidation[34]; a less common presentation consists of multiple 5 to 10 mm diffusely scattered bilateral radiopacities that have a tendency to calcify[8]
Fungal	
Actinomyces israelii (*A. israelii*)	Represents normal inhabitant of oropharynx; infection results when organism reaches devitalized tissue and proliferates; mandibular infection may complicate dental extractions; pulmonary infection develops from direct extension or aspiration of infectious debris; it appears as peripheral lower lobe airspace consolidation
Histoplasma capsulatum (*H. capsulatum*)	Endemic to the Mississippi, Ohio, and St. Lawrence River valleys and Puerto Rico; the majority of infections are asymptomatic with a past presence suggested by multiple scattered discrete calcific densities with (or without) accompanying calcified hilar and mediastinal lymph nodes; chronic involvement of the mediastinum may lead to fibrosing mediastinitis
Coccidioides immitis (*C. immitis*)	Endemic to the southwest United States (San Joaquin Valley), infected individuals may describe arthralgias and erythema nodosum (valley fever); imaging findings include well-defined segmental radiopacities, which typically resolve over time; mediastinal and hilar lymphadenopathy may be present; the chronic progressive form of the disease is similar to postprimary tuberculosis or histoplasmosis

Continued

TABLE 22-I
Characteristics of Selected Pneumonias—cont'd

Causative agent	Comments
Fungal—cont'd	
Aspergillus fumigatus (*A. fumigatus*)	Presents as aspergilloma ("fungal ball" or "mycetoma") representing mass in a preexisting pulmonary cavity; more invasive varieties of parenchymal infection are seen in the immunocompromised patient[41] (Fig. 22-5)
Blastomyces dermatitidis (*B. dermatitidis*)	Chronic systemic infection appearing as nonsegmental homogenous consolidation with a tendency to involve the upper lobes of the lung; less commonly it presents as single or multiple mass lesions[19]
Cryptococcus neoformans (*C. neoformans;* formerly *Torula histolytica*)	Worldwide distribution, infection results from inhalation of contaminated dust; a wide variety exists of radiographic presentations; it is associated with lymphomas, steroid therapy, and AIDS; meningitis and encephalitis represent the most serious complications; the most common radiographic appearance is a single well-defined nodule or mass,[18] less commonly region of consolidation[13]
Parasitic	
Pneumocystis carinii (*P. carinii*)	Significant pneumonia among immunocompromised patients (e.g., AIDS and organ transplant patients), demonstrates bilateral parahilar fine, ground-glass radiographic appearance[30]; it may progress to air-space consolidation pattern (Fig. 22-6); pleural effusion and lymphadenopathy are uncommon
Echinococcus granulosus (*E. granulosis*—infection called *hydatid disease*)	Tapeworm whose definitive host is dogs and intermediate host is sheep; when man becomes the accidental intermediate host, disease results; pulmonary involvement is marked by a well-defined, three-layered pulmonary mass[7] or cyst, most often in the lower lobes; rupture of the cyst may produce a radiodense air shadow ("crescent" sign) or noticeable floating debris on the internal fluid of the cyst ("water lily" sign)

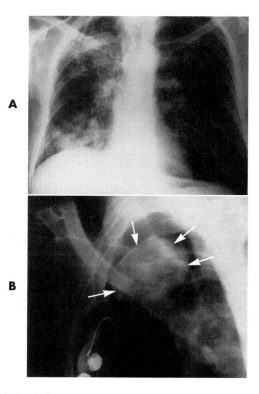

FIG. 22-3   A, Posteroanterior projection demonstrating pneumonia and volume loss of the right lung. **B,** Oblique projection demonstrating aspergillosis fungal ball within tuberculosis cavity *(arrows).* (Courtesy Steven P. Brownstein, Springfield, NJ.)

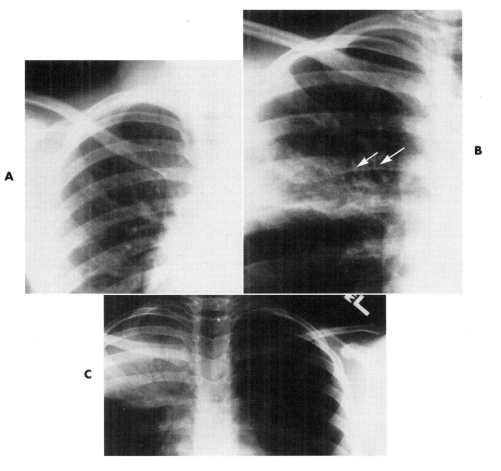

FIG. 22-4   Mycoplasma pneumonia within the right upper lobe. **A,** Posteroanterior radiograph demonstrating no abnormalities, taken when clinical symptoms began. **B,** Radiograph taken 2 weeks later demonstrating radiolucent tubular shadows representing air-filled bronchi contrasted by the surrounding fluid-filled alveoli (air-bronchogram) *(arrows)*. This appearance is indicative of an air-space pattern of pulmonary disease. **C,** Radiograph taken 2 weeks later (4 weeks from presentation), which shows resolution of pneumonia. (Courtesy Steven P. Brownstein, Springfield, NJ.)

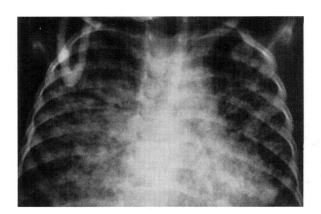

FIG. 22-5   Bilateral consolidating pulmonary radiodense areas in a 15-month-old male with primary invasive aspergillosis. (Courtesy Steven P. Brownstein, Springfield, NJ.)

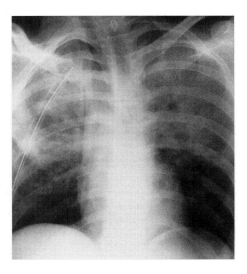

FIG. 22-6   Bilateral partially consolidating pulmonary airspace shadows in the upper and middle regions of the lungs ("hazy regions") secondary to pneumocystosis carinii pneumonia in a patient with AIDS. (Courtesy Steven P. Brownstein, Springfield, NJ.)

TABLE 22-2
Radiographic Appearance of Pneumonia

Radiographic type	Radiographic appearance
Broncho(lobular) pneumonia	Represents the most common pneumonic pattern, in which inflammatory exudate involves some and spares some of the parenchymal tissue along a large airway; it appears as fluffy, patchy, multifocal densities tracking along a large airway; because the airways are affected there may be volume loss, and air-bronchograms are more uncommon; common agents include *S. aureus, H. influenza,* gram-negative bacteria
Lobar pneumonia	Inflammatory exudate beginning in the periphery of the lung and spreading circumferentially through pores of Kohn and canals of Lambert to involve adjacent lung tissue, involving the entire bronchopulmonary segment and eventually lobe; the region of pneumonia appears homogenously radiodense and may eventually involve the entire lobe; because the airways are not involved, volume loss is rare and air bronchograms are common; common agents include *S. pneumoniae, K. pneumoniae, S. aureus*
Interstitial pneumonia	Localized or generalized thickening of the interstitium producing peribronchial or reticulonodular radiographic patterns; it is typically caused by viral or mycoplasma infections
Aspiration pneumonia	Bilateral, poorly-defined consolidation in gravity-dependent portions of the lung

TABLE 22-3
Classic Radiographic Presentations of Pneumonia

Radiographic appearance	Organisms
Consolidation of all or nearly all of a lobe	Bacteria
Consolidation with cavitation or pneumatoceles	*Staphylococcus aureus*
Consolidation with expansion of the lobe	Klebsiella (Fig. 22-7)
Spherical (nodular) pneumonia	Pneumococcal,[33] *Legionella micdadei,*[31] and Q fever[28] (Fig. 22-8)
Localized or widespread reticulonodular pattern	Viruses[10] or mycoplasma
Miliary nodules	Tuberculosis, fungi, or varicella-zoster
Patchy upper lobe consolidations	Tuberculosis, histoplasmosis, blastomycosis, cryptococcosis, etc.
Large pleural effusions	*S. aureus* and *S. pyogenes*

IMAGING FINDINGS

Chest radiography remains the primary tool to establish the presence and extent of pneumonia. Although it should be emphasized that the lack of radiographic evidence does not exclude pneumonia, nor does the presence of consolidation exclusively indicate the presence of pneumonia. It is imperative that clinical findings be correlated to the radiographic appearance.

Although large areas of crossover exist, several radiographic patterns of lung infection have been identified (Table 22-2). However, except for a few classic presentations (Table 22-3), the radiographic appearance of most lung infections is so general that radiographs offer little help in isolating a particular causative agent.[36]

The essential radiographic finding of pneumonia is partial or complete lung consolidation, often with associated pleural effusion, a silhouette sign, lung cavitation, and empyema (Fig. 22-9). Selected causative agents and their radiographic appearances are presented in Table 22-1.

CLINICAL COMMENTS

Pneumonia is the most life-threatening infectious disease.[32] Its clinical importance depends on the causative organism involved, the patient's age, and any predisposing illness. Mortality is higher for individuals with a preexisting condition or otherwise healthy children and elderly patients. Clinical findings of pneumonia typically precede radiographic evidence. Further, clinical findings resolve before imaging findings of pneumonia resolve. Serial films may help in assessing treatments. However, given the often low correlation between imaging findings and patient symptoms, it is difficult to support frequent radiographs used to follow the course of pneumonias in the general population.

Most pneumonias resolve within 4 weeks in otherwise healthy individuals. Those who remain unresponsive to conservative measures or exhibit common reoccurrence suggest misdiagnosis or the presence of an underlying condition.[40]

KEY CONCEPTS

- *Pneumonia is a commonly encountered clinical entity.*
- *It is classified by causative organism (such as viral, bacteria, mycoplasma, yeasts, and fungi), radiographic appearance (lobar, lobular or bronchostitial, interstitial, and spherical or round) or etiology (community-acquired, nosocomial, immunosuppressed, or aspiration).*
- *Radiographic findings are typically marked by partial or complete lung consolidation.*
- *Most pneumonias resolve within 4 weeks in otherwise healthy individuals; children, the elderly, and patients with comorbidity should be monitored more closely.*

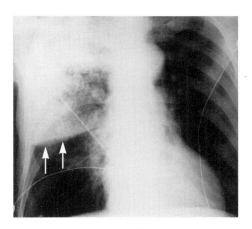

FIG. 22-7 Inferiorly bulging right horizontal fissure secondary to Klebsiella pneumonia within right upper lobe *(arrows)*. (Courtesy Steven P. Brownstein, Springfield, NJ.)

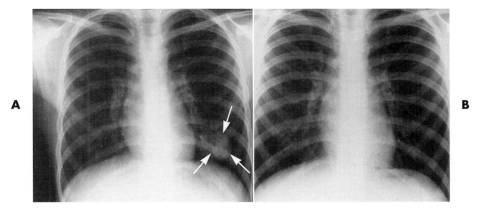

FIG. 22-8 Round pneumonia located adjacent to the left heart border, before (**A,** *arrows*) and after (**B**) antibiotic therapy. (Courtesy Steven P. Brownstein, Springfield, NJ.)

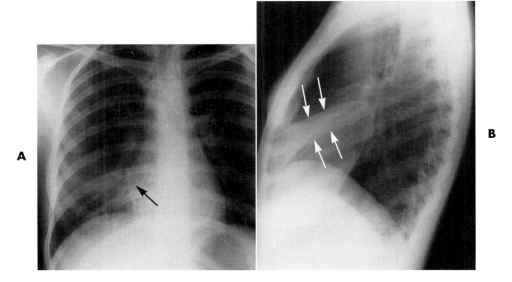

FIG. 22-9 Pneumonia of right middle lobe. **A,** Posteroanterior projection with absence of a clearly demarcated right heart border resulting from contact of the fluid-filled right middle lobe (silhouette sign) *(arrow)*. **B,** Lateral projection demonstrating a wedge-shaped consolidated right middle lobe with the apex of the consolidated segment directed toward the hilum *(arrows)*. (Courtesy Steven P. Brownstein, Springfield, NJ.)

Tuberculosis

BACKGROUND

Pulmonary tuberculosis (TB) is a chronic granulomatous disease characterized pathologically by caseating granulomas or pneumonia.[23] Although widespread at the turn of the century, tuberculosis has declined markedly throughout most of this century in developed countries. However in recent years a slight increase has been noted.[29] This is related to higher incidence among the homeless, prisoners, elderly in nursing homes, IV drug users, and AIDS patients.[1,11]

For the most part, tuberculosis infections result from inhalation of *Mycobacterium tuberculosis* sputum droplets produced by coughing of infected persons. The pathogen is disseminated by homogenous, bronchogenic, and lymphangitic mechanisms. Pulmonary infections are classified into primary and secondary (postprimary or reinfection) types based on clinical and radiographic criteria. Primary infection represents the first recorded exposure to the pathogen, in which no immunity exists. Secondary infections occur in subsequent exposures where some degree of immunity is present.

Classically, primary tuberculosis is a childhood disorder, and because of the lack of clinical symptoms, the infection often goes unnoticed. If the immune response is overcome by the inhaled bacilli, an inflammatory focus develops. The surrounding tissue response to the acute tuberculous infection results in caseous necrosis and fibrosus. The area may undergo dystrophic calcification and granuloma (tuberculoma) formation, in which the active disease and containment of the disease are balanced. Postprimary infection occurs in adults as either a reactivation of a primary infection or may represent a slow continuation of the active state of a primary infection with no intervening indolent stage.[25]

IMAGING FINDINGS

Chest radiography remains the mainstay in the radiologic evaluation of suspected or proven pulmonary tuberculosis.[27] Because tuberculosis often passes unrecognized, radiographs are not always available during the initial exposure. Lymphadenopathy, with or without parenchymal consolidation, is the hallmark imaging finding of primary tuberculosis (Fig. 22-10).[26] Hilar lymphadenopathy represents lymphangitic spread from the parenchymal lesion. Alternatively, no radiographic evidence of infection may be present.[26] The right side is more commonly involved, and no predilection for the upper or lower lobes exists.

In otherwise healthy individuals, the imaging findings typically resolve completely. Occasionally a characteristic primary complex

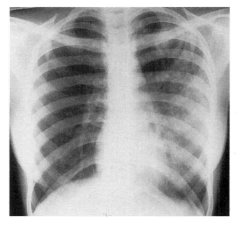

FIG. 22-10 Primary tuberculosis presenting as incomplete pulmonary consolidation in the middle left lung field. (Courtesy Steven P. Brownstein, Springfield, NJ.)

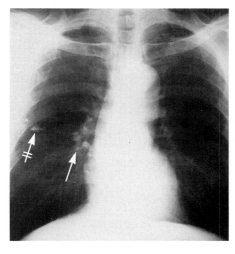

FIG. 22-11 Calcific granulomas in the right hilum *(arrow)* with associated parenchymal focus of calcification peripherally *(crossed arrow)*. Together this configuration is known as a *Ranke complex* indicative of healed tuberculosis infection.

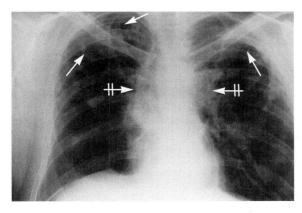

FIG. 22-12   Secondary (reinfection) tuberculosis presenting as bilateral hilar adenopathy (*crossed arrows*) and linear radiodense lines (*arrows*) in the upper lung fields. (Courtesy Steven P. Brownstein, Springfield, NJ.)

(Ranke complex) provides residual evidence of a primary infection, as seen in Fig. 22-11. A Ranke complex is the combination of a calcified region of parenchymal involvement (known as a *Ghon tubercle*) and corresponding hilar lymph node calcification.

Reinfection tuberculosis produces a progressive infection with predilection of the posterior and apical segments of the upper lobes and, like primary infections, is more common on the right. Lymphadenopathy is a less common manifestation than the primary form of the disease. Parenchymal involvement appears as subsegmental, poorly defined, incomplete consolidations, which have a tendency to coalesce into strandlike radiopacities (Fig. 22-12). The presence of cavitation indicates reinfection tuberculosis and suggests disease is active.

Calcified hilar lymph nodes may erode adjacent airways to become broncholiths, which may lead to obstructive atelectasis. Also, bronchogenic spread of tuberculosis may produce a widespread lung infection. Hematogenous spread of tuberculosis results in discrete miliary nodules widely scattered throughout both lungs as well as systemic foci of disease. Pleural effusion may occur in response to either primary or postprimary infections and are more common when parenchymal involvement is present.

CLINICAL COMMENTS

Predisposing conditions for primary infection include alcoholism, corticosteroids, and diabetes mellitus. Symptoms of cough and productive sputum are rarely present. As with other infections the presence of a single opacity without a confirmed history of TB is presumed to be a solitary pulmonary nodule or "coin lesion" of undetermined etiology. Postprimary infections are more likely associated with symptoms. Typically the patient exhibits cough, night sweats, weight loss, and pleuritic chest pain. Hematogenous spread of TB is an uncommon but serious problem resulting in multiple systemic sites of infection, necessitating immediate attention.

KEY CONCEPTS

- *Persons at risk for tuberculosis infection include homeless, prisoners, elderly in nursing homes, IV drug users, and AIDS patients.*
- *Infections are classified into primary and secondary (postprimary or reinfection) types based on clinical and radiographic criteria.*
- *Primary findings present with no or limited imaging findings; secondary infections exhibit predilection for the upper lung regions and appear as lung scarring and possible cavity formations.*

References

1. Agrons GA, Markowitz RI, Kramer SS: Pulmonary tuberculosis in children, *Sem Roentgenol* 28:58, 1993.
2. Alfageme I et al: Empyema of the thorax in adults: etiology, microbiologic findings, and management, *Chest* 103:839, 1993.
3. Barnhard HJ, Kniker WT: Roentgenologic findings in pertussis with particular emphasis on the "shaggy heart" sign, *AJR* 4:445, 1960.
4. Bartlett JG: Anaerobic bacterial pneumonitis, *Am Rev Respir Dis* 119:19, 1979.
5. Basiliere JL, Bistrong HW, Spence WF: Streptococcal pneumonia: recent outbreaks in military recruit populations, *Am J Med* 44:580, 1968.
6. Bates JH: The role of infection during exacerbations of chronic bronchitis, *Ann Intern Med* 97:130, 1982.
7. Beggs I: The radiology of hydatid disease, *Am J Roentgenol* 145:639, 1985.
8. Brunton FJ, Moore ME: A survey of pulmonary calcification following adult chicken-pox, *Br J Radiol* 42:256, 1969.
9. Cameron DC, Borthwick RN, Philip T: The radiographic patterns of acute *Mycoplasma pneumonitis, Clin Radiol* 28:173, 1977.
10. Conte P, Heitzman EK, Markarian B: Viral pneumonia: roentgen pathological correlations, *Radiology* 95:267, 1970.
11. Couser JI, Glassroth J: Tuberculosis: an epidemic in older adults, *Clin Chest Med* 14:491, 1993.
12. Fairbank JT, Patel MM, Dietrich PA: Legionnaire's disease, *J Thorac Imag* 6:6, 1991.
13. Feigin DS: Pulmonary cryptococcosis: Radiologic-pathologic correlation of its three forms, *Am J Roentgenol* 141:1263, 1983.
14. Felson LB, Rosenberg LS, Hamburger M: Roentgen findings in acute Friedlander's pneumonia, *Radiology* 53:559, 1949.
15. Foy HM et al: Radiographic study of Mycoplasma pneumoniae pneumonia, *Am Rev Respir Dis* 108:469, 1973.
16. Fraser RG, Wortzman G: Acute pneumococcal lobar pneumonia: the significance of nonsegmental distribution, *J Can Assoc Radiol* 3:37, 1959.
17. Frommhold W, Lagemann K, Wolf KJ: Die akute Klebsiellen-pneumonie, *Fortschr Geb Romtgellstr* 121:25, 1974.
18. Gordonson J et al: Pulmonary cryptococcosis, *Radiology* 112:557, 1974.
19. Halvorsen RA et al: Pulmonary blastomycosis: radiologic manifestations, *Radiology* 150:1, 1984.
20. Hanna JW, Reed JC, Choplin RH: Pleural infections: clinicoradiologic review, *J Thorac Imag* 6:68, 1991.
21. Holmes RB: Friedlander's pneumonia, *AJR* 75:728, 1956.
22. Iannini PB, Claffey T, Quintiliani R: Bacteremic Pseudomonas pneumonia, *JAMA* 230:558, 1974.
23. Im JG et al: CT-pathology correlation of pulmonary tuberculosis, *Crit Rev Diagn Imaging* 36:227, 1995.
24. Krysl J et al: Radiologic features of pulmonary tuberculosis: an assessment of 188 cases, *Can Assoc Radiol J* 45:101, 1994.
25. Lee KS et al: Adult-onset pulmonary tuberculosis: findings on chest radiographs and CT scans, *Am J Roentgenol* 160:753, 1993.
26. Leung AN, Muller NL, Pineda PR, FitzGerald JM: Primary tuberculosis in childhood: radiographic manifestations, *Radiology* 182:87, 1992.
27. McAdams HP, Erasmus J, Winter JA: Radiologic manifestations of pulmonary tuberculosis, *Radiol Clin North Am* 33:655, 1995.
28. Millar JK: The chest film findings in Q fever—a series of 35 cases, *Clin Radiol* 29:371, 1978.
29. Nainar HS: Tuberculosis: revisited, *ASDC J Dent Child* 59:450, 1992.
30. Peters SG, Prakash UB: Pneumocystis carinii pneumonia. Review of 53 cases, *Am J Med* 82:73, 1987.
31. Pope TL et al: Pittsburgh pneumonia 3 agent: chest film manifestations, *AJR* 138:237, 1983.

32. Putnam JS, Tuazon CU: Symposium on infectious lung diseases: foreword, *Med Clin North Am* 64:317, 1980.

33. Rose RW, Ward BH: Spherical pneumonias in children simulating pulmonary and mediastinal masses, *Radiology* 106:179, 1973.

34. Sargent EN, Carson MJ, Reilly ED: Roentgenographic manifestations of varicella pneumonia with postmortem correlation, *Am J Roentgenol* 98:305, 1966.

35. Smith CB, Overall IC: Clinical and epidemiologic clues to the diagnosis of respiratory infections, *Radiol Clin North Am* 11:261, 1973.

36. Tew J, Calenoff L, Berlin BS: Bacterial or nonbacterial pneumonia: accuracy of radiographic diagnosis, *Radiology* 124:607, 1977.

37. Trollfors B et al: Incidence, predisposing factors and manifestations of invasive Haemophilus influenzae infections in adults, *Eur J Clin Microbiol* 3:180, 1984.

38. Vessal K et al: Radiological changes in inhalational anthrax: a report of radiological and pathological correlation in two cases, *Clin Radiol* 25:471, 1975.

39. Wiedemann HP, Rice TW: Lung abscesses and empyema, *Sem Thorac Cardiovasc Surg* 7:119, 1995.

40. Winterbauer RH, Bedon GA, Ball WC Jr: Recurrent pneumonia: predisposing illness and clinical patterns in 158 patients, *Ann Intern Med* 70:689, 1969.

41. Young RC et al: Aspergillosis: the spectrum of the disease in 98 patients, *Medicine* 49:47, 1970.

chapter 23

Thoracic Neoplasms

DENNIS M MARCHIORI*

Bronchial Carcinoid Tumors
Bronchogenic Carcinoma
Hamartoma

Lymphoma
Metastatic Lung Disease
Pleural Mesothelioma

Teratomas
Thymic Masses

Bronchial Carcinoid Tumors

BACKGROUND

Bronchial carcinoid tumors are uncommon pulmonary tumors, formerly termed *bronchial adenomas*. The term *adenoma* to describe these lesions is a misnomer resulting from their locally invasive nature, tendency for recurrence, and occasional metastasis to extrapulmonary tissues. They typically occur in patients at least 40 years of age but represent the most common primary lung tumors under the age of 16 years. These tumors arise from neuroectodermal cells[49,68] and are hormonally active, known to produce symptoms similar to Cushing's disease.[22,25] Overall, 75% arise in the lobar bronchi, 10% in the mainstem bronchi, and 15% in the periphery of the lung.[18] Ninety percent of bronchial carcinoids are well-differentiated lesions. Atypical carcinoids are less common but exhibit a higher malignancy rate than well-differentiated lesions.

IMAGING FINDINGS

Often a solitary nodule can be seen on plain films. This is more likely if the lesion is peripherally located. Bronchial carcinoids are commonly discovered by recognizing associated findings of bronchial obstruction. If the airway obstruction is partial, a check-valve obstruction may result in overexpansion of the distal airspace. If obstruction is complete, atelectasis results. Recurrent pneumonia, bronchiectasis, and calcification of the lesion also may occur.[6] Computed tomography (CT) is helpful in confirming suspected lesions (Fig. 23-1).

CLINICAL COMMENTS

Because bronchial carcinoid tumors are commonly centrally located in the lobar divisions of bronchi, they often present with findings related to bronchial obstruction (recurrent atelectasis and pneumonia). Clinical findings of hemoptysis, wheezing, cough, and atypical asthma may be noted. A small percentage of patients remain asymptomatic. Resection is typical, with a 5-year survival rate of 95%. The prognosis is usually excellent and is more specifically determined when the pathological grade and stage of the tumor is known.

---

*Special thanks to James C. Reed for his contribution as a reviewer of this material.

KEY CONCEPTS

- *Bronchial carcinoid tumors are low-grade malignancies most commonly arising in the lobar bronchi.*
- *Well-differentiated carcinoid tumors represent almost 90% of all bronchial carcinoids.*
- *Lesions may be directly seen on radiographs or are often found by recognizing concurrent findings of airway obstruction. Usually, resection is associated with an excellent prognosis.*

Bronchogenic Carcinoma

BACKGROUND

Risk factors. Bronchogenic carcinoma (lung cancer) was a relatively uncommon tumor at the beginning of the century. It has grown to become the leading cause of cancer-related deaths among men and women. Lung cancer accounts for 20% of cancer deaths among men and 10% among women, replacing breast cancer as the most common cause of cancer death among women.[44] Cancer rates correlate positively with population density, urbanization, industrialization, cigarette smoking, and carcinogenic inhalants (such as asbestos, nickel, uranium, and chromates).

Cigarette smoking is probably the most common important risk factor for developing lung cancer. Its development is related to both the duration and dose of cigarette smoking.[21,69] Although rates of smoking among men appear to have leveled off, smoking among women has increased[7] and is likely to be responsible for the contemporary increase in lung cancer rates among women.

Categorization. Bronchogenic carcinomas develop from the airways, not the lung parenchyma. Parenchymal neoplasms are represented by leiomyomas, fibromas, chondromas and other mesenchymal derivatives.[60] Bronchogenic tumors are divided into four groups, based on histology: squamous cell (epidermoid) carcinoma, adenocarcinoma, large cell carcinoma, and small (oat) cell carcinoma[33,51] (Table 23-1). Bronchoalveolar carcinoma is a subtype of the adenocarcinoma cell type.[14]

Lesions are often divided by location into central (near the hilum) or peripheral (lateral to the hilum) location. Peripheral lesions appear as masses (greater than 3 cm diameter) or nodules (less than or equal to 3 cm diameter)[26] in the lateral lung field arising from the third or fourth order bronchi and beyond. Central lesions arise from the main stem, lobar, or segmental bronchi and appear as hilar enlargements or present with secondary findings

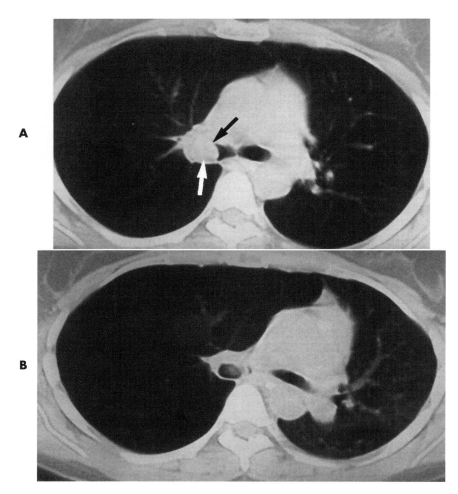

FIG. 23-1 **A,** CT shows an endobronchial tumor in the right mainstem bronchus *(arrows)*. CT performed after exhalation **(B)** shows a significant mediastinal shift to the patient's left as a result of air trapping on the right. (From Swenson SJ: *Radiology of thoracic diseases: a teaching file,* St Louis, 1993, Mosby.)

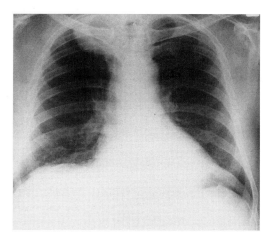

FIG. 23-2 Opacification of the lung above the right first rib caused by a bronchogenic carcinoma (Pancoast tumor). (Courtesy Steven P. Brownstein, Springfield, NJ.)

TABLE 23-1
Radiographic Appearance of Bronchogenic Carcinoma Types

Type	Radiographic appearance*
• Squamous cell (epidermoid) carcinoma	Most often a central lesion with locally invasive hilar and mediastinal involvement, often presenting as lobar collapse; peripheral presentation appears as nodule, mass, or cavity
• Adenocarcinoma	Most common cell type, nearly always presents as peripheral mass, smaller in size than large cell type
Alveolar cell carcinoma (bronchoalveolar cell carcinoma)	Subtype of adenocarcinoma, most commonly presents as a nodule, but it is more noted for its presentation of diffuse or localized air-space disease pattern
• Small (oat) cell carcinoma	Classically presents as a hilar or mediastinal metastasis while the primary tumor remains occult; it is the most aggressive cell type, having the worst prognosis; central involvement may lead to atelectasis and/or superior vena cava syndrome
• Large cell carcinoma	Like adenocarcinoma, presents in a peripheral location, but it is most often larger in size than adenocarcinoma cell type

*Considerable crossover exists in radiographic appearance, making distinction between types difficult.

related to airway obstruction. Approximately 60% of lesions are central and 40% are peripheral.[4] Sixty percent of lesions (peripheral and central) are right-sided. Similarly, 60% of peripheral lesions are in the upper lung (Fig. 23-2), 30% in the lower, and the remaining 10% in the middle and lingual segments. The average age of patients with recently recognized lung cancer is 53 years, with 80% of lesions developing between the ages of 40 to 70 years.[66]

IMAGING FINDINGS

The radiographic features of a nodule or mass are extremely important to the clinical management of the patient. When considered with the patient age, the growth rate, calcification, size, and location of the lesion are important indicators of a benign versus malignant lesion (Fig. 23-3). Associated bone destruction is a strong indicator of malignancy (Fig. 23-4).

Location. Central tumors demonstrate radiographic changes related to airway obstruction. Airway obstruction leads to volume changes presenting as atelectasis or overinflation (if a check-valve mechanism develops), both of which may displace the mediastinum, heart shadow, diaphragm, or other anatomical borders. A consolidated radiographic pattern may result from postobstructive pneumonitis, which refers to marked retention of lung secretions in the alveolar spaces secondary to airway obstruction.[9]

An enlarged hilum is a common finding of central tumors.[56] The enlarged hilum represents the tumor mass itself or associated lymph node involvement. A classic radiographic appearance, known as the *S-sign of Golden,* develops when the hilar mass is found with concurrent radiopacity of the right upper lobe secondary to either atelectasis or postobstructive pneumonitis resulting from airway obstruction (Fig. 23-5). The inferior border of the parenchymal radiopacity appears as a smooth, reversed S-shape. The radiographic appearance appears S-shaped when present on the patient's left side.

Pancoast (superior sulcus) tumors are defined as dense, homogenous masses with smooth borders located in the lung apex (Fig. 23-6). Lesions often demonstrate adjacent rib or vertebral destruction (Fig. 23-7). Most Pancoast tumors are caused by squamous cell carcinomas, although other types of bronchogenic tumors may be reponsible. Alternatively, Pancoast tumors may appear with little more than subtle pleural thickening.

Size. Peripheral lesions often present as only a spherical radiopacity (Fig. 23-8).[10] Lesions present in variable sizes, but they

are difficult to detect on plain films if less than 1 cm in diameter.[28,42] The average diameter at the time of discovery is 5 cm.[66] Lesions greater than 3 cm in diameter are malignant 85% of the time.[53] Most solitary pulmonary nodules (lesions less than or equal to 3 cm in diameter) are indeterminate at the time of discovery. Further procedures (CT, biopsy, and thoracotomy) are needed to reach a definitive diagnosis.[30]

Nipple shadows, moles, and other body wall lesions may mimic pulmonary nodules, particularly in the periphery of the lung. Repeating the radiograph with metallic markers over the area in question is a simple method to exclude such body wall lesions (Fig. 23-9).

Borders. The appearance of the outer border of the lesion has been emphasized in the past. Circumferential strandlike radiopacities radiating from the outer border of the tumor (corona radiata) have been described[71] as characteristic but not specific to bronchogenic tumor.[35] The irregular outer border is believed to represent tissue fibrosis or radial spread of the tumor. A lobulated appearance of the outer border, representing areas of rapid growth, is found in 50% of peripheral tumors. Cavitation has been described in 16% of peripheral lesions,[66] most often seen in the squamous cell type.

Calcification. Calcification of bronchogenic tumors is rarely demonstrated on plain film studies (Fig. 23-10). Computed tomography demonstrates calcification in 6% to 7% of lesions.[45,73] As depicted in Fig. 23-11, certain patterns of calcification strongly suggest a benign etiology. Central, laminated, or total homogeneous calcification is typical of granulomas. A "comma-shaped" or "popcorn" calcification pattern suggests a hamartoma. Eccentric calcification is associated with bronchogenic carcinoma, representing calcium produced by the tumor, dystrophic calcification of ischemic tissue, or a granuloma that has been engulfed by the growing tumor mass. Patients who demonstrate masses and nodules with no calcification or calcification only in the periphery of the lesions should be vigorously studied for the possibility of malignancy (Fig. 23-12).

Growth rate. It has been estimated that on average bronchogenic tumors double in volume every 1 to 18 months (Fig. 23-13).[27,34] Doubling in volume is equal to a 25% increase in diameter. Lesions that double in size more rapidly or more slowly than normal suggest another cause (infection, edema, etc.). Lesions known to be stable over a 2-year period can be assumed to be benign.

Text continued on p. 870

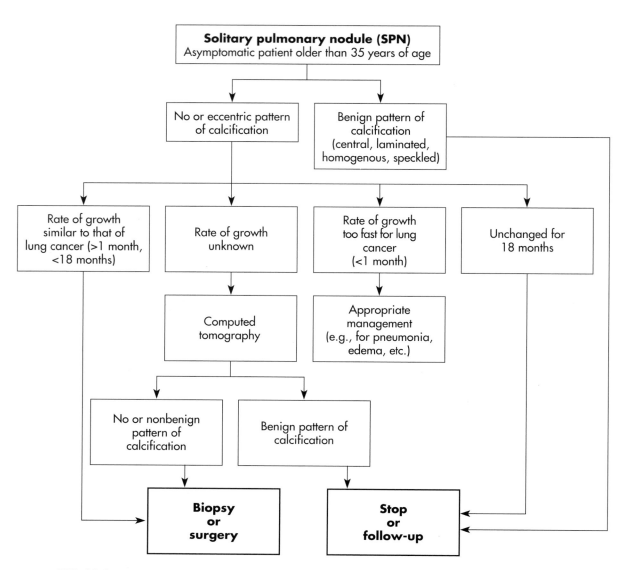

FIG. 23-3 Management algorithm of solitary pulmonary nodules of patients in cancer age group, based on imaging findings.

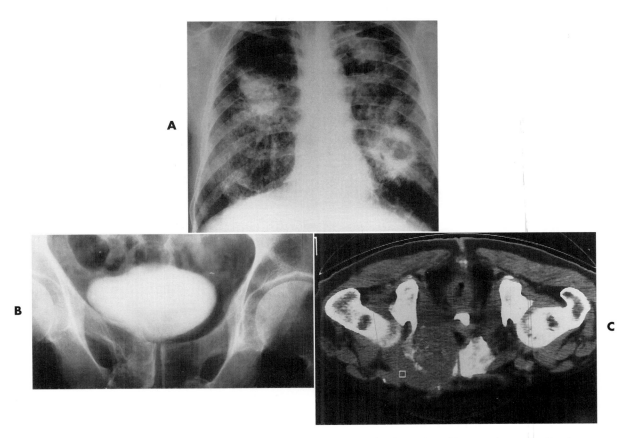

FIG. 23-4 **A,** Cavitating squamous cell carcinoma of the left lower lung field in a patient with progressive massive fibrosis noted by the bilateral, asymmetrical radiodensities in the upper lung fields. Plain film radiograph **(B)** and CT scan **(C)** revealing lytic bone destruction of the right pubis resulting from metastasis of the lung carcinoma. (Courtesy Steven P. Brownstein, Springfield, NJ.)

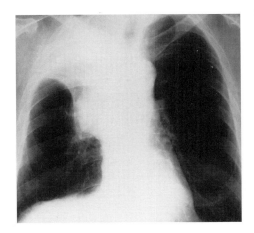

FIG. 23-5 Bronchogenic carcinoma presenting as a right hilar mass producing obstructive atelectasis of the right upper lobe. The serpentine configuration of the horizontal fissure contouring the atelectatic lung and hilar mass is known as the (reversed) *S-sign of Golden.*

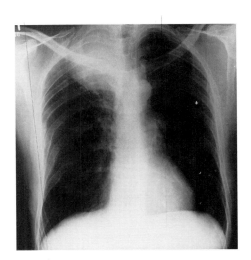

FIG. 23-6 Bronchogenic carcinoma presenting as a mass in the right lung apex (Pancoast tumor). (Courtesy Steven P. Brownstein, Springfield, NJ.)

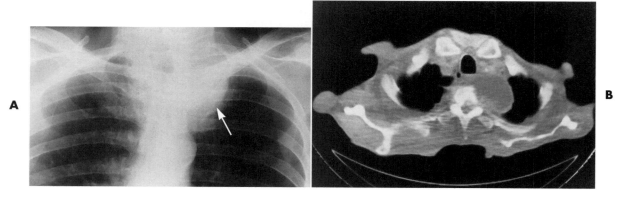

FIG. 23-7   A, Bronchogenic carcinoma within the medial portion of the patient's left lung apex (Pancoast tumor) *(arrow).* **B,** CT reveals the tumor mass with associated vertebral body destruction. (Courtesy Steven P. Brownstein, Springfield, NJ.)

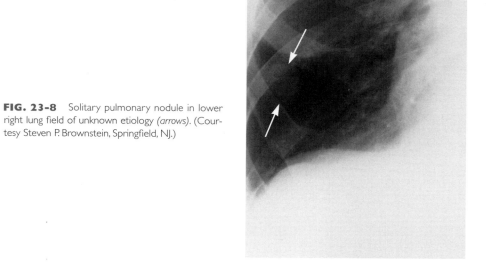

FIG. 23-8   Solitary pulmonary nodule in lower right lung field of unknown etiology *(arrows).* (Courtesy Steven P. Brownstein, Springfield, NJ.)

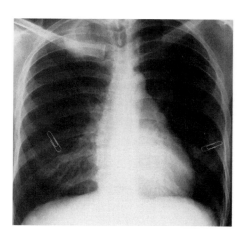

FIG. 23-9   Paper clips confirming that nipple shadows represent the bilateral symmetrical pulmonary nodules. In addition, a bronchogenic carcinoma is in the apex of the patient's right lung (Pancoast tumor). (Courtesy Steven P. Brownstein, Springfield, NJ.)

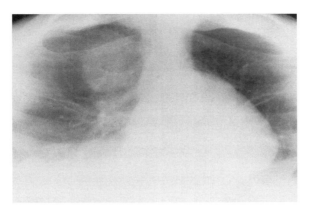

FIG. 23-10 Apical lordotic projection demonstrating noncalcific mass in the right lung apex, consistent with bronchogenic carcinoma. (Courtesy Steven P. Brownstein, Springfield, NJ.)

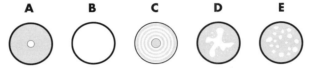

FIG. 23-11 Benign patterns of nodule calcification. **A,** Central. **B,** Homogenous (total). **C,** Laminated. **D,** Amorphous. **E,** Speckled.

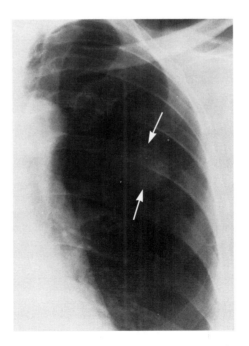

FIG. 23-12 Squamous cell bronchogenic carcinoma presenting as a noncalcified solitary pulmonary nodule at the level of the posterior angle of the sixth left rib (arrows). (Courtesy Steven P. Brownstein, Springfield, NJ.)

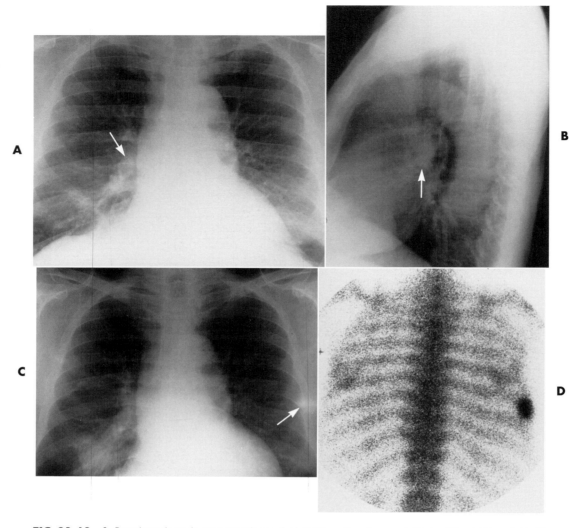

FIG. 23-13   A, Bronchogenic carcinoma presenting on the initial film with pulmonary infiltrate of the right lung field with enlargement of the right hilum *(arrow).* **B,** Lateral projection revealing radiodense region in the aortic pulmonary window corresponding to the right hilum *(arrow).* **C,** 13 months later, the pulmonary infiltrate has consolidated into a mass. Also of interest is an unrelated fracture of the lateral margin of the seventh left rib *(arrow).* **D,** Radionuclide bone scan demonstrating radionuclide uptake at the fracture site. (Courtesy Steven P. Brownstein, Springfield, NJ.)

Growth rate is most often assessed by comparing the appearance of a lesion to its appearance on earlier radiographs of the same patient that may be available. If the past radiographs reveal a stable lesion, no further work-up may be necessary. However, if past studies do not reveal the lesion, or if the lesion appears to have grown, further work-up is necessary to exclude aggressive pathology (Fig. 23-14).

CLINICAL COMMENTS

Twenty-five percent of lung cancer patients are asymptomatic at the time of diagnosis.[58] When clinical findings are present, they are nonspecific and of little diagnostic value. When carcinoma is still confined to the lung, clinical findings of cough, wheezing, and hemoptysis are common clinical manifestations. Mediastinal involvement is suggested with hoarseness, chest pain, brachial plexus neuropathy, Horner's syndrome, superior vena cava obstruction, and dysphagia. Recurrent, unresolving, or persistent (unchanged over 2 weeks) patterns of pneumonia suggest underlying airway obstruction.

Because of their anatomical location, Pancoast tumors are often associated with clinical findings of Horner's syndrome (ptosis, miosis, anidrosis, and enophthalmos) and brachial plexus neuropathy.

Treatments for lung cancer are disappointing with a 5-year survival rate of less than 10%[55] to 13%[23]. The poor prognosis is in part due to the advanced stage of the disease at the time of initial recognition. By the time clinical symptoms are noted, the tumor is in its later stages.[70] The formation of lung tumors predates their initial identification by 8 to 17 years.[53] Peripheral lesions have a slightly better prognosis, owing to the more diverse surgical techniques available to these lesions, when compared with central lesions. Because 90% of cases are related to smoking, a preventive approach to the disease is crucial.[50]

Patients with a solitary pulmonary nodule on the chest radiograph should be vigorously investigated for the possibility of ma-

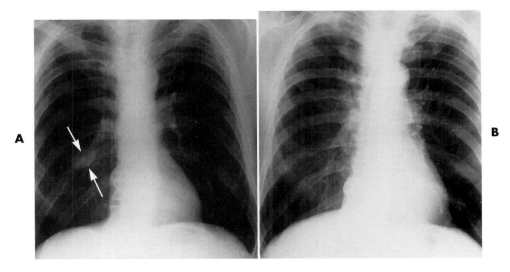

FIG. 23-14 **A,** Bronchogenic carcinoma presenting as solitary pulmonary nodule adjacent to the anterior end of the fifth right rib *(arrows)*. **B,** Radiograph of 8 years earlier without tumor nodule. (Courtesy Steven P. Brownstein, Springfield, NJ.)

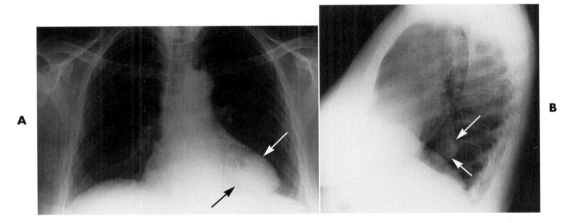

FIG. 23-15 Noncalcific hamartoma presenting as pulmonary mass overlying the apex the heart shadow **(A)** in the frontal projection *(arrows)* and in the retrocardiac clear space **(B)** in the lateral projection *(arrows)*. (Courtesy Steven P. Brownstein, Springfield, NJ.)

lignancy. The patient's age, size and borders of the lesion, presence of calcification, and growth over time (evaluated by previous radiographs) may be helpful in determining malignancy.

KEY CONCEPTS

- *The majority of lung cancers appear as either a solitary parenchymal nodule/mass or a hilar mass that demonstrates progressive growth with time.*
- *Plain film radiology may reveal the tumors themselves or, as is often the case with central lesions, abnormalities related to bronchial obstruction by the tumor (e.g., postobstructive pneumonitis or obstructive emphysema).*
- *A lesion's size, pattern of calcification, borders, and growth over time are helpful criteria in differentiating a benign versus malignant etiology.*

Hamartoma

BACKGROUND

Hamartomas are focal tissue malformations representing faulty tissue development at the organ level. Lung hamartomas are com-

posed of fibrous, cartilaginous, muscle, fatty, and epithelial tissues normally found in lung, but the quantity, proportions, and arrangement of the tissues are abnormal.

Hamartomas represent the most common type of benign lung tumor, representing 5% of all solitary pulmonary nodules.[5] The average age at discovery is 58 years, with a range of 14 to 76 years reported.[32]

IMAGING FINDINGS

Hamartomas grow at the same rate as their parent organ, and therefore do not exhibit neoplastic pressure erosion of adjacent tissues. Hamartomas are typically peripheral, presenting as well-defined pulmonary nodules.[5] Peripheral lesions are equally distributed among the lobes. Hamartomas may appear very large (Fig. 23-15)[17] but are typically less than 4 cm in diameter; an average diameter of 2.2 cm has been reported.[32] Typically calcification is demonstrated in 25%[5] to 30% of patients, with rates as high as 75% reported.[61] When present, the pattern of calcification often has a pathognomonic "popcorn" or "comma-shaped" appearance. Approximately 8% of hamartomas are in an endobronchial location,[52] possibly leading to airway obstruction.

CLINICAL COMMENTS

Most lesions are clinically asymptomatic. Occasionally, hemoptysis, cough, and chest pain are present. Surgical resection is considered for expanding lesions found in young and middle-age patients and in patients with clinical symptoms.

KEY CONCEPTS

- *Pulmonary hamartomas result from faulty tissue differentiation at the organ level. They appear as peripheral pulmonary nodules.*
- *Calcification is often present, characteristically appearing with a "popcorn," or "comma-shaped," pattern.*
- *Endobronchial and growing lesions are associated with greater clinical significance resulting from potential bronchial obstruction.*

Lymphoma

BACKGROUND

Lymphomas are malignant tumors composed of lymphocytes and less commonly histiocytes that arise in the lymph nodes, spleen, or other sites of lymphoid tissue elsewhere in the body. Lymphomas are classified by cell type, degrees of differentiation, and nodular or diffuse pattern of distribution. Hodgkin's disease (HD) is a distinctive form of lymphoma, separated from the larger spectrum of non-Hodgkin's lymphoma (NHL) on the basis of a characteristic appearance of cellular morphology (Reed-Sternberg cells). When disseminated, lymphomas, especially the lymphocytic type, may invade the peripheral blood and manifest as leukemia.

HD has a bimodal age distribution, 15 to 34 years and over 45 years. It has a propensity toward involvement of the mediastinum, hilum, or lung parenchyma. Intrathoracic disease is more common in HD than NHL.[24] HD involves the mediastinum in 67% to 87% of cases.[11,24]

NHL is seen in patients from 30 to 70 years of age. Thoracic involvement is seen in less than half of patients. Pulmonary involvement is much less common than lymphadenopathy of the hilum or mediastinum.

IMAGING FINDINGS

Moderate-to-extensive adenopathy is easily demonstrated with conventional radiographs, CT is more sensitive to early or more subtle presentations. Both HD and NHL demonstrate hilar and mediastinal lymph node enlargement.

Mediastinal lymph nodes from the thoracic inlet to the diaphragm may be involved. Involvement may be extensive, exhibiting huge conglomerate masses, or more subtle limited nodal masses. In the mediastinum, the pattern of involvement is contiguous for HD, spreading from one node to another. In contrast, adenopathy resulting from NHL may be noncontiguous. Rarely is hilar involvement noted without concurrent involvement of the mediastinum (Fig. 23-16). Typically, lymphoma spreads from mediastinal or hilum involvement along the bronchovascular lymphatics to involve the pulmonary tissue.

Pulmonary parenchymal involvement with HD is usually associated with hilar and mediastinal nodal disease[24,39]; virtually never are the pulmonary tissues involved alone. This is not the case for NHL, in which the pattern is more unpredictable and pulmonary involvement may be seen without hilar or mediastinal adenopathy.

Parenchymal involvement is typically nodular, sometimes

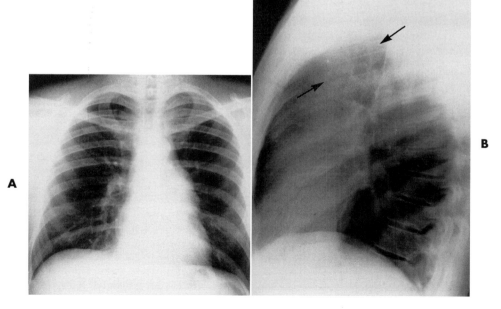

FIG. 23-16 A, Wide mediastinum. **B,** It is most pronounced the anterior portion *(arrows)* in a patient with non-Hodgkin's lymphoma. (Courtesy Michael Whitehead, Kansas City, Mo.)

demonstrating poorly defined borders. The appearance may be very similar to metastatic lung disease. An interstitial pulmonary pattern is rare. Often seen are patterns of consolidation and atelectasis of a lobe or segment. This is due to either extrinsic bronchial compression by enlarged lymph nodes or endobronchial tumors.[59,62]

Pleural effusions are noted in 7% to 10% of cases.[24] Less commonly, solid pleural[62] and pericardial masses are seen. Chest wall lesions are most often anterior, resulting from direct extension of anterior mediastinal disease. Occasionally, posterior nodes will invade adjacent vertebrae or the spinal canal.

CLINICAL COMMENTS

The clinical presentation of lymphoma is variable. Both HD and NHL may present with either an indolent or rapidly progressing course. Indolent disease presents with painless lymphadenopathy, whereas the progressive course is marked by constitutional symptoms such as fever, drenching night sweats, or weight loss. Once the pathological diagnosis is established, the patient should be evaluated to determine the extent of disease. Staging will determine whether regional therapy such as surgery or radiation therapy is appropriate or whether the disease must be approached in a systemic fashion with chemotherapy.

KEY CONCEPTS

- *Lymphoma is separated into Hodgkin's and non-Hodgkin's types. Each type is further classified by cell type, degrees of differentiation, and nodular or diffuse pattern of distribution.*
- *Both Hodgkin's disease and non-Hodgkin's lymphoma are marked by hilar and mediastinal lymphadenopathy; parenchymal involvement is less common.*
- *Clinically both Hodgkin's disease and non-Hodgkin's lymphoma may demonstrate either an indolent or rapidly progressing course.*

Metastatic Lung Disease

BACKGROUND

Reflecting their rich vascularity and central location in the vascular system, the lungs are a very common location for metastasis.[15,63] At autopsy, 30% to 50% of cancer patients have pulmonary metastasis. Both carcinomas and sarcomas arising anywhere in the body may spread to the lungs via the blood, lymphatics, or direct extension of a contiguous lesion.

Most lung metastases are blood-borne arising from mesenchymal tumors, melanomas, sarcomas, and primary renal and thyroid tumors. Lymphangitic carcinomatosis refers to pulmonary dissemination and tumor growth in the lymphatics, most commonly related to primaries of the stomach, pancreas, prostate, and breast.[37] Growth of contiguous tumors of the lungs occurs most often with esophageal and thyroid carcinomas[67] and mediastinal lymphomas.

IMAGING FINDINGS

Blood-borne metastasis typically presents as multiple well-defined nodules ranging from 1 to 5 cm in size located in the peripheral lung fields.[16,19,54] Nodules tend to involve the basal portions of lungs, possibly related to preferential blood flow.[16] Larger lesions are termed "cannonball" metastasis. Lymphangitic spread of metastasis presents with Kerley's lines, discrete nodules, and linear shadows denoting a reticulonodular interstitial pattern of pulmonary disease.

The pattern is typically bilateral, as in Fig. 23-17, with a unilateral presentation suggesting a bronchogenic primary lesion. Radiographs of other skeletal sites may reveal bone destruction as in Fig. 23-18. Abnormal radiographic findings may occur in less than 2 years after normal radiographic studies (Fig. 23-19). Cavitation is present in 6% to 7%,[20] and more common with squamous cell carcinoma than adenocarcinomas. The uterus, cervix, colon, head, and neck are common sites of origin.[12]

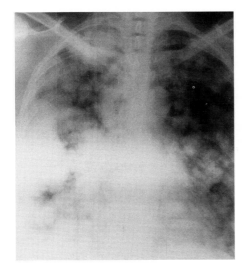

FIG. 23-17 Multiple mass and nodule presentation of pulmonary metastasis from primary adenocarcinoma. (Courtesy Steven P. Brownstein, Springfield, NJ.)

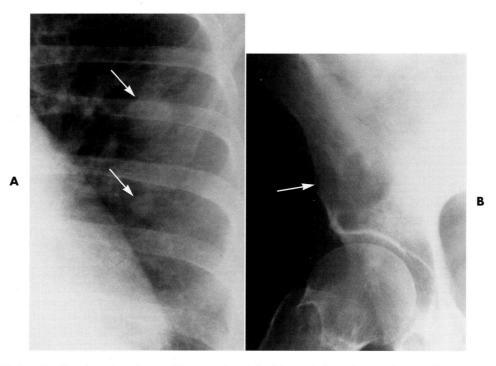

FIG. 23-18 Bronchogenic carcinoma with metastasis to skeletal sites and other pulmonary sites. **A,** Multiple nodules in left lung *(arrows)*. **B,** Osteolytic bone destruction in right supraacetabular region *(arrow)*. (Courtesy Steven P. Brownstein, Springfield, NJ.)

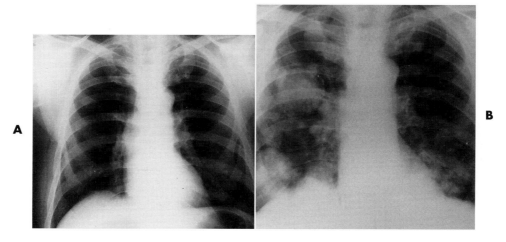

FIG. 23-19 Pulmonary metastasis developing from adenocarcinoma of the colon. **A,** Initial film with no abnormalities. **B,** Film taken 16 months later, demonstrating multiple bilateral masses and nodules characteristic of pulmonary metastasis. (Courtesy Steven P. Brownstein, Springfield, NJ.)

Calcification is unusual unless the metastasis is from osteosarcoma or chondrosarcoma. The higher contrast resolution and fewer blind spots make CT the most sensitive imaging technique for detecting pulmonary metastasis.

Pleural effusion is a common manifestation accompanying lung metastasis or may signify pleural metastasis. It most often accompanies carcinoma of the lung, breast, stomach, and pancreas.[1,13,46]

CLINICAL COMMENTS

Pulmonary metastases are a devastating complication for the cancer patient. Their presence usually signals a lethal outcome. Often no signs or symptoms are present at the time of discovery, and although helpful when known, a reported history of primary tumor elsewhere in the body may not exist. Pleural involvement may cause dyspnea on exertion. The disease is mostly limited to those over the age of 50 years.

KEY CONCEPTS

- *The lungs are common recipients of metastatic disease.*
- *Hematogenous metastasis results in multiple well-delineated peripheral nodules; lymphangitic metastasis appears as an interstitial pattern resulting from engorgement of the axial interstitial space; and direct extension most often results from tumors of the esophagus and mediastinal lymphoma.*
- *Pleural effusion is common.*

Pleural Mesothelioma

BACKGROUND

Primary tumors of the pleura are much less common than metastatic pleural disease, which typically arises from breast or lung primary tumors. Mesotheliomas are the most common primary tumors of the pleura,[3,31] arising from either the visceral or parietal pleura.[38] Two forms are recognized: localized benign (pleural fibroma) and diffuse malignant. The localized form, typically seen in patients between 45 and 65 years of age, is rare and not related to asbestos exposure. It arises most often from the visceral pleura and often is not recognized until it grows very large.

The malignant variety is recognized in patients between 40 and 70 years of age and is more common in men. It is caused primarily by asbestos exposure, with the duration and intensity of exposure relating to the risk of developing the disease.[2] The lifetime risk of developing mesothelioma with heavily exposed individuals is around 10%. The incidence is rising because the disease's 15-year latent period is resulting in current cases from asbestos exposures of recent past.

IMAGING FINDINGS

The localized form appears as a solitary mass in the lung periphery,[57] or occasionally in the lung fissure. It may be attached to the pleura by a pedicle. Calcification and accompanying pleural effusion are rare.

Malignant mesotheliomas begin as nodules on the visceral or parietal pleura that progress widely through the pleural space and form a thick rind encasing and constricting the lung. A shift of the mediastinum toward the involved side is seen in advanced cases. The radiographic appearance is that of multiple areas of pleural thickening or pleural masses with or without pleural effusion (Fig. 23-20). The main differential diagnostic considerations are metastatic tumor and lymphoma.

CLINICAL COMMENTS

Unless very large, the benign localized form is typically clinically silent. The diffuse malignant variety may demonstrate presenting complaints of chest pain, shortness of breath, cough, weight loss, fever, and recurrent pleural effusions.[2]

KEY CONCEPTS

- *Localized benign (pleural fibroma) and diffuse malignant forms are recognized.*
- *The malignant variety is closely related to asbestos exposure.*
- *The benign localized form is typically clinically silent; the diffuse malignant variety is most often associated with clinical symptoms.*

PART THREE Chest

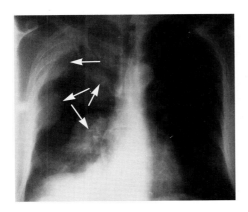

FIG. 23-20 Malignant mesothelioma involving right lung *(arrows)*. (Courtesy Steven P. Brownstein, Springfield, NJ.)

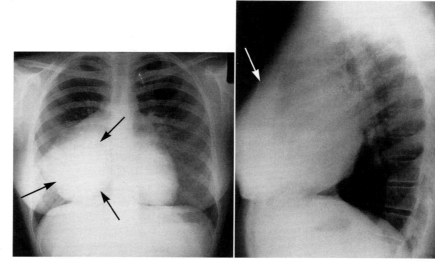

FIG. 23-21   Large teratoma in the anterior portion of the mediastinum (arrows).

Teratomas

BACKGROUND

Teratomas are neoplasms composed of multiple tissues derived from all three germ cell layers, including tissues not normally found in the lung.[41] Within the mass, it is not uncommon to find such elements as skin, teeth, hair, muscle, bone, cartilage, and fat. The thorax represents the third most common site for teratomas, following gonadal and sacrococcygeal locations. Nearly all intrathorax lesions are mediastinal, accounting for 10% of mediastinal tumors.[72] Grossly, they appear as benign cystic or solid malignant lesions.[29,40]

IMAGING FINDINGS

Teratomas are most frequently anterior mediastinal lesions, arising near the junction of the heart and great vessels (Fig. 23-21). Benign lesions are well-defined, malignant lesions that appear lobulated and often asymmetrical. Peripheral calcification may be noted, similar to thymomas. On average they are larger than thymomas. Rarely, an intrapulmonary location has been described.[48]

CLINICAL COMMENTS

Teratomas usually cause no symptoms, although large lesions may cause shortness of breath and coughing. Some patients relate a feeling of fullness or pain in the retrosternal area. Those lesions presenting later in life are more often malignant than those presenting in younger individuals. Malignant teratomas are usually highly aggressive lesions, often resulting in patient death within a short period of diagnosis.

KEY CONCEPTS

- *Teratomas are lesions containing tissue from all three germ cell layers.*
- *They are most commonly found in the anterior mediastinum, although intrapulmonary location has been identified.*
- *Most are benign and produce few symptoms; the less common malignant variety is highly aggressive.*

Thymic Masses

BACKGROUND

Thymomas may be benign or malignant. Appearing most commonly during the Middle Ages, thymomas represent 10%[47] of anterior mediastinal lesions and follow lymphoma as the second most common primary tumor to affect the mediastinum.[36] Thymolipomas are uncommon anterior mediastinal tumors consisting of an admixture of fat and thymic epithelial and lymphoid tissue of unknown etiology.[65] Thymic cysts are uncommon, accounting for less than 3% of anterior mediastinal lesions. Thymic hyperplasia is also rare overall, but it represents the most common anterior mass among infants and children.

IMAGING FINDINGS

All the lesions present as anterior mediastinal masses (Figs. 23-22 and 23-23). Thymomas are typically located near the junction of the heart and great vessels and are 5 cm to 10 cm in diameter. If large they may displace the heart or great vessels posteriorly. Thymolipomas extend inferiorly from the base of the heart, creating an enlarged appearance of the heart shadow.

CLINICAL COMMENTS

Patients with thymomas typically experience symptoms related to either pressure from an anterior mediastinal mass, producing cough, chest pain, and shortness of breath,[43] or myasthenia gravis, which is noted in 35% of those with thymomas.[8,72] Thymolipomas cause few symptoms and are typically discovered incidentally.

KEY CONCEPTS

- *Tumors, cysts, and hyperplasia of the thymus are common anterior mediastinal lesions.*
- *Clinical symptoms typically depend upon the size of the mass.*
- *Clinical data and radiographic appearance may assist in differentiating various thymic lesions.*

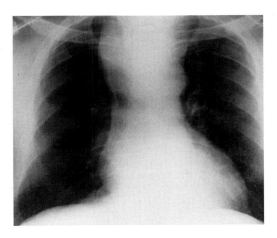

FIG. 23-22   Substernal thyroid presenting as a mass in the upper anterior mediastinum. (Courtesy Steven P. Brownstein, Springfield, NJ.)

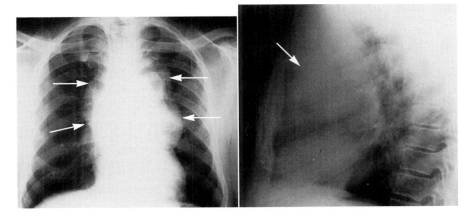

FIG. 23-23   Thymoma presenting as a solid mass in the anterior portion of the mediastinum *(arrows)*. (Courtesy Steven P. Brownstein, Springfield, NJ.)

References

1. Anderson CB, Philpott GW, Ferguson TB: The treatment of malignant pleural effusions, *Cancer* 33:916, 1974.

2. Antman C: Malignant mesothelioma, *N Engl J Med* 303:200, 1981.

3. Antman KH: Natural history and epidemiology of malignant mesothelioma, *Chest* 103(suppl 4):373, 1993.

4. Auerbach 0, Garfinkel L: The changing pattern of lung carcinoma, *Cancer* 68:1973, 1991.

5. Bateson EM: An analysis of 155 solitary lung lesions illustrating the differential diagnosis of mixed tumors of the lung, *Clin Radiol* 16:51, 1965.

6. Bateson EM, Whimster WF, Woo-Ming M: Ossified bronchial adenoma, *Br J Radiol* 43:570, 1970.

7. Beamis JR, Stein A, Andrews JL: Epidemiology of lung cancer, *Med Clin N Am* 59:315, 1975.

8. Benjamin SP et al: Critical review: "primary tumors of the mediastinum," *Chest* 62:297, 1972.

9. Burke M, Fraser R: Obstructive pneumonitis: a pathologic and pathogenetic reappraisal, *Radiology* 166:699, 1988.

10. Byrd RB et al: The roentgenographic appearance of squamous cell carcinoma of the bronchus, *Mayo Clin Proc* 43, 1968.

11. Castellino RA et al: Hodgkin's disease: contributions of chest CT in the initial staging evaluation, *Radiology* 160:603, 1986.

12. Chaudhuri MR: Cavitary pulmonary metastases, *Thorax* 25:375, 1970.

13. Chernow B, Sahn SA: Carcinomatous involvement of the pleura, *Am J Med* 63:695, 1977.

14. Clayton F: The spectrum and significance of bronchoalveolar carcinoma, *Pathol Annu* 23(part 2):361, 1988.

15. Coppage L, Shaw C, Curtis AM: Metastatic disease to the chest in patients with extrathoracic malignancy, *J Thorac Imag* 2:24, 1987.

16. Crow J, Slavin G, Kreel L: Pulmonary metastasis: a pathologic and radiologic study, *Cancer* 47:2595, 1981.

17. Darke CS et al: The bronchial circulation in a case of giant hamartoma of the lung, *Br J Radiol* 45:147, 1972.

18. Davila DG et al: Bronchial carcinoid tumors, *Mayo Clin Proc* 68:795, 1993.

19. Davis SD: CT evaluation for pulmonary metastases in patients with extrathoracic malignancy, *Radiology* 180:1, 1991.

20. Dodd GD, Buyle JS: Excavating pulmonary metastases, *AJR* 85:277, 1961.

21. Doll R: The age distribution of cancer; implications for models of carcinogenesis, *J Roy Stat Sco Series A,* Part 2, 133:66, 1971.

22. Doppman JL et al: Ectopic adrenocorticotrophic hormone syndrome: localization studies in 28 patients, *Radiology* 172:115, 1989.

23. Epstein DM: The role of radiologic screening in lung cancer, *Radiol Clin North Am* 28:489, 1990.

24. Filly R, Blank N, Castellino RA: Radiographic distribution of intrathoracic disease in previously untreated patients with Hodgkin's disease and non-Hodgkin's lymphoma, *Radiology* 120:277, 1976.

25. Findling JW. Tyrell B: Occult ectopic secretion of corticotropin, *Arch Intern Med* 146:929, 1986.

26. Fleischner Society: Glossary of terms for thoracic radiology: recommendations of the nomenclature committee of the Fleischner Society, *AJR* 143:509, 1984.

27. Geddes DM: The natural history of lung cancer: a review based on rates of tumor growth, *Br J Dis Chest* 73:1, 1979.

28. Goldmeier E: Limits of visibility of bronchogenic carcinoma, *Am Rev Respir Dis* 91:232, 1955.

29. Gonzales-Crussi F: Extragonadal teratomas. In *Atlas of tumor pathology,* Washington, DC, 1982, Armed Forces Institute of Pathology.

30. Gurney JW: Determining the likelihood of malignancy in solitary pulmonary nodules with bayesian analysis, *Radiology* 186:405, 1993.

31. Hammar SP: The pathology of benign and malignant pleural disease, *Chest Surg Clin N Am* 4:405, 1994.

32. Hansen CP et al: Pulmonary hamartoma, *J Thorac Cardiovasc Surg* 104:674, 1992.

33. Haque AK: Pathology of carcinoma of lung: an update on current concepts, *J Thorac Imag* 7:9, 1991.

34. Hayabuchi N, Russell WJ, Murakami J: Slow-growing lung cancer in a fixed population sample: radiologic assessments, *Lancet* 52:1098, 1983.

35. Heitzman ER et al: Pathways of tumor spread through the lung: radiologic correlations with anatomy and pathology, *Radiology* 144:3, 1982.

36. Ingels GW et al: Malignant schwannomas of the mediastinum, *Cancer* 27:1190, 1971.

37. Janower ML, Blennerhassett JB: Lymphangitic spread of metastatic cancer to the lung: a radiologic-pathologic classification, *Radiology* 101:267, 1971.

38. Kannerstein M et al: Asbestosis and mesothelioma, *Pathol Annu* 13(part 1):81, 1978.

39. Kaplan HS: Contiguity and progression in Hodgkin's disease, *Cancer Res* 31:1811, 1971.

40. Keslar PJ, Buck JL, Suarez ES: Germ cell tumors of the sacrococcygeal region: radiologic-pathologic correlation, *Radiographics* 14:607, 1994.

41. Kountakis SE et al: Teratomas of the head and neck, *Am J Otolaryngol* 15:292, 1994.

42. Kundel HL: Predictive value and threshold detectability of lung tumors, *Radiology* 139:25, 1981.

43. Lewis JE et al: Thymoma. A clinicopathologic review, *Cancer* 60:2727, 1987.

44. Loeb LA et al: Smoking and lung cancer: an overview, *Cancer Res* 44:5942, 1984.

45. Mahoney MC et al: CT demonstration of calcification in carcinoma of the lung, *AJR* 154:255, 1990.

46. Matthay RA et al: Malignancies metastatic to the pleura, *Invest Radiol* 25:601, 1990.

47. Meza MP, Benson M, Slovis TL: Imaging of mediastinal masses in children, *Radiol Clin North Am* 31, 1993.

48. Morgan DE et al: Intrapulmonary teratoma: a case report and review of the literature, *J Thorac Imag* 7:70, 1992.

49. Muller NL, Miller RR: Neuroendocrine carcinomas of the lung, *Semin Roentgenol* 25:96, 1990.

50. Petty TL: What to do when an x-ray film suggests lung cancer, *Postgrad Med J* 89:101, 1991.

51. Pietra GG: The pathology of carcinoma of the lung, *Semin Roentgenol* 25:25, 1990.

52. Poirier TJ, Van Ordstrand HS: Pulmonary chondromatous hamartoma: report of seventeen cases and review of the literature, *Chest* 59:50, 1971.

53. Pugatch RD: Radiologic evaluation in chest malignancies: a review of imaging modalities, *Chest* 107(suppl):294, 1995.

54. Remy-Jardin M et al: Pulmonary nodules detection with thick-section spiral CT versus conventional CT, *Radiology* 187:513, 1993.

55. Ries LG, Pollack ES, Young JL: Cancer patient survival: surveillance, epidemiology, and end results program, 1973-79 *J Natl Cancer Inst* 70:693, 1983.

56. Rigler LG: The roentgen signs of carcinoma of the lung, *AJR* 74:415, 1955.

57. Robinson LA, Reilly RB: Localized pleural mesothelioma. The clinical spectrum, *Chest* 106:1611, 1994.

58. Rosenow EC, Carr DT: Bronchogenic carcinoma, *CA Cancer J Clin* 29:233, 1979.

59. Samuels ML et al: Endobronchial malignant lymphoma: report of five cases in adults, *AJR* 85:87, 1961.

60. Sargent EN, Barnes RA, Schwinn CP: Multiple pulmonary fibroleiomyomatous hamartomas, *Am J Roentgenol* 110:694, 1970.

61. Shin MS, McElvein RB, Ho KJ: Radiographic evidence of calcification in pulmonary hamartomas, *J Natl Med Assoc* 84:329, 1992.

62. Stolberg HO et al: Hodgkin's disease of the lung: roentgenologic-pathologic correlation, *AJR* 92:96, 1964.

63. Suster S, Moran CA: Unusual manifestations of metastatic tumors to the lungs, *Semin Diagn Pathol* 12:193, 1995.

64. Suzuki Y: Diagnostic criteria for human diffuse malignant mesothelioma, *Acta Pathol Jpn* 42:767, 1992.

65. Teplick JG, Nedwich A, Haskin ME: Roentgenographic features of thymolipoma, *AJR* 117:873, 1973.

66. Theros EG: Varying manifestations of peripheral pulmonary neoplasms: a radiologic-pathologic correlative study, *AJR* 128:893, 1977.

67. Tsumori T et al: Clinicopathologic study of thyroid carcinoma infiltrating the trachea, *Cancer* 56:2843, 1985.

68. Warren WH, Gould VE, Faber LP: Neuroendocrine neoplasms: a clinicopathologic update, *J Thorac Cardiovasc Surg* 98:321, 1989.

69. Weiss W: Cigarette smoke as a carcinogen, *Am Rev Respir Dis* 108:364, 1973.

70. Weiss W: Tumor doubling time and survival in men with bronchogenic carcinoma. *Chest* 65:3, 1974.

71. Wenckebach KF: The radiology of the chest, *Arch Roentgen Ray* 18:169, 1913.

72. Wychulis AR et al: Surgical treatment of mediastinal tumors, *J Thorac Cardiovasc Surg* 62:379, 1971.

73. Zwirewich CV et al: Solitary pulmonary nodule: high-resolution CT and radiologic-pathologic correlation, *Radiology* 179:469, 1991.

chapter 24

Miscellaneous Chest Diseases

DENNIS M MARCHIORI*

Adult Respiratory Distress Syndrome
Extrinsic Allergic Alveolitis

Pneumoconioses
Pneumothorax

Sarcoidosis

Adult Respiratory Distress Syndrome

BACKGROUND

Adult respiratory distress syndrome (ARDS) is a condition in which the pulmonary system is affected as a result of more generalized, multiorgan capillary damage.[14] The pathogenic sequence appears to

---

BOX 24-1

Partial List of Factors Associated with Adult Respiratory Distress Syndrome[2,26,31]

- Amniotic fluid embolism
- Arterial embolism
- Aspiration
- Drug abuse
- Eclampsia
- Fat embolism
- Fractures
- Heat stroke
- High-altitude pulmonary edema
- Pancreatitis
- Pulmonary contusions
- Radiation pneumonitis
- Shock
- Smoke inhalation
- Transplantation

---

be related to inappropriate activation of the complement cascade,[32,18] resulting in increased capillary permeability and pulmonary edema. Eventually, fluid spills into the alveolar spaces, leading to hemorrhaging, reduced surfactant levels, and a resultant smaller functional area for gas exchange. A wide range of factors and conditions is associated with the development of ARDS (Box 24-1).

IMAGING FINDINGS

During the initial stage of ARDS, no changes are detectable radiographically unless the ARDS is caused by pneumonia, aspiration, or another pulmonary condition, in which case the pulmonary findings of the concurrent disease may be noted. The latter stages of the disease are marked by alveolar filling. At first, patchy areas of incomplete lung consolidation are noted (Fig. 24-1), which eventually become more uniform, generalized, and homogenous. During the ensuing weeks, the radiographically detectable features gradually resolve. Pleural effusion is rare.

CLINICAL COMMENTS

ARDS is characterized by rapidly progressing respiratory distress.[2,12] Alveolar filling is followed by acute respiratory failure that

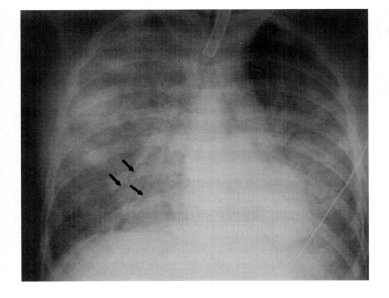

FIG. 24-1 Diffuse pulmonary consolidations with air bronchograms (*arrows*) are the result of ARDS following viral pneumonia. This appearance is radiologically indistinguishable from pulmonary alveolar edema and diffuse pneumonia. (From Reed JC: *Chest radiology: plain film patterns and differential diagnosis*, ed 4, St Louis, 1997, Mosby.)

---

*Special thanks to James C. Reed for his contribution as a reviewer of this material.

necessitates mechanical ventilation and oxygen administration. The eventual clinical outcome depends heavily on whether the patient develops a nosocomial infection, a hemorrhage, sepsis, lung barotrauma, or another major complication.[18]

KEY CONCEPTS

- *Adult respiratory distress syndrome (ARDS) involves increased capillary permeability that is caused by a wide variety of systemic and pulmonary insults.*
- *The radiographic features are related to excessive fluid accumulation in the alveolar spaces and present as varying degrees of lung consolidation.*

TABLE 24-1
Selected Provocative Agents of Extrinsic Allergic Alveolitis

Disease	Provocative agent
Bagassosis	Moldy sugar cane
Bird fancier's lung	Avian excreta
Farmer's lung	Moldy hay
Humidifier lung	Contamination from humidifying, heating, and air conditioning systems
Malt worker's lung	Moldy malt
Maple bark stripper's lung	Moldy maple bark
Mushroom worker's lung	Mushroom spores
Sequoiosis	Redwood dust
Suberosis	Moldy cork dust

Extrinsic Allergic Alveolitis

BACKGROUND

Extrinsic allergic alveolitis (EAA), also known as hypersensitivity pneumonitis, is a nonatopic, nonasthmatic allergic lung disease. EAA manifests as an occupational lung disease caused by the inhalation of organic dusts, which produces granulomatous and interstitial lung changes. Several etiological agents are listed in Table 24-1.

IMAGING FINDINGS

The radiographic presentation of EAA is the same regardless of the type of organic dust inhaled,[43] but it does vary according to the intensity of the exposure.[30] The early stages of EEA are usually characterized by reversible, multiple, small (1 to 3 mm), nodular radiodensities[10,31] that are scattered bilaterally throughout the lung zones[42,43]; although it is less common, the lung apices may be spared (Fig. 24-2).[15] Repeated exposures may result in a chronic interstitial (honeycomb) pattern[3,42] with upper lobe predominance.

CLINICAL COMMENTS

Acute EAA is characterized by sudden onset of malaise, chills, fever, cough, dyspnea, and nausea within hours after exposure to the offending agent. Subacute and chronic forms are characterized by a chronic cough and slowly progressing dyspnea, anorexia, and weight loss. The patient's history of exposure preceding the clinical symptoms is important for a proper diagnosis.

KEY CONCEPTS

- *Extrinsic allergic alveolitis (EAA) comprises a group of diseases caused by the inhalation of organic dusts.*
- *The radiographic appearance is marked by the presence of small radiopaque nodules scattered throughout the lung fields.*
- *Chronic forms of the disease often develop a chronic interstitial pattern.*

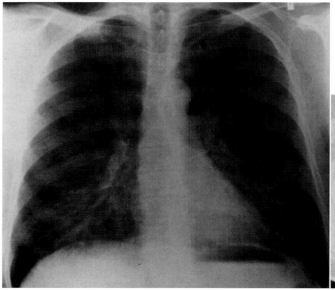
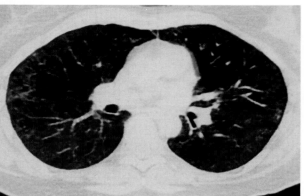

FIG. 24-2 EAA presenting with bilateral diffuse infiltrate **(A)** and small pulmonary nodules on a computed tomogram **(B)** following exposure to pigeon droppings. (From Swensen SJ: *Radiology of thoracic diseases: a teaching file,* St Louis, 1993, Mosby.)

Pneumoconioses

BACKGROUND

Pneumoconioses are a group of diseases caused by inhalation of inorganic dust and its accumulation in the lung.[30] The dust deposits cause a nonneoplastic lung reaction that is often seen on radiographs. Asbestos, silicon, and coal dust incite a fibrogenic tissue reaction throughout the lung. Tin, barium, iron, and other inert particles do not incite fibrogenic changes but do cause particle-laden macrophages to accumulate in the lung[4]. Because these reactions are less aggressive, they are called *benign pneumoconioses* (even though their radiographic appearance can be dramatic).

IMAGING FINDINGS

The chest radiograph is the primary means of determining the presence and extent of pneumoconiosis.[45] The International Labor Office (ILO) has established a classification system for the radiographic appearance of pneumoconioses,[20,39] which focuses on the size and shape of the lung nodules. The classification also includes a detailed categorization of pleural thickening.

The radiographic appearance of pneumoconiosis depends on the type and amount of dust inhaled and on individual immunological lung reactions (Table 24-2).[5,22] In general the nonfibrogenic pneumoconioses show nodular opacities. A fibrogenic lung response is associated with lymphadenopathy; interstitial parenchymal patterns; and pleural thickening, calcification (Figs. 24-3 and 24-4), and effusion.

CLINICAL COMMENTS

Radiographic and clinical findings are often not consistent. Extensive changes may be seen in radiographs of relatively asymptomatic patients. Occasionally dyspnea and rales are present. The treatment is supportive.

▌ KEY CONCEPTS

- *Pneumoconioses are a group of occupational lung diseases that develop in response to repeated inhalation of inorganic dust particles.*
- *Pneumoconioses are divided into fibrogenic and nonfibrogenic (benign) categories.*
- *The resulting radiographic appearance depends on the type and quantity of dust inhaled and on the patient's immunological characteristics.*

TABLE 24-2
Selected Pneumoconioses

Condition and causative agent	Comments
Nonfibrogenic (benign)	
Stanosis: tin	Stannosis is caused by deposits of tin in the lung that lead to formation of very opaque nodules.
Baritosis: barium	Baritosis is caused by inhalation of barium sulfate, which produces small, rounded opacities that exceed the attenuation of calcium.
Siderosis: iron	Siderosis develops in workers who inhale fumes containing iron oxide particles, which produces scattered radiopacities in the lung fields.
Fibrogenic	
Asbestosis: asbestos	Construction workers, insulation workers, pipe fitters, ship builders, and asbestos miners may be exposed to asbestos fibers of varying levels of pathogenicity (e.g., crocidolite>amosite>anthophyllite> chrysotile), causing interstitial lung disease (asbestosis), pleural thickening (asbestos-related pleural disease), and malignancies. Asbestosis appears as linear radiopacities in the lung bases progressing to the apex. Asbestos-related pleural disease may be focal (plaques) or diffuse and usually appears in a posterolateral location. It is assumed to be the result of asbestos fibers that have pierced the visceral pleura.[29] Asbestos exposure increases the risk of developing mesothelioma[1,7] and lung cancer.[6,23]
Silicosis: silicon dioxide	Silicosis results from exposure to silicon dioxide,[40] which is abundant in the earth's crust and commonly encountered in mining, quarrying, sandblasting, and ceramic work. Small, radiopaque nodules are seen throughout the parahilar and apical regions. The nodules coalesce to form large (i.e., greater than 2 cm) conglomerate masses that progressively migrate toward the hilum in a bilateral but asymmetrical pattern known as *progressive massive fibrosus (PMF)*. Occasionally, hilar lymphadenopathy with possible peripheral "eggshell" calcifications of the hilar lymph nodes are present.
Coal worker's pneumoconiosis (CWP): coal	Coal miners are almost the only inidividuals who inhale enough carbon-containing inorganic material to cause a reaction. Carbon deposits in the lung form coal dust macules that are seen as round, 1- to 5-mm nodules scattered throughout the upper lung fields.[33] This feature is the hallmark of simple CWP and is radiographically indistinguishable from silicosis. Complicated CWP develops when the simple pattern is complicated by the formation of PMF similar to that seen in silicosis. Caplan's syndrome is CWP in patients who also have rheumatoid arthritis; Erasmus syndrome is CWP in patients who also have progressive systemic sclerosis.

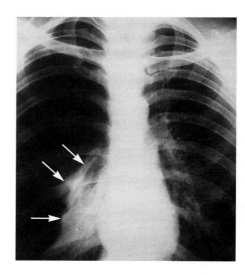

FIG. 24-5 Atelectasis of right lung with tension pneumothorax maintaining the midline position of the mediastinum and heart. The collapsed lung remains as a radiodense mass along the right heart border *(arrows).* (Courtesy Steven P. Brownstein, Springfield, NJ.)

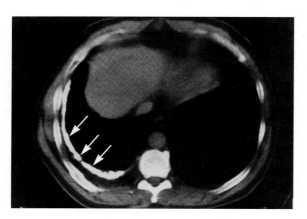

FIG. 24-3 Computed tomogram demonstrating calcific asbestosis-related pleural plaques in the right posterior region *(arrows).* (Courtesy Steven P. Brownstein, Springfield, NJ.)

Their etiology probably involves a pleural "flap" defect. In a patient with a flap defect, the flap opens during inspiration and allows air to enter the pleural space; during expiration, the flap closes and traps the air in the space. Each respiratory cycle pumps air into the over-expanded pleural space. Tension pneumothoraces may become large and lead to atelectasis (Fig. 24-5), impairing venous return to the heart and displacing the mediastinum and hemidiaphragm.

IMAGING FINDINGS

On a chest radiograph of a patient in the upright position, trapped air in the pleural space usually appears as a crescent-shaped radiolucent shadow between the lung and chest wall in the upper chest (Figs 24-6, 24-7). The absence of lung markings indicates that the air is extrapulmonary. The subjacent visceral pleura is contrasted by air on both sides and is seen as a thin, curvilinear, radiodense line (Figs. 24-8 and 24-9). A pneumothorax is difficult to detect on radiographs taken with the patient in the supine position.[41] Suspected pneumothorax may be more easily seen on radiographs of patients in a state of full expiration. Full expiration decreases the radiolucent appearance of the lung, leading to greater contrast between the lung and pleural air of the pneumothorax.

CLINICAL COMMENTS

Pneumothoraces typically present with a sudden onset of ipsilateral chest pain and dyspnea. A tension pneumothorax is characterized by tachypnea, tachycardia, cyanosis, and hypotension. A tension pneumothorax is a medical emergency that requires immediate action to alleviate the progressive lung collapse.

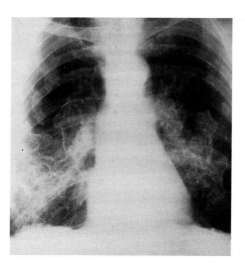

FIG. 24-4 Asbestosis with calcific pleural plaques and an interstitial parenchymal pattern.

Pneumothorax

BACKGROUND

A pneumothorax is a collection of air in the pleural space that has a spontaneous or traumatic etiology. A traumatic pneumothorax results from blunt or penetrating injuries and is often iatrogenic. A pneumothorax is caused by rupturing of the parietal or visceral pleura, which permits air from outside the body or in the lung to collect in the pleural space.

A spontaneous pneumothorax has primary and secondary forms. The primary form most often develops in young or middle-aged males.[35] A primary spontaneous pneumothorax is thought to result from rupturing of subpleural air collections that are known as *blebs.*[25] A spontaneous pneumothorax may also be secondary to chest diseases that produce cysts and cavities in the lung (e.g., chronic obstructive pulmonary disease,[26] cystic fibrosis, Ehlers-Danlos syndrome,[9] histiocytosis X, Marfan syndrome[19]).

Tension pneumothoraces develop in a small percent of patients.

KEY CONCEPTS

- *A pneumothorax is classified as either traumatic or spontaneous based on its etiology.*
- *The spontaneous variety is further subdivided into primary and secondary types based on the presence of underlying disease.*
- *A radiograph of the patient in the upright position is most helpful for recognizing pneumothorax.*
- *Tension pneumothoraces are uncommon, but when they develop they require immediate medical attention to alleviate the intrathoracic pressure and halt progressive lung collapse.*

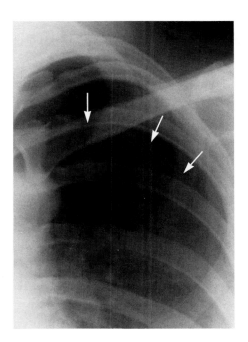

FIG. 24-6 Pneumothorax with displaced visceral pleura in the fourth posterior rib interspace *(arrows)*.

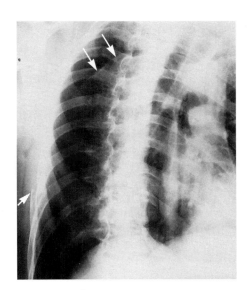

FIG. 24-8 Rib fracture with lateral offset of the distal fragment and associated pneumothorax *(arrows)*. (Courtesy Steven P. Brownstein, Springfield, NJ.)

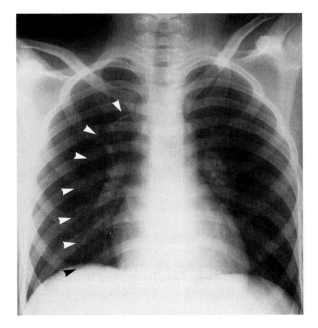

FIG. 24-7 Clothing artifact caused by emblem on shirt. Appearance mimics a pneumothorax in the right lung *(arrowheads)*. (Courtesy Steven P. Brownstein, Springfield, NJ.)

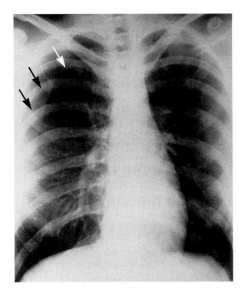

FIG. 24-9 Pneumothorax with characteristic linear density in the right upper lung field representing the displaced visceral pleura *(arrows)*.

Sarcoidosis

BACKGROUND

Sarcoidosis is a multisystem disease of unknown etiology that is characterized by the formation of noncaseating epithelioid granulomas. Intrathoracic involvement occurs in nearly all patients. Sarcoidosis typically presents between the ages of 20 and 40 years,[21,24] is more common in females,[17,38] and is 10 to 20 times more common in blacks.[13,28]

IMAGING FINDINGS

Sarcoidosis is staged according to its radiographic appearance.[11] Stage 0 has no radiographic changes present. Stage 1 is characterized by the formation of extensive bilateral hilar, paratracheal, tracheobronchial, and azygous lymphadenopathy (Fig. 24-10). In stage 2, radiography shows bilateral hilar adenopathy with parenchymal radiopacities, usually in a diffuse nodular or reticulonodular pattern. The presence of parenchymal opacities with no associated hilar lymphadenopathy defines stage 3 (Fig. 24-11). Radiographs of

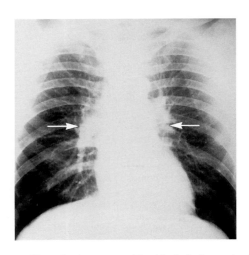

FIG. 24-10   Bilateral enlargement of the hila, indicating early stage I sarcoidosis (arrows). (Courtesy of Steven P. Brownstein, Springfield, NJ.)

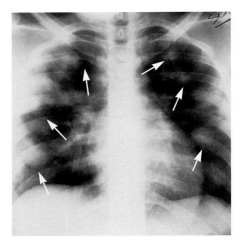

FIG. 24-11   Multiple mass and nodule presentation of alveolar (stage 3) sarcoidosis (arrows). (Courtesy Steven P. Brownstein, Springfield, NJ.)

patients in stage 4 show pulmonary fibrosis without concurrent lymphadenopathy or parenchymal opacities. Patients may not necessarily progress sequentially through all four stages.

Endobronchial involvement is common, and physiological evidence of airway obstruction may be present in up to 63% of patients.[8] In rare cases, lobar atelectasis may develop as a result of endobronchial obstruction or extrinsic bronchial compression by adjacent adenopathy.[37] Pleural effusion and "eggshell" calcifications of the hilar lymphadenopathy are occasionally present.

In addition to the intrathoracic changes, about 15% of patients with sarcoidosis develop lacelike or honeycombed osteolytic bone lesions predominantly in the small tubular bones of the hands. Arthritis is also an uncommon finding. The majority of patients with bone involvement also have skin lesions and intrathoracic involvement.

CLINICAL COMMENTS

Patients with sarcoidosis are usually initially asymptomatic, but up to 50% may develop pulmonary symptoms including a nonproduc-

tive cough, dyspnea, chest pain, and hemoptysis. Extrathoracic manifestations of the disease include osteolytic bone lesions, hepatosplenomegaly, erythema nodosum, and cutaneous granulomas.

Sarcoidosis is considered as a diagnosis only after neoplastic and infectious diseases with similar radiographic presentations have been considered. Definitive diagnosis is aided by biopsy or the less accurate Kveim skin test.[34] Spontaneous regression of the thoracic sarcoidosis will occur in 80% of cases, with the remaining progressing to extensive tissue fibrosis and the end stages of lung disease.

KEY CONCEPTS

- *Sarcoidosis is a condition of unknown etiology characterized by non-caseating granulomatous deposits in multiple organ systems.*
- *The thorax is the most common site of involvement.*
- *The radiographic appearance of sarcoidosis is typically characterized by small or massive bilateral hilar lymphadenopathy.*

References

1. Andersen HA, Lilis R, Daum SM: Household-contact asbestos neoplastic risk, *Ann N Y Acad Sci* 271:310, 1976.
2. Balk R, Bone RC: The adult respiratory distress syndrome, *Med Clin North Am* 67:685, 1983.
3. Braun SR et al: Farmer's lung disease: long-term clinical and physiologic outcome, *Am Rev Respir Dis* 119:185, 1979.
4. Brooks SM: An approach to patients suspected of having an occupational pulmonary disease, *Clin Chest Med* 2:271, 1981.
5. Burrell R: Immunological aspects of coal workers' pneumoconiosis, *Ann N Y Acad Sci* 200:94, 1972.
6. Casey KR, Rom WN, Moatamed F: Asbestos-related diseases, *Clin Chest Med* 2:179, 1981.
7. Chen W, Mattet NK: Malignant mesothelioma with minimal asbestos exposure, *Hum Pathol* 9:253, 1978.
8. Cieslicki J, Zych D, Zielinski J: Airway obstructions in patients with sarcoidosis, *Sarcoidosis* 8:42, 1991.
9. Clark JG, Kuhn C, Uitto J: Lung collagen in type IV Ehler's-Danlos syndrome: ultrastructural and biochemical studies, *Am Rev Respir Dis* 122:971, 1980.
10. Cook PG, Wells IP, McGavin CR: The distribution of pulmonary shadowing in farmer's lung, *Clin Radiol* 39:21, 1988.
11. DeRemee RA: The roentgenographic staging of sarcoidosis, *Chest* 83:128, 1983.
12. Divertie MB: The adult respiratory distress syndrome: subject review, *Mayo Clin Proc* 1982;57:371.
13. Edmondstone WM, Wilson AG: Sarcoidosis in Caucasians, blacks and Asians in London, *Br J Dis Chest* 79:27, 1985.
14. Effros RM, Mason GR: An end to "ARDS," *Chest* 89:162, 1986.
15. Emanuel UA et al: Farmer's lung: clinical, pathologic and immunologic study of twenty-four patients, *Am J Med* 37:392, 1964.
16. Epler GR: Clinical overview of occupational lung disease, *Radiol Clin North Am* 30:1121, 1992.
17. Freundlich LM et al: Sarcoidosis: typical and atypical thoracic manifestations and complications, *Clin Radiol* 1970;21:376.
18. Greene R: Adult respiratory distress syndrome: Acute alveolar damage, *Radiology* 163:57, 1987.
19. Hall JR et al: Pneumothorax in the Marfan syndrome: prevalence and therapy, *Ann Thorac Surg* 37:500, 1984.
20. International Labour Office: *Guidelines for the use of ILO international classification of radiographs of pneumoconioses,* Geneva, 1980, International Labour Office.
21. IsraeI HL, Sones M: Sarcoidosis: clinical observation on one hundred sixty cases, *Arch Luteru Med* 102:766, 1958.
22. Jacobsen M: New data on the relationship between simple pneumoconiosis and exposure to coal mine dust, *Chest* 78:408, 1980.

23. Kipen HM et al: Pulmonary fibrosis in asbestos insulation workers with lung cancer: a radiologic and histopathological evaluation, *Br J Ind Med* 44:96, 1987.

24. Kirks DR, Greenspau RH: Sarcoid, *Radiol Clin North Am* 11:279, 1973.

25. Kjaergaard H: Spontaneous pneumothorax in the apparently healthy, *Acta Med Scand* 43(suppl):1, 1932.

26. Light RW: Management of spontaneous pneumothorax, *Am Rev Respir Dis* 148:245, 1993.

27. Matthay MA: Pathophysiology of pulmonary edema, *Clin Chest* 6:301, 1985.

28. Mayock RL et al: Manifestations of sarcoidosis: analysis of 145 patients, with a review of nine series selected from the literature, *Am J Med* 35:67, 1963.

29. McLoud TC: Conventional radiography in the diagnosis of asbestosis-related disease, *Radiol Clin North Am* 30:1177,1992.

30. McLoud TC: Occupational lung disease, *Radiol Clin North Am* 29:931, 1991.

31. Mindell HJ: Roentgen findings in farmer's lung, *Radiology* 97:341, 1970.

32. Morgan PW, Goodman LR: Pulmonary edema and adult respiratory distress syndrome, *Radiol Clin North Am* 29:943, 1991.

33. Morgan WKC, Lapp NL: Respiratory disease in coal miners, *Am Rev Respir Dis* 113:531, 1976.

34. Munro CS, Mitchell DN: The Kveim response: still useful, still a puzzle, *Thorax* 42:321, 1987.

35. Primrose WR: Spontaneous pneumothorax: a retrospective review of aetiology, pathogenesis and management, *Scott Med J* 29:15, 1984.

36. Reynold HY: Hypersensitivity pneumonitis, *Clin Chest Med* 3:503, 1982.

37. Rockoff SD, Rohatgi PK: Unusual manifestations of thoracic sarcoidosis, *AJR* 144:513, 1985.

38. Romer FK: Presentation of sarcoidosis and outcome of pulmonary changes, *Danish Medical Bulletin* 29:27, 1982.

39. Shipley RT: The 1980 ILO classification of radiographs of the pneumoconioses, *Radiol Clin North Am* 30:1135, 1992.

40. Stark P, Jacobsen F, Shaffer K: Standard imaging in silicosis and coal worker's pneumoconiosis, *Radiol Clin North Am* 30:1147, 1992.

41. Tocino IM, Miller MH, Fairfax WR: Distribution of pneumothorax in the supine and semirecumbent critically ill patient, *AJR* 144:901, 1985.

42. Uargreave F et al: The radiological appearances of allergic alveolitis due to bird sensitivity (bird fancier's lung),*Clin Radiol* 23:1, 1972.

43. Unger GF et al: A radiologic approach to hypersensitivity pneumonias, *Radiol Clin North Am* 11:339, 1973.

44. Unger J, Fink JN, Unger GF: Pigeon breeder's disease: a review of the roentgenographic pulmonary findings, *AJR* 90:683, 1968.

45. Wagner GR, Attfield MD, Parker JE: Chest radiography in dust-exposed miners: promise and problems, potential and imperfections, *Occup Med* 8:127, 1993.

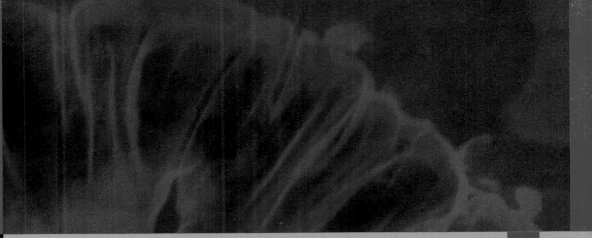

Abdomen

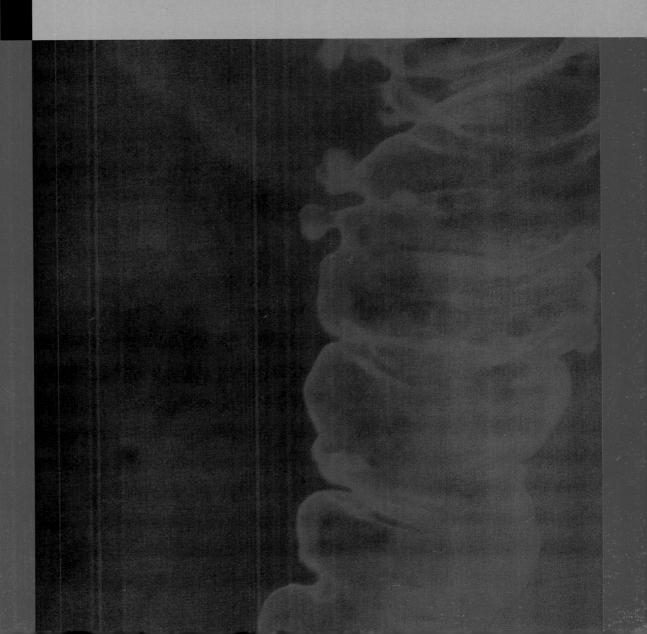

chapter 25

Plain Film Radiography of the Abdomen

BEVERLY L HARGER

LISA E HOFFMAN

RICHARD ARKLESS

Anatomy

Imaging

As an initial imaging procedure, plain film radiography of the abdomen can be useful in evaluating serious and even life-threatening conditions. Even though it may not reveal abnormalities shown by diagnostic ultrasonography and computed tomography (CT), this imaging modality can be a cost-effective method for use in diagnosing and managing abdominal pathosis. The recognition of key diagnostic features (seen incidentally on spine x-rays or noted on abdomen views used in the initial investigation of abdominal complaints) on plain film can be critical to patient management.

Obtaining a single radiograph showing a recumbent anteroposterior (AP) view of the abdomen is the first step. Upright or decubitus views may add valuable information about gas and fluid patterns, masses, and abnormal organs. Oblique views may aid in further localizing abnormal findings. The entire abdomen from the hemidiaphragms to the pubic symphysis should be visualized. An upright, posteroanterior (PA) view of the chest may reveal valuable information about the presence of infiltrates in the lung bases, pleural fluid, or free peritoneal air. Although a high peak kilovoltage is correlated with a low x-ray dose, the higher the peak kilovoltage, the less the contrast. Often a peak kilovoltage of 80 to 90 kV is optimal, depending on what type of x-ray generator is being used (single phase, three phase, high frequency). Without the aid of contrast, abdominal contents are generally seen only if they contain gas or are surrounded by fat.

Indications for plain film radiography of the abdomen include trauma, abdominal distention or pain, vomiting, diarrhea, and constipation. Abdominal masses are best evaluated with ultrasonography or CT. Complete evaluation of abdominal pathosis usually requires additional imaging, which may include barium-filled bowel or intravenous contrast studies, ultrasonography, CT, magnetic resonance imaging (MRI), and radionuclide studies. Some portions of the gastrointestinal (GI) tract can be directly visualized via fiberoptics.

Anatomy

GENERAL

Interpretation of abdominal radiographs is aided by knowledge of basic anatomical relationships. The location and relative mobility of abdominal organs are important factors in the evaluation of radiographic signs. Whether a viscus is solid or hollow can also be important. Gas in the stomach, portions of the small bowel, and most of the colon and rectum usually make identification of these structures possible. Fat surrounding the renal capsules and abutting the inferior aspect of the liver aid in their visualization.

Retroperitoneal structures are relatively fixed in position, which among other factors increases their potential for traumatic injury. Consistently retroperitoneal structures include the kidneys and adrenal glands, the second and third portions of the duodenum, the ascending and descending portions of the colon, the psoas muscles, and the abdominal aorta. Fascial planes provide channels for the spread of fluids, cells, and pathogens. Processes affecting the psoas muscle may follow the fascial sheath as far as the lesser trochanter of the femur.

Intraperitoneal structures can be categorized by their location within conceptual quadrants of the abdomen. In the right upper quadrant (RUQ) the liver location is fixed. The liver shadow is generally well outlined by intraperitoneal fat. Basic guidelines indicate that the liver should have a homogenous density and should not extend below the level of the iliac crest (although some normal anatomical variants do this) or past the midline. Liver margins may be delineated by gas in the abutting hepatic flexure of the colon. Although the gallbladder is almost always in the RUQ, closely opposed to the anteroinferior aspect of the liver, it is quite mobile in some patients and may be found in any quadrant. Much of the ascending colon is found in the RUQ. The transverse colon is quite mobile and its position may vary greatly—from running crosswise in the upper abdomen to dipping well into the pelvic area.

STOMACH

Most of the stomach is located in the left upper quadrant (LUQ), although its distal part does cross the midline into the RUQ and may extend ptotically into the lower abdomen. The stomach is identified on plain film by the gas it contains, especially the magenblase (stomach bubble) seen superiorly in the fundus on upright views (although gas may be seen throughout the stomach on supine views). The stomach is relatively fixed proximally at the gastroesophageal junction. The remainder is relatively mobile. Mucosal detail is best provided by barium contrast studies. Barium contrast studies may also reveal mass effects, ulcers, tumors, scars, strictures, swollen folds, and motility disorders. CT with diluted barium contrast may be required for processes that do not alter the lumen. The degree of contraction of the stomach at the time of imaging may markedly alter its appearance, so conclusions often cannot be drawn from one image.

SMALL BOWEL

The duodenum is primarily a fixed retroperitoneal structure, making it more vulnerable to injury in cases of blunt abdominal trauma. Although the duodenal bulb frequently contains some air, contrast material such as barium is generally required to visualize the duodenum adequately. The descending, or second, portion of the duodenum is closely associated with the head of the pancreas and is the emptying site of the pancreatic and common bile ducts. Processes affecting these structures may be identified by secondary changes involving the duodenum.

The jejunum often does not contain enough gas to serve any diagnostic purpose and requires contrast material for optimal visualization. Mucosal folds tend to be fine and "feathery." This portion of the small bowel is quite mobile; its mesenteric attachment to the posterior abdominal wall may serve as an axis for torsion.

The ileum also has the potential to be quite mobile, except when it is obstructed or paralyzed. Like other portions of the small bowel, the ileum usually contains too little gas to be used for diagnostic purposes. Differentiation between the jejunum and ileum can be difficult. The distal end of the ileum is connected to the colon by the ileocecal valve. Several diseases, including Crohn's disease and tuberculosis, tend to develop in this region.

LARGE BOWEL

The colon (which includes the cecum, appendix, ascending colon, transverse colon, descending colon, sigmoid colon, and rectum) is relatively well visualized because of its gas content, but it still requires contrast material for an adequate evaluation. The large bowel is easily recognized by haustral, or semilunar mucosal, folds that are much further apart than the closely packed small bowel folds. The cecum is usually found in the right lower quadrant (RLQ) even though it is not a fixed retroperitoneal structure. It can be quite mobile in some patients, sometimes even undergoing volvulus. The vermiform appendix is generally only filled with gas under pathological conditions. It is quite mobile and may even be retroperitoneal. The appendix may not fill during contrast studies, so in cases of suspected appendicitis, diagnostic ultrasound may be most useful. The ascending and descending portions of the colon are found retroperitoneally in the right and left lateral regions of the abdomen, respectively. The sigmoid colon is another intraperitoneal, relatively mobile portion that is usually seen in the middle or left lower region of the abdomen, although it can occasionally rise all the way up to the stomach. The rectum is relatively fixed and often contains gas or formed stool.

LIVER

The liver is seen as a relatively homogeneous density in the RUQ. The inferior and lateral margins are usually defined by very thin linings of intraperitoneal fat. The hepatic flexure of the colon may also aid in localizing liver margins. Gas overlying the liver shadow should be considered a possible abnormality and be carefully evaluated. Occasionally a normal bowel will be between the liver and anterior abdominal wall. CT is the imaging modality of choice for evaluating liver pathoses. Diagnostic ultrasound is extremely useful

in evaluating the liver and gallbladder and should be the next step after using plain film radiography. Occasionally nuclear medicine or MRI can reveal even more information.

GALLBLADDER

The gallbladder is closely associated with the anteroinferior aspect of the liver, although in some patients it is attached by mesentery and may be mobile. This is one of the more common sites in which abdominal calcifications are visualized even though only a modest percentage of gallstones are calcified. Ultrasonography often provides adequate information for diagnosing gallbladder pathoses. In cases requiring contrast for visualization, endoscopic retrograde cholangiopancreatography (ERCP) or percutaneous transhepatic cholangiography (PTHC) is often used.

PANCREAS

The pancreas is one of the more difficult organs to visualize. The head of the pancreas lies in the duodenal sweep, with the tail extending posteriorly and to the left. CT with contrast in the adjacent bowel generally provides the best images of the pancreas, but in some cases meticulous ultrasonography may be all that is needed. ERCP provides images of the ductal system but is invasive.

SPLEEN

The spleen is located in the LUQ, lateral and somewhat posterior to the stomach. The lower pole of the spleen may be seen when contrasted with intraperitoneal fat. Images of the spleen may be obtained by CT or diagnostic ultrasound. Gas shadows overlying the spleen should be considered possible abnormalities and evaluated further.

KIDNEYS

The kidneys are outlined by pericapsular fat, and their profiles are seen in many patients. Failure to visualize the renal outline is not necessarily abnormal. The kidneys are retroperitoneal and therefore relatively fixed. Regardless, a few centimeters of excursion are normally seen between images of the upright and recumbent views. During respiration, the right kidney will occasionally drop into the bony pelvis on the image of the upright view, making it difficult to find. The normal renal shadow spans two to three vertebral body heights. The kidneys are located at approximately the L1 to L3 levels, with the left being positioned slightly more cephalad than the right. The normal axis of the kidney extends from a medial position of the superior pole to a more lateral position caudally. The intravenous pyelogram (IVP) is sometimes the initial imaging modality used, but ultrasound (including Doppler ultrasound) can often answer many questions regarding scars, tumors, stones, blockages, etc. The IVP procedure provides somewhat crude information about the functional capacity of the kidneys and also can reveal tumors, cysts, and blockages. Ultrasonography may provide adequate information when the clinical picture is strongly indicative of certain pathoses. CT provides the most detailed anatomical information, particularly of the renal parenchyma, but newer Doppler ultrasound evaluations can sometimes be used instead of CT.

ADRENALS

The adrenal glands are bilateral, V-shaped organs seen superior and somewhat anterior to the superior poles of the kidneys. Cross-sectional imaging modalities such as CT or MRI (but only occasionally ultrasound) is required to evaluate the adrenal glands adequately.

URETERS

The ureters can be difficult to visualize completely even with the use of intravenous contrast material that is excreted by the kidneys. They extend from their junction with the renal pelvis anteriorly along the psoas muscles to their posterior junction with the bladder. Few pathoses affect primarily the ureters, but they are the site of most symptomatic calculi. Three common sites for calculi to lodge are the normal ureter constriction sites, where they exit the renal pelvis, the point at which the ureter crosses the iliac crest, and the ureter's junction with the bladder. Clinical symptoms, especially pain in the kidney or groin area, usually develop as a calculus passes along a ureter. Microscopic (or macroscopic) hematuria is virtually always present. It must be remembered that if a small blood clot is passed (e.g., from a kidney cancer), it may present with signs and symptoms mimicking a stone.

BLADDER

The bladder is often seen as a water density immediately superior to the pubic symphysis. In females the uterus may lay against the superior aspect of the bladder, causing an indentation. Other indentations may be fluid- or partially gas-filled loops of bowel. The mucosal surface of the bladder is best defined with contrast material, although even moderately sized tumors may not be seen on an intravenous urogram. Although CT is a better way to evaluate abnormalities, the most definitive way to search for potentially serious abnormalities is still cystoscopy.

UTERUS

The uterus is located in the pelvic bowl between the bladder and the rectum and is only seen on plain films if it indents the bladder, is grossly enlarged, or contains calcifications of uterine fibroids. The best way to evaluate the uterus with imaging studies is by ultrasound, although for certain problems CT (or MRI) can be quite helpful.

OVARIES

The ovaries are considered to be contents of the pelvic bowl, but their exact location can vary significantly. If they are large, benign or malignant ovarian tumors may extend well into the abdomen. Ultrasound is the most useful technique for locating and evaluating ovaries. CT or MRI may be occasionally required to clarify abnormalities.

PROSTATE

The prostate gland lies just above the pubic symphysis and is not normally seen on plain film radiographs unless it has calcifications from prior inflammation. Prostate enlargement may be shown by displacement of the bladder and its ureter insertions superiorly after intravenous contrast is given. Transrectal ultrasound provides the best imaging of the prostate with CT or MRI sometimes used to evaluate the full extent of lesions and spread of cancers.

BLOOD VESSELS

The abdominal aorta runs along the left anterolateral aspect of the lumbar spine and bifurcates into common iliac arteries at approximately the L3-L4 level. Calcification within the walls is more common in the elderly; younger persons with calcification often have a history of smoking. Ultrasound is the imaging modality of choice for evaluating aortic diameter and searching for aneurysms, occlusion, or stenosis. CT (especially after a rapid bolus of intravenous contrast) or MRI may reveal valuable information (e.g., concerning a leaking aneurysm and whether renal arteries are involved).

The common iliac arteries branch from the aortic bifurcation and extend downward and outward to the groin. Like the aorta, they are common sites of calcification. The inferior vena cava runs parallel to the right side of the abdominal aorta. Calcification in the walls of abdominal venous structures is rare. Ultrasound can be used to determine the presence of blood clots, extension of kidney or other cancers, and obstructions.

Imaging

Abdominal pathologies are diagnosed using the patient's history, physical examination findings, and laboratory investigations. Although not always necessary, diagnostic imaging usually adds an integral part of the evaluation of abdominal disease and abnormality. Table 25-1 lists some common abdominal pathoses and the procedures that may be used to diagnose, evaluate, or follow their disease process. All listed modalities may not be required in each case, and some uncomplicated conditions requre no imaging studies whatsoever.

Many organ diseases refer pain to the musculoskeletal system. Table 25-2 lists the more common sites of pain referral.

TABLE 25-1
Diagnostic Imaging Modalities Applied to Selected Conditions

Suspected condition	Diagnostic procedure
Abdominal abscess	CT—abdomen and pelvis with IV contrast* Ultrasound Plain film radiography Nuclear medicine MRI
Abdominal trauma (blunt)	Plain film radiography—upright chest, supine, abdomen, and upright abdomen* CT—abdomen and pelvis Ultrasound
Appendicitis	Ultrasound CT—abdomen and pelvis
Ascites	Ultrasound* CT Laparoscopy

*Usual first imaging modality.   *Continued*

TABLE 25-1
Diagnostic Imaging Modalities Applied to Selected Conditions—cont'd

Suspected condition	Diagnostic procedure
Bladder cancer	Intravenous urography* CT MRI Cystoscopy, cystourethroscopy
Cervical cancer	CT, MRI (for staging)
Cholecystitis, cholelithiasis	Ultrasound* Oral cholecystography Percutaneous cholangiography CT—abdomen and pelvis
Cirrhosis	Ultrasound CT Plain film radiography (may show enlargement) MRI
Colitis, antibiotic associated	Plain film radiography—abdomen* Contrast enema Sigmoidoscopy
Colorectal cancer	Colonoscopy Barium enema Endorectal ultrasound CT—abdomen and pelvis Radiography—chest (for metastases)
Constipation, colon obstruction	Plain film radiography—supine and upright abdomen films* Barium enema Colonoscopy/sigmoidoscopy
Crohn's disease	Upper GI with small bowel follow-through* Barium enema Colonoscopy
Diarrhea • Acute • Chronic	• Sigmoidoscopy • Radiography—abdomen Upper GI barium study with small bowel follow-through CT —abdomen and pelvis Sigmoidoscopy
Diverticulitis	Plain film radiography—abdomen Sigmoidoscopy Barium enema CT—abdomen and pelvis Nuclear medicine (for occult bleeding)
Dysmenorrhea, secondary	Ultrasound* Laparoscopy MRI Hysteroscopy Hysterogram
Dyspepsia	Upper GI study (UGI)* Endoscopy Ultrasound (gallbladder and pancreas)
Endometrial carcinoma	Intravenous urography (IVU), cystoscopy, sigmoidoscopy, ultrasound, MRI, chest radiography to determine extent
Endometriosis	Ultrasound MRI Barium enema Laparoscopy
Gastric tumors	Upper GI barium study endoscopy*
Gastritis	Upper GI barium study endoscopy*
Gastroesophageal reflux, esophagitis, dysphagia	Barium swallow* Endoscopy

*Usual first imaging modality.

TABLE 25-1

Diagnostic Imaging Modalities Applied to Selected Conditions—cont'd

Suspected condition	Diagnostic procedure
GI bleeding	
• Lower, acute	• Sigmoidoscopy/colonoscopy
	Barium enema
• Upper, acute	• Endoscopy
	Upper GI barium study
• Occult	• Upper GI and barium enema*
	Colonoscopy and endoscopy
Hemochromatosis	MRI, CT (not diagnostic alone)
Hepatic abscess	Ultrasound*
	CT
	MRI
	Radiography—chest
Hepatic tumor	CT*
	MRI
	Arteriography
Infertility	Hysterosalpingography*
	Laparoscopy
Irritable bowel syndrome	Barium enema*
	Sigmoidoscopy, colonoscopy
Jaundice	Ultrasound*
	CT
	MRI
	Endoscopic retrograde cholangiopancreatography (ERCP)
	Percutaneous transhepatic cholangiography (PTHC)
Nausea and vomiting	Plain film radiography—upright and recumbent abdomen
	Ultrasound, CT (for hepatic origin)
	Upper GI barium study
Ovarian tumors	Ultrasound*
	CT—abdomen and pelvis
	Laparoscopy
	Plain film radiography—chest (to check for metastasis)
Pancreatic tumors	CT*
	MRI
	ERCP
Pancreatitis, acute or chronic	CT*
	Plain film radiography (often nondiagnostic)
	ERCP (chronic)
Pelvic inflammatory disease	Ultrasound*
	Hysterosalpingogram
Peptic ulcer	Upper GI barium study*
	Endoscopy
Polyps	Barium enema, especially double contrast
	Sigmoidoscopy, colonoscopy
Prostate mass/enlargement	IVU*
	Ultrasound
	MRI
Renal calculi	Plain film radiography—abdomen (KUB)
	Ultrasound
	IVU with tomograms
Renal function abnormalities	Radionuclide studies
	Ultrasound
	IVU, CT (not performed if blood BUN or creatinine are too high or rising)
	MRI
	Arteriography, renal venography
Renal tumors	Ultrasound*
	IVU
	CT
	MRI

*Usual first imaging modality.

Continued

TABLE 25-1
Diagnostic Imaging Modalities Applied to Selected Conditions—cont'd

Suspected condition	Diagnostic procedure
Scrotal tumors	Ultrasound* CT
Small bowel obstruction	Plain film radiography—supine and upright abdomen* Small bowel barium study CT—abdomen and pelvis
Small bowel tumors (rare)	Upper GI barium study with small bowel follow-through or enteroclysis
Ulcer perforation	Plain film radiography—upright or decubitus abdomen Upper GI study with water-soluble contrast
Ulcerative colitis	Sigmoidoscopy Plain film radiography—abdomen
Uterine bleeding, abnormal	Ultrasound MRI Hysteroscopy Hysterosalpingogram
Uterine fibroids	Ultrasound* MRI Hysteroscopy, hysterography

*Usual first imaging modality.

TABLE 25-2
Musculoskeletal Pain Referral Sites Associated
with Organ Disease

Diseased organ or disease process	Site of pain referral
Aorta	Lumbar spine
Colon	Midlumbar spine
Gallbladder	Inferior scapula, interscapular
Gynecological disorders	Lumbar spine—rarely above L4, pelvis
Kidneys, ureters	Groin
Pancreas	Lower thoracic spine
Peptic ulcer	Midthoracic spine
Rectum	Sacral region Left lumbar paraspinal region
Sigmoid colon	Sacral region

chapter 26

Abdominal Disease Patterns

BEVERLY L HARGER
LISA E HOFFMAN
RICHARD ARKLESS

PART FOUR
Abdomen

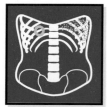

AB1 | Abdominal Calcifications

Numerous pathological processes in the abdomen may cause soft tissue calcification. A pattern approach that evaluates the morphological features, location, and mobility of an abnormal opacity often provides sufficient information for a definitive diagnosis or, at the very least, narrows the etiological considerations to a few possibilities.[3] Almost all abdominal calcifications fall into four major morphological categories. Each one of the four categories possesses characteristic roentgen features based on shape, border sharpness, marginal continuity, and internal architecture.[3] The four morphological categories are concretions, conduit wall calcification, cystic calcification, and solid mass calcification (Table 26-1).[3]

Several limitations of classification according to radiographic morphology exist. When a calcification is very small, it is difficult to categorize. Furthermore, very faint calcification cannot be classified if no information about margins or internal matrix can be ascertained.[3]

Following is a brief presentation of each of the four major morphological categories (AB1a through AB1d) with the most common etiological considerations.

TABLE 26-1
Comparison of Roentgen Features of Abdominal Calcifications[3]

	Concretion	Conduit	Cyst	Mass
Shape	Varied	Tracklike, ring, or annular	Round or oval	Varied
Border	Smooth	Irregular	Smooth	Irregular
Margin	Continuous	Interrupted	Interrupted	Interrupted
Matrix	Laminations uniform	None	Less dense	Speckled, mottled, whorled, or streaky

AB1a Concretions

A concretion (also called a *stone* or *calculus*) is a calcified mass that forms in a tubular or hollow structure such as the lumen of a vessel or hollow viscus. A fairly constant appearance of concretions is a sharp, clearly defined external margin that is almost always continuous.[3] This continuity may help differentiate a concretion—in a hollow viscus (e.g., renal pelvis, gallbladder, and urinary bladder)—from a calcified cyst. Discontinuity of the outer margin makes a diagnosis of a stone unlikely. The internal architecture of concretions may vary in appearance. Concretions may have concentric laminations, may contain a slightly eccentric area of lucency, or may be homogenously dense. Generally, concretions are seen in association with anatomical structures and do not pass through the vascular or visceral wall. Concretions appearing outside of common, expected anatomical locations is unusual.

CONCRETION	COMMENTS
Appendicolith (FIG. 26-1)	Frequently associated with current or future appendiceal perforation, especially in children[18]; it is most commonly seen in the right lower quadrant but location may vary

Continued

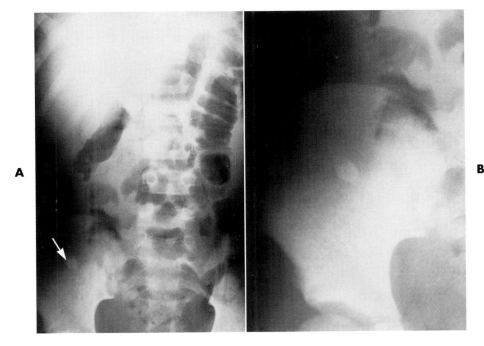

FIG. 26-1 Appendicolith. **A,** A concretion in the right lower quadrant in a child *(arrow).* Appendicolith may indicate appendicitis with perforation and abscess. **B,** Close-up. Notice the sharp, continuous external margin characteristic of a concretion. The concretion in this case is uniformly dense.

CONCRETION	COMMENTS
Cholelithiasis (FIG. 26-2) [p. 963]	10% to 15% are calcified and therefore visible on plain film[30,62]; cholelithiasis occurs more frequently in the elderly and obese, predominantly in females[30]; typically cholelithiasis occurs in the right upper quadrant, but location may vary
Pancreatic calculi (FIG. 26-3)	Most commonly associated with chronic pancreatitis secondary to alcoholism[61]; the typical appearance is multiple, tiny, dense, discrete opacities that cross the midline at the level of L1-L2

Phleboliths (FIG. 26-4)	Most commonly encountered calcification in pelvis[3]; they are frequently multiple and bilateral; sometimes a concentric or slightly eccentric interior lucency occurs; they can be confused with urinary tract stones
Prostatic calculi (FIG. 26-5)	Multiple concretions of varied sizes clustered behind pubic symphysis in males usually more than 40 years of age[3]; this condition results from prior prostatitis; protastatic calculi is often asymptomatic

Continued

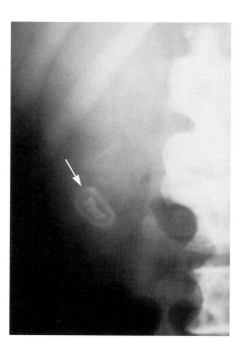

FIG. 26-2   Cholelith. A laminated gallstone with continuous outer margin typical of a concretion *(arrow)*.   (Courtesy John A.M. Taylor, Portland, Ore.)

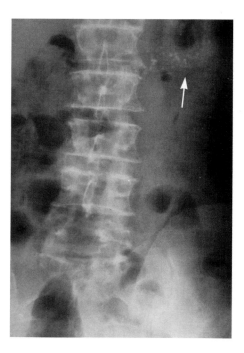

FIG. 26-3   Pancreatic calculi and chronic pancreatitis in a patient suffering from alcoholism. This is the typical appearance of numerous dense, discrete opacities that cross midline at the level of L1-L2 *(arrow)*. The normal pancreas is not visible on abdominal plain films.

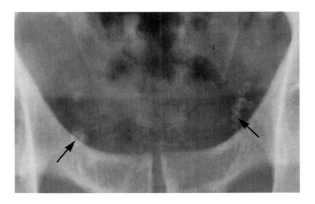

FIG. 26-4   Numerous phleboliths. Phleboliths are frequently multiple and bilateral, and they are asymptomatic. They are inconsequential concretions of thrombi attached to the walls of veins. Observe the concentric interior lucency of the phleboliths *(arrows)*. These should not be confused with ureteral stones or calcifications of a pelvic mass.

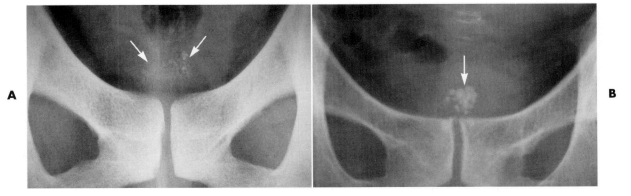

A   B

FIG. 26-5   Prostatic calculi in two different patients. Intraductal calculi may form in a chronically inflamed prostate. These multiple concretions are from prior prostatitis. **A,** Numerous tiny, discrete calculi project above the symphysis pubis *(arrows)*. **B,** Multiple larger calculi are clustered in a midline location *(arrow)*. *(A, Courtesy Cynthia Peterson, Bournemouth, England; B, Courtesy John A.M. Taylor, Portland, Ore.)*

CONCRETION	COMMENTS
Urinary tract calculi (FIG. 26-6, 26-7, AND 26-8)	May be seen in the renal calyces or pelvis, ureters, and bladder; they are uncommon in the urethra[52]; sometimes urinary tract calculi are associated with conditions producing hypercalcemia or hypercalciuria[3]

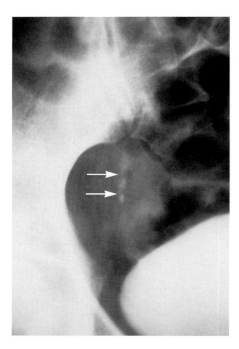

FIG. 26-7 Ureteral stones. Intravenous urogram demonstrates multiple small opacities located within the lower segment of the ureter *(arrows)*.

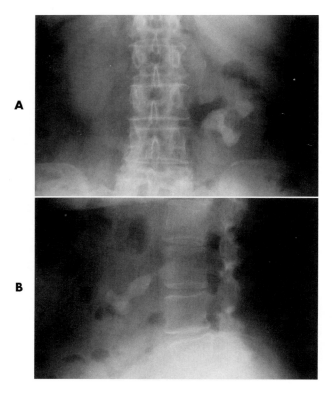

FIG. 26-6 Staghorn calculus. **A,** AP projection shows a concretion taking the shape of the pelvicalyceal system (staghorn calculus). **B,** Lateral view. Superimposition of the concretion over the vertebral body indicates the retroperitoneal location. (Courtesy Cynthia Peterson, Bournemouth, England.)

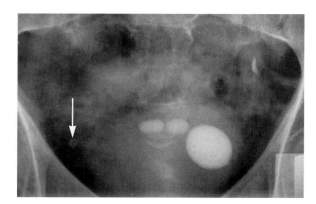

FIG. 26-8 Bladder calculi. Three homogeneously dense bladder stones with a continuous rim of calcification typical of concretions. Incidentally noted is a phlebolith with the diagnostic concentric lucency that should not be mistaken for a ureteral stone *(arrow)*.

ABIb | Conduit Wall Calcification

Conduits are channels or tubular structures through which fluids are conducted.[3] Conduit wall calcifications are confined to only the tubular walls, which are seen radiographically as parallel, linear opacities or, when seen end on, as ringlike calcifications.[3] Therefore, any internal radiopacity indicates another class of calcification.

The calcification in conduit walls is not homogeneous. The most common site is in the walls of arteries, where one sees interrupted but basically linear calcifications.[3] This feature helps differentiate them from concretions, which usually have a continuous calcified external margin. The calcification can also outline a vessel's branching pattern.[3]

LOCATION	COMMENTS		
Aorta and iliac arteries (FIG. 26-9)	Occurs mostly as a result of atherosclerosis; patients younger than 40 years of age are rarely affected; this may be associated with smoking or diabetes; patients can be hypertensive or have coronary artery disease	**Renal arteries**	Arise from abdominal aorta at or near L1 and usually extend laterally or infralaterally; calcification occurs primarily as a consequence of atherosclerosis or diabetes[2,59]; this is often accompanied by aortic calcification

Continued

PART FOUR Abdomen

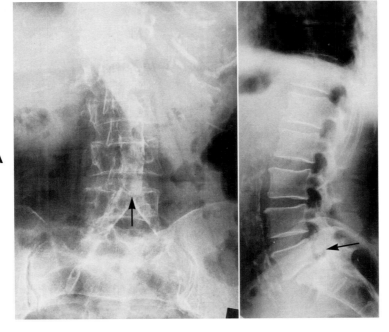

FIG. 26-9 Abdominal aorta and iliac arteries calcification. **A,** AP projection. Tubular appearance characteristic of conduit wall calcification. The aortic bifurcation is clearly seen (*arrow*). **B,** Lateral view. Notice that the anterior and posterior walls are parallel and the abdominal aorta diameter does not exceed 3.5 cm. Aneurysm should be suspected if the diameter of the abdominal aorta exceeds 3.5 cm. A spondylolytic spondylolisthesis of L5 is also visible (*arrow*). (Courtesy John A.M. Taylor, Portland, Ore.)

LOCATION

Splenic artery (FIG. 26-10)

Iliac veins and inferior vena cava

COMMENTS

Frequently calcifies and has a characteristic serpentine course in the left upper quadrant

Veins not subjected to either high pressure or pulsatile flow and are therefore relatively protected from the risk of intimal layer damage[3]; see Figs. 26-4 and 26-68

Gallbladder wall (FIG. 26-11)

Vas deferens (FIG. 26-12)

Also known as *porcelain gallbladder,* can resemble a large gallstone; a significant percentage of these patients will also develop gallbladder cancer, usually adenocarcinoma*

Most often in diabetic patients, rarely secondary to infection[11,23,35]; most often it is bilateral, curved, symmetrical, and paralleling the pubic rami

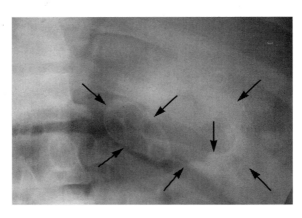

FIG. 26-10   Splenic artery calcification. A convoluted and tubular appearance is typical of splenic artery *(arrows).*

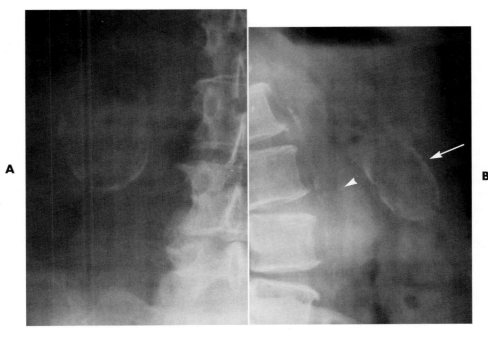

FIG. 26-11 Calcification within the wall of the gallbladder. **A,** AP projection. Calcification within the wall of the gallbladder mimics a cyst. This condition is important to recognize, because a common complication is adenocarcinoma. **B,** Lateral view confirms the intraperitoneal location *(arrow).* Also visible is conduit calcification of the abdominal aorta *(arrowhead).* (Courtesy John A.M. Taylor, Portland, Ore.)

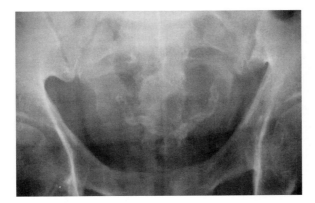

FIG. 26-12 Vas deferens calcification. Tramlike calcification paralleling the superior pubic rami is typical of vas deferens calcification. Location helps differentiate this from arterial calcification.

ABIc | Cystic Calcification

Calcium deposition in the wall of an abnormal fluid-filled structure defines cystic calcification.[3] Calcium around the surface of a tumor can occasionally mimic this appearance. Examples of cystic calcification include epithelial-lined cysts, pseudocysts that have fibrous integument, and artery aneurysms. Calcification shows up as a smooth, curvilinear rim of opacity.[3] This rimlike appearance is usually larger than that of conduit wall calcification; however, in both types, calcification may be interrupted in spots, appearing as an incomplete circle. Single, incomplete calcified margins likely represent a cystic density, in contrast to a concretion where one should expect a continuous margin of calcification.[3] The external border of the cyst is usually smooth, whereas the internal aspect is irregular, reflecting the interface with the contained fluid.[3] In contrast to a solid mass type pattern, the outer margin of a cystic structure usually exhibits a relatively well-defined margin. Adjacent organs or vessels may be displaced or distorted by either solid masses or cystic structures.

CYST	COMMENTS
Left upper quadrant (above L3)	
Spleen **(FIG. 26-13)**	Two thirds of splenic cysts caused by *Echinococcus granulosis* (rare in the United States)[60]; other possibilities include hemorrhagic and serous cysts, usually secondary to trauma[13]; cystic changes may be secondary to subcapsular hematoma and metastatic mucinous adenocarcinoma of the ovary[47]; occasionally an aneurysm of splenic artery may mimic a cyst; see also Renal and Adrenal sections that follow

Right upper quadrant (above L3)	
Liver	Rare hepatic cysts except those associated with *Echinococcus granulosis;* occasionally gallbladder carcinoma calcification can be inside the liver and high[7,21]
Right or left upper quadrant	
Renal **(FIG. 26-14)**	Benign and malignant neoplasms of the kidney and renal cysts; renal cysts are more common with advancing age, but usually they do not calcify[31,34,50]; renal artery aneurysm and subcapsular hematoma may also present as cystic calcifications
Adrenal **(FIG. 26-15)**	Infrequent; pseudocysts are the most common cysts to calcify[46]; calcified cystic pheochromocytomas and other benign and malignant tumors are rare[20,54,68]
Midabdomen *Pancreas*	Rare calcification of the wall of a pancreatic pseudocyst[36]; cystic calcifications may be seen in benign and malignant tumors[19]
Right lower quadrant (below L3)	
Appendix	Mucocele calcification rarely appearing as a calcified cyst; it occurs primarily in middle age and is slightly more common in males[14]
Left lower quadrant (below L3)	Least likely of the abdominal regions to contain calcific densities; when present, they are likely to be ureteral stones, vascular densities, and leiomyomas; these are rarely cystic in appearance

Continued

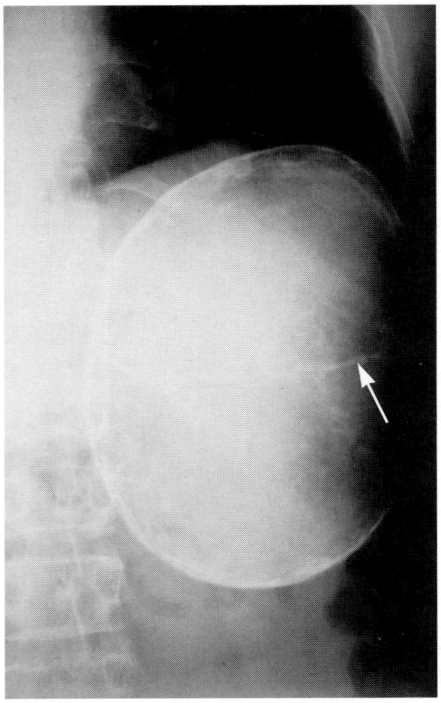

FIG. 26-13　Calcified splenic cyst. Observe the smooth, curvilinear rim of opacity in the wall of the cyst, although continuous in this case, most cysts will have an interrupted rim of calcification. A central, horizontal line of calcification indicates septation (*arrow*).

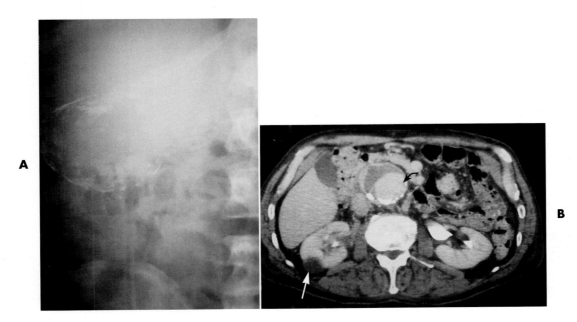

FIG. 26-14 **A,** Renal cell carcinoma. This cystic lesion proved to be a malignant neoplasm of the kidney. Note the rim calcification characteristic of a cyst. **B,** CT of a non-calcified benign renal cyst *(arrow)*. This would not be visible on plain film. Note the calcification in the wall of an abdominal aortic aneurysm *(curved arrow)*.

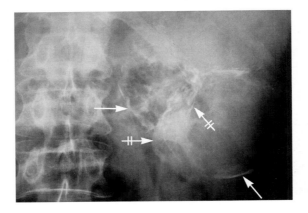

FIG. 26-15 Massive adrenal cyst with septations. This massive lesion proved to be adrenal carcinoma *(arrows)*. Contrast opacification of the pelvicalyceal system and proximal ureter is noted *(crossed arrows)*.

CYST	COMMENTS
Pelvic bowl	
Bladder	Schistosomiasis of the bladder, worldwide, is the most common cause of mural calcification and is seen as a thin, continuous curvilinear calcification of cyst type; it is rare in the United States[65]
Ovary	Most common ovarian lesion: cystic teratoma (dermoid cyst)[67]; about 10% of cystic teratomas show calcification of cyst type[12,67]; benign cystadenomas and cystadenocarcinomas may appear as curvilinear calcifications of cystic type[45]; any cystic calcification in this area must be considered a possible malignancy unless proven otherwise
Any location	
Mesentery and omentum	Cysts resulting from inflammation, trauma, or congenital rests[3]; they can move on sequential films; they are located anterior to pancreas, kidney, spleen, and adrenal glands
Cystic calcifications that cross midline	
Aorta **(FIG. 26-16)**	Abdominal aortic aneurysm: most common abnormality with the radiographic appearance of the cystic calcification in this location[3]

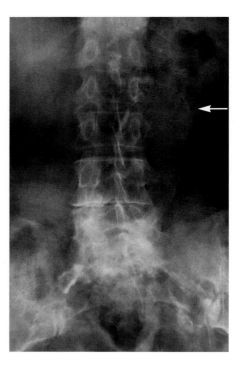

FIG. 26-16   Abdominal aortic aneurysm. Curvilinear calcification of the wall of an abdominal aortic aneurysm presenting as a cystic calcification *(arrow)*.

ABId | Solid Mass Calcification

This category comprises the most diverse presentation of the four. Irregularly calcified borders and complex internal architecture are characteristic of solid mass calcification.[3] Prominent but irregular and inhomogeneous calcification in the more central portion of the mass and discontinuity of the outer border are frequently encountered.[3]

MASS	COMMENTS
Left upper quadrant	
Spleen (FIG. 26-17)	Splenic densities most often resulting from calcium deposition in granulomas, often from histoplasmosis if multiple or occasionally from tuberculosis[22,58]

Right upper quadrant	
Liver	Most common universal cause of solid calcifications: tuberculosis and histoplasmosis[1,16]; calcified metastases (usually from colon and ovary) and benign neoplasms, such as cavernous hemangioma, may cause solid calcifications[40]

Continued

PART FOUR Abdomen

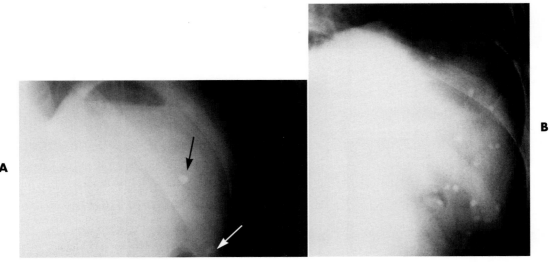

FIG. 26-17 Splenic mass calcifications—two different patients **A,** Splenic granulomas are seen as solid mass calcification in the left upper quadrant *(arrows).* **B,** Multiple calcified granulomas. These are most often from histoplasmosis.

MASS

Right or left upper quadrant

Adrenal
(FIG. 26-18)

COMMENTS

In the adult, a normal-sized adrenal gland with calcification seen secondary to tuberculosis, Addison's disease, and old neonatal hemorrhage; solid adrenal calcification in an enlarged gland may be due to cortical carcinoma; adenomas rarely calcify[6]

Right or left upper quadrant—cont'd

Renal
(FIG. 26-19)

Hypernephromas making up 90% of all solid mass type calcification involving the kidney[15]; among inflammatory diseases, tuberculosis most frequently shows calcification[64]; solid mass calcification can occur in other primary malignancies, metastases (rare), and hamartomas[53]

Midabdomen

Pancreas
(FIG. 26-20)

Pancreatic cystadenoma and cystadenocarcinoma solid mass calcification varying from a large stellate to closely aggregated solid masses to scattered clumps[28,48]

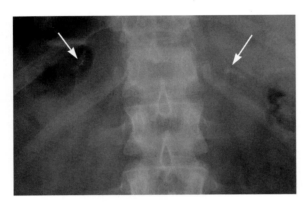

FIG. 26-18 Bilateral adrenal gland calcification. The size and location of the adrenal glands are visible because of calcification *(arrows)*. These normal-sized adrenal glands show calcification most likely secondary to tuberculosis, Addison's disease, or old neonatal hemorrhage.

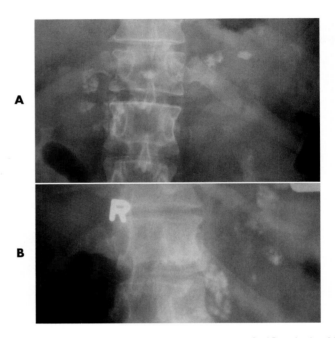

FIG. 26-20 Solid mass calcification of the pancreas. **A,** AP projection. Notice the calcifications are close to the midline on the right and extend far to the periphery to the left. **B,** RAO view. These scattered clumps of calcification of the pancreas may indicate benign or malignant lesions. Pancreatic lithiasis associated with pancreatitis typically will present as small, discrete opacities (concretions).

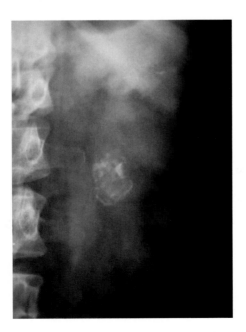

FIG. 26-19 Solid mass calcification. This was proven renal mass calcification from tuberculosis. Solid calcifications share the common feature of a nongeometric inner architecture and irregular, often incomplete margins.

Pelvic bowl

Bladder

Detectable calcifications seen in only 0.5% of bladder tumors[43]; bladder calcification is rare with urinary tuberculosis[27]; schistosomiasis can calcify but is rare in the United States

Uterine
(FIG. 26-21)

Coarse, granular calcifications resembling popcorn or cauliflower, developing within necrotic areas of uterine leiomyoma (very common) and leiomyosarcoma (rare)[56]

Ovary

Two thirds of all ovarian malignancies: papillary serous cystadenocarcinomas that may calcify at the primary site and in metastatic deposits[8,63]; the calcification, known as *psammomatous* calcification, can vary from a flocculent, sharply demarcated focus to a less well-defined density and sometimes are throughout the abdomen

Any location

Intestinal tract

Adenocarcinomas or colloid carcinomas of the intestinal tract characteristically mottled, speckled, or granular pattern calcification; however, calcified small bowel tumors are rarely seen on x-rays; when seen, carcinoid tumors are more common[32]

Subcutaneous
(FIG. 26-22)

Extensive calcification resulting from scleroderma, dermatomyositis, and subcutaneous fat necrosis; this calcification can project over the abdomen and seem as if it is intraabdominal[26]

Continued

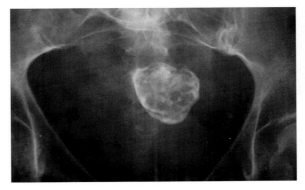

FIG. 26-21 Uterine leiomyoma. Mass calcification associated with uterine leiomyoma is very common. Location and pattern of calcification are helpful in determining the diagnosis.

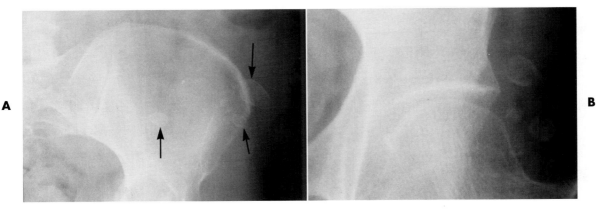

FIG. 26-22 Subcutaneous fat necrosis with calcium in two patients. **A,** Subcutaneous fat necrosis following injections can produce calcification that can project over the abdomen and seem as if it is intraabdominal *(arrows).* **B,** Close-up view. (Courtesy John A.M. Taylor, Portland, Ore.)

MASS	COMMENTS
Any location— cont'd	
Lymph node **(FIG. 26-23; SEE ALSO FIG. 26-28, A)**	Mesenteric lymph nodes: most common abdominal nodes to calcify[57]; they are one of the more common types of abdominal calcifications seen; healed tuberculosis is sometimes the cause of these calcifications, with exposure usually occurring several decades previously[57]
Peritoneal	Psammomatous calcifications appearing within ovarian cystadenocarcinoma and its peritoneal implants; they may be widespread[63]
Scars **(FIG. 26-24)**	Occasionally peculiar shape calcifications, often located in abdominal wall

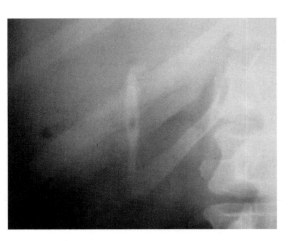

FIG. 26-24   Abdominal scar. Scars may on occasion give a peculiar pattern of calcification. Perpendicular views may indicate their surface location.

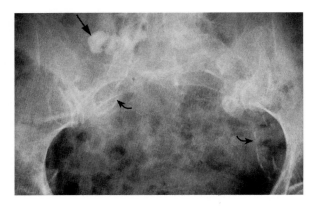

FIG. 26-23   Calcified mesenteric nodes. Mesenteric nodes are the most common abdominal nodes to calcify and present as mass calcification *(arrow)*. Observe the conduit pattern of arterial calcification *(curved arrows)*.

AB2 Pneumoperitoneum

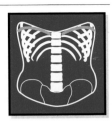

Sources of free air in the peritoneal cavity are numerous. In some patients this is a benign, inconsequential finding, but in others it indicates such grave conditions as perforation of a hollow viscus.

AB2a Most Common Causes of Pneumoperitoneum

DISEASE	COMMENTS
Recent laparotomy	Usually present for 3 to 7 days after laparotomy, occasionally longer[55]; the volume of air decreases daily; faster resorption is seen in young adults[25]
Trauma	Can be secondary to diagnostic studies such as peritoneoscopy and culdoscopy or from perforation during double-contrast barium enema or with colonoscopy; pneumoperitoneum may occur after severe external trauma
Spontaneous	Most common cause: perforation of gastric or duodenal ulcer; rarely, air enters peritoneum via uterus and fallopian tubes (from puberty on)

AB2b | Plain Film Technique for Detection of Pneumoperitoneum

A complete series to detect free air includes erect and decubitus abdomen and upright PA chest views.[42] This approach may occasionally require up to 30 minutes to allow air to migrate between views, although larger amounts migrate faster and smaller amounts usually do not need more than a few minutes to migrate.

PROJECTION

COMMENTS

Left lateral decubitus

Should be performed first[43]; patient is placed in left lateral decubitus position for 10 or 20 minutes (if the condition affecting the patient permits); lower right lung field is included in the film; chest technique is used[42]

Upright view **(FIG. 26-25)**

Patient placed in sitting or standing position a few minutes, 5 to 10 if possible; film is centered at thoracolumbar junction area[42]

Supine film

May be only film taken in acutely ill patients; however, smaller amounts of air will usually not be seen; it is crucial to be familiar with these subtle signs of pneumoperitoneum on the supine film if the condition is to be recognized[42]

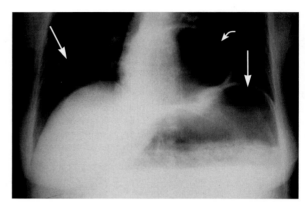

FIG. 26-25 Free air in abdomen. Air beneath both hemidiaphragms is seen in this upright view of the lower thorax and upper abdomen *(arrows)*. A large hiatal hernia is demonstrated as a mass with an air-fluid level superimposed over the cardiac silhouette *(curved arrow)*.

AB2c | Signs of Pneumoperitoneum on Supine Abdominal Films

The complete series for detection of intraperitoneal gas may not be possible, such as with debilitated patients and for those who suffer from acute abdominal pain. In such cases, recognition of free air on the supine radiograph is essential, recognizing that smaller amounts (which can be just as ominous) will not be seen.

SIGN	COMMENTS
Gas-relief or double-wall sign (FIG. 26-26)	Intraluminal and extraluminal air outlining both surfaces of the bowel wall; usually, at least 1 L of gas is required to demonstrate this sign[9]
Falciform ligament sign	Falciform ligament: lies just to the right and parallel to the spine at the inferior aspect of the liver; the sign may appear as a linear density when surrounded by air[24]
Urachus sign	Triangular soft tissue density with its base at the urinary bladder seen in midline below the umbilicus; urachus represents a remnant of the fetal allantois and may have its own peritoneal reflection to contrast pneumoperitoneum[29]
Inverted "V" sign	Visualization of the lateral umbilical ligaments[66]
Football sign	Large amounts of air forming a dome over free intraperitoneal fluid in the central part of the abdomen; this has an ellipsoidal shape, resembling a football; the football sign is seen most frequently in children[3]
Morison's pouch sign	A triangular gas density projected over the superior margin of the right kidney, representing air trapped dorsally under the liver[41]
Parahepatic air	Air may be trapped under the tip of the right lobe of the liver, presenting as an oblique, linear gas density[39]
Triangle sign	A triangular collection of free contrasted between three loops of bowel[39]
Air in the fissure for ligamentum teres	Air possibly confined to the fissure for the ligamentum teres; this will appear as a vertically directed area of hyperlucency in the right upper quadrant[9]

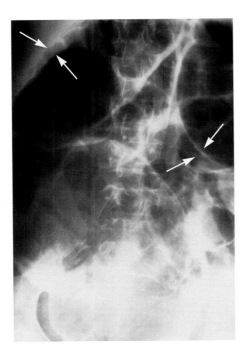

FIG. 26-26 Gas-relief sign (double-wall sign). Massive pneumoperitoneum from rupture of a duodenal ulcer allows clear demarcation of the inner and outer walls of many intestinal loops (arrows).

AB2d | Pseudopneumoperitoneum

Many processes may stimulate free air in the peritoneal cavity (pseudopneumoperitoneum).

DISEASE	COMMENTS
Double-wall finding	Two closely approximated gas-filled bowel loops, one of which may mimic free air
Chilaiditi syndrome (FIG. 26-27)	Gas-filled intestine between liver and diaphragm; intestine is examined for haustra and continuity with other bowel loops
Subdiaphragmatic fat	Fat in the posterior pararenal space may extend between the diaphragm and peritoneum; its appearance as a thin black stripe can mimic free subdiaphragmatic air
Extraperitoneal air	Streaky or bubbly air collections that do not change on decubitus views; if abutting the diaphragm this structure appears too thick; it is also seen at the edge of the abdomen in the abdominal wall
Situs inversus	Stomach bubble appearing under right diaphragm resembling free air; however, the usual position of the stomach is devoid of gas, being occupied by the liver

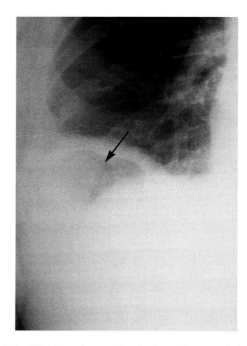

FIG. 26-27   Chilaiditi syndrome. AP projection of the upper abdomen reveals the colon interposed between the liver and the diaphragm. Cirrhosis and ascites predispose to Chilaiditi syndrome. Demonstration of haustra *(arrow)* will help in differentiating this from pneumoperitoneum.

AB3 | Abnormal Localized Intraperitoneal Gas Collections

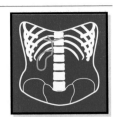

B esides free air in the peritoneal cavity, localized intraperitoneal gas collections may also be seen in the biliary ducts, the gallbladder, the portal veins, the renal pelvis, the urinary bladder, in an abscess, and in a pancreatic pseudocyst.[3]

LOCATION	COMMENTS		
Gas in the biliary tract (pneumobilia) (FIG. 26-28)	Often a result of surgery on Oddi's sphincter during stone removal for the common duct; this surgery often allows gas to subsequently occupy the biliary tree for years; a fistula secondary to erosion of a gallstone into the intestine is the most common nonsurgical cause of pneumobilia[4]; sometimes the gallstones can be seen obstructing a loop of small bowel	**Gas in the gallbladder (emphysematous cholecystitis)**	Emphysematous cholecystitis, of infectious etiology, resulting in gas either in the lumen or in the wall of the gallbladder; the fatality rate is 15%, independent of patient age[38]

Continued

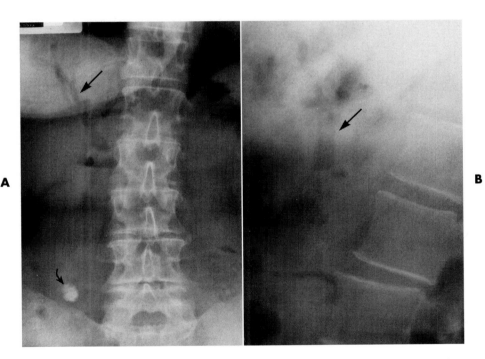

FIG. 26-28 Pneumobilia secondary to surgical creation of a fistula between the bile duct and the duodenum (choledochoduodenostomy). **A,** AP projection shows branched, tubular areas of lucency in the central portion of the liver characteristic of gas in the biliary tree *(arrow).* Incidentally noted is calcification of a lymph node in the right lower quadrant *(curved arrow).* **B,** Lateral view demonstrates air within the biliary duct *(arrow).* (Courtesy Cynthia Peterson, Bournemouth, England.)

LOCATION	COMMENTS		
Gas in the portal vein system	May present with multiple tubular lucencies that extend to the periphery of the liver; this usually results from bowel wall necrosis or infection, and therefore the mortality of these patients can be as high as 75%[37]	Small bubbles in an abscess (FIG. 26-29)	Bubbly gas seen within some abscesses; often a history exists of diabetes, pancreatitis, or recent surgery; CT scan with oral contrast is the best imaging modality to differentiate abscess from bowel gas

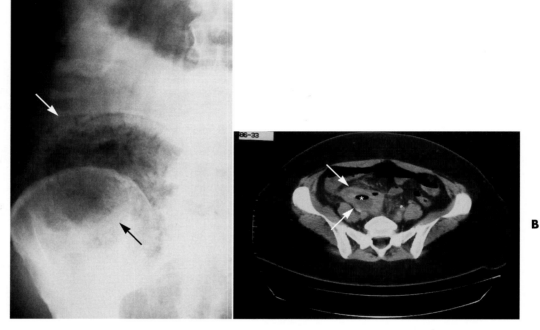

FIG. 26-29   **A,** Abnormal intraperitoneal gas collection. Bubbly gas within an abscess can be seen in this patient that recently had abdominal surgery *(arrows)*. **B,** Appendiceal abscess *(arrows)* containing air *(asterisk)*. CT scan is the best imaging modality to differentiate abscess from bowel gas.

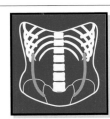

AB4 | Pneumoretroperitoneum

Pneumoperitoneum may also be simulated by air in the retroperitoneal space and its lateral and anterior continuations on supine films. Retroperitoneal and intraperitoneal air may exist simultaneously, producing even more confusing signs. The markedly different etiology, clinical course, and treatment of pneumoperitoneum and pneumoretroperitoneum make differentiation of the two crucial to patient evaluation.[3] Pneumoretroperitoneum is quite uncommon. The most common causes are listed below.

ETIOLOGY	COMMENTS
Trauma	Commonly trauma from penetrating wounds, following surgery, after diagnostic procedures such as barium enema or endoscopy, and perforation by pelvic fracture fragments[3]
Spontaneous colon perforation	Frequently caused by perforation of colonic diverticula or carcinoma in the ascending or descending colon (which are retroperitoneal); rupture of the sigmoid colon within or posterior to the peritoneal cavity secondary to volvulus may also be a cause[3]
Extension from pneumomediastinum	Various posterior and midline openings in the diaphragm providing a route for communication of free air in the mediastinum with the retroperitoneal space[3]
Gas-containing retroperitoneal abscess **(FIG. 26-30)**	Infection by gas-forming organisms occurring in any retroperitoneal compartment; communication from the perirenal space may occur inferiorly to the anterior and posterior pararenal spaces[3]; this type may be caused by a recent back or kidney surgery, pancreatitis, or penetrating injury

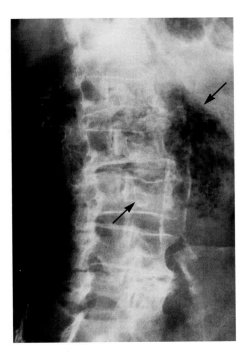

FIG. 26-30 Gas-containing retroperitoneal abscess. Infection by gas-forming organisms may occur in any retroperitoneal compartment and on plain film the abscess may be seen as an extraluminal collection of gas (arrows).

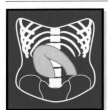

AB5 | Abnormal Bowel Gas Resulting from Obstruction

Identification of bowel obstruction on plain film can be difficult. The hallmark findings are noted involving the small bowel. Prominent valvulae conniventes can be identified by their contrast against the gas in the lumen. Several adjacent or continuous distended loops are usually identified. The overall appearance of these tubular lucencies are affected by the site, duration, and degree of obstruction. Measuring the relative amounts of gas and liquid within the occluded segment also helps determine the radiographic presentation. Often the distended bowel loop in obstruction has a "tight" or hairpin appearance, rather than the flaccid appearance of inflamed or paralyzed bowel.

The stomach can be altered drastically in caliber and volume. Because stomach contents can vary depending on what was recently ingested, whether the patient recently vomited or had fluid aspirated through a stomach tube, and whether stomach emptying is rapid or slow, the appearance of the stomach can be misleading.

The colon presents with a variety of normal configurations. Obstruction will also have a variety of presentations determined by the site and duration of blockage, the liquid versus solid versus gaseous nature of the luminal contents, the competency of the ileocecal valve, and the possible concomitant dilatation of small loops. Typically, with mechanical obstruction, dilatation of the lumen proximal to the obstructed point will be seen.[3]

Intestinal dilatation is noted secondary to many diseases. Diseases or injuries that directly or reflexively affect bowel motility or transport may lead to this appearance. Signs of nonobstructive dilatation include diffuse, symmetrical, predominately gaseous distention of the bowel in a patient who has little in the way of symptoms. With nonobstructive dilatation a point of abrupt disruption is usually not identified. Differentiation of mechanical from functional obstruction may require an oral barium study of the stomach, small bowel follow-through, and barium enema of the colon. Possible causes would include reaction to medications such as narcotics, peritonitis, recent enemas, and (rarely) diseases such as scleroderma.

SITE	COMMENTS		
Gastric obstruction	Occlusion of the gastric outlet sometimes caused by a chronic ulcer scar or antral carcinoma; a dilated, fluid-filled stomach may be imaged as a large water and/or gas density mass displacing the transverse colon downward[3]	Small bowel obstruction **(FIGS. 26-31 AND 26-32)**	Identified by distention of small bowel, which normally should not exceed 3 cm in diameter; adhesions from prior surgery is the most common cause, but external and internal hernias, masses, and volvulus can also cause obstruction[3]

Continued

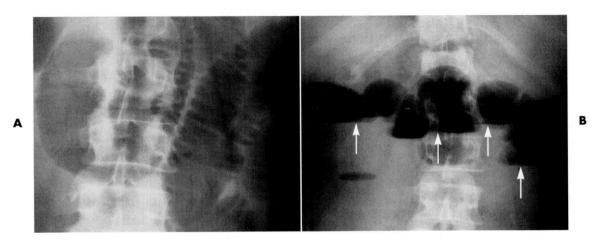

FIG. 26-31   Small bowel obstruction. **A,** The supine film demonstrates dilated small bowel in the abdomen. Note that the mucosal folds of the small bowel are much narrower than the haustral folds of the colon. **B,** The upright view shows multiple air-fluid levels *(arrows).*

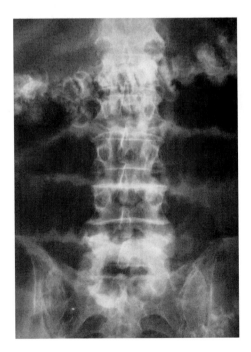

FIG. 26-32   Small bowel obstruction. The supine film reveals dilated small bowel loops greater than 3 cm diameter. Most small bowel obstructions are caused by postoperative adhesions.

SITE

Large bowel ob-
struction
(FIGS. 26-33
AND 26-34)

COMMENTS

The diameter of the colon, with the exception of the cecum, normally less than 6 cm; the cecum can safely be somewhat larger, sometimes up to 8 cm; the most common cause is a distal obstruction either from colon cancer or diverticulitis, but other causes to be considered are cecal volvulus, obstruction distally by peritoneal metastases (especially ovarian cancer), by pressure from a massively distended bladder or other large pelvic mass, and by adhesions[3]

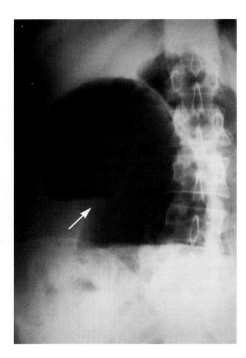

FIG. 26-34   Cecal volvulus. Erect film reveals a dilated cecum with a single air-fluid level. The ileocecal valve *(arrow)* produces a soft tissue indentation so that the gas-filled cecum has the appearance of a coffee bean or kidney.

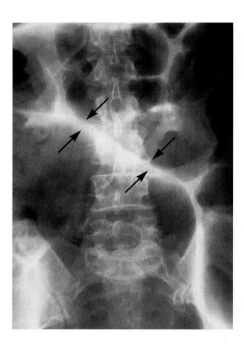

FIG. 26-33   Sigmoid volvulus. Recumbent plain film of the abdomen shows the massively dilated "inverted U" of gas-filled colon pointing toward the right upper quadrant. Opposed inner walls of the sigmoid colon form a dense white line *(arrows)*. This finding should not be confused with the double-wall sign of pneumoperitoneum.

AB6 | Ascites

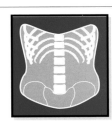

The importance of plain abdomen films in the evaluation of ascites has diminished in recent years with the introduction of ultrasound and computerized tomography (CT) (Fig. 26-35). Most plain radiographic signs have limited reliability since usually large amounts of fluid need to be present for identification, whereas CT and ultrasonography can accurately detect small amounts.

SIGN	COMMENTS		
Loss of hepatic angle (inferior lateral tip of liver) (FIG. 26-36, A)	Normally, the liver is contrasted by the adjacent fat; one pitfall is that adhesions may slow the flow of fluid along the right paracolic gutter, thereby preserving the hepatic angle	**Dog ears (FIGS. 26-36, B AND 26-36, C)**	Pelvic accumulation of ascites; peritoneal fluid may accumulate as symmetrical bulges above the bladder resembling the contour of dog ears; smaller amounts of fluid can be seen here; upright abdomen film is best
Widening of paracolic gutter	Large effusions increasing the distance, which is normally 2 to 3 mm, between the flank stripe and gas in the ascending or descending colon; supine films are more likely to show this if obtained on inspiration	**Ground glass sign**	Ascites sometimes extensive enough to produce this overall increase in density; in such cases, other imaging and physical exam findings are normally present

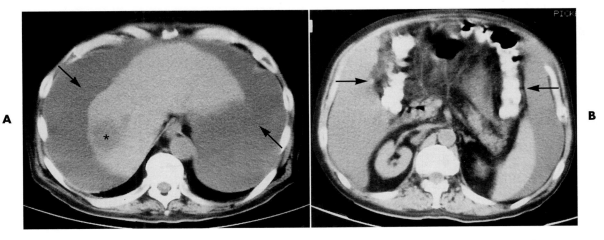

FIG. 26-35 Ascites. Ultrasound and CT may detect small amounts of ascitic fluid. To detect ascites on plain films a larger amount of fluid, more than 500 mL is required. **A,** CT scan shows the presence of a fluid-filled peritoneum (*arrows*). A lesion within the liver is also visible (*asterisk*). **B,** Centralization of bowel loops is occurring (*arrows*) because of the large amount of fluid in the paracolic gutters.

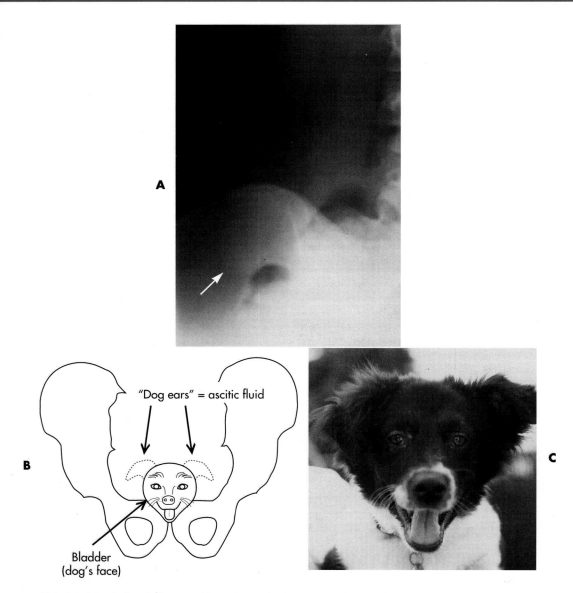

FIG. 26-36　Ascites. **A,** The normal liver edge is visible in this patient *(arrow).* With ascites, the normal liver edge may be obscured **B,** Symmetrical bulges above the bladder resembling the contour of dog ears represent intraperitoneal fluid accumulation in the pouch of Douglas with central indentation from the bladder or rectum. **C,** Chiro Woller demonstrating dog ears sign of ascites.

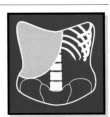

AB7 | Enlarged Organ Shadows

Radiographic evidence of enlarged organs is generally the recognition of displacement of adjacent structures. Structures (such as the stomach, transverse and sigmoid colon, small bowel, and urinary bladder) that are mobile can be easily pushed by enlarging masses. Adjacent normal structures move as they accommodate themselves to the growth of the organ. The direction of this movement is particularly useful in the localization of small to moderate-size masses. Especially with retroperitoneal masses such as tumors or aortic aneurysm, the kidneys may also be displaced.

AB7a | Hepatomegaly

The liver fills the right upper abdomen and extends transversely from the right lateral abdominal wall to the left of the midline. On the right side the liver extends sagittally from the diaphragm to about the inferior costal margin. The usual causes of generalized hepatomegaly are fatty infiltration, congestive heart failure, primary neoplasms, leukemia, lymphoma, abscesses, hepatitis, metastases, and cystic or storage disease.

STRUCTURE DISPLACED WITH HEPATOMEGALY	DIRECTION OF DISPLACEMENT
Hepatic flexure—anterior liver	Pushed inferiorly
Proximal transverse colon—anterior liver (FIG. 26-37)	Displaced below right renal shadow
Hepatic shadow—anterior liver	Displaced across right psoas margin
Right kidney—posterior liver (FIG. 26-37)	Displaced inferiorly
Stomach—left lobe of liver	Displaced laterally; depressed lesser curvature
Right hemidiaphragm	Elevated

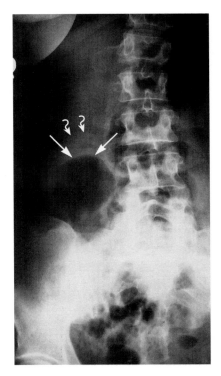

FIG. 26-37 Hepatomegaly. The proximal transverse colon and hepatic flexure *(arrows)* are displaced below the right renal shadow *(curved arrows)*. The right kidney is displaced downwardly as well.

PART FOUR
Abdomen

AB7b | Gallbladder Enlargement

The gallbladder normally lies in a fossa on the anteroinferior surface of the right liver lobe and when normal cannot be identified. It is situated cephalad and slightly dorsal to the right transverse colon and anteriorly and slightly lateral to the descending duodenum. Gallbladder enlargement may be secondary to hydrops, acute cholecystitis, carcinoma of the gallbladder, or acute obstruction (Courvoisier gallbladder).

STRUCTURE DISPLACED WITH GALLBLADDER ENLARGEMENT	DIRECTION OF DISPLACEMENT
Proximal transverse colon	Depressed inferiorly
Hepatic flexure	Pushed inferiorly
Duodenal loop	Pushed medially

AB7c | Spleen Enlargement

The spleen is usually about 10 cm in length, although up to 13 cm is considered normal. It lies in the posterior left upper abdomen. Causes of splenomegaly include leukemia, lymphoma, infection, storage diseases, portal hypertension from hepatitis or cirrhosis, and hematologic abnormalities.

STRUCTURE DISPLACED WITH SPLEEN ENLARGEMENT	DIRECTION OF DISPLACEMENT
Splenic flexure (FIG. 26-38, FIG. 26-40)	Depressed inferiorly
Left kidney	Displaced inferiorly
Greater curvature of stomach	Lateral impression
Gastric lumen (FIGS. 26-39 AND 26-40)	Displaced medially
Left hemidiaphragm	Rarely elevated except when spleen is huge

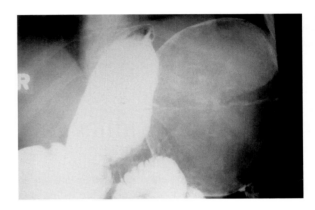

FIG. 26-39 Splenomegaly. Displacement of stomach medially is noted from a large calcified splenic cyst.

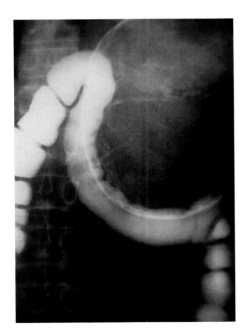

FIG. 26-38 Splenomegaly from a calcified posttraumatic cyst. Inferior displacement of the distal transverse colon and splenic flexure is seen.

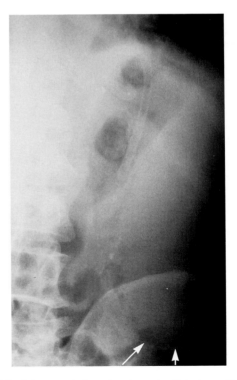

FIG. 26-40 Splenomegaly from chronic myelocytic leukemia. Plain film findings of splenomegaly include medial displacement of the stomach (with nasogastric tube) and inferior tip of the spleen projected over the iliac wing *(arrows)*. Downward depression of the splenic flexure is also observed.

AB7d | Gastric Distension

The stomach and first portion of the duodenum occupy the anterior left upper quadrant. The stomach is quite distensible and may vary widely in size and shape.

STRUCTURE DISPLACED WITH GASTRIC DISTENTION	DIRECTION OF DISPLACEMENT
Transverse colon	Depressed inferiorly
Small bowel	Depressed inferiorly

AB7e | Right Kidney Enlargement

After abdominal aortic aneurysms, renal lesions are the largest group of retroperitoneal masses identified on abdominal plain film radiographs.

STRUCTURE DISPLACED WITH RIGHT KIDNEY ENLARGEMENT	DIRECTION OF DISPLACEMENT
Proximal transverse colon (lower pole enlargement)	Elevated – *lower pole of kidneys are at level of transverse colon.*
Proximal transverse colon (upper pole enlargement)	Usually not displaced *because upper pole of kidneys are above transverse colon*
Ascending colon and/or hepatic flexure	Displaced anteriorly and laterally or medially
Descending duodenum	Indented or displaced medially and anteriorly

AB7f | Left Kidney Enlargement

STRUCTURE DISPLACED WITH LEFT KIDNEY ENLARGEMENT	DIRECTION OF DISPLACEMENT
Transverse colon (FIG. 26-41)	Displaced inferiorly
Descending colon (SEE FIG. 26-41)	Pushed laterally
Duodenal-jejunal junction	Displaced anteriorly and medially
Posterior gastric wall	Indented

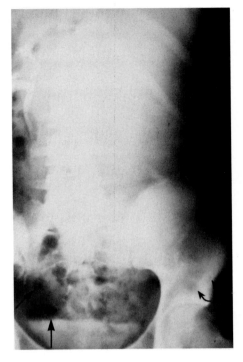

FIG. 26-41 Left kidney enlargement. The transverse colon is displaced inferiorly *(arrow)* and the distal colon is pushed laterally *(curved arrows)*.

AB7g | Adrenal Enlargement

The adrenal gland rests on the superior medial border of the adjacent, with the right gland more caudally situated than the left. Normally, the adrenal glands are not longer than 3 cm or wider than 2.5 cm. Common adrenal masses include congenital or posttraumatic cysts, neuroblastoma, pheochromocytoma, adenoma, and carcinoma (primary or metastatic). Smaller masses will not be seen on plain films unless they are calcified or contain fat.

STRUCTURE DISPLACED WITH ADRENAL ENLARGEMENT	DIRECTION OF DISPLACEMENT
Subjacent kidney	Elevated but rarely affected

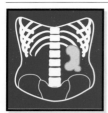

AB8 | Abdominal Masses

With the expanding role of advance imaging modalities, the abdominal radiograph often is most useful as a guide to further studies. Abdominal and pelvic masses are recognized by both direct and indirect signs. The direct signs include visualization of the actual mass or an alteration in the size, contour, or density of an abdominal or pelvic organ, or identifying gas, fat, or calcium in them. The indirect signs are displacement of normal structures, and obliteration of normal fat lines of the organ interfaces with adjacent fat.

Determining if the mass is intraperitoneal or extraperitoneal narrows the diagnostic possibilities. The lateral radiograph may be a useful supplement to the routine study if displacement of the retroperitoneal segments of the intestinal tract can be seen. A retroperitoneal mass can cause anterior displacement of the kidneys, ureters, duodenum, or vertical colon segments. However, if a mass is retroperitoneal and anterior to the kidneys, the kidneys will be displaced posteriorly. Intraperitoneal masses are more mobile and changes in position may be seen on sequential films. Fat can surround extraperitoneal masses and provide a sharp outline. This is rarely true of intraperitoneal masses.

AB8a | True Abdominal Masses

MASS	COMMENTS
Right upper quadrant (above L3)	
Liver—right lobe **(FIG. 26-42)**	Usual causes of generalized hepatomegaly: fatty infiltration, congestive heart failure, primary neoplasms, leukemia, lymphoma, abscesses, hepatitis, metastases, and cystic or storage disease
Gallbladder	Most common causes: hydrops, acute cholecystitis, carcinoma of gallbladder, and a Courvoisier's gallbladder
Duodenum/gastric antrum **(FIG. 26-43)**	Large mass produced by gastric leiomyoma or leiomyosarcoma; adenocarcinoma rarely displaces structures but may cause obstruction of the gastric outlet

MASS	COMMENTS
Left upper quadrant (above L3)	
Liver—left lobe	Focal masses caused by congenital or acquired cystic lesions as well as benign or malignant neoplasms; these masses may also involve the right lobe of the liver
Spleen **(FIG. 26-44)**	Most common causes for enlargement: traumatic or spontaneous hemorrhage, portal hypertension, infiltrative diseases, sickle cell anemia, malaria, septicemia, and kala-azar

Continued

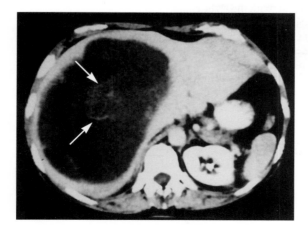

FIG. 26-42 Hepatic mass. Enhanced CT scan demonstrates a large cystic-appearing lesion occupying the right lobe of the liver. Subtle areas of higher density *(arrows)* indicate that this is not a simple cyst. A malignant lesion that has undergone massive necrosis must be considered.

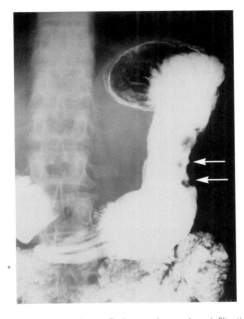

FIG. 26–43 Gastric carcinoma. Barium study reveals an infiltrating mass producing an irregular narrowing with nodularity of the mucosa of the greater curvature of the stomach (arrows).

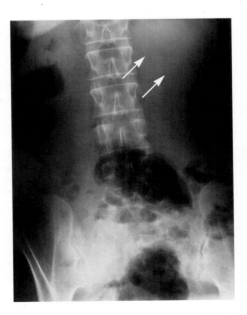

FIG. 26–44 Splenomegaly. Plain film demonstrates marked splenic enlargement with the inferior tip of the spleen extending a significant distance below the twelfth rib (arrows).

MASS

COMMENTS

Right and/or left upper quadrant (above L3)

Adrenal **(FIG. 26-45)**

Most common adrenal mass: an adenoma; these may be found as a normal variant, but they are usually only a few centimeters in size and therefore would not be seen on plain x-rays; plain film identifiable lesions are uncommon but include congenital or posttraumatic cysts, neuroblastoma, pheochromocytoma, adenoma, and carcinoma (metastatic, especially from the lung, and primary)

Right and/or left upper quadrant (above L3)— cont'd

Kidney **(FIG. 26-46)**

Cystic masses, including polycystic disease, multicystic kidney, simple renal cyst (found in up to 10% of older patients, but often small), inflammatory cyst, and in alcoholics, pancreatic pseudocyst; solid masses include pseudotumor, Wilm's tumor, renal cell carcinoma, and metastases

Pancreas **(FIG. 26-47)**

With the exception of a pseudocyst, pancreatic masses rarely reach sufficient size to be identified on abdominal radiographs

Continued

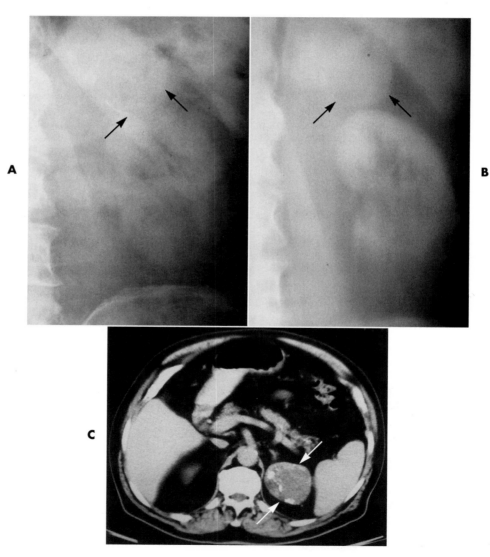

FIG. 26-45 Adrenal carcinoma. **A,** Plain film demonstrates a faint calcified mass with a cystic pattern of calcification *(arrows)*. **B,** Conventional tomography confirms the suprarenal location of this mass *(arrows)*. **C,** CT shows a large adrenal mass with rim calcification *(arrows)*.

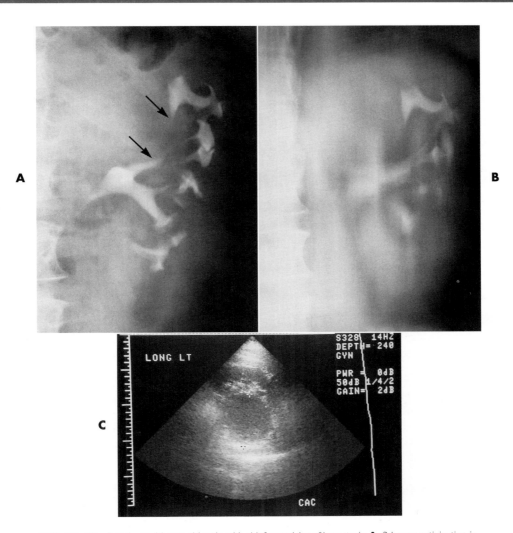

FIG. 26-46 Renal cyst. 64-year-old male with chief complaint of hematuria. **A,** 3-hour postinjection intravenous urogram (IVU). Note the displacement and stretching of the upper and middle calyces of the left kidney around a mass *(arrows)*, which proved at ultrasonography to be a cyst. **B,** Conventional tomography reveals similar findings as the IVU. **C,** Sonography shows an echolucent (black) round mass characteristic of a fluid-filled cyst (margins noted by cursors). Ultrasound can usually differentiate between a fluid-filled cyst and a solid renal tumor.

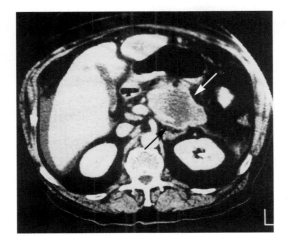

FIG. 26-47 Carcinoma of the pancreas. This mass was not visible on abdominal radiographs. CT scan demonstrates a pancreatic mass with a central zone of decreased attenuation *(arrows)*.

MASS	COMMENTS
Right lower quadrant (below L3)	
Appendix **(FIG. 26-48)**	Appendiceal abscess common; the usual peri-appendiceal abscess indents the tip of the cecum and displaces local loops of ileum away from the abscess
Cecum	Cecal carcinoma sometimes appearing as a mass or obstruction of the appendix, resulting in acute appendicitis; sometimes it can be seen as a filling defect in a gas-filled cecum

Left lower quadrant (below L3)	
Rectosigmoid colon	Common inflammatory mass produced by diverticulitis with abscess; this mass most frequently involves the descending and sigmoid portions of the colon, but usually it is too small to show up on plain films; colon carcinoma occurs most commonly in the rectosigmoid but also does not commonly present as a radiographically visible mass, except when outlined by bowel gas in a dilated loop
Midline	
Abdominal aorta **(FIG. 26-49)**	Aneurysm possibly presenting as an abdominal mass; ultrasound is the procedure of choice in determining the presence, size, and extent of an abdominal aortic aneurysm
Any location	
Colon **(FIG. 26-50)**	Inflammatory masses possibly resulting from diverticulitis, granulomatous colitis, amebiasis, and tuberculosis; colon carcinoma seldom presents as a mass; herniation of peritoneal structures, most occurring in the groin, may present as a palpatory mass
Small bowel mesentery **(FIG. 26-51)**	Masses arising in the small bowel mesentery most commonly inflammatory, from regional enteritis; mesenteric cysts can also occur and can be quite large; curvilinear calcifications may be seen in the cyst wall
Small bowel	Jejunal or ileal masses classified as congenital, inflammatory, or neoplastic; except for the rare duplication of this area, they usually are not seen as masses on radiographs; volvulus of the bowel (especially in children) and dilated fluid-filled small bowel secondary to distal obstruction from regional enteritis especially in young adults should both be considerations

Continued

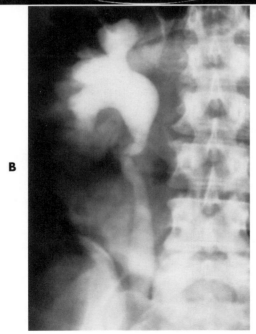

FIG. 26-48 Appendiceal abscess. **A,** Enhanced CT demonstrates an air-containing abdominal mass *(arrows)* within the right lower quadrant. The left ureter *(arrowhead)* is visible, the right ureter is obscured by the mass. **B,** IVU shows dilation of the pelvicalyceal system and ureter from obstruction secondary to this appendiceal abscess.

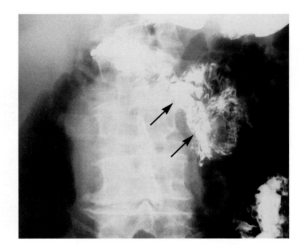

FIG. 26-49 Huge noncalcified abdominal aneurysm. Upper gastrointestinal study demonstrates displacement of the duodenum *(arrows)* from the large abdominal aneurysm.

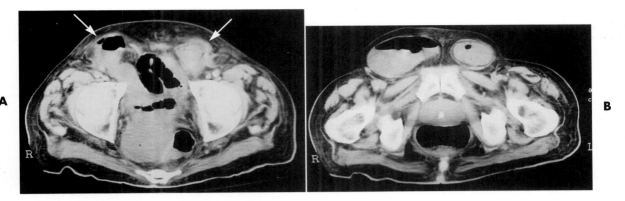

FIG. 26-50 Inguinal hernias: CT appearance. **A,** The peritoneal sac containing bowel loops is seen protruding through both inguinal canals *(arrows)*. **B,** The same patient showing right and left well-defined groin masses produced by bowel loops.

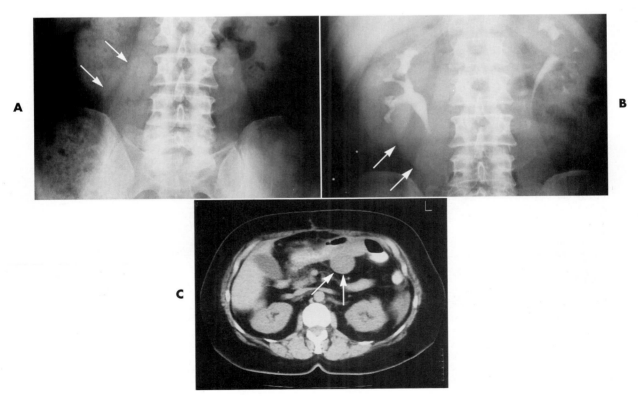

FIG. 26-51 Mesenteric cyst. 57-year-old female with palpable abdominal mass. **A,** Abdominal plain film demonstrates a large mass *(arrows)*. **B,** IVU shows that the mass is not involving the kidneys. The margin of the mass has changed position with the patient now recumbent *(arrows)*. **C,** CT of a different patient. This mesenteric cyst would not be visible on plain films *(arrows)*.

MASS	COMMENTS
Pelvic	
Prostate **(FIG. 26-52)**	Elevated base of bladder possible result of enlarged prostate; benign prostatic hypertrophy may appear as a soft tissue mass behind the symphysis pubis; prostatic carcinoma is more irregular but cannot be differentiated from the more common benign prostatic hypertrophy
Uterus	Enlargement most commonly caused by pregnancy; other causes include pregnancy complications (including molar pregnancy), benign neoplasm (leiomyoma), and malignancy; in a child, if there is no exit point for uterine blood and debris, the uterus can become rather large
Ovaries **(FIG. 26-53, 26-54 AND 26-55)**	Approximately 20% of ovarian tumors: dermoid cysts; these can be quite large and sometimes fat or teeth can be seen within them[3]; other common ovarian masses include follicular cysts, corpus luteum cysts, serous or mucinous cystadenomas and cystadenocarcinomas; endometriosis can cause cystic and/or solid ovarian enlargement, as can tubular ovarian abscesses (both are somewhat common)
Bladder **(FIG. 26-56)**	Commonly carcinoma and leiomyosarcoma; unless they become quite large, these cannot be seen on plain radiographs; contrast material in the bladder is needed to see them; a large bladder diverticulum may stimulate pelvic fluid or a pelvic mass
Congenital lesions	Including urachal cyst, mesenteric cyst, pelvic kidney, and choledocal cyst

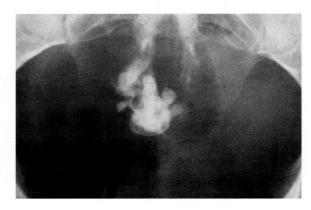

FIG. 26-53 Dermoid cyst. A radiolucent mass containing several teeth characteristic of a dermoid cyst.

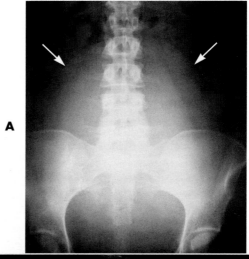

A

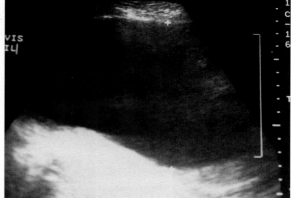

B

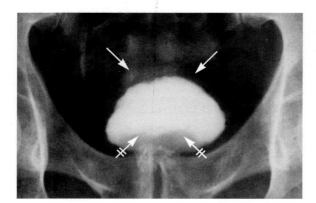

FIG. 26-52 Enlarged prostate. An enlarged prostate elevates the base of this contrast-filled bladder *(crossed arrows)*. Also, numerous calculi clustered over the symphysis pubis are seen, which are characteristic of prostatic concretions. Note the thickened bladder wall from the increased contractions required to overcome urethral constrictions by the enlarged prostate *(arrows)*. (Courtesy John A.M. Taylor, Portland, Ore.)

FIG. 26-54 Huge cystadenoma. A 36-year-old female reporting a feeling of fullness in her abdomen for 6 weeks. **A,** Plain film of the abdomen demonstrates a huge soft tissue mass extending out of pelvis to the level of L2 *(arrows)*. **B,** Ultrasound shows an echolucent mass typical of a fluid-filled cyst. Cursors delineate walls of the lesion.

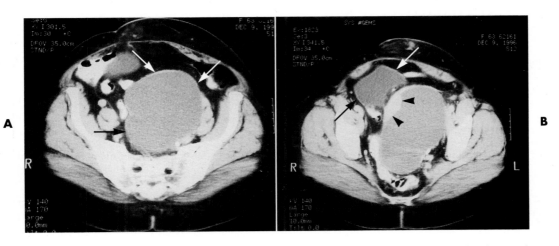

FIG. 26-55 Endometrioma. **A,** CT demonstrates a large soft tissue mass in the pelvis of lower attenuation than muscle *(arrows)*. **B,** A more caudal section shows the urinary bladder *(arrows)* displaced to the right by the lesion. A thickened area in the wall of this lesion is also seen *(arrowheads)*.

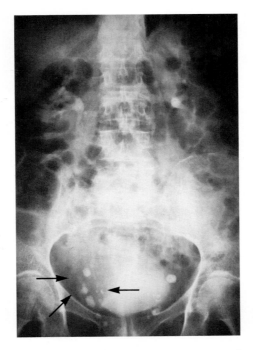

FIG. 26-56 Bladder carcinoma. IVU demonstrates a mass creating a filling defect of the bladder *(arrows)*.

AB8b | Pseudomasses

O n occasion, a fluid-containing viscus or a normal solid organ may simulate an abdominal mass. Listed below are the more common pseudomasses.

STRUCTURE	COMMENTS	STRUCTURE	COMMENTS
Stomach (FIG. 26-57)	Dilated, fluid-filled stomach projecting as a smooth homogeneous left upper quadrant mass	Dilated bowel loops	In intestinal obstruction a dilated, fluid-filled loop of bowel may simulate an abdominal mass
Dilated urinary bladder (FIG. 26-58)	Dilated bladder appearing as a smooth, round mass in the lower midline pelvis; occasionally with chronic obstruction it can fill much of the abdomen	Ectopic kidney and anomalies (FIG. 26-59)	Pelvic kidney and other renal anomalies appearing as an abdominal or pelvic mass

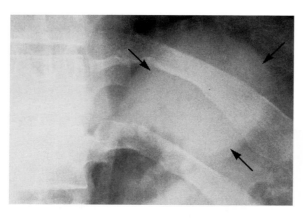

FIG. 26-57 A fluid-filled stomach in the left upper quadrant simulating a mass *(arrows)*.

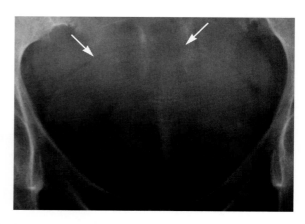

FIG. 26-58 A fluid-filled bladder may simulate a pelvic mass *(arrows)*. Note the rim of pelvic fat that defines the margin.

A

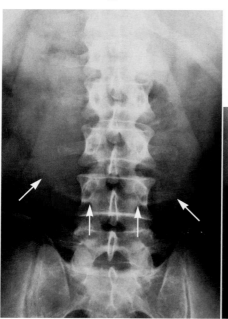

B

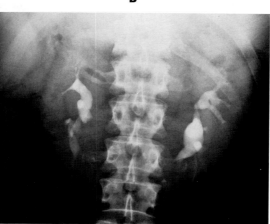

FIG. 26-59 Anomalous, conjoined horseshoe kidneys. **A,** Plain film findings simulate an abdominal mass *(arrows)*. **B,** On this intravenous pyelogram, the inferior aspects of the right and left kidneys are joined, a characteristic of horseshoe kidneys.

AB9 | Diseases of the Gallbladder

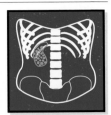

The gallbladder can change its volume and configuration rapidly. Nevertheless, its location next to the liver and its lack of adjacent, contrasting fat makes it rarely identifiable on plain radiograph.

DISEASE	COMMENTS		
Acute cholecystitis	Most frequently caused by obstruction of the cystic duct by a gallstone[49]; gallbladder distention (hydrops) may result, a round to oval right upper quadrant (RUQ) mass may be seen	Cholelithiasis **(FIGS 26-60 AND 26-61)** [p. 963]	Gallstones containing enough radiodense material to be visible on plain films in only 10% to 15% of patients[30, 62]; most stones, however, can be easily demonstrated with ultrasound

Continued

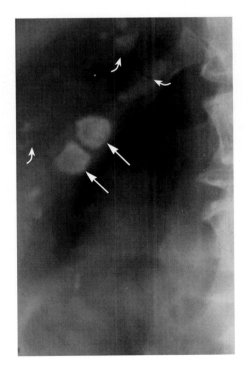

FIG. 26-60 Calcified gallstones *(arrows)* and costal cartilage calcification *(curved arrows).*

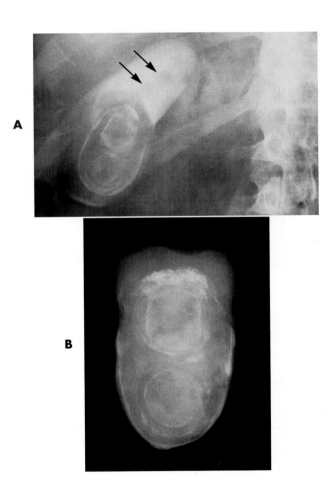

FIG. 26-61 **A,** This oral cholecystogram shows a large filling defect of the inferior half of the gallbladder created by a large partially calcified stone with two stones within it. Note: two nonopaque stones creating filling defects of upper half of gallbladder *(arrows).* **B,** Surgical specimen.

DISEASE	COMMENTS
Milk of calcium (FIG. 26-62)	Numerous, minute, calcific stones are in suspension in bile; an upright or lateral decubitus film frequently produces a fluid level with the heavier calculi in the dependent portion and a layer of bile above

Calcification of wall (FIG. 26-63)	Also known as *porcelain gallbladder;* affected individuals are usually asymptomatic; five times as many women as men are affected[5]; the frequency of gallbladder carcinoma increases, so prophylactic cholecystectomy is generally performed
Gallbladder carcinoma	Uncommon; this neoplasm rarely calcifies

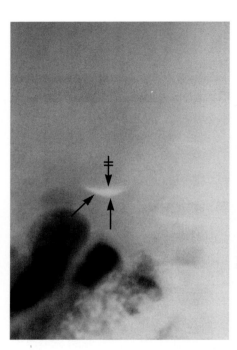

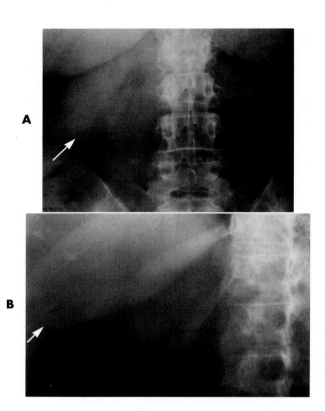

FIG. 26-62 Milk of calcium gallbladder. Upright film demonstrates radiopaque substance that layers dependently within the fundus of the gallbladder *(arrows).* The horizontal cephalad surface on the upright film indicates a fluid *(crossed arrow).* This most likely is calcium carbonate material.

FIG. 26-63 Porcelain gallbladder. **A,** AP plain film shows a cystlike calcification of the gallbladder *(arrow).* **B,** Calcifications of the gallbladder move further away from the spine during the right posterior oblique view *(arrow).* (Courtesy Cynthia Peterson, Bournemouth, England.)

Gallstone ileus (FIG. 26-64)	Obstruction of the intestine by a gallstone that has eroded through the gallbladder and is in the small bowel; the typical patient is an obese, elderly female, often diabetic, who complains of vague and poorly localized symptoms; classic plain film triad is small-bowel obstruction, biliary tract air, and an opaque concretion in the small bowel	Emphysematous cholecystitis	Acute infection of the gallbladder caused by gas-forming organisms; air resulting from perforation is five times more common than routine acute cholecystitis; gas fills the lumen first, then the gas infiltrates the gallbladder wall; air within the gallbladder is a serious sign indicating advanced gallbladder disease

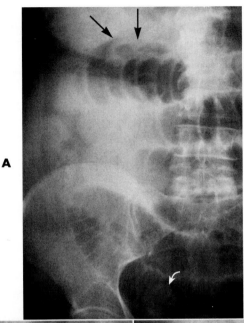

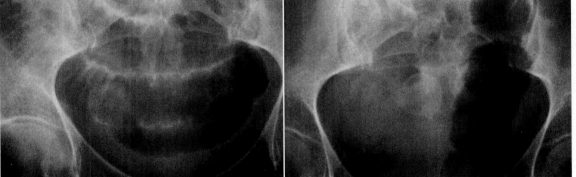

FIG. 26-64 Gallstone ileus. **A,** The classic triad of air in the biliary tree (pneumobilia) *(arrows)*, small bowel obstruction evidenced by the dilated, gas-filled loops, and an ectopic gallstone *(curved arrow)* is virtually diagnostic of gallstone ileus. Observe the gallstone remaining within the right upper quadrant. **B,** Close-up view of the ectopic gallstone and small bowel obstruction. **C,** A second opaque gallstone has eroded into the gastrointestinal tract. These gallstones often create a mechanical obstruction.

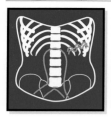

AB10 Vascular Calcifications

This is a very common finding in middle-aged and elderly patients. Typically, linear, parallel calcifications are seen along the path of the major arteries.

VASCULAR STRUCTURE	COMMENTS
Aorta (FIG. 26-65)	Frequently calcification in the walls of the aorta observed in radiographs of middle-aged and elderly patients; similar calcifications can also be seen in young persons, especially those suffering from diabetes
Iliac artery (FIG. 26-66)	Fragmentary calcification of an iliac artery just below the sacroiliac joint can be mistaken for a ureteral calculus
Splenic artery (FIG. 26-67)	Located in the left upper quadrant and can be recognized by its extreme tortuosity
Renal artery	Occasionally calcify
Celiac and superior mesenteric arteries	Can occasionally be seen coming off a calcified aorta on a lateral spine film that includes the L1 and L3 area

Phlebolith (FIG. 26-68)	Common in the pelvic veins and have no clinical significance; they are usually round, 1-mm to 5-mm calcifications and may have a lucent center; easily confused with a ureteral stone
Portal vein	Rare imaging finding, occurring almost always in patients with portal hypertension or thrombosis
Lymph nodes (SEE FIG. 26-23)	(Mesenteric or paravascular) may be affected by granulomatous diseases, especially histoplasmosis or tuberculosis, with subsequent calcification; rarely other entities such as lymphoma or sarcoid occur

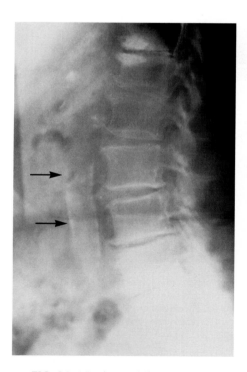

FIG. 26-65   Aorta calcification *(arrows)*.

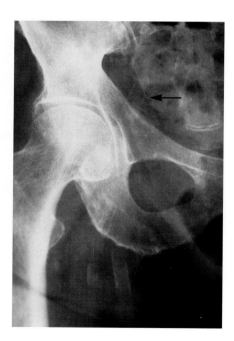

FIG. 26-66   Iliac artery calcification *(arrow)*.

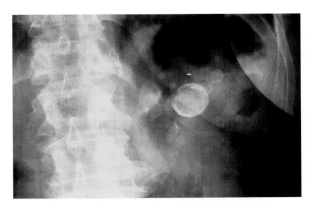

FIG. 26-67 Splenic artery calcification. Multiple ringlike calcifications represent portions of the tortuous splenic artery projected on end. The largest ring indicates aneurysmal dilation.

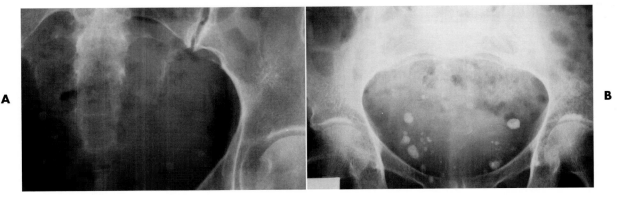

FIG. 26-68 Phleboliths. Two different patients. **A,** Multiple small, round calcifications with a central lucency, which should not be confused with urinary tract calculi. **B,** Larger phleboliths found in a pattern consistent with pelvic veins.

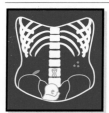

AB11 | Miscellaneous Radiopacities and Abdomen Artifacts

A variety of miscellaneous radiographic densities can simulate calcification on abdominal radiographs (Figs. 26-69 through 26-80).

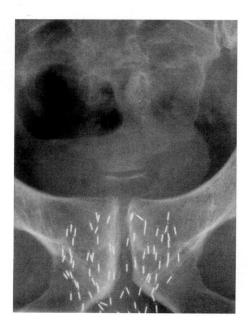

FIG. 26-69   Treatment for prostate carcinoma. Multiple metallic implants that contain radioactive material have been injected into the prostate gland.

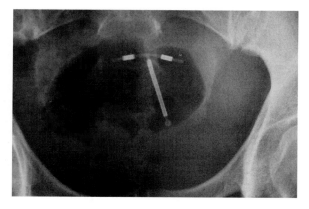

FIG. 26-70   Intrauterine device (IUD). A T-shaped metal and plastic density in the region of the uterus. Note the eyelet in the caudal end for the removal.

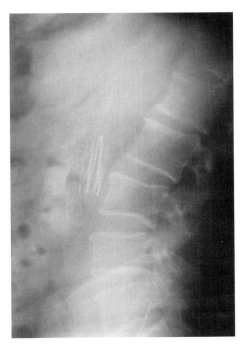

FIG. 26-71 Thrombi filter. Basketlike devices may be placed in the inferior vena cava of patients with a propensity to produce thromboemboli. (Courtesy Cynthia Peterson, Bournemouth, England.)

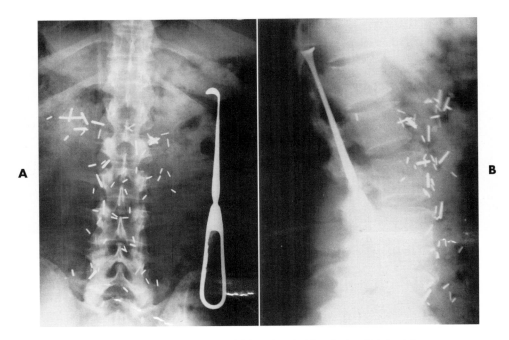

FIG. 26-72 Surgical retractor left in patient. **A,** AP projection. **B,** Lateral view.

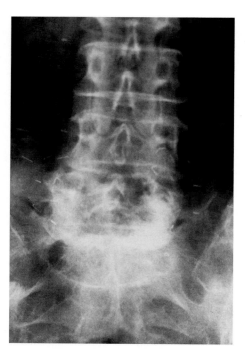

FIG. 26-73   Acupuncture needles. Hari, a Japanese form of acupuncture, consists of placement of many gold needles into the subcutaneous tissues. They are cut off at the skin surface and remain in place permanently.

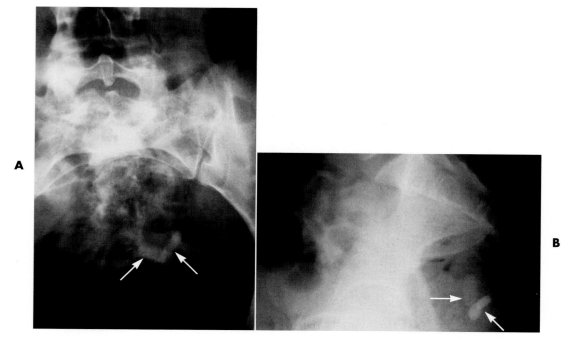

FIG. 26-74   Ingested tablets. Undigested tablets may mimic abdominal calcifications. **A,** AP projection (arrows). **B,** Lateral view (arrows).

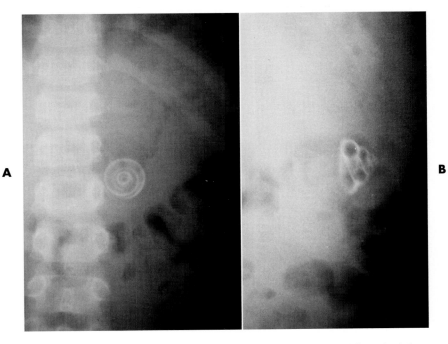

FIG. 26-75 Ingested snail shell. The characteristic spiral makes this unusual diagnosis obvious. **A,** AP projection. **B,** Lateral view.

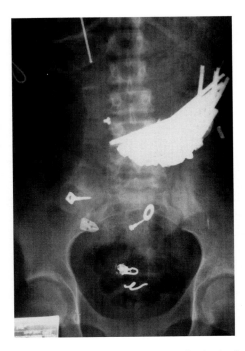

FIG. 26-76 Ingested metallic objects. Metallic foreign bodies are seen throughout the gastrointestinal tract.

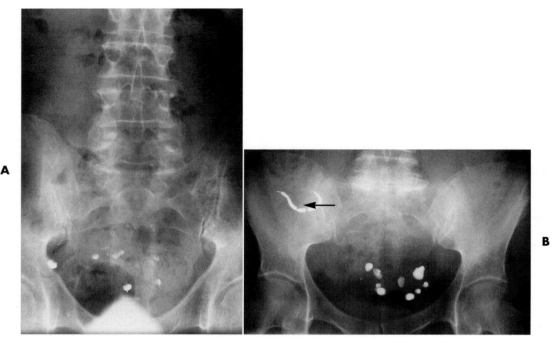

FIG. 26-77　**A,** Barium retained in diverticula following barium enema. Note their dense, homogeneous metallic opacification that can usually be distinguished from calcifications. Most diverticula occur in the sigmoid. **B,** Barium retained in appendix *(arrow)* and diverticula. Barium is present in multiple, left-sided diverticula and the appendix.　(*A,* Courtesy John A.M. Taylor, Portland, Ore.; *B,* Courtesy Cynthia Peterson, Bournemouth, England.)

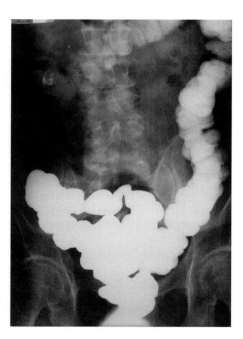

FIG. 26-78　Impaction of ingested barium occurred in the colon because of dehydration of retained barium by the colonic mucosa. (Courtesy Cynthia Peterson, Bournemouth, England.)

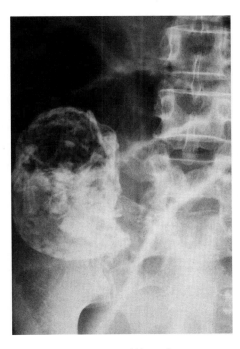

FIG. 26-79 Lithopedion.

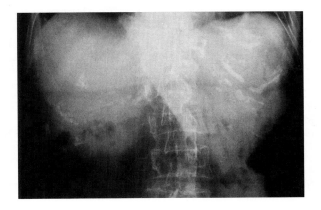

FIG. 26-80 Costal cartilage.

References

1. Astley R, Harrison N: Miliary calcification of the liver: report of a case, *Br J Radiol* 22:723, 1949.
2. Azimi T, Cameron DD: Calcification of the intrarenal branches of the renal arteries, *Clin Radiol* 28:217, 1977.
3. Baker SR: *The abdominal plain film*, ed 1, Norwalk, Conn, 1990, Appleton & Lange.
4. Balthazar EJ, Gurkin S: Cholecystoenteric fistulas: significance and radiographic diagnosis, *Am J Gastroenterol* 65:168, 1976.
5. Berk RN, Armbuster TG, Saltzstein SL: Carcinoma in the porcelain gallbladder, *Radiology* 106:29, 1973.
6. Boise CL, Sears WN: Calcification in adrenal neoplasms, *Radiology* 56:731, 1951.
7. Caplan LN, Simon M: Non-parasitic cysts of the liver, *AJR* 96:421, 1966.
8. Castro JR, Klein EW: The incidence and appearance of roentgenologically visible psammomatous calcification of papillary cystadenocarcinoma of the ovaries, *AJR* 88:886, 1962.
9. Cho KC, Baker SR: Air in the fissure for the ligamentum teres: new sign of intraperitoneal air on plain radiographs, *Radiology* 178:489, 1991.
10. Cornell CM, Clarke R: Vicarious calcification involving the gallbladder, *Ann Surg* 149:267, 1959.
11. Culver GJ, Tannenhaus J: Calcification of the vas deferens: its relation to diabetes mellitus and arteriosclerosis, *N Engl J Med* 245:321, 1951.
12. Cusmano JV: Dermoid cysts of the ovary: roentgen features, *Radiology* 66:719, 1956.
13. Dachman AH et al: Non-parasitic splenic cysts: a report of 52 cases with radiologic-pathologic correlation, *Am J Roentgenol* 147:537, 1986.
14. Dachman AH, Lichtenstein JE, Friedman AC: Review: mucocele of the appendix and pseudomyxoma peritonei, *Am J Roentgenol* 144:923, 1985.
15. Daniel WW Jr et al: Calcified renal masses: a review of ten years' experience at the Mayo Clinic, *Radiology* 103:503, 1972.
16. Darlak JR, Moskowitz M, Kattan KE: Calcifications in the liver, *Radiol Clin N Am* 18:209, 1981.
17. Etala E: Cancer de la vesicula biliar, *Prensa Med Argent* 49:2283, 1962.
18. Fagenberg D: Fecaliths of the appendix, incidence of significance, *Am J Roentgenol* 89:572, 1963.
19. Friedman AC, Lichtenstein JE, Dachman AH: Cystic neoplasms of the pancreas, *Radiology* 149:45, 1983.
20. Grainger RG, Lloyed GAS, Williams JL: Eggshell calcification: a sign of phaeochromocytoma, *Clin Radiol* 18:282, 1967.
21. Gonzalez LR et al: Radiologic aspects of hepatic echinococcosis, *Radiology* 130:21, 1979.
22. Gray EF: Calcifications of the spleen, *Am J Roentgenol* 61:336, 1944.
23. Hafiz A, Melnick JC: Calcification of the vas deferens, *J Can Assoc Radiol* 19:56, 1968.
24. Han SY: Variations in falciform ligament with pneumoperitoneum, *J Can Assoc Radiol* 31:171, 1980.
25. Harrison I, Litwer H, Gerwig WH: Studies on the incidence and duration of post-operative pneumoperitoneum, *Ann Surg* 145:591, 1957.
26. Hilbrish TF, Bartler FC: Roentgen findings in abnormal deposition of calcium in tissues, *Am J Roentgenol* 87:1128, 1962.
27. Holman CC: Urinary tuberculosis with extensive calcification of the bladder, *Br J Surg* 40:90, 1952.
28. Imhof H, Frank P: Pancreatic calcification in malignant islet cell tumors, *Radiology* 122:333, 1977.
29. Jelasco DV, Schultz EH: The urachus: an aid to the diagnosis of pneumoperitoneum, *Radiology* 92:295, 1969.
30. Johnston DE, Kaplan MM: Pathogenesis and treatment of gallstones, *N Engl J Med* 328:412, 1993.
31. Jonutis AJ, Davidson AJ, Redman HC: Curvilinear calcifications in four uncommon benign renal lesions, *Clin Radiol* 24:468, 1973.
32. Kaude JV: Calcification in carcinoid tumors, *N Engl J Med* 289:921, 1973.
33. Kazmierski RH: Primary adenocarcinoma of gallbladder with intramural calcification, *Am J Surg* 82:248, 1951.

34. Kikkawa K, Lasser ER: Ringlike or rimlike calcifications in renal cell carcinoma, *AJR* 107:737, 1969.

35. King JC Jr, Rosenbaum HD: Calcification of the vasa deferentia in nondiabetics, *Radiology* 100:603, 1971.

36. Komaki S, Clark JM: Pancreatic pseudocyst: a review of 17 cases with emphasis on radiologic findings, *AJR* 122:385, 1974.

37. Liebman PR et al: Hepatic-portal venous gas in adults: etiology, pathophysiology, and clinical significance, *Ann Surg* 107:281, 1978.

38. Mentzer RM et al: A comparative appraisal of emphysematous cholecystitis, *Am J Surg* 129:10, 1973.

39. Menuck L, Siemers PT: Pneumoperitoneum: importance of right upper quadrant features, *AJR* 127:753, 1976.

40. Miele AJ, Edmonds HW: Calcified liver metastases: a specific roentgen diagnostic sign, *Radiology* 80:779, 1963.

41. Miller RE: Perforated viscus in infants: a new roentgen sign, *Radiology* 74:65, 1960.

42. Miller RE: The technical approach to the acute abdomen, *Semin Roentgenol* 8:267, 1973.

43. Miller SW, Pfister RC: Calcification in uroepithelial tumors of the bladder: report of 5 cases and survey of the literature, *AJR* 121:827, 1974.

44. Milner LR: Cancer of the gallbladder. Its relationship to gallstones, *Am J Gastroenterol* 39:480, 1963.

45. Moncada R, Cooper RA, Garces M: Calcified metastases from malignant ovarian neoplasm: review of the literature, *Radiology* 113:31, 1974.

46. Parker JM: Calcified cyst of the adrenal gland, *Mil Med* 138:791, 1970.

47. Papavasiliou CG: Calcification in secondary tumors of the spleen, *Acta Radiol* 51:278, 1959.

48. Parientes RA et al: Cystadenoma of the pancreas: diagnosis by computed tomography, *J Comput Asst Tomogr* 4:364, 1980.

49. Phemister DB, Rewbridge AG, Rudisill H Jr: Calcium carbonate gallstone following cystic duct obstruction, *Ann Surg* 94:493, 1931.

50. Phillips TL, Chin FG, Palubinskas AJ: Calcification in renal masses: an eleven-year survey, *Radiology* 80:786, 1963.

51. Polk HC Jr: Carcinoma and the calcified gallbladder, *Gastroenterology* 50:582, 1966.

52. Roth CS, Bowyer BA, Berquist TH: Utility of the plain film abdominal radiograph for diagnosing urteral calculi, *Ann Emerg Med* 14:311, 1985.

53. Salik JO, Abeshouse BS: Calcification, ossification and cartilage formation in the kidney, *AJR* 88:125, 1962.

54. Samuel E: Calcification in suprarenal neoplasms, *Br J Radiol* 21:139, 1948.

55. Samuel E et al: Radiology of the post-operative abdomen, *Clin Radiol* 14:133, 1963.

56. Schabel SI, Burgener FA, Reynolds J: Radiographic manifestations of malignant mixed uterine tumors, *J Can Assoc Radiol* 26:176, 1975.

57. Schechter S: Calcified mesenteric lymph nodes: their incidence and significance in routine roentgen examination of the gastrointestinal tract, *Radiology* 27:485, 1936.

58. Schwarz J et al: The relationship of splenic calcifications to histoplasmosis, *N Engl J Med* 252:887, 1955.

59. Sheshanarayana KN, Keats TS: Intrarenal arterial calcifications: roentgen appearance and significant, *Radiology* 95:145, 1970.

60. Soler-Bechara J, Soscia JL: Calcified echinococcus (hydatid) cyst of the spleen, *JAMA* 187:62, 1964.

61. Steer ML et al: Chronic pancreatitis, *N Engl J Med* 332:1492, 1995.

62. Tait N, Little JM: The treatment of gallstones, *BMJ* 311:99, 1995.

63. Teplick JG, Haskins ME, Alavi A: Calcified intraperitoneal metastases from ovarian carcinoma, *AJR* 127:1003, 1976.

64. Tonkin AK, Witten DM: Genitourinary tuberculosis, *Semin Roentgenol* 14:305, 1979.

65. Umerah BC: The less familiar manifestations of schistosomiasis of the urinary tract, *Br J Surg* 50:105, 1977.

66. Weiner CI, Diaconis JN, Dennis JM. The inverted V: a new sign of pneumoperitoneum, *Radiology* 107:47, 1973.

67. Wollin E, Ozonoff MB: Dermoid development of teeth in an ovarian teratoma, *N Engl J Med* 265:890, 1961.

68. Wood JC: A calcified adrenal tumor, *Br J Radiol* 25:222, 1952.

chapter 27

Genitourinary System Diseases

BEVERLY L HARGER

LISA E HOFFMAN

RICHARD ARKLESS

PART FOUR
Abdomen

Angiomyolipoma (Hamartoma)

BACKGROUND

Angiomyolipoma (AML) is the most common benign renal neoplasm diagnosed radiologically. It is a hamartomatous tumor containing varying amounts of fat, smooth muscle, and vascular tissues, and it may range in size from a few millimeters to more than 20 cm.[21] AMLs are found in young adults to elderly patients and are four and a half times more common in women.[10,21] Multiple, bilateral, small AMLs that may be symptomatic are found in up to 80% of patients with tuberous sclerosis, an uncommon heritable condition.[10,13,21] However, most angiomyolipomas arise sporadically.

IMAGING FINDINGS

The radiolucent fatty tissue of these tumors is seldom appreciated on plain film radiographs. The AML may be revealed by its mass effect after contrast injection on an intravenous pyelogram but cannot be differentiated from other masses. Attenuation of the collecting system with displacement and focal dilation of the calyces may be visible.[21]

A renal tumor containing fat density tissue is essentially diagnostic for AML. Unenhanced computed tomographic (CT) scans, use of small areas for attenuation measurements, and use of thin sections may be required to detect small amounts of fat.[3,12,21]

Sonography characteristically shows a very hyperechoic lesion compared with adjacent renal parenchyma.[6,7,14,21,26,27] The high fat content, heterogeneous cellular architecture, and presence of multiple vessels all contribute to the marked echogenicity, but still this lesion cannot accurately be separated from renal cell carcinoma on ultrasound, and therefore computed tomography is necessary.[14,21]

CLINICAL COMMENTS

Angiomyolipomas are generally asymptomatic and usually are identified during evaluation for unrelated genitourinary conditions.

Flank pain, hematuria, and palpable mass are classic symptoms and are usually seen in otherwise healthy patients with isolated, unilateral lesions.[21] Parenchymal, subcapsular, or perirenal hemorrhage may lead to hypotension.[21]

Embolization or partial excision is usual for large and/or symptomatic lesions. Overall, treatment for AMLs is usually conservative with follow-up alone being sufficient for most small, asymptomatic tumors.[10,21]

KEY CONCEPTS

- *Angiomyolipoma is the most common radiologically diagnosed benign renal neoplasm.*
- *Classic symptoms, when present, are flank pain, hematuria, and palpable mass.*
- *Fatty attenuation seen on CT is virtually diagnostic for AML.*

Bladder Calculi

BACKGROUND

Ninety-eight percent of bladder calculi identified in the United States occur in elderly males.[16] The instigating factor in their formation is usually urinary retention with high residual urine. Superimposed infections add to susceptibility. The presence of bladder stones is associated with an increased incidence of carcinoma.[16]

IMAGING FINDINGS

Bladder calculi are often nonopaque or only faintly opaque, allowing them to be frequently overlooked. Fecal material and gas in the rectosigmoid colon and the sacrum itself also overlie the area and may further obscure them. Bladder calculi usually are located centrally in the pelvis (Fig. 27-1). Those that are found more laterally may lie in a bladder diverticulum.[16]

CLINICAL COMMENTS

Bladder calculi may abrade and irritate the mucosa and predispose to infection. Bladder infections are more difficult to treat when cal-

951

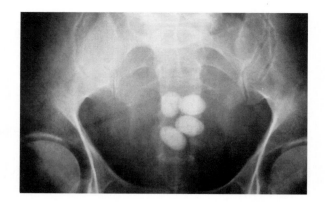

FIG. 27-1   Multiple bladder calculi. Four oval radiopaque bladder stones are visible centrally in the pelvis. Most bladder calculi are round or oval but they may be amorphous, laminated, or even spiculated.

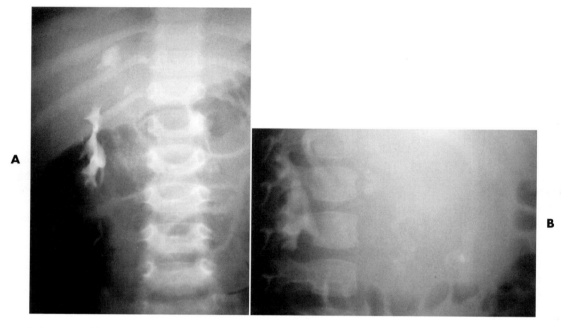

FIG. 27-2   Nephroblastoma (Wilms' tumor). **A,** Intravenous urogram AP projections show diffuse amorphous calcification of a large right upper quadrant mass in a pediatric patient. **B,** Intravenous urogram lateral view of this same patient demonstrates the retroperitoneal location of this mass. Nephroblastoma is the most common abdominal malignancy of children with 80% occurring between 1 and 5 years of age.

culi are present. Ureteral or bladder outlet obstruction may also be present.[16] Approximately 15% of patients with gout, as well as hyperuricemic patients, produce uric acid stones.[16]

Standard treatment of bladder stones consists of endoscopic visualization and fragmentation by electrohydraulic probe.[31] Massive calculi may require open surgery.[31]

KEY CONCEPTS

- *Urinary retention with a high residual urine is common cause for formation. It may be difficult to detect on plain radiographs.*
- *Bladder calculi usually lie centrally in the pelvis on plain radiographs.*
- *The incidence of carcinoma of bladder increases in presence of stones.*

Nephroblastoma (Wilms' Tumor)

BACKGROUND

Nephroblastoma (Wilms' tumor) is the most common abdominal malignancy in childhood.[8,13] Overall, leukemia-lymphoma, brain tumors (astrocytoma and medulloblastoma), and neuroblastoma have a higher incidence in pediatric populations when other sites of the body are also considered.[19] The highest incidence occurs in 3- and 4-year-olds with 80% of Wilms' tumors occurring between the ages of 1 and 5 years.[2,5,19]

IMAGING FINDINGS

Wilms' tumor appears radiographically as a complex renal mass (Fig. 27-2). Approximately 5% to 10% of these lesions show areas of calcification, but calcium, when seen in a mass in this area, is much more likely to be in a neuroblastoma of the adrenal or other similar tissue.[19] Intravenous pyelogram will show either a displaced and/or a nonfunctioning kidney. Ultrasound typically reveals a well-defined tumor, often surrounded by a hyperechoic halo of compressed normal renal tissue.[13,17] Noncontrast CT usually reveals a large intrarenal mass of lower attenuation than the adjacent normal kidney. Cystic spaces or areas of tumor necrosis appearing as inhomogeneous, low-density areas are seen in most tumors.[13]

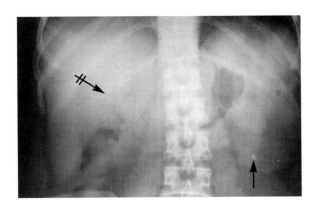

FIG. 27-3   Nephrocalcinosis. Cortical (*arrow*) and medullary (*crossed arrow*) nephrocalcinosis.

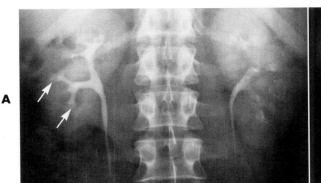
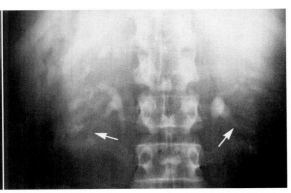

A   B

FIG. 27-4   Medullary sponge kidney. **A,** Faint calculi are seen in the renal pyramids (*arrows*). Medullary sponge kidney is characterized by ectatic collecting ducts and associated small cysts communicating with these ducts. **B,** Renal tubular acidosis. This parenchymal renal calcification results from renal tubular acidosis. The calcifications occur within the tubules surrounding the calyces (*arrows*).

CLINICAL COMMENTS

Patients with Wilms' tumor present with an abdominal mass in more than 90% of cases.[13] Approximately 50% of patients experience hypertension and/or fever. Hematuria is relatively uncommon.[13,19] No male or female predominance is noted.[13] Up to 30% with the rare condition of aniridia (congenital absence of the iris) develop nephroblastoma.[19] Four to five percent of cases show bilateral tumors.[19]

▌ KEY CONCEPTS
- *Wilms' tumor is the most common abdominal malignancy of children.*
- *Abdominal mass is the most common clinical presentation.*
- *Radiographically, Wilms' tumor is seen as a complex renal mass; 5% to 10% have internal calcification.*

Nephrocalcinosis

BACKGROUND

Based on its location, calcification in the kidney can be classified broadly into two categories: calcification within the pyelocalyceal lumina or nephrolithiasis, and intraparenchymal calcification or nephrocalcinosis. Nephrocalcinosis can also be categorized with respect to its predominant location. A limited group of diseases, cortical nephrocalcinosis, may produce calcification confined to, or predominantly located in, the renal cortex. Other conditions, such as medullary nephrocalcinosis, spare the cortex and cause calcium salt deposition in the medullary, interstitium, or lumina of the nephrons.

IMAGING FINDINGS

Radiographically, cortical nephrocalcinosis can be differentiated from the medullary variety by the peripheral location of the calcification (Fig. 27-3). Medullary calcification is typically that of bilateral, diffuse, fan-shaped clusters of stippled calcifications, primarily in the renal pyramids (Fig. 27-4).

CLINICAL COMMENTS

The two most common etiologies of *cortical* nephrocalcinosis are acute cortical necrosis and chronic glomerulonephritis, although radiographically evident calcification is rare in both conditions. Persons on chronic dialysis may have similar calcifications.

Roughly 40% of cases of *medullary* nephrocalcinosis are attributable to primary hyperparathyroidism, another 20% to renal tubular acidosis, and the remaining 40% are divided among many other causes.

▌ KEY CONCEPTS
- *Renal intraparenchymal calcification is known as nephrocalcinosis.*
- *Two categories of nephrocalcinosis are cortical and medullary.*
- *Peripheral location is seen with cortical nephrocalcinosis.*

- *Cortical nephrocalcinosis is rare.*
- *Bilateral, diffuse, fan-shaped clusters of stippled calcifications are typically seen with medullary nephrocalcification.*
- *Primary hyperparathyroidism and renal tubular acidosis are the most common causes of medullary nephrocalcinosis.*

Nephrolithiasis (Renal Calculi)

BACKGROUND

Nephrocalcinosis is calcification in renal parenchyma, whereas nephrolithiasis is concretion calcification in the luminal portion of the urinary tract (Fig. 27-5). The composition of renal stones varies with geography. In the United States, about 75% of renal stones are calcium oxalate. The remaining 25% of renal calculi are noncalcareous and are composed of either uric acid, struvite, or cystine.

IMAGING FINDINGS

Ultrasonographically, most stones bigger than a few millimeters will show shadowing. However, ultrasound is not the procedure of choice in diagnosis, because too many false-negative studies exist. In intravenous pyelography, the radiolucent stones can be difficult to differentiate from blood clots or sloughed tissue. (All of these can obstruct drainage from the kidney.) With computed tomography, all stones are denser than unenhanced renal parenchyma and urine.

Segments of the urinary tract proximal to the stone may show varying degrees of dilation depending on the degree and chronicity of occlusion created by the stone (Fig. 27-6). Not all dilated drainage systems are from stones and other intrinsic filling defects, because crossing bands of vessels or congenital narrowings can give the same appearance on intravenous pyelograms. Up to 90% of renal calculi are opaque enough to be seen on plain film radiographs.

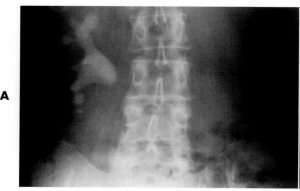
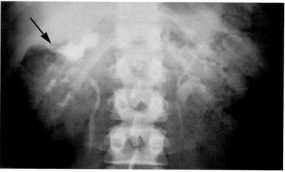
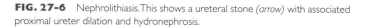

FIG. 27-5   Staghorn calculus in two different patients. **A,** Plain film of the abdomen demonstrates a calculus that conforms to the shape of the calyces, infundibulum, and pelvis. **B,** Intravenous pyelogram showing bilateral duplication of the collecting systems with a staghorn calculus obstructing the upper collecting system on the right *(arrow).*

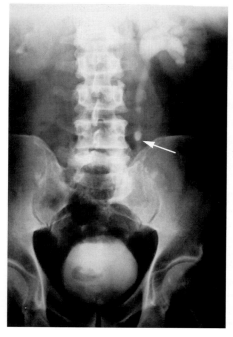

FIG. 27-6   Nephrolithiasis. This shows a ureteral stone *(arrow)* with associated proximal ureter dilation and hydronephrosis.

CLINICAL COMMENTS

Low urine volume and stasis contribute to formation of both calcareous and noncalcareous stones by increasing the urinary concentration of stone-forming constituents.

Renal calculi in the ureters cause renal colic, which has a dramatic clinical presentation, often with severe flank pain. Stones remaining in the renal pelvis may lead to obstruction. If they pass into the bladder, on unusual occasions, they may act as the nidus of a bladder calculus.

KEY CONCEPTS

- *Nephrolithiasis is produced in conditions causing urinary stasis or providing a nidus for stone formation.*
- *Symptoms are usually produced by obstruction.*
- *Nearly 90% are opaque enough to be seen on plain film radiographs.*

Ovarian Dermoid Cysts

BACKGROUND

Approximately 80% of ovarian tumors are benign. Most are discovered in women of reproductive age. In patients between 20 and 45 years old, approximately 30% to 50% of benign ovarian neoplasms are mature teratomas (dermoid cysts). Dermoid cysts represent only 10% of benign tumors in patients over 45 years.[23] Without complete tissue diagnosis, however, malignancy can never be ruled out.

IMAGING FINDINGS

The radiographic image of teratomas is influenced by the presence of tissues from all three germ layers. Characteristic densities frequently aiding in the diagnosis of these tumors include fat and teeth (Figs. 27-7 and 27-8). Both fat and calcium result in high-level reflective echoes on ultrasound, creating a relatively high degree of specificity for this imaging modality. Calcium also results in acoustical shadowing. Cystic type calcification is seen in the walls of about 10% of cystic teratomas. High signal foci on T1-weighted MRIs reflect the characteristic fat content.

CLINICAL COMMENTS

Dermoid cysts are usually found incidentally in young women. Although usually asymptomatic, they are prone to torsion, perforation, and infection (often salmonella). The complication rate for dermoid cysts is high compared with other ovarian tumors. Sudden rupture can result in chemical peritonitis and shock.[23] Benign teratomas are usually surgically removed to avoid these complications. Up to 25% of dermoid cysts are bilateral. Malignant transformation is rare, but it cannot be excluded by imaging studies alone.[11]

KEY CONCEPTS

- *80% of ovarian tumors are benign.*
- *In women between 20 and 45 years of age, 30% to 50% of benign neoplasms are mature teratomas; only 10% occur in patients over 45 years of age.*

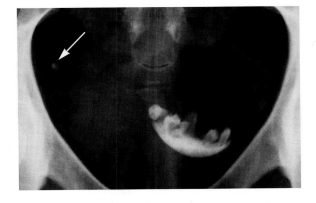

FIG. 27-7   Dermoid cyst containing a partial mandible with multiple well-formed teeth. The speck of calcification on the opposite side most likely represents another dermoid cyst *(arrow).*

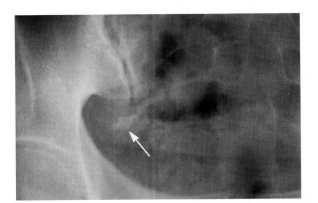

FIG. 27-8   Single well-formed tooth in the pelvis indicative of a dermoid cyst *(arrow).* The wall of the cyst is not visible.

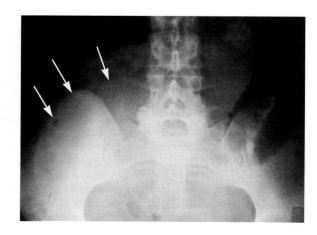

FIG. 27-9 Cystadenoma of the ovary. An extremely large cystadenoma occupying the majority of the pelvis *(arrows)*.

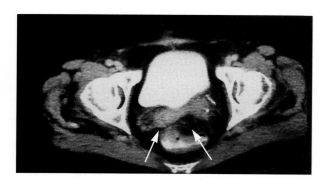

FIG. 27-10 Ovarian carcinoma. CT exam reveals an anexal mass that was proven to be ovarian carcinoma *(arrows)*.

- *The radiographic appearance of teratomas reflects its composition from all three germ cell layers; the presence of teeth and fat are particularly helpful.*
- *Dermoid cysts are usually found incidentally in young women and are typically asymptomatic.*

Other Ovarian Lesions

BACKGROUND

Approximately 80% of ovarian neoplasms are benign, and the majority occur in patients of reproductive age.[23] Approximately one half to two thirds of lesions considered suspicious based on ultrasound, physical exam, and laboratory findings are determined to be benign (Fig. 27-9).

Ovarian cancers are more common in peri- and postmenopausal women (Figs. 27-10 and 27-11). The odds of an ovarian lesion being malignant increase to 1 in 3 for patients over the age of 45. Only 10% of benign tumors are seen in patients more than 45 years old. The most common malignant ovarian tumors are adenocarcinoma, serous or mucinous cystadenocarcinoma, and endometrioid carcinoma.[23]

IMAGING FINDINGS

Ultrasound is used extensively as the initial imaging modality for evaluation of the adnexa.[23,28] Ultrasound findings are usually ade-quate to differentiate functional cysts, dermoids, some endometriomas, ectopic pregnancies, and more complex masses that require additional evaluation. The usefulness of ultrasound is limited by obesity, the presence of gas and bone in the area of concern, and the experience of the operator.[28] Transvaginal ultrasound offers better spatial resolution than transabdominal, but it has a more limited field of view.[25,28]

CT is appropriate for identifying fat or calcium within lesions and is recommended for staging ovarian carcinoma.[23] Magnetic resonance imaging (MRI) is capable of distinguishing adnexal from uterine masses as well as identifying fat or hemorrhage within lesions. MRI is additionally useful in identifying metastatic lesions.[23,25]

Irregular walls, thick septations and papillary projections are characteristic of malignant lesions.[23] Other findings suggestive of malignancy include large size, complex architecture, solid components, and cystic lesions that fail to resolve on serial ultrasound exams.[25] Solid portions of the lesion typically enhance and may show signs of necrosis.

No demonstrable difference in sensitivity or specificity in the detection of malignancy has been reported between MRI and CT, but MRI with contrast does provide better detail of the internal architecture of lesions.[23] CT has been recommended as the preferred modality for staging to assist in surgical and chemotherapeutic planning.[23]

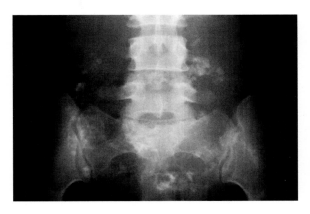

FIG. 27-11 Calcification in a hemangiopericytoma of the ovary. This represents a rare primary tumor of the ovary. This pattern of calcification is similar to the psammomatous calcifications associated with ovarian malignancy.

CLINICAL COMMENTS

Nonneoplastic cysts, or functional cysts, rarely cause symptoms unless they become quite large, rupture, or hemorrhage. Malignancies of the ovaries are notorious for their presentation of minimal symptoms such as abdominal distention.[23]

KEY CONCEPTS

- *Ovarian cancers are more common in peri- and postmenopausal women.*
- *Only 10% of benign tumors are seen in patients over 45 years old.*
- *Ultrasound (US) is the initial imaging modality of choice.*
- *Patients with malignancies often experience minimal symptoms.*

Pheochromocytoma

BACKGROUND

Pheochromocytoma is a rare, potentially life-threatening neoplasm characterized by its marked production of catecholamines. Approximately 85% to 95% occur in the adrenal medulla. The remainder occur in parts of the sympathetic nervous system in other abdominal locations, the thorax, or the neck, and are referred to as *paragangliomas*. Most cases occur sporadically, but in 10% an association is seen with other neuroectodermal disorders such as simple familial pheochromocytoma, von Recklinghausen's neurofibromatosis, MEN (multiple endocrine neoplasm) type II syndromes, Sturge-Weber syndrome, and von Hippel-Lindau disease.[4,18,29]

IMAGING FINDINGS

The role of diagnostic imaging is to localize the tumor. Computed tomography is 85% to 95% accurate in detecting adrenal masses larger than 1 cm in diameter, but it cannot accurately differentiate between pheochromocytoma and other adrenal masses such as adenomas or metastasis (see Fig. 26-45). Nuclear medicine scanning with met-iodobenzylguanidine (MIBG) specifically localizes adrenergic tissue and is recommended if CT is negative with the appropriate clinical and laboratory findings.[29] Magnetic resonance imaging is less sensitive than CT, but it may differentiate pheochromocytoma from other adrenal tumors by its marked enhancement on T2-weighted images.[18,29] These tumors tend to be encapsulated and highly vascular. Larger tumors often contain hemorrhagic and necrotic areas. Diffuse or nodular adrenal hyperplasia often is seen before or with development of pheochromocytoma.[29]

CLINICAL COMMENTS

The presenting signs and symptoms of pheochromocytoma reflect the tumor's marked production of catecholamines (epinephrine and norepinephrine). Adrenocorticotropic hormone (ACTH) and other renal and vasoactive hormones may be produced as well. The hallmark symptom is sustained or paroxysmal hypertension. Abnormalities of glucose regulation also occur.[29] The classic clinical triad of headache, sweating, and palpitations occurs only in approximately 40% of patients.[18] Laboratory detection of serum or urinary catecholamines and their metabolites provides the diagnosis. Surgery is the only effective treatment.

Identification of malignant pheochromocytoma cannot be made on the basis of clinical presentation, biochemical assay, or histological evaluation. Surgical identification of local tissue invasion or the presence of metastasis or recurrence after resection indicates malignancy. Approximately 10% prove to be malignant.[4,18,29]

KEY CONCEPTS

- *Pheochromocytoma is a rare tumor characterized by marked production of catecholamines.*
- *Catecholamines primarily affecting blood pressure and glucose regulation produce presenting symptoms.*
- *Pheochromocytoma is occasionally associated with genetic neuroectodermal syndromes.*
- *CT and MIBG scans localize tumor for surgical resection.*

Renal Cell Carcinoma

BACKGROUND

Renal cell carcinoma accounts for 80% to 90% of primary malignant renal neoplasms and approximately 3% of all malignancies in the adult population. The median age at diagnosis is 57 years, although renal cell carcinoma may occur at any age.[2,20] Renal cell carcinoma is about twice as common in men as in women. Most of these tumors occur sporadically, and the etiology is unknown.[20]

IMAGING FINDINGS

Radiologic identification of a renal mass requires differentiation of renal cell carcinoma from simple cyst, abscess, hematoma, lymphoma, renal metastasis, oncocytoma, or angiomyolipoma.[24]

Several excretory urography findings may suggest renal cell carcinoma, although this procedure cannot fully characterize a renal mass. Calcification occurs in approximately 13% of renal cell carcinomas, and it is usually amorphous and centrally located.[9,20] The calcification may simulate a calcified simple cyst and appear as a peripheral or central curvilinear or annular calcification (Figs. 27-12 and 27-13).[1,20,30]

Size, vascularity, and the extent of necrosis or cystic change affect the CT appearance. On unenhanced CT scans the neoplasm may appear hypodense, isodense, or hyperdense as compared with the normal renal parenchyma (Fig. 27-14).[20,32] Tumor calcification is readily identified and characterized on CT. On ultrasound, the mass will appear solid with or without cystic components to its walls. Any cystic component is not as thin as a pencil line, as is typical of a benign cyst.

Unenhanced MRI spin-echo (SE) sequences vary based on the

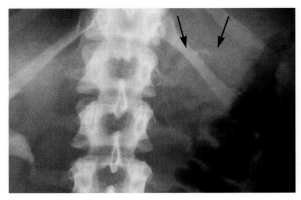

FIG. 27-12   Renal cell carcinoma. Calcification is present within the wall of a renal mass simulating a cyst but proven at biopsy to be a renal cell carcinoma *(arrows)*.

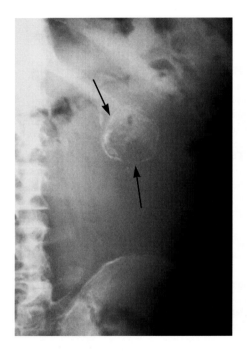

FIG. 27-13   Renal cell carcinoma. Mottled calcification within a renal cell carcinoma *(arrows)*.

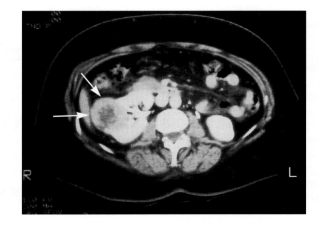

FIG. 27-14   CT of renal cell carcinoma *(arrows)*.

homogeneity of the lesion. Signal intensity of renal cell carcinoma is comparable to normal renal parenchyma on both T1- and T2-weighted images. Areas of hemorrhage and necrosis result in a heterogeneous appearance on unenhanced images.[15,20] Unenhanced SE images detect only 63% of tumors less than 3 cm in diameter.[15,20] MRI is somewhat limited in usefulness in evaluating renal masses because of the difficulty of appreciating calcification on almost any MRI pulse sequence.

CLINICAL COMMENTS

Renal cell carcinoma produces signs and symptoms in as few as 5% of patients. Metastatic spread is present at initial presentation in up to 45% of patients (Fig. 27-15). Classic presenting symptoms include flank pain sometimes because of a subcapsular bleed, flank mass, and hematuria.[22]

KEY CONCEPTS

- *Renal cell carcinoma accounts for 80% to 90% of primary malignant renal neoplasms.*
- *Radiologic identification of a renal mass requires differentiation from simple cyst, abscess, hematoma, lymphoma, renal metastasis, oncocytoma, or angiomyolipoma.*
- *Classic presenting symptoms include flank pain, flank mass, and hematuria, but patients often have only some or none of these findings.*

Uterine Fibroma (Leiomyoma)

BACKGROUND

Leiomyomas are seen in approximately 40% of women over 35 years of age and are the most common benign uterine tumor. They can be intramural, subserosal, or submucosal. Sometimes they are associated with infertility. Subserosal and submucosal types may be pedunculated, and the uterus may be deformed by these tumors. A unique characteristic of leiomyomas is their ability to detach from the uterus and develop a new blood supply from another organ. Tumor growth is affected primarily by estrogen. Estrogen levels increased by pregnancy or oral contraceptives can lead to tumor growth. Growth ceases after menopause without estrogen replacement therapy.[11]

IMAGING FINDINGS

Most uterine fibroids are identified either by pelvic examination, by palpation of a uterine enlargement or mass, or by discovering them on plain x-ray exam done for other purposes (by seeing either a mass or calcifications). Pelvic ultrasound is the most useful tool for evaluating these masses. The appearance of leiomyomas may vary, but common findings include general enlargement of the uterus (longer than 10 cm and wider than 5 cm), focal bulges in the uterine contour, and areas of inhomogeneous mural echoes.[11] Acoustic shadowing usually occurs when calcifications are present. Obviously, however, tissue diagnosis cannot be definitively made with ultrasound alone.

Plain radiographs or computed tomographs may reveal "popcorn-like" or "cauliflower-like" mass-type calcifications, which develop in necrotic areas of leiomyomas (Figs. 27-16 through 27-18).

Leiomyomas without areas of degeneration produce an MRI signal isointense with myometrium on T1-weighted and hy-

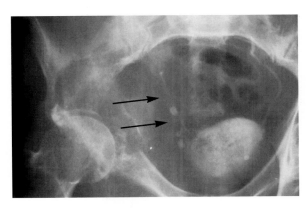

FIG. 27-15   Renal cell metastasis. Osteolytic metastasis. Osteolytic destructive lesions of left ilium and superior pubic rami, acetabulum, and ischium Note: Phleboliths are displaced toward midline *(arrows)*.

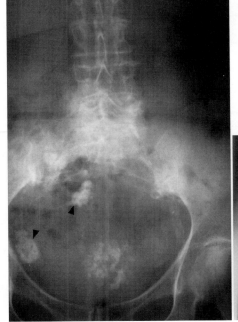
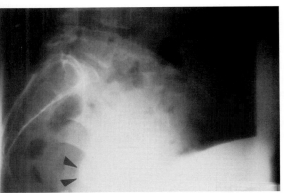

FIG. 27-16   Uterine leiomyoma. **A,** AP projection demonstrating the characteristic stippled or whorled calcific appearance *(arrowheads)*. **B,** On the lateral view the calcifications are more difficult to visualize *(arrowheads)*.

PART FOUR   Abdomen

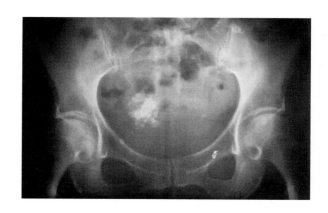

FIG. 27-17 Uterine leiomyoma. This is the typical stippled calcification of a uterine fibroid.

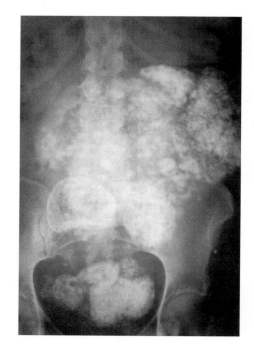

FIG. 27-18 Uterine leiomyomas. Massive uterine fibroids are extending out of the pelvis.

pointense on T2-weighted images. Degeneration of leiomyomas produces heterogenicity of signal and a wide range of intensities.[11] Again, diagnosis cannot be 100% definitive with imaging studies alone.

CLINICAL COMMENTS

More than 50% of uterine fibroids are asymptomatic and are not a health concern for women. Abnormal bleeding presenting as heavier and longer menses is the most common chronic symptom. Acute degeneration occurs in approximately one third of cases. Infertility is an occasional result. Symptoms secondary to pressure on adjacent abdominal contents and an increase in abdominal girth may

occur as the tumor increases in size. Malignant degeneration occurs in less than 3% of cases of leiomyoma.[11]

KEY CONCEPTS

- *Leiomyoma is the most common benign uterine tumor; it occurs in approximately 40% of women over 35 years of age.*
- *Tumor growth is affected by estrogen.*
- *Most uterine fibroids are identified first by pelvic examination or on x-ray alone for other reasons.*
- *More than 50% are asymptomatic.*
- *"Popcorn-like" or "cauliflower-like" mass calcification may be seen on plain film.*

References

1. Arkless R: Cyst-like calcification in renal cell carcinomas, *Clin Radiol* 17:397, 1966.
2. Bennington JL, Beckwith JB: Tumors of the kidney, renal pelvis and ureter. In *Atlas of tumor pathology,* Washington, DC, 1975, Armed Forces Institute of Pathology.
3. Bosniak MA et al: CT diagnosis of renal angiomyolipoma: the importance of detecting small amounts of fat, *AJR* 151:497, 1988.
4. Bravo EL: Evolving concepts in the pathophysiology, diagnosis, and treatment of pheochromocytoma, *Endocr Rev* 15:356, 1994.
5. Breslow N et al: Age distribution of Wilms' tumor study, *Cancer Res* 48:1653-1657, 1988.
6. Bret PM et al: Small, asymptomatic angiomyolipomas of the kidney, *Radiology* 154:7, 1985.
7. Charboneau JW et al: Spectrum of sonographic findings in 125 renal masses other than benign simple cyst, *AJR* 140:87, 1983.
8. Cris WM, Kun LE: Common solid tumors of childhood, *N Engl J Med* 324:461, 1991.
9. Daniel WW et al: Calcified renal masses: a review of ten years' experience at the Mayo Clinic, *Radiology* 103:503, 1972.
10. Earthman WJ, Mazer MJ, Winfield AC: Angiomyolipomas in tuberous sclerosis: subselective embolotherapy with alcohol, with long-term follow-up study, *Radiology* 160:437, 1986.
11. Hall DA, Hann LE: Gynecologic radiology: benign disorders. In Taveras JM, Ferrucci JR, editors: *Radiology-diagnosis-imaging-intervention,* vol 4, Philadelphia, 1996, Lippincott-Raven.
12. Hansen GC et al: Computed tomography diagnosis of renal angiomyolipoma, *Radiology* 128:789, 1978.
13. Hartman DS: Pediatric renal tumors. In Taveras JM, Ferrucci JR, editors: *Radiology-diagnosis-imaging-intervention,* vol 4, Philadelphia, 1996, Lippincott-Raven.
14. Hartman DS et al: Angiomyolipoma: ultrasonic-pathologic correlation, *Radiology* 139:451, 1981.
15. Hricak H et al: Detection and staging of renal neoplasms: a reassessment of MR imaging, *Radiology* 166:643, 1988.
16. Imray TJ, Kaplan P: Lower urinary tract infections and calculi in the adult, *Semin Roentgenol* 18: 267, 1983.
17. Jaffe MH et al: Wilms' tumor: ultrasonic features, pathologic correlation, and diagnostic pitfalls, *Radiology* 140:147, 1981.
18. Kazantsev GB, Prinz RA: Functioning tumors of the adrenal gland, *Compr Ther* 19:232, 1993.
19. Kissane JM, Dehner LP: Renal tumors and tumor-like lesions in pediatric patients, *Pediatr Nephrol* 6:365, 1992.
20. Levine E: Renal cell carcinoma: clinical aspects, imaging diagnosis, and staging, *Semin Roentgenol* 30:128, 1995.
21. Meilstrup JW et al: Other renal tumors, *Semin Roentgenol* 30:168, 1995.
22. Mevorach RA et al: Renal cell carcinoma: incidental diagnosis and natural history: review of 235 cases, *Urology* 39:519, 1992.
23. Occhipinti KA, Frankel SD, Hricak H: The ovary, *Radiol Clin North Am* 31:1115, 1993.
24. O'Toole KM, Brown M, Hoffmann P: Pathology of benign and malignant kidney tumors, *Urol Clin North Am* 20:193, 1993.
25. Outwater EK, Dunton CJ: Imaging of the ovary and adnexa: clinical issues and applications of MR imaging, *Radiology* 194:1, 1995.
26. Raghavendra BN, Bosniak MA, Megibow AJ: Small angiomyolipoma of the kidney: sonographic-CT evaluation, *AJR* 141:575, 1983.
27. Scheible W et al: Lipomatous tumors of the kidney and adrenal: apparent echographic specificity, *Radiology* 129:153, 1978.
28. Scott LM, McCarthy SM: Imaging of ovarian masses: magnetic resonance imaging, *Clin Obstet Gynecol* 34:443, 1991.
29. Werbel SS, Ober KP: Pheochromocytoma: update on diagnosis, localization, and management, *Med Clin N Am* 79:131, 1995.
30. Weyman PJ et al: CT of calcified renal masses, *AJR* 138:1095, 1982.
31. Wickman JEA: Treatment of urinary tract stones, *BMJ* 307:1414, 1993.
32. Zagoria RJ et al: CT features of renal cell carcinoma with emphasis on relation to tumor size, *Invest Radiol* 25:261, 1990.

PART FOUR Abdomen

chapter 28

Gastrointestinal System Diseases

BEVERLY L HARGER

LISA E HOFFMAN

RICHARD ARKLESS

Cholelithiasis (Gallstones)
Colon Polyps
Colorectal Carcinoma

Crohn's Disease
Diverticular Disease
Hiatal Hernia

Pancreatic Lithiasis
Peptic Ulcer Disease
Ulcerative Colitis

Cholelithiasis (Gallstones)

BACKGROUND

The incidence of gallstones in patients in the United States approaches 20% of men and 35% of women by the age of 75 years.[24] Thus, gallstones exhibit a greater prevalence in women and in older age groups. Obesity and certain diseases are also associated with the development of gallstones (Table 28-1).

IMAGING FINDINGS

Ultrasonography is generally the preferred imaging modality for evaluating patients for possible gallstones or biliary duct obstruction. Gallstones produce hyperechoic foci with acoustic shadowing, and mobility of the stone is usually apparent (Fig. 28-1).[5,15] Because these stones can be missed in a contracted gallbladder, the patient should be fasting for 4 or more hours.[25]

These stones may be incidentally imaged on plain film radiographs even in asymptomatic patients, but only 10% to 15% of them contain enough calcium to be visible (Fig. 28-2).[11,32] Oral cholecystography (OCG) requires the patient to take an oral contrast agent, which is absorbed from the bowel, excreted by the liver, and concentrated in the gallbladder (except when the gallbladder cystic duct is blocked or sometimes when the gallbladder is inflamed). The gallbladder will also not be seen in cases of a lack of absorption or significant liver damage.

However, OCG does demonstrate most gallstones, but since the development of ultrasound to accomplish this task, it is thought by some to be most useful for providing information about the functional status of the gallbladder (Fig. 28-3).[7] The clinical usefulness of this is still controversial, however.

CLINICAL COMMENTS

Cholelithiasis is usually discovered incidentally during other studies. In the first 5 years following diagnosis, only approximately 10% of patients experience symptoms resulting from gallstones.[32] Right upper quadrant pain is the most commonly reported symptom.[32] The pain is usually steady, lasting for several hours. Radia-

tion to the lower abdomen, the back, and/or to the tip of the right scapula is not uncommon; vomiting may occur.[5]

Complications seen with gallstone disease include cholecystitis, choledocholithiasis, pancreatitis (migration of a stone to the distal common duct where the pancreatic duct enters), cholangitis, stone perforation of the duodenum or colon, and gallstone ileus. (Table 28-2).[2,3,5,19,32] Symptomatic gallbladder disease may require surgical intervention if nonsurgical techniques such as lithotripsy (using strong ultrasound waves to break up the stone) are ineffective, unsuitable, or unavailable.[32]

KEY CONCEPTS

- *The prevalence of cholelithiasis increases with age.*
- *It is more common in women.*
- *Obesity is a risk factor.*
- *Symptoms vary and clinical correlation is required.*
- *Ultrasound is the most common and most useful imaging test.*
- *Plain film radiography plays a minor role.*

Colon Polyps

BACKGROUND

Colon polyps are found in up to 12% of the population.[34] The adenomatous polyp is considered the precursor to colorectal cancer.[16] Therefore detection of colonic polyps is extremely important. The incidence of malignancy increases with increased size of the polyp (Table 28-3). Most polyp development is incidental, but polyps also appear as part of familial polyposis syndromes (not common). Table 28-4 reviews the characteristics of several polyposis conditions.

IMAGING FINDINGS

The barium examination and endoscopy are the most important methods for detecting polyps.[33] Polyps appear as discrete masses, sessile or pedunculated, which protrude into the lumen of the gut (Figs. 28-4, 28-5, and 28-6). Recent investigations report up to 98% accuracy in identification of polyps by double-contrast barium enema. Older studies report less accuracy, but the accuracy depends

TABLE 28-1
Associated Factors for Gallstone Formation

Associated factors	Comments
Obesity	Rapid weight loss resulting in increased risk of symptomatic gallstone formation[11,17]
Increasing age	Associated with increased cholesterol secretion[11]
Northern European ethnic group	Associated with increased cholesterol secretion[11]
Estrogen replacement therapy and oral-contraceptive use	Increases biliary output of cholesterol and also reduces synthesis of bile acid in women[11]
Pregnancy	Associated with increased risk of gallstones and symptomatic gallbladder disease[11,32]
Sickle cell anemia or other hemolytic conditions	Hemolysis increases bilirubin excretion[11]
Crohn's disease	Disease of the terminal ileum causing disruption of bile acid reabsorption[11]

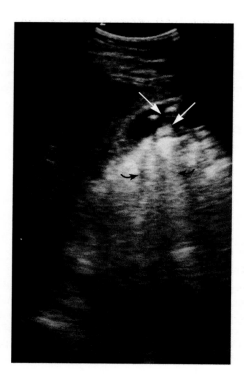

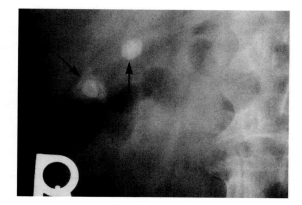

FIG. 28-1   Choleliths. Ultrasound image shows multiple echogenic foci within the gallbladder lumen *(arrows)* with posterior acoustic shadowing *(curved arrows)*. (Courtesy John A.M. Taylor, Portland, Ore.)

FIG. 28-2   Choleliths. Two laminated and faceted calculi in the gallbladder characteristic of concretion calcifications *(arrows)*.

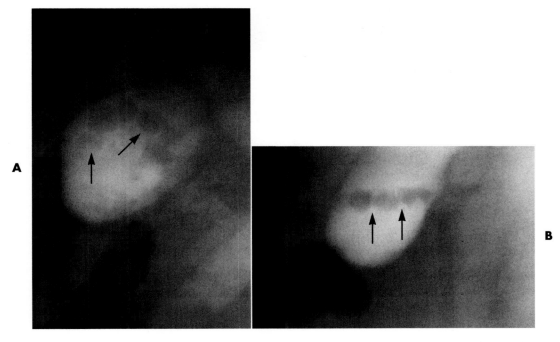

FIG. 28-3   Oral cholecystographic appearance of gallstones. **A,** Oral cholecystogram with the patient in the recumbent position demonstrates several nonopaque stones within the gallbladder *(arrows).* **B,** With the patient in the upright position, the stones float just above the fundus *(arrows).* (Courtesy John A.M. Taylor, Portland, Ore.)

PART FOUR
Abdomen

TABLE 28-2
Complications Associated with Gallstones

Complications	Comments
Acute cholecystitis	May remit temporarily, but sometimes progresses to gangrene and perforation[11]
Choledocholithiasis	Gallstones obstructing the common bile duct[11]
Cholangitis	Infection of the bile ducts following obstruction possible[11]
Acute pancreatitis	Probably secondary to transient obstruction of the main pancreatic duct[11]
Gallstone ileus	Follows perforation of the duodenum or bowel by gallstone: classic plain film triad: small bowel obstruction, biliary tract air, and an opaque concretion in the small bowel

TABLE 28-3
Incidence of Malignancy in Relation to Polyp Size[33]

5 mm or less	5mm to 10 mm	10 mm to 20 mm	More than 20 mm
Less than 0.5%	1% to 2.5%	10%	46%

TABLE 28-4
Review of Polyposis Conditions

Complications	Comments
Nonfamilial adeonomatous polyps	Present in 30% of adults over 50 years of age; malignancy correlates with polyp size, villous features, and degree of dysplasia[12]
Familial adenomatous polyposis	Autosomal dominant; it begins to appear between ages of 10 and 35 years; colon cancer usually occurs by age 50[12]
Gardner's syndrome	Variant of familial adenomatous polyposis; it is characterized by extraintestinal osteomas, fibromas, and desmoid tumors[12]
Familial juvenile polyposis	Autosomal dominant; most common—colon
Peutz-Jehgers syndrome	Autosomal dominant; mucocutaneous pigmented macules appear on lips, buccal mucosa, and skin; 50% of patients develop malignancies in GI and nonintestinal organs[12]
Turcot's syndrome	Autosomal recessive; central nervous system neoplasm[12]

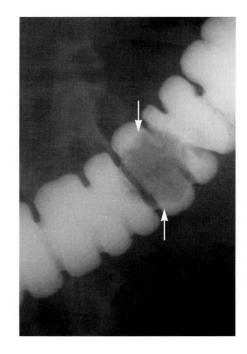

FIG. 28-4 Sessile polyp. Filling defect of a sessile-based polyp is well demonstrated (arrows).

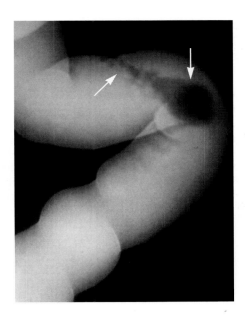

FIG. 28-5   Polyp with stalk. A pedunculated polyp is visualized within this contrast-filled bowel *(arrows)*.

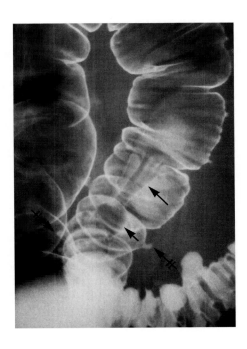

FIG. 28-6   Polyp with stalk. Double contrast (air and barium) study reveals a pedunculated polyp *(arrows)*. Diverticulae are also seen with this study *(crossed arrows)*.

on the meticulousness and quality of the exam. Lesions smaller than 1 cm in diameter are more difficult to detect.

In general, the inner margin of a polyp will appear sharper than the outer margin because it is an intraluminal mass surrounded by barium. On occasion a diverticulum coated with barium and filled with air can mimic a polyp on one or more x-rays, but with meticulous evaluation it should not be misdiagnosed.

CLINICAL COMMENTS

Most patients with multiple small polyps or even small carcinomas have no overt symptoms. Chronic occult blood loss from polyps may lead to iron deficiency. Occasionally, symptoms from large polyps are related to complications such as intussusception or colonic obstruction.[33] Polyps measuring 1 cm or larger should definitely be removed and histologically examined, although some experts believe even smaller ones should also be removed.

KEY CONCEPTS

- *Colonoscopy and barium enema are two possibly equal modalities in evaluating the colon for polyps.*
- *Adenomatous polyps may be a precursor to colonic cancer.*
- *The incidence of malignancy increases with increased size of the polyp.*

Colorectal Carcinoma

BACKGROUND

Colorectal cancer is second only to lung cancer in men and breast and lung cancer in women as a cause of death.[39] The incidence of colorectal cancer increases after 35 to 45 years of age; however,

TABLE 28-5
High-Risk Groups for Colorectal Carcinoma

Risk factors	Comments
Familial polyposis	100% risk of cancer if untreated[26]
Gardner's syndrome	Characterized by precancerous colorectal polyps, associated with osteomas, fibromas, soft tissue desmoids, and lipomas[26]
Ulcerative colitis	Patients with longstanding and extensive ulcerative colitis at high risk[26]
Crohn's disease	Risk not as high as for those with ulcerative colitis[26]
Family history	Positive family history for colorectal cancer or polyps[26]
Hereditary cancer of multiple anatomical sites	Autosomal dominant syndrome, such as breast, endometrium, ovary, and colon[26]

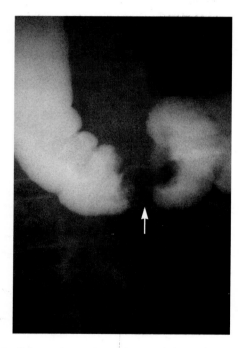

FIG. 28-7   Colon carcinoma. An annular constricting carcinoma can be seen as a narrowed segment of bowel with a markedly narrowed lumen, abrupt transition, and overhanging edges known as "napkin-ring" or "applecore" lesion *(arrow).*

high-risk persons (Table 28-5) develop colorectal cancer at a much younger age.[26,35] Most colorectal cancers are thought to arise from malignant transformation of an adenomatous polyp.[35]

IMAGING FINDINGS

Colorectal cancer may produce changes that are imaged as infiltration, mucosal destruction, and masses (Fig. 28-7). Colonoscopy demonstrates these changes and is the preferred diagnostic procedure when patient history is suggestive of colon cancer or barium enema has demonstrated abnormalities consistent with colon cancer. Any large, broad-based polyp with an irregular surface is highly suggestive of carcinoma.[29] The classic appearance on barium enema is the annular "napkin-ring" or "applecore" lesion produced by an infiltrating tumor, which causes narrowing of the lumen,

thickening of the wall, and rigidity. However, this is an advanced stage and the cancer is obviously best discovered when much smaller. Mucosal destruction and overhanging edges are also components of this appearance.

CLINICAL COMMENTS

Clinical features do not consistently reflect tumor size, so some quite large carcinomas may remain clinically silent. However, patients presenting with rectal bleeding or hemoccult-positive stools must be evaluated for colorectal cancer.[18,29,36] In individuals older than 40 years of age, a change in bowel habits or particularly constipation, weight loss, and unexplained anemia are other clinical features that suggest possible colorectal cancer.[29]

■ KEY CONCEPTS
- *Colorectal cancer is suspected in any patient over 40 years of age with change in bowel habits, weight loss, and unexplained anemia.*
- *Characteristic findings on barium enema include narrowing of bowel lumen, thickening of bowel wall, and rigidity.*
- *Colonoscopy with biopsy establishes diagnosis.*

Crohn's Disease

BACKGROUND

Crohn's disease is an idiopathic inflammatory process primarily affecting the distal small intestine and the colon; however, any portion of the alimentary tract (from mouth to anus) potentially may be involved. The terminal ileum and adjacent proximal ascending colon are the only sites of involvement in approximately half of the cases, but Crohn's disease can involve the small bowel alone (30% to 40%) or the colon alone (25%).[13,14] This disease most commonly affects adolescents and young adults.[13,14] Symptoms are sometimes present for years before the patient is bothered enough to seek medical attention.

IMAGING FINDINGS

The preferred imaging procedure is an upper gastrointestinal barium study with small bowel follow-through. Hyperperistalsis of the bowel, mucosal and submucosal edema with thickening of mucosal folds, and a finely granular mucosal pattern are the earliest radiologic changes.[13,14] Advanced imaging findings include ulcerations, separation of bowel loops, strictures, and fistulas (Figs. 28-8 through 28-11).[13,14] Approximately 10% to 15% of cases of Crohn's disease cannot be adequately differentiated from ulcerative colitis even under the microscope.[13,14] Significant findings that help differentiate Crohn's from ulcerative colitis include "rose thorn" ulcerations, cobblestone mucosal appearance, skip areas, severe anorectal disease or fistulas, non-bloody diarrhea, and fissures. Major complications such as mass, abscess, thickening of bowel wall, and obstruction of the right distal ureter with hydronephrosis may be demonstrated with ultrasonography or computed tomography.

CLINICAL COMMENTS

Intermittent episodes of low-grade fever, diarrhea, abdominal distention, and right lower quadrant pain are suggestive of Crohn's disease, although the symptoms and signs can be quite varied.[13,14] Presence of a perineal fistula demands search for possible Crohn's disease, and it may be the presenting symptom. Laboratory findings include normal or elevated white blood cell count, increased erythrocyte sedimentation rate, iron-deficiency anemia, macrocytic anemia, and decreased total proteins and albumin.[13,14] A partial list of complications of Crohn's disease is provided in Table 28-6. Over the long term, a small percentage of patients will

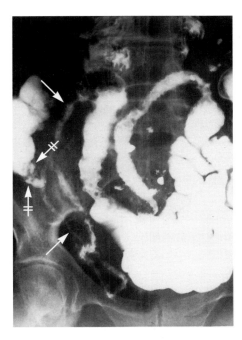

FIG. 28-8 Crohn's disease. Marked narrowing of the ileum is typical of the "string" sign *(arrows)* and the "cobblestone" pattern of the cecum is a feature of advanced Crohn's disease *(crossed arrows).*

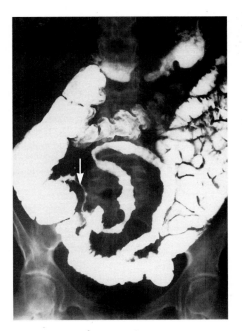

FIG. 28-9 Narrowed terminal ileum of Crohn's disease *(arrow).*

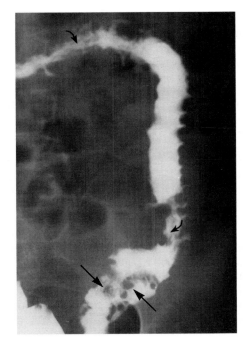

FIG. 28-10 Crohn's disease. Large inflammatory polyps *(straight arrows)* and fissures *(curved arrows)* in narrowed segments of bowel are characteristics of Crohn's disease.

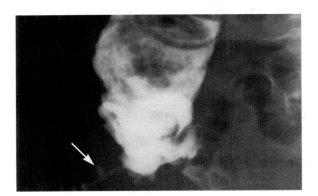

FIG. 28-11 Crohn's disease. A fistula that forms a communication between the cecum and the skin is barely visible *(arrow).*

TABLE 28-6
Complications of Crohn's Disease

Complications	Comments
Nutritional deficiencies	Decreased intake of food, excessive loss of protein and nutrients resulting from diarrhea and intestinal bleeding, drug interference, bacterial overgrowth, and malabsorption are all factors that may possibly lead to nutritional deficiencies[13,14]
Bone complications	Nondeforming migrating polyarthritis (usually knees, ankles), sacroiliitis and ankylosing spondylitis, osteopenia and osteomalacia are possibly associated with Crohn's disease. Osteonecrosis (e.g., of the femoral heads) as a complication of steroid therapy may also be seen[13,14]
Carcinoma	Risk increases with extent and duration of the disease. Approximately 1% to 2% develop carcinoma[13,14]
Growth complications	Cessation of linear growth, lack of weight gain, and delayed bone and sexual maturation occur in 20% to 30% of affected children[13,14]

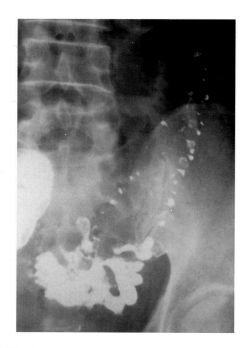

FIG. 28-12   Diverticulosis. Postevacuation study demonstrates diverticulae. (Courtesy John A.M. Taylor, Portland, Ore.)

develop colon and occasionally small bowel cancer, ascending cholangitis, lymphoma, or sacroiliitis. In addition, a familial tendency exists, and the disease is more commonly seen in individuals who smoke.

KEY CONCEPTS
- *Crohn's disease is marked by an insidious onset.*
- *The patient experiences intermittent bouts of low-grade fever, diarrhea, bloating, and/or right lower quadrant pain.*
- *Ulceration, stricturing, or fistula of small intestine or colon are advanced imaging findings.*
- *Perineal fistula or fissure may cause the initial complaint.*

Diverticular Disease

BACKGROUND

Diverticular disease of the colon refers to a group of related diseases comprising diverticulosis and diverticulitis. The known incidence of colonic diverticular disease in patients over 60 years of age exceeds 30%, but it is probably much higher.[23,38] Dietary deficiency of fiber is related to its development.[23,38]

Diverticula are most common in the sigmoid colon, where higher intraluminal pressure is a cofactor in development, but they may occur anywhere in the length of the colon.[38] These outpouchings of mucosa through the muscular layer occur at sites of weakness in the bowel wall, generally where the nutrient artery penetrates the wall.[38] Connective tissue diseases such as Ehlers-Danlos syndrome, Marfan's syndrome, and scleroderma can reduce the integrity of the bowel wall and predispose patients to the development of diverticula.[38]

IMAGING FINDINGS

Characteristic findings of diverticulosis include the presence of diverticula, muscular hypertrophy, and spasm (Figs. 28-12 and 28-13). Diverticulitis is suspected when fistula (more common with Crohn's disease and occasionally seen with colon cancer), abscess producing an extrinsic mass, or extravasation is noted (Fig. 28-14).[10,37] Plain film of the abdomen, ultrasound, and computed tomography may be helpful if an abscess, obstruction, or perforation is suspected.[21]

CLINICAL COMMENTS

Uncomplicated disease with no symptoms, except perhaps chronic small stool size or tenesmus, represents more than two thirds of cases of diverticulosis.[38] Chronic constipation, abdominal pain, or fluctuating bowel habits are some of the nonspecific complaints that have been reported. Inflammation (diverticulitis) and hemorrhage are the two most common pain complications in diverticular disease of the colon.[38] Patients with diverticulitis usually experience fever, left lower quadrant tenderness, and an abdominal mass.[35] Rectal bleeding may occur intermittently or may be continuous for several days. This bleeding is usually from right colon diverticulitis without symptoms of diverticulitis. A colon cancer or vascular malformation can give similar bleeding. Characteristically, rectal bleeding associated with right colon diverticulitis has a sudden onset, is painless, and is often severe and may require surgical intervention.

KEY CONCEPTS
- *Diverticulae become more numerous toward the distal end of the colon.*
- *It is most common in individuals with a diet low in fiber.*
- *Fever, left lower quadrant pain, tenderness, and abdominal mass are characteristics of acute diverticulitis.*
- *Rectal bleeding from right-sided diverticulae may occur suddenly and be severe enough to require surgical intervention.*

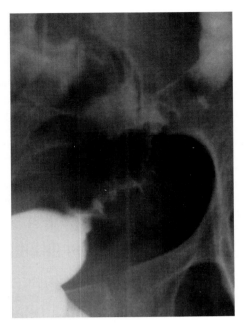

FIG. 28-13   Diverticulitis. Contrast enema depicts spasm of a portion of the sigmoid. This finding is indicative of diverticular disease but not diagnostic for diverticulitis.

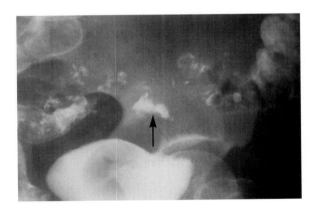

FIG. 28-14   Diverticulitis. Extravasation of contrast material is noted (*arrow*). With this finding a specific diagnosis of perforated diverticulitis can be made.

Hiatal Hernia

BACKGROUND

Hiatal hernia is the most common diagnostic entity identified on radiographic examination of the upper gastrointestinal tract. The sliding or axial hiatal hernia, in which the esophagogastric junction and a portion of the gastric fundus herniates into the chest, comprises more than 95% of hiatal hernias.[1] At least 10% of the adult North American population have a sliding hiatal hernia, but with Valsalva's maneuver one can demonstrate at least a tiny hiatal hernia in many, if not most, people.[1] The paraesophageal type, in which the junction remains fixed below the diaphragmatic hiatus but a portion of the gastric fundus herniates into the chest alongside the lower esophagus, represents about 1% of all hiatal hernias.[6] A mixed type represents the third type of hiatal hernia. Presence or absence of this hernia is not nearly as important as presence or absence of gastroesophageal reflux, which can occur even in the absence of a hernia and may not occur even with a large hernia.

IMAGING FINDINGS

Identification of the esophagogastric junction at least 2 cm above the diaphragm, usually seen with the aid of barium contrast, is needed. Identification of a mucosal web is helpful but often is not present. A soft tissue mass and/or an air-fluid level in the posterior mediastinum on a plain film chest radiograph may indicate hiatal hernia (Fig. 28-15). Use of barium esophagram allows differentiation from other posterior mediastinal masses (Fig. 28-16).

CLINICAL COMMENTS

Hiatal hernias are common and the associated symptoms of reflux are usually their only clinical significance. Endoscopic evidence of reflux esophagitis is absent in most patients with hiatal hernia.[22,32] However, hiatal hernia can be imaged in 90% of patients with gastroesophageal reflux disease.[22] The more severe forms of reflux esophagitis are less common in patients without hiatal hernia, but normal esophagogastric junction does not rule out reflux esophagitis.[22] A rare but potentially life-threatening complication of massive hiatal hernia is volvulus of the stomach ("upside-down stomach") with strangulation.[8]

KEY CONCEPTS

- *Hiatal hernia commonly occurs in adults.*
- *The presence or absence of hiatal hernia poorly predicts presence of gastroesophageal reflux disease.*
- *Most are sliding (axial) hernias.*
- *With massive hiatal hernia, volvulus of stomach with strangulation can be life-threatening.*

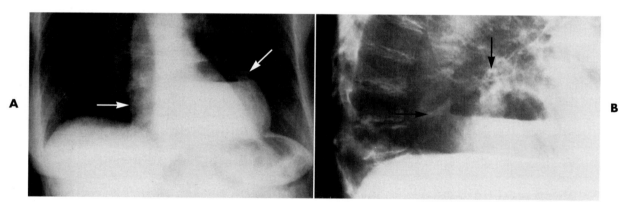

FIG. 28-15   Hiatal hernia. **A,** PA projection. A mass with an air-fluid level within can be seen behind the heart *(arrows)*. **B,** Lateral view of hiatal hernia *(arrows)*.

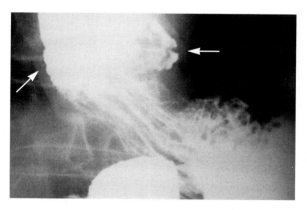

FIG. 28-16   Hiatal hernia. Upper gastrointestinal study demonstrates a sliding hiatal hernia *(arrows)*.

Pancreatic Lithiasis

BACKGROUND

Relative obstruction of the pancreatic ductal system is the likely underlying mechanism for pancreatic calculus development.[20,28] The calculi primarily represent calcified masses of inspissated secretions.[20,28] A history of high alcohol intake is elicited in nearly 90% of patients with pancreatic calculi.[27] Table 28-7 lists other conditions that may lead to pancreatic calculus formation.

IMAGING FINDINGS

Pancreatic calculi secondary to alcoholic pancreatitis usually appear as small, irregular concretions, commonly numerous and scattered throughout the gland. These concretions are seen on the abdominal films at the level of L1-L2 and conform to the shape of the pancreas. On the right side, the densities are close to the midline, but on the left the calcifications may extend far peripherally (Figs. 28-17 and 28-18). In approximately 25% of cases the calcifications are seen in only the head or tail of the pancreas.[27]

CLINICAL COMMENTS

Patients with pancreatic calcifications secondary to alcoholic pancreatitis usually have a 5- to 10-year history of episodic abdominal pain.[27]

KEY CONCEPTS

- *Alcohol pancreatitis is the most common cause of pancreatic lithiasis.*
- *It appears as numerous irregular, tiny concretions widely scattered throughout the pancreas.*
- *Calcification usually develops after 5 to 10 years of episodic abdominal pain.*
- *Pancreatitis is usually seen on plain film radiographs.*

TABLE 28-7
Conditions That May Lead to Pancreatic Calcification

Condition	Pattern	Comments
Alcoholic pancreatitis	Small concretions widely scattered throughout gland	Usually develops after 5 to 10 years of pain[27]
Pseudocysts	Widely scattered or rim calcification usually in or near pancreas	Up to 20% of cases exhibit calcification similar to chronic pancreatitis[27]
Pancreatic cancer	Diffusely present throughout gland; however, most pancreatic cancers do not calcify	Higher incidence of pancreatic cancer in patients with chronic pancreatitis
Hyperparathyroidism	Pancreatic and renal calcification	Pancreatitis occurs as a complication of hyperparathyroidism in 10% of cases[27]
Cystadenoma or cystadenocarcinoma	Sunburst pattern—pathognomonic, but not common	Tumor calcification in 10% of patients[27]

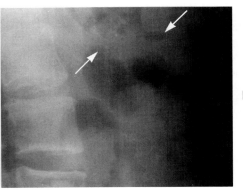

FIG. 28-17 Pancreatic lithiasis. **A,** AP projection demonstrates faint discrete calculi superimposed over and near the L2 vertebral body (*arrows*). **B,** Lateral view reveals multiple, tiny, dense, discrete opacities typical of pancreatic lithiasis (*arrows*).

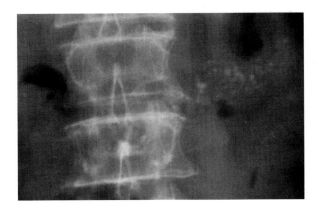

FIG. 28-18 Pancreatic lithiasis. AP projection. On the right side the stippled opacities are close to midline, but on the left the calcification extends far peripherally conforming the shape of the pancreas. (Courtesy Cynthia Peterson, Bournemouth, England.)

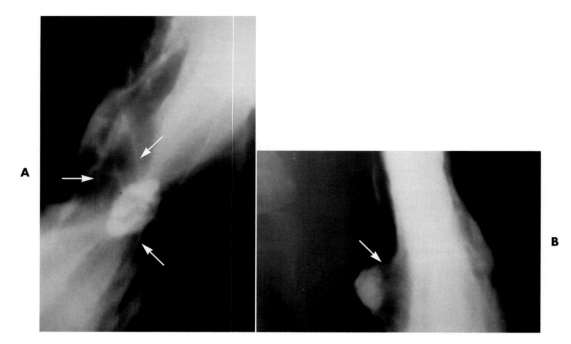

FIG. 28-19   Benign gastric ulcer. **A,** View of the ulcer end on shows that the mucosal folds are thin and regular and extend up to the margin of the ulcer crater *(arrows)*. **B,** Tangential view demonstrating the ulcer collar *(arrow)*. Moderately edematous tissue at the ulcer mouth produces a lucent mound when seen in profile. A large ulcer is seen along the lesser curvature of the stomach. Notice the ulcer projects beyond the normal expected lesser curvature, a sign suggesting benignancy.

Peptic Ulcer Disease

BACKGROUND

Peptic ulcer disease is the result of erosion of the gastric or duodenal mucosa. Although the etiology of peptic ulcer disease can be complex, the presence of *Helicobacter pylori* bacteria in the stomach is thought to be a major factor.[4] *Helicobacter pylori* infection is identified in more than 90% of patients with duodenal ulcers and more than 80% of patients with gastric ulcers.[4] The vast majority of peptic ulcers are benign. Ninety-five percent occur in the duodenum with virtually no association with malignancy.[12] Only 5% of gastric ulcers are associated with malignancies.[12]

IMAGING FINDINGS

Although debate continues regarding the best imaging method, double-contrast studies have shown a sensitivity of 95% for lesions identified by endoscopy.[30]

Small gastric ulcers produce a defect that is filled by barium or air. This niche is persistent in multiple images and usually projects beyond the gastric mucosa margin. Slight notching (incisura) may be visible along the wall opposite the ulcer. As gastric distension from barium or air decreases, the edematous collar of tissue around the ulcer will become visible (Fig. 28-19).[30] When the ulcer crater is seen on profile, a 1-mm thin lucent line traversing the orifice of the ulcer crater, known as *Hampton line*,

may be seen. Table 28-8 identifies the criteria for benign gastric ulcers.

Imaging of the duodenal ulcers does not differ significantly from gastric ulcers. A constant, reproducible collection of barium must be seen, and folds radiating to the crater are characteristic.[12] Duodenal bulb is more often deformed by changes from prior ulcers than is the stomach.[12] The so-called "clover-leaf" deformity is one created by marked contraction of tissues toward the site of a present or prior ulcer (Fig. 28-20).

CLINICAL COMMENTS

Epigastric pain (dyspepsia) is present in 90% of patients.[9] The more common pain pattern includes increased pain between meals and at night. Ulcer penetration or perforation should be suspected if pain becomes constant or radiates to the back or shoulders. Most patients will experience symptomatic periods lasting up to several weeks with intervening pain-free months to years.[9] Gastric outlet obstruction (or gastric malignancy) should be suspected if significant vomiting or weight loss is noted.[12]

KEY CONCEPTS

- *Epigastric pain occurs in 90% of patients with peptic ulcer disease.*
- *Duodenal ulcers are virtually never malignant.*
- *5% of gastric ulcers occur in malignancies.*
- *Upper gastrointestinal study is the procedure of choice for diagnosis of duodenal and gastric ulcers.*

TABLE 28-8
Roentgen Findings of Benign Gastric Ulcers

Roentgen findings	Comments
Radiation of folds	Gastric folds connecting to the ulcer crater[40,41]
Crater beyond lumen	When viewed in profile, a benign ulcer typically penetrating beyond the expected margin of the lumen[40,41]
Hampton's line	A thin (1 to 2 mm), lucent line occasionally visible crossing the base of the ulcer[40,41]
Ulcer collar	Moderately edematous tissue at the ulcer mouth producing a lucent band when seen in profile[40,41]
Ulcer mound	Lucent mound produced by a large amount of edema surrounding an ulcer, especially when seen in profile[40,41]; it indicates some retraction from prior scarring
Incisura	Indrawing of the wall opposite the ulcer is a sign of a benign ulcer[40,41]
Peristalsis	Peristalsis continuing normally through the region of the ulcer, and the area should be pliable[40,41]

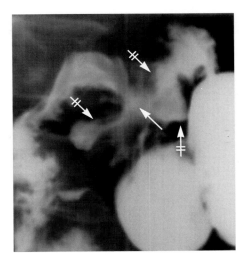

FIG. 28-20 Duodenal ulcer. A small ulcer (arrow) is seen in the central portion of the bulb. Note the radiating folds (crossed arrows) and bulbar deformity associated with the ulcer.

Ulcerative Colitis

BACKGROUND

Ulcerative colitis is an idiopathic inflammatory condition affecting the mucosal surface of the colon and resulting in diffuse friability and erosions with bleeding. This disease involves only the rectosigmoid region in roughly half of patients.[35] In approximately 30% of patients, ulcerative colitis extends to the splenic flexure and in less than 20% it extends more proximally.[35] Alternating episodes of exacerbations and remissions characterize this process.[35]

IMAGING FINDINGS

Plain radiographs of the abdomen are utilized to identify significant colonic dilation (in excess of 6.5 cm) associated with toxic megacolon (a very serious and potentially life-threatening condition) in patients with severe colitis.[35] Barium enema may reveal variable loss of the haustra pattern, a coarse granular appearance of the mucosa, collar button ulcerations, pseudopolyps, decreased rectal distensibility, and frequent shortening of the colon (Fig. 28-21).[13] As opposed to Crohn's disease, the colon is involved continuously without skip areas; also, no strictures, fistulae, or fissures are present, unlike Crohn's disease.

CLINICAL COMMENTS

In contrast to Crohn's disease, bloody diarrhea is the hallmark finding in patients with ulcerative colitis.[35] Other symptoms include abdominal cramping, rectal urgency, anorexia, and weight loss.[13] Sec-

ondary colon cancer becomes an increasingly significant concern the longer the disease is present. Complications of ulcerative colitis are listed in Table 28-9.[14]

▌KEY CONCEPTS

- *Bloody diarrhea is the hallmark of ulcerative colitis.*
- *About one half of patients have disease limited to rectosigmoid region.*
- *Plain films are obtained to look for toxic megacolon.*
- *Barium enema reveals distinctive findings including a loss of haustra pattern and coarse, granular appearance of the mucosa.*

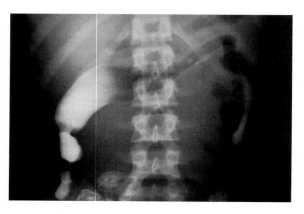

FIG. 28-21   Chronic ulcerative colitis. The colon is shortened, tubular, lacks haustra, and is narrow.   (Courtesy John A.M. Taylor, Portland, Ore.)

TABLE 28-9
Complications of Ulcerative Colitis

Complications	Comments
Colorectal cancer	Occurs in approximately 3% of patients[14]
Complications involving bone	Nondeforming migratory polyarthritis of large joints, sacroiliitis and ankylosing spondylitis, osteonecrosis in patients receiving steroids[14]
Hepatobiliary abnormalities	Fatty liver; hepatitis; cirrhosis; ascending cholangitis; portal hypertension[14]
Gallbladder abnormalities	Increased incidence of cholelithiasis, sclerosing cholangitis[14]
Toxic dilatation	Diameter of transverse colon exceeding 6.5 cm[14]

References

1. Aronson MR, Szucs RA, Turner MA: Gastrointestinal tract abnormalities related to diaphragmatic disorders, *Postgrad Radiol* 16:3, 1996.
2. Ashur H et al: Calcified gallbladder, *Arch Surg* 113:594, 1978.
3. Aucott JN et al: Management of gallstones in diabetic patients, *Arch Intern Med* 153:1053, 1993.
4. Brooks MJ, Maxson CJ, Rubin W: The infectious etiology of peptic ulcer disease: diagnosis and implications for therapy, *Prim Care* 23:443, 1996.
5. Cohen SM, Kurtz AB: Biliary sonography, *Radiol Clin North Am* 29:1171, 1991.
6. Dodds WJ: Esophagus and esophagogastric region including diaphragm. In Margulis AR and Burhenne HJ, editors: *Alimentary tract radiology,* St Louis, 1989, Mosby.
7. Gelfand DW et al: Oral cholecystography vs gallbladder sonography: a prospective, blinded reappraisal, *AJR* 151:69, 1988.
8. Gerson DE, Lewicki AM: Intrathoracic stomach: when does it obstruct?, *Radiology* 171:385, 1989.
9. Glick SN: Duodenal ulcer, *Radiol Clin North Am,* 32:1259, 1994.
10. Homer MJ, Danford RO: Acute diverticulitis in the young adult, *Radiology* 125:623, 1977.
11. Johnston DE, Kaplan MM: Pathogenesis and treatment of gallstones, *N Engl J Med* 328:412, 1993.
12. Jones B, Braver JM: Ulcer disease. In *Essentials of gastrointestinal radiology,* Philadelphia, 1982, WB Saunders.
13. Kirsner JB: Inflammatory bowel disease part I: nature and pathogenesis, *Disease-a-Month,* 37:605, 1991.
14. Kirsner JB: Inflammatory bowel disease part II: clinical and therapeutic aspects, *Disease-a-Month,* 37:669, 1991.
15. Laing FC: Ultrasound diagnosis of choledocholithiasis, *Semin Ultrasound CT MR* 8:103, 1987.
16. Levine MS et al: Atypical hyperplastic polyps at double-contrast barium enema examination, *Radiology* 175:691, 1990.
17. Liddle RA, Goldstein RB, Saxton J: Gallstone formation during weight-reduction dieting, *Arch Intern Med* 149:1750, 1989.
18. Mandel JS et al: Reducing mortality from colorectal cancer by screening for fecal occult blood, *New Engl J Med* 328:1365, 1993.
19. Milner LR: Cancer of the gallbladder: its relationship to gallstones, *Am J Gastroenterol* 39:480, 1963.
20. Minagi H, Margolia FR: Pancreatic calcifications, *Am J Gastroenterol* 57:139, 1972.
21. Norman DC, Yoshikawa TT: Intra-abdominal infections: diagnosis and treatment in the elderly patient, *Gerontology* 30:327, 1984.
22. Ott DJ: The esophagus: diaphragmatic hernias. In Traveras JM and Ferrucci JT, editors: *Radiology diagnosis-imaging-intervention,* vol 4, Philadelphia, 1996, Lippincott-Raven.
23. Painter NS: Diverticular disease of the colon: a disease of Western civilization, *Br Med J* 2:450, 1971.
24. Ranshohoff DF, Gracie WA: Treatment of gallstones, *Ann Intern Med* 119:606, 1993.
25. Raptopoulos V et al: Comparison of real-time and gray scale static ultrasonic cholecystography, *Radiology* 140:153, 1981.
26. Realini JP: Screening for colorectal cancer: issues for primary care physicians, *Prim Care* 15:63, 1988.
27. Ring EJ, Ferrucci JT, Short WF: Differential diagnosis of pancreatic calcification, *Am J Roentgenol* 117:446, 1973.
28. Sarles H, Sahel J: Pathology of chronic calcifying pancreatitis, *Am J Gastroenterol* 66:117, 1976.
29. Skucas J, Gasparaitis AE: Colon cancer. In Traveras JM and Ferrucci JT, editors: *Radiology diagnosis-imaging-intervention,* vol 4, Philadelphia, 1996, Lippincott-Raven.
30. Stevenson GW: Gastric ulcers. In Traveras JM and Ferrucci JT, editors: *Radiology diagnosis-imaging-intervention,* vol 4, Philadelphia, 1996, Lippincott-Raven.
31. Reference deleted in proofs.
32. Tait N, Little JM: The treatment of gallstones, *BMJ* 311:99, 1995.
33. Thoeni RFL, Bischof TP: Colonic polpys. In Traveras JM and Ferrucci JT, editors: *Radiology diagnosis-imaging-intervention,* vol 4, Philadelphia, 1996, Lippincott-Raven.
34. Thoeni RFL, Menuck L: Comparison of barium enema and colonoscopy in the detection of small colonic polyps, *Radiology* 124:631, 1977.
35. Tierney, Jr LM, McPhee SJ, Papadakis MA, editors: The alimentary tract. In *Current medical diagnosis and treatment 1997,* ed 36, Stanford, 1997, Appleton and Lange.
36. Toribara NW, Sleisenger MH: Screening for colorectal cancer, *New Engl J Med* 332:861, 1995.
37. Williams I, Fleischchner FG: Diverticular disease of the colon. In Margulis AR and Burhenne HJ, editors: *Alimentary tract roentgenology,* ed 2, St Louis, 1973, Mosby.
38. Wilson JM: Diverticular disease of the colon, *Prim Care* 15:111, 1988.
39. Wingo PA, Tong T, Bolden S: Cancer statistics 1995, *CA Cancer J Clin* 45:8, 1995.
40. Wolf BS: Observations of roentgen features of benign and malignant gastric ulcers, *Semin Roentgenol* 6:140, 1971.
41. Zboralske FF, Stargardter FL, Harell GS: Profile roentgenographic features of benign greater curvature ulcers, *Radiology* 127:63, 1978.

chapter 29

Miscellaneous Abdomen Diseases

BEVERLY L HARGER

LISA E HOFFMAN

RICHARD ARKLESS

Abdominal Aortic Aneurysm

Hydatid Disease

Abdominal Aortic Aneurysm

BACKGROUND

Abdominal aortic aneurysm (AAA) affects approximately 3% to 6% of the population. Incidence increases rapidly in men after age 55 and in women after age 70. Overall incidence and deaths resulting from AAA are more common in men.[4,5] The underlying cause of AAA is multifactorial, including such factors as smoking, hypertension, and processes affecting the integrity of the vessel wall collagen and elastin.

An individual's risk is increased 12-fold if a first-degree relative has an abdominal aortic aneurysm.[4] Although impossible to predict for a given individual, the risk of AAA rupture increases with larger initial aneurysm diameter, hypertension, and chronic obstructive pulmonary disease (COPD). Rupture of AAA is considered essentially inevitable if the patient lives long enough.[5]

IMAGING FINDINGS

Ultrasonography (US) reaches almost 100% accuracy in detecting abdominal aortic aneurysm, making it ideal for screening, diagnosis, and follow-up studies in suspected cases.[2] Obesity and excessive bowel gas may interfere with US imaging.[5] Approximately 50% of AAAs may be seen as cystic structures on plain film radiography resulting from the calcium content of atherosclerotic plaques (Figs. 29-1 and 29-2).[5]

Computed tomography (CT) provides better anatomical detail, especially regarding the aneurysm's relationship to the renal arteries (Fig. 29-3). Magnetic resonance imaging (MRI) demonstrates excellent anatomical detail and sizing of aneurysm but provides no distinct advantage and is more expensive than CT. Aortography, although not appropriate for diagnosis, is often ordered for surgical planning.[5] It may significantly underestimate the width of the aneurysm, however, because large areas of thrombus can fill an aneurysm and aortography will show only the residual central canal (which can resemble a normal-size aorta).

For the majority of patients, diagnosis is made by ultrasound, and preoperative planning is based on aortography. Ultrasound, which is faster and less expensive than other methods, and CT are ways to follow up nonsurgical cases. These are those cases in which the diameter is less than 5 cm (some surgeons feel this is too large a dividing point, however).[5]

CLINICAL COMMENTS

Most abdominal aortic aneurysms are asymptomatic and are discovered on routine physical examination or via imaging for other complaints.[6] A pulsatile abdominal mass may be palpated. Leakage, rapid expansion, or rupture may produce mild to severe flank, back, or abdominal pain. Hypovolemic shock may follow rupture.

The death rate increases 12-fold in patients experiencing rupture versus patients undergoing elective surgery. Surgical repair is recommended for all symptomatic or ruptured AAAs, and for asymptomatic AAAs measuring over 5 cm, unless strong contraindications to surgery are identified.[2] Surgery is not commonly recommended for AAAs measuring less than 4 cm.[2] Those measuring 4 cm to 5 cm represent a gray area, in which case the risk of surgery is weighed against the risk of rupture.[2,4] All saccular AAAs should be treated because of an increased risk of rupture. Screening programs may be useful in patients 55 to 80 years old, and patients with hypertension, aneurysms of the popliteal or femoral arteries, or a family history of AAAs.[5]

KEY CONCEPTS

- The incidence of AAAs increases in men after age 55 and women after age 70.
- Risk is increased in patients with a first-degree relative who has AAA, patients with a history of smoking, patients with hypertension, and patients with a connective tissue disease.
- Most patients are asymptomatic.
- Fifty percent of AAAs can be seen on plain film.

Hydatid Disease

BACKGROUND

Hydatid cysts represent infestation by the *Echinococcus granulosus* or *Echinococcus multilocularis* (tapeworm) parasite. Sheep, cattle, hogs, and deer are the common intermediate hosts for *E. granulosus;* dogs often play an important role in transmitting this parasite to humans. Rodents are the primary intermediate host for *E. multilocularis.*[1,3] Hydatid cysts are slow growing and may affect the liver, lungs, muscle, bone, kidney, and brain. Echinococcus infestation is most common in ranching areas of Australia, South America, and Mediterranean countries. In North America, the disease is

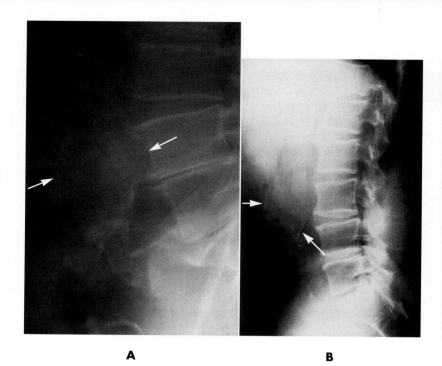

A   **B**

FIG. 29-1 Abdominal aortic aneurysm in two different patients. **A,** Lateral view demonstrates a calcified wall of a fusiform abdominal aorta *(arrows)*. Plain film visualization is possible because of the calcium content of atherosclerotic plaques. **B,** Lateral view shows an abdominal aortic aneurysm *(arrows)*. Most abdominal aortic aneurysms occur between the renal artery and iliac bifurcation.

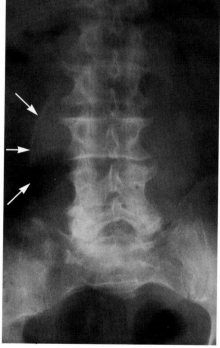

FIG. 29-2 Abdominal aortic aneurysm in AP projection. Note the characteristic thin rim of curvilinear calcification *(arrows)*. The location to the right of the spine indicates an extremely large aneurysm. (Courtesy Cynthia Peterson, Bournemouth, England.)

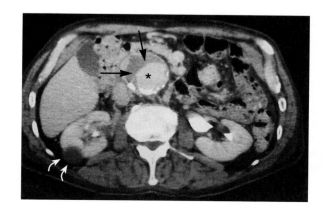

FIG. 29-3 Abdominal aortic aneurysm: computed tomography with intravenous contrast. This scan shows a large, partially calcified abdominal aortic aneurysm anterior to the spine. Within the aneurysm is a region of increased density *(asterisk)* that corresponds to the functional lumen of the aneurysm; the remaining low-attenuated region represents a large thrombus *(arrows)*. Note the renal cyst *(curved arrows)*.

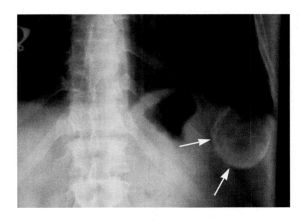

FIG. 29-4   Hydatid cyst. Plain film demonstrates a cystic calcific abdominal mass in the left upper quadrant *(arrows).* This was proven to be a hydatid cyst of the spleen.

rare but occasionally is seen in sheepherders of Basque descent in California and Idaho and sheep ranchers of Utah, New Mexico, and Arizona. It is more often seen in immigrants who bring the disease with them. Cases in Alaska have been linked to caribou.[3]

IMAGING FINDINGS

Hydatid cysts may be seen involving the liver, peritoneum, kidney, spleen, or bladder on abdominal imaging. The liver is more commonly involved, with multiple cysts occurring in about 20% of cases.[3] These cysts average 5 cm in diameter but may grow to 50 cm. Cystic calcification may be seen on plain film (Fig. 29-4). Computed tomography shows well-defined, round masses with or without internal septations. The cyst wall and septations are visible with contrast. Ultrasound most commonly demonstrates a complex heterogeneous mass. Well-defined anechoic cysts are another common presentation. Identification of "daughter cysts" within a cyst is pathognomonic but rare.[7]

CLINICAL COMMENTS

Most hydatid cysts are asymptomatic when discovered. Symptoms are produced most commonly by mass effect or are a result of leakage or rupture of the cyst. Eosinophilia may result from allergic reaction to slow leaks. Anaphylaxis and death can result from acute rupture.[1,3] The only treatment is surgical excision, which is recommended for liver cysts over 5 cm and all pulmonary cysts. Cysts located in nonvital areas may be monitored.[1,3] Aspiration is contraindicated because of the potentially life-threatening allergic reaction to leakage.[3]

KEY CONCEPTS

- *Sheep, cows, and pigs are intermediate hosts with dogs providing a route to humans.*
- *Most cysts are asymptomatic; mass effect, leakage, or rupture produces symptoms.*
- *Cystic calcification may be seen.*
- *Aspiration is contraindicated because of potential anaphylactic response to rupture.*

References

1. Altamura RF: Children, pets, and disease, *J Am Osteopath Assoc* 81:334, 1982.
2. Desforges JF: Abdominal aortic aneurysm, *New Engl J Med* 328:1167, 1993.
3. Elliot DL et al: Pet-associated illness, *New Engl J Med* 313:985, 1985.
4. Fine LG: Abdominal aortic aneurysm: grand round, *Lancet* 341:215, 1993.
5. Rose III WW, Ernst CB: Abdominal aortic aneurysm, *Compr Ther* 21:339, 1995.
6. Tierney LM, Messina LM: Blood vessels and lymphatics. In Tierney LM, McPhee SJ, Papdakis MA, editors: *Current medical diagnosis and treatment,* ed 36, Stanford, Conn, 1997, Appleton and Lange.
7. Tierney LM, Messina LM: Infectious diseases: protozoal & helminthic. In Tierney LM, McPhee SJ, Papdakis MA, editors: *Current medical diagnosis and treatment,* ed 36, Stanford, Conn, 1997, Appleton and Lange.

PART FOUR
Abdomen

PART FIVE

Brain and Spinal Cord

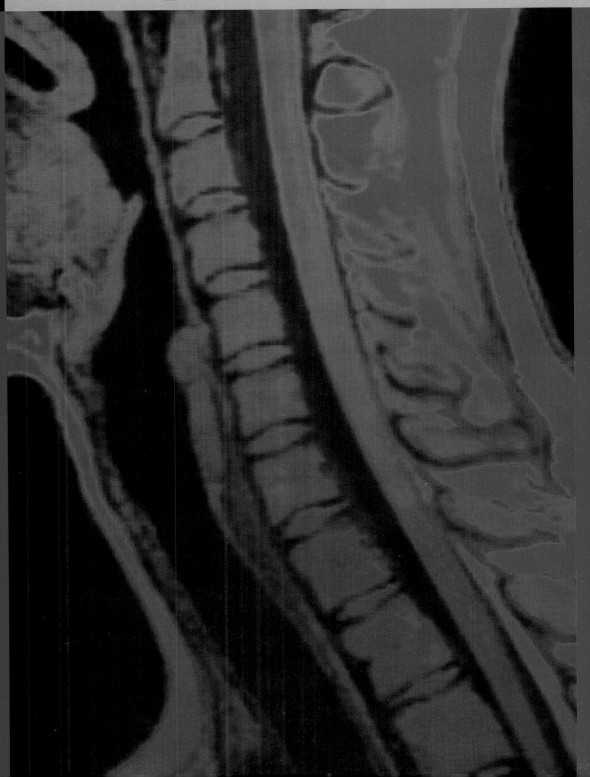

chapter 30

Brain and Spinal Cord

RAJIV SHAH
RUTH G RAMSEY

Trauma
Vascular Disorders

Infections and Inflammatory Processes of the
Central Nervous System
Tumors

Selected Tumors
Miscellaneous Selected Conditions

Trauma

BACKGROUND

Trauma is the leading cause of morbidity and mortality in people under the age of 30 years in the United States. This section briefly outlines the clinical approach, application of diagnostic imaging, and description of various injuries in the evaluation of the trauma patient. A full discussion of the topic is beyond the scope of this text; the list of suggested readings at the end of this chapter includes sources of additional information.

CLINICAL COMMENTS

The assessment of critically injured patients begins at the site of injury by trained paramedics. Initial quick assessment of airway, breathing, and circulation is made followed by protection of the neck for possible cervical spine injury. Most critically injured patients are brought to specially equipped and staffed trauma centers at major hospitals designated as level I trauma centers.

In regard to brain and spine injury, a quick neurological assessment is made with respect to appropriate level of consciousness and evaluation of any motor or sensory deficit. This is accomplished by patient scoring using the Glasgow coma scale. Essentially, this scale provides an index of the injury sustained to the brain.

IMAGING FINDINGS

Spinal trauma. Plain films of the spine are initially obtained in patients with suspected spine trauma. For cervical spine trauma, the following views should be obtained: AP, lateral, open-mouth, and obliques. If all seven cervical bodies are not visualized, a swimmer view with slight overexposure is obtained to visualized the lower cervical spine. If this is still unsuccessful because of technical or patient-related factors, a computed tomography (CT) scan is suggested.

It is imperative that all seven cervical bodies as well as their alignment be examined in suspected spine injury. If abnormality is noted on the initial views of the cervical spine series, this should be confirmed on the other views. If an abnormality is seen only on one view but not seen on other views, further examination with CT should be accomplished. Even in neurologically intact patients, any questionable findings should be further investigated after the collar is removed. It has been repeatedly shown that features may be iden-

tified by CT that are not visible on plain film evaluation. The addition of flexion and extension views assists the evaluation of post-traumatic segmental instability.

In terms of importance of the view, a properly obtained lateral view is most crucial. If all the views are negative and no neurological deficits exist, further study is usually not indicated. However, soft tissue and ligamentous injury cannot be excluded on plain films. Furthermore, if the patient's symptoms warrant further study, magnetic resonance imaging (MRI) of cervical spine is the preferred method for evaluation of soft tissues, ligaments, and disc herniation. Increasingly, trauma centers have MRI machines compatible with life-support equipment, which are capable of handling the patients with acute injuries. CT is not well-suited for evaluation of soft tissue and ligaments; however, in the assessment of bony injury, CT it is the modality of choice. CT is particularly adept at evaluating the spinal canal, the possibility of repulsed fragments, and further delineating the vertebral arch, including the facet joints. Axial CT data can be reformatted, giving excellent lateral, coronal, and oblique views that can further aid in the management of complex fractures. The evaluation of injury to the thoracic and lumbar spine is similar as described above for cervical injury. The difference, of course, is the level of deficit suffered by the patients.

Plain films, CT, and MRI all play a vital role in the management and assessment of spinal injury. For evaluation of the spinal cord, MRI is clearly superior. The entire cord can be well seen with MRI, and abnormalities including cord contusion, transection, and edema are clearly visible on MRI. MRI also provides a clear view of blood products and compromise of the canal and pressure or mass effect on the cord.

Skull trauma. Following clinical evaluation of the injured patient, a decision is made in regard to the urgency of a particular imaging study. For trauma related to the brain and skull, CT is the preferred method of study. This differs from suspected spinal injury, where plain films of the spine provide the initial study. CT is the preferred method in the assessment of brain or skull injury because it has the following characteristics:

1. Readily available. Nearly all hospitals in the United States have CT available.
2. Quick. Modern helical scanners can scan the entire brain in less than 10 seconds. This enables the trauma team to quickly

assess the patient for other possible life-threatening injuries. Motion artifacts resulting from respiratory and cardiac movement, which often plague MRI, are almost nonexistent with fast CT scanning.

3. Compatibility. Unlike MRI, life-support devices can be safely brought in the CT room.

4. Evaluation of acute hemorrhage and bony injuries. CT is far superior to MRI in the detection of subarachnoid hemorrhage and acute parenchymal hemorrhage.

5. Evaluation of spinal injury. Acute bony trauma to the spine as well as compromise of the spinal canal by bony fragment is easily imaged on CT scans. However, the evaluation of cord injury and involvement of the adjacent soft tissues is better seen with MRI.

Limitations to the use of CT include the following:

1. Beam-hardening artifact secondary to bone limits the use of CT to image CNS tissue of the posterior fossa, brainstem, and regions close to bone (i.e., frontal and temporal regions).

2. CT provides poor soft tissue contrast in comparison with MRI. Nonhemorrhagic contusions, subtle white matter shear injuries, vascular dissections/occlusions, and spinal cord injuries are clearly better studied with MRI.

3. MRI provides multiplanar capability, direct three-dimensional imaging (i.e., axial, sagittal, and coronal). CT is limited to direct imaging in the axial plane. Images in the sagittal and coronal plane must be reformatted from the axial information, leading to degradation of the image quality.

4. Vascular structures are poorly seen without the use of iodinated contrast agents. Visualization of these structures is often not needed in the acute trauma patient. However, if necessary, analysis for vascular injury will necessitate either magnetic resonance angiography (MRA) or conventional angiography.

SELECTED INJURIES

Acute cortical contusion. A cortical contusion describes a direct injury suffered by the brain. It is usually seen as areas of increased attenuation (density) compared with normal grey matter. This appearance is often best seen near rough, bony ridges in the frontal and temporal lobes. Cortical contusions may appear anywhere in the brain and their importance depends on particular location and associated clinical symptoms. CT is the study of choice for acute hemorrhagic contusion. MRI is better for nonhemorrhage contusion and shear injury involving the white matter.

Acute epidural hematoma. An acute epidural hematoma is typically due to an arterial rupture of the meningeal arteries feeding the dura. These arteries are located in bony grooves of the inner calvarium and are external to the tough, fibrous dura mater constituting the outer envelope of the brain. During high-impact injury to the skull, bony fracture may rupture and transect the branches of meningeal arteries, resulting in rapid accumulation of blood, which may press on the adjacent brain. The pooled blood usually does not cross suture lines and does not follow the dural foldings.

Epidural hematomas appear as lentiform-shaped areas of increased attenuation near the inner table of the skull (Fig. 30-1). Epidural hematomas, depending on the size and location, are surgical emergencies. CT is the preferred method of study in the detection of hematomas and associated bony fractures of the skull.

Acute subdural hematoma. The subdural space lies between the inner layer of the dura and arachnoid membranes. Cortical veins that drain the brain tissue traverse the subdural space before reaching the major sinuses in the dura mater.

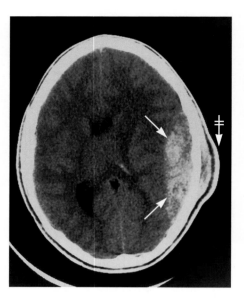

FIG. 30-1 Epidural hematoma. Axial noninfused CT at the level of the thalamus demonstrates a large extraaxial lentiform-shaped area of increased attenuation, displacing the brain and causing mass effect (*arrows*). Note the soft tissue swelling overlying the calvarium (*crossed arrow*). The CT bone window (not shown) revealed a nondisplaced fracture of the temporal bone. This appearance is characteristic of acute epidural hematoma.

Acute subdural hematoma is often the result of venous bleeding. Because venous bleeding is slow, most small subdural hematomas are self-limiting. If they do cause compression of adjacent brain and are not symptomatic, they may be treated conservatively. However, if large they may produce a mass effect on the adjacent brain and lead to death secondary to cerebral edema.

CT is the study of choice for acute hematomas. On CT scans they appear as areas of increased density that follow the outer surface of the brain in the subdural space (Fig. 30-2). Classically they cross suture lines and dural foldings such as the interhemispheric fissures.

Acute subarachnoid hemorrhage. Subarachnoid hemorrhage (SAH) occurs below the inner layer of the arachnoid and above the pia-lined cortical surface (Fig. 30-3). This space is clinically important because it contains the arteries that feed the brain. In the setting of trauma, SAH is usually due to either transgression of blood from the subdural space into the subarachnoid space or occult injury of the small penetrating arteriole.

Most cases of traumatic SAH are not treated unless complication secondary to vasospasm develops. Vasospasm is vessel narrowing that results from the irritant effect of acute blood on the vessel's wall. Vasospasm may lead to brain ischemia. Nontraumatic SAH may occur and is discussed later in this chapter.

Vascular injury. The paired internal carotid and vertebral arteries provide the major blood supply to the brain. Although uncommon, vascular injury involving the extra- and intracranial portions of the carotid and vertebral arteries can lead to serious ischemic injury to the brain parenchyma. Therefore early detection and treatment are vital.

A typical blood vessel is composed of three closely bound layers. The inner (intimal, endothelial) layer is a single-cell layer firmly attached to the thicker, muscular (media) middle layer. The outer (adventitia) layer is largely composed of connective tis-

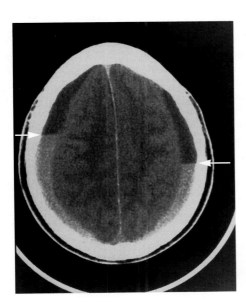

FIG 30-2 Acute subdural hematoma. This 62-year-old patient is on Coumadin and recently fell. Axial noninfused CT demonstrates bilateral extraaxial hematoma with fluid level. Note the high-density portion of the blood, mainly RBCs and protein, layering in the dependent portion with the serum on top *(arrows)*. No fracture nor significant soft tissue swelling occurred. All of these features are suggestive of acute subdural hematoma. Note the shape of this hematoma as opposed to the lentiform-shaped epidural hematoma. Subdural hematomas are usually venous in origin because of the tearing of dural veins and are confined between the arachnoid and outer dura layer. Epidural hematomas, in contrast, are a result of shearing of a branch of the middle meningeal artery associated with skull fracture.

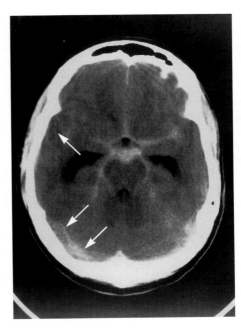

FIG 30-3 Acute subarachnoid hemorrhage (SAH). Axial noninfused head CT in a 41-year-old female with acute onset of headache and nausea. The study demonstrates massive hemorrhage within the subarachnoid space *(arrows)* and acute communicating hydrocephalus. Subsequent conventional angiogram showed a right posterior communicating aneurysm responsible for the hemorrhage. CT is the preferred method of study in the detection of acute SAH.

sue and contains the vasa vasorum (i.e., vessel of vessel). During high-impact trauma to the vessel, the intimal layer may rupture, creating a conduit for high pressure blood to dissect through to the media. Intimal tears initiate arterial dissection. Following arterial dissection, high pressure blood is contained by only the media and minuscule adventitia layers of the vessel. The vessel is weakened and dissecting aneurysms and rupture of the vessel may develop.

Before the advent of MRI, conventional catheter angiography was the preferred study of the evaluation of traumatic injury to the vessel wall. Presently, MRI is well suited for noninvasive study of the extra- and intracranial vessel injury. Dissection is demonstrated by MRI when the true lumen with normal flow "void" is separated from the false lumen by a intimal flap. The false lumen usually contains areas of increased signal secondary to subacute hemorrhage, or slow flow. Alteration of a particular MRI pulse sequence can lead to acquisition of thin axial images of the vessel. Reformatting the images gives an "angiographic" appearance of the vasculature. Therefore MRA can be obtained in a noninvasive matter in the evaluation of major extra- and intracranial vessels.

Traumatic pseudoaneurysms. Traumatic pseudoaneurysms occur as a result of injury to the vessel wall that leads to rupture of the vessel wall. Frank extravasation of blood does not occur immediately, because the thin adventitia overlies a focal bulge. This often occurs at major bifurcation points and within large distal vessels. These types of aneurysms are prone to rupture, and treatment usually involves surgical clipping.

Vascular Disorders

SELECTED CONDITIONS

Stroke

Background. The brain, unlike other organ systems, requires a continuous source of oxygen and vital nutrients such as glucose for its proper function. The brain receives about 5% of the cardiac output throughout the cardiac cycle. The perfusing pressure is well maintained by the unique vasculature of the brain. Any prolonged interruption of the blood supply can lead to irreversible damage to the brain parenchyma with varying neurological outcome, depending on the volume and location of brain involved.

A stroke, like a heart attack, results from an acute occlusion of a cortical or a subcortical vessel. Many causes of stroke exist, but the most common cause is an embolus arising from the heart and carotid artery bifurcation. Other causes include atherosclerosis, vasculitis, coagulopathy disorders, and trauma. Regardless of the cause, the appearance on imaging is stereotypical.

Imaging findings. Clinically, most acute strokes are recognized by altered mental status or focal neurological deficit related to the ischemic brain tissue involved. Initially the imaging study starts with a CT scan performed without contrast. Most strokes are not seen within the first 24 hours on CT scan. The study is performed to rule out hemorrhage related to the stroke or other abnormality that may clinically mimic stroke. This is important to recognize, because the presence of hemorrhage precludes anticoagulation therapy. With evolution of the stroke, follow-up CT scan (after 24 to 48 hours) will show the manifestations of brain injury.

Initially, the findings are related to swelling of the brain as demonstrated by loss of cortical sulci and mass effect. The prognosis of the patients depend on not only the size of the stroke but also location.

A large stroke involving the entire middle cerebral artery distribution may eventually lead to death secondary to extreme mass effect and transtentorial herniation. A small stroke in the pons or anterior limb of the internal capsule may lead to permanent and disabling neurological deficits. Subsequent CT scans (after 72 hours) will show regions of hypodensity affecting both grey and white matter and following vascular territory. Injection of contrast at this time may show enhancement of the affected cortex in a gyriform matter. Chronic stroke will show areas of encephalomalacia with loss of grey and white matter and ex vacuo dilatation of the adjacent ventricle (Fig. 30-4).

Although CT is widely used for cortical strokes, MRI is beginning to play a dominant role in the evaluation and management of stroke. MRI can detect abnormal signals in the region of ischemia after as few as 6 hours (Fig. 30-5). The brainstem and posterior fossa structures are visible without the degrading beam-hardening artifacts seen on the CT scans. The use of MRA is a valuable screening test in the evaluation of major intracranial vessels in the setting of acute strokes. The multiplanar capability of MRI characterizes the vascular territory as well as gives confidence to the vascular etiology of the patient's neurological deficit. The disadvantages of MRI include time involved in the study and problems related to patient motion. In the acute setting of stroke, patients may be critically ill or may not tolerate a lengthy procedure.

In summary both CT and MRI play valuable roles in the diagnosis and management of patients with ischemic insults to the brain tissues.

Nontraumatic subarachnoid hemorrhage. The most common cause of nontraumatic subarachnoid hemorrhage is a ruptured berry aneurysm. An aneurysm is a bulge in the vessel wall

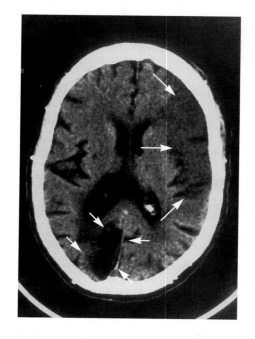

FIG 30-4 Stroke infarct. Axial noninfused study in a 72-year-old patient with acute onset of right hemiparesis. The study demonstrates two infarcts of differing ages. Note the old infarct involving the patient's right occipital cortex (short arrows). Note the density of the lesion (similar to cerebrospinal fluid in the ventricle) and also the lack of mass effect on adjacent sulci and gyri. This appearance with the additional finding of an enlarged appearance of the trigone suggests a chronic process, likely from chronic stroke. Note the subacute stroke in the left suprainsular region (long arrows). Both grey and white matter are involved; it follows a specific vascular distribution (branches of the left middle cerebral arteries), and the adjacent mass effect as seen by effacement of sulci and compression of gyri. Note that the density is unlike the old infarct in that it is more dense than CSF. These findings, in addition to the acute onset of clinical symptoms, favor an acute vascular insult. In this case, the patient had a history of atrial fibrillation with showering of emboli from the heart.

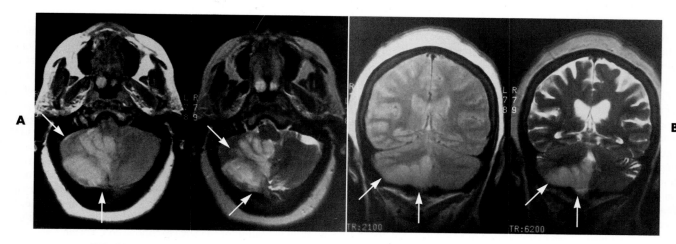

FIG. 30-5 Acute stroke. Axial (**A**) and coronal (**B**) MRIs demonstrating an acute stroke involving the right posterior inferior cerebellar artery. The corresponding CT scan (not shown) demonstrated only subtle mass effect on the fourth ventricle without any structural abnormality. The MRI clearly shows the abnormality (arrows). MRI is extremely sensitive to minute alteration of water content in the brain and is much more sensitive than CT in characterizing early changes in tissue water.

occurring at bifurcation points or at the origin of a branch vessel. Clinically a patient usually complains of having the "worst headache of my life." The clinical status of the patient depends on the quantity of hemorrhage in the subarachnoid space.

The study of choice in the detection of SAH is a noncontrast CT scan (Figs. 30-6 and 30-7). CT is highly sensitive in the detection of SAH. If CT is positive, the patient is taken to the angiographic suite for immediate evaluation of all the intracranial vessels to look for the aneurysms responsible for the bleeding, and in 15% of cases, to look for multiple aneurysms. All the vessels, including both internal carotid and vertebral arteries, are evaluated. Common sites of aneurysms in-clude the anterior communicating artery, posterior communicating artery (Fig. 30-8), basilar artery, and vessels of the posterior fossa.

Early complications of SAH include acute hydrocephalus resulting from interruption of cerebrospinal fluid (CSF) absorption by the arachnoid granulations embedded in the dura. Late complications (usually 24 to 48 hours) include vasospasm, infarcts, and death. Most aneurysms are treated as emergencies because of the high rate of rebleeding and late complications of vasospasm.

Vascular malformation. Vascular malformations of the brain and spinal cord can be divided into four basic types: arterio-venous malformation, cavernous hemangioma, venous angiomas,

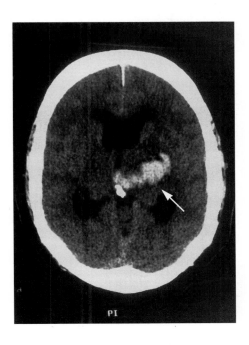

FIG. 30-6 Cerebral hemorrhage. Axial noninfused CT in a 63-year-old hypertensive male. The study demonstrates an irregular area of hemorrhage in the left basal ganglia with rupture into the third ventricle *(arrow)*. The appearance is classic for typical hypertensive bleed. The hemorrhage is theorized to be a result of rupture of lenticulostriate artery secondary to chronic effect of hypertension on small vessels. CT is the preferred method of study for detection of acute hemorrhage within the brain or within the extraaxial spaces of the brain.

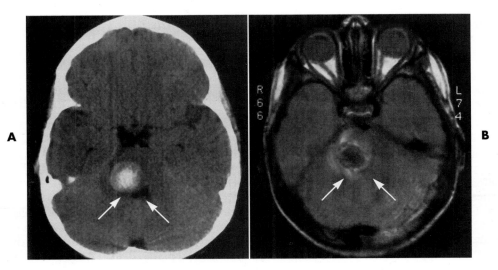

FIG. 30-7 Acute cerebral hemorrhage. Axial noninfused head CT **(A)** and proton density weighted MRI **(B)** in a 9-year-boy who fell off his bicycle. The noninfused head CT shows acute hemorrhage in the right side of pons *(arrows)*. The axial MRI shows acute hemorrhage as dark signal occupying the right side of the pons *(arrows)*. The appearance of blood on MRI is highly variable and depends not only on the age of the hematoma but also on extrinsic parameters such as particular sequences on MRI. In this case the hematoma is dark on MRI because of the deoxyhemoglobin content of the hematoma. As the hematoma ages and resolves so will the MRI appearance. MRI is more sensitive in the detection of blood breakdown products than CT, although in the acute state CT is better as demonstrated in this case.

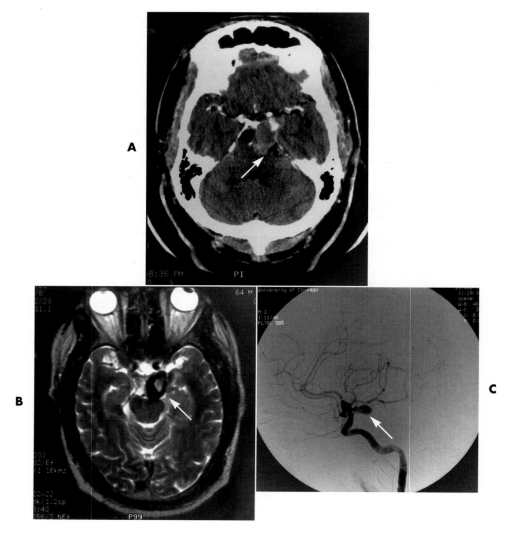

FIG 30-8 Posterior communicating artery aneurysm. Axial infused CT **(A)** and a T2-weighted MRI **(B)** with left internal carotid conventional angiogram **(C)** in another patient. Both patients reveal a left posterior communicating artery aneurysm *(arrows)*. Note the dark area surrounding area of increase signal on the T2-weighted image, which represents chronic hemosiderin-laden thrombus in the wall of the aneurysm. On the CT scan this area does opacify with contrast. In this particular case, the conventional angiogram underestimated the size of the aneurysm; it only fills the patent portion of the aneurysm **(C).** Conventional angiogram remains the gold standard in the diagnosis and treatment of cerebral aneurysms.

and capillary telangiectasia. The former two are more important clinically, because they often present with intracranial hemorrhage. Arteriovenous malformations (AVMs) are abnormal communication between arteries and veins with no normal capillary network between the two. They are easily seen with postinfused study using CT or MRI (Fig. 30-9). However, the gold standard for accurate characterization of arterial supply and venous drainage as well as possible emboli therapy requires conventional catheter angiography.

Imaging studies usually begin with noninfused CT, which may show hemorrhage or demonstrate abnormally dilated vessels on the surface of the brain. Contrast injection results in bright and serpiginous enhancement of the vessel, rendering the diagnosis easily. Cavernous hemangiomas, formerly known as *occult vascular malformations,* are important causes of parenchymal hemorrhage. They

are often found in the brainstem, pons, and posterior fossa. They are abnormal collections of venous sinusoid, which have a high propensity of repeated hemorrhage. Unlike AVM they do not have feeding arteries and draining veins.

Before the advent of MRI, most patients underwent catheter angiogram. Lesions were often "occult," because the angiogram was often negative. However, on MRI cavernous hemangiomas have a characteristic appearance. MRI is the preferred method for their evaluation. On MRI they appear as bright signal intensity, centrally surrounded by darkly stained rings. This appearance is seen on all MRI sequences. The dark rings represent areas of hemosiderin from chronic repeated hemorrhage, and the central bright area represents more subacute hemorrhage. CT scan often shows calcification in this region. Venous angiomas and capillary telangiectasia are other vascular malformations of less importance clinically.

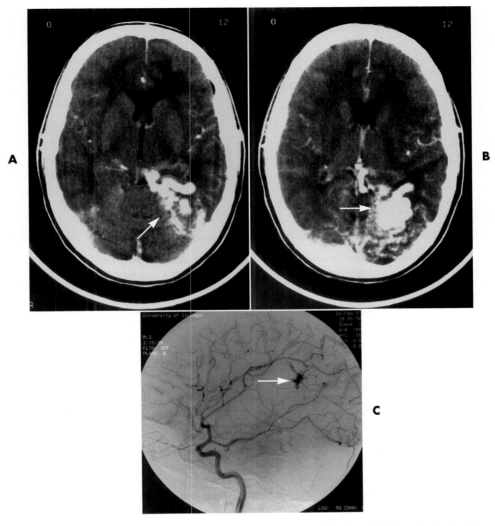

FIG. 30-9 Arteriovenous malformation (AVM). **A** and **B,** Axial infused head CT in a patient with left temporooccipital AVM. The study demonstrates enlarged serpiginous vascular channels highly suggestive of an AVM *(arrows)*. **C,** Angiogram from another patient demonstrates a small AVM fed by the branches of posterior division of the middle cerebral arteries with early draining veins *(arrow)*. The conventional angiogram remains the gold standard in the evaluation and treatment of AVM of the brain and spinal cord.

Infections and Inflammatory Processes of the Central Nervous System

BACKGROUND

Central nervous system infections are uncommon but potentially life-threatening conditions. In the antibiotic era, most are easily treatable and cured without permanent sequelae, but prompt treatment must be instituted.

Bacteria, viruses, protozoa, and other parasites can involve the brain and spine. The most common entry into the nervous system is hematogenous spread. This occurs secondary to pathogens gaining access to the vascular system from a primary source. Common primary sources include pneumonia, limb abscess, heart valve infection, or infections of the abdomen or pelvis. Another mode of entry

is a direct penetrating injury to the brain or spine, usually with concomitant contamination of the injury site.

A common way to evaluate infections of the brain or spine is to compartmentalize the site of infection. Infections can involve the brain parenchyma or any of its coverings. Infections may be confined to only bone, potentiating different imaging and clinical presentations. Infection can spread locally from one compartment to another, which may change the clinical management and patient outcome.

SELECTED CONDITIONS

Abscess

Background. An abscess is a walled-off collection of pus. The formation of a brain abscess gradually evolves from an initial focus of infection within brain tissue. The most common etiology of brain abscess is bacterial infection. Other organisms such as protozoa and

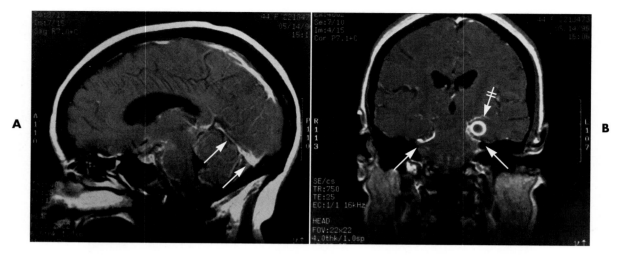

FIG. 30-10 Brain abscess. Sagittal **(A)** and coronal **(B)** postinfused T1-weighted images in patient with tuberculous meningitis and parenchymal abscess. Note the dense and irregular enhancement of the basilar meninges *(arrows),* including the optic and oculomotor nerves. Note also the enhancement of the ependymal surface of the roof of the fourth ventricle. Coronal image shows temporal lobe abscess on the left side *(crossed arrow).*

parasites are less common. Because most infections involving the brain are hematogenous, the initial site of infection is typically the highly vascular grey-white matter interface.

The initial infection incites an intense inflammatory response generated by the host tissue. Increased blood flow creates leakage of fluid and proteins into the interstitial tissue of the brain. This is called *vasogenic edema.* Depending on the immune status of the patient, marked or little vasogenic edema may be present. At this stage the infection is not walled off and it is in what is referred to as *early cerebritis stage.* Imaging at this point may not show the classic appearance of infection. Instead, vasogenic edema confined to the white matter with mass effect may be seen. The overlying grey matter is relatively intact. Injection of contrast does not show any enhancement; however, there may be slowed flow in adjacent vessels and arteries, demonstrating prominent vascular enhancement.

After the cerebritis stage, early capsule formation occurs. As the inflammatory process continues, a thick layer of granulation tissue comprising macrophage, fibroblasts, and collagen attempts to contain the infection and inflammatory responses. It is this layer that shows intense enhancement with contrast on CT and MRI studies. The central area of nonenhancement represents inflammatory exudate.

Imaging findings. A brain abscess proceeds from an early cerebritis stage to later capsule formation. CT and MRI are equally adept at demonstrating the thick rind of enhancement associated with abscess ring. However, MRI is particularly advantageous because it may demonstrate smaller abscesses and multiple abscess and generally provides better views of difficult areas to image with CT, such as the temporal lobe and subfrontal regions (Fig. 30-10).

Clinical comments. The treatment of abscess was previously surgical drainage; however, more and more smaller abscesses are now treated with intravenous antibiotics and follow-up imaging. The follow-up study of abscess can be performed by either MRI or CT with an intravenous contrast agent.

Meningeal infections

Background. Infections of the pia and arachnoid appear similar and are termed *meningitis.* Infection involving the dura of the brain exhibits different clinical and radiographic presentations.

Imaging findings. Imaging plays an important role in the evaluation of meningitis (Fig. 30-11). MRI is the preferred modality in the evaluation of the leptomeninges (arachnoid and pia). The leptomeninges are best evaluated with the use of intravenously injected paramagnetic MRI contrast. Normal leptomeninges enhance to a minimal degree in a somewhat focal and patchy fashion reflective of the blood-brain barrier. Diffuse and thickened meningeal enhancement, especially if it appears nodular, is considered abnormal. It is important to note that any infiltrating event can lead to abnormal enhancement of the pia-arachnoid matter, whether it is because of infection, neoplastic process, or granulomatous process.

In addition to bacteria, viruses can also infect the meninges. Viral infections cause a different clinical and CSF analysis. Granulomatous processes such as TB and sarcoid can also involve the leptomeninges. These process tend to involve the base of the brain and often show dense and thick enhancement of the basilar cisterns. Metastatic diseases from breast, lung, and leukemia can also inflame the leptomeninges.

Clinical comments. Clinically patients with meningitis often experience nonspecific symptoms, including neck pain, headache, nausea, and vomiting. With bacterial involvement, patients may exhibit associated fever and increased white blood cell counts in the peripheral blood smear. Definitive diagnosis is made following lumbar tap and evaluation of the drawn CSF for bacteria, white blood cell, glucose, and protein content.

One of the most feared complications of acute bacterial meningitis is acute cortical stroke. This occurs often secondary to spasm of arteries that travel through severe inflammatory exudate of the subarachnoid space. Vessel spasm may lead to ischemia and/or anoxia of the involved brain supplied by the artery. Other potential complications include acute communicating hydrocephalus and subdural empyema.

Encephalitis. Encephalitis is inflammation of the brain parenchyma. This devastating condition is uncommon but important to recognize clinically and radiologically. Imaging plays a vital role in the diagnosis of encephalitis, although the definitive diagnosis is made by brain biopsy. Presumptive diagnosis can be

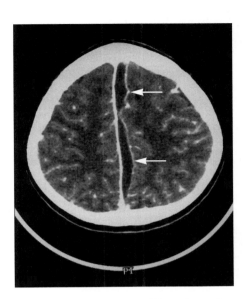

FIG. 30-11 Meningitis. Axial postinfused CT scan in a patient with streptococcus meningitis demonstrated left-sided subdural empyema near the falx cerebri *(arrows)*. This is a well-known complication of bacterial meningitis. Note the extraaxial nature of this collection with dense enhancement of the falx and reactive enhancement along the left cortical surface.

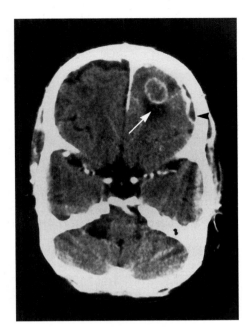

FIG. 30-12 Epidural abscess. Axial postinfused CT scan of a 9-year-old achondroplastic dwarf with frontal sinusitis demonstrates a ring enhancing mass with minimal vasogenic edema in the left frontal lobe *(arrow)* and a small irregular enhancing extraaxial fluid collection *(arrowhead)* near the inner table on the left. This case demonstrates the potential complication of frontal sinusitis, which included brain and epidural abscess. Both were confirmed and drained at surgery.

made clinically and by evaluation of the cerebrospinal fluid. MRI is the preferred imaging modality for revealing areas of increased signal on T2-weighted images.

In the newborn many viruses can cause encephalitis, including herpes, cytomegalovirus, and rubella. The latter two are often introduced through transplacental passage from maternal blood. The former is due to passage through an infected birth canal. In the adult, herpesvirus type 1 is often the most common cause of encephalitis. MRI may suggest the diagnosis in the adult, especially if the classic appearance of temporal lobe involvement is noted. Signal changes on MRI involve both the grey and white matter and may be bilateral.

Because of the potentially devastating outcome, patients are often treated with antiviral drugs before they undergo imaging. Imaging findings may also reveal occult infections not yet uncovered clinically or through laboratory studies. In the newborn either CT or MRI may demonstrate diffuse and extensive global cerebral edema in cases of acute encephalitis. Chronic changes include extensive areas of encephalomalacia and cortical atrophy. Periventricular calcification can also be seen.

Epidural abscess. Epidural abscess is a collection of pus located external to the dura but confined within the skull (Figs. 30-12 and 30-13). It most often occurs as a complication of sinus infection with retrograde thrombophlebitis of diploic veins and seeding of bacteria in the epidural space. If epidural abscess is not recognized and treated early, contiguous involvement of the brain parenchyma or the leptomeninges can occur. The latter, as discussed earlier, can have devastating complications. Both CT and MRI with contrast will show the epidural abscess; however, CT may be superior in regard to any adjacent bony involvement.

Spinal infections. With the advent of MRI, the presence and location of infections of the spinal axis can be established. In-

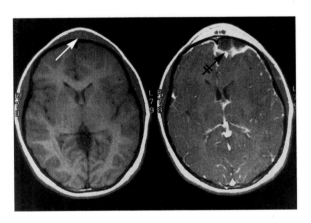

FIG. 30-13 Epidural abscess. Another case of frontal sinusitis and adjacent epidural abscess. Axial pre- and postcontrast T1-weighted MRIs demonstrate soft tissue inflammation in the frontal sinus *(arrow)* and extraaxial fluid collection with dense reactive enhancement of the adjacent dura *(crossed arrow)* typical of epidural abscess.

fections may involve the intervertebral disk, vertebral body, or may extend into the epidural space. Sagittal MRI often shows the inflamed disk as a region of low signal on T1-weighted images compared with the normal adjacent disks. On the T2-weighted images the region appears hyperintense. Diskitis or inflammation of the intervertebral disk shows enhancement on contrast MRI. MRI is superior to CT and plain films in diagnosing diskitis.

Infection of the vertebral bodies or involvement of epidural space is also clearly visible on MRI. Accurate characterization of the extent of involvement as well as assessment of the spinal canal and neural foramina are clearly visible with MRI. CT has a limited role; how-

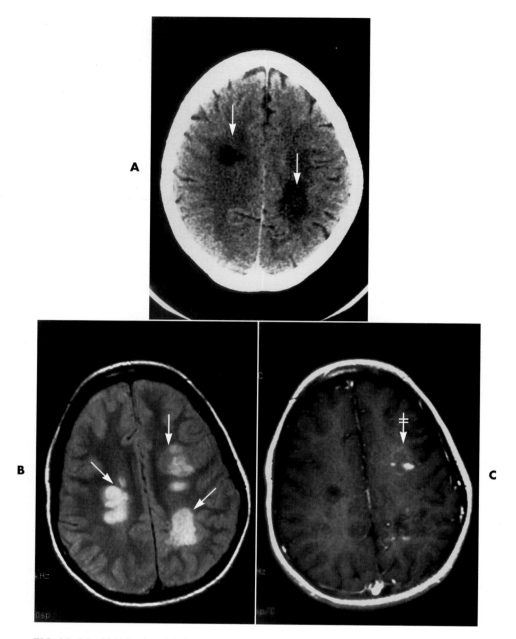

FIG. 30-14 Multiple sclerosis. Axial noninfused CT **(A)**, axial T2-weighted **(B)**, and axial post-gadolinium T1-weighted **(C)** MRI of a 23-year-old female with clinical history of multiple sclerosis. Note the multiple hypodense lesions on CT *(arrows)* in the deep white matter, which are much better characterized on MRI. Note the enhancement of one of the lesions *(crossed arrow)* suggesting an active lesion and breakdown of the blood brain barrier. MRI is a better study than CT in the evaluation of white matter abnormalities.

ever, bony destruction and calcification are better seen on CT than MRI. In addition, CT does play a complementary role to MRI in many situations involving the diagnosis of spinal axis infections.

Noninfectious inflammatory conditions

Multiple sclerosis. Multiple sclerosis is the prototype of autoimmune noninfectious inflammatory conditions of the brain and spinal cord. The etiology is unknown but the condition is defined by a demyelinating process involving the white matter of the brain and spinal cord. MS is a clinical diagnosis and imaging plays a limited, although important supportive role.

MRI is the preferred modality in the evaluation of the white matter of the brain and spinal cord (Fig. 30-14). MS is seen classically as patchy areas of increased signal deep within the white matter ad-

jacent to the lateral ventricles. Presumably this abnormal signal represents areas of gliosis that develop secondary to the demyelinating event. Enhancement is usually not seen unless the lesions are active. Any portion of the brain can be involved. MS has the potential to mimic many other pathological processes, including tumors, infections, and rarely stroke. Involvement of the spine is not uncommon.

Sarcoidosis. Sarcoidosis is a systemic disease with rare involvement of the brain and spinal cord. The disease is characterized by noncaseating granulomatous involvement of the leptomeninges or the brain and spinal cord. Classically it involves the basilar meninges in the region of the suprasellar, interpeduncular, and pontine cistern. MRI with contrast is the preferred modality in the evaluation of sarcoid in the brain.

Tumors

BACKGROUND

The following section introduces the imaging findings of patients with tumors of the central nervous system. A very brief description of tumors and their differential diagnosis is presented.

Understanding the radiological approach relies upon comprehension of the basic terminology used by the neuroradiologist to describe various tumors of the brain and spinal cord. A common way of narrowing the differential diagnosis is to determine if a tumor is intra- or extraaxial in location. Intraaxial tumors are tumors originating from, or metastasizing to, the brain parenchyma or spinal cord. Extraaxial tumors are located outside the brain parenchyma but inside the bony calvarium or vertebral canal. These tumors may originate from the arachnoid, dura, bone, or metastasize to these tissues from distant origins. They may also represent congenital tumors that develop from inclusion of cellular rests during embryogenesis.

IMAGING FINDINGS

General. Imaging plays an important role in determining if a tumor is intra- or extraaxial in origin. MRI, with its multiplanar capability, depicts the tumor in three planes, which aids in the localization of the lesion. Intraaxial tumors are easy to differentiate from extraaxial tumors based on morphology, mass effect on the adjacent brain, and pattern of enhancement. Adjacent bony changes and the effects on adjacent CSF pathways are additional clues in determining the location of the tumor.

Extraaxial lesions will displace the grey-white matter interface and produce buckling of the white matter toward the deeply located ventricles. The interface between enhancing vessels on the surface of the cortex and lesion is well seen with extraaxial masses especially on MRI with intravenous contrast agent (i.e., gadolinium). The lack of a blood-brain barrier often makes detection of extraaxial lesions much easier because they are homogenously enhanced following administration of intravenous contrast. Once the location is judged to be intraaxial, the differential diagnosis is narrowed between primary brain tumor versus metastatic diseases. In general, metastatic disease is more common than primary tumors of the brain. No distinctive features exist that allow for differentiating primary from individual metastatic deposits; however, the presence of appropriate clinical history of cancer as well as multiplicity of lesions favor metastatic disease.

MRI or CT. MRI and CT are complementary tools in the evaluation of brain and spinal tumors. Both have advantages and disadvantages. In general MRI is superior to CT in the evaluation of tumors of brain and spine. MRI has direct multiplanar capability, enabling visualization of the tumor in three planes. Multiplanar capabilities not only verify an intra- or extraaxial location but also help to further define the location of the tumor with respect to other anatomy. This capability is not possible with CT. The soft tissue resolution and characterization of MRI are far superior to that of CT.

Because of its inherent capabilities, MRI is able to visualize vascular structures without the use of contrast agent. However, the use of contrast agent in MRI effectively aids in the specificity of diagnosis of various central nervous system tumors and tumorlike conditions. Breakdown of blood products is also much better appreciated on MRI, as described in previous sections of this chapter.

The disadvantage of MRI is in the evaluation of bone and calcification. Certain tumors have a high propensity to calcify: ependymoma, craniopharyngioma, and oligodendrogliomas, for example. The characterization of the calcification associated with a tumor is

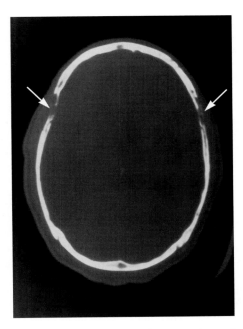

FIG. 30-15   Multiple myeloma. Axial CT scan filmed at bone window in a 61-year-old male with multiple myeloma. This scan shows multiple lytic lesions (*arrows*) located in the frontal bones bilaterally. Generally CT is a better study than MRI in the detection of bony lesions whether due to trauma, tumor, or infection. CT is much better in the evaluation of subtle cortical destruction and calcification. This patient did not have any parenchymal lesions in the brain.

better accomplished by CT. Acute hemorrhage within tumor is also better appreciated on CT. Metastatic tumors are more likely to be hemorrhagic than primary brain tumors. CT is superior in the assessment of bony calvarium (Fig. 30-15). Meningiomas, because of their slow growth, may cause reaction of adjacent inner table of the skull, a feature that is far better appreciated with CT.

Selected Tumors

PRIMARY TUMORS

General

Cell types.   The brain parenchyma consists of neurons and supporting glial tissue. The neurons form seven layers of cells constituting the bulk of the grey matter. The white matter contains a vast network of glial cells and tissue supporting the long axon processes of cortical neurons. These axons form bundles of tracts that cross the midline of the brain; they are the major connecting pathways that link the two cerebral hemispheres as well as the brain with the spinal cord. These include the corpus callosum, anterior and posterior commissure, and various tracts from the brain into the deep nuclei of the basal ganglia, pons, and spinal cord. The predominant glial cell type is called the *astrocytes;* these are the cells from which most primary brain tumors arise. Other glial cells that also can transform into malignant tumors are cells that line the ventricles, primitive cell rests found in the cerebellum, cells of the choroid plexus, and rare tumors of the cortical neurons.

As already stated, most primary tumors of the brain are astrocytic in origin. However, not all astrocytomas behave the same. Astrocytomas are histologically graded (examination of a sample of tumor tissue under the microscope by an experienced pathologist) as low, intermediate, anaplastic, or high-grade (or glioblastoma multiforme). The patient's prognosis is closely related to the grade of the tumor. In general, low-grade tumors are often found in the pediatric population, whereas high-grade tumors occur most commonly in the elderly.

Blood-brain barrier. The normal brain and spinal cord, unlike other organs, have a unique vascular quality called the *blood-brain barrier (BBB).* The BBB prevents large macromolecules such as high-molecular-weight protein from entering the brain tissue. This includes contrast agents used in CT and MRI. The BBB is a unique aspect of the microvasculature of the brain and is not replicated in other systems. The presence of the BBB is important to the neuroradiologist because injected contrast agent normally does not cross the intact blood-brain or blood-spine barrier and remains in the intravascular compartment.

Tumors, on the other hand, whether primary or metastatic, usually do not possess the normal blood-brain capillaries. Therefore, the injection of a contrast agent will often enhance tumors as compared with normal adjacent brain. This aids in the detection and characterization of various tumors of the brain. The breakdown of blood-brain barrier is not limited to tumors but can occur in a variety of pathologies, including infection and inflammatory, demyelinating, and traumatic conditions involving the brain and spine.

Differential diagnosis. After determining the intraaxial location of the tumor, it is useful to localize the tumor to a particular location within the brain. Certain tumors arise from or within the ventricles of the brain. Some have locations so unique that a confident diagnosis can be prospectively accomplished. The patient's age also aids in narrowing the differential list of diagnoses. In general, pediatric brain tumors are biologically not as aggressive as those in the adult population. Also certain tumors are almost invariably found in the young population (i.e., pilocystic astrocytoma).

Once it has been confidently determined that the tumor is intraaxial and the location and age have been taken into consideration, further characterization of the tumor can proceed. The presence of calcification, hemorrhage, and enhancement pattern aid in narrowing the differential diagnosis. Calcification is present in high proportions in certain tumors, whereas other tumors lack internal calcification. Some tumors are prone to hemorrhage. The pattern of enhancement can sometimes help in the differential diagnosis.

Astrocytoma. The most common primary tumor of the brain is an astrocytoma. Most low-grade astrocytomas are found in the pediatric population. An example is the pilocytic astrocytoma, often found in the posterior fossa among children. This tumor is a relatively benign tumor with a classic appearance of a cyst; it demonstrates a characteristic mural nodule. The mural nodule is defined by a vividly enhancing portion of the tumor following the administration of intravenous contrast.

High-grade astrocytomas are found predominantly in adults. High-grade tumors are marked by their infiltration into adjacent brain parenchyma. Surgery with radiation treatment prolongs survival, but the life span is usually less than 5 years. High-grade tumors contain areas of hemorrhage and necrosis that can be appreciated on imaging. Hemorrhage on MRI will be of high or low signal intensity, depending on the chronicity and local tissue environment. Necrosis is often seen after injection of contrast as areas of nonenhancement surrounded by tumor enhancement. Calcifications are usually not found in high-grade tumors of astrocytic origin but are often seen in low-grade tumors such as oligodendrogliomas.

Ependymoma. This is a relatively uncommon tumor found in the posterior fossa of children arising from the ependymal surface of the fourth ventricle. This tumor often exhibits calcification and appears heterogenous on both CT and MRI. Ependymomas are often infiltrative tumors that can grow via normal foramina in the fourth ventricle (i.e., foramen of Luschka and Magendie) into the cisternal subarachnoid space, metastasize to the subarachnoid space, and invade other parts of the brain and spine.

Hemangioblastoma. This is the most common primary tumor of the posterior fossa in the adult. It represents a benign tumor of endothelial origin and often occurs in patients with von Hippel-Lindau disease. Classically this tumor is described as having a hypervascular core of neoplastic vessels associated with tumoral cysts that do not enhance. The nidus often vividly enhances with contrast and abuts the pial surface of the cerebellum (Fig. 30-16).

Medulloblastoma. This tumor occurs in the posterior fossa of children and young adults. It arises from primitive cell rests located in the floor of the fourth ventricle and adjacent cerebellum (Fig. 30-17). Medulloblastomas have a high propensity to invade the subarachnoid space and have high rates of recurrence. If completely removed, and with adjunctive chemotherapy and radiation therapy, long-term survival is approximately 70%.

This tumor often appears hyperdense on noninfused CT scans and enhances following the administration of an intravenous contrast agent. MRI with gadolinium is most accurate to characterize the tumor and look for subarachnoid spread. Drop metastasis into the spinal column is not uncommon, and often develops after treatment of primary tumor. MRI is the preferred imaging study for detecting spinal leptomeningeal metastasis, with CSF analysis remaining the gold standard to confirm the diagnosis.

Meningioma. Tumors originating from the meninges of the brain are histologically and radiologically different tumors than those that arise within the parenchyma of the brain. The most common tumors arising from the covering of the brain are meningiomas. Meningiomas arise from rests of arachnoid cells in the dura mater. As described previously, the dura mater is a tough, mesenchymal-derived tissue covering the entire brain. It not only serves as protective barrier but also houses the major sinuses, which drain the venous blood from the brain. In general, meningiomas are histologically benign tumors with slow or indolent growth. Complete resection is often but not always a permanent cure. However, some meningiomas, because of their location may not be amenable to surgical cure and often lead to death of the patient.

Meningiomas are the most common intracranial tumor. They arise from meningothelial cell rests in the dura mater and are usually slow-growing tumors. Histologically they represent a diverse group although on imaging they often appear stereotypical. They are extraaxial tumors that compress the adjacent brain and often are found incidentally on imaging. Symptoms are usually due to their size and resultant compression of adjacent vital brain parenchyma. They may occur in many locations, although more common locations include the parasagittal convexity, sphenoid wing, posterior fossa, and sellar and suprasellar regions.

Because they do not contain a blood-brain barrier, tumors often enhance homogeneously with contrast (Fig. 30-18). They are often difficult to detect on noninfused studies, especially if the lesion is small and does not contain calcification. Large meningiomas can encase adjacent vessels such as the dural sinuses and the internal carotid artery. MRI with gadolinium is superior to CT in characterizing the location of the tumor as well as in assessing adjacent involvement of vessels and brain parenchyma. CT can display adjacent bony reaction and calcification to better advantage than MRI. CT and MRI may be complementary.

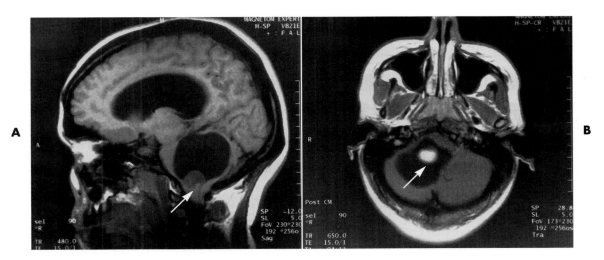

FIG 30-16   Hemangioblastoma. Sagittal precontrast T1-weighted **(A)** and axial postcontrast T1-weighted **(B)** MRIs of a 32-year-old male who demonstrates a large cystic mass with enhancing nodule *(arrows)*. Note the obstructive hydrocephalus resulting from compression of the fourth ventricle. Findings are suggestive of hemangioblastoma, which was confirmed at surgery.

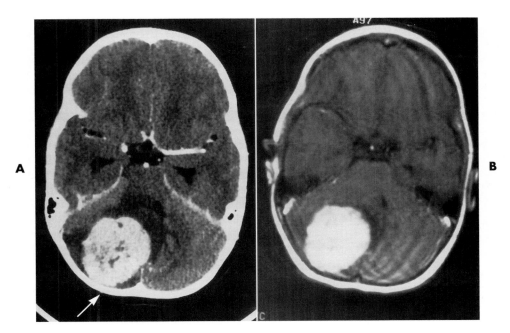

FIG. 30-17   Medulloblastoma. Axial postinfused CT **(A)** and postinfused MRI **(B)** of a 5-year-old boy with history of ataxia and headache. The studies demonstrate a large homogeneously enhancing mass in the right cerebellar hemisphere with compression of the fourth ventricle *(arrow)*. Differential diagnosis include medulloblastoma and ependymoma. Surgery revealed medulloblastoma.

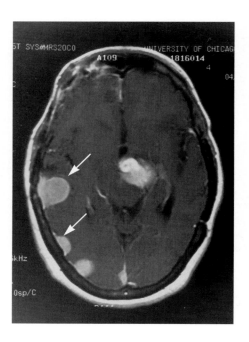

FIG. 30-18 Multiple meningiomas. Axial postinfused T1-weighted MRI of a patient with neurofibromatosis type II, who demonstrates a multiple extraaxial enhancing mass abutting the dural surfaces *(arrows)*. Note the sharp demarcation of the lesions from the adjacent brain. These findings are highly suggestive of multiple meningiomas.

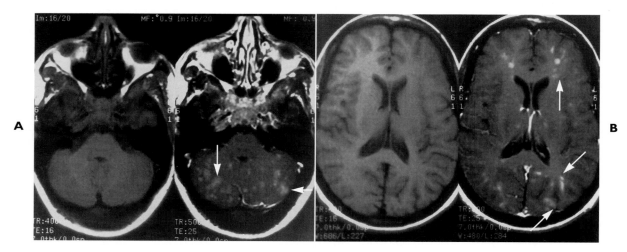

FIG. 30-19 Metastasis. Axial preinfused and postinfused T1-weighted MRI scans at two different levels (**A** and **B**) of a 33-year-old female with breast carcinoma. The studies demonstrate innumerable small enhancing nodules scattered throughout the brain consistent with metastatic disease *(arrows)*. Note how the use of contrast agent is indispensable in detecting small lesions.

SECONDARY TUMORS

Metastasis. The brain is a common site for metastatic disease from distant organs. Although virtually any tumor can metastasize to the brain, those from breast, lung, kidney, and thyroid are common. Others include melanoma, prostate carcinoma, and sarcomas.

No distinguishing features appear on imaging of metastatic tumors, although multiplicity and history of malignancy often favor a diagnosis of metastatic process. Both CT and MRI with contrast are efficacious in detecting metastasis, although MRI can often detect smaller lesions to better advantage (Fig. 30-19).

The appearance of metastatic deposit in the brain is generic. On noninfused MRI or CT scans, areas of vasogenic edema adjacent to the tumor are often seen. The tumor, if not hemorrhagic, is often iso- or hypodense on CT studies. On MRI the tumor may be of iso-, hypo-, or hyperintense signal, depending on its cellularity, calcification, hemorrhage, and cell type. After contrast injection, almost all tumors enhance markedly with areas of nonenhancement that represent areas of necrosis or tumoral cyst formation. Often these areas are multiple and are located near the cortical grey matter-white matter junction. MRI may demonstrate more lesions than CT and may more accurately show invasion of the subarachnoid space.

Metastatic tumor can also involve the arachnoid, dura, and the bony calvarium. Examples include leukemia and lymphoma. Tumor invasion of bony marrow of the calvarium is seen with tumors with lung, breast, multiple myeloma, and leukemia. MRI with gadolinium is superior in the evaluation of leptomeningeal carcinomatosis.

Miscellaneous Selected Conditions

ARNOLD-CHIARI MALFORMATION

Background. The Chiari type I malformation is marked by inferior displacement of the cerebellar tonsils from 3 to 5 mm below the foramen magnum. The inferior displacement is associated with a wedge-shape appearance. Inferior displacement of the cerebellar tonsils of up to 5 mm without a wedged appearance is noted in normal individuals. Chiari type I malformations occur in children and adults and are often (about 50% of cases) associated with hydrosyringomyelia.

Chiari type II malformation represents the most common major malformation of the posterior fossa. It is more common among children. Findings include caudally displaced fourth ventricle and brainstem with herniation of the cerebellar tonsils and vermis through the foramen magnum. It is nearly always associated with obstructive hydrocephalus and lumbar myelomeningocele.

Chiari type III malformations are rare, consisting of osseous defects of the occiput and upper cervical spine with an occipital encephalocele or meningoencephalocele.

Imaging findings. MRI is the preferred imaging modality for evaluating Chiari malformations and associated syringohydromyelia or myelomeningocele. In general MRI is far superior to CT for evaluating the posterior fossa.

Clinical comments. Symptoms vary depending on the severity of the defect. Chiari I malformation is often associated with vague symptoms, which often mimic cervical radiculopathy. Chiari type II and III are much more serious and debilitating conditions, the latter usually leading to death during infancy.

SYRINGOHYDROMYELIA

Background. Syringohydromyelia (or simply syrinx) is a primary (congenital) or secondary (i.e., posttraumatic, postinflammatory, or tumorous), fluid-filled cavitation of the central canal (hydromyelia) or substance of the spinal cord (syringomyelia).

Imaging findings. MRI is the preferred imaging modality of choice and reveals cystic areas of low signal intensity on the T1-weighted scans, which increase on the T2-weighted scans. The spinal cord appears enlarged, and the central canal often reveals a septated appearance (Fig. 30-20).

Clinical comments. Patients experience loss of pain and temperature sensation secondary to involvement of the spinothalamic tracts. Joints may become neurotrophic, particularly the shoulder. Muscle atrophy may develop, most often in the hands.

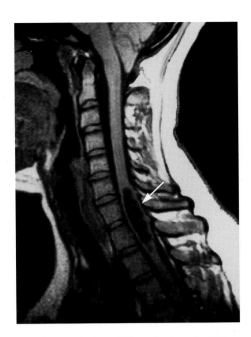

FIG. 30-20 Syringomyelia. Sagittal T1-weighted cervical MRI revealing a focal signal hypointense cavitation of the internal substance of the spinal cord consistent with CSF within a syringomyelia *(arrow)*. (Courtesy Ian D. McLean, Davenport, Iowa.)

Suggested Readings

Grossman RI, Yousem DM: *Neuroradiology: the requisites,* St Louis, 1994, Mosby.

Osborn AG: *Diagnostic neuroradiology: a text atlas,* St Louis, 1993, Mosby.

Osborn AG: *Handbook of neuroradiology: brain and skull,* St Louis, 1996, Mosby.

Ramsey RG: *Neuroradiology,* Philadelphia, 1994, WB Saunders.

Glossary

a-, an- a prefix meaning without or lack of.

ab-, abs- a prefix meaning away, departure, or draw away from (i.e., away from the median axis of the body).

abscess a circumscribed collection of pus that results from acute or chronic localized infection secondary to tissue necrosis.

acanthion the center point at the base of the anterior nasal spine.

accessory supplementary, auxiliary, or additional to some major structure.

acid phosphatase an enzyme that is found in many tissues including the liver, bone marrow, red blood cells, and most notably the prostate gland. It is most useful clinically to diagnose prostatic carcinoma and monitor the effectiveness of treatments for this disease. Levels increase as the carcinoma metastasizes beyond the prostate capsule. Normal levels in the adult patient are between 0.11 and 0.6 U/L.

acute sudden, brief, short-term onset; running a short, often severe course.

ad- a prefix meaning toward (i.e., toward the median axis of the body).

adenocarcinoma any one of a large group of malignant epithelial cell tumors of glands or glandlike tissues.

ALARA principle the use of ionizing radiation in diagnostic imaging should be *a*s *l*ow *a*s *r*easonably *a*chievable.

aliasing artifact an artifact in magnetic resonance images caused by inadequate sampling. It most often occurs when the field of view is smaller than the part being imaged, and protons outside the field of view are excited. The artifact appears to be a portion of the anatomy outside the field of view being folded into the image (e.g., wraparound).

alkaline phosphatase a nearly ubiquitous enzyme found in highest concentrations in the kidneys, liver, intestine, teeth, and bone. Levels are elevated in patients who have liver and bone abnormalities. Normal levels in the adult are between 42 and 128 U/L.

Andersson lesion an irregularly shaped vertebral endplate found in patients who have ankylosing spondylitis who have sustained fractures of ankylosed segments and resultant intersegmental hypermobility.

anemia any condition in which the hemoglobin in 100 ml of blood, number of red blood cells per cubic millimeter of blood, and volume of packed red blood cells per 100 ml of blood are less than normal. Anemia results from blood loss, decreased red blood cell production, or increased red blood cell destruction. Clinical manifestations include pallor of the skin and mucous membranes, shortness of breath, exertional dyspnea, dizziness, palpitations, headaches, soft systolic murmurs, and lethargy.

angiography radiography of the heart, arteries (arteriogram), or veins (venogram) using a radiopaque contrast agent.

ankylosis an abnormal bony or fibrous union across a joint; joint immobility.

anomaly a deviation from average or normal; usually pertains to a structure.

apophysis a nonpathological outgrowth or projection, usually of bone; commonly functions as an attachment site for ligaments and tendons on nonarticular bone surfaces. They do not contribute to bone length.

arachnodactyly a congenital condition characterized by long, slender, spiderlike fingers and, in some cases, toes; characteristic of Marfan syndrome.

Arnold-Chiari malformation congenital inferior displacement of the brain stem and lower cerebellum through the foramen magnum into the cervical vertebral canal. The defect may be associated with spina bifida and meningoceles in the upper cervical spine and lower occiput. The degree of displacement and associated defects are staged together into four types (type I-IV).

arteriosclerosis hardening of the arteries. Three types are generally recognized: atherosclerosis, Mönckeberg's arteriosclerosis, and arteriolosclerosis.

arthritis mutilans a form of advanced, severe, and destructive arthritis marked by osteolysis and pronounced changes of the joints surfaces; usually develops in the hands and feet of patients who have chronic rheumatoid arthritis.

arthrodesis surgical stiffening or fixation of joint.

arthrography radiography in which the introduction of air or contrast medium into a joint is used to enhance visibility of the joint's anatomy.

asterion defect a radiolucent defect of the skull found adjacent to the lambdoidal suture and just posterior to the parietomastoid and occipitomastoid sutures.

atrophy a wasting, or diminution in size, of tissues, organs, or the entire body.

axial (transverse) plane the plane located at right angles to both the sagittal and coronal planes. The axial plane divides a standing patient into upper and lower sections.

Baastrup's (kissing spines) syndrome a syndrome characterized by sclerosis and interspinous pseudoarthrosis caused by approximation of spinous processes; often develops in patients who have excessive lordosis.

Baker's cyst a large collection of synovial fluid in a synovial-lined sac, which extends into the popliteal space between the medial gastrocnemius tendon and the semimembranosus tendon; associated with rheumatoid arthritis.

balanitis xerotica obliterans a chronic skin disease characterized by inflammation of the glans penis and white indurated area around the meatus.

balanorrhagia a condition characterized by inflammation of the glans penis and discharge of a large amount of pus from the penis.

bamboo spine (poker spine) a term used to describe the appearance of syndesmophytes and ankylosis of multiple contiguous vertebrae in patients who have ankylosing spondylitis.

Bankart lesion avulsion of a fragment of cartilage and/or bone from the anterior glenoid rim. Bankart lesions are associated with recurrent anterior shoulder dislocations.

bare area a region of intraarticular bone that is not covered by articular cartilage or a joint capsule; a common nidus for rheumatoid arthritis bone involvement.

bare orbit a region that develops as a result of agenesis or hypoplasia of the posterior wall of the orbit; develops in patients who have neurofibromatosis.

barium (Ba) a chemical element with an atomic weight of 137.327 and atomic number of 56; belongs to the alkaline earth metals. Barium sulfate ($BaSO_4$) is used as a contrast medium in radiography because of its high radiopacity.

barium enema a rectal infusion of barium sulfate; a radiopaque contrast medium used for imaging studies of the gastrointestinal tract.

barium meal ingestion of barium sulfate, a radiopaque contrast medium used for imaging studies of the gastrointestinal tract.

basion the midpoint on anterior margin of the foramen magnum of the occipital bone, opposite the opisthion.

Bence Jones proteins lightweight, unusually thermosoluble immunoglobulins that are made by the plasma cells of patients who have multiple myelomas. They are rapidly filtered from the blood by the kidneys and are therefore best detected in the urine. Normally no Bence Jones proteins are present in urine.

benign mild in character (i.e., a mild illness); nonmalignant (i.e., a nonmalignant tumor).

berry aneurysm a small (usually less than 2 cm in diameter) saccular aneurysm resembling a berry; most often develops at vessel junctions of the circle of Willis. Frequent rupture leads to subarachnoid hemorrhage.

blade-of-grass (candle flame) sign V-shaped radiolucent defect caused by the osteolytic progression of Paget's disease moving through the tibia.

B$_o$ the symbol used to designate the main magnetic field of a magnetic resonance imaging system; expressed in tesla (T).

bolus a round mass, especially one of masticated food; a dose of intravenous medication delivered all at once.

bone window a computed tomographic image at a window level and width that emphasize bone anatomy and make it easy to distinguish between cortical and cancellous bone. Soft tissues appear dark gray.

Boston brace a brace worn over the lower trunk used to decrease lordosis and increase pelvic flexion. The brace is worn by individuals with spondylolisthesis who still want to maintain motion.

boutonnière deformity also called the *buttonhole defect;* proximal interphalangeal joint flexion and concurrent distal interphalangeal joint hyperextension; a result of rupture of the extensor hood at the proximal interphalangeal joint—proximal phalanx head protrudes through the resulting defect.

bowline of Brailsford (inverted Napoleon's hat sign, Gendarme's cap) the inferiorly bowed radiodense line created by the anterior vertebral body of L5 on a- frontal radiographic projection of a patient with spondylolisthesis.

brim sign cortical thickening along the pelvic brim or iliopectineal line secondary to Paget's disease.

brown tumor (osteoclastoma) a mass of fibrous tissue containing hemosiderin-pigmented macrophages and multinucleated giant cells that develop in patients who have hyperparathyroidism and replace bone; appear as small, slightly expansile, radiolucent lesions mimicking a destructive process.

Bucky the moveable housing of the film and grid used in plain film radiography.

buffalo hump an accumulation of fat seen posteriorly above the upper thoracic vertebrae; associated with Cushing's disease or prolonged use of glucosteroids.

Bywater's-Dixon syndesmophyte a nonmarginal, incompletely bridging syndesmophyte that does not appear to attach to either a superior or inferior vertebra; develops in some patients who have Reiter's syndrome or psoriatic arthritis.

cachexia a physical state characterized by weight loss, emaciation, and weakness; caused by malnutrition or the poor health associated with serious illnesses.

café au lait spots light to dark brown cutaneous hyperpigmentations that develop normally or are cutaneous manifestations of neurofibromatosis and fibrous dysplasia.

calcitonin a peptide hormone that is an antagonist to parathormone (PTH); increases calcium and phosphate deposition in bone and lowers serum calcium levels by reversing parathormone effects on bone, the kidneys, and the intestine.

calculus a concretion formed in any part of the body; usually composed of the salts of inorganic or organic acids or of cholesterol; often found in the biliary and urinary tracts.

cancer a general term indicating the presence of a malignant growth or tumor, especially a carcinoma.

canthus angle of the eye; point at which the eyelids meet.

Caplan's syndrome intrapulmonary nodules that develop in coal workers who have pneumoconiosis with rheumatoid arthritis.

carcinoma any one of the various types of malignant tumors originating from epithelial tissue.

cardiac gating a process used to reduce the number of cardiac-cycle–related motion artifacts on magnetic resonance imaging scans. The patient's heart rate is synchronized to the magnetic resonance imaging signal acquisition.

central ray the center of the x-ray beam, which is approximated by the cross marks of the light localizer.

centric pertaining to the center.

Charcot's joint the classic term for a joint with neuropathic joint disease, especially when the disease is caused by tabes dorsalis (tabetic neurosyphilis).

chemical shift artifact an artifact on magnetic resonance imaging scans that is found at fat-water tissue interfaces along the frequency encoding the axis; develops because of the similar Larmor frequencies of fat and water tissues.

Chopart's (transverse tarsal) joint the synovial joint between the talus and navicular bones medially and the calcaneus and navicular bones laterally.

chronic continuing for a prolonged period of time; long-term, protracted course of disease, often of low intensity.

cicatrix scar; contracted fibrous tissue.

Clutton's joint a joint, especially the knee, with bilateral arthrosis secondary to syphilis.

coalition a fibrous or osseous union between two or more bones.

codfish vertebra an exaggerated biconcave endplate deformity associated with advanced osteopenia.

Codman's sign, triangle, angle (periosteal cuff) a subperiosteal extension of a lesion causing subperiosteal new bone growth and elevation of the free margin of the disrupted periosteum at the interface of normal bone and a growing bone tumor.

cold spots (photopenia) a term used in scintigraphy to describe areas of decreased gamma emission caused by a lack of radioisotope absorption.

collimator an apparatus placed on the front of the x-ray tube to limit the field of exposure.

complete blood count (CBC) the number of red and white blood cells per cubic millimeter of blood.

concretion the aggregation or formation of a solid, stony mass by succeeding layers of mineral salts surrounding a foreign body.

coniosis a disease or morbid condition caused by dust.

consolidation a disease process marked by solidification of a normally porous tissue into a firm, dense mass; often applied to lung tissue infections.

contralateral related to the opposite side.

core decompression a surgical procedure used to treat avascular necrosis of the femoral head. A core of bone marrow is removed to reduce intraosseous pressure and facilitate revascularization of the head.

coronal plane the vertical plane located at right angles to the sagittal plane. The coronal plane divides a standing patient into front and back sections.

cotton-wool skull an osteosclerotic skull with fuzzy, poorly defined edges that develop during the osteoblastic phase of Paget's disease.

coxa the hip or hip joint.

craniosynostosis premature skull ossification and suture fusion.

C-reactive protein (CRP) test a nonspecific test that detects acute inflammatory conditions such as bacterial infections or rheumatoid arthritis. The test is sensitive but not specific. It is thought to be more sensitive and responsive than the erythrocyte sedimentation rate (ESR).

crepitus crackling, fine bubbling sound produced by bone or irregular cartilage surfaces rubbing together.

dagger sign the appearance of ossified interspinous and supraspinatus ligaments in the midline of the lumbar radiograph of some patients who have ankylosing spondylitis.

deciduous temporary; that which falls off or is shed.

decubitus lying down.

dextro- a prefix meaning right.

diploë the central layer of cancellous osseous tissue in the space between the inner and outer tables of the skull.

dissecting aneurysm splitting or dissection of an arterial wall by a localized extravasation of blood from the true lumen of the vessel—longitudinal dissection between the outer and middle layers of the vessel creates a second lumen (double barrel lumen); most often occurs in the aorta and often rupture through the outer wall.

distal away from (i.e., away from the body or the origin or beginning of some part of the body).

diverticulitis inflammation of a diverticulum.

diverticulosis the presence of multiple diverticula (abnormal).

diverticulum a blind sac or pouch extending from a main cavity or lumen.

dolicho- a prefix meaning long.

dolichostenomelia long, narrow limbs characteristic of patients who have Marfan syndrome.

dorsal the back (i.e., the back of the body or a structure); opposite of ventral.

dys- a prefix meaning difficult or painful, abnormal or impairment; opposite of eu-.

dysplasia abnormal development of an organ or tissue.

dyspnea difficult or impaired breathing.

dysraphism incomplete closure of a raphe; dorsal fusion defect of the neural tube.

dysuria difficult or painful urination.

eburnation (subchondral sclerosis) increased radiodensity of the subarticular bone; caused by degeneration and increased mechanical forces applied to the bone that make it dense and smooth like ivory.

ec- a prefix meaning out or outside of.

eccentric off center, away from midline; opposite of concentric.

echo time (TE) one-half the time interval between successive 90-degree and 180-degree pulses in a spin-echo magnetic resonance imaging sequence—the primary determinant of differences in contrast of T2-weighted images.

ecto- a prefix meaning outside, external, or without.

-ectomy a suffix meaning surgical removal.

edema abnormal accumulation of fluid in tissues or body spaces.

effusion escape of fluid from vessels into tissues or body spaces.

elephantiasis chronic condition in which the affected body part becomes enlarged and overlying skin thickens, resembling an elephant's hide.

elephantiasis neuromatosa large soft tissue mass that causes the overlying skin to appear undulated; seen in patients who have neurofibromatosis.

em-, en- a prefix meaning in or enclosed by.

emaciation a wasted appearance associated with a chronic disease state.

embolism obstruction of a blood vessel by an embolus.

embolus a detached thrombus, air bubble, fatty fragment, or other obstructive plug that is carried by the bloodstream and lodges in small vessels.

emphysema a lung condition characterized by increased air space size distal to the terminal bronchiole, with destructive changes in the alveolar walls and reduction in the number.

empty vertebra a horizontal radiolucent lumbar vertebra defect seen on frontal radiographic projections; results from a horizontal fracture through both pedicles and transverse processes.

empyema accumulation of pus in a body cavity.

endo- a prefix meaning within.

endoscopy examination of the interior of a canal or hollow viscus with a fiberoptic scope.

enteritis inflammation of the intestines, especially the small intestines.

enthesis the insertion site of tendons and ligaments into bone, specifically the zone in which tendon and ligament fibers blend with the periosteum of bone.

enthesopathy a disease process occurring at the insertion site of tendons and ligaments into bones.

epi-, ep- a prefix meaning on, upon, over, or on the outside of.

epidural hematoma an intracranial hemorrhage that results in a collection of blood outside the dura mater of the brain and spinal cord.

epiphysial plate the cartilage plate between the metaphysis and the epiphysis of an immature bone; the site of lengthening bone growth.

epiphysis the end of a bone; develops from a center of ossification distinct from that of the bone's shaft; develops before mature bone is separated from the shaft by a cartilage plate.

Erlenmeyer flask deformity a splayed deformity caused by failure of metaphyseal modeling.

erythema an abnormal state skin redness associated with inflammation and vasodilatation.

erythrocyte sedimentation rate (ESR) test a nonspecific test for inflammatory, neoplastic, necrotic, or infectious diseases. The test measures the amount (millimeters) of red blood cells that settle in saline in 1 hour. The C-reactive protein test may be helpful if the ESR test results are equivocal.

etiology the science of causation.

eu- a prefix meaning well or normal; opposite dys-.

eventration protrusion of the intestine or omentum from the abdomen.

eventration of the diaphragm elevation of half or part of the diaphragm. The elevated portion is usually atrophic, abnormally thin, or poorly innervated.

evert to turn outward.

ex- a prefix meaning out, out of, or away from; outside of

exostosis a cartilage-capped bony outgrowth from a bone.

extravasation the escape of material from space or compartment into surrounding tissues.

exudate any proteinaceous fluid that has exuded from injured or inflamed tissues or vessels.

fabella a sesamoid bone within the tendon of the lateral head of the gastrocnemius.

facet tropism a condition in which the zygapophyseal joint planes of the spine are oriented asymmetrically; one joint plane is sagittal and the other is coronal.

Faraday shield an electrical conductor such as copper mesh or an aluminum sheet that is used to block out electromagnetic radiation. Most magnetic resonance imaging rooms are surrounded by a Faraday shield to keep extraneous radiowaves from entering the room.

Felty's syndrome rheumatoid arthritis with leukopenia and splenomegaly.

fibroma a benign fibrous neoplasm.

fibroma molluscum multiple, soft, nonpainful, cutaneous nodules; the cutaneous manifestation of neurofibromatosis.

fibrosis the proliferation of fibrous material in any organ or tissue.

field of view the anatomy contained within the area imaged.

fissure a narrow cleft, furrow, or slit.

fistula an abnormal passage leading from one hollow organ to another.

flaccid without firmness or tone.

FLASH *f*ast *l*ow *a*ngle *sh*ot; magnetic resonance imaging gradient echo protocol in which a short repetition and echo time with a flip angle of less than 90 degrees are used. As the flip angle moves toward 0 degrees, the resulting image appears more T2 weighted. The gradient echo protocol is a way to quickly obtain images that appear T2 weighted. Gradient images also show joints well, but their major disadvantage is that they do not show bone marrow well.

flip angle the angle of hydrogen atom deflection resulting from the atoms' equilibrium orientation after an applied radiofrequency pulse.

flocculent the appearance of fluid containing soft flakes or shreds that resemble tufts of cotton or wool.

focal giantism enlargement of the skin and underlying bone; seen in patients who have neurofibromatosis.

focal plane the plane of tissue in maximum focus on a tomogram.

focal plane level the distance from the tabletop to the focal plane.

fossa a pit, cavity, or depression; usually longitudinal in shape.

fovea a pit or cup-shaped depression.

frog-leg projection a frontal projection of the hip in which the femur is flexed and externally rotated.

functional scoliosis a nonstructural lateral curvature that is compensatory or positional.

fusiform aneurysm an elongated, spindle-shaped, progressive dilation of a vessel.

gadolinium (Gd) a rare earth metallic element with an atomic number of 64 and an atomic weight of 157.25. Its paramagnetic properties make it a widely used contrast media in magnetic resonance imaging.

gallium Ga 67 citrate a cyclotron-produced radionuclide (the ^{67}Ga citrate salt) used as a radiotracer to localize tumor and inflammation.

gamma camera a scintigraphic camera that uses gamma emissions emanating from the patient to produce an image.

gangrene tissue necrosis caused by an insufficient blood supply to an organ or a tissue.

Gardner's syndrome a syndrome characterized by a triad comprising multiple osteomas, colonic polyposis, and soft tissue fibromas.

Garré's osteomyelitis a chronic, low-grade form of osteomyelitis that appears densely sclerotic and is associated with proliferative periostitis.

gavage feeding by a stomach tube.

geode a large, subarticular, degenerative cyst.

giant bone island a bone island greater than 1 cm in diameter.

gibbus an acute or sharply angled kyphosis

glioma a malignant tumor in the supporting or connective tissues of the central nervous system.

gradient echo sequence any one of a number of magnetic resonance imaging pulse sequences that lack the 180-degree radiofrequency refocusing pulse used in the more commonly used spin-echo sequence. Examples include fast field echo (FFE), fast imaging with steady state precession (FISP), and gradient recalled acquisition in the steady state (GRASS).

gradient magnetic coils coils used to produce a magnetic field gradient that allows "slicing" of the patient's anatomy into sagittal, coronal or transverse planes. During the examination, these coils switch on and off very rapidly, which produces the characteristic and sometimes quite loud tapping noise associated with the magnetic resonance imaging scan.

gravid pregnant.

grid a plate consisting of a series of lead strips that is placed on the front of the Bucky between the patient and the radiographic film. A grid increases film quality by reducing the scatter radiation that reaches the film.

Guillain-Barré syndrome acute idiopathic peripheral polyneuritis that develops between 1 and 3 weeks after a mild viral infection or an immunization.

gumma a soft, gummy, necrotic mass with surrounding inflammatory and fibrotic zones that develops in patients who have tertiary syphilis.

gyromagnetic ratio a constant for a given nucleus expressed in megahertz/tesla; the ratio of the magnetic moment to the angular momentum of the nucleus.

habitus bodily appearance; form and structure of the body.

hamartoma a malformation that resembles a tumor but is composed of a tissue or a mixture of tissues normally found in its region.

Haygarth's nodes periarticular nodules found at the dorsal aspect of the metacarpophalangeal joints.

hemoptysis expectoration of blood in sputum.

hernia a rupture or protrusion of part of an organ through the tissue in which it is normally contained.

heterogeneous differing in kind or nature; composed of unlike elements.

high signal intensity indicated by bright pixels on an magnetic resonance image. Fat demonstrates a high signal intensity on T1-weighted images, and water demonstrates a high intensity on T2-weighted images.

hilum, hilus a depression on a gland or organ marking the entrance and exit of vessels and nerves to and from the structure; root of an organ or gland.

hitchhiker's thumb a characteristic of diastrophic dwarfism in which the thumb is malpositioned and tilted laterally because of a short first metacarpal.

homogeneous same in kind or nature; composed of like elements.

honeycomb lung the radiological and gross appearance of the lung during end stage diffuse interstitial fibrosus.

hot spots a term used in scintigraphy to designate areas of increased gamma emission caused by increased radioisotope absorption.

Hounsfield number (CT number) the normalized value of a pixel's (picture element's) x-ray attenuation during computed tomography. The attenuation is expressed in Hounsfield units.

Hounsfield unit a normalized scale of x-ray attenuation used in computed tomography were -1000 (air) to $+1000$ or more (bone) and water is 0.

hydrocephalus a condition marked by an excessive amount of cerebrospinal fluid in cerebral ventricles; accompanied by ventricle dilation and brain atrophy.

hydromyelia a pathological accumulation of fluid in the central canal of the spinal cord.

hydronephrosis an accumulation of urine in the kidney pelvis caused by obstructed urine flow.

hydrosyringomyelia a condition in which the patient has coexisting syringomyelia and hydromyelia; the term applied when the location of a fluid accumulation cannot be pinpointed to the central canal or the cord.

hyper- a prefix meaning over, beyond, or excessive; opposite of hypo-.

hyperplasia a nonneoplastic increased number of cells in a tissue or organ.

hypertrichosis excessive hair growth. The localized form often accompanies spinal dysraphism and is known as *faun's tail.*

hypertrophy a nonneoplastic increased body part size caused by increased cell size.

hypo- a prefix meaning under, below, or deficient; opposite of hyper-.

-iasis a suffix meaning diseased state.

iatrogenic caused or induced by treatment; a term typically used to describe unsuccessful results of treatment.

incontinence involuntary discharge of any excretion, particularly urine or feces.

indium-111 (^{111}In) a radionuclide bone marrow and tumor-localizing tracer.

infarct an area of tissue necrosis caused by an obstructed local blood supply.

inferior situated lower or nearer the bottom.

infiltration a term commonly used to describe any shadow on a chest radiograph, especially an ill-defined opacity.

inflammation the vessel and tissue response to injury. The cardinal signs of redness (*rubor*), heat (*calor*), swelling (*tumor*), pain (*dolor*), and loss of function (*functio laesa*) are usually noted.

insufflation the act of blowing air or gas into a body cavity.

intervertebral chondrosis degeneration of the intervertebral disc; usually manifests primarily at the inner regions of the disc and is seen as reduced disc height on the radiograph.

invert to turn inward.

involucrum a sheath of new bone that surrounds a sequestrum.

involuntary independent of will.

ipsilateral on the same side.

-itis a suffix denoting inflammation.

ivory vertebra a densely radiopaque vertebra.

jaundice a morbid condition caused by obstruction of the biliary tract and characterized by a yellow discoloration, particularly of the skin and eyes.

jelling phenomenon articular stiffness caused by periods of inactivity.

joint mouse a small moveable calcific body in or near a joint.

kilovolts peak (kVp) a measurement of peak potential difference between the cathode (filament) and anode voltage. The kilovolts peak determines the penetrability or quality of the x-ray beam.

Kirner's deformity congenital medial curvature of the distal fifth finger.

knife-clasp defect an elongated L5 spinous process with a concurrent cleft defect of the S1 sacral arch.

KUB the abbreviation for kidney, ureter, and bladder; the recumbent frontal radiograph of the abdomen.

Kveim reaction a reaction in which noncaseating granuloma develops after an intradermal injection of an antigen derived from a known sarcoidosis-containing lymph node. The reaction indicates the presence of sarcoidosis.

Kveim test an intradermal test used to confirm the diagnosis of sarcoidosis by a positive Kveim reaction.

kyphoscoliosis lateral and posterior curvature of the spine.

kyphosis sagittal curvature of the spine with posterior convexity.

labrum any lip-shaped structure, especially the cartilaginous structure that outlines the perimeter of the acetabular and glenoid cavities.

lamina a thin, flat plate or layer; lamina of vertebrae is flat section extending between the pedicles and the midline at the base of the spinous process.

laminectomy the excision of the vertebral lamina or posterior region of the vertebral arch.

Larmor equation the basis of magnetic resonance imaging physics, which states that the frequency of spin/precession of the hydrogen nuclei is proportional to the strength of the magnetic field and depends on the gyromagnetic ratio of the atom imaged.

Lanois deformity fibular deviation of the digits with dorsal subluxation at the metatarsal phalangeal joints, sometimes seen in advanced rheumatoid arthritis.

latent not apparent or manifest.

lateral pertaining to the side, opposite of midline; in radiography, a projection taken with the patient facing perpendicular to the central ray.

leptomeningeal cyst a cyst formed by cerebrospinal fluid accumulations in a dural sac extending into a skull fracture.

Lhermitte's sign sudden, transient, shocklike or lighteninglike sensations extending into the extremities and occurring when the head is flexed forward; often seen in patients who have multiple sclerosis, cervical cord neoplasms, radiation myelopathy, trauma, and advanced spondylosis.

licked-candy-stick bone tapered distal bone ends caused by atrophic bone resorption.

limbus bone a small ossicle located at the edge or corner of a vertebra that results from an intravertebral herniation of nuclear material separating the secondary growth center of the vertebral endplate from the primary growth centers of the vertebral body.

lipo- a prefix meaning fat.

lipohemarthrosis the leakage of fat and blood into joint spaces as a result of intraarticular fractures; creates a fat-blood interface (FBI sign) on radiographs taken of limbs in a gravity-dependent position.

Lisfranc's joint a tarsometatarsal joint.

-lith a suffix meaning concretion or calculus.

Lofgren's syndrome an acute onset of sarcoidosis with high fever, arthralgia, lymphadenopathy, and erythema nodosum.

long (tall) vertebra a vertebral body that appears taller than normal vertebrae as a result of altered mechanical stresses; usually found caudal to a gibbus formation.

lordosis sagittal curvature of the spine with anterior convexity.

low signal intensity indicated by dark pixels on a magnetic resonance image. Fat demonstrates a low signal intensity on T2-weighted images, water demonstrates a low signal intensity on T1-weighted images, and cortical bone demonstrates a low signal intensity on all images.

lumbarization a congenital anomaly of the lumbosacral junction in which the first sacral segment develops as a lumbar vertebra, producing a total of six lumbar vertebrae.

Magnavist trade name for gadopentetate dimeglumine, an intravenous magnetic resonance imaging contrast agent that lowers T1 and T2 resulting in decreased signal intensity on T2-weighted images and increased signal intensity on T1-weighted images.

magnetic resonance imaging (MRI) a diagnostic imaging modality based on magnetic nuclei (especially protons), which become aligned in a strong magnetic field, absorb energy from pulsed radiofrequency, and emit radiofrequency signals as the excitation decays. These signals vary according to proton density and the relaxation times of the tissue. A tomographic image that can be three-dimensional is constructed from the signal information.

mal- a prefix meaning ill or bad.

malignant resistant to treatment; tending to cause death; virulent.

mallet deformity a flexion abnormality of the distal interphalangeal joint of a finger or toe.

mallet finger chronic flexion deformity of the distal interphalangeal joint caused by rupture or avulsion of the extensor digitorum common tendon at base of the distal phalanx.

Marjolin's ulcer a squamous cell carcinoma in or around the sinus draining an osteomyelitis.

McCune-Albright syndrome a syndrome characterized by a triad comprising polyostotic fibrous dysplasia, precocious puberty, and skin pigmentations.

medial situated in or pertaining to the midline.

median central position; midline.

median sagittal plane a vertical plane that passes through the center of the body and divides the subject into right and left halves.

mediastinum the space between the pleural sacs of the lungs, sternum, and thoracic spine.

medulla the soft material in the center of a part; marrow of bones.

metaphysis the section of long bone between epiphysis and diaphysis.

metastasis a transfer or seeding of disease from one part of the body to another.

milliampere-seconds (mAs) measurement of filament current over time; determines the number or quantity of x-rays produced in the beam.

Mitchell markers lead markers used in radiography to orient interpreters to the patient's anatomy. By convention the side of the patient closest to the film is usually marked. Either side may be marked for frontal projections.

monoarticular involving one joint.

Morton's disease a disease in which the metatarsal arch is flattened, causing pressure neuropathy of the lateral plantar nerve's digital branches.

Morton's foot (metatarsalgia) pain in the forefoot caused by shortening of the first metatarsal.

myelitis inflammation of spinal cord or bone marrow.

myoma a benign tumor in the muscle tissue.

myxoid (mucoid) degeneration degeneration of connective tissue into a gelatinous or mucoid substance.

myxoma a benign neoplasm of connective tissue found in the subcutaneous tissues, bones, genitourinary tract, and retroperitoneal area.

nasion the midpoint of the frontonasal suture.

negative ulnar variance an offset at the articular surfaces of the ulna and radius because of a short ulna.

nephrolithiasis accumulation of calculi in the kidney.

nephroptosis abnormal dropping or downward movement of the kidney.

nidus the central point, origination, or focus of a disease process, especially an infection.

nonspondylolytic spondylolisthesis forward displacement of one vertebrae over the one immediately below resulting from an etiology other than unilateral or bilateral disruption of the pars interarticularis at the same level; usually caused by degeneration of the posterior vertebral joints.

nuclear magnetic resonance (NMR) the phenomenon of absorption or emission of radiofrequency by atomic nuclei precessing about an axis of a strong external magnetic field at a certain frequency (the Larmor frequency). The frequency can be predicted from a specific atomic constant (the gyromagnetic frequency) and the strength of the external magnetic field.

occult fracture a fracture not detected immediately; may become detected in the future.

Omnipaque trademark name for a water-soluble nonionic myelographic contrast agent that is commonly used; less toxic than fat-soluble agents (e.g., Pantopaque).

opera-glass hand (main en lorgnette) a hand deformity associated with destructive arthritis in which the fingers and wrist are shortened and the overlying skin undulates into transverse folds. The fingers appear telescoped like an opera glass.

opisthion the midpoint of the posterior margin of the occipital bone's foramen magnum.

Oppenheimer's erosions pressure erosions from an enlarged abdominal aortic mass seen as erosive gouge defects occurring along the anterior margin of the middle lumbar vertebrae.

Oppenheimer's ossicle a nonunion of the secondary growth center of the inferior articular process of a vertebra.

Ortolani's test an orthopedic maneuver used to evaluate the hip stability in infants. With the infant supine in a supine position, the knees and hips are flexed 90 degrees and abducted. While abducted, the femur is rotated internally and externally. Asymmetry of movement or a palpatory clicking (Ortolani's sign) constitutes a positive test, suggesting lateral dislocation of the femoral head from the acetabulum.

-osis suffix denoting a state or condition (usually an abnormal one).

osteolysis degeneration and destruction of bone caused by disease.

osteomyelitis inflammation of bone marrow and the medullary portion of bone.

osteopenia a condition in which the bone is subnormally mineralized. The term does not imply causality.

osteophyte a bony outgrowth or bone protuberance at a joint margin caused by degeneration.

osteoporosis circumscripta cranii a localized, geographical resorption of the skull that develops in patients in the osteolytic phase of Paget's disease; most predominately develops in the frontal and occipital areas.

otosclerosis a hereditary condition in which the bony labyrinth of the inner ear is ossified, especially the stapes.

overhanging margin sign an extensive osseous erosion with an overhanging bone margin that develops in patients who have tophaceous gout.

pachy- a prefix meaning thick or dense.

pannus the granulation tissue affecting the joint during chronic inflammation, especially rheumatoid.

paramedian sagittal plane a plane situated near but not at the midline, dividing the subject into right and left sections.

parathyroid hormone (parathormone, PTH) a hormone produced by the parathyroid glands that increases serum calcium by promoting bone, kidney, and intestinal calcium resorption.

parenchyma the essential, specific, or functional cells of a gland or organ.

pars interarticularis the part of the vertebral arch located between the ipsilateral superior and inferior articular processes, especially in the lumbar spine.

patent open; not occluded; exposed.

pauciarticular involvement of a few joints.

pectus carinatum an outward deformity of the middle of the anterior chest wall.

pectus excavatum an inward deformity of the middle of the anterior chest wall.

Pelken's spurs perpendicular bony outgrowths from metaphyseal margins of patients who have scurvy.

Pellegrini-Stieda disease ossification of the upper portion of the medial collateral ligament.

permanent magnets a magnet system in which the magnetic field is created using ferromagnetic material that is permanently magnetized.

pes cavus foot deformity characterized by an excessively high arch with concurrent toe hyperextension.

pes equinus (talipes equinus) foot deformity characterized by extreme foot hyperextension.

pes planus foot deformity characterized by a flattened longitudinal plantar arch.

phakomatosis (phacomatosis) a group of hereditary neuroectodermal disorders characterized by benign, tumorlike nodules (hamartomas) of the skin, bones, eyes, and brain. Four diseases are recognized: tuberous sclerosis, neurofibromatosis, Sturge-Weber syndrome, and von Hippel-Lindau disease.

Phemister's triad the radiographic findings of tuberculous arthritis: progressive loss of joint space, juxtarticular osteoporosis, and peripheral erosive defects of the joint surfaces.

phlebolith a stone formation in a vein; often seen in the lower pelvis on frontal radiographs.

picture frame vertebra a vertebral body with a squared, enlarged appearance because of thickening of its cortical perimeter as a result of Paget's disease.

pilonidal cyst a cyst most often found in the skin of the sacrococcygeal region. Although this type of cyst is not usually clinically significant, a chance of infection arises if the cyst connects to the surface of the skin by a pilonidal fistula.

Pitt's pit a radiolucent bone defect of the femoral neck resulting from mechanical erosion of femoral capsule irregularities.

pixel an abbreviation for *picture element,* which is a two-dimensional representation of a volume element *(voxel)* in the digital display of a computed tomographic (512 × 512 pixels) or magnetic resonance (256 × 256 pixels) image; the tiny squares that make up the image.

pleurisy inflammation of the pleura.

plica a fold.

pneumocephalus air in the cranium, especially air in the subarachnoid space secondary as a result of a fracture with dissection of air from the paranasal sinuses.

pneumoconiosis a condition in which particulate matter is permanently deposited in pulmonary tissues; lung fibrosis caused by dust inhalation.

pneumothorax an accumulation of air or other gas in a pleural cavity.

podagra gout of the great toe.

polyarticular (multiarticular) involving many joints.

polydactyly congenital anomaly characterized by more than five fingers or toes.

polydipsia a prolonged period of excessive thirst; characteristic of diabetes mellitus.

polyp any bump or projection of tissue that projects above or outward from the surface.

popliteal pertaining to the posterior area of the knee.

posterior back surface (i.e., the back surface of the body); opposite of anterior.

precession the wobbling and gyroscopiclike motion of hydrogen protons' magnetic fields in the presence of a static magnetic field.

prespondylolisthesis unilateral or bilateral disruption of the pars interarticularis without forward displacement of the vertebrae.

primary center of ossification the site at which ossification begins, either the shaft of a long bone or the body of an irregularly shaped bone.

primary magnets the assembly constituting the bulk of the magnetic resonance imaging unit and producing the strong main magnetic field, as opposed to the secondary and weaker gradient magnets.

pro- a prefix meaning forward or before.

pronation of hand medial rotation of hand so that it faces downward.

prostate-specific antigen (PSA) a glucoprotein normally found in the prostate that can be detected in all males. Its levels are increased in patients who have prostatic hypertrophy and adenocarcinoma, which often aids in early diagnosis of these diseases.

proximal toward the beginning; the source or origin of a part.

pseudo- a prefix meaning false or illusory.

pseudofracture (Looser's lines, Milkman's syndrome, increment fracture, umbau zonen) an osseous defect that is not a true fracture; often seen in patients who have Paget's disease, rickets, osteomalacia, and fibrous dysplasia

pseudogout acute or subacute arthralgia associated with calcium pyrophosphate dihydrate (CPPD) deposition disease.

pseudohemangioma appearance of diffuse osteopenia mimicking multiple levels of vertebral hemangioma.

pseudospondylolisthesis forward displacement of one vertebrae over the one immediately below as a result of posterior spinal joint degeneration and not a disruption of the pars interarticularis.

ptosis prolapse, or dropping, of an organ or part from its normal position.

purulent consisting of pus.

pyelogram a radiographic projection or series of projections taken of the kidneys and ureters after intravenous injection of radiopaque dye that collects in the urinary system and allows visualization of the urinary tract anatomy.

rachi- a prefix denoting a relationship to the spine.

radiofrequency (RF) coils RF waves excite the nuclear spins. The RF coils serve as both the transmitters and the receivers of the magnetic resonance imaging signal. Manipulation of the radiofrequencies allows for changes in the repetition times and the echo times. Radiofrequency surface coils are placed directly on the anatomical being imaged.

radiolucent offers little resistance to the passage of x-rays used in diagnostic imaging. Radiolucent substances appear black on radiographs.

radiopaque offers resistance to the passage of x-rays used in diagnostic imaging. Radiopaque substances appear white on radiographs.

radiopharmaceutical a radioisotopic particle with an unstable nucleus that undergoes radioactive decay. The consequent emission of gamma radiation is used in radionuclide imaging (i.e., gallium 67); any radioactive pharmaceutical.

Raynaud's phenomenon intermittent attacks of ischemia that are most pronounced in the fingers, toes, nose, and ears; brought on by cold or emotional stimuli and mediated by a dysfunctional sympathetic nervous system. Attacks begin with vasoconstriction and blanching and are followed by cyanosis, vasodilation, and redness.

repetition time (TR) the time interval between successive 90-degree pulses in a spin-echo sequence; represents the primary determinant of T1 relaxation. Longer repetition times reduce T1-dependent image contrast.

resistive electromagnets a system in which the magnetic field originates from current flowing through an electrical conductor, it is not supercooled.

Reynold's phenomenon the development of central vertebral endplate defects secondary to hypoperfusion of vertebral body centrum seen in sickle cell anemia; also know as "H-shaped," "Lincoln log," or "step-down" vertebrae.

rhizomelic pertaining to the root of a limb; the proximal region of the humerus and femur.

rhizotomy surgical resection of spinal nerve root.

Risser's sign used to determine skeletal maturity. The iliac crest apophysis is observed; the apophysis ossifies from lateral to medial along the superior margin of the ilium. The extent of fusion is graded by fourths, from grade I to grade IV. Grade V indicates complete fusion of the iliac apophysis.

Romanus lesion an erosion found at the insertion of the outer anulus fibrosus into the anterior corners of the vertebral bodies; seen in patients who have ankylosing spondylitis.

rotator cuff a structure comprising four muscles that arise from the scapula and insert into the humeral head. From anterior to posterior the muscles are the subscapularis, supraspinatus, infraspinatus, and teres minor. The rotator cuff provides dynamic stability for the glenohumeral joint.

rugger-jersey spine a spine in which uniform condensation occurs subjacent to the vertebral endplates; seen in patients who have hyperparathyroidism.

saber shin deformity anterior bowing of the tibia seen in patients who have Paget's disease and syphilis.

saccular aneurysm a large (usually more than 5 cm in diameter) spherical outpouching of one side of a vessel; usually caused by trauma.

sacralization the transition of the last lumbar vertebra into the first sacral segment, producing a total of four lumbar segments.

salt and pepper skull a skull that has undergone granular deossification and has a resulting finely mottled appearance; seen in patients who have hyperparathyroidism.

Salter-Harris classification a system for classifying growth plate fractures into five classes based on the appearance of the fracture.

sarcomatous transformation the malignant degeneration of benign lesion to a fibrous, osseous, or cartilaginous sarcoma.

sausage digit a single digit experiencing soft tissue swelling, which occurs during the early stages of psoriatic disease.

sausage finger fingers that appear swollen as a result of acromegaly.

Schmorl's node an intravertebral herniation of the nucleus pulposus through the vertebral body endplate into the spongiosa of the vertebra; often seen on radiographs as a focal defect of the vertebral endplate.

scoliosis abnormal lateral curvature of the spine.

Scotty dog the name given to the appearance of the vertebral arch's anatomy on an oblique lumbar radiographic projection. The shape is similar to that of a Scottish terrier (Scotty) dog. The parts of the dog are as follows: pars interarticularis—dog's neck; ipsilateral pedicle—dog's eye; superior articular process—dog's ears; inferior articular process—dog's forelimbs; lamina—dog's body.

sequestrum a necrotic fragment of tissue, especially bone, that is separated from the surrounding normal tissue.

seronegative arthritis arthritis in patients who do not contain the rheumatoid antigen in their serum (i.e., ankylosing spondylitis).

seropositive arthritis arthritis in patients who have the rheumatoid antigen in serum (i.e., rheumatoid arthritis).

serum calcium level the amount of calcium in the blood; used to monitor parathyroid function and calcium metabolism. Normally, total serum calcium levels are between 9 and 10.5 mg/dl. Although not common, increased serum calcium levels may be seen in malignancy resulting from massive osteolysis or a tumor that is producing a substance similar to parathyroid hormone. Decreased levels are associated with conditions such as hypoparathyroidism, renal failure, rickets, and osteomalacia.

serum phosphorus level the amount of phosphorus in the blood; used to indicate parathyroid function and calcium metabolism. Serum phosphorus and calcium levels are inversely related. Normally, serum phosphorus levels are between 3 and 4.5 mg/dl. Increased levels may be a result of renal dysfunction, increased dietary intake, acromegaly, or hypoparathyroidism; decreased levels may be caused by conditions such as hyperparathyroidism, dietary deficiencies, and hypercalcemia.

shepherd's crook deformity a varus deformity of the hip caused by a decreased femoral angle.

shiny corner sign bone sclerosis at the anterior vertebral margins associated with Romanus lesions in patients who have ankylosing spondylitis.

soft tissue window the window level and width in a computed tomographic study that emphasizes soft tissue anatomy. Soft tissues appear light gray, and distinguishing between cortical and medullary bone is difficult.

SPECT *single proton emission computed tomography*; creates cross-sectional radionuclide images.

spicule a small, needle-like fragment.

spin density (proton-weighted, hydrogen-weighted, balanced) image a magnetic resonance image primarily based on the number of hydrogen nuclei within the sampled volume; T1 and T2 contrast is minimized. A spin density image is obtained by utilizing long repetition time (TR) and short echo time (TE) pulse sequences.

spin-echo (SE) sequence the most common magnetic resonance imaging pulse sequence. Lengthening and shortening of pulses (spin) and "listening" (echo) times create either T1-weighted (short), T2-weighted (long), or proton-density–weighted images. Spin-echo sequences use pulse angles of 90 degrees.

spina bifida a congenital malformation of the vertebral arch of one or more levels resulting in a cleft with or without herniation of the cord and meninges.

spina bifida occulta a cleft in the vertebral arch with no associated herniation of the spinal cord or meninges.

spondylitis inflammation of the vertebral joints.

spondylolisthesis forward displacement of one vertebrae over the one immediately below. The term does not specify etiology or amount of displacement.

spondylolysis a condition in which the pars interarticularis is interrupted. Defects may be bilateral or unilateral, and most are caused by stress fractures.

spondylolytic spondylolisthesis forward displacement of one vertebrae over the one immediately below as a result of unilateral or bilateral disruption of the pars interarticularis at the same level.

spondylophyte the osteophyte of a spinal joint.

spondylosis degeneration of a vertebral joint, particularly the intervertebral disc.

spondylosis deformans degeneration of the intervertebral disc; primarily manifests at the outer regions of the disc and presents as osteophytes.

spot projection a tightly collimated projection of specific portion of the anatomy. It is smaller than a routine projection of the same area.

square vertebra a vertebra that has lost its concavity; most characteristic of ankylosing spondylitis.

Srb's anomaly dysplasia of the first rib(s) with synostosis to the second rib.

stroma supportive, connective, non-functional tissue of an organ.

structural scoliosis a fixed lateral curvature that is not compensatory or positional.

subarachnoid hematoma an intracranial collection of blood internal to the arachnoid and external to the pia mater of the brain and spinal cord in the space normally occupied by cerebral spinal fluid.

subdural hematoma an intracranial collection of blood between the dura mater and arachnoid mater of the brain and spinal cord.

Sudeck's atrophy (reflex sympathetic dystrophy) an exaggerated neurovascular-mediated response to trauma or other stimulus resulting in pain, vasomotor instability, and trophic disturbances.

summation effect of rheumatoid arthritis a term referring to the vertical subluxation, atlantoaxial impaction, or cranial settling of the upper cervical spine that develops in patients who have advanced rheumatoid arthritis. When extensive, the effects can be fatal.

super scan a bone scan that reveals skeletal uptake that is so diffuse it may be interpreted as normal because of its lack of obvious radionuclide uptake regions. It is most often seen in patients who have a generalized skeletal metastasis. Less uptake is noted in the bladder because of the marked skeletal uptake.

superconductive magnets a magnet system that has been supercooled by cryogens such as liquid helium or liquid nitrogen.

supination of the hand lateral rotation of hand so that it faces upward.

swan-neck deformity flexion of the distal interphalangeal joint with concurrent extension of the proximal interphalangeal joint.

synchondrosis a joint between two bones that has been formed by hyaline cartilage or fibrocartilage.

syndactyly congenital webbing or fusion of adjacent fingers or toes.

syndesmophyte a radiodense ossification of the outer annulus fibrosis as a result of inflammatory joint disease (e.g., ankylosing spondylitis).

synostosis osseous union of adjacent bones.

syringomyelia a pathological longitudinal accumulation of fluid within the spinal cord.

T1 a term used in magnetic resonance imaging to denote the time for 63% of the excited hydrogen nuclei to undergo longitudinal relaxation. The time depends on the strength of the external magnet and chemical environment of the hydrogen. Fat demonstrates a bright signal on T1-weighted images. Generally, T1-weighted images provide good anatomical detail.

T2 a term used in magnetic resonance imaging to denote the time for 63% of the excited hydrogen nuclei to undergo transverse relaxation. The time depends on the strength of the external magnet and chemical environment of the hydrogen. Water demonstrates a bright signal on T2-weighted images. Generally, T2-weighted images are more "grainy"-appearing than T1-weighted images. Because most pathological conditions have associated edema (fluid accumulations), T2-weighted images are sensitive for disease processes.

Tarlov's cyst a perineural cyst in the proximal portion of the spinal nerve roots of the lower spinal cord.

technetium 99m (^{99m}Tc) an artificial radioactive element with an atomic number of 43 and an atomic weight of 99; widely used as a tracer in nuclear imaging. Technetium Tc 99m diphosphonate is one of the more common complexes used for bone scans.

tennis elbow (lateral humeral epicondylitis) pain radiating from elbow at the origin of the wrist extensors resulting from repetitive muscular strains.

theca a protective case or sheath.

thecal sac a term usually used in a radiological context referring to the dura and arachnoid mater of the spinal cord.

three-phase bone scan the common bone scan that is interpreted in three phases. The first phase, or *flow phase,* uses a radionuclide angiogram taken the first minute after injection. The second phase is the *blood pool scan,* which takes place 1 to 3 minutes after injection. The third phase is the *static bone scan,* which takes place 2 to 4 hours following injection. With increased blood flow, the first and second phases demonstrate prominent collection. Collection of radionuclide in the third phase corresponds to osteogenic activity and blood flow and is the most useful portion of the radionuclide bone scan study.

thrombus a plug or clot formed in the heart or a blood vessel that remains at its formation site.

tophus the chalky, white calculi of sodium urate deposits in and around joints of patients who have gout.

tortuous winding or curving.

trident hand a hand that has a widening space between the third and fourth digits; slight flexion of digits of nearly equal length.

trolley track sign ossification of the zygapophyseal joints bilaterally and the supraspinatus and interspinous ligaments along the median, forming three, nearly parallel, vertical lines on frontal lumbar radiographs of some patients who have ankylosing spondylitis.

tube-film distance (TFD) the distance between the x-ray tube and the film; also referred to as *focal-film distance (FFD).*

tubercle a small nodule or prominence, especially one that is non-pathological.

tuberosity a large tubercle or process on a bone extending from the surface.

turret exostosis a subperiosteal hemorrhage resulting in a bony protuberance from the ulnar and dorsal aspects of the base of the proximal or middle phalanx.

ureteric colic spasmodic pain in the abdomen caused obstruction or disease of the ureter.

urography radiographic examination of the urinary tract with contrast medium.

vacuum phenomenon (Knuttson's sign) a radiolucent defect caused by nitrogen gas accumulations in anular and nuclear degenerative fissures of the intervertebral disc. The nitrogen gas is thought to arise from the extracellular spaces. Because the gas accumulates in areas of lower pressure, they are often seen in fissures of the anterior portion of the disc on extension radiographs. The presence of a vacuum phenomenon virtually excludes the possibility of an infection being the cause of a narrowed intervertebral disc space. The presence of gas-forming infections is a rare exception to this general rule. Vacuum phenomena are normal in synovial joints under slight distraction.

valgus describes the abnormal position or deviation of a part lateral to the midline.

Valsalva's maneuver the act of forcing a deep breath when the glottis is closed, a hand is over the mouth and nose, or the airway is blocked in some other way.

varix a permanently dilated and tortuous vessel, especially a vein.

varus describes the abnormal position or deviation of a part medial to the midline.

ventral pertaining to the front or anterior side (i.e., the front side of the body).

vertebra plana a flattening compression deformity of the vertebral body height.

vertex the top or highest part of the head.

voxel an abbreviation for volume element; a three-dimensional version of a pixel; the basic unit of computed tomography or magnetic resonance imaging reconstruction.

wedged vertebra compression deformity of the vertebra in which the vertebra has a decreased anterior body height but maintains its posterior body height.

Wilkinson's syndrome unilateral disruption of the pars interarticularis with contralateral sclerosis of the pedicle.

Wimberger's sign (ring epiphysis) the radiodense appearance of the epiphyseal circumference that is seen in patients who have scurvy.

window level the midpoint of the window width; expressed in Hounsfield units. The window level determines which tissues are displayed. For example, a window level of -500 Hounsfield units excludes bone and soft tissues and emphasizes pulmonary anatomy.

window width the range of computed tomography numbers, expressed in Hounsfield units, that are included in the gray scale image.

xanthoma a benign plaque, nodule, or tumor of fatty and fibrous origin found in the subcutaneous layer of skin, often around tendons.

xeroradiography a diagnostic imaging technique in which an image is produced electrically rather than chemically using a specially coated charged plate instead of x-ray film. It requires less exposure time and lower radiation doses than radiography and provides inherent edge enhancement. It is used primarily for mammography.

zone of provisional calcification a thin line of increased radiodensity at the junction of the physis and metaphysis representing the region of physis cartilage calcification.

Index

C

F

G

O

V

Y

Z

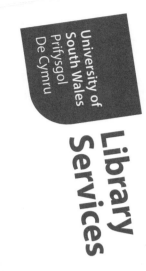

Radiology Mnemonics

Acronyms and mnemonics are useful aids for learning and remembering differential diagnoses for particular radiographic presentations. Most of the following mnemonics are from Wolfgang Dähnert's *Radiology Review Manual.** Many of these differential lists vary from those provided in the pattern chapters of this book—certain items have been added, and others have been omitted. Although differences exist among sources, the most important entries remain constant.

Bone

Basilar invagination: "COOP"
Congenital, Osteogenesis imperfecta, Osteomalacia, Paget's disease

Solitary lytic defect in the skull: "TORMENT"
Tuberculosis, Osteomyelitis, Radiation, Metastasis/Multiple myeloma, Epidermoid/dermoid, Neurofibromatosis/Necrosis (radiation), Trauma

Multiple lytic defects in the skull: "BAMMAH"
Brown tumor, Arteriovenous malformation, Multiple myeloma, Metastases, Amyloidosis, Histiocytosis

Button sequestrum of the skull: "TORE ME"
Tuberculosis, Osteomyelitis, Radiation, Eosinophilic granuloma, Metastasis, Epidermoid

Hair-on-end appearance of the skull: "SHITE"
Sickle cell disease, Hereditary spherocytosis, Iron deficiency anemia, Thalassemia major, Enzyme deficiency (glucose-6-phosphate dehydrogenase)

Absent greater wing of the sphenoid: "M FOR MARINE"
Meningioma, Fibrous dysplasia, Optic glioma, Relapsing hematoma, Metastasis, Aneurysm, Retinoblastoma, Idiopathic, Neurofibromatosis, Eosinophilic granuloma

Wormian (sutural) bones: "PORK CHOPS"
Pyknodysostosis, Osteogenesis imperfecta, Rickets (healing phase), Kinky hair syndrome, Cleidocranial dysplasia, Hypothyroidism/Hypophosphatasia, Otopalatodigital syndrome, Pachydermoperiostosis/Primary acro-osteolysis, Syndrome of Down

Increased skull thickness: "HIPFAM"
Hyperostosis frontalis interna, Idiopathic, Paget's disease, Fibrous dysplasia, Anemia, Metastasis

Atlantoaxial subluxation: "JAP LARD"
Juvenile rheumatoid arthritis, Ankylosing spondylitis, Psoriatic arthritis, Lupus erythematosus, Accident (trauma), Retropharyngeal abscess/Rheumatoid arthritis, Down syndrome

Ivory vertebra: "My Only Sister Left Home On Friday Past"
Myelosclerosis, Osteoblastic metastasis, Sickle cell anemia, Lymphoma, Hemangioma, Osteoporosis, Fluorosis, Paget's disease

Vertebra plana: "FETISH"
Fracture, Eosinophilic granuloma, Tumor (metastasis, multiple myeloma), Infection, Steroids, Hemangioma

Bullet-shaped vertebra: "HAM"
Hypothyroidism, Achondroplasia, Morquio's disease

*Dähnert W: *Radiology review manual,* ed 3, Baltimore, 1996, Williams & Wilkins.

Posterior vertebral body scalloping: "HAMENTS"
Hurler's syndrome/Hydrocephalus, Achondroplasia/Acromegaly, Marfan's syndrome, Ehlers-Danlos syndrome, Neurofibromatosis, Tumor (meningioma, ependymoma), Syringomyelia

Anterior vertebral body scalloping: "MALT"
Multiple myeloma (paravertebral soft tissue mass), Aortic aneurysm, Lymphadenopathy (lymphoma), Tuberculosis

Expansile lesions in the vertebral arch: "GO APE"
Giant cell tumor, Osteoblastoma, Aneurysmal bone cyst, Plasmacytoma, Eosinophilic granuloma

Tumor predisposed to the vertebral body: "CALL HOME"
Chordoma, Aneurysmal bone cyst, Leukemia, Lymphoma, Hemangioma/Hydatid cyst, Osteoblastoma, Multiple myeloma/Metastasis, Eosinophilic granuloma

Neoplasms of the sacrum: "CAGE"
Chordoma/Chondrosarcoma, Aneurysmal bone cyst, Giant cell tumor, Ewing's tumor

Protrusio acetabuli: "PORT"
Paget's disease, Osteomalacia/Otto pelvis, Rheumatoid arthritis, Trauma

Aberrant development of the pubic bone: "CHIEF"
Cleidocranial dysostosis, Hypospadias/epispadias, Idiopathic, Exstrophy of bladder, F for syringomyelia

Widened symphysis pubis: "EPOCH"
Exstrophy of bladder, Prune belly syndrome, Osteogenesis imperfecta, Cleidocranial dysostosis, Hypothyroidism

Widened sacroiliac joint: "CRAP TRAP"
Colitis, Rheumatoid arthritis, Abscess (infection), Parathyroid disease, Trauma, Reiter's syndrome, Ankylosing spondylitis, Psoriasis

Calcification of the intervertebral disc: "DO IT"
Degeneration, Ochronosis, Idiopathic, Trauma

Chondrocalcinosis: "WHIP A DOG"
Wilson's disease, Hemochromatosis/Hemophilia/Hypothyroidism/Hyperparathyroidism/Hypophosphatasia, Idiopathic, Pseudogout, Amyloidosis, Diabetes mellitus, Ochronosis, Gout

Premature osteoarthritis: "COME CHAT"
Calcium pyrophosphate dihydrate crystal deposition, Ochronosis, Marfan's syndrome, Epiphyseal dysplasia, Charcot (neurotrophic) arthropathy, Hemophilic arthropathy, Acromegaly, Trauma

Arthritis with demineralization: "HORSE"
Hemophilia, Osteomyelitis, Rheumatoid arthritis/Reiter's syndrome, Scleroderma, Erythematosus (systemic lupus)

Arthritis without demineralization: "PONGS"
Psoriatic arthritis, Osteoarthritis, Neuropathic joint, Gout, Sarcoidosis

Continued

Arthritis involving distal interphalangeal joints: "POEM"
Psoriatic arthritis, Osteoarthritis, Erosive osteoarthritis, Multicentric reticulohistiocytosis

Premature closure of the epiphyseal plate: "JB HIT"
Juvenile rheumatoid arthritis, Battered child syndrome, Hemophilia, Infection, Trauma

Epiphyseal lesions: "CAGGIE"
Chondroblastoma, Aneurysmal bone cyst, Giant cell tumor, Geode, Infection, Eosinophilic granuloma/Enchondroma

Epiphyseal lesions: "GELCO"
Giant cell tumor, Eosinophilic granuloma/Enchondroma, Lipoma, Chondroblastoma/Cyst (degenerative), Osteomyelitis

Diaphyseal tumors: "FEMALE"
Fibrous dysplasia, Ewing's sarcoma, Metastasis, Adamantinoma, Lymphoma/Leukemia, Eosinophilic granuloma

Frayed metaphyses: "CHARMS"
Congenital infections (rubella, syphilis), Hypophosphatasia, Achondroplasia, Rickets, Metaphyseal dysostosis, Scurvy

Rhizomelic dwarfism: "MA CAT"
Metatrophic dwarfism, Achondrogenesis, Chondrodysplasia punctata, Achondroplasia (heterozygous),Thanatophoric dysplasia

Short fourth metacarpal: "TOP"
Turner's syndrome/Trauma, Osteomyelitis, Pseudohypoparathyroidism

Radiolucent metaphyseal bands: "SLING"
Systemic illness (rickets, scurvy), Leukemia, Infection (congenital syphilis), Neuroblastoma metastasis/Normal variant, Growth lines

Dense metaphyseal bands: "Heavy Cretins Sift Scurrilously through Rickety Systems"
Heavy metal poisoning (lead, bismuth), Cretinism, Syphilis (congenital), Scurvy, Rickets (healed), Systemic illness

Periosteal reaction in child: "PERIOSTEAL SOCKS"
Physiological/Prostaglandin, Eosinophilic granuloma, Rickets, Infantile cortical hyperostosis, Osteomyelitis, Scurvy, Trauma, Ewing's sarcoma, A-hypervitaminosis, Leukemia, Syphilis, Osteosarcoma, Child abuse, Kinky hair syndrome, Sickle cell disease

Expansile rib lesion: "THELMA"
Tuberculosis, Hematopoiesis, Eosinophilic granuloma/Ewing's sarcoma/Enchondroma, Leukemia/Lymphoma, Multiple myeloma/Metastasis, Aneurysmal bone cyst

Destruction of the medial end of the clavicle: "FEMALE"
Fibrous dysplasia, Ewing's sarcoma, Metastasis, Adamantinoma, Lymphoma/Leukemia, Eosinophilic granuloma

Thick heel pad: "MAD COP"
Myxedema, Acromegaly, Dilantin therapy, Callus, Obesity, Peripheral edema

Acro-osteolysis: "RADISH"
Raynaud's phenomena, Arteriosclerosis, Diabetes, Injury (thermal), Scleroderma/Sarcoidosis, Hyperparathyroidism

Cystic bone lesions: "FEGNOMASHIC"
Fibrous dysplasia, Enchondroma, Giant cell tumor, Nonossifying fibroma, Osteoblastoma, Multiple myeloma/Metastasis, Aneurysmal bone cyst, Simple bone cyst, Hyperparathyroidism/Hemophilic pseudotumor, Infection, Chondroblastoma

Multiple lytic lesions: "FEEMHI"
Fibrous dysplasia, Enchondroma, Eosinophilic granuloma, Metastasis/Multiple myeloma, Hyperparathyroidism (brown tumors)/Hemangioma, Infection

Lytic lesion surrounded by sclerosis: "BOOST"
Brodie's abscess, Osteoblastoma, Osteoid osteoma, Stress fracture, Tuberculosis

Generalized bone sclerosis: "3 M's PROF"
Metastasis (blastic), Mastocytosis, Myelofibrosis, Paget's disease, Rickets, Osteopetrosis, Fluorosis

Moth-eaten bone destruction: "LEMON"
Lymphoma, Ewing's sarcoma/Eosinophilic granuloma, Metastasis/Multiple myeloma, Osteomyelitis, Neuroblastoma

Avascular necrosis: "PLASTIC RAGS"
Pancreatitis/Pregnancy, Lupus erythematosus, Alcoholism, Sickle cell anemia, Trauma, Idiopathic, Caisson disease, Rheumatoid arthritis/Radiation, Atherosclerosis, Gaucher's disease, Steroids

Failed back surgery: "ABCDEF"
Arachnoiditis, Bleeding, Contamination (infection), Disc (residual, recurrent, new level), Error (wrong level or side), Fibrosis (scar formation)

Chest

Diffuse air-space disease: "AIRSPACED"
Aspiration, Inhalation, Renal disease, Swimming (near drowning), Pneumonia, Alveolar proteinosis, Cardiovascular disease, Edema, Drug reaction

Diffuse air-space disease: "BEPT"
Blood, Edema, Pus, Tumor

Opacification of hemithorax: "FAT CHANCE"
Fibrothorax, Adenomatoid malformation, Trauma (hematoma), Collapse/Cardiomegaly, Hernia, Agenesis of lung, Neoplasm (mesothelioma), Consolidation, Effusion

Perihilar (bat-wing) infiltrates: "Please, Please, Please, Study Light, Don't Get All Uptight"
Pulmonary edema, Proteinosis, Periarteritis, Sarcoidosis, Lymphoma, Drugs, Goodpasture's syndrome, Alveolar cell carcinoma, Uremia

Interstitial lung disease: "LIFE lines"
Lymphangitic spread, Inflammation/Infection, Fibrosis, Edema

Interstitial lung disease: "SHIPS & BOATS"
Sarcoidosis, Histiocytosis, Idiopathic, Pneumoconiosis, Scleroderma, Bleomycin/Busulfan, Oxygen toxicity, Arthritis (rheumatoid)/Amyloidosis/Allergic alveolitis, Tuberous sclerosis/Tuberculosis, Storage disease (Gaucher's disease)

Acute interstitial lung disease: "HELP"
Hypersensitivity, Edema, Lymphoproliferative, Pneumonitis (viral)

Chronic infiltrates in child: "ABC'S"
Asthma/Agammaglobulinemia/Aspiration, Bronchiectasis, Cystic fibrosis, Sequestration (intralobular)

Advanced interstitial lung disease (honeycomb lung): "B CHIPS"
Bronchiectasis, Collagen vascular disease, Histiocytosis X, Interstitial pneumonia (viral), Pneumoconiosis, Sarcoidosis